D0866124

NETTER'S NEUROLOGY

3rd EDITION

NETTER'S NEUROLOGY

Editors:

Jayashri Srinivasan, MD, PhD, FRCP
Division of Neurology
H. Royden Jones Chair of Neuroscience
Lahey Hospital and Medical Center
Burlington, Massachusetts

Claudia J. Chaves, MD
Division of Neurology
Lahey Hospital and Medical Center
Burlington, Massachusetts

Brian J. Scott, MD
Department of Neurology
Stanford University Medical Center
Palo Alto, California

Juan E. Small, MD
Division of Neuroradiology
Lahey Hospital and Medical Center
Burlington, Massachusetts

Illustrations by:

Frank H. Netter, MD

Contributing Illustrators:

Carlos A. G. Machado, MD

John A. Craig, MD

Tiffany Slaybaugh Davanzo, MA, CMI

James A. Perkins, MS, MFA

Anita Impagliazzo, MA, CMI

ELSEVIER

NETTER'S NEUROLOGY, THIRD EDITION ISBN: 978-0-323-55476-3

Copyright © 2020 by Elsevier, Inc. All rights reserved.

No part of this publication may be reproduced or transmitted in any form or by any means, electronic or mechanical, including photocopying, recording, or any information storage and retrieval system, without permission in writing from the publisher. Details on how to seek permission, further information about the Publisher's permissions policies and our arrangements with organizations such as the Copyright Clearance Center and the Copyright Licensing Agency, can be found at our website: www.elsevier.com/permissions.

This book and the individual contributions contained in it are protected under copyright by the Publisher (other than as may be noted herein).

Permission to use Netter Art figures may be sought through the website *NetterImages.com* or by emailing Elsevier's Licensing Department at H.Licensing@elsevier.com.

Notice

Practitioners and researchers must always rely on their own experience and knowledge in evaluating and using any information, methods, compounds or experiments described herein. Because of rapid advances in the medical sciences, in particular, independent verification of diagnoses and drug dosages should be made. To the fullest extent of the law, no responsibility is assumed by Elsevier, authors, editors or contributors for any injury and/or damage to persons or property as a matter of products liability, negligence or otherwise, or from any use or operation of any methods, products, instructions, or ideas contained in the material herein.

Previous editions copyrighted 2012 and 2005.

International Standard Book Number: 978-0-323-55476-3

Content Strategist: Marybeth Thiel
Publishing Services Manager: Catherine Jackson
Senior Project Manager: Daniel Fitzgerald
Designer: Patrick Ferguson

Printed in China.

Last digit is the print number: 9 8 7 6 5 4 3 2 1

ELSEVIER

1600 John F. Kennedy Blvd.
Ste 1600
Philadelphia, PA 19103-2899

 Working together
to grow libraries in
developing countries

www.elsevier.com • www.bookaid.org

*To our patients, students, residents, fellows, and colleagues
for everything they have taught us.*

And

*To our wonderful families for their love and support,
which makes it all worthwhile.*

Jayashri Srinivasan, MD, PhD, FRCP, grew up in Chennai, India, where she graduated from Stanley Medical College. She initially pursued her postgraduate training in Cardiff, Wales, where she received a doctorate in neurophysiology, as well as completing a residency in internal medicine and becoming a Fellow of the Royal College of Physicians (FRCP), United Kingdom. Jayashri moved to Boston to train at the Tufts neurology program; subsequently she completed a fellowship in neuromuscular disorders at Brigham & Women's Hospital and Harvard Medical School. She briefly returned to the Tufts faculty at Tufts Medical Center but soon thereafter moved to the Lahey Clinic in 2003. Jayashri is an associate professor of neurology at Tufts University School of Medicine. Jayashri was appointed the H. Royden Jones Chair of Neuroscience in 2015 and runs a very busy clinical neurology division. She is also the Vice Chair of Department of Medicine, a position she has held since 2012.

At Lahey Dr. Srinivasan specializes in neuromuscular medicine, where she is a very skillful clinical neurophysiologist with particular interests in electromyography and autonomic disorders. When she is not practicing neurology, Jayashri devotes almost all of her free time to her family—her husband, VS Balakrishnan, Chair of Nephrology at St. Elizabeth's Medical Center, and their 2 children.

Claudia J. Chaves, MD, grew up in Brazil and received her medical degree from the Uberlândia School of Medicine. She completed her first residency in neurology at The University of São Paulo, Brazil, and after moving to the United States, she completed an additional neurology residency at the New England Medical Center, Boston. She did a research fellowship at the New England Medical Center and a clinical fellowship at the Beth Israel Deaconess Medical Center in Boston, both in cerebrovascular disease. In addition, she did subspecialty training in multiple sclerosis at the Southwestern Medical Center, Dallas, Texas, and is a graduate of the Global Clinical Scholar Research Training Program through Harvard Medical School.

After her fellowship training, she worked at the Beth Israel Deaconess Medical Center for a few years as a stroke neurologist and was an Instructor in Neurology at the Harvard Medical School. Subsequently, she moved to the Lahey Clinic in 2000. She is currently an associate professor of neurology at Tufts University School of Medicine.

Dr. Chaves is the medical director of the Multiple Sclerosis Center at the Lahey Clinic and co-director of the neurology research program at the Lahey Clinic. She is board certified in neurology and cerebrovascular disease and is a Fellow of the American Academy of Neurology.

Her main interest over the years has been clinical research and she has participated in multiple clinical trials and studies involving both cerebrovascular and demyelinating disorders. Outside neurology, she enjoys spending time with her husband, Steven Gans, a psychiatrist at McLean's Hospital, and with her three teenage children. She also enjoys learning French, traveling, and jogging.

Brian J. Scott, MD, grew up in Chagrin Falls, Ohio. He received a BA in biology from Colby College, Waterville, Maine, and an MD from Wright State University School of Medicine, Dayton, Ohio. He completed neurology training in the Tufts/New England Medical Center residency program. From the earliest points in training, Dr. Royden Jones proved an influential presence as a memorable consult attending and mentor. Following residency, Dr. Scott trained as a fellow in neuro-oncology at the combined Massachusetts General Hospital/Dana-Farber Cancer Institute program before taking his first faculty position at Lahey.

Dr. Scott went on to complete a second clinical fellowship in Neurohospitalist Medicine at the University of California, San Francisco, where he remained on faculty before returning to Lahey as Director of the Neurology Inpatient Service and Medical Director of Neuro-oncology. In this role, he directed the transition to a neurohospitalist service model, attended in the neurovascular group, and assisted in the creation of the Lahey neurocritical care team and service. He has subspecialty board certification in neuro-oncology and neurocritical care and has served as principal investigator for several treatment trials for glioblastoma and acute ischemic stroke.

Dr. Scott is currently a member of the neurohospitalist division at Stanford University Medical Center. He attends on the general inpatient neurology ward and consult services and is involved in teaching and mentoring medical students, residents, and fellows. Outside the hospital, Brian enjoys spending time to his wife, Candace Kim, an acute care geriatrician at UCSF, and 3 children. He can often be found rooting for and/or defending his favorite Cleveland sports teams.

Juan E. Small, MD, is the Section Head of the Neuroradiology Division at Lahey Hospital and Medical Center in Burlington, Massachusetts. Dr. Small earned a Bachelor of Science degree in Psychology from the University of Miami, a Master's in Neuroscience degree from the University of Oxford, and a Doctor of Medicine degree from Harvard Medical School. He continued on at Harvard Medical School to complete a Radiology Residency at Brigham and Women's Hospital and a Neuroradiology Fellowship at Massachusetts General Hospital. Dr. Small has authored and edited several books including *Neuroradiology: Key Differential Diagnoses and Clinical Questions, Neurorradiologia: Diagnosticos Diferenciales Claves y Preguntas Clinicas, Neuroimaging Pharmacopoeia,* and *Neuroradiology: Spectrum and Evolution of Disease.* Dr. Small lives in Newton, Massachusetts, with his wife and two sons.

The second edition of *Netter's Neurology* speaks to the perpetuity of Frank Netter's incomparable artistic genius and educational vision. During my first year at Northwestern University Medical School we were forewarned as to how difficult the introductory neuroanatomy course was going to be, "the toughest one" that we would face. A few upperclassmen told me to purchase the *Netter Atlas of Neurosciences* and it would all fall into place. Indeed it did, and I became interested in a career in neurology.

Having continued to be impressed with Dr. Netter's skillful renditions of many medical subjects, as presented in his semimonthly Ciba Symposia, some years later I enquired at an AMA meeting, where these were on display, as to whether he might have interest in illustrating the various mononeuropathies. Never did I think this suggestion would be transmitted directly to Dr. Netter. However, less than a year later, in 1982, I received a letter from him asking me to elaborate my ideas. I soon found myself visiting Dr. Netter at his new studio in Palm Beach. This was an undreamed of opportunity, especially as one of my hobbies includes rather amateur attempts at oil and water color painting. After a few visits with Frank, who was a very gracious and kind gentleman, he asked me to help him revise his *Neurologic and Neuromuscular Disorders* of his two-volume *Netter Nervous System* atlas, the very one that had so impressed me during my first-year neuroanatomy course. We spent many 3-day weekends together as he listened to my ideas as to how best illustrate each subject. The typical Netter day began in his studio at 7 AM … Frank always had a cigar going, and in self-defense I kept a pipe well stoked. With much help from some dear colleagues, this was published in 1986.

We planned to update this text every 6 to 8 years; however, with Frank's death in 1991 and CIBA Pharmaceutical's merging into Novartis, ongoing revisions seemed to be relegated to the publishing tundra. Much to my delight in 2000 Icon Publishers contacted me after they had purchased the rights to use the Netter paintings. Their vision led to the development of a number of more traditional, specialty oriented textbooks, and I had the honor of editing the first neurology edition in this more classic format.

As Frank Netter often stated to me "a picture is worth a thousand words." Indeed they are, and his magnificent plates provide the foundation for this monograph. However, when conceiving the overall format for the first edition of *Netter's Neurology* it was very important for me not only to include an overview of a neurologic condition but also to use clinical case vignettes, particularly since these are my most effective means of teaching. Case-based methodologies are currently used at a number of medical schools; we have aimed this volume to complement such for both the undergraduate medical student as well as residents. My first neuroscience teachers at Northwestern very effectively used patient presentations to bring life to the complexities of basic neurologic anatomy and physiology. This didactic approach was very well received by the beginning student and resident alike in the first edition of *Netter's Neurology*. We also think that the practicing clinical neurologist will find this combination of basic anatomy and clinical neurology to be a refreshing alternative to the various forms of clinical review now available for our required recertification process.

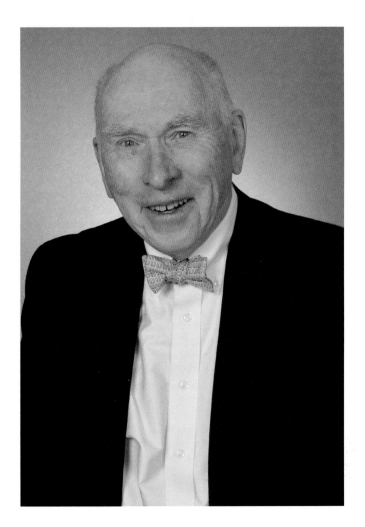

The 3rd edition of *Netter's Neurology* is the first that has been completed since the death of its principal architect, Dr. H. Royden Jones. The editors would like to acknowledge the tremendous passion, creative energy, and tireless effort that Dr. Jones devoted to writing and editing the previous editions. His commitment to this work, dedication to the practice of fundamentally sound medicine, and clinical neurology are embedded within its pages. Having had the privilege to work with him, we miss him often and are greatly indebted to him for the example he provided. To us, Dr. Jones embodied the highest standard for clinical acumen, professionalism, and education in clinical neurology.

One of the most tangible legacies left by Dr. Jones is the enduring impression he left on his patients. All of us in the neurology department at Lahey have had encounters that start with a patient's proud declaration that "I was a patient of Dr. Jones'" immediately followed by their vivid and memorable description of his time with them. He was gifted in his ability to impress upon his patients the value of their experience and his commitment to their well-being. It is our hope by continuing his work in this 3rd edition of *Netter's Neurology* that we honor his legacy and that readers will be equipped and inspired to follow Dr. Jones' model of excellence in the practice of clinical neurology.

Frank H. Netter, MD

Frank Netter was born in 1906 in New York City. He studied art at the Art Student's League and the National Academy of Design before entering medical school at New York University, where he received his medical degree in 1931. During his student years, Dr. Netter's notebook sketches attracted the attention of the medical faculty and other physicians, allowing him to augment his income by illustrating articles and textbooks. He continued illustrating as a sideline after establishing a surgical practice in 1933, but he ultimately opted to give up his practice in favor of a full-time commitment to art. After service in the United States Army during World War II, Dr. Netter began his long collaboration with the CIBA Pharmaceutical Company (now Novartis Pharmaceuticals). This 45-year partnership resulted in the production of the extraordinary collection of medical art so familiar to physicians and other medical professionals worldwide.

In 2005 Elsevier, Inc., purchased the Netter Collection and all publications from Icon Learning Systems. There are now over 50 publications featuring the art of Dr. Netter available through Elsevier (in the US: www.us.elsevierhealth.com/Netter and outside the US: www.elsevierhealth.com).

Dr. Netter's works are among the finest examples of the use of illustration in the teaching of medical concepts. The 13-book *Netter Collection of Medical Illustrations*, which includes the greater part of the more than 20,000 paintings created by Dr. Netter, became and remains one of the most famous medical works ever published. *The Netter Atlas of Human Anatomy*, first published in 1989, presents the anatomical paintings from the Netter Collection. Now translated into 16 languages, it is the anatomy atlas of choice among medical and health professions students the world over.

The Netter illustrations are appreciated not only for their aesthetic qualities, but also, more important, for their intellectual content. As Dr. Netter wrote in 1949, "…clarification of a subject is the aim and goal of illustration. No matter how beautifully painted, how delicately and subtly rendered a subject may be, it is of little value as a *medical illustration* if it does not serve to make clear some medical point." Dr. Netter's planning, conception, point of view, and approach are what inform his paintings and what makes them so intellectually valuable.

Frank H. Netter, MD, physician and artist, died in 1991.

Learn more about the physician-artist whose work has inspired the Netter Reference collection: http://www.netterimages.com/artist/netter.htm.

Carlos A. G. Machado, MD

Carlos Machado was chosen by Novartis to be Dr. Netter's successor. He continues to be the main artist who contributes to the Netter collection of medical illustrations.

Self-taught in medical illustration, cardiologist Carlos Machado has contributed meticulous updates to some of Dr. Netter's original plates and has created many paintings of his own in the style of Netter as an extension of the Netter collection. Dr. Machado's photorealistic expertise and his keen insight into the physician-patient relationship informs his vivid and unforgettable visual style. His dedication to researching each topic and subject he paints places him among the premier medical illustrators at work today.

Learn more about his background and see more of his art at: http://www.netterimages.com/artist/machado.htm

CONTRIBUTORS

Michael Adix II, MD
Interventional Neuroradiologist
Premier Radiology
Kalamazoo, Michigan
United States

Lloyd M. Alderson, MD
Division of Neurosurgery
Lahey Hospital and Medical Center
Burlington, Massachusetts
United States

Gregory J. Allam, MD
Department of Neurology
Brigham and Women's Hospital
Boston, Massachusetts
United States

Timothy D. Anderson, MD
Division of Otolaryngology
Lahey Hospital and Medical Center
Burlington, Massachusetts
United States

Diana Apetauerova, MD
Division of Neurology
Lahey Hospital and Medical Center
Burlington, Massachusetts
United States

Patrick R. Aquino, MD
Division of Psychiatry and Behavioral
   Medicine
Lahey Hospital and Medical Center
Burlington, Massachusetts
United States

Jeffrey E. Arle, MD, PhD
Department of Neurosurgery
Beth Israel Deaconess Medical Center
Boston, Massachusetts
United States

Geetha K. Athappilly, MD
Division of Ophthalmology
Lahey Hospital and Medical Center
Burlington, Massachusetts
United States

Ritu Bagla, MD
Division of Neurology
Lahey Hospital and Medical Center
Burlington, Massachusetts
United States

Joseph D. Burns, MD
Division of Neurology
Lahey Hospital and Medical Center
Burlington, Massachusetts
United States

Ted M. Burns, MD
Department of Neurology
University of Virginia Heath Sciences
Charlottesville, Virginia
United States

Ann Camac, MD
Division of Neurology
Lahey Hospital and Medical Center
Burlington, Massachusetts
United States

Claudia J. Chaves, MD
Division of Neurology
Lahey Hospital and Medical Center
Burlington, Massachusetts
United States

G. Rees Cosgrove, MD
Department of Neurosurgery
Brigham and Women's Hospital
Boston, Massachusetts
United States

Donald E. Craven, MD
Division of Infectious Diseases
Lahey Hospital and Medical Center
Burlington, Massachusetts
United States

Allison Crowell, MD
Department of Neurology
University of Virginia
Charlottesville, Virginia
United States

Carlos A. David, MD
Division of Neurosurgery
Lahey Hospital and Medical Center
Burlington, Massachusetts
United States

Peter K. Dempsey, MD
Division of Neurosurgery
Lahey Hospital and Medical Center
Burlington, Massachusetts
United States

Robert A. Duncan, MD
Division of Infectious Disease
Lahey Hospital and Medical Center
Burlington, Massachusetts
United States

Khaled Eissa, MD
Division to Pulmonary & Critical Care
   Medicine
Lahey Hospital and Medical Center
Burlington, Massachusetts
United States

Stephen R. Freidberg, MD
Division of Neurosurgery
Lahey Hospital and Medical Center
Burlington, Massachusetts
United States

Paul T. Gross, MD
Division of Neurology
Lahey Hospital and Medical Center
Burlington, Massachusetts
United States

Jian Guan, MD
Department of Neurosurgery
Clinical Neurosciences Center
University of Utah
Salt Lake City, Utah
United States

Jose A. Gutrecht, MD
Division of Neurology
Lahey Hospital and Medical Center
Burlington, Massachusetts
United States

Kelly G. Gwathmey, MD
Department of Neurology
Virginia Commonwealth University
Richmond, Virginia
United States

Gisela Held, MD
Division of Neurology
Lahey Hospital and Medical Center
Burlington, Massachusetts
United States

Doreen T. Ho, MD
Division of Neurology
Lahey Hospital and Medical Center
Burlington, Massachusetts
United States

Obehi Irumudomon, MD
Department of Pediatric Neurology
Cohen Children's Medical Center
New Hyde Park, New York
United States

H. Royden Jones, Jr., MD[†]
Division of Neurology
Lahey Hospital and Medical Center
Burlington, Massachusetts
United States

Samuel E. Kalluvya, MD
Division of Infectious Diseases
Lahey Hospital and Medical Center
Burlington, Massachusetts
United States

Ian Kaminsky, MD
Interventional Neuroradiologist
RIA Neurovascular LLC
Englewood, Colorado
United States

Johannes B. Kataraihya, MD
Division of Infectious Diseases
Lahey Hospital and Medical Center
Burlington, Massachusetts
United States

Mara M. Kunst, MD
Division of Neuroradiology
Lahey Hospital and Medical Center
Burlington, Massachusetts
United States

Kenneth Lakritz, MD
Division of Psychiatry and Behavioral
    Medicine
Lahey Hospital and Medical Center
Burlington, Massachusetts
United States

Julie Leegwater-Kim, MD, PhD
Division of Neurology
Lahey Hospital and Medical Center
Burlington, Massachusetts
United States

David P. Lerner, MD
Division of Neurology
Lahey Hospital and Medical Center
Burlington, Massachusetts
United States

Sui Li, MD
Department of Neurology
Mount Auburn Hospital
Cambridge, Massachusetts
United States

Caitlin Macaulay, PhD
Division of Neurology
Lahey Hospital and Medical Center
Burlington, Massachusetts
United States

Subu N. Magge, MD
Division of Neurosurgery
Lahey Hospital and Medical Center
Burlington, Massachusetts
United States

Ippolit C. A. Matjucha, MD
Former Neuro-ophthalmologist
Lahey Hospital and Medical Center
Burlington, Massachusetts
United States

Michelle Mauermann, MD
Consultant in Neurology
Assistant Professor of Neurology
Mayo Clinic
Rochester, Minnesota
United States

Daniel P. McQuillen, MD
Division of Infectious Diseases
Lahey Hospital and Medical Center
Burlington, Massachusetts
United States

Carol L. Moheban, MD
Division of Neurology
Lahey Hospital and Medical Center
Burlington, Massachusetts
United States

Winnie W. Ooi, MD, DMD, MPH
Division of Infectious Diseases
Lahey Hospital and Medical Center
Burlington, Massachusetts
United States

Joel M. Oster, MD
Department of Neurology
Tufts Medical Center
Boston, Massachusetts
United States

Robert Peck, MD
Division of Infectious Diseases
Lahey Hospital and Medical Center
Burlington, Massachusetts
United States

Dana Penney, PhD
Division of Neurology
Lahey Hospital and Medical Center
Burlington, Massachusetts
United States

Pooja Raibagkar, MD
Division of Neurology
Lahey Hospital Medical Center
Burlington, Massachusetts
United States

Anil Ramineni, MD
Division of Neurology
Lahey Hospital and Medical Center
Burlington, Massachusetts
United States

Haatem M. Reda, MD
Department of Neurology
Massachusetts General Hospital
Harvard Medical School
Boston, Massachusetts
United States

James A. Russell, DO
Division of Neurology
Lahey Hospital and Medical Center
Burlington, Massachusetts
United States

Monique M. Ryan, MB BS, M Med, FRACP
Royal Children's Hospital
Murdoch Children's Research Institute
Melbourne
Australia

Brian J. Scott, MD
Department of Neurology
Stanford University Medical Center
Palo Alto, California
United States

Juan E. Small, MD
Division of Neuroradiology
Lahey Hospital and Medical Center
Burlington, Massachusetts
United States

[†]Deceased.

Jayashri Srinivasan, MD, PhD, FRCP
Division of Neurology
H. Royden Jones Chair of Neuroscience
Lahey Hospital and Medical Center
Burlington, Massachusetts
United States

Sujit Suchindran, MD, MPH
Division of Infectious Diseases
Lahey Hospital and Medical Center
Burlington, Massachusetts
United States

Joanna Suski, MD
Division of Neurology
Lahey Hospital and Medical Center
Burlington, Massachusetts
United States

Matthew E. Tilem, MD
Division of Neurology
Lahey Hospital and Medical Center
Burlington, Massachusetts
United States

Elizabeth Toh, MD, MBA
Division of Otolaryngology-Head and Neck
    Surgery
Lahey Hospital and Medical Center
Burlington, Massachusetts
United States

Daniel Vardeh, MD
Division of Neurology and Anesthesia
Lahey Hospital and Medical Center
Burlington, Massachusetts
United States

Barbara Voetsch, MD, PhD
Division of Neurology
Lahey Hospital and Medical Center
Burlington, Massachusetts
United States

Michal Vytopil, MD, PhD
Division of Neurology
Lahey Hospital and Medical Center
Burlington, Massachusetts
United States

Kenneth M. Wener, MD
Division of Infectious Diseases
Lahey Hospital and Medical Center
Burlington, Massachusetts
United States

Robert G. Whitmore, MD
Division of Neurosurgery
Lahey Hospital and Medical Center
Burlington, Massachusetts
United States

Yuval Zabar, MD
Medical Director, PSP
Biogen Idec
Cambridge, Massachusetts
United States

Visit www.ExpertConsult.com for the following printable patient education brochures from Ferri's Netter Patient Advisor, 3rd edition

CONTENTS

Clinical Evaluation

Jayashri Srinivasan

Clinical Neurologic Evaluation

Brian J. Scott, Claudia J. Chaves, Jayashri Srinivasan

The neurologic sciences are the most intellectually challenging, unequivocally fascinating, and tremendously stimulating of the various clinical disciplines. Initially, the vast intricacies of basic neuroanatomy and neurophysiology often seem overwhelming to both medical student and neuroscience resident alike. However, eventually the various portions of this immense knowledge base come together in a discernible pattern, not unlike a Seurat canvas. Often one is expanding or revisiting our neurologic base as we are challenged by variations on the theme of our previous experiences. It is the keen observation and coding of these clinical experiences that lead the astute neurologic physician to solve new patient challenges.

One must first and foremost be an astute historian initially listening very carefully to the patient. Most often the intricacies, as well as the subtleties, of the neurologic history provide the essential foundation leading to a rational and structured neurologic examination allowing the neurologist to answer two basic questions: WHERE is the lesion and WHAT is the likely etiology. This will guide the clinician in ordering the appropriate diagnostic testing.

Although it is easy to define the requisite methodology to examine the neurologic patient, it is much more challenging to similarly address the history acquisition other than making a few generalities. One of the most important elements of neurologic training is the opportunity for the student and the resident to observe senior neurologists evaluate a patient. As a resident, this was absolutely one of our most important learning experiences. Too often the student does not appreciate the elegance illustrated by a carefully derived neurologic clinical history. A major attribute of a skillful and successful neurologist is being an astute listener. This requires the neurologist to bring together various seemingly disparate and subtle data from the patient's various concerns and then focus on this information with specific questions to decide on its relevance to the issues at hand. Understanding the temporal profile of the patient's symptoms is crucial; was the symptoms' onset acute and stable, or has it followed an ingravescent course? Very often, this information provides a most important perspective that is one of the very important keys to diagnosis.

CLINICAL VIGNETTE *A 42-year-old woman with juvenile autoimmune diabetes mellitus came for further investigation of her extremely painful neuropathy initially presumed secondary to diabetes, or possibly to recent chemotherapy for breast cancer. However, her temporal profile was the final clue to her diagnosis. On careful review of the onset of her symptoms, it was found that she had never had the slightest hint of intolerable paresthesia until awakening from her mastectomy. Her pain had begun precipitously in the recovery room. It was steady from its inception and totally incapacitating in this previously vigorous woman whose favorite pastime was backpacking in mountainous national forests. This temporal profile was in total contradistinction to any symmetric diabetic or antineoplastic chemotherapy-related polyneuropathy. These disorders always have a clinical course of subtle onset and gradual evolution.*

With this information, we investigated what transpired at the time of her breast surgery when she awakened with this extremely limiting painful neuropathy. In fact, she had had a general anesthetic with nitrous oxide (N_2O) induction. This N_2O uncovered a second autoimmune disorder, namely vitamin B_{12} deficiency. The anesthetic had precipitously led to symptoms in this previously clinically silent process. Fortunately, vitamin B_{12} replacement led to total resolution of her symptoms.

Comment: In this instance, her initial physicians had let themselves be trapped by what was familiar to them because diabetes is the most common cause for a painful neuropathy. However, only rarely does it lead to a precipitous onset of symptoms. The fine-tuning of this patient's temporal profile, especially the abrupt onset of symptoms, led us to seek a more detailed history as to whether some toxic process was operative. Review of the operative records per se led to the diagnosis when the suspicion of N_2O intoxication was confirmed.

Most neurologic disorders follow a well-defined clinical paradigm. However, it is their very broad clinical perspective that continually challenges the astute neurologic clinician to maintain a vigilant intellectual posture. When these specific clinical subtleties are appreciated, the clinician is rewarded with the knowledge of having done the very best for his or her patient, as well as having the intellectual reward for being on the cutting edge of the clinical neurosciences. The skillful clinician, taking a very careful history, is the one most able to recognize the attributes of something quite uncommon presenting in a fashion more easily confused with more mundane afflictions.

For example, numbness or tingling in a patient's hand most commonly represents entrapment of the median nerve at the wrist, reflecting the presence of a very common disorder known as the *carpal tunnel syndrome*. However, symptoms of this type may occasionally represent early signs of a pathologic lesion at the level of the brachial plexus, nerve root, spinal cord, or brain per se. It is imperative for the clinician to always consider a broad anatomic perspective in each patient evaluation. When this approach is not carefully followed, less common and potentially treatable disorders may not be diagnosed in a timely fashion. It is absolutely imperative that no compromise be made in obtaining a thorough and accurate history when first meeting the patient. This is the most important interchange the physician will have. It needs to be taken in a relaxed, hopefully uninterrupted setting allowing for privacy. In addition, it is very important to invite the spouse, parent, or significant other into the room. Rarely will a patient object to this; having another close observer of a patient's difficulties available can provide insights that may be essential to diagnosis. A thorough initial evaluation engenders a patient-family sense of trust in the physician as a detailed history, with a careful examination demonstrates a major commitment. Once developed, this clinical setting encourages patients to communicate openly with their physician as they outline their diagnostic plans and eventually a treatment formulation. This chapter provides a foundation that will serve as an anchor for both the student and resident as they learn the art and science of the performance of detailed neurologic evaluations.

NEUROLOGIC HISTORY AND EXAMINATION

An accurate history requires paying attention to detail, often observing the patient's demeanor while reading the patient's body language, having the opportunity to witness the patient's difficulties, and interviewing family members. History taking is a special art and science in its own right. It is a skill that requires ongoing additions to one's own interviewing techniques. Listening to the patient is a most important part of this exercise; it is something that can be more time consuming than current clinical practice "time allowed guidelines" provide for within various patient settings. This approach provides the diagnostic keystone that often distinguishes an astute clinician's ability to find a diagnosis where others have failed.

A complete neurologic examination also requires carefully honed clinical skills. For example, the ability to decide whether the patient is truly weak and not giving way, or similarly does or does not have a Babinski sign present, is key to arriving at a correct diagnosis. The ability to define a sensory loss at a spinal cord level is another very crucial exercise.

One challenging clinical scenario occurs with patients who have seen other clinical neurologists and no diagnosis was made. The patient is frustrated, as often is the prior neurologist. To be fair to the patient, as well as oneself, when evaluating such an individual seeking a second neurologic opinion, it is important to gain one's own initial and totally unbiased history and examination. Furthermore, to prevent unwelcome bias, the new neurologist should avoid reading other colleagues' notes or looking at previous neurologic images prior to gaining his or her own history and performing the examinations.

Although time consuming, the history is the most important factor leading to accurate diagnoses. One of the essential attributes of a skillful neurologist is the ability to be a good listener so as not to miss crucial historic points. It is important to begin the initial meeting by asking patients why they have come; this offers them the opportunity to express concerns in their own words. If at all possible, the neurologist should not interrupt, thus providing the patient the opportunity to provide their primary concerns to the neurologist, emphasizing the symptoms of greatest importance. Rarely, anxious or compulsive patients may speak of their concerns at great length; with experience, physicians learn to make discreet interjections to maintain control of the evaluation and draw the patient back from extraneous tangents.

When the patient's primary concerns are established, specific issues can be explored. In addition, making careful observations during the review of history allows better focus for subsequent questions. An accurate baseline assessment of mental status and language can be obtained from listening to the patient and observing responses to questions. It is through listening that the clinician gains insight into the patient's real concerns. For example, it is not unusual to see a patient referred to a neurologist for evaluation of headaches, which only became exacerbated with the recent discovery of a brain tumor in someone known to the patient.

Unfortunately, the economics of modern health care has forced primary care physicians and specialists to shorten visit times with patients and their families. One must be fastidious not to use diagnostic tools, such as magnetic resonance imaging (MRI), as substitutes for careful clinical history and examination. The current detailed medical information available on the internet, in conjunction with sophisticated basic health education, has indeed enhanced patients' knowledge, although not always in a balanced format. Patient expectations may affect the diagnostic approach of physicians. In this environment, it is not surprising that imaging techniques such as MRI and computed tomography (CT) have replaced or supplemented a significant portion of clinical judgment. However, even the most dramatic test findings may prove irrelevant without appropriate clinical correlation. To have patients unnecessarily undergo surgery because of MRI findings that have no relation to their complaints may lead to a tragic outcome. Therein lies the importance of gaining a complete understanding of the clinical issues.

Although neurology may seem in danger of being subsumed by overreliance on highly sophisticated diagnostic studies, this needs to be kept in perspective because many of these innovations have greatly improved our diagnostic skills and therapeutic capacities. For example, much knowledge regarding the early recognition, progression, and response to treatment of multiple sclerosis (MS) depends on careful MRI imaging.

It is essential to make patients feel comfortable in the office, particularly by fostering a positive interpersonal relationship. Taking time to gather information about patients' lives, education, and social habits often provides useful clues. A careful set of questions providing a general review of systems may lead to the key diagnostic clue that focuses the evaluation. When the patient develops a sense of confidence and rapport with an empathetic physician, he or she is more willing to return for follow-up, even if a diagnosis is not made at the initial evaluation. Sometimes a careful second or third examination reveals a crucial historic or examination difference that leads to a specific diagnosis. Follow-up visits also allow the patient and physician to have another conversation regarding the symptoms and concerns. Some patients may come to their first office visit with an exhaustive list of concerns and symptoms, whereas others provide minimal information. Subsequent visits are intended not only to discuss the results of tests but also to clarify the symptoms and/or response to treatment. If patients feel rushed on their first visit, they may not return for follow-up, thus denying the neurologist a chance at crucial diagnostic observations. The physician-patient relationship must always be carefully nurtured and highly respected.

APPROACH TO THE NEUROLOGIC EVALUATION

Throughout training, examination skills are continually being amplified as the resident is exposed to an ever-evolving clinical experience. One important learning opportunity is the observation of the varied skill sets demonstrated by academic neurologists as they approach different types of patients. One of the essentials of the neurologic evaluation is learning how to elicit important, sometimes subtle, clues to diagnosis; in addition, an appreciation of what is "normal" at different ages is also important. A hasty history and examination can be misleading. For example, briskly preserved ankle reflexes in an elderly patient is not normal, whereas moderately diminished vibration sense at the ankles is normal. A diagnosis of early MS may be missed by not asking about such things as previous problems with visual function, shooting electric paresthesia when bending the neck (Lhermitte sign), or sphincter problems manifested by increasing urgency to urinate.

Even though carpal tunnel syndrome is the most common cause of a numb hand, one must always be fastidious not to overlook other pathoanatomic sites that could result in the same symptoms, such as the more proximal median nerve, brachial plexus, or cervical nerve root. In another instance, the failure to perform a thorough neuromuscular examination (including asking the patient to change into a gown and inspecting muscle bulk and tone) may preclude the examining physician from recognizing the presence of an unexpected subtle spasticity, reflex asymmetry, and/or a Babinski response indicative of a central nervous system (CNS) lesion. Similarly, identifying a sensory level is indicative of a myelopathy as the pathophysiologic explanation for the patient's numb hand. Lastly the finding that the sensory loss in the fingers primarily involves position sense and stereognosis becomes the entrée to examine the cerebral cortex as the site for these complaints.

Another important outcome from performing a complete neurologic examination at the initial evaluation in almost every patient is that this not only establishes the patient's current status but will also provide a baseline for future comparison. There are certain "normal" asymmetries in many individuals, often not previously appreciated by the patient or relatives. These may include a patient's slightly asymmetric smile, somewhat irregular pupils, or hint of ptosis. However, at times such findings do take on significant meaning. As an example, a middle-aged woman was thought to have benign tension headaches. This was based on a "normal" neurologic exam elsewhere. However, she had an asymmetric smile that previously had not been appreciated. Imaging studies identified a frontal lobe tumor contralateral to her facial weakness. Thus the careful observation of seemingly subtle clinical findings may prove to have significant bearing on the issue at hand. Even when these findings are proven to be "normal variants," clear documentation may often be very helpful during the course of the patient's illness or later on when new concerns occur. In that setting, the prior definition of what proves to be a normal asymmetry will prevent erroneous conclusions from being developed.

Formulation

One of the most intellectually challenging aspects of neurology relates to the neurologist's ability to amalgamate the historical and physical findings into a unitary hypothesis. One needs to first consider the multiple neuroanatomic sites that can potentially explain the patient's clinical presentation (Where is the lesion?). Subsequently, this is placed in the perspective of the patient's past medical and family history, as well as the clinical temporal profile of the symptom's occurrence (What is the etiology?). Did all of the patient's symptoms begin abruptly, as is usually seen with a stroke? Or was there an evolution of degree of clinical loss or did new features gradually get added to the patient's findings as is characteristic of certain neoplastic lesions and sometimes more diffuse vasculitides? Formulation can be hindered by the patient's inability to provide an accurate history or participate in the neurologic examination. One of the more subtle and difficult conditions to recognize is anosognosia to one's illness, as may occur in patients with right parietal brain injury. Under these circumstances, the patient may not have sensory, visual, or motor neglect, but unawareness of cognitive, emotional, and other functional limitations. Family interview is most important in this setting.

Overview and Basic Tenets

The neurologic examination begins the moment the patients get out of their seat to be greeted, the character of their smile or lack thereof, and subsequently as they walk to enter the neurologist's office. An excellent opportunity to judge the patient's language function and cognitive abilities occurs during the acquisition of the patient's history. Concurrently, the neurologist is always attuned to carefully making observations to identify various clinical signs. Some are overt movements (tremors, restlessness, dystonia, or dyskinesia); others are subtler, for example,

vitiligo, implying a potential for a neurologic autoimmune disorder. Equally important may be the lack of normal movements, as seen in patients with Parkinson disease. By the time the neurologist completes the examination, she or he must be able to categorize and organize these historical and examination findings into a carefully structured diagnostic formulation.

The subsequent definition of the formal examination may be subdivided into a few major sections. Speech and language are assessed during the history taking. The cognitive part of the examination is often clearly defined with the initial history and often does not require formal mental status testing. However, there are a number of clinical neurologic settings where this evaluation is very time consuming and complicated; Chapter 25 is dedicated to this aspect of the patient evaluation.

Here the multisystem neurologic examination provides a careful basis for most essential clinical evaluations. Neurologists in training and their colleagues in practice cannot expect to test all possible cognitive elements in each patient they evaluate. Certain basic elements are required; most of these are readily observable or elicited during initial clinical evaluation. These include documentation of language function, affect, concentration, orientation, and memory. When concerned about the patient's cognitive abilities, the neurologist must elicit evidence of an apraxia or agnosia and test organizational skills. Once language and cognitive functions are assessed, the neurologist dedicates the remaining portion of the exam to the examination of many functions. These include cranial nerves (CNs) (Fig. 1.1), muscle strength, muscle stretch reflexes (MSRs), plantar stimulation, coordination, gait, and equilibrium, as well as sensory modalities. These should routinely be examined in an organized fashion in order not to overlook an important part of the examination. The patient's general health, nutritional status, and cardiac function, including the presence or absence of significant arrhythmia, heart murmur, hypertension, or signs of congestive failure, should be noted. If the patient is encephalopathic, it is important to search for subtle signs of infectious, hepatic, renal, or pulmonary disease.

CRANIAL NERVES: AN INTRODUCTION

The 12 CNs subserve multiple types of neurologic function (see Fig. 1.1). The CNs are formed by afferent sensory fibers, motor efferent fibers, or mixed fibers traveling to and from brainstem nuclei (Fig. 1.2).

The special senses are represented by all or part of the function of five different CNs, namely, olfaction, the olfactory (I); vision, the optic (II); taste, the facial (VII) and the glossopharyngeal (IX); and hearing and vestibular function, the cochlear and vestibular (VIII) nerves. Another three CNs are directly responsible for the coordinated, synchronous, and complex movements of both eyes; these include CNs III (oculomotor), IV (trochlear), and VI (abducens). CN VII is the primary CN responsible for facial expression, which is important for setting the outward signs of the patient's psyche's representation to his or her family and close associates, or signs of paralysis from a brain or CN lesion. Facial sensation is subserved primarily by the trigeminal nerve (V); however, it is a mixed nerve also providing primary motor contributions to mastication. The ability to eat and drink depends on CNs IX (glossopharyngeal), X (vagus), and XII (hypoglossal). The hypoglossal and recurrent laryngeal nerves are also important to the mechanical function of speech. Last, CN XI, the accessory, contains both cranial and spinal nerve roots that provide motor innervation to the large muscles of the neck and shoulder.

Disorders of the CNs can be confined to a single nerve such as the olfactory (from a closed-head injury, early Parkinson disease, or meningioma), trigeminal (tic douloureux), facial (Bell palsy), acoustic

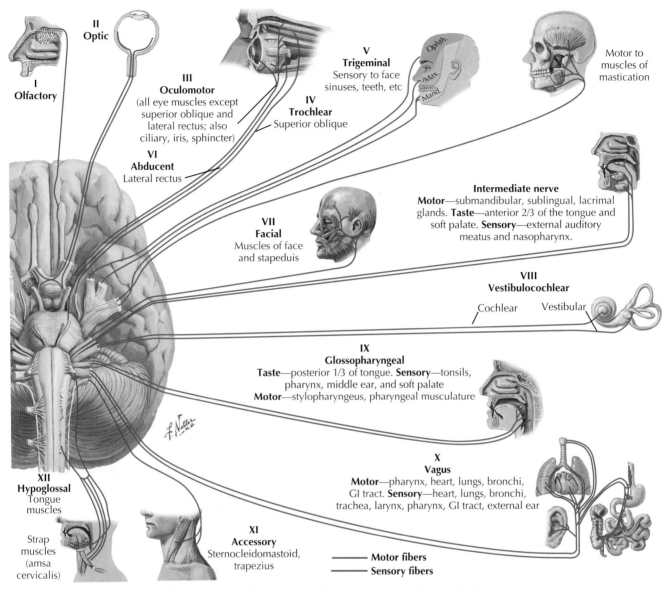

Fig. 1.1 Cranial Nerves: Distribution of Motor and Sensory Fibers. *GI*, Gastrointestinal.

(schwannoma), and hypoglossal (carotid dissection). There is a subset of systemic disorders with the potential to infiltrate or seed the base of the brain and the brainstem at the points of exit of the various CNs from their intraaxial origins. These processes include leptomeningeal seeding of metastatic malignancies originating in the lung, breast, and stomach, as well as various lymphomas, or granulomatous processes such as sarcoidosis or tuberculosis, each leading to a clinical picture of multiple, sometimes disparate cranial neuropathies. Many times, a stuttering onset occurs. The various symptoms are related to individual CNs. These typically develop within just weeks or no more than a few months.

CN dysfunctions will commonly bring patients to medical attention for a number of clinical limitations. These include ophthalmic difficulties, such as diminished visual acuity or visual field deficits (optic nerve and pericavernous chiasm) and double vision, either horizontal, vertical, or skewed (oculomotor, trochlear, and abducens nerves). Other CN presentations include facial pain (trigeminal nerve), evolving facial weakness (facial nerve), difficulty swallowing (glossopharyngeal and vagus nerves), and slurred speech (hypoglossal nerves).

CRANIAL NERVE TESTING

I: Olfactory Nerve

The sense of smell is a very important primordial function that is much more finely tuned in other animal species. Here, other mammals are able to seek out food, find their mates, and identify friend and foe alike because of their finely tuned olfactory brain. In the human, the loss of this function can still occasionally have very significant consequences primarily bearing on personal safety. If the human being cannot smell fires or burning food, their survival can be put at serious risk. The loss of smell also affects the pleasure of being able to taste, even though, as later noted, taste per se is primarily a function of CNs VII and IX.

Olfactory nerve function testing is relevant despite its only occasional clinical involvement. This may be impaired after relatively uncomplicated head trauma and in individuals with various causes of frontal lobe dysfunction, especially an olfactory groove meningioma. Loss of olfaction is sometimes an early sign of Parkinson disease. Clinical evaluation of olfactory functions is straightforward. The examiner has the patient sniff and attempt to identify familiar substances having specific odors

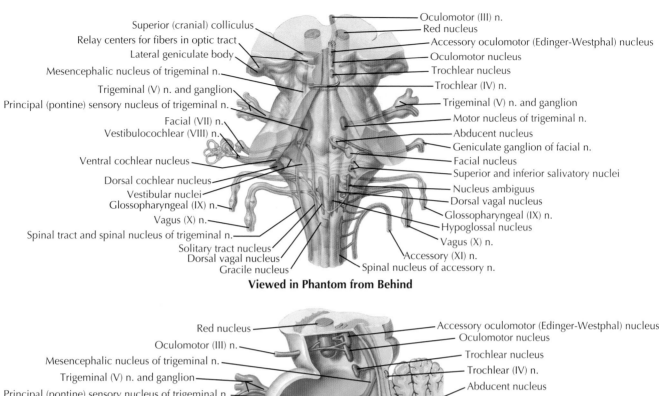

Superior (cranial) colliculus
Relay centers for fibers in optic tract
Lateral geniculate body
Mesencephalic nucleus of trigeminal n.
Trigeminal (V) n. and ganglion
Principal (pontine) sensory nucleus of trigeminal n.
Facial (VII) n.
Vestibulocochlear (VIII) n.
Ventral cochlear nucleus
Dorsal cochlear nucleus
Vestibular nuclei
Glossopharyngeal (IX) n.
Vagus (X) n.
Spinal tract and spinal nucleus of trigeminal n.
Solitary tract nucleus
Dorsal vagal nucleus
Gracile nucleus

Oculomotor (III) n.
Red nucleus
Accessory oculomotor (Edinger-Westphal) nucleus
Oculomotor nucleus
Trochlear nucleus
Trochlear (IV) n.
Trigeminal (V) n. and ganglion
Motor nucleus of trigeminal n.
Abducent nucleus
Geniculate ganglion of facial n.
Facial nucleus
Superior and inferior salivatory nuclei
Nucleus ambiguus
Dorsal vagal nucleus
Glossopharyngeal (IX) n.
Hypoglossal nucleus
Vagus (X) n.
Accessory (XI) n.
Spinal nucleus of accessory n.

Viewed in Phantom from Behind

Red nucleus
Oculomotor (III) n.
Mesencephalic nucleus of trigeminal n.
Trigeminal (V) n. and ganglion
Principal (pontine) sensory nucleus of trigeminal n.
Motor nucleus of trigeminal n.
Spinal tract and spinal nucleus of trigeminal n.
Facial (VII) n.
Vestibulocochlear (VIII) n.
Abducent (VI) n.
Glossopharyngeal (IX) n.
Hypoglossal (XII) n.
Vagus (X) n.
Accessory (XI) n.
Spinal nucleus of accessory n.

Accessory oculomotor (Edinger-Westphal) nucleus
Oculomotor nucleus
Trochlear nucleus
Trochlear (IV) n.
Abducent nucleus
Facial nerve loop
Facial nucleus
Vestibular nuclei
Ventral and dorsal cochlear nuclei
Superior and inferior salivatory nuclei
Solitary tract nucleus
Dorsal vagal nucleus
Hypoglossal nucleus
Nucleus ambiguus

■ Efferent fibers
■ Afferent fibers
■ Mixed fibers

Viewed in Lateral Dissection

Fig. 1.2 Cranial Nerves: Nerves and Nuclei.

(coffee beans, leaves of peppermint, lemon). Inability or reduced capacity to detect an odor is known as anosmia or hyposmia, respectively; inability to identify an odor correctly or smell distortion is described as parosmia or dysosmia. Bilateral olfactory nerve disturbance with total loss of smell, typically from head trauma, chronic upper airway infections, or medication, is usually a less ominous sign than unilateral loss, which raises the concern for a focal infiltrative or compressive lesion such as a frontal grove meningioma.

II: Optic Nerve

Of all the human sensations, the ability to see one's family and friends, read, and appreciate the beauties of nature is supreme; therefore it is difficult to imagine life without vision. Obviously, many individuals, such as Helen Keller, have vigorously and successfully conquered the challenge of being blind; however, given the choice, vision is one of the most precious of all animal sensations. "Blurred" vision is a common but relatively nonspecific symptom that may relate to dysfunction anywhere along the visual pathway (Fig. 1.3). When examining optic nerve function, it is important to identify any concomitant ocular

abnormalities such as proptosis, ptosis, scleral injection (congestion), tenderness, bruits, and pupillary changes.

Visual acuity is screened using a standard Snellen vision chart that is held 14 inches from the eye. Screening must be performed in proper light, as well as to the patient's refractive advantage, using corrective lenses or a pinhole when indicated. A careful visual field evaluation is the other important means to assess visual function. These tests are complementary, one testing central resolution at the retinal level and the other to evaluate peripheral visual field defects secondary to lesions at the levels of the optic chiasm, optic tracts, and occipital cortex. Visual fields are evaluated by having the patient sit comfortably facing the examiner at a similar eye level. First, each eye is tested independently. The patient is asked to look straight at the examiner's nose. The examiner extends an arm laterally, equidistant from himself or herself and the patient, and asks the patient to differentiate between one and two fingers. The patient's attention must always be directed back to the examiner because most patients will reflexively look laterally at the fingers. This will require repeated testing. Each quadrant of vision is evaluated separately. After individual testing, both eyes are tested

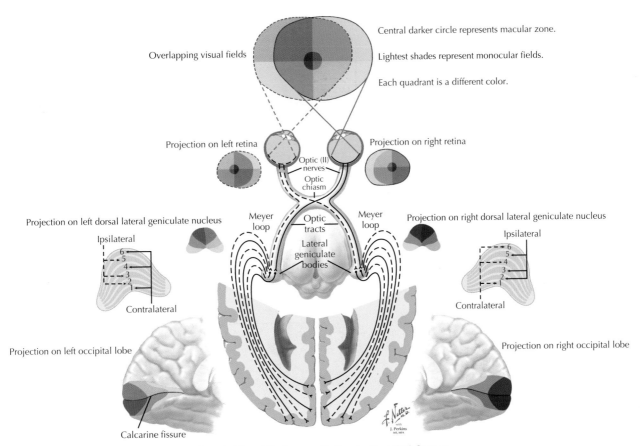

Fig. 1.3 Visual Pathways: Retina to Occipital Cortex.

simultaneously for visual neglect, as may occur with right hemispheric lesions. Progressively complex perimetric devices have the advantage of providing valuable data on the health of the visual system.

In *kinetic perimetry,* a stimulus is moved from a nonseeing area (far periphery or physiologic blind spot) to a seeing area, with patients indicating at what point the stimulus is first noticed. Testing is repeated from different directions until a curve can be drawn connecting the points at which a given stimulus is seen from all directions. This curve is the isopter for that stimulus for that eye. The isopter plot has been likened to a contour map, showing "the island of vision in a sea of darkness." The Goldmann perimeter, a half-sphere onto which spot stimuli are projected, is the premiere device for this mapping. The normal visual field extends approximately 90 degrees temporally, 45 degrees superiorly, 55 degrees nasally, and 65 degrees inferiorly. Practically, this geographic shape mimics the oblique teardrop shape of aviator-style sunglass lenses.

In *static perimetry,* the test point is not moved but turned on in a specific location. Typically automated, computer testing preselects locations within the central 30 degrees of field. Stimuli are dimmed until they are detected only intermittently on repetitive presentation—this intensity level is called the threshold. The computer then generates a map of numeric values of the illumination level required at every test spot, or the inverse of this level, often called a sensitivity value. Values may also be displayed as a grayscale map, and statistical calculations can be performed—by comparing to adjacent spots or precalculated normal values or noting sudden changes in sensitivity—to detect abnormal areas.

Most visual field changes have localizing value: specific location of the loss, its shape, or border sharpness (i.e., how quickly across the field the values change from abnormal to normal). Its concordance with the visual field of the other eye tends to implicate specific areas of the visual system. Localization is possible because details of anatomic organization at different levels predispose to particular types of loss (see Chapter 5).

When one examines the pupils, their shape and size need to be recorded. A side-to-side difference of no more than 1 mm in otherwise round pupils is acceptable as a normal variant. Pupillary responses are tested with a bright flashlight and are primarily mediated by the autonomic innervation of the eye (Fig. 1.4). A normal pupil reacts to light stimulus by constricting with the contralateral constriction of the unstimulated pupil as well. These responses are called the *direct* and *consensual reactions,* respectively, and are mediated through parasympathetic innervation to the pupillary sphincter from the Edinger-Westphal nucleus along the oculomotor nerve. The pupils also constrict when shifting focus from a far to a near object (*accommodation*) and during convergence of the eyes, as when patients are asked to look at their nose.

The sympathetic innervation of the pupillary dilator muscle involves a multisynaptic pathway with fibers ultimately reaching intracranially along the course of the internal carotid artery. Branches innervate the eye after traveling through the long and short ciliary nerves. The *ciliospinal reflex* is potentially useful when evaluating comatose patients. In this setting, if the examiner pinches the patient's neck, the ipsilateral pupil should transiently dilate. This provides a means to test the integrity of ipsilateral pathways to midbrain structures.

The short ciliary nerve, supplying parasympathetic inputs to the pupil, may be damaged by various forms of trauma. This results in a unilateral dilated pupil with preservation of other third nerve function.

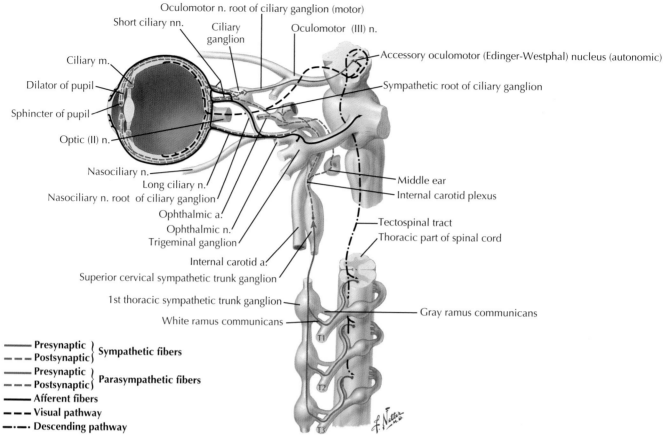

Fig. 1.4 Autonomic Innervation of Eye.

TABLE 1.1   Pupillary Abnormalities

	Argyll Robertson	**Horner**	**Holmes Adie**
Response to light	None	Yes	None
Other responses	Brisk reaction to near stimulus Converge	Normal	Tonic reaction to near stimulus Accommodation
Margins	Irregular	Regular	Regular
Associated changes	Iris depigmentation	Ptosis	Loss of muscle stretch reflex
Causes	Tabes dorsalis	Carotid dissection Carotid aneurysm Pancoast tumor Syringomyelia	Ciliary ganglion
Anatomy	Unknown (tectum of midbrain likely)	Loss of sympathetic	Loss of parasympathetic

Significant unilateral pupillary abnormalities are usually related to innervation changes in pupillary muscles.

A number of pathophysiologic mechanisms lead to mydriasis (pupillary dilatation) (Table 1.1). Atropine-like eye drops, often used for their ability to produce pupillary dilation, inadvertent ocular application of certain nebulized bronchodilators, and placement of a scopolamine anti-motion patch with inadvertent leak into the conjunctiva are occasionally overlooked as potential causes for an otherwise asymptomatic, dilated, poorly reactive pupil. Other medications may also lead to certain atypical light reactions. The presence of bilateral dilated pupils, in an otherwise neurologically intact patient, is unlikely to reflect significant neuropathology. In contrast, the presence of prominent pupillary constriction most likely reflects the use of narcotic analogs or parasympathomimetic drugs, such as those typically used to treat glaucoma.

Horner Syndrome

The classic findings include miosis (pupillary constriction), subtle ptosis, and an ipsilateral loss of facial sweating. Here the constricted pupil develops secondary to interference with the sympathetic nerves at one of many different levels along its long intramedullary (brain and spinal cord) and complicated extracranial course.

Sympathetic efferent fibers originate within the hypothalamus and traverse the brainstem and cervical spinal cord, then exit the upper thoracic levels and course rostrally to reach the superior cervical ganglia (see Fig. 1.4). Subsequently, these sympathetic fibers track with the carotid artery within the neck to reenter the cranium and subsequently reach their destination innervating the eye's pupillodilator musculature. Typically, patients with Horner syndrome (Fig. 1.5) have an ipsilateral

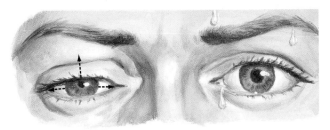

Interruption of the sympathetic fibers outside the brain causes ipsilateral ptosis, anhidrosis, and miosis without abnormal ocular mobility.

Fig. 1.5 Right Horner Syndrome.

loss of sweating in the face (anhidrosis), a constricted pupil (miosis), and an upper lid droop from loss of innervation to Müller muscle, a small smooth muscle lid elevator (ptosis). The levator palpebra superioris, a striated muscle innervated by the oculomotor nerve CN III, is not affected.

Optic Fundus

The ability to peer into the patient's eye is a very unique and fascinating experience because it provides an opportunity to directly examine not only the initial portion of the optic nerve but also tiny arterioles and veins. This is the only portion of human anatomy that provides the physician with such an opportunity. Here one may find signs of increased intracranial pressure or evidences of the effects of poorly controlled hypertension or diabetes mellitus. Currently all of these various lesions are much less commonly observed because of much better treatment of systemic illnesses that affect the smaller blood vessels. Similarly, the development of MRI and CT scanning makes it easier to identify intracerebral mass lesions at a much earlier stage of illness. Currently, as brain tumors no longer reach a critical size, obstructing cerebrospinal fluid flow, creating the increased intracranial pressure that leads to papilledema, this is now a relatively rare finding but one that still demands recognition.

A careful optic funduscopic examination is essential in the evaluation of very many neurologic disorders. This evaluation is best performed in a relatively dark environment that leads to both a reflex increase in pupillary size and improvement in contrast of the posterior chamber structures. Findings that should be documented include optic nerve margins, venous pulsations, and the presence of hemorrhages, exudates, or any obvious obstruction to flow by embolic material (such as cholesterol plaque in patients complaining of transient visual obscuration), and pallor of retinal fields that may reflect ischemia.

Papilledema is characterized by elevation and blurring of the optic disk, absence of venous pulsations, and hemorrhages adjacent to and on the disk (Fig. 1.6). The finding of papilledema indicates increased intracranial pressure of any cause, including brain tumors, subarachnoid hemorrhage, metabolic processes, pseudotumor cerebri, and venous sinus thrombosis.

III, IV, VI: Oculomotor, Trochlear, and Abducens Nerves

Our ability to acutely focus our eyes on an object of interest depends on being able to move the eyes together in a conjugate fashion; this requires three related CNs that take their origin from various juxta midline midbrain and pontine nuclei. These provide us with the ability to astutely focus on an object of interest without concomitantly moving our head. Whether it is a detective watching a suspect or a teenager taking a furtive glance at a new classmate, these CNs provide us with a broad sweep of very finely tuned motor function. There is no other group of muscles that is so finely innervated as these. Their innervation ratio is approximately 20:1, in contrast to those of large muscles of the

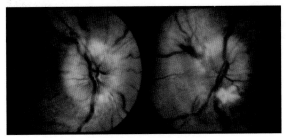

Optic fundus with papilledema

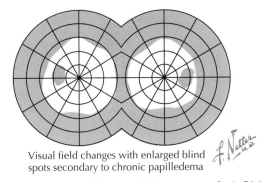

Visual field changes with enlarged blind spots secondary to chronic papilledema

Fig. 1.6 Effects of Increased Intracranial Pressure on Optic Disk and Visual Fields.

extremities with ratios between 400:1 and 2000:1. Certainly, this accounts for the fact that one of the earliest clinical manifestations of myasthenia gravis relates to the extraocular muscles (EOMs), where the interruption of just a few neuromuscular junctions affects the finely harmonized EOM function, leading to a skewed operation and thus double vision.

To identify isolated EOM dysfunction, it is most accurate to test each eye individually, describing the observed specific loss of EOM function. For example, when the eye cannot be turned laterally, the condition is labeled as an *abduction paresis,* as opposed to CN VI palsy. This is because the responsible lesion can be at any one of three sites, namely, CN, neuromuscular junction, or muscle per se. A more detailed assessment of these CNs is available in Section II, Chapter 6.

The medial longitudinal fasciculus (MLF) is responsible for controlling EOM function because it provides a means to modify central horizontal conjugate gaze circuits. The MLF connects CN III on one side and CN VI on the opposite side. Understanding the circuit of horizontal conjugate gaze helps clinicians to appreciate the relation between the frontal eye fields and the influence it exerts on horizontal conjugate gaze, as well the reflex relation between the ocular and vestibular systems (Fig. 1.7).

The connection of the vestibular system to the MLF can be tested by two different means. One is the doll's-eye maneuver. Here the patient's head is rotated side to side while the examiner watches for rotation of the eyes. Passive movement of the head to the left normally moves the eyes in the opposite direction, with the left eye adducting and the right eye abducting. The opposite occurs when the head is rotated to the right.

Ice-water caloric stimulation provides another option to study vestibular ocular MLF pathways. This is primarily used for the examination of comatose patients; on very rare occasions, it is extremely helpful for rousing a patient presenting with a suspected nonorganic coma. Patients' heads are placed at an elevation of approximately 45 degrees. Next, the tympanic membranes are checked for intactness, and then 25–50 mL of ice water is gradually infused into each ear. A normal response in the awake patient, after left ear stimulation, is to observe slow deviation

Excitatory endings → → → → → →
Inhibitory endings →
Indeterminate endings ⇢

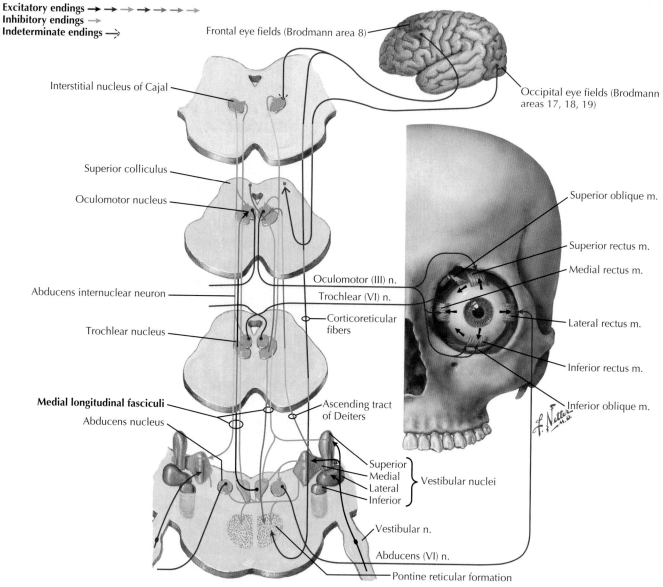

Frontal eye fields (Brodmann area 8)

Occipital eye fields (Brodmann areas 17, 18, 19)

Interstitial nucleus of Cajal

Superior colliculus

Oculomotor nucleus

Superior oblique m.

Superior rectus m.

Medial rectus m.

Oculomotor (III) n.

Trochlear (VI) n.

Corticoreticular fibers

Abducens internuclear neuron

Trochlear nucleus

Lateral rectus m.

Inferior rectus m.

Inferior oblique m.

Medial longitudinal fasciculi

Ascending tract of Deiters

Abducens nucleus

Superior
Medial
Lateral
Inferior

Vestibular nuclei

Vestibular n.

Abducens (VI) n.

Pontine reticular formation

Fig. 1.7 Control of Eye Movements.

of the eyes to the left followed by rapid movement (nystagmus) to the right (see Fig. 1.8). In contrast, the comatose patient with an intact brainstem has a persistent ipsilateral deviation of the eyes to the site of stimulation with loss of the rapid eye movement component to the opposite side.

The center for vertical conjugate gaze and convergence is also located within the midbrain, although the underlying circuit is not well delineated. The vertical conjugate gaze centers can be tested by flexion of the neck while holding the eyelids open and watching the eye movements. When CNS processes affect conjugate gaze, such as with MS, a prominent nystagmus is often defined. The nystagmus is thought to result from an attempt to maintain conjugate function of the eyes and minimize double images.

V: Trigeminal Nerve

Our ability to perceive various stimuli applied to the face depends almost entirely on this nerve; whether as a warning to protect oneself from subzero cold, something potentially threatening to our eyesight, or the pleasurable sensation from the kiss of a beloved one, all forms

of sensations applied to the face are tracked to our brain through the trigeminal nerve (Fig. 1.9). The primary sensory portion of this nerve has three divisions, ophthalmic, maxillary, and mandibular; they respectively supply approximately one-third of the face from top to bottom, as well as the anterior aspects of the scalp. The angle of the jaw is spared within the trigeminal mandibular division lesions. This provides an important landmark to potentially differentiate patients with conversion disorders, because they are not anatomically sophisticated and may report they have lost sensation in this region.

The clinical testing of trigeminal nerve function includes both appreciation of a wisp of cotton and a sharp object on the facial skin, as well as the corneal reflex. To evaluate the broad spectrum of facial sensation (i.e., touch, pain, and temperature), the examiner uses a cotton wisp; the tip of a new, previously unused safety pin; and the cold handle of a tuning fork. In a symmetric fashion, the physician asks whether the patient can perceive each stimulus in the three major divisions of the trigeminal nerve supplying the face.

The *corneal reflex* depends on afferents from the first division of the trigeminal nerve combined with facial nerve efferents. This is also best

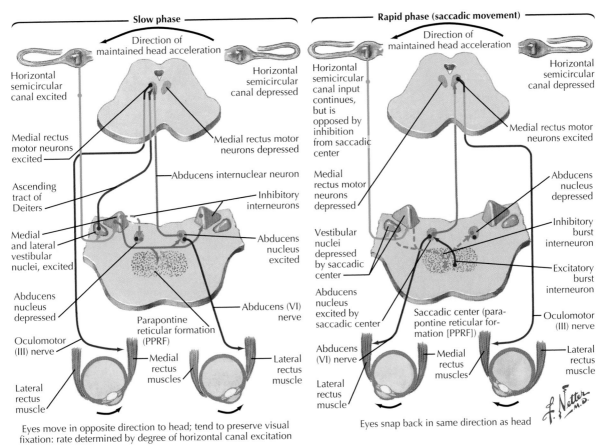

Fig. 1.8 Vestibular Eighth Nerve Input to Horizontal Eye Movements and Nystagmus.

tested using a wisp of cotton approaching the patient from the side while she or he looks away. Normally, both eyelids close when the cornea on one side is stimulated; this is because this reflex involves multisynaptic brainstem pathways.

Lastly, there is a primary motor portion that is part of the trigeminal nerve. It primarily supplies the muscles of mastication. It is best assessed by having the patient bite down and by trying to open the mouth against resistance.

VII: Facial Nerve

Facial expression is one of our very important innate human attributes, allowing one to demonstrate a very broad spectrum of human emotions, especially happiness and sorrow; these are primarily dependent on the facial nerve (Fig. 1.10). The motor functions of CN VII are tested by asking patients to wrinkle their forehead, close their eyes, and smile. Whistling and puffing up the cheeks are other techniques to test for subtle weakness. When unilateral peripheral weakness affects the facial nerve after it leaves the brainstem, the face may look "ironed out," and when the patient smiles, the contralateral healthy facial muscle pulls up the opposite half of the mouth while the affected side remains motionless. Patients often cannot keep water in their mouths, and saliva may constantly drip from the paralyzed side. With peripheral CN VII palsies, patients are also unable to close their ipsilateral eye or wrinkle their foreheads on the affected side. However, although the lid cannot close, the eyeball rolls up into the head, removing the pupil from observation. This is known as the Bell phenomena.

In addition, there is another motor branch of the facial nerve; this innervates the stapedius muscle. It helps to modulate the vibration of the tympanic membrane and dampens sounds. When this part of the facial nerve is affected, the patient notes hyperacusis; this is an increased, often unpleasant perception of sound when listening to a phone with the ipsilateral ear.

Lastly, the facial nerve has a few other functions. These include prominent autonomic function, sending parasympathetic fibers to both the lacrimal and the salivary glands. It also subserves the important function of taste, another function providing both safety from rancid food and pleasure from a delightful wine. There is also a tiny degree of routine skin sensation represented for portions of the ear.

VIII: Cochlear and Vestibular Nerves (Auditory Nerve)

Many mornings some of us are blessed by a virtual ornithologic symphony in our backyards. This always makes one pause and give thanks once again for this marvelous primary sensation. Here, yet another CN, the cochlear, provides for the emotional highs that auditory sensations bring to the human brain. Whether it is the first cry of a newborn, the reassuring words of a loved one, or Beethoven's seventh symphony, this unique sensation of higher animal life is tracked through this one CN.

Beyond the simple test of being able to hear, more sophisticated clinical evaluation of CN VIII is often challenging for the neurologist. Fortunately, our otolaryngologist colleagues are able to precisely measure the appreciation of specific auditory frequencies in a very sophisticated manner. Barring the availability of these formal audiometric evaluations, simple office-based hearing tests sometimes help to demonstrate diagnostically useful asymmetries. Using a standard tuning fork, it is possible to differentiate between *nerve (perceptive) deafness* caused by cochlear nerve damage and that caused by *middle ear (conduction) deafness,* with two different applications of the standard tuning fork. We are able to test both air and bone conduction.

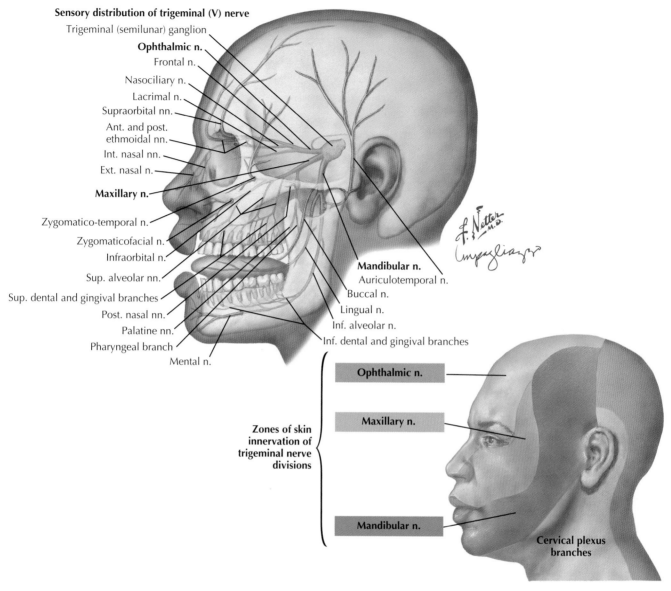

Sensory distribution of trigeminal (V) nerve

Trigeminal (semilunar) ganglion

Ophthalmic n.

Frontal n.

Nasociliary n.

Lacrimal n.

Supraorbital nn.

Ant. and post. ethmoidal nn.

Int. nasal nn.

Ext. nasal n.

Maxillary n.

Zygomatico-temporal n.

Zygomaticofacial n.

Infraorbital n.

Sup. alveolar nn.

Sup. dental and gingival branches

Post. nasal nn.

Palatine nn.

Pharyngeal branch

Mental n.

Mandibular n.

Auriculotemporal n.

Buccal n.

Lingual n.

Inf. alveolar n.

Inf. dental and gingival branches

Zones of skin innervation of trigeminal nerve divisions

Ophthalmic n.

Maxillary n.

Mandibular n.

Cervical plexus branches

Fig. 1.9 Trigeminal Nerve Neuralgia.

Initially a vibrating tuning fork is placed on the vertex of the skull, *Weber test,* allowing bone conduction to be assessed. Here the patient is asked to decide whether one ear perceives the sound created by the vibration better than the other (Fig. 1.11). If the patient has nerve deafness, the vibrations are appreciated more in the normal ear. In contrast, with conduction deafness, the vibrations are better appreciated in the abnormal ear.

The *Rinne test* is carried out by placing this vibrating instrument on the mastoid process of the skull. Here the patient is asked to identify the presence of sound. As the vibrations of the tuning fork diminish, eventually the patient is unable to appreciate the sound. At that instant, the instrument is moved close to the external ear canal to evaluate air conduction. If the individual has normal hearing, air conduction is longer than bone conduction. When a patient has nerve (perceptive) deafness, both bone and air conductions are diminished, but air conduction is still better than bone conduction. In contrast with *conduction deafness,* secondary to middle ear pathology, these findings are reversed. Here, when the patient's bony conduction has ceased, air conduction is limited by the intrinsic disorder within the middle ear. Therefore the

sound can no longer be heard; that is, it cannot pass through the mechanoreceptors that amplify the sound and thus cannot reach the auditory nerve.

Vestibular Nerve

The vestibular system can be tested indirectly by evaluating for nystagmus during testing of ocular movements or by positional techniques, such as the Barany maneuver (aka Dix-Hallpike test), that induce nystagmus in cases of benign positional vertigo (BPV) in which inner ear dysfunction is caused by otolith displacement into the semicircular canals (Fig. 1.12). Here the patient is seated on an examining table and the eyes are observed for the presence of spontaneous nystagmus. If none is present, the examiner rapidly lays the patient back down, with the head slightly extended and concomitantly turning the head laterally. If, after a few seconds' delay, the patient develops the typical symptoms of vertigo with a characteristic delayed rotary, eventually fatiguing nystagmus, the study is positive.

Eye movements depend on two primary components, the induced voluntary frontal eye fields and the primary reflex-driven vestibular-ocular

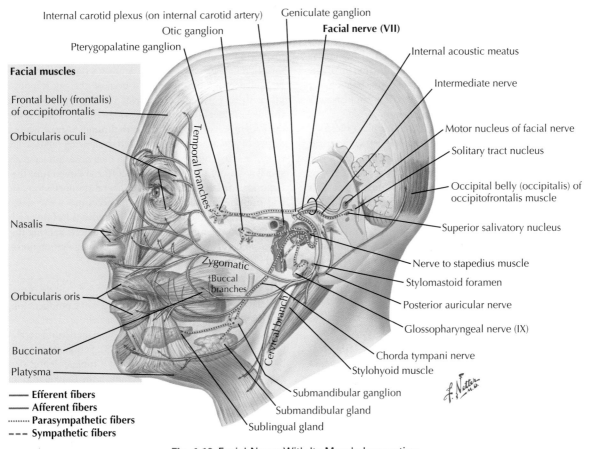

Internal carotid plexus (on internal carotid artery)
Otic ganglion
Pterygopalatine ganglion
Geniculate ganglion
Facial nerve (VII)
Internal acoustic meatus
Intermediate nerve

Facial muscles

Frontal belly (frontalis) of occipitofrontalis
Orbicularis oculi
Nasalis
Temporal branches
Motor nucleus of facial nerve
Solitary tract nucleus
Occipital belly (occipitalis) of occipitofrontalis muscle
Superior salivatory nucleus
Zygomatic
Buccal branches
Orbicularis oris
Buccinator
Platysma
Cervical branch
Nerve to stapedius muscle
Stylomastoid foramen
Posterior auricular nerve
Glossopharyngeal nerve (IX)
Chorda tympani nerve
Stylohyoid muscle
Submandibular ganglion
Submandibular gland
Sublingual gland

—— **Efferent fibers**
—— **Afferent fibers**
········ **Parasympathetic fibers**
--- **Sympathetic fibers**

Fig. 1.10 Facial Nerve With Its Muscle Innervation.

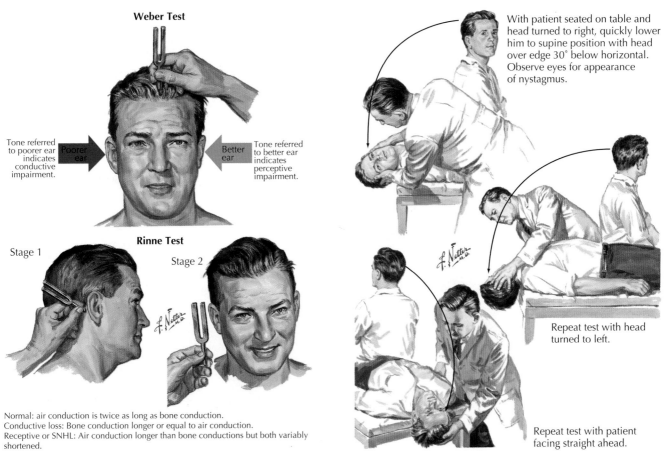

Weber Test

Tone referred to poorer ear indicates conductive impairment.
Poorer ear
Better ear
Tone referred to better ear indicates perceptive impairment.

With patient seated on table and head turned to right, quickly lower him to supine position with head over edge 30° below horizontal. Observe eyes for appearance of nystagmus.

Rinne Test

Stage 1   Stage 2

Repeat test with head turned to left.

Normal: air conduction is twice as long as bone conduction.
Conductive loss: Bone conduction longer or equal to air conduction.
Receptive or SNHL: Air conduction longer than bone conductions but both variably shortened.

Repeat test with patient facing straight ahead.

Fig. 1.11 Auditory Nerve Testing: Weber and Rinne Testing.

Fig. 1.12 Test for Positional Vertigo.

movement controlled by multiple connections (see Fig. 1.8; and also Fig. 1.7). The ability to maintain conjugate eye movements and a visual perspective on the surrounding world is an important brainstem function. It requires inputs from receptors in muscles, joints, and the cupulae of the inner ear. Therefore, when the patient has dysfunction involving any portion of the vestibular-ocular or cerebellar axis, the maintenance of basic visual orientation is challenged. Nystagmus is a compensatory process that attempts to help maintain visual fixation.

Traditionally, when one describes nystagmus, the fast phase direction becomes the designated title (see Fig. 1.8). For example, left semicircular canal stimulation produces a slow nystagmus to the left, with a fast component to the right. As a result, the nystagmus is referred to as right beating nystagmus. Direct stimulation of the semicircular canals or its direct connections (i.e., the vestibular nuclei) often induces a torsional nystagmus. This is described as clockwise or counterclockwise, according to the fast phase.

A few beats of horizontal nystagmus occurring with extreme horizontal gaze is normal in most individuals. The most common cause of bilateral horizontal nystagmus occurs secondary to toxic levels of alcohol ingestion or some medications (i.e., phenytoin and barbiturates).

IX, X, XI: Glossopharyngeal, Vagus, and Accessory Nerves

The most common complaints related to glossopharyngeal-vagal system dysfunction include swallowing difficulties (dysphagia) and changes in voice (dysphonia). A patient with a glossopharyngeal nerve paresis presents with flattening of the palate on the affected side. When the patient is asked to produce a sound, the uvula is drawn to the unaffected side (Fig. 1.13). Indirect mirror examination of the vocal cords may demonstrate paralysis of the ipsilateral cord. The traditional test for gag reflex, placing a tongue depressor on the posterior pharynx, is of equivocal significance at best because the gag response varies significantly and patients can display wide varieties of tolerance to this stimulus. Preservation of swallowing reflexes is best tested by giving the patient 30 mL of fluid to drink through a straw while seated at 90 degrees. Patients with compromised swallowing reflexes develop a "wet cough" and regurgitate fluids through their nose. Intracranial or proximal spinal accessory nerve damage limits the ability to turn the head to the opposite side (weakness of the ipsilateral sternocleidomastoid muscles and trapezius muscle). More distal accessory nerve damage is most commonly seen following surgical misadventures during lymph node biopsy from the posterior triangle of the neck, sparing the sternocleidomastoid but affecting the trapezius, causing dysfunction and winging of the scapula.

XII: Hypoglossal Nerve

Damage to the hypoglossal nucleus or its nerve produces tongue atrophy and fasciculations. The fasciculations usually are seen best on the lateral aspects of the tongue. If the nerve damage is unilateral, the tongue often deviates to that side (see Fig. 1.13). Subtle weakness can be tested by asking the patient to push against a tongue depressor held by the examiner or by having the patient push the tongue into the cheek.

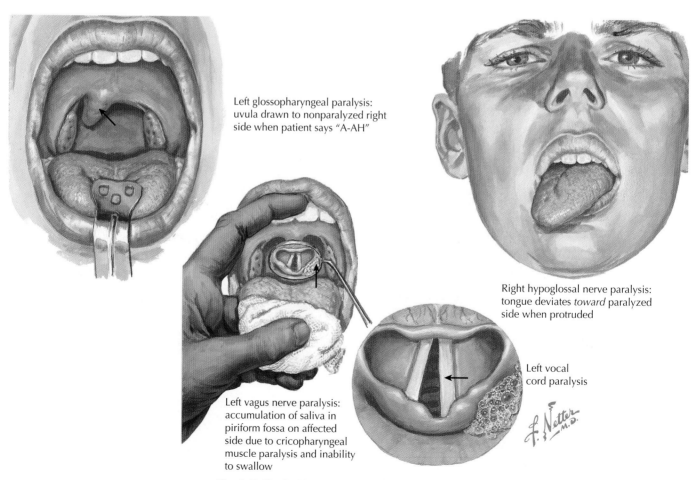

Left glossopharyngeal paralysis: uvula drawn to nonparalyzed right side when patient says "A-AH"

Left vagus nerve paralysis: accumulation of saliva in piriform fossa on affected side due to cricopharyngeal muscle paralysis and inability to swallow

Right hypoglossal nerve paralysis: tongue deviates *toward* paralyzed side when protruded

Left vocal cord paralysis

Fig. 1.13 Uvula, Tongue, and Vocal Cord Weakness.

CRANIAL NEUROPATHIES AND SYSTEMIC DISEASE

When one evaluates a patient presenting with any cranial neuropathy, it is important to search for signs of other neurologic and systemic disorders. The patient with recently discovered anosmia may have early Parkinson disease. An acute painful, but pupil-sparing, third nerve palsy may be a tip-off to the diagnosis of diabetes mellitus. When one meets an individual with unilateral or bilateral facial nerve palsies, Lyme disease and sarcoidosis are in the differential diagnosis. When one evaluates patients having multiple cranial neuropathies, leptomeningeal infiltration from metastatic carcinoma or lymphoma, sarcoidosis, or chronic infectious processes, such as tuberculosis, always require diagnostic consideration.

CEREBELLAR DYSFUNCTION

Evaluation of posture and gait provides the opportunity to observe the most dramatic clinical manifestations of cerebellar dysfunction. The patient presenting with *midline cerebellar lesions* affecting the vermis characteristically assumes a broad-based stance when walking that typically mimics an inebriated individual. At the extreme, these individuals are unable to maintain a stance. In contrast, when there is a *cerebellar hemisphere problem,* the patient has a tendency to veer to the affected side. With midline lesions, gait is usually unchanged whether the eyes are open or closed, suggesting that this is not the result of disruption of proprioceptive inputs. Patients with unilateral lesions are often able to compensate with their eyes open but deteriorate when they lose visual inputs.

Loss of limb coordination in cerebellar disorders is the result of an inability to calculate inputs from different joints and muscles and coordinate them into smooth movements. This is best observed by testing *finger-to-nose* and *heel-to-shin* movements and making bilateral comparisons. When performing the finger-to-nose test, the examiner provides his or her finger as the target; it is sequentially moved to different locations. The patient in turn keeps the arm extended and tries to touch the examiner's finger at each location. When unilateral cerebellar dysfunction is present, the patient *overshoots* the target, so-called *past pointing.* It is important not to misinterpret such findings as always of cerebellar origin, because patients with focal motor or sensory cerebral cortex lesions may present with mild arm weakness and proprioceptive sensory loss affecting that limb. In this setting, a degree of focal limb dysmetria may develop; this is sometimes difficult to distinguish from primary cerebellar dysfunction. One clinical means to distinguish cerebellar from cerebral cortical dysfunction is that the patient with cerebellar hemisphere lesions will have these movements improve after a few trials. In contrast, with cerebral cortical dysmetria, repeated trials lead only to further deterioration in the attempted action.

Dysdiadochokinesia is a sign of cerebellar dysfunction that occurs when the patient is asked to rapidly change hand or finger movements (i.e., alternating between palms up and palm down). Patients with cerebellar dysfunction typically have difficulties switching and maintaining smooth, rapid, alternating movements.

Tremor, nystagmus, and *hypotonia* are other important indications of potential cerebellar dysfunction. *Tremors* may develop from any lesion that affects the cerebellar efferent fibers via the superior cerebellar peduncle. This is characterized by coarse, irregular movement. *Nystagmus* may occur with unilateral cerebellar disease; the nystagmus is most prominent on looking to the affected side. *Hypotonia* may be present but is often difficult to document. This is best observed when testing a patient's MSRs at the quadriceps tendon knee jerk. Here the normal "check" does not occur after the initial movement, so the leg on the affected side swings back and forth a few times after the initial patellar tendon percussion.

GAIT EVALUATION

Whenever possible, the neurologic clinician is encouraged to personally greet the patients, watching them arise from their chair and initiate their gate. Next, before moving to the examination room the patient needs to be observed walking in the hallway. On occasion it is important to observe the patient on stairs, particularly if there is a query about proximal weakness. A smooth gait requires multiple inputs from the cerebellum and primary motor and sensory systems. Gait disorders provide a very broad differential diagnostic challenge that results from lesions in any part of the neuraxis (Fig. 1.14).

Frontal lobe (see Fig. 1.14D) processes including tumors and normal-pressure hydrocephalus lead to apraxia, spasticity, and leg weakness. *Spasticity* is a nonspecific marker of corticospinal tract disorders that may arise with various neurologic lesions between the frontal lobe and the distal spinal cord (Fig. 1.15). Various *neurodegenerative* conditions, particularly those affecting the basal ganglia, such as *Parkinson disease* (see Fig. 1.14A1–3), are some of the most common causes of gait difficulties. These are typically manifested by slowness initiating gait, small steps, and eventually gait festination, wherein once patients begin to accelerate their walking, they take increasingly more rapid but paradoxically smaller steps. There is an innate, almost waxlike rigidity to their stooped body carriage, including the frozen posture of one or both arms that usually lacks the normal arm swing. Very occasionally, a change in posture from the seated position to attempted gait will be manifested by a dystonic posturing, which may be indicative of another genetic disorder, dystonia musculorum deformans, or paroxysmal choreoathetosis.

Cerebellar disorders related to midline anterior cerebellar *vermis* lesions or various *heredofamilial spinocerebellar* entities lead to a broad-base gait ataxia (see Fig. 1.14C1–2). The patient is asked to walk in tandem, with one foot in front of the other. It is an effective means to elicit a subtle disequilibrium often related to midline cerebellar dysfunction such as with simple entities, including alcohol intoxication.

Myelopathies with posterior column dysfunction, such as vitamin B_{12} deficiency, present with loss of proprioception function. These particularly affect the patient's gait in dark environments, as do some of the *peripheral neuropathies, especially those with a primary sensory ganglionopathy* (see Fig. 1.14F1). Testing for the presence of a Romberg sign is an excellent clinical marker for these disorders. Here, patients are asked to stand in place with their eyes open, gain their equilibrium, and then close their eyes. Individuals with various proprioceptive disorders are unable to maintain their balance when visual clues are withdrawn; such a condition is referred to as a positive Romberg sign. One of the earliest signs, and at times a prominent sign of a myopathy, is the need to push off the arms of a chair when arising to walk. When these individuals do walk, their gait may be a broad-based gait mimicking an anterior cerebellar lesion. When viewed from the side, the curve of their low back is accentuated (i.e., hyperlordotic). Both the wide base and the hyperlordosis are representative of weakness of the most proximal muscle groups—the iliopsoas, quadriceps, and glutei—as well as the paraspinal axial musculature.

An often-overlooked cause of gait difficulties is orthopedic and musculoskeletal problems. A perhaps simplistic perspective on the contribution of this system to gait is the analogy that the musculoskeletal system functions similar to an axle on a car, maintaining alignment and proper, symmetric rotation of the wheels. Our vertebral column is a sophisticated axle that, with time, loses some of its alignment. The

A Parkinson Disease

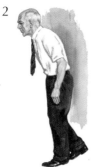

1

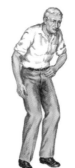

2

3

Stage 1: unilateral involvement; blank facies; affected arm with tremor

Stage 2: bilateral involvement with stooped posture; slow, shuffling gait with short steps (petit pas)

Stage 3: pronounced gait disturbances, moderate generalized disability; postural instability with tendency to fall

B Spastic Corticospinal

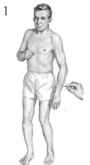

1

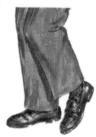

2

Right hemiparesis with flexed right arm secondary to a corticospinal tract lesion

Typical spastic gait, circumduction of the leg at the hip and scuffling the toe on affected leg.

C Cerebellar Gait

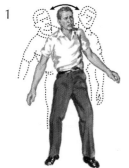

1

2

Wide-based gait of midline cerebellar tumor or other lesion

Typical wide-based gait of drug intoxication

D Apraxic, Frontal Gait

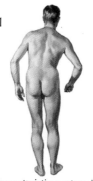

Apraxic gait of normal-pressure hydrocephalus

E Lumbar Spine Disease

1

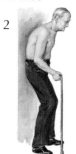

2

Characteristic posture in left-sided lower lumbar disc herniation

Patient with lumbar spinal stenosis with forward flexion gait

F Peripheral Neuropathies

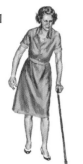

1

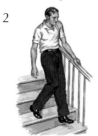

2

3

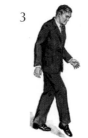

Patient walks gingerly due to loss of position sense and/or painful dysesthesia

Sudden buckling of knee while going down stairs (femoral nerve)

Sudden occurrence of foot drop while walking (peroneal nerve)

f. Netter M.D.

G Myopathy

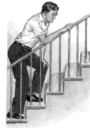

Severe myopathy or NMJ lesion with proximal weakness

Fig. 1.14 Gait Disorder Characteristics and Etiology. *NMJ,* Neuromuscular junction.

attached muscles, to a misaligned chain of vertebrae, ultimately generates aberrant feedback loops to the spinal cord and the brain.

Many of our *senior citizens* gradually lose precise control of their gait, initially manifested by subtle changes on neurologic exam. Healthy older individuals often have limited ability to perform tandem gait. The very important message here is that this finding in isolation should not be considered abnormal per se among patients living into their eighth decade. Nevertheless, older patients become increasingly limited by a dwindling ability to walk independently.

Very often, in this setting there is not one specific mechanism either operative or identifiable. A number of patients have a multifaceted

source related to the gradual *aging* (graying) of multiple neurologic systems. One source that always requires consideration is the possibility of *orthostatic hypotension*. Most commonly, this relates to medications; however, one of the neurodegenerative disorders, multiple system atrophy (see Chapter 29), may present in this fashion. Thus it is important to carefully check blood pressures in the supine posture, when seated, then immediately on standing, and then every 30 seconds thereafter until the pressure is stabilized. A persistent drop in blood pressure of 20–30 mm Hg is usually regarded as significant in this setting.

It is important to ask about the circumstances accompanying the gait decline. Does the individual scuff a foot because of a spastic leg

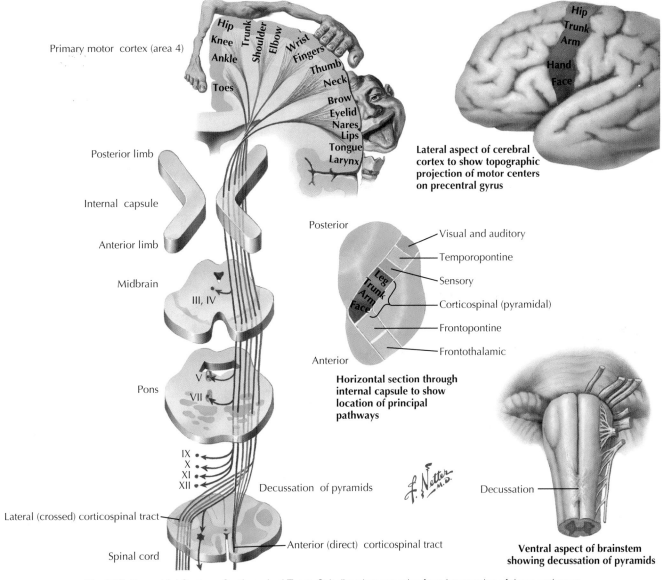

Fig. 1.15 Pyramidal System, Corticospinal Tract. Gait disorders can arise from interruption of these pathways at any level.

that interferes with a smooth alteration of individual legs? What settings lead to a fall? Does one catch one's toe on a rug as with subtle spasticity (see Fig. 1.14B1–2) or feel a leg give out going downstairs secondary to weakness of the quadriceps femoris muscle (see Fig. 1.14F2)? Having such information, the examiner can then easily try to reproduce the circumstances that lead to the falls.

Typically, gait function is tested under several conditions, including walking straight, walking at least 10 yards in open space, making turns, maneuvering through a tight corridor, attempting tandem gait, or in low light settings, as well as on the stairs. The normal degree of foot separation (the base) is widened when proprioception or midline cerebellar vermis function is compromised. Occasionally, having the patient climb stairs reveals a subtle degree of iliopsoas weakness as found in various peripheral motor unit disorders (particularly myopathies) and, less commonly, neuromuscular junction or proximal peripheral neuropathies (see Fig. 1.14G). Finally, the appearance of spasticity may be enhanced by having the patient walk longer distances and even asking him or her to walk several blocks and return to the clinic. Rarely, this

uncovers an unsuspected corticospinal tract lesion. Chapter 38 expands on the clinical evaluation of gait disorders.

ABNORMAL ADVENTITIOUS MOVEMENTS

Neurologists are frequently consulted to evaluate various adventitious movements, including tremors, chorea, dyskinesias, and ballismus. The most common movement disorder encountered in the office is "essential tremor," usually a "benign" hereditary condition that generally does not herald a progressive neurodegenerative process. These patients often seek medical attention because they are concerned that their tremors are a sign of Parkinson disease. Therefore differentiating between different types of tremors is a common and important concern. An essential tremor characteristically occurs during certain voluntary actions, such as when bringing a cup of coffee to the mouth. In contrast, with classic Parkinson disease, the pill-rolling tremor is primarily evident at rest and when the patient is seated or walking and disappears with the spontaneous use of the extremity. A subtle fidgeting may represent the

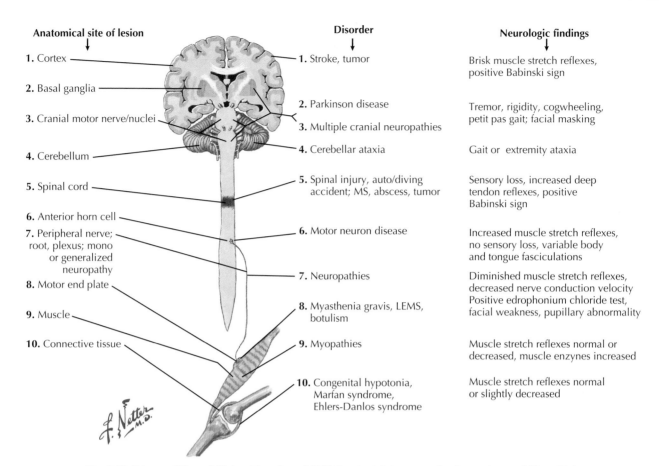

Anatomical site of lesion

1. Cortex
2. Basal ganglia
3. Cranial motor nerve/nuclei
4. Cerebellum
5. Spinal cord
6. Anterior horn cell
7. Peripheral nerve; root, plexus; mono or generalized neuropathy
8. Motor end plate
9. Muscle
10. Connective tissue

Disorder

1. Stroke, tumor
2. Parkinson disease
3. Multiple cranial neuropathies
4. Cerebellar ataxia
5. Spinal injury, auto/diving accident; MS, abscess, tumor
6. Motor neuron disease
7. Neuropathies
8. Myasthenia gravis, LEMS, botulism
9. Myopathies
10. Congenital hypotonia, Marfan syndrome, Ehlers-Danlos syndrome

Neurologic findings

Brisk muscle stretch reflexes, positive Babinski sign

Tremor, rigidity, cogwheeling, petit pas gait; facial masking

Gait or extremity ataxia

Sensory loss, increased deep tendon reflexes, positive Babinski sign

Increased muscle stretch reflexes, no sensory loss, variable body and tongue fasciculations

Diminished muscle stretch reflexes, decreased nerve conduction velocity Positive edrophonium chloride test, facial weakness, pupillary abnormality

Muscle stretch reflexes normal or decreased, muscle enzymes increased

Muscle stretch reflexes normal or slightly decreased

Fig. 1.16 Primary Sites of Motor Disorders. *LEMS,* Lambert-Eaton myasthenic syndrome; *MS,* multiple sclerosis.

earliest sign of Huntington or Sydenham chorea. Very rarely a patient will present with a more energetic, purposeless, wing-beating movement of an extremity, referred to as hemiballismus. A full discussion of movement disorders and their presentation is found in Section IX.

MUSCLE STRENGTH EVALUATION

Weakness is one of the most common complaints of patients seeking neurologic care. The motor pathways encompass multiple anatomic areas within the CNS, including the cerebral cortex and important subcortical structures such as the basal ganglia, brainstem, cerebellum, spinal cord, and peripheral motor unit (Fig. 1.16). Although complaints of generalized weakness, fatigue, or both often are not caused by a specific neurologic condition, the possibility of MS in younger individuals and Parkinson disease in older patients always needs to be considered. When the patient is significantly overweight or has a neuromuscular disorder, sleep apnea needs consideration as a cause of fatigue or a feeling of "weakness." Peripheral motor unit disorders are important considerations for the differential diagnosis of a patient with generalized weakness. These include processes affecting the anterior horn cell (i.e., amyotrophic lateral sclerosis [ALS]), peripheral nerve (i.e., Guillain-Barré syndrome or chronic inflammatory demyelinating disorders), neuromuscular junction (including Lambert-Eaton myasthenic syndrome [LEMS]), or muscle cells (various myopathies).

Partial limb weakness is referred to as *monoparesis*. Total limb paralysis is referred to as *monoplegia*. Unilateral weakness of the limbs is referred to as hemiparesis or *hemiplegia*. Paraparesis refers to involvement of both legs; if no motor function remains, this is considered *paraplegia*. Similarly, *quadriplegia* relates to total paralysis of all four extremities.

Focal weakness often has a subtle character that frequently is not recognized by the patient as loss of motor strength. Dropping objects or clumsy handwriting may represent a single peripheral nerve lesion, such as a radial neuropathy leading to a wrist drop. Tripping on rugs or steps may be the expression of a peroneal nerve lesion causing a foot drop (see Fig. 1.14F3). In contrast, dramatic whole limb weakness is obvious and of greater patient concern, often leading to immediate medical attention, as occurs with a stroke. Bilateral motor loss without cognitive or visual difficulties is most commonly due to lesions affecting the spinal cord or the peripheral nervous system and muscles.

When analyzing the complaint of weakness, the physician must consider the presence or absence of associated neurologic complaints or difficulties, such as language, speech, and visual changes; gait dysfunction; difficulty with rising from chairs and associated movements; and alteration in sensation. The neurologist testing for strength must search for evidence of atrophy and fasciculations or spasticity. Equally important is the need to note the degree of patient effort and cooperation, as well as to consider associated problems that may compromise the testing, such as pain or orthopedic lesions. Formal strength testing must be conducted in a systematic manner evaluating successive areas of the motor unit, beginning at the brain and proceeding distally to the individual muscles per se (see Fig. 1.16). Here one places an initial focus on the major muscle groups, such as the flexors and extensors, to seek out any areas of weakness. More specific muscle testing is particularly useful when distinguishing between lesions of the nerve root, plexus, or mononeuropathies (Table 1.2).

When individual muscle testing does not demonstrate specific weakness, other techniques sometimes uncover more less-obvious functional loss. If the patient is instructed to extend the arms with the palms up

TABLE 1.2   Muscle Testing in a Routine Neurologic Examination

Muscle	Action	Nerve	Root
Infraspinatus	External rotation of arm	Suprascapular	C5
Biceps	Flexion of forearm	Musculocutaneous	C5–6
Deltoid	Abduction of arm	Axillary	C5
Triceps	Extension of forearm	Radial	C7
Extensor digitorum	Extension of fingers	Posterior interosseous of radial	C7
Flexor digitorum	Grip	Median	C7–8
Abductor pollicis brevis and opponens pollicis	Abducting thumb	Median	T1
Dorsal interossei	Spread fingers apart	Ulnar	C8
Iliopsoas	Flexion of thigh	Femoral	L2–3
Quadriceps	Extension of leg	Femoral	L3–4
Hamstring	Flexion of knee	Sciatic	S1
Gluteus medius	Abduction of thigh	Superior gluteal	L5
Gluteus maximus	Extension of thigh	Inferior gluteal	S1
Tibialis anterior	Dorsiflexion of foot	Deep peroneal	L5
Tibialis posterior	Inversion of foot	Tibial	L5
Peroneus longus	Eversion of foot	Superficial peroneal	L5, S1
Gastrocnemius	Plantar foot flexion	Tibial	S1–2

TABLE 1.3   Grading System for Clinical Documentation of Degree of Weakness

Grade	Clinical Findings
0	No movement (complete paralysis)
1	Able to move a muscle but no movement of limb
2	Minor movement of limb but inability to overcome gravity
3	Moderate weakness; movement of limb against gravity
4	Mild weakness; some resistance against mild pressure
5	Normal; resistance against moderate pressure

Adapted from The Guarantors of Brain. *Aids to the Examination of the Peripheral Nervous System.* 4th ed. Philadelphia: WB Saunders; 2000.

and the eyes closed, subtle arm weakness may manifest as a pronating downward or lateral drift of the affected extremity. Similarly, moving the fingers as if playing piano or rapidly tapping may demonstrate a subtle incoordination. Subtle proximal lower extremity weakness may not be appreciated with individual muscle testing. Watching the patient rise from a chair may demonstrate use of furniture arms to "push off" and is a good means to identify early proximal leg weakness. One particularly effective means to uncover proximal leg weakness is to observe the patient climb stairs or squat and attempt to rise without using his or her arms. Also asking the patient to walk on the heels or the tips of the toes is helpful in uncovering distal leg weakness.

Grading Weakness

The traditional, most widely used British system for quantifying degrees of weakness is based on a scoring range of 0–5, with 5 being normal. The extremes of grading are easy to understand, although the subtle grading between 4 and 5 (i.e., 4 minus, 4, 4 plus, or 5 minus) may be slightly different depending on the examiner's own strength (Table 1.3). Other systems judge the patient to have mild (<1), moderate (<2), severe (<3), or total paralysis (<4) strength, and this grading is viewed by some of us to be a simpler and more reproducible methodology. When testing individual muscles of the patient, the examiner must recognize that this is not an athletic match but rather a determination of whether the patient has normal strength. There is a significant range of normal, and a sense of that latitude can be gained only by examining multiple individuals.

The examiner assesses the symmetry of function and coexisting changes in tone to formulate appropriate conclusions regarding the significance of subtle changes. The patient's degree of effort also needs to be assessed to distinguish organic disorders from feigned weakness in those with somatoform disorders or individuals with potential for secondary gain, as may occur with workers' compensation or other litigation. One of the most useful methods here is to ask the patient to very briefly put all of his or her effort into just one muscle. Most patients with various emotional nonorganic causes for "weakness" will not move the limb at all or produce very inconsistent (consistently inconsistent) efforts in contrast to a normal person's very firm, persistent motor output. The individual with nonorganic weakness classically "*gives way*," after just a very brief effort.

In the setting of possible "give way" weakness, one also needs to consider whether there is evidence of posttetanic facilitation, where the patient's initial effort suggests weakness but on a few more tries seemingly normal motor strength is achieved. This is the classic feature of a presynaptic defect in neuromuscular transmission as seen in LEMS. Occasionally, one sees something like this with early Guillain-Barré syndrome or MS. This is an important and occasionally difficult differentiation. One must always listen carefully to the patient; when one is uncertain, the best study is sometime a careful reexamination of the patient. Currently the findings of normal neuroimaging and neurophysiologic modalities are reassuring when considering diagnosis of a functional nonorganic disorder. It is very important to recognize that this is a diagnosis of exclusion. Furthermore, there is no urgency to make such a psychological-based diagnosis. Repeated, careful evaluations may uncover definitive findings leading to an organic diagnosis or, when normal, reassure both physician and patient alike that there is less concern about a serious illness.

Motor Lesions

Cerebral Cortex

When evaluating patients with *focal weakness due to brain lesions,* one should document the evolution of symptoms and any associated changes in sensation or pain. Sudden onset of localized weakness, without preceding trauma or associated pain, suggests ischemic or hemorrhagic cerebral damage. CNS processes cause preferential weakness of the arm extensors and leg flexors. Pure motor weakness of the arm and leg, with slurring of speech, is the hallmark of a stroke in the posterior limb of the internal capsule. Strokes involving the brainstem typically have corticospinal weakness associated with CN findings. Language deficits usually point to left hemispheric processes. Neglect of the affected arm or hand, in association with variable degrees of left-sided weakness, often occurs with pathologic processes in the right hemisphere. Visual field deficits may also develop, depending on whether there is concomitant involvement of the optic nerve, chiasm, tract, radiation, or optic cortex.

Brainstem Bulbar Weakness

Rarely, the weakness may be confined to the *brainstem bulbar musculature,* leading to difficulty speaking, chewing, swallowing, or even breathing. Infarction of the lateral medulla, also called Wallenberg syndrome, often presents with these symptoms, accompanied by vertigo and crossed body sensory loss. Lesions at the *motor neuron* levels such as bulbar ALS, or hypoglossal nerve injury from carotid artery dissection, also require consideration in this setting. Similar symptoms are rarely presenting signs of peripheral *nerve* lesions, including Guillain-Barré and tick paralysis, the *neuromuscular junction,* such as myasthenia gravis and botulism, and rarely *inflammatory myopathies.* Poliomyelitis and

diphtheria are always suspected in the rare geographic areas where these disorders are still endemic. Fortunately, these are now more of historical interest where modern immunization programs are successful.

Myelopathies

It is necessary to differentiate weakness caused by *spinal cord* lesions from brain disorders. Primary lesions affecting the spinal cord include compressive lesions from progressive spondylosis (thickening of the bony spinal canal), metastases, trauma, demyelinating processes, particularly MS or transverse myelitis, and spinal epidural abscess. Depending on the location and temporal profile, spinal cord lesions often begin with subtle symptoms of gait disturbance, weakness, or both. Concomitantly, spinal cord lesions are usually associated with sensory findings and urinary bladder difficulties. Pain frequently accompanies acute spinal cord lesions; localized spine and/or radicular pain from concomitant nerve root involvement is typical of metastatic cancer, epidural abscess, or transverse myelitis. These disorders can rapidly lead to paraplegia.

A very careful examination is crucial to define the presence of a sensory level; this is often best documented by using pin and temperature modalities. One must either sit patients up or turn them on their side, carefully moving the sensory stimulus from the buttocks to the neck to see if there is a sudden change in degree of perception characteristic of a "sensory level." Failure to perform this evaluation may lead to missing a treatable spinal cord lesion. Detailed knowledge of the specific sensory territories of the nerve root dermatomes (Fig. 1.17) is very helpful when assessing potential spinal cord lesions. Looking for a sweat level is also sometimes helpful because the skin below the level of a significant spinal cord lesion will be noticeably drier from loss of autonomic sympathetic innervation. Acute lower extremity weakness

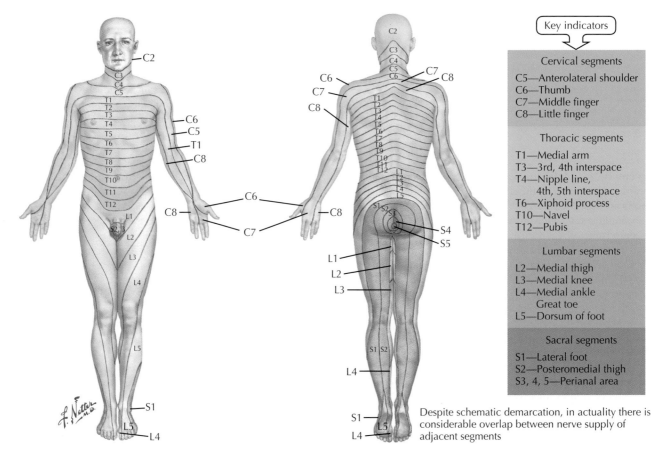

Key indicators

Cervical segments

C5—Anterolateral shoulder
C6—Thumb
C7—Middle finger
C8—Little finger

Thoracic segments

T1—Medial arm
T3—3rd, 4th interspace
T4—Nipple line,
     4th, 5th interspace
T6—Xiphoid process
T10—Navel
T12—Pubis

Lumbar segments

L2—Medial thigh
L3—Medial knee
L4—Medial ankle
     Great toe
L5—Dorsum of foot

Sacral segments

S1—Lateral foot
S2—Posteromedial thigh
S3, 4, 5—Perianal area

Despite schematic demarcation, in actuality there is considerable overlap between nerve supply of adjacent segments

Fig. 1.17 Dermatomal Levels.

is also seen with Guillain-Barré syndrome or other acute generalized polyneuropathies. These disorders may mimic a primary spinal cord lesion.

Patients with *painless asymmetric weakness* typically have primary motor neuron, or very occasionally motor nerve root, motor nerve demyelinating lesions. Fasciculations, spontaneous firing of small groups of muscle fibers innervated by a single motor axon (a motor unit), commonly accompany lower motor neuron weakness. Although often perceived by the patient as twitching or jumping, fasciculations may not be easily seen with the naked eye. Sometimes it may be necessary to observe a specific muscle for several minutes to see these signs. Fasciculations are quite common and often benign; when present in isolation with no motor weakness or muscle atrophy and the patient has a normal electromyogram (EMG), there is little chance that the individual has primary motor neuron disease. Typically, lower motor nerve lesions have a concomitant diminution of specific MSRs; however, with ALS the MSRs are exaggerated and often accompanied by Babinski signs.

Nerve Root, Plexus, or Peripheral Nerve

The presence of cervical or lumbosacral pain with concomitant focal extremity numbness or weakness is characteristic of a radiculopathy. Interspinal disc herniation and spinal stenosis are the most common processes affecting individual nerve roots. Because sensory examination is the most subjective part of the neurologic examination, occasionally it is difficult to clearly define. Sometimes the patient can provide the most accurate assessment by using his or her finger to outline the area of diminished sensation. It often then becomes clear that the pattern of sensory loss specifically fits the distribution of a particular peripheral nerve or nerve root dermatome. Knowledge of the cutaneous sensory supply of peripheral nerves is essential to perform an accurate and useful clinical sensory examination (Fig. 1.18).

Some peripheral mononeuropathies, or rarely multifocal motor neuropathies, present with unilateral peripheral weakness; in particular, the wrist drop of radial nerve lesions and foot drop of peroneal nerve lesions are mistaken for processes above the foramen magnum, often mimicking a stroke. Understanding the motor distribution of the major peripheral nerves ultimately aids in the correct diagnosis. Although a peroneal nerve lesion causes a foot drop, an L5 nerve root lesion also presents with a foot drop but usually with associated low back pain. In addition, the L5 lesion also produces weakness of the posterior tibial muscle innervated by the tibial nerve; this provides the means to make a clinical distinction from a common peroneal nerve lesion. Rarely, lesions as high as the parasagittal frontal lobe within the brain may also present with foot weakness.

Atrophy of muscles innervated by the involved nerve occurs when there is significant denervation. Measuring extremity circumference may document significant side-to-side asymmetries and, by inference, muscle atrophy secondary to anterior horn cell, nerve root, or peripheral nerve damage. It is most important also to carefully search for sensory loss, such as one finds with the ulnar nerve lesion often presenting with painless intrinsic hand muscle atrophy mimicking ALS or syringomyelia.

Muscle Disorders

Most *myopathic* processes lead to *symmetric proximal weakness,* although such can occur with other disorders, particularly chronic inflammatory demyelinating polyneuropathy or rare neuromuscular transmission defects, such as LEMS. Neck flexor and arm extensor weakness may provide early signs of a myopathic process, especially with myasthenia gravis and the inflammatory myopathies. At its most extreme, these patients may present with a floppy head. On rare occasions, primary myopathies have an asymmetric distribution, particularly inclusion body myositis, that mimics ALS or facioscapulohumeral muscular dystrophy.

MOTOR TONE

The motor system depends on multiple inputs to provide precise, well-synchronized, and smooth muscle function. These include positive inputs from the cerebrum, basal ganglia, cerebellum, brainstem, and spinal cord through the corticospinal tracts. Projections from the pontine reticular formation and reticulospinal tract also have direct connections with motor neurons innervating the proximal and axial body musculature. These fibers also originate from the cerebrum and cerebellum and have a primary inhibitory function that serves to decrease motor tone.

Four primary types of changes in tone are found in patients with primary CNS disease: hypotonia, flaccidity, spasticity, and rigidity. It is important to place these observed changes in motor tone within the context of the complete neurologic examination rather than in isolation. The patient's *body tone* is best evaluated when the individual is fully relaxed. Sometimes, it is useful to check tone more than once during the examination. *Tone* is described as the patient's primary level of muscular tension. To become comfortable with this part of the examination, it is important, as with other portions of the neurologic evaluation, to routinely check these parameters in healthy individuals to establish one's normal base of observations.

Hypotonia

This is occasionally demonstrable in patients with cerebellar hemispheric lesions. For example, the distal part of the ipsilateral extremity may not be able to perform rapid alternate movements (called dysdiadochokinesia) because of the inability to maintain a stable posture. Similarly, the smooth, straight pursuit seen when one elicits the knee MSR loses the out-and-back motion that typically has an inhibitory cerebellar check. Instead, on return, there is overshoot with no check, leading to a repetitive pendular response. This classic hypotonic cerebellar tone is a relatively uncommon finding.

A more generalized loss of normal tone is most commonly seen among infants with either central or peripheral motor unit disorders, classically spinal muscular atrophy (Werdnig-Hoffmann disease), or the various congenital myopathies. Although a similar example is seen in adults, rarely a floppy head syndrome develops in an older patient.

Flaccidity

This is the term for a total loss of tone and is seen in various disease processes affecting the upper motor neurons. Most commonly, this occurs in acute settings such as with a recent stroke or a sudden spinal cord injury (i.e., spinal shock). However, with both of these, the flaccidity is temporary and tone increases later to present in the form of varying degrees of spasticity.

Spasticity

Extremes of muscle tone that are maximal at the initiation of the physician's attempt to move the limb and then suddenly release partway through the movement (a clasp-knife, spastic release) are the typical findings seen with a spastic limb. Significant degrees of spasticity are easily elicited with any reasonable stimulation of muscles that induces the stretch reflex. More subtle spasticity may be obvious only with stretching the muscle in a specific direction and at a specific rate. Increased tone, such as may occur with stroke or spinal cord injury, evolves from a flaccid state to spasticity over a matter of days to weeks subsequent to the initial neurologic injury.

Rigidity

Increasing tone from basal ganglia disorders, as may occur with Parkinson disease, is known as rigidity. Rigidity creates a continuous sense

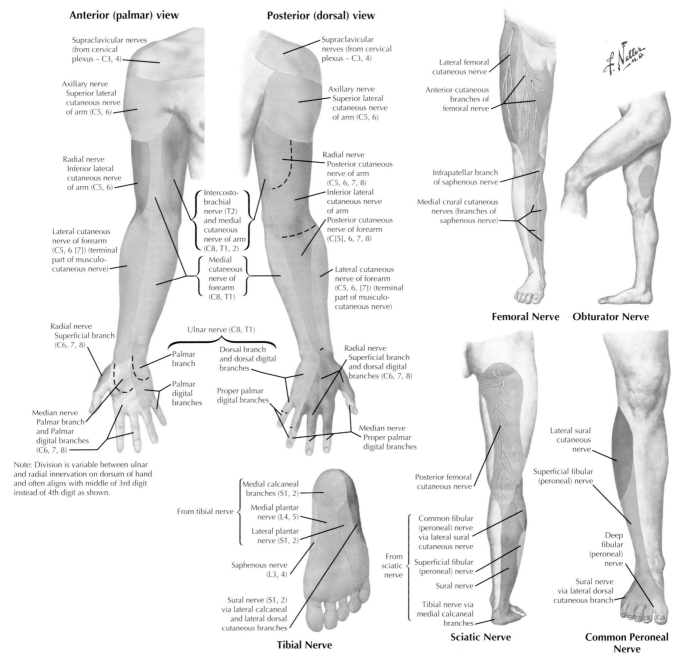

Fig. 1.18 Cutaneous Innervations.

of tightness in the attempt to move the joint through a full excursion from extension to flexion.

Decerebrate Rigidity

When there is total loss of a motor neuron inhibition, as may occur with an upper brainstem injury, the syndrome of decerebrate rigidity develops. Here a simple noxious stimulus leads to bilateral extension in unison of all four extremities, with the arms pronated and the legs adducted (Fig. 1.19) rotated inward. Most commonly, one sees this in the setting of cardiac arrest or from shear injuries to the brainstem resulting from severe head injuries, most typically from automobile accidents or battlefield injuries. When these patients survive more than 3 months, and are otherwise totally unresponsive, they are said to be in a *persistent vegetative state*.

MUSCLE STRETCH REFLEXES, CLONUS, AND THE BABINSKI SIGN

Both Ia and Ib peripheral sensory nerve afferents join the posterior columns of the spinal cord, entering through the dorsal root ganglia. Their primary function is to convey information from touch and pressure receptors. Therefore, although the muscle spindles and Golgi tendon organs cannot be specifically tested, some of their spinal cord connections can be clinically evaluated by testing position and vibration sensory modalities. In addition, the Ia and Ib afferents convey similar information to the cerebellum via the posterior spinocerebellar tract that travels into the cerebellum through the inferior cerebellar peduncle (Fig. 1.20). In isolation, it is difficult to assess the contribution of each tract specifically to motor control.

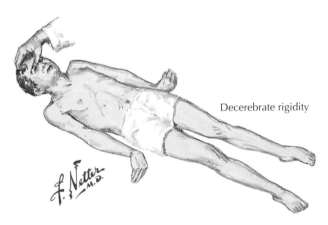

Decerebrate rigidity

Fig. 1.19 Motor Tone Abnormality.

With simple passive stretching, such as occurs with tapping the patellar tendon at the knee, the intrafusal muscle spindle is activated, leading to a direct stimulus to the large alpha motor neurons. These in turn stimulate the extrafusal skeletal muscle fibers, leading to the clinically observed muscle contraction (Fig. 1.21). If the afferent sensory or efferent motor limb of this nerve supply is damaged, the MSR is affected and may be diminished or lost, as occurs with many peripheral neuropathies. These reflexes are sometimes inappropriately referred to as deep tendon reflexes (DTRs) when in fact their physiologic basis primarily depends on the intrafusal muscle spindle fibers, not the Golgi tendon organs. MSR is a more accurate term.

During the neurologic examination, MSRs (named for the specific muscle stretched) are usually readily elicited by tapping lightly over the muscle insertion tendon or while palpating the tendon and then percussing the palpating digit. Occasionally, it is difficult to obtain MSRs

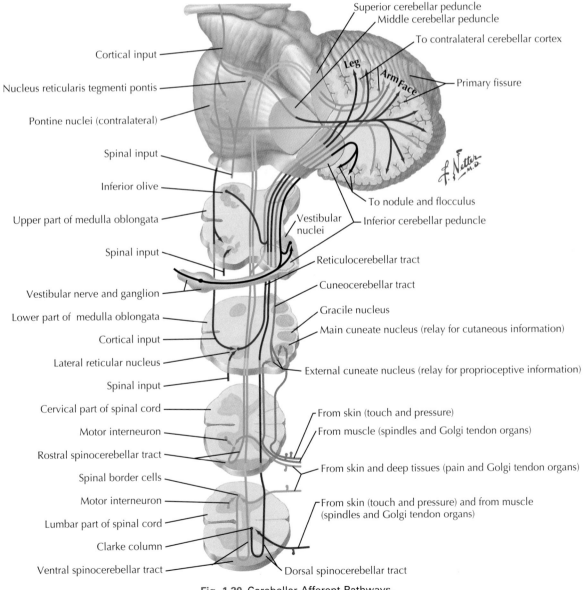

Fig. 1.20 Cerebellar Afferent Pathways.

Muscle and joint receptors

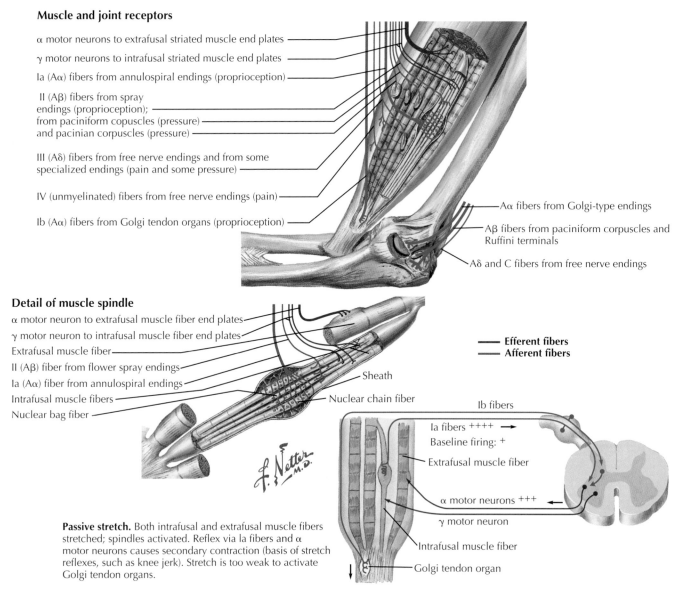

α motor neurons to extrafusal striated muscle end plates

γ motor neurons to intrafusal striated muscle end plates

Ia (Aα) fibers from annulospiral endings (proprioception)

II (Aβ) fibers from spray
endings (proprioception);
from paciniform copuscles (pressure)
and pacinian corpuscles (pressure)

III (Aδ) fibers from free nerve endings and from some
specialized endings (pain and some pressure)

IV (unmyelinated) fibers from free nerve endings (pain)

Ib (Aα) fibers from Golgi tendon organs (proprioception)

Aα fibers from Golgi-type endings

Aβ fibers from paciniform corpuscles and
Ruffini terminals

Aδ and C fibers from free nerve endings

Detail of muscle spindle

α motor neuron to extrafusal muscle fiber end plates

γ motor neuron to intrafusal muscle fiber end plates

Extrafusal muscle fiber

II (Aβ) fiber from flower spray endings

Ia (Aα) fiber from annulospiral endings

Intrafusal muscle fibers

Nuclear bag fiber

Sheath

Nuclear chain fiber

——— Efferent fibers
——— Afferent fibers

Ib fibers

Ia fibers ++++ →

Baseline firing: +

Extrafusal muscle fiber

α motor neurons +++

γ motor neuron

Intrafusal muscle fiber

Golgi tendon organ

Passive stretch. Both intrafusal and extrafusal muscle fibers
stretched; spindles activated. Reflex via Ia fibers and α
motor neurons causes secondary contraction (basis of stretch
reflexes, such as knee jerk). Stretch is too weak to activate
Golgi tendon organs.

Fig. 1.21 Muscle and Joint Receptors and Muscle Spindles.

in healthy individuals. In this setting, it is sometimes useful to distract the patient or apply techniques that reinforce the reflex to potentiate the appearance of the MSRs. The most common method is the Jendrassik maneuver, wherein patients flex their fingers, interlocking one hand with the other and pulling on the count of three while the clinician percusses the appropriate tendon at the knee or ankle. For the upper extremities, the patient may be asked to clench the contralateral fist as the neurologist percusses over the arm tendons, activating the intrafusal muscle spindle.

When grading MSRs, the extremes are easy to appreciate and range from 0 to 4. A reflex grading of 0 is indicative of complete lack of MSR. A generalized loss of reflexes is pathologic and is known as areflexia; this typically occurs in Guillain-Barré syndrome. Briskly responding MSRs are graded as 4 and are typical of a prior stroke or spinal cord lesion. When the patient has brisk MSRs, a single Achilles tendon percussion sometimes elicits a repetitive series of dorsi and plantar movements in the foot. This is known as *clonus.* This does not commonly occur spontaneously, but clonus may be elicited by giving a quick snap to the dorsiflexed foot as it is held in the palm of the hand. This also occurs, rarely, at the quadriceps tendon. Here the reflex is graded as

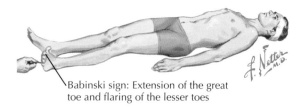

Babinski sign: Extension of the great
toe and flaring of the lesser toes

Fig. 1.22 Elicitation of the Babinski Sign.

4+. The remainder of the grading is very logical. A reflex of 1 is a mere contraction of the muscle; 2 is a normal contraction, and 3 is a brisk reflex but not as exaggerated as grade 4.

The *Babinski sign* is an important pathologic reflex that is elicited at the lateral, plantar surface of the foot using subtle, very careful stroking with a tongue depressor or the base of a key. The great toe extends, and the remaining toes fan out (Fig. 1.22). A more exaggerated response, known as *triple flexion,* includes flexion of the hip, knee, and foot, often with a Babinski response. Because this reflex primarily depends on sensory stimulation of the foot, a kind, gentle, nonirritating stimulus is best to obtain an accurate response. It absolutely does not require excessive or painful pressure. With sensitive or ticklish patients, appropriate responses can usually be obtained from a careful stimulation of the lateral outside, not plantar, surface of the foot. However, some patients have a withdrawal response wherein the foot and entire set of toes dorsiflex. This is often overcome by separately pulling down on the middle toe while carefully stimulating the sole in traditional fashion.

The clinical circumstance where there is a combination of brisk MSRs, clonus, and a Babinski sign indicates an *upper motor neuron lesion*. These abnormalities result from various pathophysiologic mechanisms originating in the brain or spinal cord. The many possibilities include destructive cerebral lesions, such as stroke, tumor, encephalitis, and spinal cord trauma, or demyelinating disorders such as MS affecting the spinal cord, the brain, or both. In addition, signs of upper motor neuron lesions are sometimes observed in patients during the postictal period after a seizure or in patients who have toxic or metabolic encephalopathies. Therefore, although brisk MSRs and a Babinski sign are nonspecific regarding the anatomic setting of the CNS abnormality, their presence provides unequivocal evidence of anatomic persistent upper motor neuron pathology, with the exception of the postictal or encephalopathic setting.

SENSORY EXAMINATION

A carefully designed sensory system evaluation is essential to define the presence or absence of normal sensation and, if abnormal, to define the specific anatomic patterns of loss for the affected modalities. Because part of the sensory examination is fairly subjective, the examiner should analyze the consistency of responses. In addition, the relevance of sensory changes to the patient's complaints and other findings needs to be carefully evaluated. Initially, the examination needs to focus on defining the presence or loss of sensation. One must avoid having the patient be overly zealous trying to define the most subtle differences in sensory appreciation. This often leads to an exhausted patient and a frustrated clinician.

In most clinical settings, it is best to separate the sensory examination into two major categories (i.e., those derived from superficial skin receptors or deeper mechanoreceptors). The former are small, unmyelinated, slowly conducting type C fibers or larger, slightly myelinated, somewhat more rapidly conducting type A-delta fibers. These small fibers primarily subserve *pain and temperature* (respectively tested using a pin point or a cold object such as the handle of a tuning fork) and gross touch modalities. The large, well-myelinated type A-alpha and A-beta fibers carry the kinesthetic modalities of *position sense* studied by the examiner's passively moving the patient's finger or toe in the vertical plane and asking the patient which direction the digit was moved, either up or down.

Fine tactile discrimination is evaluated by using a pair of calipers to check their ability to recognize whether one or two points are applied to the digit. *Vibratory sensation* depends on both deep afferent and cutaneous sensory modalities subserved by type A-alpha fibers. It is best tested by a 128-Hz tuning fork that typically has a low frequency rate and longer duration of action. This modality is the one that most commonly diminishes in sensitivity with aging.

Classic Syndromes of Peripheral Sensory Dysfunction

Generalized polyneuropathies typically present with symptoms of numbness and tingling at the tips of the toes and, later, fingers (i.e., a stocking-glove distribution) (Fig. 1.23). Eventually, this loss will gradually spread proximally past the ankles and wrists into the legs and forearms but usually not above the knees and elbows. On examination with a cold object, a pin (for small fiber function), a tuning fork, and

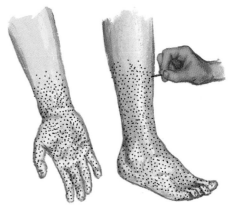

Graduated glove-and-stocking hypesthesia to pain and/or temperature

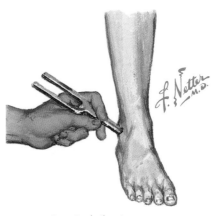

Impaired vibration sense

Fig. 1.23 Documentation of Various Types of Sensory Modalities in a Peripheral Neuropathy.

position sense (if large fibers are also involved), the examiner notes a distal loss that is maximum in the periphery and gradually reaches normal at a more proximal site.

Individual mononeuropathies are typified by symptoms and findings specific to a single peripheral nerve (see Fig. 1.18). For example, the patient notes numbness in the thumb, index, middle fingers, and adjacent lateral aspect of the fourth finger if the median nerve is involved. In carpal tunnel syndrome with entrapment of the median nerve at the wrist, the examination results are often subtly abnormal, only with loss of fine discriminatory function with two-point discrimination. Sometimes, one can use a reflex hammer to percuss directly over the entrapment site. If there is a focal area of peripheral nerve injury, this action commonly elicits brief paresthesia distal to the percussion site and within the specific distribution of the sensory fibers of that nerve, in this case the median. This maneuver is known as the Tinel sign; the name applies to instances wherein this simple provocative test defines the lesion site for any mononeuropathy.

Plexopathies are usually unilateral in distribution, affecting the brachial or lumbosacral groups of nerves. Typically, these are characterized by combined motor and sensory loss involving multiple peripheral nerves within the affected limbs. These lesions have a broader distribution of motor and sensory loss than do single nerve root or mononeuropathy lesions. Therefore, when a clinical examination demonstrates findings not exclusively defined by one specific peripheral nerve or nerve root, a plexus lesion is likely to be present.

Radiculopathies frequently are characterized by more subjective, often intermittent but sometimes persistent, symptoms confined to the dermatomal patterns of one specific nerve root (see Fig. 1.17). Pain is the most common symptom, starting in the neck, shoulder, and low back, often radiating down along the limb in a specific dermatomal distribution. The most common and classic example in the cervical region is at the C7 nerve root where there is paresthesia primarily involving the index and middle fingers. Often there is a concomitant diminution in triceps muscle strength, as well as loss of the triceps reflex. In the low back, the L5 nerve root is the classic example, with numbness in the first and second toes and the lateral calf and accompanying weakness of both the tibialis anterior and tibialis posterior muscles. However, as the knee jerk relates to the L4 nerve root, and the ankle jerk to the S1 root, the examiner has to test a less commonly used reflex, namely the internal hamstring that has an L5 root innervation. When there is sensory involvement along the lateral aspect of the foot and the small toe with absence of the Achilles reflex, an S1 root lesion is most likely.

SPINAL CORD SYNDROMES

Transverse Complete

The site of a spinal cord lesion is defined by identifying the exact distribution of specific motor and sensory deficits (Fig. 1.24). A *complete lesion* of the spinal cord leads to total loss of function distal to the site of the abnormality. A distinct level of sensory loss can be discerned with tests for loss of pain and/or temperature sensations, associated with loss of sweating below the lesion level. Concomitantly, all muscles subserved by anterior horn cells distal to the site of the lesion experience paralysis. Distinct partial cord syndromes are briefly described later and discussed further in Section XVI.

Brown-Séquard

A lesion in the anterior lateral aspect of the spinal cord causes contralateral loss of pain and temperature sensation. If the lesion is more extensive, leading to damage of the anterior and posterior aspects of

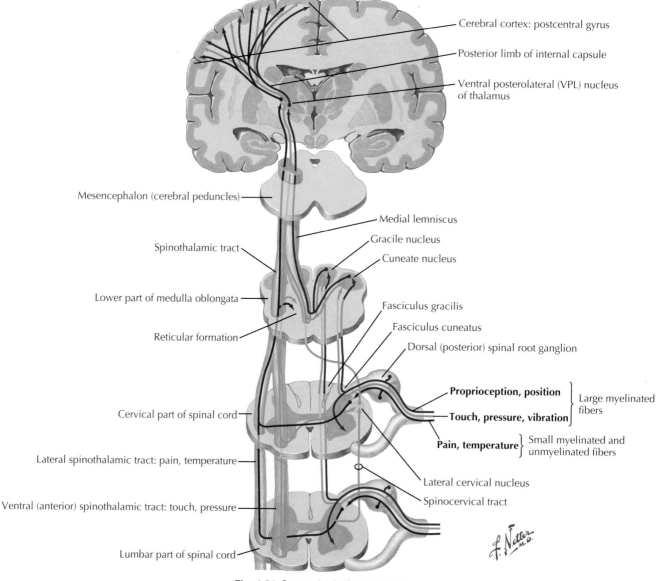

Fig. 1.24 Somesthetic System: Body.

the cord on one side, *Brown-Séquard syndrome* occurs; it is characterized by contralateral loss of pain and temperature sensation, ipsilateral loss of position and vibration sensation, and ipsilateral upper motor neuron weakness.

Central Cord

Syringomyelia or a lesion such as a central spinal cord hemorrhage leads to another anatomically specific lesion referred to as the *central cord* syndrome. The pathology occurs at the center of the cord, destroying fibers carrying pain and temperature sensation from both sides as they cross in the anterior commissure. Fibers carrying vibration and position sense are spared in this syndrome because they do not cross at their entry level into the spinal cord and ascend within the posterior columns. This leads to a dissociated sensory loss with isolated loss of pain and temperature sensation, usually in a "cape" distribution, while concomitantly, vibration and position sense are preserved.

Anterior Spinal Artery

A patient with an infarction within the territory of this essential artery presents another classic sensory picture. This is related to the inherent territory of supply of the anterior spinal artery; namely, it supplies the anterior two-thirds of the cord. Here, there is bilateral damage to the spinothalamic and corticospinal tracts while the posterior columns are spared because of their dependence on the posterior spinal artery system. Although the patient is paralyzed and has total loss of pain and temperature sensation, position and often vibratory sensory modalities are preserved.

THALAMIC INVOLVEMENT

The ventral posterior lateral and ventral posterior medial thalamic nuclei are the two major sensory relay nuclei (Fig. 1.25). Lesions in these areas can cause loss of sensation to all modalities involving the entire contralateral half of the body. This most commonly occurs in patients with lacunar or hemorrhagic infarcts. Initially presenting with a relatively tolerable numbness, eventually the damage incurred from the stroke may produce an unpleasant, sometimes disabling, hyperpathic sensory alteration known as the thalamic pain syndrome. Rarely, this loss of sensation can lead to a limb deafferentiation sensory ataxia. Lesions within the corona radiata, undercutting the parietal cortex, can cause similar, although often less extensive, findings.

CORTICAL SENSORY INVOLVEMENT

The parietal lobe receives topographically organized sensory inputs from the thalamic nuclei, brainstem, spinal cord, and peripheral nerves (see Fig. 1.24). An important function of the parietal lobe is the integration of this information with other sensory and motor information to formulate body awareness. In the purest form of cortical sensory dysfunctions, patients are unable to differentiate the location of their toes or fingers in space, make a distinction between one and two points, or use stereognostic discrimination to allow differentiation of various objects placed in their hands, such as differing coin sizes. In addition, these individuals are unable to recognize numbers traced on the palm (graphesthesia).

Many other sensory abnormalities occur, including "neglect," wherein the patient with a right, nondominant, parietal lesion is unaware of paralysis or sensory loss of the contralateral limbs. These are especially obvious with double simultaneous stimulation (extinction). Here, one or two sides of the body are variably stimulated, and the patient is asked to identify the stimulus location. Individuals with a more subtle parietal sensory loss cannot identify the contralateral stimulus when bilateral

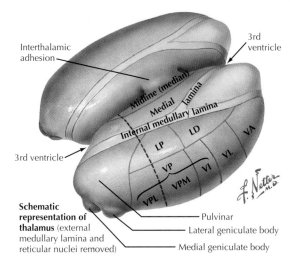

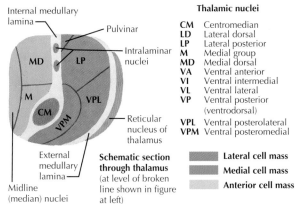

Fig. 1.25 Thalamus and Its Multiple Nuclei.

Thalamic nuclei	
CM	Centromedian
LD	Lateral dorsal
LP	Lateral posterior
M	Medial group
MD	Medial dorsal
VA	Ventral anterior
VI	Ventral intermedial
VL	Ventral lateral
VP	Ventral posterior (ventrodorsal)
VPL	Ventral posterolateral
VPM	Ventral posteromedial

stimuli are applied. At the extreme a patient sustaining very large hemisphere and subcortical stroke presents with a complete loss of sensation of the contralateral body.

ADDITIONAL RESOURCES

Bates B. A guide to physical examination and history taking. 4th ed. Baltimore, MD: JB Lippincott Co; 1987.

Bear MF, Connors BW, Paradiso MA. Neuroscience, exploring the brain. Baltimore, MD: Lippincott Williams & Wilkins; 2007.

Benarroch EE, Daube JR, Flemming KD, et al. Mayo Clinic medical neurosciences: organized by neurologic systems and levels. 5th ed. St. Helier, NJ: Informa; 2008.

Brazis P, Masdeau J, Biller J. Localization in clinical neurology. 5th ed. Baltimore, MD: Lippincott Williams & Wilkins; 2006.

Kandel ER, Schwartz JH, Jessell TM. Principles of neural science. 4th ed. New York, NY: McGraw-Hill, Health Professions Division; 2000.

Luria AR. Higher cortical functions in man. 2nd ed. New York, NY: Basic Books, Inc; 1980.

Mayo Clinic Department of Neurology. Mayo clinic examinations in neurology. 7th ed. St. Louis, MO: Mosby; 1998.

Miller NR, Newman NJ, Biousse V, et al. Walsh & Hoyt's clinical neuro-ophthalmology: the essentials. Baltimore, MD: Lippincott Williams & Wilkins; 2007.

O'Brien M. Aids to the examination of the peripheral nervous system. 5th ed. Philadelphia, PA: WB Saunders; 2010.

Parent A. Carpenter's human neuroanatomy. 9th ed. Baltimore, MD: Williams & Wilkins; 1996.

Peters A, Jones EG, editors. Cerebral cortex: vol 4. Association and auditory cortices. New York, NY: Plenum Press; 1985.

Laboratory Testing in Neurology

Brian J. Scott, Claudia J. Chaves, Jayashri Srinivasan

CLINICAL VIGNETTE *A 45-year-old woman presents to clinic with episodic left-sided weakness, dysarthria, and gait imbalance. The first episode occurred 9 months ago upon awakening and resolved gradually over 2 days. She had no associated headache, visual symptoms, or nausea. She has had three additional episodes of increasing severity over the following 8 months and has had incomplete recovery following the two most recent episodes. She has begun to use a wheelchair for the past 4 weeks, due to persistent left-sided weakness. Ischemic stroke/transient ischemic attack (TIA) was initially suspected. Noncontrast head computed tomography (CT) was negative, and a brain Magnetic resonance imaging/angiography (MRI/A) showed no acute ischemic stroke, demyelinating lesions, and no large vessel occlusion. A screen for hypercoagulability (factor V Leiden, prothrombin gene mutation, protein C, protein S, homocysteine) was performed and was negative. Following the third episode, a repeat brain MRI was performed, which showed areas of enhancement and T2 hyperintensity within the basis pontis (Fig. 2.1). A serum rheumatologic screen (antinuclear antibody, angiotensin converting enzyme, rheumatoid factor, and Anti-Ro/Anti-La antibodies) was negative. Serum C-reactive protein was elevated at 11.9 mg/dL (normal < 6.3). Cervical and thoracic spine imaging were unrevealing, and a body PET/CT revealed a thyroid nodule and multiple FDG-avid hepatic and splenic lesions. Ophthalmologic evaluation including slit lamp was unremarkable. Cerebrospinal fluid (CSF) studies were as follows: white blood cell count 11 per high power field, red blood cell count 5 per high power field, glucose 59 milligrams per deciliter, protein 45 mg/dL, immunoglobulin index 0.42 (normal < 0.6), no oligoclonal bands present. CSF cytology and flow cytometry were negative. Follow-up neuroimaging revealed an increase in the enhancement and T2 hyperintense pontine abnormality. The patient was offered empiric corticosteroids versus diagnostic brain biopsy and referred for neurosurgical consultation.*

Comment: This case illustrates a challenging diagnostic quandary, with early presenting symptoms suggestive of cerebrovascular disease but imaging and clinical evolution that did not confirm this suspicion. This unexpected result led to additional diagnostic testing and forced the caregivers over time to reframe the problem more broadly and to investigate both neurologic and systemic infectious, inflammatory, and neoplastic disorders. Ultimately a comprehensive analysis of blood, CSF, and imaging were inconclusive. The patient declined biopsy due to the risk of neurologic morbidity yet had gradual clinical improvement with time and corticosteroids, leading to a presumed diagnosis of chronic lymphocytic inflammation with pontine perivascular enhancement responsive to steroids (aka CLIPPERS).

GENERAL PRINCIPLES

It cannot be overstated that a careful and skilled neurologic history and physical examination are the cornerstones of the neurologic evaluation (see Chapter 1). To successfully navigate a challenging case, these must be completed, synthesized, and reflected upon before ordering tests.

The selection of diagnostic testing of all types (serum, cerebrospinal fluid [CSF], imaging, neurophysiology, and tissue studies) must be driven by the unanswered questions that arise from the clinical history and examination findings. To embark on laboratory investigations with an inadequate understanding of the patient's problem or incomplete neurologic examination invites waste and error. This is not to say that there is no role for a heuristic approach, but the best clinicians listen carefully to their patients and modify their diagnostic approach when new information challenges their heuristics.

Hypothesis-driven testing based on a prioritized differential diagnosis is the most effective strategy. It is important to be as familiar as possible with the strengths and limitations of each diagnostic test and to anticipate potential results. When considering a test, some questions to consider include:

- Is this the best test to answer my clinical question?
- Is there a less invasive, quicker, or less costly testing option?
- What is/are the potential result(s) of the test?
- How long will it take to get results? For a test with long processing time, will the result still be helpful?
- How will the result(s) impact my next steps/recommendations?

Another consideration is whether to acquire tests in series or in parallel. Ordering tests in series is a strategy by which the clinician orders a single or small number of tests and then awaits the results before proceeding to additional testing. This strategy optimizes accuracy and minimizes waste. The clinician may begin with test(s) related to the most likely diagnosis and move in a strategic fashion to test for successively less common possibilities based on each test result as it becomes available. The disadvantage to this approach is that it takes considerably longer to complete a diagnostic evaluation when ordering tests in series. It is most appropriate when there is a highly reliable test that can be obtained and interpreted quickly (such as head CT scanning to evaluate for acute intracranial hemorrhage), or when the pace of illness is subacute to chronic and there is less pressure to make a quick diagnosis, or if there is a highly reliable test that takes a long time to get results or is highly costly (such as genetic testing).

Testing in parallel takes the approach of ordering multiple tests simultaneously. Parallel testing is useful for conditions in which there are numerous potential causes for a clinical condition. For example, a clinician seeing a patient with a sensory neuropathy may identify specific risk factors (such as hyperglycemia or exposure to chemotherapy) but ultimately may not be able to exclude a handful of other potential causes. Rather than scheduling multiple return visits and phlebotomy sessions, one may opt to send a group of tests in parallel to efficiently screen for numerous common causes in a matter of days with a single trip to the lab. The hypercoagulability screen and rheumatologic laboratories in the previous case are also examples of parallel testing. A potential disadvantage to parallel testing is added cost if expensive or extraneous tests are ordered.

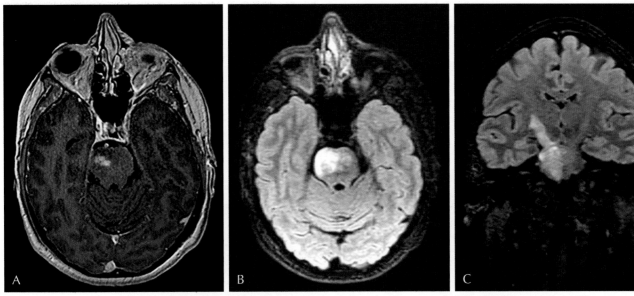

Fig. 2.1 Brain MRI with gadolinium demonstrating abnormal enhancement of the rights pons on axial T1 postcontrast images (A); T2 hyperintense signal within the body of the pons (B). The abnormality extends cranially along the corticospinal tract (C).

Another important factor in ordering clinical tests is the logistical burden and the invasiveness of the test. Clinicians tend to think of diagnostic testing in terms of the ways that it is helpful to us (how reliably a test or tests will achieve the diagnosis). However, this is not the only consideration for patients. The discomfort associated with a blood draw or electromyography (EMG) procedure, claustrophobia in a scanner, procedural risk associated with a biopsy, and individual or cultural beliefs and attitudes about medical care all factor into a patient's willingness to pursue diagnostic testing and influence their "compliance" with our recommendations. It is therefore important when ordering tests to ensure that our patients understand and accept the reasoning for the test and have a realistic picture of what they will experience. This conversation is particularly essential prior to diagnostic lumbar puncture and electrophysiology testing, because patients often have strong perceptions about the discomfort associated with these tests. For biopsies, or other invasive procedures such as ventriculostomy, it is appropriate for the proceduralist to explain the rationale and associated risks of the procedure and to answer any related questions.

A challenging situation that arises with diagnostic testing occurs when patients are convinced that they need a specific test, but the clinician does not agree or favors pursuing an alternative diagnosis. Increasingly, with online medical resources and community- and web-based sharing of information and experiences, patients enter the examination room with an element of "self-diagnosis." For example, a patient being seen for tingling of the dominant hand may have a history and exam that confirms a diagnosis of carpal tunnel syndrome. The clinician recommends appropriate therapy and potentially EMG testing, yet the patient may be insistent that he or she has a brain MRI because he or she is convinced that a stroke, brain tumor, or multiple sclerosis is the cause for his or her symptoms. These situations required careful listening, skilled redirection, explanation of the clinical evidence to support or refute a diagnosis, reassurance, and confidence. Often it is useful to ask, "Why do you think these symptoms are due to a stroke?" Explicitly addressing, rather than avoiding, these concerns often leads to useful insights. Through this process, clinicians ideally learn more about their patients' values, fears, and communication styles, and patients ultimately come to trust their clinicians' judgment and recommendations.

LUMBAR PUNCTURE

There is no exact substitute for CSF analysis in many neurologic disorders, such as acute or chronic meningoencephalitis, autoimmune central nervous system (CNS) disorders, and acute and chronic inflammatory demyelinating polyneuropathies. Head CT imaging has a greater than 95% sensitivity in subarachnoid hemorrhage, but there is still a role for CSF analysis in clinically suspected cases with negative head CT, especially when presenting more than 24 hours after symptom onset, because sensitivity of imaging decreases with time.

The widespread availability of CT scanners in acute care settings makes it uncommon for one to perform a lumbar puncture without neuroimaging. Neuroimaging is crucial to confirm that there is no mass lesion for which lumbar drainage of CSF could produce or worsen a herniation syndrome. Specifically, patients with a history of cancer, immunosuppression (human immunodeficiency virus [HIV] or organ transplant), focal neurologic deficits, fever, trauma, or depressed level of consciousness need head imaging prior to the procedure. It may also be necessary to repeat brain imaging prior to lumbar puncture in cases in which there has been a neurologic decline since the previous neuroimaging.

The main risks of lumbar puncture are bleeding or infection (cutaneous or epidural) at the site of puncture, post-lumbar puncture (LP) headache, or nerve root injury. Use of the atraumatic "Sprotte" spinal needle is associated with a significantly lower incidence of post-LP headache than cutting spinal needles (1%–2% vs. 15%–20%, respectively) (Fig. 2.2). Cellulitis involving the lumbar puncture site or suspected epidural abscess is an absolute contraindication to lumbar puncture. Coagulopathy is a relative contraindication due to potentially increased risk for hemorrhagic complications, although there is no high-quality evidence to quantify the risk, and specific coagulation parameters under which lumbar puncture is acceptably safe are not well established. It is best to perform the procedure after all antiplatelet and anticoagulant medications have been discontinued long enough that normal coagulation may occur.

CSF is produced at a rate of 0.2–0.7 mL/min, or 600–700 mL/day, with an average total circulating volume in adults of 125–150 mL. The majority of CSF is produced by the choroid plexus within the lateral

Headache is orthostatic, worse in an upright position; often aggravated by exertion, bending over, or Valsalva maneuver

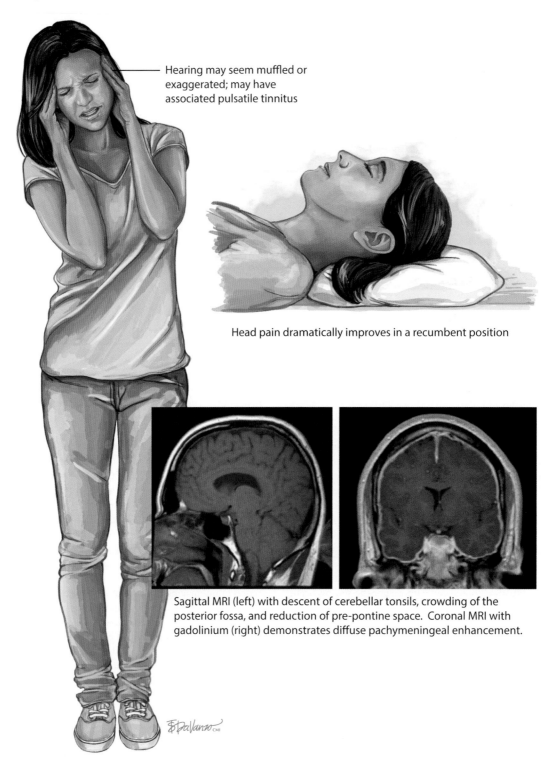

Hearing may seem muffled or exaggerated; may have associated pulsatile tinnitus

Head pain dramatically improves in a recumbent position

Sagittal MRI (left) with descent of cerebellar tonsils, crowding of the posterior fossa, and reduction of pre-pontine space. Coronal MRI with gadolinium (right) demonstrates diffuse pachymeningeal enhancement.

Fig. 2.2 Post-Lumbar Puncture Headache.

ventricles, but approximately 80% of CSF volume is outside the ventricular system (Fig. 2.3). A typical LP involves removal of 10–30 mL of fluid, which the body replaces under normal physiologic conditions in 1–3 hours.

Personal protective equipment, sterile technique, and local anesthesia minimize the risk of complications for the patient and the proceduralist. The lateral decubitus position tends to be most comfortable for the patient and allows for easier measurement of CSF opening pressure. LP may be performed in the seated position if it is difficult to identify landmarks in the lateral decubitus position or if the patient has severe orthopnea and cannot lie flat for the duration of the procedure. However, once the needle enters the CSF space, the seated patient must then be transitioned onto his or her side if opening pressure measurements are desired. Normal CSF opening pressure in the lateral decubitus position with legs straightened is between 8 and 15 cm H_2O and may be slightly higher in intubated patients.

CEREBROSPINAL FLUID STUDIES

Certain CSF studies require prompt processing to ensure accurate results. For example, CSF xanthochromia is a measure of red blood cell breakdown that can be diagnostic for subarachnoid hemorrhage in the appropriate clinical context (Fig. 2.4). However, if there is a delay in CSF processing, even red blood cells introduced at the time of the procedure from local tissue injury start to break down and may produce a false-positive result. Delays in processing CSF for cytology or flow cytometry may result in degradation of the specimen, making it more difficult to diagnose a CSF malignancy.

The most common CSF study is a red blood cell count, and white cell count with differential, total protein, and glucose measurements (often referred to as a CSF basic profile). CSF is typically acellular. However, peripheral blood contamination of a CSF sample due to local trauma during the procedure may result in an elevated red and white blood cell count. To distinguish CSF inflammation from trauma, it is useful to consider the number of red blood cells (RBCs) in a specimen and determine if the elevated white blood cell (WBC) count is proportionate. The ratio of RBC to WBC in someone with a normal peripheral WBC count is 500–1000 : 1. For example, if a CSF sample has 12 WBCs and 9000 RBCs, the RBC to WBC ratio is 750 : 1, which is within what would be expected with peripheral blood contamination. By contrast, if the WBC count was 12 and the RBC count was 150, this is suggestive of a CNS inflammatory process. The WBC differential may provide a diagnostic clue. A normal CSF differential will be mostly lymphocytic (70%) with approximately 30% monocytes. Neutrophilic predominance is a common initial feature of CNS bacterial infection, whereas viral infections characteristically produce a lymphocytic pleocytosis. The presence of eosinophils in CSF is uncommon and abnormal, raising concern for a fungal or parasitic meningitis.

CSF protein elevation is nonspecific but generally indicative of an inflammatory process. Mild elevation, especially in elderly individuals, may be normal. Elevated CSF protein in isolation may be seen in acute inflammatory demyelinating polyneuropathy, due to autoantibody production. Additional testing may help to clarify the nature of an elevated CSF protein. Measuring CSF to serum immunoglobulin index and CSF to serum electrophoresis will determine whether the inflammation is a systemic process or in some way CNS specific. The immunoglobulin index is elevated in the presence of a CNS inflammatory process. Protein electrophoresis can compare serum and CSF antibodies. A small number of serum antibodies passively diffuse into CSF; however, it is abnormal for unique antibodies to be present in CSF and not in serum. The presence of "oligoclonal bands" in CSF indicates intra-CSF synthesis of antibodies that are not present in serum and

may be seen in multiple sclerosis and autoimmune encephalitides. CSF protein, immunoglobulin index, and serum to CSF protein electrophoresis are useful screening tests for CNS inflammation, due to their high sensitivity. More specific molecular testing has become available to identify the presence of specific antibodies in serum and/or CSF. For example, antiganglioside (GM1) antibodies are found in some cases of Guillain-Barré syndrome, GQ1b antibodies in Miller Fisher variant Guillain Barré, and paraneoplastic/autoimmune antibodies in cases of noninfectious encephalitis (see Chapter 51). Bacterial (16S ribosomal ribonucleic acid [rRNA]) and viral polymerase chain reaction (PCR) studies, metagenomics, and proteomics are improving the diagnostic power of CSF investigation for CNS infections. For example, in Creutzfeldt-Jakob disease, one test for prions in CSF using the second-generation real-time quaking-induced conversion (RT QuIC) test; this has autopsy-verified data that indicate 98.5% specificity and 89%–92% sensitivity for detection of all human prion diseases.

CSF glucose is normally greater than two-thirds serum glucose. It is useful to obtain a serum glucose or fingerstick near the time of CSF acquisition to make an accurate comparison. A low CSF glucose (<50% of serum) may be extremely useful diagnostically because it is associated with a relatively small number of disease states. These include bacterial meningitis, fungal meningitis, neoplastic meningitis, neurosarcoidosis, CNS lymphoma, and neurosyphilis.

BRAIN BIOPSY

Although serum and CSF studies are often adequate to reach a diagnosis and treatment plan, the case at the beginning of the chapter illustrates a situation in which there is still diagnostic uncertainty even after all of the imaging and testing have been completed. Brain biopsy allows for direct examination of meningeal and parenchymal brain pathology that may not be evident by less invasive means. It is a requisite procedure in neuro-oncology for primary brain tumors and brain masses in individuals without a history of cancer to devise appropriate therapy. The diagnostic sensitivity of brain biopsy for CNS tumors is 95%. The yield is slightly less in rapidly progressive neurologic conditions or dementia (~65%). The risk associated with the procedure varies depending on the location of the biopsy and the patient's perioperative and anesthesia risk. In general, there is an estimated 5% risk of permanent neurologic deficit and 0.5% mortality associated with the procedure and higher for brainstem and spinal cord procedures.

The main alternative to brain biopsy is empiric therapy or observation, often with periodic imaging studies. If an individual has a high surgical risk (severe medical comorbidities, advanced age), a mild or indolent clinical course, or a brain lesion in a high-risk area, it is reasonable to consider a nonsurgical plan with close follow-up.

ELECTROENCEPHALOGRAPHY

Electroencephalography (EEG) is a powerful tool that provides a noninvasive measurement of brain physiology over time. It was developed in the first half of the 20th century and has technologically advanced with modern digital recording capabilities, refined software, and advanced surgical techniques.

Routine EEG consists of placement of 20 scalp electrodes in a standardized method (Fig. 2.5). Typically, an EEG recording will proceed for 30–60 minutes and often includes maneuvers such as brief hyperventilation or photic stimulation. These may bring out subtle EEG abnormalities such as spikes or sharp waves. Routine EEG can help to localize specific electrophysiologic abnormalities and assess for abnormal interictal discharges, which help to guide anticonvulsant medication decisions or may indicate an increased risk of seizure.

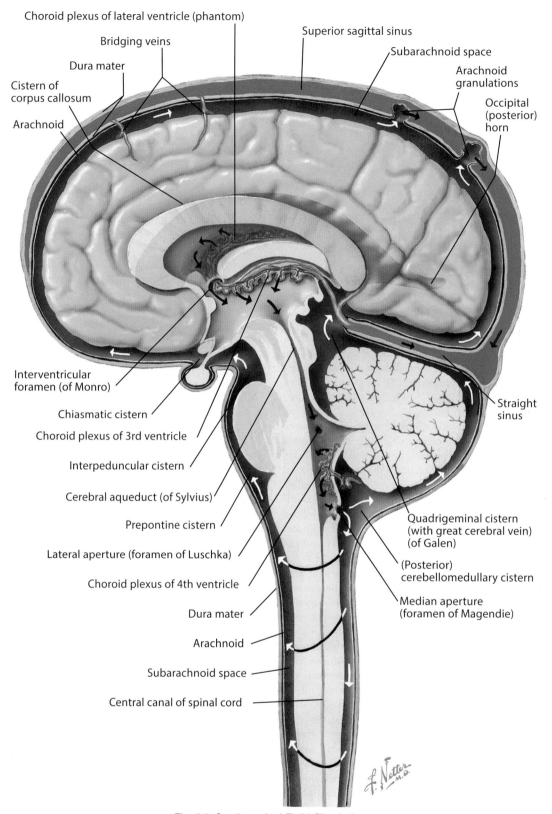

Choroid plexus of lateral ventricle (phantom)

Bridging veins

Dura mater

Cistern of corpus callosum

Arachnoid

Superior sagittal sinus

Subarachnoid space

Arachnoid granulations

Occipital (posterior) horn

Interventricular foramen (of Monro)

Chiasmatic cistern

Choroid plexus of 3rd ventricle

Interpeduncular cistern

Cerebral aqueduct (of Sylvius)

Prepontine cistern

Lateral aperture (foramen of Luschka)

Choroid plexus of 4th ventricle

Dura mater

Arachnoid

Subarachnoid space

Central canal of spinal cord

Straight sinus

Quadrigeminal cistern (with great cerebral vein) (of Galen)

(Posterior) cerebellomedullary cistern

Median aperture (foramen of Magendie)

Fig. 2.3 Cerebrospinal Fluid Circulation.

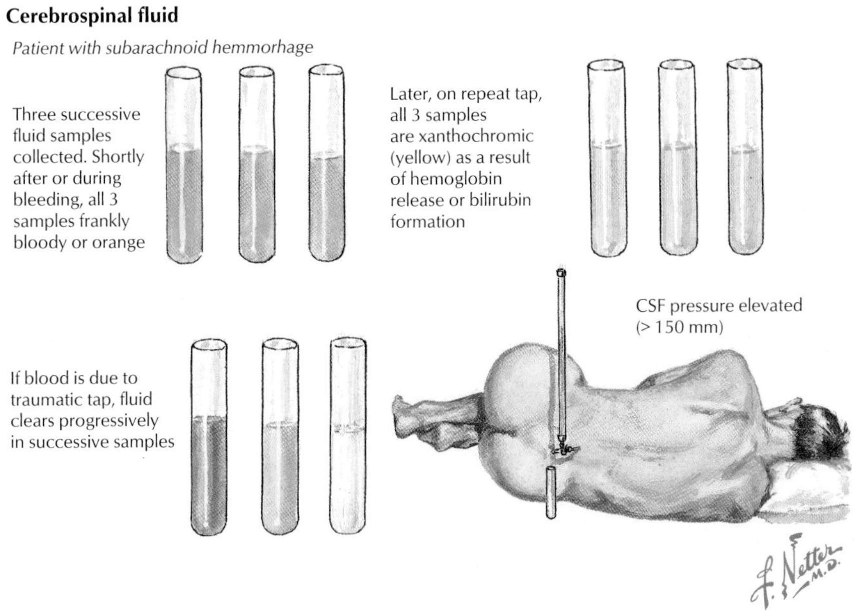

Cerebrospinal fluid

Patient with subarachnoid hemmorhage

Three successive fluid samples collected. Shortly after or during bleeding, all 3 samples frankly bloody or orange

Later, on repeat tap, all 3 samples are xanthochromic (yellow) as a result of hemoglobin release or bilirubin formation

If blood is due to traumatic tap, fluid clears progressively in successive samples

CSF pressure elevated (> 150 mm)

Fig. 2.4 Cerebrospinal Fluid (CSF) Xanthochromia.

More extended monitoring with concurrent video is extremely useful for specific clinical applications such as during high-risk anticonvulsant medication changes in the hospital for those with medically refractory epilepsy or for detection of nonconvulsive status epilepticus in hospitalized patients with altered mental status. In cases of medically refractory localization-related epilepsy, continuous video EEG monitoring, ictal single photon emission computed tomography (SPECT) or placement of subdural electrodes may pinpoint the seizure focus and create an opportunity for surgical epilepsy treatments.

Continuous video EEG is also diagnostically helpful for differentiating epilepsy from psychogenic nonepileptic seizure (PNES). Individuals having events that are suspicious for nonepileptic seizures often benefit from longer-duration EEG monitoring. The finding of one or more characteristic event(s) on monitoring without any change in the normal awake EEG background is diagnostic for PNES. Making a diagnosis of PNES is useful because it may lead to additional attention and resources directed toward treatment (such as cognitive behavioral therapy) for an underlying psychological trigger. It is critical not to form a bias in these patients against a diagnosis of epilepsy because a nonepileptic seizure on EEG does not exclude the possibility of epilepsy, and it is possible to have both.

EEG is the mainstay of diagnosis in sleep disorders such as sleep apnea, narcolepsy, and rapid eye movement (REM) sleep behavior disorder (see Chapter 24). Visual-evoked potentials may be useful to detect optic nerve demyelination. Somatosensory-evoked potentials, when absent, are associated with a worse neurologic prognosis when assessed 3 days after cardiac arrest.

ELECTROMYOGRAPHY/NERVE CONDUCTION STUDIES

As EEG provides physiologic insight into the function of the cerebral cortex, EMG and nerve conduction studies (NCSs) provide a dynamic interrogation of the function of the peripheral nervous system. Disorders of the peripheral nerve (Section XVII–XXI), neuromuscular junction (Section XXII), and muscle (Section XXIII) are covered in detail later in the book, including specific EMG findings.

A basic understanding of the components of EMG/NCS and the strengths and limitations of the study help the clinician to better understand when to order EMG/NCS and how to interpret the results. Not all peripheral nerve disorders require EMG/NCS. For example, radiculopathy is usually diagnosed by clinical history and exam, with confirmatory imaging when necessary. EMG/NCS are characteristically normal in radiculopathy, and the study is most useful to exclude an alternative localization such as a plexopathy if there is diagnostic uncertainty. EMG/NCS may also be limited in the diagnosis of small fiber peripheral sensory neuropathy because the study is unable to detect small fiber sensory nerve pathology.

The electromyographer is tasked with lesion localization and characterization, much in the same way as the clinician but with the added ability to interrogate the function of the peripheral nervous system at multiple levels (Fig. 2.6). The nature of the clinical complaint and history dictates how focused or comprehensive the study will be and which levels of the nervous system to investigate. Motor and sensory symptoms in the fourth and fifth digits of the right upper extremity with diminished grip strength, for example, could raise suspicion for an ulnar neuropathy. However, it may be difficult to determine whether this is due to a focal compression, and sometimes it can be challenging to differentiate from a C8 radiculopathy. NCS stimulates motor and sensory nerves and enables the electrophysiologist to calculate conduction velocities and peak amplitudes for each response. Stimulation of a motor nerve generates a compound motor action potential (CMAP), and stimulation of a sensory nerve generates a smaller amplitude response known as a sensory nerve action potential (SNAP). The examiner must compare the recorded conduction velocities and response amplitudes with known reference normal values. The conduction velocities reflect the physiologic state of myelination over the segment of nerve being studied. Amplitudes reflect the population of axons within the sensory or motor nerve, and motor amplitudes are reduced in conditions in which the lower motor neuron axon is injured or destroyed. Careful attention to the distance between stimulus and recording site and maintenance of normal limb temperature ensure accurate results. When a limb being tested becomes cooler than body temperature, the conduction velocities become prolonged, potentially leading to false abnormal findings.

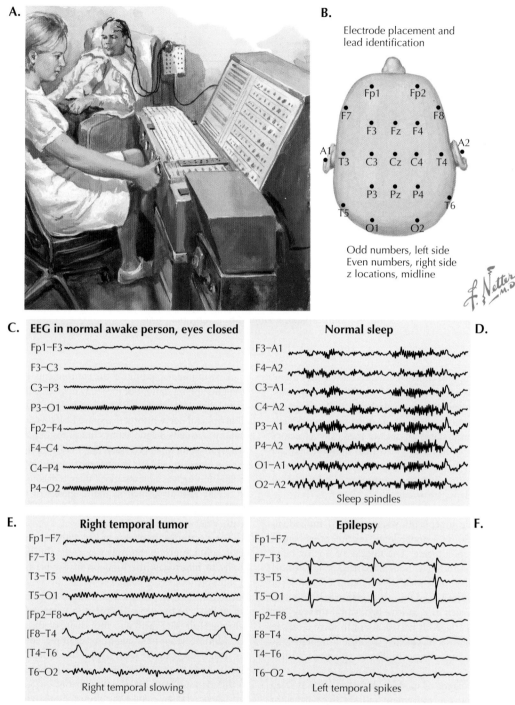

A.

B. Electrode placement and lead identification

Fp1 Fp2
F7   F8
F3 Fz F4
A1
T3 C3 Cz C4 T4
A2
P3 Pz P4
T5   T6
O1   O2

Odd numbers, left side
Even numbers, right side
z locations, midline

C. EEG in normal awake person, eyes closed

Fp1–F3
F3–C3
C3–P3
P3–O1
Fp2–F4
F4–C4
C4–P4
P4–O2

Normal sleep D.

F3–A1
F4–A2
C3–A1
C4–A2
P3–A1
P4–A2
O1–A1
O2–A2

Sleep spindles

E. Right temporal tumor

Fp1–F7
F7–T3
T3–T5
T5–O1
[Fp2–F8
[F8–T4
[T4–T6
T6–O2

Right temporal slowing

Epilepsy F.

Fp1–F7
F7–T3
T3–T5
T5–O1
Fp2–F8
F8–T4
T4–T6
T6–O2

Left temporal spikes

Fig. 2.5 Electroencephalography (EEG).

In cases in which focal demyelination is suspected, measurement of conduction velocity above and below the level of suspected compression may reveal an area of delayed or blocked conduction. NCSs of the limbs measure the nerve physiology over the segment of nerve between the stimulator and the recording electrode (Fig. 2.7). However, the function of the nerve root can be measured by assessing so-called late responses, the F-wave and H-reflex. Late responses are obtained by stimulating a limb and measuring the small delayed electrical potential that is conducted proximally and reaches the recording electrode after synapsing in the spinal cord. Conditions such as acute demyelinating inflammatory polyneuropathy may produce demyelination injury to the most proximal

segment of the nerve, which will manifest on NCSs as an absent or delayed F-wave or H-reflex.

Lastly, NCS can be configured to deliver a repeated stimulus to the same peripheral nerve as a useful way to investigate problems within the neuromuscular junction. In myasthenia gravis, repetitive stimulation at a rate of 3 Hz results in progressive decrement in the CMAP amplitudes because of acetylcholine receptor (postsynaptic) dysfunction. A decrement of greater than 20% in amplitude with repetitive stimulation is consistent with a diagnosis of myasthenia gravis (Fig. 2.8). Presynaptic disorders of the neuromuscular junction such as Lambert-Eaton myasthenic syndrome are physiologically different. With repetitive

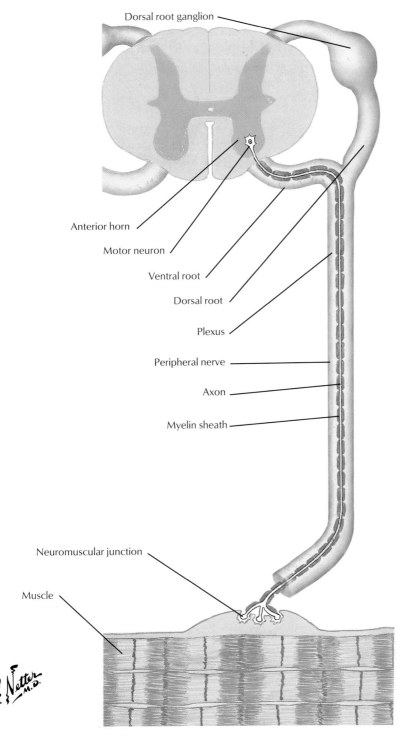

Motor neuron
Primary motor neuron diseases
Progressive muscular atrophy
Primary bulbar palsy
Amyotrophic lateral sclerosis
Werdnig-Hoffman disease
Poliomyelitis
Tetanus

Dorsal root ganglion
Herpes zoster
Friedreich ataxia
Hereditary sensory neuropathy

Spinal nerve (dorsal and ventral roots)
Disc extrusion or herniation
Tumor

Plexus
Tumor
Trauma
Idiopathic plexopathy
Diabetic plexopathy

Peripheral nerve
Metabolic, toxic, nutritional,
idiopathic neuropathies
Arteritis
Hereditary neuropathies
Infectious, postinfectious,
inflammatory neuropathies
(Guillain-Barré syndrome)
Entrapment and compression
syndromes
Trauma

Neuromuscular junction
Myasthenia gravis
Lambert-Eaton syndrome
Botulism

Muscle
Duchenne muscular dystrophy
Myotonic dystrophy
Limb-girdle muscular dystrophy
Congenital myopathies
Polymyositis/dermatomyositis
Potassium-related myopathies
Endocrine dysfunction myopathies
Enzymatic myopathies
Rhabdomyolysis

Labels on figure:
Dorsal root ganglion
Anterior horn
Motor neuron
Ventral root
Dorsal root
Plexus
Peripheral nerve
Axon
Myelin sheath
Neuromuscular junction
Muscle

Fig. 2.6 Peripheral Nerve and Muscle.

high-frequency (20–50 Hz) stimulation, more acetylcholine is released, resulting in a dramatic increase in CMAP known as facilitation (Fig. 2.9).

Needle EMG is the second portion of the peripheral nerve electrophysiologic study. The clinical history, examination, and results of NCSs all frame the approach to the needle EMG in terms of which muscles to test and how comprehensive the examination must be to answer the clinical question. Needle EMG requires an in-depth understanding of peripheral nerve anatomy, muscle innervation patterns, and anatomic variants. The EMG needle contains an active recording thread surrounded by a metal shaft, which, when placed within a muscle, detects the activity of a small population of motor units in the vicinity. The EMG is performed with the recording needle within the muscle at rest, with slight activation and with full activation to assess the relationship between the nerve and the muscle. Disorders of the peripheral nerve and muscle manifest with characteristic EMG changes:

- Denervation injury—fibrillation potentials, fasciculations, positive sharp waves
- Reinnervation—large polyphasic motor units
- Myopathy—small motor units, myotonic discharges

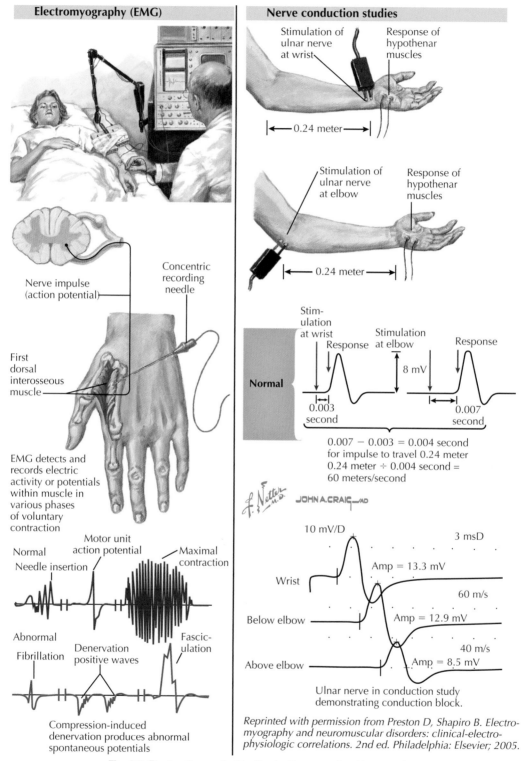

Electromyography (EMG)

Nerve impulse (action potential)

Concentric recording needle

First dorsal interosseous muscle

EMG detects and records electric activity or potentials within muscle in various phases of voluntary contraction

Normal | Motor unit action potential | Maximal contraction

Normal Needle insertion

Abnormal

Fibrillation | Denervation positive waves | Fascic-ulation

Compression-induced denervation produces abnormal spontaneous potentials

Nerve conduction studies

Stimulation of ulnar nerve at wrist

Response of hypothenar muscles

0.24 meter

Stimulation of ulnar nerve at elbow

Response of hypothenar muscles

0.24 meter

Normal

Stim-ulation at wrist

Response

Stimulation at elbow

Response

8 mV

0.003 second

0.007 second

0.007 − 0.003 = 0.004 second for impulse to travel 0.24 meter
0.24 meter ÷ 0.004 second = 60 meters/second

10 mV/D   3 msD

Wrist   Amp = 13.3 mV

                                              60 m/s

Below elbow   Amp = 12.9 mV

                                              40 m/s

Above elbow   Amp = 8.5 mV

Ulnar nerve in conduction study demonstrating conduction block.

Reprinted with permission from Preston D, Shapiro B. Electro-myography and neuromuscular disorders: clinical-electro-physiologic correlations. 2nd ed. Philadelphia: Elsevier; 2005.

Fig. 2.7 Electrodiagnostic Studies in Compression Neuropathy.

Thymus gland abnormality in myasthenia gravis

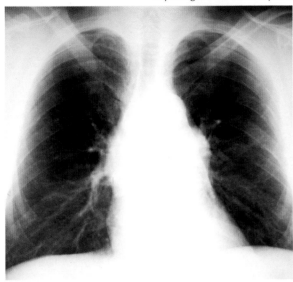

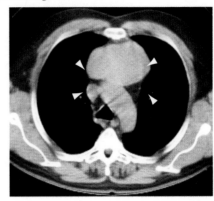

CT scan clearly demonstrates same large tumor anterior to aortic arch (arrowheads)

X-ray film shows large mediastinal tumor, which localized to anterior compartment (view not shown)

Repetitive nerve stimulation

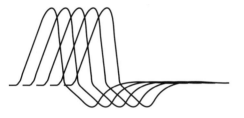

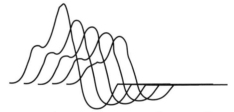

No decremental response is seen to slow rates of stimulation (1,2,3,5,Hz) in normal individuals

Decremental responses are seen to slow rates of stimulation in patients with abnormal synaptic transmission

Single fiber electromyography

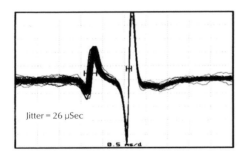

Jitter = 26 µSec

0.5 ms/d

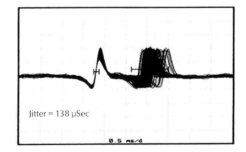

Jitter = 138 µSec

0.5 ms/d

Normal neuromuscular jitter (variation in single action potential intervals) in normal individuals

Increased neuromuscular jitter in patients with abnormal synaptic transmission

Fig. 2.8 Complementary Exams: Thymus Gland Abnormality in Myasthenia Gravis.

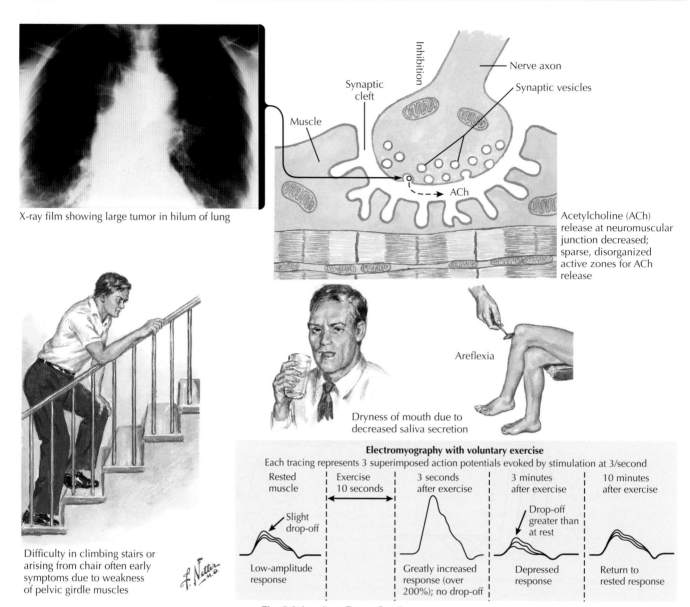

X-ray film showing large tumor in hilum of lung

Inhibition

Nerve axon

Synaptic vesicles

Synaptic cleft

Muscle

ACh

Acetylcholine (ACh) release at neuromuscular junction decreased; sparse, disorganized active zones for ACh release

Areflexia

Dryness of mouth due to decreased saliva secretion

Difficulty in climbing stairs or arising from chair often early symptoms due to weakness of pelvic girdle muscles

Electromyography with voluntary exercise

Each tracing represents 3 superimposed action potentials evoked by stimulation at 3/second

Rested muscle	Exercise 10 seconds	3 seconds after exercise	3 minutes after exercise	10 minutes after exercise
Slight drop-off			Drop-off greater than at rest	
Low-amplitude response		Greatly increased response (over 200%); no drop-off	Depressed response	Return to rested response

Fig. 2.9 Lambert-Eaton Syndrome.

The electromyographer uses the pattern of NCS/EMG changes to determine the lesion localization within the peripheral nervous system or potentially to exclude a peripheral nervous system disorder if the study results do not explain the clinical presentation.

ADDITIONAL RESOURCES

Ellenby MS, Tegtmeyer K, Lai S, et al. Videos in clinical medicine. Lumbar puncture. N Engl J Med 2006;355:e12. doi:10.1056/NEJMvcm054952.
Lumbar puncture technique.

Preston DC, Shapiro BE. Electromyography and neuromuscular disorders. 3rd ed. Elsevier; 2012.
A thorough introductory text with a focus on clinical applications.

Arevalo-Rodriguez I, Muñoz L, Godoy-Casasbuenas N, et al. Needle gauge and tip designs for preventing post-dural puncture headache (PDPH). Cochrane Database Syst Rev 2017;(4):CD010807. doi:10.1002/14651858. CD010807.pub2.
Systematic review of traumatic versus citraumatic spinal needles as well as needle gauge and the risk of postdural puncture headache.

Pittock SJ, Debruyne J, Krecke KN, et al. Chronic lymphocytic inflammation with pontine perivascular enhancement responsive to steroids (CLIPPERS). Brain 2010;133(9):2626–34.
The initial case series reporting clinical, radiographic, and neuropathologic description of CLIPPERS.

Burns JD, Cadigan RO, Russell JA. Evaluation of brain biopsy in the diagnosis of severe neurologic disease of unknown etiology. Clin Neurol Neurosurg 2009;111(3):235–9.
Case series of diagnostic yield and complications in brain biopsy for unknown progressive neurologic disorders.

Josephson SA, Papanastassiou AM, Berger MS, et al. The diagnostic utility of brain biopsy procedures in patients with rapidly deteriorating neurological conditions or dementia. J Neurosurg 2007;106:72–5.
Case series of diagnostic yield and complications in brain biopsy for unknown progressive neurologic disorders.

Magaki S, Gardner T, Khanlou N, et al. Brain biopsy in neurologic decline of unknown etiology. Hum Pathol 2015;46:499–506.
Case series of diagnostic yield and complications in brain biopsy for unknown progressive neurologic disorders.

3

Neuroimaging in Neurologic Disorders

Juan E. Small, Mara M. Kunst

The armamentarium of neuroimaging techniques includes: computed tomography (CT), magnetic resonance imaging (MRI), ultrasound, x-ray, fluoroscopy, and nuclear medicine (NM). Of these, CT and MRI have found the most use in daily practice and are frequently used as first-line neuroimaging, with the remaining modalities providing important, often ancillary, functions. The strength of CT lies in its high spatial resolution, speed of acquisition, and lack of required patient prescreening, making it the ideal tool for rapid cross-sectional evaluation of the emergency patient. CT uses radiation to create images, whereas MRI depends on strong magnetic fields, radiofrequency waves, and field gradients. Individual sequences can probe the physiology of various common neurologic disease states, including stroke, hemorrhage, and tumors. Ultrasound is a cost-effective imaging technique that uses sound waves to produce both dynamic and static cross-sectional imaging, ideal for evaluating soft tissues and vessels. X-ray, with its unparalleled spatial resolution and ability to capture large areas, is ideal for investigating bony anatomy, the integrity of surgical hardware, and ventricular shunts. Fluoroscopy capitalizes on the high spatial resolution of x-ray but is used in real time to assess cerebrovascular anatomy and flow and to conduct various imaging-guided neurointerventional procedures. Finally, NM uses minute amounts of radiotracers to assess varying disease states ranging from infection and inflammation to neurodegenerative disease and neoplasia.

With such a variety of available imaging modalities, often with overlapping or complementary applications, knowing which exam to order becomes an important clinical skill. The ideal exam will answer the clinical question, provide potential alternative diagnoses, and keep detection of incidental, often distracting, findings to a minimum. For each modality, a fundamental understanding of image acquisition, strengths and limitations, and established clinical applications will help guide the clinician to the correct diagnostic exam and potentially aid in management and treatment.

COMPUTED TOMOGRAPHY

A CT image constitutes a gray-scale map of the body's attenuation of x-rays. The images are produced by moving the patient through a gantry while a thin, fan-shaped x-ray beam rotates. On the opposite side of the x-ray beam, detectors measure the attenuated x-rays that are able to pass through the patient. Via the process of "filtered back projection," computer software is then able to reconstruct an image based on the attenuation properties of the tissues imaged. The attenuation factor at each point in image space is a unitless number known as the Hounsfield unit (HU). For the purposes of image display, each HU is assigned a grayscale value which determines the brightness/darkness of each pixel within the display matrix. Therefore CT images are a map of tissue density or absorption at each voxel, expressed in HU, which ultimately represents the attenuation of x-rays at each point in space within the

patient. CT's ability to discriminate small differences in tissue x-ray attenuation rapidly and with a high degree of spatial resolution is the basis of its diagnostic strength (Fig. 3.1).

Once CT images have been acquired, several postprocessing tools can be used to improve and enhance the images for display and interpretation. A digital CT image has a dynamic range of 4096 shades of gray, which is well beyond what a monitor can display (256) and the human eye can distinguish (32). Therefore prior to interpretation, each image must be digitally manipulated to augment the gray scale of the tissue in question, whether this be air, fat, water, muscle, or bone. Common reconstruction algorithms include bone windows for accentuated visualization of bone, bone matrix, and osseous abnormalities; and soft tissue windows for accentuated visualization of soft tissues, muscle, water, and fat (Fig. 3.2).

Each postprocessed series can then be "windowed and leveled," which refers to window width and level selection. The window width is the range of HU displayed. The window level is the center point of the width. Only the tissues within the window width are assigned a variety of gray levels within the spectrum of display. Tissues displaying HU greater than the window level are assigned white pixels, and HU levels less than the lower range of the window level are assigned black pixels. Although the window width and level can be dynamically manipulated, commonly used "set points" include Brain Windows for accentuated visualization of the brain parenchyma, Narrow Brain Windows for accentuated visualization of gray-white matter differentiation, and Subdural Windows for accentuated visualization of hyperdense blood products adjacent to the inner table of the skull (Figs. 3.3 and 3.4).

Postprocessing methods can also be used to reformat axially acquired data into two-dimensional (2D) images in other planes (coronal and sagittal) and three-dimensional (3D) data sets including volume-rendered and surface-rendered displays. The reformatting process does not alter the CT voxels; it simply displays the data in an orientation or configuration different than the way in which they were originally acquired (Fig. 3.5).

Once acquired and postprocessed, CT imaging of the brain allows for rapid exclusion or evaluation of intracranial hemorrhage, mass effect, midline shift, or hydrocephalus, making it the ideal first-line imaging tool to examine the neurologically compromised patient. Exclusion of hemorrhage and signs of completed infarction with CT are required prior to administration of tissue plasminogen activator (tPA) in the clinical setting of acute stroke. Although less sensitive than MRI in the detection of early infarction, subtle signs are often present on CT and can help confirm the diagnosis. The high spatial resolution of CT is also ideal for visualizing bony anatomy and detecting fractures, whether in the head or spine.

By administering intravenous iodinated contrast immediately prior to or during imaging, the capabilities of CT can be extended further. If given before imaging, contrast allows us to evaluate the integrity of the blood-brain barrier, thereby aiding in the detection of infection,

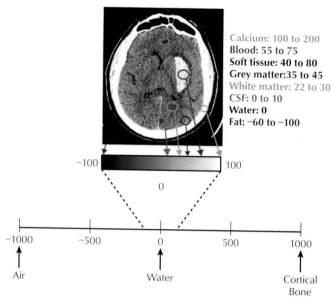

Calcium: 100 to 200
Blood: 55 to 75
Soft tissue: 40 to 80
Grey matter:35 to 45
White matter: 22 to 30
CSF: 0 to 10
Water: 0
Fat: −60 to −100

−100   100

0

−1000   −500   0   500   1000

Air   Water   Cortical
                                   Bone

Fig. 3.1 Hounsfield Units (HU) and Brain Imaging. HU are based on the arbitrary definitions of air (−1000 HU) and water (0 HU) *(bottom of figure)*. The range of HU between −100 and 100 is the most clinically useful in neurologic imaging *(grayscale bar in the middle of the figure)*. One of the most common clinical applications is the assessment of intracranial hemorrhage *(top of figure)*. Being well acquainted with the density of calcium, blood, soft tissue, gray matter, white matter, cerebrospinal fluid (CSF), and fat forms the basis of computed tomography interpretation.

inflammation, and neoplasia. Contrast administration during imaging can be used to visualize arterial (CT angiography [CTA]) and venous (CT venography [CTV]) anatomy. Axial, postprocessed 2D and 3D images can be used for the planning of aneurysm, arteriovenous malformation, and carotid stenosis intervention or surgery, or for the detection of vascular pathology, including stenosis, dissections, and vasculitis. Additional postprocessing techniques such as maximum intensity projections (MIPs) provide useful depictions of the often-tortuous vasculature. In addition, CT perfusion (CTP) allows for real-time dynamic data acquisition during contrast bolus administration and therefore provides quantitative and qualitative information in regard to cerebral perfusion (Fig. 3.6).

The speed of the CT image acquisition (just a few seconds for a head CT) not only expedites diagnosis, but it also reduces the likelihood of image degradation related to patient motion. The speed, combined with widespread availability and lack of required prescreening for implanted devices, makes CT extremely accessible for patients. The high spatial resolution of CT is particularly useful when imaging bone architecture or vasculature. Although catheter angiography remains the "gold standard" for evaluation of the vessels, the ability of CTA to rapidly and noninvasively image the vasculature has made this the modality of choice for initial assessment. Unfortunately, all the benefits of CT come at the expense of radiation, concerns about which are well reported in the medical and lay literature. The imaging industry is actively addressing these concerns with new and better dose-reduction techniques. Individual radiology departments endeavor to achieve the best imaging for the patient at the lowest possible radiation dose.

MAGNETIC RESONANCE IMAGING

Instead of using radiation, MRI creates images of the human body based on hydrogen protons, which are abundantly present as water in the human body. Normally, these hydrogen nuclei are randomly aligned. However, when placed in a magnetic field, a small percentage of them align along the axis of that field. An applied external radiofrequency (RF) pulse disrupts this magnetization and creates two magnetization vector components: longitudinal magnetization (in the direction of the magnetic field) and transverse magnetization (perpendicular to the magnetic field). When the RF pulse is turned off, the net magnetization vector realigns with the MR magnetic field—therefore longitudinal magnetization starts to increase (T1 recovery), and transverse magnetization starts to decrease (also called T2 or T2* decay). Different tissues relax and decay at different rates, resulting in characteristic T1, T2, and T2* values that define their appearance on MR imaging (Fig. 3.7).

Although tissues and organs have a characteristic MR imaging appearance, tissue injury or disease, leading to even small differences in the biochemical composition, will result in often-detectable MR imaging changes. By adjusting MR imaging parameters (such as RF excitation, switching of spatial encoding gradients, relaxation waiting times, and signal measurements), different MR sequences are produced, which accentuate these differences. The most common sequences used currently for neurologic imaging include T1, T2, inversion recovery (IR), gradient echo (GRE), and diffusion-weighted imaging (DWI). T1 imaging is used to visualize anatomic detail and highlight specific disease entities, such as fat, protein, melanin, hemorrhage, and MR contrast (gadolinium) that are hyperintense on MR imaging. On T2-weighted imaging, fluid is hyperintense, enabling visualization of the cerebrospinal fluid (CSF)-containing structures, and highlighting smaller entities, such as vessels, cranial nerves, and spinal nerve roots that traverse that fluid. IR sequences alter these basic T1 and T2 images by suppressing signal from fat (called short tau inversion recovery [STIR]) or fluid (fluid attenuation inversion recovery [FLAIR]), respectively. STIR is excellent at highlighting disease states that replace fat, such as metastases or infection in fatty bone marrow. FLAIR is excellent at highlighting brain parenchymal disease which may be isointense to CSF on routine T2, such as tumor, infection, inflammation, and hemorrhage in certain stages. GRE sequences are more sensitive to magnetic susceptibility effects, which result in faster T2* relaxation and, in turn, reduction in signal. It is this prominent reduction in signal which makes GRE sequences particularly sensitive for the detection of blood products, iron deposition, and calcification. DWI sequences are based on the detection of the random motion of water molecules within tissue. Pathologic processes such as infarction or abnormal viscous fluids such as pus will exhibit restricted diffusion and appear bright on DWI and dark on ADC images. Diffusion tensor imaging (DTI) is an extension of DWI which allows for the depiction of white matter tracts. A 3D representation of white matter tracts is referred to as diffusion tractography (Fig. 3.8).

Similar to iodinated contrast with CT, the administration of paramagnetic gadolinium as intravenous contrast markedly improves our sensitivity to pathologic areas of breakdown of the blood-brain barrier, including tumors, infection, and inflammation. Imaging of vessels with MR can be performed without intravenous contrast by using pulse sequences to "label" flowing blood while at the same time suppressing the background tissue signal. These time-of-flight (TOF) techniques can be performed in both 2D and 3D and are particularly useful in patients requiring vessel imaging who cannot receive contrast due to renal insufficiency or allergy. Postcontrast vessel imaging is also used and is usually preferred because is it less prone to flow-related artifact than the TOF techniques.

MR spectroscopy (MRS) is used to determine the concentration of metabolites within the tissue in question. The main central nervous system (CNS) metabolites include N-acetyl aspartate (NAA), choline (Cho), creatine (Cr), and lactate. NAA is a marker of neuronal integrity

Brain algorithm   Bone algorithm

Brain window

Bone window

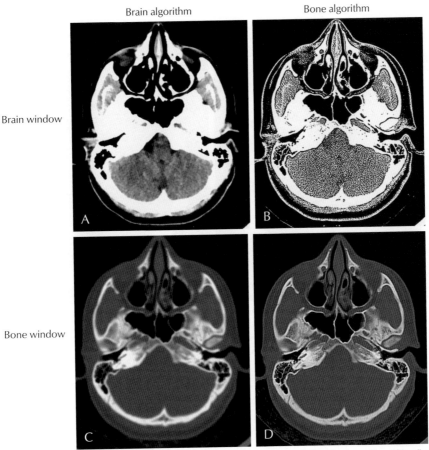

Fig. 3.2 Computed Tomography (CT) Reconstruction Algorithm and CT Window. The "filter" or "algorithm" used in CT image reconstruction affects image quality by altering the image noise and spatial resolution. A smoother algorithm produces images with lower noise but with reduced spatial resolution. A sharper algorithm produces images with higher spatial resolution but with increased noise. Therefore the selection of each is based on the needed application. For instance, a smoother brain algorithm (A and C) enhances low-contrast detectability as required for detection of infarcts. Although the cerebellum is optimally evaluated (A), evaluation of the bone is suboptimal (C). The sharper bone algorithm (B and D) is used for the assessment of bony structures with superior depiction of bony trabeculation (D) as a result of improved spatial resolution. However, notice the increased cerebellar noise of this algorithm (B).

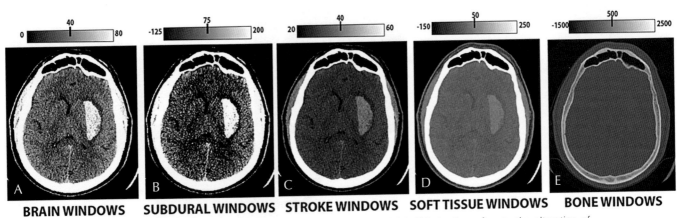

BRAIN WINDOWS   SUBDURAL WINDOWS   STROKE WINDOWS   SOFT TISSUE WINDOWS   BONE WINDOWS

Fig. 3.3 Computed Tomography (CT) Window Level and Width. Windowing refers to the alteration of the gray scale of a CT image, which in turn will alter the appearance of the picture. The window width is the range of CT numbers that an image displays. The window level (or window center) is the midpoint of the range of the window. Commonly used brain CT window levels are as follows: Brain Windows (A): Width: 70–80 Center 35–40; Subdural Windows (B): Width: 130–300 Center 50–100; Narrow (Stroke) Windows (C): Width 40 Center 40; Soft Tissue Windows (D): Width 350–400 Center: 20–60; and Bone Windows (E): Width 4000 Center 500.

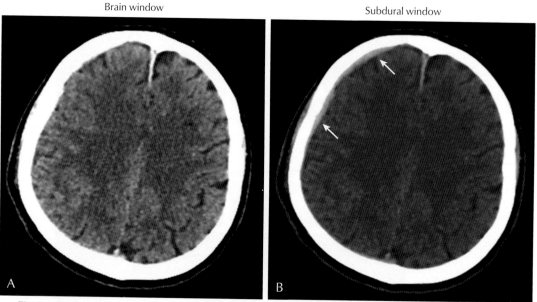

Brain window

Subdural window

Fig. 3.4 Clinical Example of the Value of Windowing. Axial brain window image (A) appears normal because both hemorrhage and the adjacent skull table are assigned white pixels in this window. However, changing to subdural windows (B) reveals a thin right frontal subdural hematoma because elevating the top of the window allows for differentiation of adjacent bone from hemorrhage *(arrows)*.

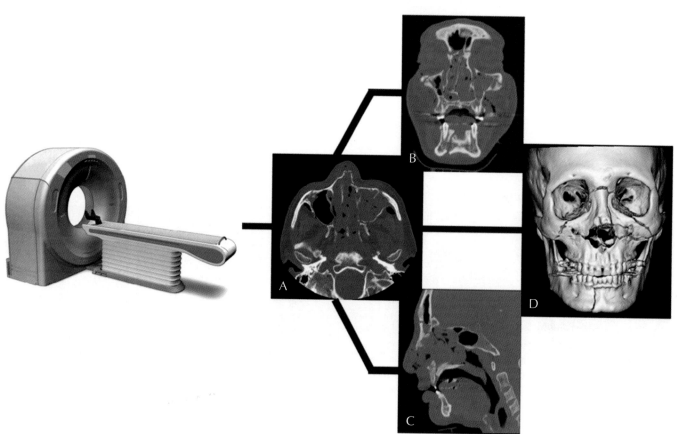

Fig. 3.5 Computed Tomography Postprocessing. Axially acquired data (A) can be reformatted into two-dimensional images in other planes such as coronal (B) and sagittal (C). In addition, three-dimensional data sets including surface rendered images (D) can be created.

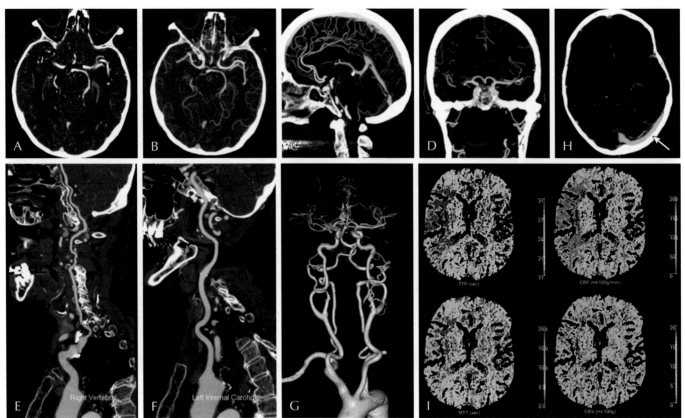

Fig. 3.6 Computed Tomography Angiography (CTA), Computed Tomography Venography (CTV), and Computed Tomography Perfusion (CTP). Contrast administration during imaging can be used to visualize arterial anatomy (CTA). Axial acquisition postcontrast CTA images (A) can then be reformatted and postprocessed into thick section images, maximum intensity projections, curved reformatted (CR), and three-dimensional images (B, C, D, E, F, G) to better visualize vessels. Venous phase CTV (H) images provide excellent visualization of venous anatomy *(arrow)* and can also be reformatted and postprocessed in a variety of ways. CTP images (I) generated from real-time dynamic data acquisition during contrast bolus flow injection provide quantitative and qualitative information regarding cerebral perfusion.

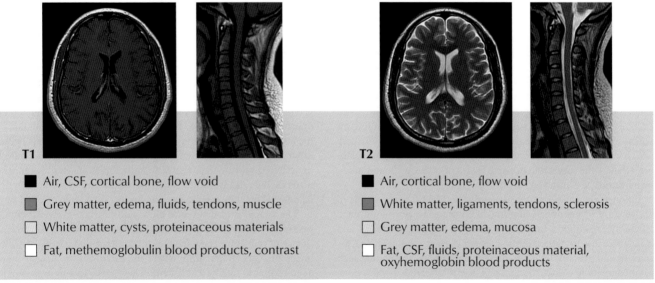

T1
- ■ Air, CSF, cortical bone, flow void
- ■ Grey matter, edema, fluids, tendons, muscle
- □ White matter, cysts, proteinaceous materials
- □ Fat, methemoglobulin blood products, contrast

T2
- ■ Air, cortical bone, flow void
- ■ White matter, ligaments, tendons, sclerosis
- □ Grey matter, edema, mucosa
- □ Fat, CSF, fluids, proteinaceous material, oxyhemoglobin blood products

Fig. 3.7 Substances and Tissues Have Characteristic T1 and T2 Signal Intensities. MRI of brain and cervical spinal cord.

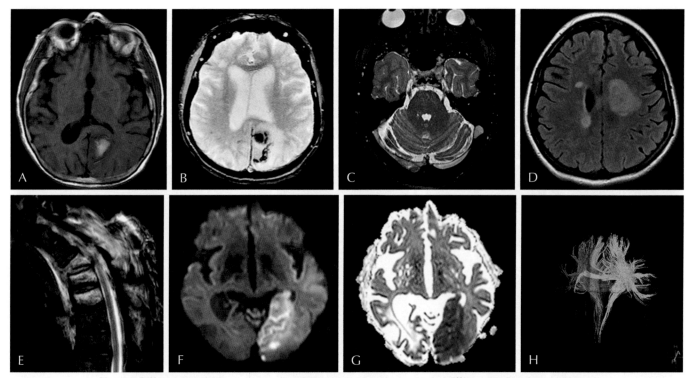

Fig. 3.8 Different magnetic resonance imaging sequences accentuate the differences that tissue injury or disease creates within the central nervous system. Subacute parenchymal hemorrhage in the left parieto-occipital lobe is hyperintense on axial T1-weighted images (A) and shows dark susceptibility artifact due to methemoglobin on gradient echo sequences (B). High-resolution T2-weighted images, as shown here at the level of the trigeminal nerves (C), is useful for evaluating vessels and cranial nerves which are surrounded by T2 hyperintense cerebrospinal fluid. Fluid attenuation inversion recovery sequences are very useful for evaluating the white matter, as seen in this patient with multiple sclerosis, "tumefactive" on the left (D). Short tau inversion recovery images are very useful for evaluating marrow edema in the background of marrow fat, as in this case of several compression fractures in the thoracic spine (E). Diffusion-weighted imaging (F) and apparent diffusion coefficient (G) maps are invaluable for early assessment of acute infarction, as seen in this acute left posterior cerebral territory infarct. Lastly, information obtained using diffusion tensor imaging can be used to create a three-dimensional model of white matter tracts, a process called diffusion tractography (H).

and therefore is the tallest peak in normal brain. Cho is a marker of membrane turnover. Cr is a marker of cellular metabolism. Neoplastic processes with high cellular turnover frequently exhibit elevated Cho peaks (Fig. 3.9).

Functional MRI (fMRI) measures brain activity by detecting minute changes in blood flow by exploiting the blood oxygen level–dependent (BOLD) contrast method. Detecting transient changes in blood flow related to neuronal activity helps localize cerebral function and therefore noninvasive assessment of brain function. fMRI is performed while the patient is engaged in neurocognitive tasks which in turn places increased metabolic demands on the activated parts of the brain. This allows us to measure the minute differences in local perfusion and therefore map activity. fMRI has found particular clinical utility in preoperative planning, to allow the surgeon to preserve eloquent cortex while still maximizing tumor resection (Fig. 3.10).

Although the superior contrast resolution of MRI is invaluable in the detection of neurologic abnormalities, the comparatively limited availability, in addition to the time-intensive imaging protocols and degradation due to patient motion, are important considerations for clinicians and patients. In addition, contraindications to scanning such as noncompatible cardiac pacemakers, metallic foreign bodies, noncompatible surgical clips, and monitoring systems are important considerations. The strong magnetic field of an MRI scanner can cause

implanted medical devices with metal to malfunction (e.g., pacemakers). Implanted medical devices that are ferromagnetic (such as some aneurysm clips or skin staples) may be dislodged or cause burns secondary to heating.

ULTRASOUND

Ultrasound uses sound waves with higher frequencies than those audible to humans (>20,000 Hz) to create a sonographic image. A sound wave is typically produced by a piezoelectric transducer encased in a plastic housing which is applied to the skin, allowing direct transmission into the body. The sound wave is partially reflected from the layers between different tissues or scattered from smaller structures. These reflected or scattered sound waves return to and vibrate the transducer, which turns the vibrations into electrical pulses that travel to the ultrasonic scanner, where they are processed and transformed into a digital image.

The strengths of diagnostic ultrasound include its availability and ease of use, its excellent depiction of soft tissues and vascular flow, and its lack of radiation. These features make ultrasound particularly useful in the pediatric population, where the brain can be imaged though open sutures to safely exclude hemorrhage, mass lesions or mass effect, hydrocephalus, and even ischemia. However, the inability of ultrasound to penetrate bone limits its utility in evaluation of the adult intracranial

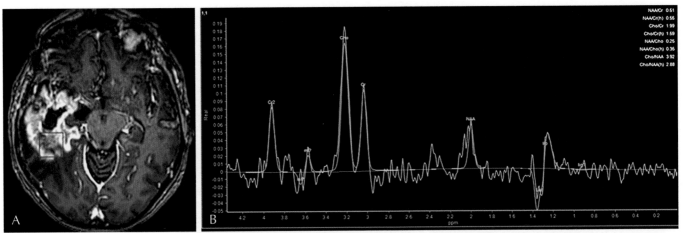

Fig. 3.9 Magnetic Resonance Spectroscopy (MRS). Axial magnetic resonance imaging postcontrast image (A) in a patient with a history or right temporal glioblastoma multiforme treated with resection and radiation therapy. MRS was performed to help distinguish between recurrent tumor and radiation necrosis, which can appear identical on conventional sequences. A single voxel placed along the posterior enhancing margin of the tumor (A, *red box*) demonstrates a pattern consistent with recurrent tumor (B), including an elevated choline peak (Cho), suppressed NAA peak (NAA), and a lactate doublet (Lac).

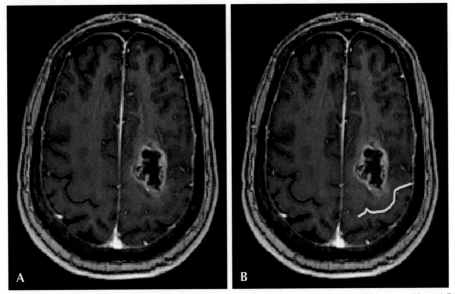

Fig. 3.10 Functional Magnetic Resonance Imaging (MRI). Axial postcontrast MRI images (A and B) in a patient with a rim-enhancing, left-sided lesion for preoperative planning prior to biopsy/resection. Functional magnetic resonance imaging performed with a right-hand finger tapping paradigm shows increase blood oxygen level–dependent signal along the posterolateral aspect of the lesion (*red area* in A), corresponding with the right-hand motor area, allowing preoperative mapping of the precentral gyrus and central sulcus (*yellow line* in B).

compartments, where sutures are closed. Nonetheless, ultrasound can be used intraoperatively to image a resection cavity through an open craniotomy. It is most commonly used to evaluate neck vessels particularly carotid stenosis, with data that closely correlate with other, often more costly, imaging modalities (Fig. 3.11). Ultrasound is also preferred for evaluation of superficial soft tissue, including lymph nodes, salivary glands, and thyroid tissue.

X-RAY

Similar to CT, x-rays are generated by a vacuum tube that uses a high voltage to accelerate the electrons released by a hot cathode to a high velocity. The high velocity electrons collide with a metal target, the anode, creating the x-rays. However, unlike CT, which uses multiple rows of detectors, x-rays are then absorbed by a single image plate or detector panel. The result is a very high spatial resolution 2D image with overlapping structures.

Because of this, many applications historically reserved for x-ray have been supplanted by CT. Nonetheless, x-ray is still preferred for imaging that requires broad coverage, such as with retained foreign body evaluation, or assessing the integrity of ventricular shunts and catheters. The high spatial resolution and absence of some CT-specific hardware-related artifacts make it very useful for imaging of bony anatomy and spine hardware (Fig. 3.12).

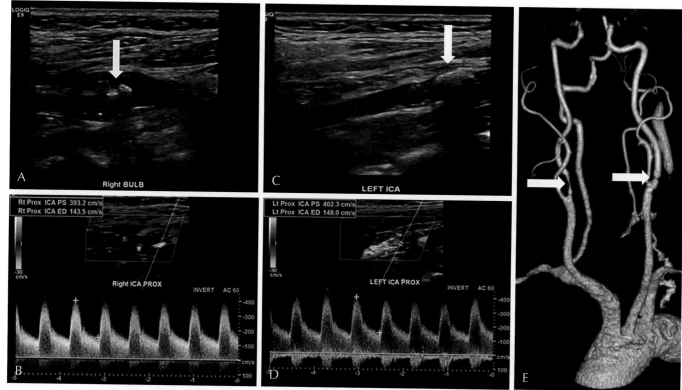

Fig. 3.11 Vascular Ultrasound of the Carotid Bifurcations. Ultrasound grayscale image A shows a gray scale image of the right carotid bifurcation, with the *vertical arrow* pointing to a focus of densely calcified atherosclerotic plaque. Corresponding M-mode Doppler ultrasound (B) shows elevated peak systolic flow velocities in the range of a greater than 70% stenosis. Figures C and D show similar findings at the left carotid bifurcation in gray scale (C) and M-mode (D). A volume-rendered reformatted computed tomography angiography reconstruction (E) demonstrates severe stenoses of bilateral proximal internal carotid arteries (*horizontal arrows*).

FLUOROSCOPY/DIGITAL SUBTRACTION ANGIOGRAPHY

Digital subtraction angiography (DSA) uses fluoroscopy to specifically evaluate the vasculature in a bony or dense soft tissue environment, making it ideal for CNS applications. Fluoroscopy is an imaging technique that uses x-rays to obtain real-time images able to detect moment-to-moment changes. In its simplest form, a fluoroscope consists of an x-ray source and a fluorescent screen, between which a patient is placed. Modern fluoroscopes couple the screen to an x-ray image intensifier and charge coupled device (CCD) video camera allowing the images to be recorded and played on a monitor. Angiography combines fluoroscopy with the injection of intravenous contrast for high-resolution, real-time vascular imaging. Although traditional angiography is limited by overlapping bone or soft tissues, DSA removes these by obtaining mask images which then can be subtracted from the contrast-enhanced image, leaving only intravascular contrast behind.

The spatial resolution of DSA surpasses that of CTA, making it the gold standard for vessel imaging. As opposed to the static images of CTA and magnetic resonance angiography (MRA), the dynamic capabilities of DSA offer a greater understanding of flow through often complex vascular lesions which are needed to plan for surgery or intervention. Beyond diagnostic imaging, DSA is the modality that guides neurointervention, ranging from mechanical thrombectomy and thrombolysis for stroke therapy, embolization of aneurysm and arteriovenous malformation, and many spine procedures (Fig. 3.13).

NUCLEAR MEDICINE

NM is a branch of diagnostic imaging that uses small amounts of radiotracers to both diagnose and treat disease. In contrast to the imaging modalities described previously, the emphasis of NM is on physiology and function rather than anatomic detail. To create images, small amounts of radiotracer are either ingested or injected, then allowed to metabolize, and localize to a particular organ or disease entity. These localized radiotracers emit small amounts of radiation which then pass through the body and can be detected by an overlying camera.

NM exams can be used to image nearly every organ system, with a commonly used study being positron emission tomography (PET). PET is used to image metabolic processes in the body by using a positron emitting nucleotide tracer that can be tied to any number of radiotracers. Three-dimensional images of tracer concentration are then constructed by computer analysis and can be combined with CT imaging to provide simultaneous physiologic and anatomic detail.

If the radiotracer chosen for PET is fluorodeoxyglucose (FDG), an analog of glucose, the concentrations of tracer imaged will indicate tissue metabolic activity as it corresponds to the regional glucose uptake. The most common application is detection of hypermetabolic tumor cells in the search for metastatic disease. Because the background brain metabolism of glucose is so high and the spatial resolution of PET is so low, there is little routine use of PET brain to evaluate CNS malignancy. However, brain tissue uptake can be used as a marker of relative cerebral blood flow and regional brain activity, which is particularly

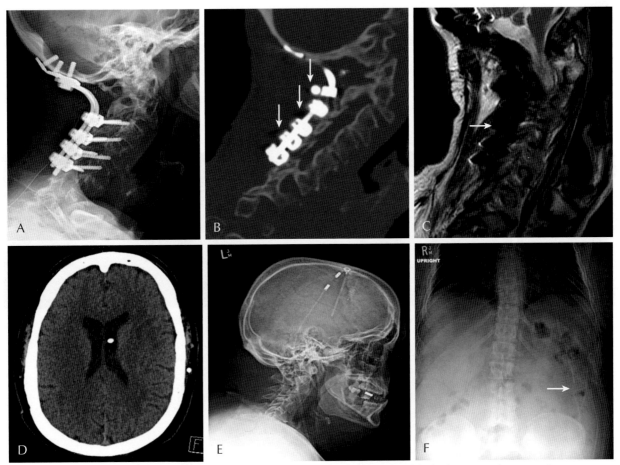

Fig. 3.12 X-ray images are useful due to their high spatial resolution and lack of computed tomography (CT)- and magnetic resonance imaging (MRI)-related artifacts. Figures A, B, and C are from the same patient who had undergone posterior suboccipital/cervical fusion for a C2 pathologic fracture. X-ray (A) enables visualization of the entire metal construct with high spatial resolution and absence of associated artifact. CT (B) is also useful for hardware evaluation but is limited by lower spatial resolution and beam hardening artifact, resulting from photon starvation adjacent to metal *(thin, white arrows)*. On MRI (C), metal produces a large amount of susceptibility artifact *(white arrow)* and is therefore not useful for hardware evaluation. Figures D, E, and F are from the same patient. Axial head CT (D) shows the position of the catheter in relation to the ventricles. X-rays (E and F) show the length of the shunt catheter, with subtle multifocal irregularity along the catheter tract, and a focal disruption in the left mid abdomen (F, *white arrow*).

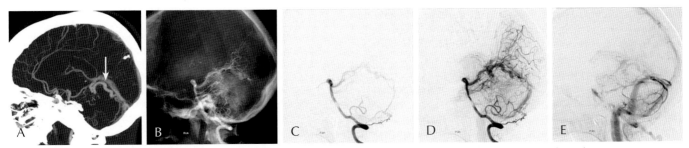

Fig. 3.13 Digital Subtraction Angiography. A sagittal computed tomography angiography maximum intensity projection (A) demonstrates the presence of an anomalous posterior fossa venous structure *(arrow)*. A sagittal angiographic image (B) shows the presence of contrast in vessels but is limited by the presence of overlying bone. Digital subtraction angiography images showing isolated intravascular contrast in the arterial (C), parenchymal (D), and delayed venous (E) phases, allowing full characterization for the arterial supply, venous drainages, and flow patterns in this arteriovenous malformation prior to embolization.

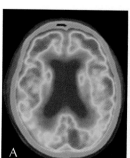
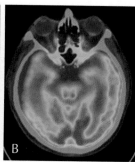
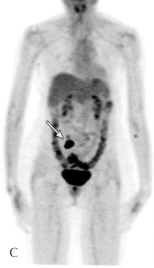
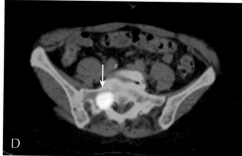

Fig. 3.14 Nuclear Medicine. Figures A and B: An 82-year-old male with memory impairment. Positron emission tomography (PET) brain images show decreased glucose uptake *(yellow-green areas)* in right greater than left parietal lobes (A) and temporal lobes (B), a pattern consistent with Alzheimer dementia. Figures C and D: A 72-year-old female with multiple myeloma status postautologous stem cell transplant, in remission for 6 years, now with slow increase in low-level M spike. X-rays showed no new lytic lesions. PET computed tomography (CT) shows a hypermetabolic focus in the right sacrum *(arrows)*. Biopsy showed plasmacytoma. A technetium-99m bone scan is frequently negative in multiple myeloma due to the prevalence of bony destruction and absence of bone formation. PET/CT is therefore the imaging modality of choice in this disease.

useful in the evaluation of epilepsy, Parkinson, Alzheimer, and various neurodegenerative disorders (Fig. 3.14).

FUTURE DIRECTIONS

Many new exciting frontiers in neuroimaging are being explored. As with computing, imaging equipment continues to be refined with promising advances in speed, sensitivity, and safety.

On the MRI front, development and refinement of MRI sequences continues. In particular, faster acquisitions are being developed, many of which promise to markedly reduce acquisition times and therefore significantly improve patient access. Rapid MRI acquisition times promise to improve our understanding of physiologic processes such as brain perfusion, CSF flow, and even motion tracking. Magnets operating at 7 or 9.4 T and ultra-high systems operating up to 26.8 T are being refined and developed. In addition, novel structural and functional techniques are areas of intense research and interest. Advanced methods aiding visualization and display are also in the works. Hybrid imaging techniques look to combine imaging modalities and promise to aid in detection and identification via data fusion. Examples of this include PET/MR, electroencephalogram (EEG)/MR, and intraoperative MR/CT. Artificial intelligence promises to automate several processes. Furthermore, the trend toward physiologic and metabolic imaging continues. Molecular imaging in particular focuses on detecting and visualizing cellular function and molecular processes. Some molecular imaging targets currently in use are amyloid beta (Abeta) peptide and tau protein.

Advances in CT technology have included the addition of multiple rows of detectors (16, 64, 128, 256, and 320), which allows for ever increasing coverage per rotation and therefore even more rapid image acquisition. In the past decade, dual energy and spectral CT technology has emerged as a powerful tool that targets some known limitations of CT. The ability of this new technology to utilize the full energy spectrum of the x-ray beam has resulted in notable metal artifact reduction, improved soft tissue contrast, and the ability to evaluate tissue, not just based on density, but also on atomic number. Clinically, this tool has found relevance in helping distinguish contrast from hemorrhage in postintervention cases, hemorrhage from calcium in trauma, or tumor imaging, with several additional applications still emerging.

ADDITIONAL RESOURCES

Kunst MM, Schaefer PW. Ischemic stroke. Radiol Clin North Am 2011;49(1):1–26.
Overview of stroke imaging with an emphasis on CT and MRI imaging.
Potter CA, Sodickson AD. Dual-energy CT in emergency neuroimaging: added value and novel applications. Radiographics 2016;36(7):2186–98.
Excellent review of the basic applications of dual energy CT in emergency neuroimaging.
Fritz JV. Neuroimaging trends and future outlook. Neurol Clin 2014;32(1):1–29.
Overview of recent advances in speed, sensitivity, safety, and workflow of various neuroimaging modalities including hybrid modalities and with emphasis on the increasing trend toward physiologic imaging and quantitation.
Radue EW, Weigel M, Wiest R, et al. Introduction to magnetic resonance imaging for neurologists. Continuum (Minneap Minn) 2016;22(5, Neuroimaging):1379–98.
Basic and straightforward introduction to the technical aspects of MRI by introducing the basics of MRI physics, technology, image acquisition, protocols, and image interpretation.
Tsai LL, Grant AK, Mortele KJ, et al. A practical guide to MR imaging safety: what radiologists need to know. Radiographics 2015;35(6):1722–37.
Review of the safety risks associated with MRI. Safety risks including translational force and torque, projectile injury, excessive specific absorption rate, burns, peripheral neurostimulation, interactions with active implants and devices, and acoustic injury are covered.

SECTION II

Cranial Nerves

Jayashri Srinivasan

4

Cranial Nerve I: Olfactory

Michal Vytopil, H. Royden Jones, Jr.[†]

CLINICAL VIGNETTE *A 64-year-old woman, a retired music teacher and a food and wine connoisseur, was driving to the airport to catch a flight to Spain when she noted she could not smell the characteristic skunk odor her friend was complaining about. She thought it had something to do with her recent cold. While traveling in Spain, she gradually became more alarmed as she realized that she had lost her sense of taste and was unable to distinguish the aromas of different wines. She now believed that her sense of smell had never fully recovered from the cold. She was less sure about her taste because she had limited herself to eating "bland and healthy" foods in the aftermath of the illness. Unable to enjoy food and wine in Spain, and preoccupied about the cause of her symptoms, depression started to set in. She had an appointment with an ear, nose, and throat (ENT) specialist, who concluded after evaluation that she had postviral anosmia. Computed tomography (CT) scan of the sinuses and a neurology consultation were recommended. Within 3 months of the viral illness, her taste gradually normalized. Recovery of her smell was slower and, unfortunately, incomplete. She struggled to distinguish coffee from chocolate, but her neurologic examination was otherwise normal. The neurologist agreed the story was characteristic of postviral hyposmia. On follow-up 3 months later, our patient reported her smell had improved to approximately 70% but plateaued thereafter. A natural optimist, however, she was quick to point out that her smell was good enough to distinguish different wines and that she had begun plans for a trip to Tuscany the following spring.*

Comment: Damage of olfactory neuroepithelium during a viral illness is one of the most common causes of olfactory dysfunction in neurologically healthy people. Olfactory dysfunction is commonly accompanied by loss of taste because taste depends largely on volatile particles from food and beverages reaching the olfactory receptor cells via the nasopharynx. A majority of patients improve, but many have residual deficits.

The olfactory nerve (CN I) provides for the sense of smell. Humans rely on proper olfactory function every day. This important sensory modality provides a warning system, enabling the identification of potentially toxic foods or noxious chemicals. Individuals with decreased smell, particularly those who are elderly and live alone, are at increased risk of nutritional problems, such as eating spoiled food, but are also in danger from gas explosion or fire. Smell also contributes to quality of life because this sensory modality provides awareness of many pleasurable sensations, including appreciation of certain foods and beverages, as well as playing an important role in subtle attractions between humans that are important for sexual desire and reproduction.

Smell disturbance is common, and its prevalence increases with age; when systematically tested, it has been estimated that 50% of adults older than the age of 60 years have a decreased sense of smell. Often a patient is not aware of or dismisses as unimportant the loss of the sense of smell. This may be particularly true in an elderly individual with concomitant dementia, as seen in Alzheimer or Parkinson disease (PD), or in an occasional patient with potentially treatable olfactory groove meningioma that compromises frontal lobe function. In such cases, it is essential to evaluate olfactory function by asking the patient to identify familiar odors such as coffee, perfumes or tobacco, or to perform one of the standardized smell tests.

ANATOMY

When identifying odors, humans rely on volatile substances entering their nasal cavity to excite receptors. *Olfactory receptor cells* are bipolar sensory neurons whose dendrites form a delicate sensory carpet, olfactory epithelium, on the superior aspect of the nasal cavity (Fig. 4.1). Basal cells within the epithelium are stem cells that serve as a source of new olfactory cells during regeneration. This unique mechanism, during which the dead olfactory cells are continually being replaced by new ones, represents the best-known example of neuronal regeneration in humans. The thin, unmyelinated axons of the bipolar sensory cells collectively form the olfactory nerve. These axons travel through the cribriform plate into the olfactory bulb at the base of the fronto-orbital lobe. Within the bulb, olfactory nerve fibers synapse with the dendrites of large mitral cells, whose axons constitute the olfactory tract passing along the base of the frontal lobe and projecting directly into the primary olfactory cortex within the temporal lobe. In contrast to all other sensory modalities, olfactory sensation does not have a central processing site within the thalamic nuclei. The human primary olfactory cortex includes the uncus, hippocampal gyrus, amygdaloid complex, and entorhinal cortex (Fig. 4.2). This direct pathway to the cerebral limbic structures may have an important evolutionary function.

Cortical representation of smell is bilateral. Although most of the olfactory tract fibers supply the ipsilateral olfactory cortex, some fibers decussate in the anterior commissure and terminate in the opposite hemisphere. Consequently, a unilateral lesion distal to the decussation rarely produces olfactory dysfunction.

CLINICAL EVALUATION AND DIAGNOSTIC APPROACH

Traditionally, olfactory function is tested by relatively crude methods such as asking a patient to sniff and identify a series of nonirritating odorants (e.g., coffee, cinnamon, chocolate, etc.). Irritating substances such as ammonia are to be avoided because their irritative effects on trigeminal nerve endings can overshadow stimulation of olfactory receptors. Several commercially available standardized and reliable methodologies are available for more precise olfactory definition. The most

---

[†]Deceased.

A. Distribution of olfactory epithelium
(blue area)

B. Schema of section through olfactory mucosa

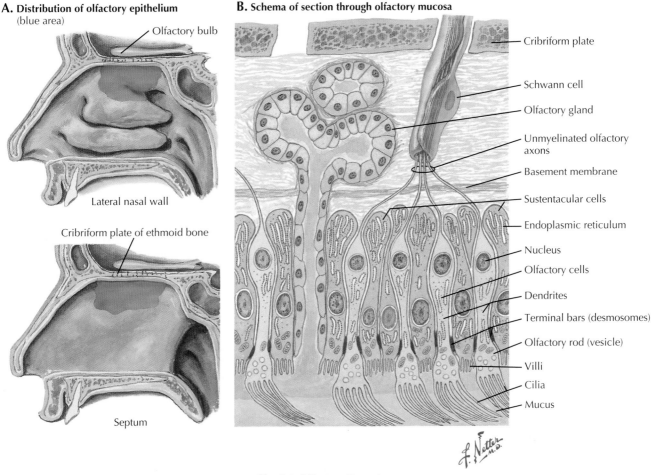

Fig. 4.1 Olfactory Receptors.

widely used of these tests is the University of Pennsylvania Smell Identification Test (UPSIT) consisting of 40 microencapsulated odorants. A shorter version, Brief Smell Identification Test (B-SIT) uses 12 common daily odorants such as banana, chocolate, or paint thinner and takes only 5 minutes to administer.

Gadolinium-enhanced brain magnetic resonance imaging (MRI) is the modality of choice for the evaluation of intracranial causes of olfactory dysfunction. Head CT with contrast is reliable when MRI cannot be performed or if a bony lesion of the anterior fossa is suspected. Laboratory studies are not very useful, with possible exception of anti-Ro/SSA and anti-La/SSB autoantibodies in a rare patient with Sjögren syndrome.

DIFFERENTIAL DIAGNOSIS

Smell dysfunction can result from disruptions at any site along the olfactory pathway. Therefore impaired olfaction is not necessarily equivalent with olfactory nerve injury. Nasal and paranasal sinus diseases (in which there is mechanical obstruction preventing volatile odorants from reaching the receptor cells) are common conditions that interfere with olfactory function without causing olfactory nerve damage. Olfactory nerve is damaged in head trauma, and olfactory receptors are commonly affected by viral infections. In fact, these three processes (nasal and paranasal disease, viral conditions, and head trauma) account for most cases of olfactory disturbance. In contrast, smell loss due to primary olfactory bulb, tract, or entorhinal cortex lesions are uncommon.

In general, most patients experiencing olfactory dysfunctions have bilateral loss of function. The rare diagnosis of unilateral anosmia is an important sign that signals the need for an MRI of the brain to exclude an olfactory groove tumor.

Congenital Disorders
Kallmann Syndrome

In this condition, anosmia results from a congenital hypoplasia or even absence of the olfactory bulbs. This occurs in conjunction with hypogonadotropic hypogonadism. Although most instances are sporadic, familial cases are reported, with variable inheritance patterns: X-linked, autosomal dominant, or autosomal recessive. Occasionally, Kallmann syndrome is associated with other congenital deficits, including cleft palate, lip/dental agenesis, color blindness, and neural hearing loss.

Acquired Disorders

Upper respiratory viral infections lead to olfactory dysfunction by destroying receptor cells in the olfactory neuroepithelium. Recovery of smell depends on the degree of concurrent damage to the stem (basal) cells; if the stem cells are relatively preserved, regeneration of the receptor cells can occur. Although most patients improve, residual deficit is common, as described in the previous vignette.

Nasal and paranasal sinus diseases account for approximately 40% of olfactory disturbances. These intranasal processes mechanically prevent volatile chemical stimuli from reaching the olfactory sensory epithelium and activating the receptors. Intranasal obstruction due to hypertrophy and hyperemia of the mucosa, rather than direct damage to the

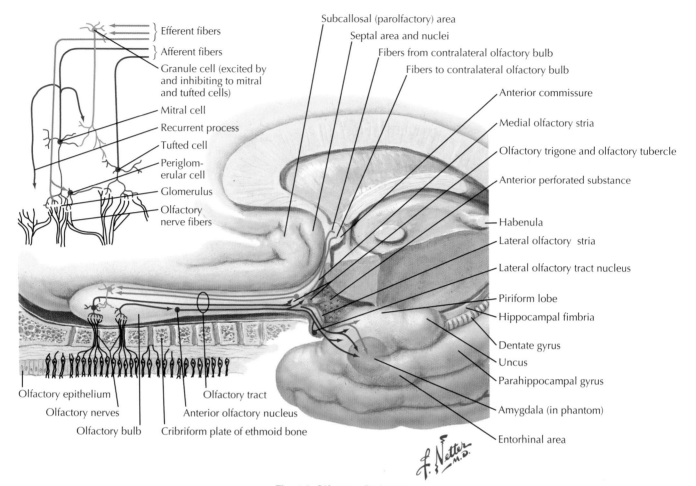

Fig. 4.2 Olfactory Pathways.

olfactory nerve pathways, is the responsible mechanism. History of fluctuating olfactory dysfunction correlating with nasal congestion provides the most important clinical clue to this diagnosis. In contrast, the presence of persistent smell disturbance is suggestive of direct damage to the olfactory nerve pathways.

Head trauma is responsible for approximately 20% of all cases of smell dysfunction. Most often, the jostling movement of the brain within the skull leads to shearing off of the olfactory axons as they pass through the cribriform plate. Direct occipital and lateral injuries to the head are more dangerous to olfaction than are frontally directed blows. More substantial damage, such as is seen in severe head trauma with anterior fossa fracture, may lead to contusion of the olfactory bulb or the olfactory area of the brain. Depending on the severity of the blunt head injury, the incidence of posttraumatic anosmia varies between 7% and 30%. This is often a permanent deficit; a small minority of patients may notice some return of their sense of smell.

Olfactory groove meningiomas are quite infrequent; however, these histologically benign tumors may lead to significant morbidity unless treated early. Meningiomas are slow-growing tumors; olfactory groove lesions comprise 8%–18% of all intracranial meningiomas (Fig. 4.3). Although unilateral or bilateral olfactory dysfunction is often their first symptom, very few patients present with just a disturbance in their sense of smell. This is probably because their slow growth leads to a very gradual decline in olfactory function that may not be noticed by the patient. Furthermore, because most meningiomas are unilateral, they often lead to unilateral anosmia and thus patients still retain olfactory function on the contralateral side. Consequently, most orbital

meningiomas are often not diagnosed until the tumor is large enough (e.g., >4 cm in diameter) to cause other symptoms resulting from pressure on the frontal lobes and optic tracts. These include headache, visual disturbances, personality changes, and memory impairment. Early diagnosis of olfactory groove meningiomas remains challenging. At times, the behavioral changes can be profound and may create a sense the patient is demented or mentally unbalanced.

Very large olfactory groove tumors, typically meningiomas, rarely lead to the development of Foster-Kennedy syndrome. This is characterized by unilateral optic atrophy and contralateral papilledema. Optic atrophy results from direct pressure of the neoplasm on the optic nerve, whereas increased intracranial pressure produces contralateral papilledema.

Esthesioneuroblastoma is a rare tumor that originates in the olfactory epithelium and presents with anosmia, epistaxis, and nasal obstruction.

Hyposmia or anosmia is often an early feature of *neurodegenerative disorders* such as *Parkinson disease (PD), Alzheimer disease, or dementia with Lewy bodies.* Olfactory dysfunction can precede the classical clinical manifestations of these diseases, sometimes by years. Idiopathic olfactory loss in cognitively normal individuals may be a marker for future cognitive decline, particularly in individuals with one or more apolipoprotein (APOE) epsilon 4 alleles. Similarly, difficulty with sense of smell may precede the onset of classic motor manifestations of PD by 4 to 8 years. Abnormal olfactory function in PD is nearly universal; in fact, normal sense of smell in a PD patient is such a rare occurrence that it should prompt review of this diagnosis. Decreased sense of smell can also be seen in Huntington disease, vascular dementia, pure

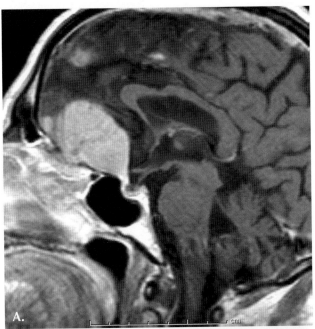

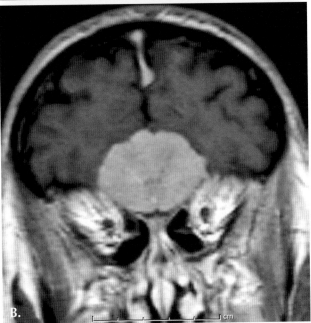

T1-weighted, gadolinium-enhanced sagittal and coronal MR images show a large enhancing mass on the skull base displacing and compressing the olfactory apparatus.

Fig. 4.3 Subfrontal Meningioma. *MR,* Magnetic resonance.

autonomic failure, and rapid eye movement sleep behavior disorder. Interestingly, progressive supranuclear palsy, corticobasal degeneration, and multiple system atrophy are associated with no or minimal loss of smell. In fact, significant olfactory dysfunction in these patients should lead one to revisit these diagnoses.

Other Entities

Autoimmune inflammation with ultimate destruction of exocrine glands in *Sjögren syndrome* may lead to xerostomia with taste and smell dysfunction.

Olfactory hallucinations are important considerations in the differential diagnosis of anyone with positive olfactory symptoms. These events do not occur with primary olfactory nerve disorders per se; most often such symptoms form the aura that precedes a focal seizure disorder—*uncinate* seizures. The typical patient initially experiences an unpleasant smell of very foul nature such as burning garbage. This classically precedes a temporal or fronto-orbital lobe focal seizure wherein the patient briefly loses contact with the environment, as characterized by staring and various automatisms. Certain patients with psychiatric conditions (e.g., severe depression, psychosis) or during alcohol withdrawal may also experience unusual olfactory symptoms.

Olfactory discrimination is also adversely affected by many *medications and drugs,* including opiates (codeine, morphine), antiepileptic drugs (carbamazepine, phenytoin), and immunosuppressive agents, that, similar to radiation, disrupt the physiologic turnover of receptor cells. Cocaine abuse, via intranasal snorting, is particularly prone to cause septal perforation that eventually leads to direct trauma to the olfactory nerve and loss of smell.

PROGNOSIS AND TREATMENT

No specific treatment is available for most causes of olfactory dysfunction. We rely on the unique ability of the olfactory neuroepithelium and olfactory bulb to regenerate. Most patients with smell dysfunction due to nasal sinus disease and postviral mechanisms can expect improvement, but in some there may be incomplete recovery. Unfortunately, smell loss due to head trauma carries a much worse prognosis, with only 10% of patients achieving meaningful recovery.

ADDITIONAL RESOURCES

Yaffe K, Freimer D, Chen H, et al. Olfaction and risk of dementia in a biracial cohort of older adults. Neurology 2017;88:456–62.
In this prospective study, it was found that poor olfactory function was associated with increased risk of dementia among both black and white older adults.

Doty RL. Olfactory dysfunction in neurodegenerative diseases: is there a common pathological substrate? Lancet Neurol 2017;16:478–88.
Introduction into theories of pathophysiological processes leading to olfactory loss in neurodegenerative diseases.

Lee DY, Lee WH, Wee JH. Prognosis of postviral olfactory loss: followup study for longer than one year. Am J Rhinol Allergy 2014;28:419–22.
In this retrospective study, it was found that over 80% of patients with postviral loss of smell reported subjective improvement but only 30% normalization.

Haehner A, Hummel T, Reichmann H. Olfactory function in Parkinson's disease. Eur Neurol Rev 2010;5(1):26–9.
This article summarizes the available literature on olfactory function in PD.

Ross Webster G, Petrovitch H, Abbott RD, et al. Association of olfactory dysfunction with risk for future Parkinson's disease. Ann Neurol 2007;63:167–73.
This prospective study suggests that olfactory disturbance can precede the classic features of Parkinson disease by years.

Reden J, Mueller A, Mueller C, et al. Recovery of olfactory function following closed head injury or infections of the upper respiratory tract. Arch Otolaryngol Head Neck Surg 2006;132:265–9.
This retrospective study found that only 10% of patients improve following olfactory loss after trauma, whereas the prognosis of postviral anosmia is better.

Doty RL, Shaman P, Dann M. Development of University of Pennsylvania Smell Identification Test. Physiol Behav 1984;32:489–502.
Authors describe development of the first standardized olfactory test battery (UPSIT). The UPSIT provided the needed scientific basis for many subsequent studies.

5

Cranial Nerve II: Optic Nerve and Visual System

Geetha K. Athappilly, Ippolit C. A. Matjucha

INTRAOCULAR OPTIC NERVE

> **CLINICAL VIGNETTE** *A 48-year-old man was referred for sudden loss of vision in the left eye. He had noted that morning while shaving that he could not see the lower half of his chin with the right eye closed. He had no pain and had no preceding systemic symptoms. His past medical history was noteworthy for mild diet-controlled hypercholesterolemia and untreated labile hypertension. The affected eye had 20/40 central acuity and an inferior central field loss that extended nasally but did not cross into the superior field. The left optic nerve showed acquired elevation and swelling, with mild peripapillary hemorrhages. The right optic nerve was small in diameter, had no physiologic cup, and had mild congenital elevation. The diagnosis of idiopathic (nonarteritic) anterior ischemic optic neuropathy (AION) was made. Over the next 6 weeks, the left optic nerve swelling abated and was replaced by mild pallor noted superiorly. He did not recover his vision in the left eye.*

The optic nerve is not a peripheral nerve but rather a central nervous system (CNS) tract containing central myelin formed by oligodendrocytes. It is composed of long axons, whose cell bodies comprise the ganglion cell layer of the inner retina (Figs. 5.1 and 5.2). The axons run in the retina's nerve fiber layer to gather at the optic disk.

The optic nerve nominally begins when the axons of the ganglion cells (the nerve fiber layer of the retina) turn 90 degrees, changing orientation from horizontal along the inner retinal surface to vertical, passing through the outer retina via the scleral canal (Fig. 5.3). The gathering of axons at the canal forms the optic disk (also, *optic nerve head*) of the fundus. Myelin is usually absent from the nerve fiber layer where the nerve exits the globe.

Vascular supply of the retina comes from the ophthalmic artery off the internal carotid artery. Proximal branches from this artery and branches off the muscular arteries constitute the posterior ciliary arteries that form a plexus of vessels around the lamina cribrosa and supply the optic disk, the adjacent optic nerve, and the outer layers of the retina. Cilioretinal branches from this plexus often also supply the macula. Another branch of the ophthalmic, the central retinal artery, enters the distal optic nerve and emerges out of the disc, dividing into four arteriolar branches to supply each quadrant of retina. The proximal part of the optic nerve is supplied by a series of small vessels of the ophthalmic artery, whereas the posterior optic nerve and the chiasm have additional supply from the anterior cerebral and the anterior communicating arteries.

The shape of visual field deficits due to vascular compromise of the inner retina is predictable, being consistent with the specific location of the arterial occlusion. Visual field defects are inverted in relation to the pathologic location: for example, a superior branch occlusion of the retinal artery will cause an inferior field defect. When retinal arteriolar occlusions affect the nerve fiber layer, field defects typically extend beyond the local occlusion in an arcuate or sectoral pattern, following the arc of the nerve fiber layer. Disease of the anterior optic nerve is an important healthcare problem. Glaucoma alone is suspected to affect 3 million patients, accounting for 120,000 cases of blindness in the United States, with an annual governmental cost of $1.5 billion in expenditures and lost revenue.

Clinical Presentations

Primary open-angle glaucoma (POAG) is a chronic, progressive, degenerative disease of the optic nerve. Its usual hallmark is high intraocular pressure (IOP; greater than 21 mm Hg), but glaucoma without high IOP (*normal pressure* or *low-tension* glaucoma) is occasionally seen, especially in the elderly. The typical optic nerve finding is cupping atrophy (i.e., enlargement of the disk's central cup as nerve fibers are lost), coupled by progressive visual field loss that often starts nasally, progresses superiorly and inferiorly, and finally extinguishes the central and temporal fields (Fig. 5.4). POAG is usually bilateral and asymmetric and the visual loss is permanent. The time course is measured in years, and because of the slow pace and the late involvement of the central field, patients may remain asymptomatic until the disease is quite advanced. It is essential that all standard eye examinations include screening IOP measurements and optic disk inspection.

Glaucoma has other forms besides POAG; it may be congenital, secondary to systemic disease (e.g., diabetes), or other acquired eye conditions (e.g., trauma). Among these, **acute narrow-angle glaucoma** (also, *acute angle-closure glaucoma*) may present dramatically with nausea, unilateral headache, and ipsilateral monocular visual loss. The diagnosis and treatment of glaucoma forms a significant subspecialty within ophthalmology, but treatment efforts revolve around lowering of IOP, whether by medical or surgical means. There are no restorative or neuroprotective treatments available for this condition at the present time.

Central retinal artery occlusion (CRAO) results from interruption of the central retinal artery circulation with resultant ischemia to the entire retina. If only a portion of the inner retinal circulation is affected, a more limited version, **branch retinal artery occlusion (BRAO),** is present. BRAO and CRAO are in effect retinal strokes, affecting the nerve fiber and ganglion cell layers. The presentation is one of sudden, painless, complete, or partial monocular visual loss often described as a "curtain" obscuring the involved area. Retinal infarcts are commonly caused by emboli, and in BRAO the embolus is typically visible in the affected retinal vessel. Episodes of temporary monocular visual loss (TMVL) or transient monocular blindness (TMB or *amaurosis fugax*)

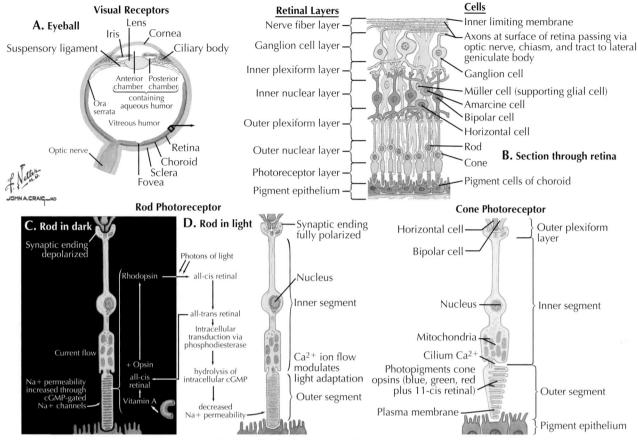

Visual Receptors

A. Eyeball

Lens
Iris
Cornea
Suspensory ligament
Ciliary body
Anterior chamber
Posterior chamber
containing aqueous humor
Ora serrata
Vitreous humor
Optic nerve
Retina
Choroid
Sclera
Fovea

Retinal Layers

Nerve fiber layer
Ganglion cell layer
Inner plexiform layer
Inner nuclear layer
Outer plexiform layer
Outer nuclear layer
Photoreceptor layer
Pigment epithelium

Cells

Inner limiting membrane
Axons at surface of retina passing via optic nerve, chiasm, and tract to lateral geniculate body
Ganglion cell
Müller cell (supporting glial cell)
Amarcine cell
Bipolar cell
Horizontal cell
Rod
Cone

B. Section through retina

Pigment cells of choroid

Rod Photoreceptor

C. Rod in dark
Synaptic ending depolarized
Current flow
Na+ permeability increased through cGMP-gated Na+ channels

D. Rod in light
Synaptic ending fully polarized
Photons of light
Rhodopsin
all-cis retinal
all-trans retinal
Intracellular transduction via phosphodiesterase
+ Opsin
all-cis retinal
hydrolysis of intracellular cGMP
Vitamin A
decreased Na+ permeability
Nucleus
Inner segment
Ca^{2+} ion flow modulates light adaptation
Outer segment

Cone Photoreceptor

Horizontal cell
Bipolar cell
Outer plexiform layer
Nucleus
Inner segment
Mitochondria
Cilium Ca^{2+}
Photopigments cone opsins (blue, green, red plus 11-cis retinal)
Plasma membrane
Outer segment
Pigment epithelium

Fig. 5.1 The Retina and the Photoreceptors.

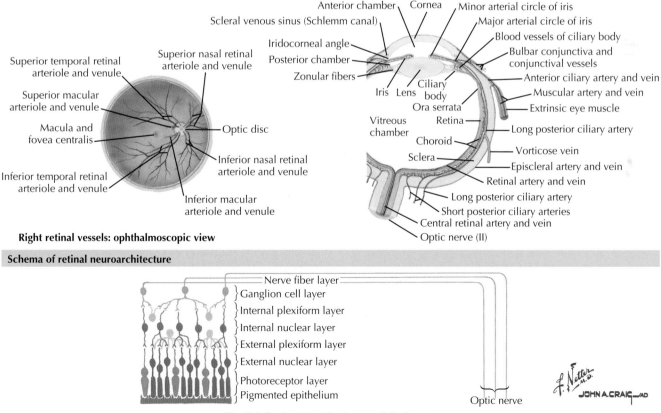

Superior temporal retinal arteriole and venule
Superior macular arteriole and venule
Macula and fovea centralis
Inferior temporal retinal arteriole and venule
Superior nasal retinal arteriole and venule
Optic disc
Inferior nasal retinal arteriole and venule
Inferior macular arteriole and venule

Right retinal vessels: ophthalmoscopic view

Anterior chamber
Cornea
Scleral venous sinus (Schlemm canal)
Minor arterial circle of iris
Major arterial circle of iris
Iridocorneal angle
Posterior chamber
Zonular fibers
Blood vessels of ciliary body
Bulbar conjunctiva and conjunctival vessels
Iris Lens
Ciliary body
Ora serrata
Vitreous chamber
Retina
Choroid
Sclera
Anterior ciliary artery and vein
Muscular artery and vein
Extrinsic eye muscle
Long posterior ciliary artery
Vorticose vein
Episcleral artery and vein
Retinal artery and vein
Long posterior ciliary artery
Short posterior ciliary arteries
Central retinal artery and vein
Optic nerve (II)

Schema of retinal neuroarchitecture

Nerve fiber layer
Ganglion cell layer
Internal plexiform layer
Internal nuclear layer
External plexiform layer
External nuclear layer
Photoreceptor layer
Pigmented epithelium
Optic nerve

Fig. 5.2 Retinal Architecture and Perimetry.

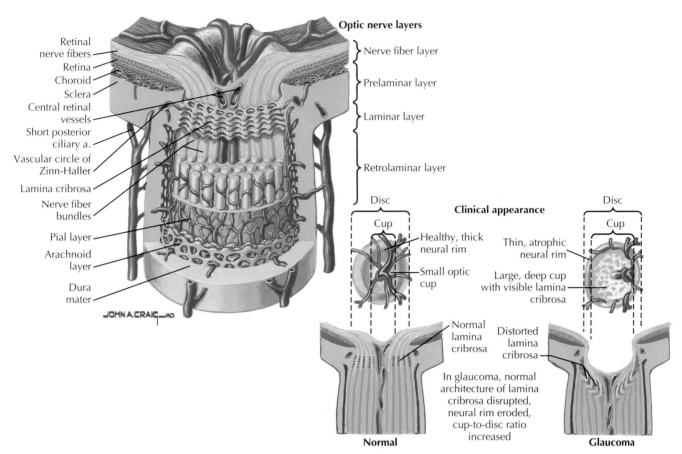

Optic nerve layers

Retinal nerve fibers
Retina
Choroid
Sclera
Central retinal vessels
Short posterior ciliary a.
Vascular circle of Zinn-Haller
Lamina cribrosa
Nerve fiber bundles
Pial layer
Arachnoid layer
Dura mater

JOHN A. CRAIG__AD

Nerve fiber layer
Prelaminar layer
Laminar layer
Retrolaminar layer

Disc
Cup

Clinical appearance

Disc
Cup

Healthy, thick neural rim
Small optic cup

Thin, atrophic neural rim
Large, deep cup with visible lamina cribrosa

Normal lamina cribrosa
Distorted lamina cribrosa

In glaucoma, normal architecture of lamina cribrosa disrupted, neural rim eroded, cup-to-disc ratio increased

Normal

Glaucoma

Fig. 5.3 Anatomy of Optic Nerve (Clinical Appearance).

often herald retinal infarcts and represent temporarily compromised flow of the inner retinal arteries usually by retinal emboli.

Patients who present within the first few hours after the onset of CRAO or large BRAO are usually treated with intermittent ocular massage and lowering of IOP (either by topical agents or by paracentesis of the anterior chamber) to promote movement of the embolus to a more distal arteriolar branch. Oxygen, alone or in combination with 5% CO_2 to promote arteriolar dilation, can also be used. Based on animal studies, it is felt that such interventions are unlikely to be helpful after 100 minutes of retinal ischemia, and in general the outlook for recovery is bleak; nevertheless, significant recovery of vision, even beyond the 100-minute window, is occasionally seen.

CRAO, BRAO, and TMVL may also serve as a warning sign of impending hemispheric stroke. Identification and treatment of the embolic source, if one can be identified, become the main focus of therapy after the window for acute treatment of the involved eye has passed. CRAO is often a sign of carotid stenosis, the appropriate management of which will significantly reduce long-term stroke risk (see Chapter 15, "Ischemic Stroke"). Cardiac embolism is another cause, and a full stroke investigation is usually required. Nevertheless, up to 40% of cases remain without a definite identifiable cause, with the presumed mechanism relating to intrinsic narrowing of the retinal artery due to atherosclerosis or, less commonly, other arteritides.

Anterior ischemic optic neuropathy can be divided into nonarteritic and arteritic (associated with temporal arteritis [TA]) and is caused by loss of blood flow in the short posterior ciliary arteries. Patients suffering vision loss from a nonarteritic ischemic optic neuropathy (NAION) usually experience sudden and severe painless monocular visual loss, often on awakening. Examination classically reveals an altitudinal

(superior or inferior) visual field loss, with a unilaterally swollen, hemorrhagic disk. The disk loses its swelling and becomes pale within weeks. The visual loss in most cases does not change following the event, but 20% may show measurable change for better or worse over days. In contrast to retinal artery occlusions, embolic NAION is extremely rare. In most cases, NAION occurs in middle-aged individuals who have a congenitally small, elevated ("crowded") optic disk or in those with one or more vascular disease risk factors, such as diabetes, hypertension, or sleep apnea. In these cases a transient fall in blood pressure causes hypoperfusion of the posterior ciliary circulation and subsequent ischemic damage to the optic nerve head. Medications may also play a role in causing NAION. Specifically, nocturnal hypotension from taking blood pressure medications at night, phosphodiesterase type 5 inhibitor medications such as sildenafil, and amiodarone have been associated with optic nerve injury as seen in NAION.

There is no proven treatment for NAION, although oral prednisone and anti-vascular endothelial growth factor (VEGF) agents such as bevacizumab have been tried. Unfortunately, there is no treatment that has been proven to be beneficial. There is a 30% risk of eventual involvement of the fellow eye. Strategies to reduce this risk have focused on identifying and treating cerebrovascular risk factors, treating sleep apnea, preventing systemic hypotension, and avoiding drugs, such as sildenafil, which may be associated with a higher risk.

In older patients, AION can be a complication, and sometimes the presenting sign, of TA (also, *giant cell arteritis*), a systemic inflammatory process of the medium-sized arteries. TA can also produce TMVL and CRAO. Funduscopic appearance in arteritic AION often consists of pallid swelling of the disk (Fig. 5.5), in contrast to the hyperemic swelling seen in NAION. In addition to an altitudinal visual loss, patients

Early

Right eye
nasal side

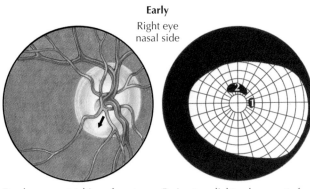

Funduscopy: notching of contour
of physiologic cup in optic disc
with slight focal pallor in area of
notching; occurs almost invariably in superotemporal or inferotemporal (as shown) quadrants

Perimetry: slight enlargment of
physiologic blind spot (1); development of a secondary, superonasal field defect (2) which corresponds to nerve fiber damage in
area of inferotemporal notching

Minimally advanced

Right eye
nasal side

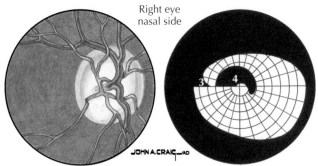

JOHN A.CRAIG—AD

Funduscopy: increased notching
of rim of cup; thinning of rim of
cup (enlargement of cup); deep-
ening of cup; lamina cribrosa
visible in deepest areas

Perimetry: localized constriction
of superonasal visual field (3)
because of progressive damage to
inferotemporal fibers; superior
arc-shaped scotoma (Bjerrum
scotoma) develops (4)

Fig. 5.4 Optic Disc and Visual Field Changes in Glaucoma.

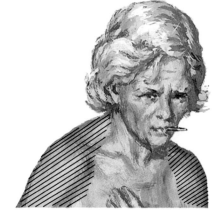

Senior citizen with sudden monocular visual blurring
or blindness, associated with malaise, scalp tenderness,
and myalgia. The erythrocyte sedimentation rate is very
elevated, usually 60 to 120 mm/hr.

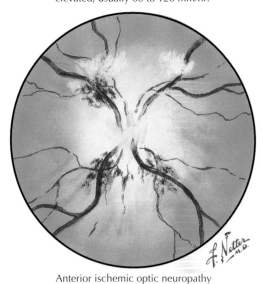

Anterior ischemic optic neuropathy

Fig. 5.5 Giant Cell Arteritis: Ocular Manifestations.

will have arteritic symptoms, including headache, scalp tenderness, jaw claudication, neck pain, malaise, loss of appetite, fevers, and morning stiffness of proximal muscles (i.e., polymyalgia rheumatica). Only rarely will a patient with arteritic AION have little or no systemic symptoms.

Untreated, TA may lead rapidly to blindness from bilateral AION or to other serious complications, including aortic dissection, myocardial infarction, renal disease, and stroke. Therefore, in any patient older than age 50 years with AION, clinical suspicion for TA is raised especially in the presence of systemic symptoms, or physical exam findings (pallid disk swelling or abnormal greater superficial temporal arteries). A high erythrocyte sedimentation rate (ESR, >45 mm/hr), high C-reactive protein (CRP, >2.45 mg/L), normocytic anemia, and thrombocytosis are supportive, but the diagnosis is established by temporal artery biopsy that reveals inflammation in the media of the arteries with disruption of the internal elastic membrane. The presence of characteristic mul-tinucleated giant cells within the affected areas is diagnostic.

TA is urgently treated with high-dose steroids, typically intravenous methylprednisolone, especially if the patient has visual symptoms. TA, once initially treated with parenteral corticosteroids, is transitioned to oral prednisone tapered over many months. Other antiinflammatory medications, especially methotrexate, have been used in those at high risk for corticosteroid complications, but the efficacy of nonsteroidal agents has been questioned. The FDA has approved the use of

tocilizumab (interleukin-6 [IL-6] inhibitor) in the management of GCA after studies have found that concomitant use with prednisone may allow for earlier steroid taper compared with patients who took placebo and prednisone. Steroid dosage is gradually reduced over time, with the patient closely monitored for disease recrudescence by following symptoms and the ESR or CRP.

Papilledema is bilateral optic nerve elevation and expansion due to high intracranial pressure (ICP). In mild cases, patients may have no visual symptoms. Moderate papilledema is typically accompanied by transient binocular visual obscurations, either spontaneously or during coughing, straining, or abrupt postural change. Other symptoms of high ICP may be present and include headaches (worse with recum-bency) and diplopia (resulting from compression of cranial nerve VI [abducens nerve] from increased ICP; see Chapter 6). When visual loss occurs, it starts with blind spot enlargement, a nonspecific and often reversible change. Visual field loss resembling that of glaucoma can ensue, often over a period of many weeks. However, papilledema due to very high ICP can progress rapidly, with severe permanent visual loss within days.

Many pathophysiologic mechanisms are associated with papilledema, including CNS tumor with mass effect or edema, obstructive hydro-cephalus, meningitis, certain medications (e.g., "cyclines" such as tetracycline, doxycycline, and minocycline, lithium, vitamin A, retinoic acid, isotretinoin, and prednisone), and intracranial venous thrombosis or obstruction. Papilledema is occasionally seen without explanation in obese women of childbearing age and is then termed **idiopathic intracranial hypertension** (IIH; also, *pseudotumor cerebri*). Treatment involves only weight loss if the condition is mild and there is no evidence of progressive visual loss or debilitating headache. In progressive IIH, in addition to weight loss, carbonic anhydrase inhibitors such as acetazolamide (typically 1–2 g/day in divided doses) are used to reduce cerebrospinal fluid (CSF) production and optic nerve edema. When medical treatment fails, three surgical options exist: optic nerve sheath fenestration, cerebral venous sinus stenting, or CSF shunting either with lumboperitoneal or ventriculoperitoneal shunts.

Papilledema can be mimicked by the rare entity of **optic perineuritis,** which consists of monocular or bilateral optic disk swelling without central visual loss or raised ICP. Its usual cause is idiopathic optic nerve sheath swelling or inflammatory orbital pseudotumor but may be due to a systemic arteritis (Wegener or giant cell arteritis) or of an infectious (syphilitic) etiology.

Optic nerve drusen are small, translucent, usually bilateral concretions within the substance of the disk that may be observed in perhaps 1% of patients. Drusen contain calcium and can therefore be demonstrated on ultrasound, autofluorescence, and computed tomographic (CT) examinations. It is speculated that a very small scleral canal may inhibit proper axonal metabolism, causing extracellular debris to be deposited as drusen over time. Drusen of the optic nerve is often associated with visual field loss; however, patients are not usually aware of the field deficit because it is usually a long-standing process. Optic nerve drusen can give the appearance of papilledema and is one of the causes of pseudopapilledema.

Drusen of the nerve head are occasionally seen in patients with certain retinal disorders, such as retinitis pigmentosa.

Congenital dysplasia of the optic nerve can be seen as an isolated monocular or binocular finding or as part of a larger disorder. The mildest form of dysplasia is "tilted" optic disks: nerve heads that are overall small with the nasal portions appearing elevated; superior temporal visual field loss (sometimes mimicking *bitemporal hemianopia*) is often encountered. Optic nerve hypoplasia, which is a congenitally smaller optic nerve, can be isolated or be part of a syndrome. Septo-optic dysplasia combines bilateral optic nerve hypoplasia with dysgenesis of midline brain structures, often with pituitary dysfunction. Children of mothers who are type 1 diabetics and up to a quarter of patients with fetal alcohol syndrome will have disk hypoplasia with associated inferior visual field loss, among other ocular manifestations. Superior segmental optic nerve hypoplasia is segmental thinning of the superior part of the optic nerve, and there is a corresponding field defect inferiorly. This is not associated with septo-optic dysplasia. Optic nerve coloboma (congenital incomplete or malfusion of the globe structures including the retina and optic nerve) can be part of Aicardi syndrome, and the "morning glory" disk anomaly has been associated with several developmental syndromes.

Diagnostic Approach

As all pathologic entities in this group display abnormalities of the disc and/or retinal vessels, careful fundus examination is the essential step in diagnosis. Visual field testing typically reveals patterns of visual loss (arcuate, altitudinal, and nasal losses with a "step" at the horizontal meridian) that localize the lesion to the anterior optic nerve but does not often guide the diagnosis. Sector losses can suggest branch arterial occlusion (any location), optic nerve hypoplasia (typically inferior), optic disk tilt, or coloboma (these last two often producing superior losses).

Additional information can be obtained by special imaging of the ocular fundus. Fluorescein angiography of the fundus reveals vascular occlusions and areas of edema caused by incompetent blood vessels. Optical coherence tomography, scanning laser ophthalmoscopy, and scanning laser polarimetry provide precise measurement of the nerve fiber layer in the peripapillary retina, ganglion cell layer, and total macular thickness. These measurements can help to define subtle cases of disk edema or atrophy and changes in disk appearance over time, along with evaluation of the macula.

ORBITAL AND INTRACANALICULAR OPTIC NERVE

> **CLINICAL VIGNETTE** *A 26-year-old woman presented with right monocular visual loss and headache after a car accident. She said she had suffered "whiplash," without bruising impact to the head. The visual loss had started 2 days after the accident. The headache was centered at the right orbit, with eye movement among its aggravating factors. Subjective visual acuity was 20/80 right eye, and visual field testing revealed nonphysiologic responses, indicating the patient was inattentive to the test, in both eyes. Fundus examination of both eyes was entirely normal; however, pupillary examination suggested a mild relative afferent papillary defect on the right. A magnetic resonance imaging (MRI) examination was obtained, revealing multiple white matter lesions. A diagnosis of multiple sclerosis (MS) presenting as optic neuritis was eventually confirmed based on spinal fluid assays and subsequent clinical course.*

After leaving the eye, the fibers of the optic nerve become myelinated. The optic nerve sheath surrounds the optic nerve, starting at the sclera and becoming contiguous with the intracranial dura. CSF is present within the sheath. The optic nerve lies in the central orbit within the extraocular muscle cone and exits the orbit through the optic canal before traveling a short distance intracranially to join the chiasm. Vascular supply is via branches of the ophthalmic artery.

Diseases that affect the orbital optic nerve give characteristic central visual field loss. It is believed that the nerve fibers corresponding to central vision, among the most metabolically active cells in the visual system, occupy a central position in the optic nerve, farthest away from the exterior blood supply. The central fibers therefore are the most prone to dysfunction or injury due to varying mechanisms, including compression, ischemia, metabolic disease, and toxic insult. Within the bony optic canal, the optic nerve is confined in a small space and is relatively immobile, making it susceptible to small tumors, and inflammatory processes, as well as shear injury produced by deceleration head trauma.

However, MS (see Chapter 39) remains the chief cause of orbital optic nerve disease and is the initial manifestation in approximately 20% of patients. An additional 20% will eventually experience it throughout the course of the disease. It is estimated that more than 90% of patients suffering "isolated" optic neuritis will eventually receive a diagnosis of MS. Diagnostic testing in optic neuritis naturally mirrors that for MS, with brain and spine MRI and CSF analysis being the primary tools.

Clinical Presentations

Optic neuritis is the clinical syndrome of subacute painful, monocular visual loss. The pain often precedes visual loss by a day or more and is a periorbital ache made worse with eye movements. Ensuing visual loss is often sudden and severe, with perceived worsening over several days. The degree of visual field loss varies, but a central scotoma is the classic finding (Fig. 5.6). Examination may also demonstrate loss of central acuity, contrast sensitivity, and color perception in the affected eye.

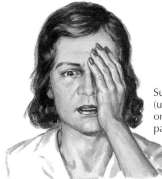

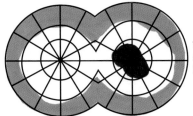

Sudden unilateral blindness, self-limited (usually 2 to 3 weeks). Patient covering one eye, suddenly realizes other eye is partially or totally blind.

Visual fields reveal central scotoma due to acute retro-bulbar neuritis.

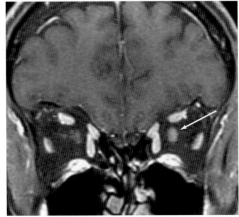

Coronal postcontrast orbital T1-weighted, fat-saturated MR image: Marked left optic nerve enlargement (arrow).

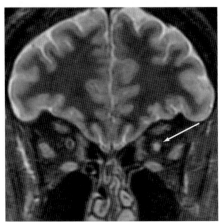

Coronal T2-weighted orbital MR image: Edematous left optic nerve (arrow).

Fig. 5.6 Multiple Sclerosis: Ocular Manifestations.

Initially, funduscopic appearance of the affected disk is normal, the presence of a relative afferent pupillary defect and visual loss confirms that optic neuropathy is present. Occasionally, mild ipsilateral disk swelling is seen and, in all cases, some degree of optic pallor, usually localized to the temporal quadrant of the disk, appears within weeks. Incomplete recovery of vision, mostly in the first 3 months, is expected, with central acuity recovering better than other parameters, often to near normal.

As with other manifestations of MS, emphasis is on early diagnosis so that patients may begin treatment with immunomodulating medications to reduce disease activity and associated morbidity. Intravenous methylprednisolone (1 g/day for 3 days, followed by an oral prednisone taper for 11 days) has been shown to accelerate visual recovery in optic neuritis, although the final level of recovery is unaffected. The same study showed a reduced risk of MS exacerbations for 2 years following methylprednisolone pulse treatment. It is unclear if the drug provides additional protection beyond 2 years and whether it affects outcome in the long run. Oral prednisone alone is contraindicated in typical demyelinating optic neuritis.

Optic neuritis can also be seen as part of Devic disease or neuromyelitis optica (NMO), once considered a more aggressive form of MS, defined by episodes of optic neuritis and transverse myelitis. The immunopathogenesis and treatment is distinct from MS, and patients with vision loss from NMO must be treated aggressively because this does affect their final visual outcome. Initial treatment recommendations for vision loss are parenteral corticosteroids, plasmapheresis, and/or intravenous immunoglobulin (IVIg), with long-term immunosuppressive agents, such as azathioprine and rituximab, used to prevent relapses. The presence of a hallmark serum immunoglobulin (NMO-IgG directed against the aquaporin-4 protein [AQP4]) is central to diagnosis. A minority of patients seronegative for AQP4 have antibodies against myelin oligodendrocyte glycoprotein (MOG) and have an overlapping clinical syndrome with NMO.

Optic neuritis can occasionally be idiopathic, with prolonged surveillance never leading to a diagnosis of MS. This is called clinically isolated syndrome. In rare cases, optic neuritis can be mimicked by treponemal infection or by inflammatory disease (e.g., sarcoidosis).

Posterior ischemic optic neuropathy presents as sudden, painless monocular visual loss without acute changes in the ocular fundus and disk. Over weeks, disk pallor becomes evident. Classically seen in chronically anemic patients after major gastrointestinal hemorrhage, it has been more recently found in these clinical settings: as bilateral visual loss after major surgery (cardiac or spine); and as unilateral visual loss, either as a complication of TA or of peripheral vascular disease. It can also occur in the setting of shock or hypotension. There is no definitive test for posterior ischemic optic neuropathy, and diagnostic workup is directed toward ruling out arteritis and occlusive carotid disease.

Indirect traumatic optic neuropathy can occur in the setting of sudden frontal head impact or deceleration. It differs from direct trauma in that no foreign object or displaced fracture has impinged upon the nerve. It is also distinct from deceleration injuries that avulse the nerve from the globe or that damage the chiasm. The exact mechanism and location of indirect nerve injury is uncertain, but interest centers on the optic canal. An international treatment trial was unable to prove benefit of either surgical decompression of the canal or parenteral corticosteroids at dosages used for spinal cord injury. Despite the lack of rigorous evidence, parenteral steroids are often still used in selected cases.

Genetic, nutritional, and toxic optic neuropathies typically affect the orbital optic nerve. The high metabolic rate of the central vision fibers and their relatively tenuous blood supply at the center of the orbital optic nerve are considered important factors placing these cells at risk.

Leber hereditary optic neuropathy (LHON) is a representative metabolic, genetic optic neuropathy. Sudden, painless monocular visual loss, typically occurring in the third or fourth decade of life, is then followed by involvement of the fellow eye after a period of weeks to years. The involved eye typically initially displays a hyperemic disk, with fluorescein angiography showing no extravasation of dye from peripapillary telangiectatic vessels. A family history of similar loss is often present: the disease, resulting from a mutation defect in one of several mitochondrial proteins, is passed maternally in the mitochondrial DNA with variable penetrance. The exact clinical presentation depends to some degree on the specific mutation involved. The most common mutations are: 11778 (which has the worst visual prognosis), 3460, 15257, and 15812. Neuronal damage is presumed to result from superoxide formation in the impaired mitochondria. Patients with first-eye involvement, or identified as having the mutation, are often advised to avoid substances (e.g., tobacco smoke, alcohol, and certain medications) that deplete systemic reductases and to consider dietary supplementation of vitamin B_{12}, which, if deficient, can precipitate LHON. Several studies have also discussed the effectiveness of idebenone. LHON is an attractive candidate for gene therapy; there are now clinical trials evaluating the effectiveness of this therapy.

Dominant optic atrophy (also, *Kjer optic atrophy*) is a dominantly inherited, progressive optic neuropathy, which presents in childhood and usually stabilizes by the third decade of life. It is also caused by defective mitochondrial metabolism, but the four known mutations are inherited in an autosomal dominant manner. Additional, related mutations can cause optic atrophies with X-linked and recessive inheritance.

Hypovitaminosis, especially thiamine (B_1), folic acid, and cyanocobalamin (B_{12}), can produce a progressive bilateral nutritional optic neuropathy. Hypovitaminosis is seen in smokers and from alcoholism with poor nutrition (there is an additive risk from the toxicity of smoking and alcohol). It is also seen from poor nutrition with gut malabsorption syndromes and occasionally in those following strict vegan diets. The drug methotrexate inhibits the metabolism of folic acid and has been associated with metabolic optic neuropathy.

Methanol (wood alcohol) poisoning occurs acutely as liver enzymes convert the ingested methanol to formaldehyde and formic acid. Exposure is usually accidental, sometimes in connection with homemade alcohol ("moonshine"). The special sensitivity of the optic nerve is not well understood, but optic neuropathy occurs at exposure levels far below those that are generally cytotoxic. Treatment consists of intravenous ethanol (to slow the conversion of methanol) and hemodialysis.

Other substances are either known or suspected to produce toxic optic neuropathies. These include the drugs ethambutol and isoniazid, both of which are increasingly used in the treatment of atypical mycobacteria, such as *mycobacterium avium-intracellulare*. Visual field monitoring and color vision testing are recommended for patients taking ethambutol or isoniazid. Amiodarone is suspected of contributing to an optic neuropathy that may mimic AION, but the association remains unclear. A larger list of medications is suspected of being able to "trigger" optic neuropathy in patients predisposed to it, such as those with an LHON mutation.

Paraneoplastic optic neuropathy is a rare disease in which autoantibodies directed against cancer cells cross-react with optic nerve proteins, such as antibodies to the collapsin response-mediator protein 5 (CRMP-5). Treatment is centered on identifying and treating the underlying cancer.

Compressive optic neuropathy is characterized by central vision loss. It can, on occasion, arise suddenly (e.g., traumatic orbital hematoma) or more commonly by slowly growing tumors. In sudden compression, urgent decompression is required to minimize permanent optic nerve injury. However, in the case of slow compression by tumor, visual loss may be reversible when compression is relieved before pallor develops. Additional findings of proptosis and limitation of extraocular movements suggest an orbital mass. If optic atrophy has not yet occurred, fundus examination may be normal but may reveal signs of scleral indentation with posterior chorioretinal folds or signs of chronic central retinal vein compression and optociliary venous shunting. MRI with gadolinium is generally preferred for imaging of orbital masses, although bone structure and abnormalities (hypertrophy with meningioma, destruction with cancers, and remodeling with large benign tumors) are better seen on CT scanning.

Typical orbital tumors compressing the optic nerve are cavernous hemangioma, optic nerve sheath meningioma, and optic nerve glioma. Cavernous hemangiomas are typically treated conservatively by observation unless there is vision loss. Optic nerve meningioma when causing vision loss can be removed surgically. Fractionated stereotactic external beam radiation can limit tumor growth. Glioma of the optic nerve cannot be easily resected without potentially compromising the optic nerve. Therefore gliomas are generally left in place, with excision indicated only if severe proptosis with eye exposure or extension of the glioma toward the chiasm, threatening vision in the other eye, occurs. Stereotactic radiation can be used. Given the possibility of rare, aggressive gliomas requiring early excision, frequent reimaging is indicated initially when following these tumors. Multiple gliomas, typically slow growing, are a common feature of von Recklinghausen neurofibromatosis (NF-1).

The enlarged extraocular muscles of *thyroid-related orbitopathy* are a common cause of proptosis but may also cause optic nerve compression. Patients with thyroid-related orbitopathy are monitored by serial central vision and visual field testing. Thyroid-related optic nerve compression is often treated initially with systemic corticosteroids, with definitive treatment of orbital decompression to quickly follow.

Orbital cellulitis produces an obvious clinical picture with acute pain, proptosis, diplopia, periorbital edema, and, if untreated, loss of sight. Because of the risk to vision posed by this acute disease, patients are often hospitalized for close monitoring and intravenous antibiotic therapy. Etiology of orbital cellulitis in adults is typically from recent penetrating periorbital trauma, from contiguous spread of facial sinusitis, or from hematogenous seeding from facial soft tissue infections. *Idiopathic orbital inflammation* (also, *orbital pseudotumor*) resembles orbital cellulitis but does not respond to antibiotic therapy and lacks clear traumatic or infectious prodrome. Pain is out of proportion to expected findings on exam, and a dramatic response to systemic corticosteroids is a key diagnostic feature. Orbital cellulitis can also be mimicked by Wegener granulomatosis or invasive fungal sinusitis.

Diagnostic Approach

The orbit represents the most anterior location where examination of the eye itself may not provide clues to the etiology of visual loss. Nevertheless, complete eye examination, with attention to central acuity, visual fields, pupil, and optic disk, remains central to diagnosis. External examination of the orbit, looking for proptosis, resistance to retropulsion of the globe, and limitation of ocular movement, may suggest an orbital tumor or mass. Details in the history of present illness (abruptness of onset, accompanying pain, etc.) will suggest the most likely etiologies.

In some diseases of the orbital optic nerve, optic disk changes may be present, as in the disk hyperemia of LHON. Additional fundus imaging may then be appropriate to better define the abnormalities

However, for the orbit—and for all more posterior etiologies of visual loss—eye examination must be coupled with appropriate imaging. MRI of the orbits is usually recommended and is done with fat suppression and gadolinium paramagnetic contrast to enhance tumors such as hemangiomas and meningiomas. Inclusion of the brain, especially fluid-attenuated inversion recovery (FLAIR) sequences, in cases of optic neuritis, helps to assess for additional white matter lesions, suggestive of MS. However, as mentioned previously, CT scanning can reveal diagnostic orbital bone changes missed by MRI. Timing of imaging is usually predicated on the acuteness of the visual loss.

When a specific diagnosis is suggested, additional studies may be indicated, such as spinal fluid analysis for optic neuritis or mitochondrial genetic testing in LHON. In cases where examination and imaging do not suggest specific etiology, screening for systemic disease may be needed.

OPTIC CHIASM

> **CLINICAL VIGNETTE** *A 51-year-old woman presented with worsening vision over many months. She reported no other significant medical history. While confirming normal central acuity, the examiner discovered that the patient could see only the left half of the eye chart with her right eye and only the right half with her left eye. A gross confrontation visual field check confirmed a dense bitemporal hemianopia. The examiner also noted that the woman had facial hypertrichosis and enlargement of her brow, nose, lips, and jaw and that the patient's rings and shoes no longer fit properly. Acromegaly, from abnormally high circulating levels of human growth hormone produced by a pituitary tumor, was diagnosed. MRI confirmed the lesion compressing the optic chiasm.*

Bitemporal hemianopia is the characteristic field abnormality of optic chiasm disease. The chiasm (from the Greek letter *x*) represents the "Great Divide" of the afferent visual system, separating clinical field defects into three anatomic areas. **Prechiasmatic** defects affect the visual field of the ipsilateral eye only and typically result from retinal or optic nerve pathology. **Chiasmatic** disorders lead to bilateral visual field loss, typically with some form of temporal field loss. Bitemporal hemianopia (also, *hemianopsia*), with loss of the right lateral field in the right eye and left lateral field in the left eye, is the most classic field defect with chiasmal compression. **Postchiasmatic** defects produce homonymous hemianopias, with defects appearing more congruous (equal for both eyes) the farther posteriorly the lesion is located.

The optic chiasm is the intersection of the optic nerves from each eye and is located above the pituitary body that lies within the sella turcica of the sphenoid bone and is covered by the diaphragm sellae (Fig. 5.7). The chiasmatic cistern is located between the chiasm and the diaphragm sella. Superior to the chiasm is the third ventricle. The internal carotid arteries flank the optic chiasm laterally and then bifurcate into the anterior and middle cerebral arteries. The anterior cerebral arteries and the anterior communicating artery are anterior to the optic chiasm.

Within the chiasm, axons from the temporal retina (nasal field) comprise its lateral aspect and remain ipsilateral as they pass through the chiasm to the optic tract. In contrast, the nasal retinal fibers decussate, carrying temporal visual field information to the contralateral side. Inferior nasal fibers decussate within the chiasm more anteriorly than superior ones. As the inferior nasal retinal fibers approach the posterior aspect of the chiasm, the fibers shift to occupy the lateral aspect of the contralateral optic tract (see Fig. 5.7).

The arterial blood supply of the optic chiasm is derived from the circle of Willis, particularly, the superior hypophyseal arteries, derived from the supraclinoid segment of the carotid arteries. A "prechiasmatic plexus," the hypophyseal portal system, and branches of the anterior cerebral arteries also contribute to the chiasmatic blood supply. Venous drainage goes to two primary areas: blood from the superior chiasm flows into the anterior cerebral veins, whereas the inferior aspect drains into the infundibular plexus and thus to the paired basal veins of Rosenthal.

The location of the chiasm renders it vulnerable to compression from vascular structures (e.g., aneurysm near the origin of the anterior communicating artery or the ophthalmic artery), from tumors of the meninges, from sphenoid sinus masses, and, most importantly, from the pituitary (Fig. 5.8).

Clinical Presentations

Chiasmal tumors produce bilateral visual field defects. Central chiasmatic lesions most commonly produce a bitemporal hemianopia (Fig. 5.9A) that ensues when the optic chiasm is compressed or damaged midsagittally at its decussation. Such lesions preferentially affect the crossing nasal retinal fibers responsible for temporal vision, as in the vignette in this chapter.

Variants of the classic bitemporal hemianopia are seen with compression of the optic nerve at its entrance to the anterior chiasm, resulting in a **junctional scotoma,** with central visual loss in the ipsilateral eye and a superotemporal defect in the other. The field loss in the contralateral eye reflects involvement of the opposite inferior nasal optic nerve fibers that swing forward into the ipsilateral anterior chiasm (Willebrand knee) before decussating to the optic tract (see Fig. 5.9B).

Posterior optic chiasm lesions lead to a **posterior junctional scotoma,** which displays the features of chiasmatic and optic tract lesions. The classic finding is **incongruous** (less dense in the ipsilateral eye) **hemianopic visual field loss** contralateral to the lesion from involvement of the anterior optic tract and an inferotemporal visual field loss in the ipsilateral eye—from pressure on the posterior chiasm affecting the late-crossing superotemporal retinal fibers (see Fig. 5.9C). Such defects occur in lesions located near the anterior aspect of the third ventricle that approach the chiasm posteromedially. The incongruous nature of the hemianopsia is caused by the incomplete intermixing of the decussating fibers entering the optic tract with their corresponding uncrossed fibers from the contralateral eye (see Fig. 5.9C).

Progressive visual field loss from an expanding sellar tumor characteristically begins in the upper temporal fields, likely from preferential compression of the inferior chiasm as the underlying pituitary tumor exerts pressure through the diaphragm sellae. Early on, the superotemporal defects may be paracentral with sparing of the far periphery. As the tumor enlarges, the superotemporal quadrantanopia extends to the periphery, and the inferotemporal field becomes affected. Later, the inferonasal quadrant, and eventually all vision, will be lost.

Most commonly, chiasmatic compression results from a benign pituitary adenoma (see Chapter 51). These are common brain tumors, visualized with high-resolution MRI. Tumors smaller than 10 mm, termed microadenomas, are generally too small to place significant pressure on the optic chiasm and are usually discovered because of the effects of excess pituitary hormone (e.g., prolactin) secretion. Small nonsecreting adenomas can be found as an incidental finding on brain MRI obtained for other reasons. Once a tumor grows sufficiently and obliterates the 10-mm distance from diaphragm sella to the chiasm, the potential for visual loss exists. Typically, the chiasm can accommodate slow-growing tumors, so that chiasmatic impingement or displacement by such tumors may be seen without any field defect. However, when the macroadenoma reaches 20–25 mm, field defects are likely. The usual

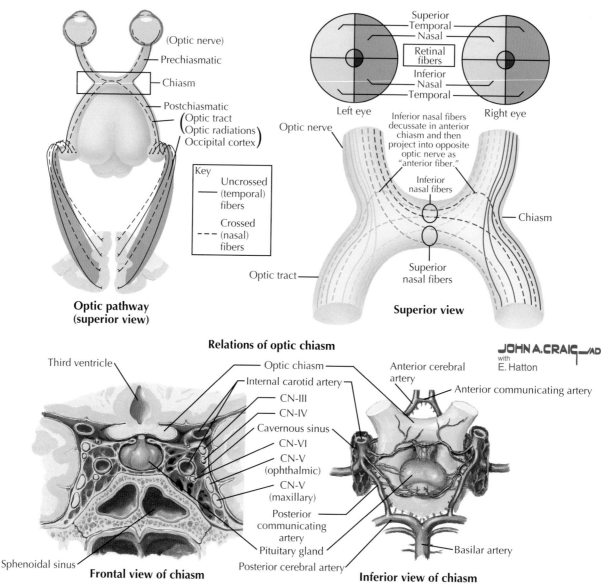

Optic pathway (superior view)

Key
—— Uncrossed (temporal) fibers
- - - Crossed (nasal) fibers

(Optic nerve)
Prechiasmatic
Chiasm
Postchiasmatic
(Optic tract
Optic radiations
Occipital cortex)

Superior
Temporal
Nasal
Retinal fibers
Inferior
Nasal
Temporal

Left eye   Right eye

Optic nerve

Inferior nasal fibers decussate in anterior chiasm and then project into opposite optic nerve as "anterior fiber."

Inferior nasal fibers
Chiasm
Superior nasal fibers
Optic tract

Superior view

Relations of optic chiasm

JOHN A. CRAIG AD
with
E. Hatton

Third ventricle
Optic chiasm
Internal carotid artery
CN-III
CN-IV
Cavernous sinus
CN-VI
CN-V (ophthalmic)
CN-V (maxillary)
Posterior communicating artery
Pituitary gland
Posterior cerebral artery
Sphenoidal sinus

Anterior cerebral artery
Anterior communicating artery
Basilar artery

Frontal view of chiasm   **Inferior view of chiasm**

Fig. 5.7 Anatomy and Relations of Optic Chiasm.

indications for surgical excision are continued tumor growth or the presence of visual compromise. Prolactinomas can often be treated medically using bromocriptine or cabergoline to shrink the tumor. Failure of medical therapy leaves the options of transsphenoidal surgical excision or precision radiotherapy (e.g., Gamma Knife).

Many other sellar masses cause bitemporal hemianopia and include benign or malignant intrinsic tumors (glioma and glioblastoma), extrinsic tumors (benign meningioma and craniopharyngioma or malignant chordoma and lymphoma), and inflammatory granulomas. Aneurysm (especially of the carotid, ophthalmic, or anterior communicating artery), demyelinating disease, and deceleration head trauma are other important etiologies that can cause injury to the chiasm.

Pituitary apoplexy is defined as sudden expansion of a pituitary tumor from infarction or hemorrhage, with subsequent edema and necrosis. Patients typically present with rapid and painful visual loss, often accompanied by alteration of consciousness and ocular motor palsy. Death from pituitary insufficiency can supervene if replacement corticosteroids are not instituted. Prompt surgical decompression of the chiasm is recommended, although improved visual outcomes have not been rigorously proven.

MRI scanning with attention to the sella is recommended in any patient presenting with bitemporal hemianopia. Patient presenting with acute bilateral visual loss should receive urgent MRI or CT scanning to look for pituitary apoplexy or aneurysm.

POSTERIOR VISUAL AFFERENT SYSTEM: OPTIC TRACTS, LATERAL GENICULATE NUCLEUS, OPTIC RADIATIONS

The axons comprising the optic tract are still those emanating from the retinal ganglion cells, which have yet to synapse. Nevertheless, after they leave the chiasm for the optic tract, they nominally become part of the "posterior visual pathway" (Fig. 5.10). Axons of the optic tract course via the anterior limb of the internal capsule, between the tuber cinereum and the anterior perforated substance, then continue posteriorly as a band of flattened fibers around the cerebral peduncles to synapse in the lateral geniculate nucleus (LGN) within the thalamus. The LGN is a thalamic relay nucleus that serves as the synapse point of the retinal ganglion cells. It comprises six gray matter layers separated by five white matter layers.

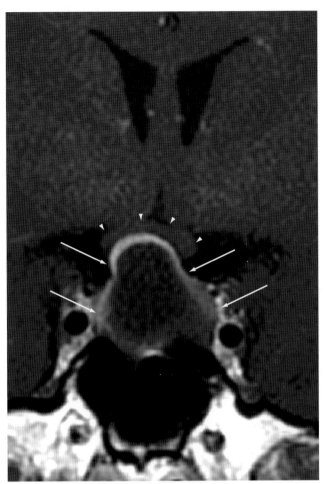

Coronal postcontrast pituitary MR: Optic chiasm (arrowheads) compressed by rim enhancing pituitary macroadenoma (arrows).

Fig. 5.8 Pituitary Macroadenoma.

The layers are folded over, forming a bend or small knee. Each layer has a retinotopic organization, creating a map of the contralateral hemifield (Fig. 5.11). The ratio of geniculate cells to retinal axons is approximately 1:1. Retinal input to the LGN comprises only one-fifth of its afferent fibers. The remainder comes from the mesencephalic reticular formation, posterior parietal cortex, occipital cortex, and other thalamic nuclei. The LGN may use these nonretinal elements to "screen" the visual input, gating certain inputs to the visual cortex while blocking other signals, depending on the relevance of the inputs.

A relatively small number of nonvisual retinal fibers within the optic tract accompany the optic nerve and chiasm but remain extrageniculate to supply the afferent stimulus to the pupillomotor center within the pretectal nucleus.

The same vessels that supply the posterior chiasm nourish the anterior one-third of the optic tract: the internal carotid, middle cerebral, and posterior communicating arteries. The blood supply of the posterior two-thirds of the optic tract is derived from the anterior choroidal artery, a branch of the internal carotid that runs posteriorly near the optic tract. The lateral geniculate body receives blood from the posterior cerebral artery and the posterior communicating arteries.

The optic radiations are myelinated axons emanating from the LGN that course to the primary visual cortex. After they leave the LGN, they continue through the posterior limb of the internal capsule. Most fibers take a fairly direct path to the calcarine cortex, following the curve of the corona radiata through the parietal lobe to the occipital lobe. However,

the most inferior axons (Meyer loop) that carry visual information from the opposite superior field detour laterally around the lateral ventricles and through the posterior temporal lobe (see Fig. 5.11). Therefore stroke or injury confined to this portion of the temporal lobe affects only this portion of the optic radiations. Meyer loop fibers rejoin the rest of the optic radiations after their detour.

Five primary arteries supply blood to the optic radiation: the anterior and posterior choroidal arteries, the middle and posterior cerebral arteries, and the calcarine artery (Fig. 5.12). The anterior choroidal artery supplies the anterior portion of the optic radiations, the optic tract, and the lateral geniculate body. The anterior optic radiations are also fed by a meshwork of branches from the posterior choroidal arteries. However, the middle portion of the optic radiations is fed via the deep optic branch of the middle cerebral artery, which lies lateral to the ventricle. The posterior portion of the optic radiation is fed by the posterior cerebral artery and one of its branches, the calcarine artery.

Clinical Presentations

Posterior to the chiasm, any insult to the afferent visual system is immediately recognizable by the resulting contralateral homonymous (same laterality and region in each eye) visual loss. It is commonly found that in pure hemianopias without optic nerve or chiasm contribution, central visual acuity for individual letters is unaffected; however, the "macular splitting" that results from total hemianopia can cause difficulty with reading text.

Optic tract lesions are unique in that they cause homonymous hemianopias combined with pupillary abnormalities and optic disk pallor. Total lesions of the optic tract affect the pupillary afferents within the tract and produce a mild relative afferent pupillary defect in the contralateral eye because more crossed fibers exist within the tract from the contralateral eye than uncrossed fibers from the ipsilateral eye. When wallerian degeneration ensues, pallor characteristic of optic tract lesions develops in the optic disks. The ipsilateral eye, losing axons from the retina temporal to the fovea, has chiefly superior and inferior polar atrophy, whereas the contralateral eye, losing the interior of the papillomacular bundle and the axons from the retina nasal to the optic nerve, has pallor in the temporal and nasal poles (**"bow-tie" atrophy**).

For the optic tract, the field loss affects both eyes and is contralateral to the affected tract. The loss depends on the extent of the tract lesion and is either a complete or incomplete homonymous hemianopia. Incomplete tract hemianopias are often incongruous (i.e., the defects in each eye do not match exactly) wedge-shaped defects, with the point of the wedge encroaching on the center, a "dagger into fixation" or "sectoranopia." As with the chiasm, neoplasms, aneurysms, and trauma are the typical lesion in this region; strokes are relatively uncommon.

Posterior to the optic tract, visual field loss is not accompanied by pupillary change or visible optic atrophy. However, specifics of the hemianopia can assist in localizing the lesion. LGN lesions produce field defects similar to those of the optic tract. Lesions confined to the temporal lobe can reach only the Meyer loop portion of the optic radiations, with the resulting visual field defect typically as a homonymous, incongruous superior wedge—one side located at the vertical meridian and the second edge being less sharp. This defect, resembling a "slice" removed from the superior visual field, has been termed the *pie-in-the-sky defect*. When encountered, it provides strong evidence of a temporal lobe pathogenesis. Often, other findings of temporal lobe dysfunction confirm the localization.

Conversely, if a parietal lesion affects the optic radiations anteriorly, an inverse lesion sparing the temporal lobe "wedge" occurs; however, such lesions are rarely encountered. Occasionally, larger or far posterior parietal lesions can affect all of the optic radiations after the Meyer loop has rejoined the other fibers, producing a complete homonymous

A. Lesions of central chiasm

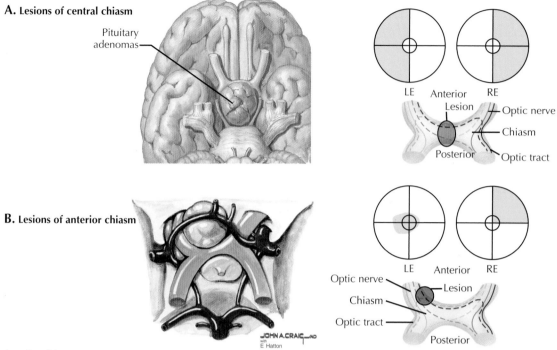

B. Lesions of anterior chiasm

Anterior chiasm tumor compressing optic nerve at its entrance to chiasm results in junctional scotoma consisting of a central visual field loss in eye ipsilateral to lesion and a superior temporal defect in the opposite eye.

C. Lesions of posterior chiasm

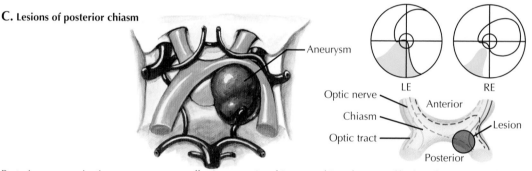

Posterior communicating artery aneurysm affecting posterior chiasm combines features of both a chiasmatic and an optic tract lesion, resulting in a posterior junctional scotoma—an incongruous (less dense in ipsilateral eye) hemianopic field loss contralateral to lesion.

Fig. 5.9 Disorders Affecting Optic Chiasm.

hemianopia. Pathologic entities affecting the posterior visual afferents are most commonly stroke, tumor, demyelination, and trauma.

Differential and Diagnostic Approach

Complete homonymous hemianopias cannot be reliably localized as to the level of the optic tract, lateral geniculate body, parietal lobe, or occipital lobe. Other than the visual fields, a broader ophthalmologic examination may provide hints to the site of the lesions. For example, optic tract lesions produce a mild contralateral relative afferent pupil defect and bow-tie atrophy of the optic disks. The parietal lobe contributes to pursuit eye movements, and patients with a complete homonymous hemianopia from a parietal lesion may show altered or absent optokinetic nystagmus in the direction of the lesion.

As with any visual loss, the diagnostic course for hemianopic visual loss includes complete eye examination, visual fields with attention to assessment of central acuity, pupillary reactions, pursuit movements, and funduscopy. The presence of additional neurologic or systemic symptoms and the speed of onset may help both localize the lesion and suggest an etiology. Review of past medical history may reveal if the patient has known risks for some etiologies, such as stroke, demyelination, or

metastasis. The most important ancillary test is diagnostic imaging. Typically, MRI examination is recommended as best able to detect, and distinguish among, the potential pathologies. Diffusion-weighted images can be particularly useful in defining recent stroke (see Chapter 54). Management and therapy are dictated by the etiology.

PRIMARY VISUAL CORTEX AND VISUAL ASSOCIATION CORTICES

CLINICAL VIGNETTE *A 64-year-old gynecologist, while operating, suddenly had difficulty seeing to the right. He had to turn his head to see the full operative field. The next day, he saw his ophthalmologist, who found evidence of a dense right homonymous hemianopia.*

A subsequent neurologic consultation was otherwise unremarkable. MRI demonstrated a positive diffusion-weighted lesion in the left occipital lobe. ECG and transesophageal echocardiography results were normal. A 48-hour Holter monitor documented seven periods of intermittent atrial fibrillation. Anticoagulation was initiated. The patient was advised to stop driving.

Axons of the optic radiations synapse with the primary visual cortex. A unique white stripe or stria (*stripe* or *line of Gennari* for the discovering anatomist) represents a myelin-rich cortical layer; it is easily seen in gross sections through the cortex and bespeaks of the layered, highly structured organization of **V1** (also known as the *primary visual cortex,* the *striate cortex,* or *Brodmann area 17*). Primarily located on the mesial surface of the occipital lobe within and surrounding the calcarine fissure, the most posterior aspect of V1 typically wraps around the posterior (occipital) pole for a short distance (Fig. 5.13).

Microscopically, the visual cortex is arranged in six laminae, running from the surface to a depth of slightly greater than 2 mm. The most superficial, layer I, primarily contains glial cells. Layers II and III contain pyramidal cells and small interneurons. The thickest stria is layer IV, comprising almost half the depth of the visual cortex. Highly branched stellate cells exist superficially within layer IVa. The Gennari stripe comprises layer IVb, containing myelinated axons from afferent visual (geniculate) cells and cortical association fibers. Pyramidal and granule cells and giant pyramidal (Meynert) cells occur more deeply at IVc. Layer V is a densely cellular region with variously sized pyramidal cells. Layer VIa is a less cellular superficial portion, and layer VIb contains a varied neuronal population.

The blood supply of the striate cortex primarily derives from the **calcarine artery,** a branch of the **posterior cerebral artery,** and sometimes the **middle cerebral artery,** or anastomoses from it (Fig. 5.14). The calcarine artery is a major supply to the visual area; however, in 75% of cases, other arteries also contribute: the posterior temporal or parietooccipital arteries and, occasionally, anastomotic connections from the middle cerebral artery.

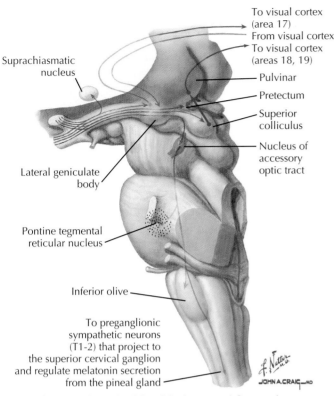

Fig. 5.10 Posterior Visual Pathway and Connections.

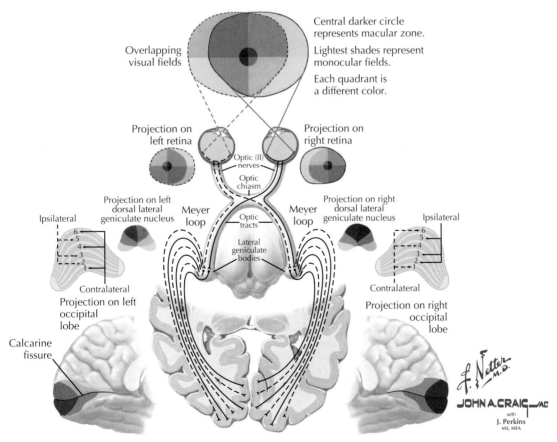

Fig. 5.11 Topographic Representation of the Visual Fields Across the Optic Pathway.

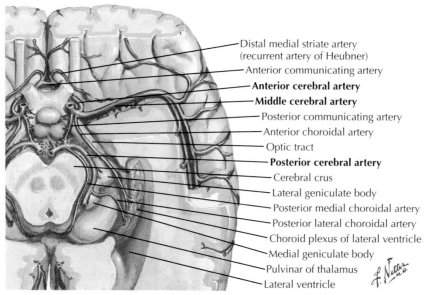

Distal medial striate artery
(recurrent artery of Heubner)
Anterior communicating artery
Anterior cerebral artery
Middle cerebral artery
Posterior communicating artery
Anterior choroidal artery
Optic tract
Posterior cerebral artery
Cerebral crus
Lateral geniculate body
Posterior medial choroidal artery
Posterior lateral choroidal artery
Choroid plexus of lateral ventricle
Medial geniculate body
Pulvinar of thalamus
Lateral ventricle

Fig. 5.12 Arteries of Brain: Inferior Views.

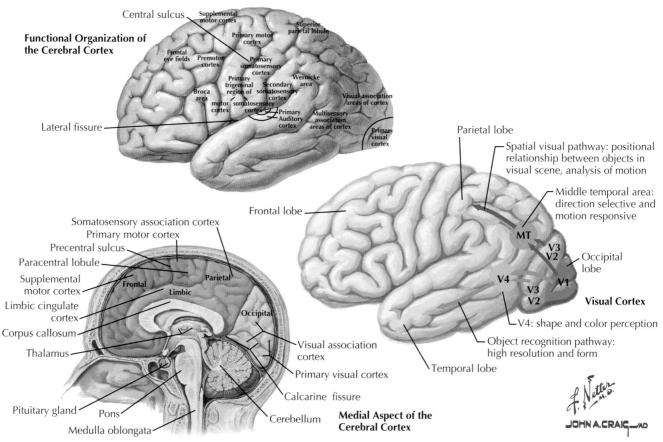

Functional Organization of the Cerebral Cortex

Central sulcus
Supplemental motor cortex
Primary motor cortex
Superior parietal lobule
Frontal eye fields
Premotor cortex
Primary somatosensory cortex
Primary trigeminal region of motor cortex
Secondary somatosensory cortex
Wernicke area
Broca area
Primary somatosensory cortex
Visual association areas of cortex
Primary Auditory cortex
Multisensory association areas of cortex
Primary visual cortex
Lateral fissure

Somatosensory association cortex
Primary motor cortex
Precentral sulcus
Paracentral lobule
Supplemental motor cortex
Limbic cingulate cortex
Corpus callosum
Thalamus
Pituitary gland
Pons
Medulla oblongata
Frontal
Parietal
Limbic
Occipital
Visual association cortex
Primary visual cortex
Calcarine fissure
Cerebellum

Medial Aspect of the Cerebral Cortex

Parietal lobe
Spatial visual pathway: positional relationship between objects in visual scene, analysis of motion
Middle temporal area: direction selective and motion responsive
Frontal lobe
MT
V3
V2
Occipital lobe
V4
V3
V2
V1
Visual Cortex
V4: shape and color perception
Object recognition pathway: high resolution and form
Temporal lobe

Fig. 5.13 Occipital Cortex and Projections.

Specific anatomic correlations are the primary clinical features pertinent to the striate cortex: visual information from the left visual field in each eye is projected to the right visual cortex (and conversely); the superior visual field is projected into the inferior half of V1 (and conversely); and the most central visual field is projected most posteriorly, whereas the peripheral field is located anteriorly within V1.

"Cortical magnification" in V1 results in much more cortex dedicated to the central area than to the periphery. Up to 50% of the cortex may correspond to the central 10 degrees of vision; in fact, the most central 1 degree of vision uses as much cortex posteriorly as the most peripheral 50 degrees. Cortical magnification is considered a reflection of the evolutionary importance of precise central vision to human survival.

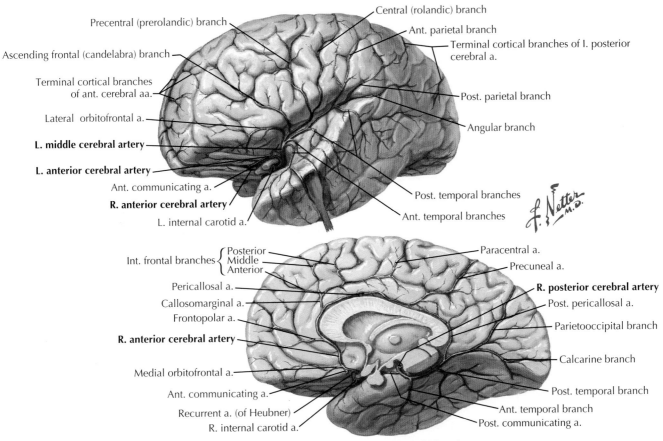

Precentral (prerolandic) branch

Ascending frontal (candelabra) branch

Terminal cortical branches
of ant. cerebral aa.

Lateral orbitofrontal a.

L. middle cerebral artery

L. anterior cerebral artery

Ant. communicating a.

R. anterior cerebral artery

L. internal carotid a.

Central (rolandic) branch

Ant. parietal branch

Terminal cortical branches of l. posterior
cerebral a.

Post. parietal branch

Angular branch

Post. temporal branches

Ant. temporal branches

Int. frontal branches { Posterior / Middle / Anterior

Pericallosal a.

Callosomarginal a.

Frontopolar a.

R. anterior cerebral artery

Medial orbitofrontal a.

Ant. communicating a.

Recurrent a. (of Heubner)

R. internal carotid a.

Paracentral a.

Precuneal a.

R. posterior cerebral artery

Post. pericallosal a.

Parietooccipital branch

Calcarine branch

Post. temporal branch

Ant. temporal branch

Post. communicating a.

Fig. 5.14 Arteries of Brain (Lateral and Medial Views).

Ocular dominance columns run at right angles to the cortical surface. Within a column, visual input is derived from one eye only; in the immediate neighboring cortical surface, perhaps 0.5 mm away, another column deriving input from the other eye is encountered.

Monocular occlusion in animal experiments during the early postnatal period demonstrates that the columns of the occluded eye grow smaller, whereas the columns of the open eye enlarge. Subsequent uncovering of the occluded eye does not restore the equality of the columns, which is considered central to understanding critical periods in visual development. The failure of that development is designated *amblyopia.*

A hierarchy exists to the processing of visual information at a cellular level. The striate cortex has different cell types that respond to increasingly specific stimuli. **Simple cells** have the same light-dark, center-surround response profile as retina and LGN cells. **Complex and hypercomplex cells** respond best to a light stimulus that is not a spot but rather a line at a particular angle or a specific length to achieve an optimal cell response.

This hierarchical structure suggests that additional cell types, probably located in extrastriate association cortices, respond to more specific and complex stimuli until, eventually, there may be "higher" association cortices, with groups of cells producing specific **patterns of neuronal activation** that represent the anatomic correlate for a specific perceptual recognition.

Brodmann areas 18 and 19, immediately adjacent to area 17, in the area surrounding the calcarine fissure, were termed the *parastriate* or *association visual cortex* on the assumption that they function to "associate" the visual data from V1 with brain areas regarding spatial orientation, recognition, and language.

The economic implications of hemianopic visual loss can be estimated by looking at its primary etiology, stroke. It has been estimated that 15% of stroke patients suffer homonymous visual loss. Overall, stroke costs in the United States will reach $2.2 trillion in the next 45 years, with hemianopia representing perhaps $300 billion.

Clinical Presentations

The vignette at the beginning of this section typifies an embolus to the left posterior cerebral artery causing a left occipital lobe infarct. Although occasionally such patients improve, often individuals have no substantial resolution of function. Driving restriction is essential in this case because of the total inability to perceive objects in the densely lost field.

Striate cortex lesions, like other neurologic lesions, can be classified into ischemic, neoplastic, demyelinating disease, and rare infections. Clinical characteristics of V1 visual field defects provide diagnostic anatomic localization even before imaging procedures are done. Incomplete hemianopias from V1 lesions show congruent deficits in each eye's visual field. The small size and close proximity of the left and right ocular dominance columns make it impossible to selectively damage the visual field of only one eye.

Features of homonymous hemianopias that suggest occipital lobe origin include extremely congruous partial defects between eyes, macular sparing, central homonymous defects, keyhole defects, and temporal crescent defects. Because of the specialized nature of V1, lesions in it affect only the vision, without other neurologic dysfunction (except, occasionally, headache). In addition to the aforementioned, striate cortex lesions produce no signs of anterior visual pathway involvement such as optic pallor or relative afferent papillary defect. Typically, central acuity in the preserve field is normal (Fig. 5.15).

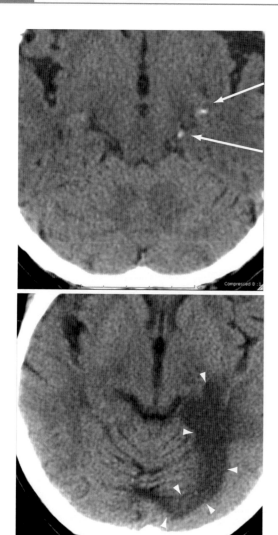

Axial noncontrast brain CT: Left posterior cerebral intraluminal thrombus (arrows) with subsequent evolution of left posterior cerebral cortically based infarct (arrowheads).

Fig. 5.15 Left Posterior Cerebral Infarction.

The extreme temporal visual field of each eye represents an exception to the previous principle of symmetric homonymous defects. Because the nasal visual field extends only approximately 65 degrees, the remaining 25% of the lateral field on each side is supplied solely by the ipsilateral eye. This "temporal crescent" of the visual field corresponds to the most anterior aspect of V1, abutting the occipitoparietal fissure, where ocular dominance columns are absent, because all input comes solely from the contralateral nasal retina. Therefore lesions of the anterior striate cortex may result in a "monocular temporal defect."

Rarely, bilateral occipital cortical lesions occur simultaneously or in quick succession. Generalized systemic hypotension, such as from a cardiac arrest or basilar or bilateral posterior cerebral artery occlusion, can cause bilateral ischemic damage. Similarly, both occipital poles can be injured by direct trauma or contrecoup mechanisms during skull injury. Initially, bilateral occipital pole lesions may be confused with bilateral optic nerve lesions because an apparent "central scotoma" is found in each eye. However, careful visual field mapping along the vertical axis demonstrates a discontinuity, or a vertical step. The vertical step is expected because cortical injuries should not be absolutely symmetric and the extent of clinical visual field loss should vary in size between the left and right hemifields. The size difference is easily recognized at the vertical meridian, resulting in a "keyhole defect." Like temporal crescent defects, keyhole defects are characteristic of occipital lobe lesions.

The most central visual field is represented widely on the posterior pole rather than only in the mesial occipital surface of V1 and is often supplied by the middle rather than the posterior cerebral artery. This means that even lesions affecting most of V1 may miss the most anterior, central vision area and produce a pattern of *macular sparing* in homonymous hemianopia with incomplete striate cortex lesions. However, when there is total loss of the cortex (e.g., surgical removal), macular sparing is not expected.

Parietal lesions differ from the isolated loss of visual field seen in V1 occipital disease in that both homonymous contralateral field loss and abnormal eye movements are usually detected. The loss of visually guided horizontal saccades to the side away from the lesion is best seen as an abnormal opticokinetic nystagmus response: when the drum is rotated toward the side of the lesion, the eyes, unable to saccade and pick up the next stripe on the drum, drift toward the affected side.

The clinical presentations of extrastriatal cortical lesions continue to be defined. Cerebral achromatopsia (impaired color perception due to occipital insult) has been described. The pathologies producing more complex visual deficits, typically termed visual agnosias, reach beyond the parastriate cortices. Prosopagnosia, for example, is typically caused by lesions encompassing the occipital and temporal lobes.

Diagnostic Approach

Visual field, ocular, and neurologic examinations will often serve to localize the visual problem to the occipital cortex. The etiology is suggested by the tempo of onset, accompanying symptoms, and presence of risk factors for a specific disease entity. However, MRI remains the standard for better specifying the pathologic process.

Cases of diffuse cerebral dysfunction may occasionally present with poor vision as the chief complaint. Electroencephalography and positron emission tomographic (PET) scanning may help in diagnosing patients with the Heidenhain variant of Creutzfeldt-Jakob disease, where visual symptoms predominate and MRI is relatively normal early in the course. However, in the visual variant of Alzheimer disease, neuropsychological testing and PET scanning with hypometabolism of the bilateral parieto-occipital cortices and the frontal eye fields probably provide the best diagnostic strategy.

TREATMENT

Treatment for most types of homonymous hemianopia is unavailing. If there is no improvement in visual deficits after the first 2 weeks, visual loss due to stroke is generally permanent. Surgical removal of an arteriovenous malformation or tumor is usually expected to leave significant residual visual loss.

Therefore mainstays of treatment are stabilization of vision (e.g., stroke prevention if stroke was the etiology) and visual rehabilitation. Rehabilitation efforts resemble those in other areas of poststroke rehabilitation, with focus on developing strategies to return to activities of daily living (e.g., reading and avoiding obstacles while ambulating) in spite of the hemianopic visual loss. Much of the improvement generally seen over time is usually attributed to increased visual scanning on the side of the blind hemifield, using saccades and head turns to that side. Protection of the patient who is unable to see obstacles in one hemifield may be improved by use of a cane on the hemianopic side and a brimmed or billed hat to detect obstacles before collision.

The possibility of "visual restoration" after stroke or traumatic brain injury using a computer-based, stimulus-detection paradigm has been explored but has not shown consistent data showing dramatic benefit.

The use of a split prismatic spectacle correction, which presents part of the "blind" hemifield to the patient's remaining vision with less head turning, may aid selected patients by providing a way to monitor the area of visual loss more easily.

FUTURE DIRECTIONS

This chapter covers a wide range of diseases that have an impact on vision. Research on improved diagnosis, prevention, treatment, genetics, and risk factors is active on all fronts.

As seen, current controversy attends the possibility of therapy for homonymous hemianopia. With the large number of patients affected by hemianopia, establishing the presence and significance of any improvement becomes an important economic, as well as medical, issue.

ACKNOWLEDGMENT

The author thanks Professor Thomas R. Hedges III, MD, for his help in organizing and clarifying this chapter.

ADDITIONAL RESOURCES

Intraocular Optic Nerve

Beck RW, Servais GE, Hayreh SS. Anterior ischemic optic neuropathy. IX. Cup-to-disc ratio and its role in pathogenesis. Ophthalmology 1987;94(11):1503–8.
Cites disk morphology as risk factor in AION.

Douglas DJ, Schuler JJ, Buchbinder D, et al. The association of central retinal artery occlusion and extracranial carotid artery disease. Ann Surg 1988;208(1):85–90.
Shows risk of ipsilateral stoke after CRAO.

Hayreh SS, Kolder HE, Weingeist TA. Central retinal artery occlusion and retinal tolerance time. Ophthalmology 1980;87(1):75–8.
Establishes retinal viability at 100 minutes after retinal artery occlusion.

Hayreh SS, Podhajsky PA, Raman R, et al. Giant cell arteritis: validity and reliability of various diagnostic criteria. Am J Ophthalmol 1997;123(3):285–96.
Offers guidance regarding confirmatory testing in giant cell arteritis.

Hayreh SS, Zimmerman MB. Non-arteritic anterior ischemic optic neuropathy: role of systemic corticosteroid therapy. Graefes Arch Clin Exp Ophthalmol 2008;246(7):1029–46.
Suggests benefit to 65-day oral steroid course in vision recovery after AION.

Salomon O, Huna-Baron R, Steinberg DM, et al. Role of aspirin in reducing the frequency of second eye involvement in patients with non-arteritic anterior ischaemic optic neuropathy. Eye 1999;13(Pt 3a):357–9.
Suggests benefit of aspirin in this context.

Orbital and Intracanalicular Optic Nerve

Alabduljalil T, Behbehani R. Paraneoplastic syndromes in neuro-ophthalmology. Curr Opin Ophthalmol 2007;18(6):463–9.
Review of available data for paraneoplastic optic neuropathy.

Beck RW, Cleary PA, Anderson MM Jr, et al. A randomized, controlled trial of corticosteroids in the treatment of acute optic neuritis. The optic neuritis study group. N Engl J Med 1992;326(9):581–8.
Established benefits of early intravenous methylprednisolone on recovery time and interval to next MS episode.

Hayreh SS. Posterior ischaemic optic neuropathy: clinical features, pathogenesis, and management. Eye 2004;18(11):1188–206.
Characteristics of 42 cases of posterior ischemic optic neuropathy (PION).

Sadda SR, Nee M, Miller NR, et al. Clinical spectrum of posterior ischemic optic neuropathy. Am J Ophthalmol 2001;132(5):743–50.
Divides 72 cases into three etiological categories.

Wallace DC, Singh G, Lott MT, et al. Mitochondrial DNA mutation associated with Leber's hereditary optic neuropathy. Science 1988;242:1427–30.
First description of mitochondrial DNA mutation in an LHON pedigree.

Wingerchuk DM, Weinshenker BG. Neuromyelitis optica. Curr Treat Options Neurol 2008;10(1):55–66.
Review of current diagnosis and treatment.

Optic Chiasm

Thomas R, Shenoy K, Seshadri MS, et al. Visual field defects in non-functioning pituitary adenomas. Indian J Ophthalmol 2002;50(2):127–30.
Relates visual field defects to tumor size.

Posterior Visual Afferent System: Optic Tracts, Lateral Geniculate Nucleus, Optic Radiations

Bowers AR, Keeney K, Peli E. Community-based trial of a peripheral prism visual field expansion device for hemianopia. Arch Ophthalmol 2008;126(5):657–64.
Showed long-term tolerance and functional improvement in 47% of patients using prismatic spectacles for hemianopic loss.

Brazis PW, Lee AG, Graff-Radford N, et al. Homonymous visual field defects in patients without corresponding structural lesions on neuroimaging. J Neuroophthalmol 2000;20(2):92–6.

Horton JC, Hoyt WF. The representation of the visual field in human striate cortex: a revision of the classic holmes map. Arch Ophthalmol 1991;109:816–24.
Discusses anatomic basis of cortical magnification, temporal crescent, etc.

Lee AG, Martin CO. Ophthalmology. Neuro-ophthalmic findings in the visual variant of Alzheimer's disease. Ophthalmology 2004;111(2):376–80, discussion 380–1.
These two articles propose diagnostic strategies for patients with visual loss and underlying progressive dementia.

Pambakian AL, Mannan SK, Hodgson TL, et al. Saccadic visual search training: a treatment for patients with homonymous hemianopia. J Neurol Neurosurg Psychiatry 2004;75(10):1443–8.
Results of 29 patients.

Pelak VS, Dubin M, Whitney E. Homonymous hemianopia: a critical analysis of optical devices, compensatory training, and NovaVision. Curr Treat Options Neurol 2007;9(1):41–7.
This reference discusses issues in the NovaVision data, tempering claims of visual improvement.

Rathore SS, Hinn AR, Cooper LS, et al. Characterization of incident stroke signs and symptoms: findings from the atherosclerosis risk in communities study. Stroke 2002;33(11):2718–21.
Showed 15% prevalence of homonymous hemianopia among 474 stroke patients.

6

Cranial Nerves III, IV, and VI: Oculomotor, Trochlear, and Abducens Nerves: Ocular Mobility and Pupils

Geetha K. Athappilly, Ippolit C. A. Matjucha

CRANIAL NERVE III: OCULOMOTOR

> **CLINICAL VIGNETTE** *A 37-year-old woman presented with a 2-day history of "blurry" vision on upward gaze and headache. One month previously, when she had experienced the same symptoms, sinusitis was diagnosed, and an antibiotic was prescribed; symptoms had resolved in 5 days.*
>
> *Examination demonstrated impaired upward, downward, and medial movement in the right eye. There was mild right-sided ptosis, and the right pupil was slightly larger and reacted poorly compared with the left.*
>
> *Magnetic resonance imaging (MRI) yielded normal results, but catheter angiography demonstrated a posterior communicating artery (p-com) aneurysm. At craniotomy the same night, the neurosurgeon reported fresh and old clot around a 10-mm aneurysm compressing the right oculomotor nerve. The aneurysm was clipped, and patient had an uneventful recovery with gradual resolution of the neuro-ophthalmologic findings.*

Oculomotor palsy is most often associated with microvasculopathy due to diabetes mellitus, hypertension, or advanced age, so that its pool of potential victims is large. It is sometimes the harbinger of urgent, dangerous disease such as an expanding berry aneurysm. Even in idiopathic cases, the diplopia it typically produces is not only distressing for the patient but also disrupts daily activities. Even in cases where ptosis is severe enough to eliminate diplopia by blocking the vision of the affected eye, the impact on patients, both on an emotional and practical level, is severe.

The oculomotor nerves course from the ventral midbrain to the orbits. CN-III provides the general somatic motor efferent innervation controlling upper lid elevation and most of the extraocular movements upward, medially, and downward. In addition, CN-III carries the general visceral motor (parasympathetic) efferent innervation responsible for pupillary constriction and accommodation (near focus) of the crystalline lens.

CN-III begins at its nucleus in the midline upper midbrain. The nucleus is a lepidopterous collection of nine subnuclei located in the center of the rostral midbrain at the level of the superior colliculi (Fig. 6.1). The most ventral of these subnuclei is the central caudate nucleus, a midline structure that innervates both levator palpebrae muscles. Uniquely, axons from the medial subnuclei or columns decussate completely to innervate the contralateral superior rectus muscles. The other six subnuclei, three left-and-right pairs, innervate ipsilateral extraocular muscles. The ventral subnucleus, intermediate column, and dorsal subnucleus, respectively, control the medial rectus (eye adduction), inferior oblique (intorsion and some elevation), and inferior rectus (depression).

Sometimes considered a subnucleus of CN-III, the Edinger-Westphal nucleus abuts the others rostrodorsally, residing at the ventral edge of periaqueductal gray matter. The Edinger-Westphal nucleus supplies the cholinergic efferents producing pupillary constriction and ciliary muscle contraction (lens accommodation). Afferents from the pretectal nuclei mediate the pupillary light reflex, whereas inputs influencing pupil constriction and lens accommodation in response to near visual stimulus originate from striate and prestriate cortex and the superior colliculus. When the pupillary fibers join the oculomotor nerve, they move exteriorly and dorsally within the nerve, a clinical continuation of the spatial relation of the Edinger-Westphal nucleus to CN-III.

The CN-III nucleus receives numerous afferents, including inputs from the paramedian pontine reticular formation for horizontal eye movement, the rostral interstitial nucleus of the medial longitudinal fasciculus (MLF) for vertical and torsional movements, and the vestibular nuclei. Other afferents come from the superior colliculi, the occipital cortex, and the cerebellum.

Axons from the CN-III nucleus gather into a fascicle that sweeps ventrally in an arc curving toward the medial surface of the cerebral peduncle, then passes through the red nucleus.

The nascent oculomotor nerve emerges from the medial surface of the cerebral peduncle to enter the interpeduncular cistern. It crosses the cistern for approximately 5 mm, passing under the posterior cerebral artery. The fibers subserving pupillary constriction are located externally at the caudal aspect of the nerve and are less prone to microvascular changes as the deeper fibers are. This arrangement is thought to explain the pupil's resilience to ischemia affecting CN-III and to its susceptibility in compression. The nerve follows beneath the p-com for 10 mm and then pierces the dura underneath the p-com before it passes the internal carotid artery (ICA) en route to the cavernous sinus.

The cavernous sinus is part of the intracranial venous system. It receives blood from the ophthalmic vein and sphenoparietal sinus, transmitting this flow to the superior and inferior petrosal sinuses. The left and right cavernous sinuses are connected via the intracavernous plexus; they also communicate with the basilar sinus and the pterygoid and foramen ovale plexuses. The cavernous sinus resides lateral to the pituitary gland, resting atop the roof and lateral wall of the sphenoid sinus. Besides venous blood, the space contains the intracavernous portions of CN-III, -IV, and -VI; the ophthalmic branch of CN-V and its maxillary nerve posteriorly; the ICA; and the sympathetic nerve fibers

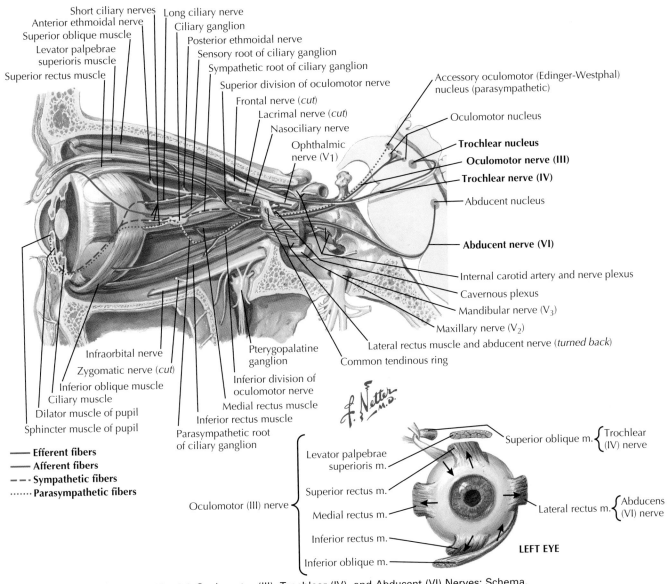

Fig. 6.1 Oculomotor (III), Trochlear (IV), and Abducent (VI) Nerves: Schema.

investing the adventitia of the ICA. CN-III, -IV, and -VI and the ophthalmic nerve all leave the cavernous sinus to enter the orbit via the superior orbital fissure.

Given the confluence of multiple structures into this relatively small sinus, cavernous lesions are prone to produce multiple cranial nerve palsies, often with pain or numbness in the ophthalmic distribution of CN-V. If the pathologic process is extensive, signs of venous obstruction in the orbit also develop (proptosis and chemosis).

CN-III typically divides into superior and inferior branches within the anterior cavernous sinus, thus entering the orbit as two distinct structures. The superior branch supplies the superior rectus and levator palpebrae muscles. The inferior branch provides somatic innervation to the medial and inferior recti and the inferior oblique, and it supplies the parasympathetic pupillary input to the ciliary ganglion, located superolaterally to the optic nerve. The parasympathetic axons from the Edinger-Westphal nucleus synapse here, with the postsynaptic neurons providing visceral motor control to the iris sphincter and the ciliary muscles via the short ciliary nerves.

Etiology and Pathogenesis

Etiologies for CN-III are broadly divided into two groups: those due to microvascular nerve infarction (e.g., diabetes mellitus) and those due to compression. There are also other, less frequent etiologies.

In the patient presenting with acute, severe headache and pupil-involved CN-III palsy, an expanding *aneurysm,* usually of the p-com, is the most important cause (Fig. 6.2). The location of these aneurysms is usually at the origin of p-com from the ICA (Fig. 6.3) and 90% of these aneurysms present with CN-III palsy. Aneurysm in other nearby arteries can likewise present as CN-III palsy, with up to 30% of acquired CN-III palsies being caused by aneurysms.

However, the majority of acquired CN-III palsies will be due to vascular compromise of some portion of CN-III, commonly affecting patients with known risk factors for vasculopathy or microvascular disease. In 60%–80% of microvascular CN-III palsy cases the pupil is spared. Typically, these palsies have a favorable prognosis and uncomplicated recovery within 2–4 months. Although common vasculopathies

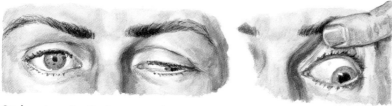

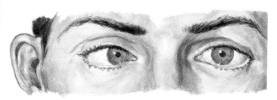

Oculomotor palsy: Ptosis, eye turns laterally and inferiorly, pupil dilated; common finding with cerebral aneurysms, especially carotid-posterior communicating aneurysms

Abducens palsy: Affected eye turns medially. May be first manifestation of intracavernous carotid aneurysm. Pain above eye or on side of face may be secondary to trigeminal (V) nerve involvement.

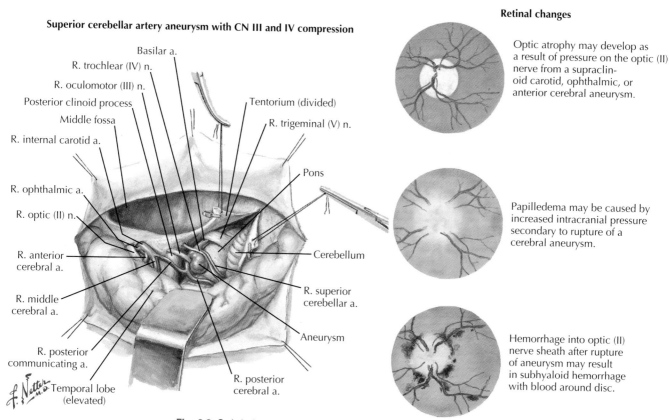

Superior cerebellar artery aneurysm with CN III and IV compression

Basilar a.
R. trochlear (IV) n.
R. oculomotor (III) n.
Posterior clinoid process
Middle fossa
R. internal carotid a.
R. ophthalmic a.
R. optic (II) n.
R. anterior cerebral a.
R. middle cerebral a.
R. posterior communicating a.
Temporal lobe (elevated)

Tentorium (divided)
R. trigeminal (V) n.
Pons
Cerebellum
R. superior cerebellar a.
Aneurysm
R. posterior cerebral a.

Retinal changes

Optic atrophy may develop as a result of pressure on the optic (II) nerve from a supraclinoid carotid, ophthalmic, or anterior cerebral aneurysm.

Papilledema may be caused by increased intracranial pressure secondary to rupture of a cerebral aneurysm.

Hemorrhage into optic (II) nerve sheath after rupture of aneurysm may result in subhyaloid hemorrhage with blood around disc.

Fig. 6.2 Ophthalmologic Manifestations of Cerebral Aneurysms.

secondary to diabetes and hypertension are seen most frequently, attention should be paid to the possibilities of other systemic vasculitides, temporal arteritis, clotting disorder, and infiltrative processes.

Third-nerve palsies due to lesions of the nucleus or fascicle within the midbrain are usually part of a larger midbrain syndrome (see below). The usual etiologies of such palsies are stroke for older patients and inflammatory or demyelinating disease (i.e., multiple sclerosis) in the young.

Open or closed head injuries may lead to *traumatic oculomotor nerve palsy.* The suspected mechanism is traction or shearing where the third-nerve root is relatively fixed at its origin and at its entrance into the dura. Typically, traumatic CN-III palsy is associated with severe frontal deceleration impact with loss of consciousness and, usually, skull fracture (e.g., unrestrained occupant in a motor vehicle accident). In cases where pupil-involving CN-III palsy is discovered after seemingly trivial injury, neurovascular imaging should be performed to detect a possible underlying skull base tumor, meningioma, or aneurysm.

Cavernous sinus thrombosis may produce a cranial polyneuropathy that features CN-III palsy. Often it is a septic complication of central facial cellulitis and a dreaded clinical entity typically producing proptosis, ophthalmoplegia, and optic neuropathy. Septic phlebitis of the facial vein or pterygoid plexus is the usual intermediary between cellulitis and infectious thrombosis.

Tolosa-Hunt syndrome is a painful ophthalmoplegia caused by idiopathic cavernous sinus inflammation, with most instances considered within the spectrum of inflammatory pseudotumor. It typically involves multiple cranial nerves and varies in degree over days. MRI of the cavernous sinus is needed to confirm the diagnosis, and treatment with high-dose corticosteroids is indicated once tumor and infection have been excluded.

Intrinsic, extrinsic, and metastatic tumors can cause third-nerve palsy. Carcinomatous or granulomatous meningitis can affect multiple cranial nerves in succession, often simulating Tolosa-Hunt syndrome.

Clinical Presentations

The classic presentation of a complete CN-III palsy is unmistakable: because of the unopposed actions of the superior oblique and lateral rectus muscles, the eye is turned outward and usually down. Upper-lid ptosis often requires that the lid be held up by the examiner to assess ocular motility.

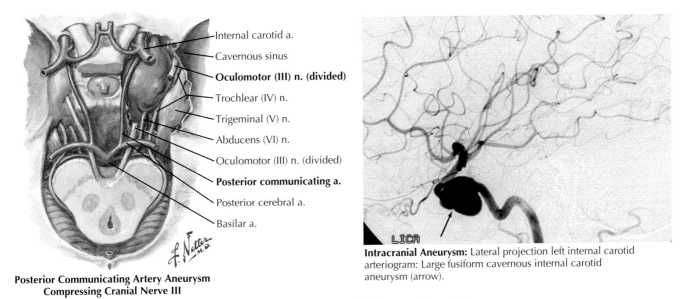

Internal carotid a.

Cavernous sinus

Oculomotor (III) n. (divided)

Trochlear (IV) n.

Trigeminal (V) n.

Abducens (VI) n.

Oculomotor (III) n. (divided)

Posterior communicating a.

Posterior cerebral a.

Basilar a.

**Posterior Communicating Artery Aneurysm
Compressing Cranial Nerve III**

Intracranial Aneurysm: Lateral projection left internal carotid arteriogram: Large fusiform cavernous internal carotid aneurysm (arrow).

Fig. 6.3 Aneurysms Causing Oculomotor Nerve Palsy.

The presence or absence of ipsilateral mydriasis ("pupil-involvement" or "pupil-sparing," respectively) has traditionally been considered a major diagnostic consideration. CN-III palsies of compressive origin have pupillary involvement in the vast majority of cases and, if acute with severe headache, strongly suggest aneurysm as the etiology. Pupil-sparing usually implies temporary CN-III palsy due to microvascular ischemia. Patients with microvascular oculomotor palsy may report a mild ache in the ipsilateral brow, but occasionally the pain can be severe.

Motor involvement of CN-III palsies are generally characterized as complete, incomplete (where the innervated muscles show subtotal palsy), and, since the CN-III divides into superior and inferior rami just before its entrance into the orbit, divisional. "Superior division" CN-III palsy involves ipsilateral dysfunction of the superior rectus and levator palpebrae muscles, whereas an "inferior division" palsy has impaired downgaze, medial gaze, and on occasion, loss of pupillary constriction. Divisional palsies would seem to imply an orbital or anterior cavernous sinus pathologic site; however, more proximal intracranial disease is often responsible. Many cases will have negative imaging and recover well and are then assumed microvascular in etiology.

Incomplete CN-III palsies show partial losses of up-, down-, and medial-gaze, along with partial ptosis with some CN-III–innervated muscles more affected than others. In such cases—as the clinical vignette illustrates—recognition that the patient's ocular misalignment is a form of third-nerve palsy can be challenging. It is generally agreed that the presence of the pupil-sparing in such cases does not rule out compressive etiology.

A patient with an *isolated medial rectus dysfunction* (inability to adduct the eye) should not be considered to have an incomplete CN-III palsy. Most often, this condition is caused by *internuclear ophthalmoplegia* (see below). It may also be seen in cases of myasthenia gravis or from orbital disease involving the horizontal rectus muscles.

When the origin of third nerve palsy is at the nucleus, the presentation is one of ipsilateral medial rectus, inferior rectus, and inferior oblique dysfunction, with contralateral superior rectus weakness because of the decussation of axons from the medial column subnucleus. Because of bilateral lid innervation by the central caudate subnucleus, the eyelids exhibit either bilateral blepharoptosis or are normal, depending on the extent of the insult. In clinical practice, such cases are exceedingly rare.

With insult to the third-nerve fasciculus, clinical localization is often aided by the presence of other signs of midbrain dysfunction. CN-III fasciculus lesions at the red nucleus present as oculomotor palsy with crossed hemitremor, *Benedikt syndrome*. If the lesion extends to the medial lemniscus, there is also contralateral hypesthesia. Similar lesions with caudal extension into the brachium conjunctivum produce ipsilateral cerebellar ataxia or *Claude syndrome*. When damage extends ventrally into the basis pedunculi and the corticospinal tract, hemiplegia contralateral to the CN-III palsy occurs *(Weber syndrome)*.

In comatose patients, unilateral mydriasis ("*blown*" or *Hutchinson pupil*) is indicative of supratentorial increased intracranial pressure (ICP), sufficient to force the uncus of the temporal lobe laterally and caudally to compress the third nerve against the anterior edge of the tentorial foramen *(uncal herniation)*. In fact, using oculocephalic maneuvers, additional evidence of compressive CN-III palsy can be uncovered. Pupil checks and oculocephalic maneuvers need to be monitored frequently in any unresponsive patient, since uncal herniation can be rapidly fatal if not detected and addressed at its earliest sign. The laterality of the blown pupil does not always correlate with the side of the lesion.

Although a few cases exist of mydriasis as a possible sign of compressive third-nerve palsy in patients who are awake and alert, this remains exceedingly unlikely without evolving signs of altered consciousness and usually indicates another etiology, such as pharmacologic pupillary mydriasis or *Adie tonic pupil* (below).

Whereas microvascular CN-III palsy is generally followed by full recovery, the prognosis for traumatic or postoperative compressive CN-III palsy is guarded. If recovery occurs, it is usually marked by aberrant regeneration and *synkinesis*. The best-known example is the pseudo–von Graefe sign: the branch of CN-III that normally innervates the inferior rectus now synkinetically innervates the levator palpebrae, causing the upper lid to lift on downward gaze (clinically simulating the lid lag, or von Graefe sign, of Graves orbitopathy). Internal motor efferents can likewise be involved, resulting in a change of pupil size as gaze is shifted.

Occasionally, *primary aberrant regeneration* (aberrant regeneration without history of prior palsy) will be encountered. This finding is due to chronic compression of the third nerve, typically within or near the cavernous sinus usually due to meningioma and occasionally from an aneurysm of the intracavernous ICA. Adie tonic pupil is another example of aberrant regeneration affecting a facet of CN-III function with a probable intraorbital location within the ciliary ganglion and is discussed further in the section pertaining to pupils.

As opposed to the preceding discussion of isolated CN-III disease, the oculomotor nerve can be involved in cranial polyneuropathies, in which case the accompanying deficits typically help localize the etiology. *Cavernous sinus syndrome* typically affects CN-III, -IV, and -VI and the ophthalmic branch of CN-V. When the intracavernous carotid artery wall is also involved, sympathetic pupil dysfunction (Horner pupil) will result, producing miosis; the Horner pupil will be unnoticeable if CN-III–related mydriasis obscures it. The clinical history in the case of slowly expanding tumor in the cavernous sinus often includes chronically increasing diplopia, sometimes with pain or numbness in the CN-V ophthalmic distribution; in cases of inflammation or infection, the onset is usually dramatic and painful. *Superior orbital fissure syndrome* is often indistinguishable from cavernous sinus syndrome.

Lesions producing diminished vision, external ophthalmoplegia, orbital pain, and corneal hypesthesia and proptosis characterize *orbital apex syndrome.* In simplified terms, this syndrome is clinically characterized by findings of superior orbital fissure syndrome with a concomitant compressive optic neuropathy. It must be distinguished from *pituitary apoplexy* where sudden, painful visual loss due to chiasmal compression by pituitary hemorrhage is often accompanied by unilateral or bilateral CN-III palsy as impingement upon the adjacent cavernous sinuses evolves.

Differential Diagnosis

Myasthenia gravis, a disorder of somatic neuromuscular junction failure that does not affect the pupil, will occasionally simulate pupil-sparing third-nerve palsy. A history of diurnal variability, findings of inducible fatigability, and resolution of the "palsy" during intravenous administration of edrophonium chloride (Tensilon) is often sufficient to expose the diagnosis, which can then be confirmed by serum antibody testing and electromyography.

Chronic, progressive external ophthalmoplegia (CPEO) presents as slowly progressive bilateral ptosis and loss of extraocular movements, usually without diplopia. CPEO has been associated with specific mutations of mitochondrial and nuclear DNA and can be part of a larger syndrome, oculopharyngeal dystrophy. The Kearns-Sayre variant of CPEO includes pigmentary retinopathy with nyctalopia, hormonal dysfunction, and most importantly cardiac conduction disorders necessitating cardiology evaluation.

The Miller Fisher variant of Guillain-Barré syndrome produces an external ophthalmoplegia that may be initially confused with CN-III palsy; the presence of viral prodrome, ataxia, areflexia, cerebrospinal fluid albuminocytologic dissociation, and in some instances positive serum anti-GQ1b IgM and IgG antibodies will confirm the diagnosis.

Patients with *internuclear ophthalmoplegia* have inability to move the ipsilateral eye into adduction when attempting horizontal gaze to the contralateral side. The responsible lesion is in the MLF, interrupting the interneurons traveling from the CN-VI nucleus to the CN-III ventral subnucleus that innervates the medial rectus (see discussion of CN-VI anatomy, below). Such patients are often assumed to have "medial rectus palsy"; however, such a variant of CN-III palsy is rarely if ever seen clinically, and the preservation of adduction during convergence to near stimulus (mediated by the mesencephalon) in internuclear ophthalmoplegia serves to confirm its central nervous system supranuclear origin.

Duane syndrome is an example of a congenital aberrant innervation. In affected individuals, prenatal abducens nerve dysgenesis or injury causes subsequent misdirected CN-III innervation of the lateral rectus. Therefore attempted lateral eye movement results in simultaneous stimulation of the medial and lateral recti, causing variable eye movement, measurable globe retraction into the orbit, and consequent pseudoptosis. In type II Duane syndrome, the combination of poor adduction and pseudoptosis during globe retraction may simulate CN-III palsy. The congenital nature of this condition is most easily deduced by the absence of symptomatic diplopia in lateral gaze despite the presence of incomitant strabismus.

Patients with isolated ptosis are often screened for the presence of CN-III palsy. The most common cause of ptosis, typically encountered in patients older than age 50 years—but occasionally seen in younger patients with a history of frequent eye rubbing—is *aponeurotic ptosis or levator dehiscence,* a lengthening of the tendon (aponeurosis) connecting the levator palpebrae muscle to the upper lid. Aponeurotic ptosis is particularly common in patients who have undergone cataract surgery. In those patients who, in addition, experienced intraoperative iris injury with postoperative mydriasis, erroneous suspicion of a partial compressive CN-III palsy can be easily prompted.

Marcus Gunn jaw-winking is a syndrome of congenital aberrant innervation of the levator palpebrae muscle by the motor neurons of CN-V that innervate the pterygoid muscles of the mandible. The typical patient will have ptosis that partially resolves with lateral and forward jaw movements with costimulation of the levator.

In the traumatic setting, ophthalmoplegia due to CN-III palsy must be distinguished from that due to orbital disease (e.g., orbital floor fracture with entrapment of the inferior rectus muscle).

Diagnostic Approach

A spared pupil in otherwise complete CN-III palsy is highly suggestive of a microvascular cause. However, in cases of a recent incomplete extraocular CN-III palsy, the absence of pupil involvement could suggest an evolving process for which imaging is required.

Once aneurysm has been excluded, in those patients without clear precipitants, testing for diabetes mellitus, hypertension, vasculitis and other inflammatory disease, clotting disorders, spirochetal disease (syphilis and Lyme disease), and myasthenia gravis is recommended. Even in patients with microvascular CN-III palsy without evidence of causative disease, consideration may be given to reevaluate already defined cerebrovascular risk factors.

Any patient presenting with diplopia, initially thought to be related to a cranial mononeuropathy, must have careful examination of the adjacent cranial nerve to exclude their involvement. Also, patients with apparently isolated CN-III palsy should be checked for signs of ataxia, areflexia, or contralateral rubral tremor, hemiparesis, or hypesthesia. Similarly, patients presenting with new upper facial pain or numbness must always be checked for impaired eye movements and corneal hypesthesia to exclude early cavernous sinus syndrome.

Management and Therapy

The management of symptomatic intracranial aneurysm is usually urgent, via endovascular or surgical intervention if the general state of the patient permits (see Chapter 56). Management of microvascular palsy usually centers on prevention of recurrent events via reduction of risk factors. Optimization of any causative disease, such as diabetes, is crucial, and daily aspirin is often recommended. Therapy for other underlying causes of CN-III palsy will vary, appropriate to etiology.

Visual management of nonhealing CN-III palsies is complicated by the number of paretic extraocular muscles involved, as ocular misalignment changes significantly depending on the direction of gaze. Prismatic spectacles are often unavailing, except in cases of minimal residual misalignment. Strabismus surgery, often involving two or three staged procedures, has the limited goal of stable relief of diplopia in primary gaze only. Often the simplest management tool, if acceptable to the patient, is occluding vision through a fogged lens or patch on the affected eye to eliminate diplopia, if the ptosis does not already accomplish that.

CRANIAL NERVE IV: TROCHLEAR

> **CLINICAL VIGNETTE** *A workman, bent over his work, sustained left occiput blunt head trauma and scalp laceration when a coworker dropped a tool from above. Diplopia and headache subsequently developed.*
>
> *Examination revealed poor depression of the right eye in leftward gaze. Prismatic spectacle lenses were prescribed to alleviate the diplopia. After a few months, the patient reported that his vision had returned to normal.*

This vignette describes isolated trochlear nerve (CN-IV) injury with relatively mild closed head trauma. Often the most benign of the cranial neuropathies, particularly those related to extraocular muscle function, it tends to recover fully over a period of weeks or months.

The CN-IV nuclei are located at the level of the inferior colliculi in the lower midbrain off the midline at the ventral edge of the periaqueductal gray. The nuclei are crossed; the left trochlear nucleus innervates the right superior oblique and vice versa.

Axons emanating from the trochlear nucleus arc dorsally around the periaqueductal gray into the tectum of the midbrain, where they cross the midline and then emerge laterally beneath the inferior colliculus at the medial border of the brachium conjunctivum as CN-IV. It then completely decussates and exits the brainstem from its dorsal aspect, a unique feature among the cranial nerves. It passes through the quadrigeminal and ambient cisterns and then runs along the free edge of the tentorium. It enters the orbit via the superior orbital fissure and innervates a single extraocular muscle, the superior oblique.

The superior oblique is chiefly a depressor of the globe and is most active when the eye is adducted and depressed. It has a secondary function of intorting the eye during ipsilateral head tilt and is a weak abductor of the eye in downgaze (Fig. 6.4). Therefore CN-IV palsy will produce ipsilateral loss of depression (hyperopia) and excyclotorsion of the globe.

Etiology and Pathogenesis

Trauma is the most frequent cause of CN-IV palsies. Traumatic palsies may be bilateral, but most often one side is spared or recovers so that

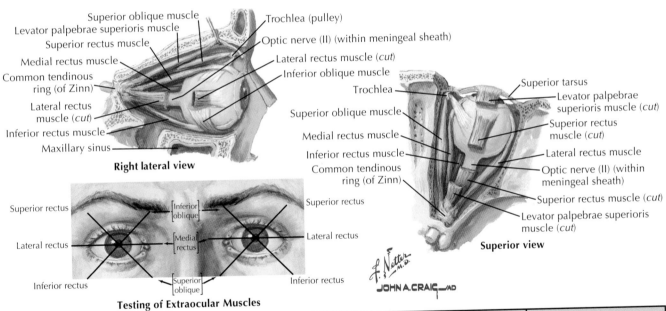

Muscle	Origin	Insertion	Innervation	Main Actions
Levator palpebrae superioris	Sphenoid bone, anterosuperior optic canal	Tarsal plate and skin of upper eyelid	Oculomotor nerve (superior tarsal muscle supplied by sympathetic fibers)	Elevates upper eyelid
Superior rectus (SR)	Common tendinous ring (annulus of Zinn)	Sclera just posterior to cornea	Oculomotor nerve	Elevates, adducts, and rotates eyeball medially
Inferior rectus (IR)	Common tendinous ring (annulus of Zinn)	Sclera just posterior to cornea	Oculomotor nerve	Depresses, adducts, and rotates eyeball medially
Medial rectus	Common tendinous ring (annulus of Zinn)	Sclera just posterior to cornea	Oculomotor nerve	Adducts eyeball
Lateral rectus	Common tendinous ring (annulus of Zinn)	Sclera just posterior to cornea	Abducent nerve	Abducts eyeball
Superior oblique (SO)	Body of sphenoid bone	Passes through a trochlea and inserts into sclera	Trochlear nerve	Medially rotates, depresses, and abducts eyeball
Inferior oblique (IO)	Floor of orbit	Sclera deep to lateral rectus muscle	Oculomotor nerve	Laterally rotates, elevates and abducts eyeball

From Hansen JH. Netter's Clincial Anatomy, 2e. Saunders, Philadelphia, 2010, p. 380.

Fig. 6.4 Extraocular Muscles and General Function.

patients are left with unilateral dysfunction. The frequent association of trauma with CN-IV palsy may imply that the thin dorsal tectum is vulnerable to traumatic forces causing shear injury between the emerging nerves and the colliculi or the cerebellar tentorium or direct injury from a hydraulic pressure wave transmitted through the aqueduct. MRI demonstration of tectal subarachnoid hematoma in traumatic trochlear palsy supports this theory. In addition, a pathologic study has shown that, with sufficient force, avulsion of the CN-IV root from the pons can occur.

The nucleus and fasciculus of the trochlear nerve lie within the pons; in this location, CN-IV palsies may result from stroke, demyelination, and tumor. Lesions of the fascicle, rarely seen clinically, produce a contralateral CN-IV palsy and an ipsilateral Horner syndrome due to coinvolvement of the descending first-order pupillary sympathetic axons passing through the pontine tegmentum. The trochlear nerve fasciculi decussate just dorsal to the sylvian aqueduct, and tumors or stroke in this area will produce bilateral trochlear palsies.

In the subarachnoid space, CN-IV can be affected by carcinomatous meningitis, by aneurysm (especially of the superior cerebellar artery; see Fig. 6.2), or by dolichoectasia of the basilar artery. The nerve itself may be the site of schwannomas. Once within the dural canal leading to the cavernous sinus, the nerve may be affected by tumors, especially meningioma. Compression of CN-IV can occur at the cavernous sinus itself, by dissections or aneurysm of the carotid artery, by extension of sellar and orbital tumors, and by metastases. Typically CN-IV, -III, -VI, and the ophthalmic branch of CN-V are involved in cavernous sinus lesions.

In cases where imaging reveals no structural cause of CN-IV palsy and where there is no history of trauma, microvascular ischemia is the usual assumed etiology. Patients with diabetes, hypertension, vasculitis, sarcoidosis, or treponemal infection may present with seemingly "idiopathic" palsies.

Clinical Presentations

Patients with trochlear palsy have hypertropia or impaired ability to depress the eye on the involved side. Weakness of depressor function of the superior oblique is exaggerated with medial downward gaze or when the head is tilted toward the side of palsy.

Normally during head tilt to one side, the ipsilateral superior oblique is activated to accomplish incyclotorsion of the eye, keeping the retina relatively level despite the head shift. The medial rectus is activated simultaneously, so that the incyclotorsion of the superior oblique is not accompanied by usual depressing of the globe. In trochlear palsy, then, when the head is tilted toward the palsied side, abnormal excyclotorsion is emphasized, magnifying both the hypertropia and diplopia. This pattern of incomitant strabismus is summarized as "hypertropia worse with gaze away and with tilt toward the affected side."

Patients with CN-IV palsy often adopt a secondary torticollis, offering a diagnostic clue. Patients prefer a chin-down posture with the head tilted away from the palsy, so that the affected eye is in up and out, where the superior oblique normally has the least action, and its palsy matters the least. Because this posture minimizes the visual consequences of CN-IV palsy, congenital CN-IV palsies are often undiagnosed for decades. A diagnosis in adulthood may be made after intermittent diplopia develops from progressive asthenopia or when treatment for torticollis is sought. The presence of the characteristic head tilt in childhood photographs often confirms the congenital nature of the palsy.

In most cases of CN-IV palsy, there is a history of trauma. A high frontal head impact with contrecoup forces at the dorsal tectum, occipital impact producing more direct injury, or coccygeal impact transmitted up a straight spinal column are all encountered. Occasionally, the appearance of vertical diplopia after frontal head trauma will prompt

suspicion of *orbital floor "blow-out" fracture* before CN-IV palsy is uncovered.

The amount of force needed to produce traumatic CN-IV palsy seems variable, and, in contradistinction to traumatic CN-III palsy, impact sufficient to produce alteration in consciousness is not required. An acquired trochlear palsy after minor head trauma should still, however, prompt suspicion of an undiagnosed mass lesion, producing a "pathologic" palsy in an already damaged nerve.

Patients with bilateral CN-IV palsy complain of rotational instead of vertical diplopia. Loss of incyclotorsion for both eyes causes images seen by the left eye to rotate clockwise compared with those seen by the right eye. Most patients with bilateral involvement will note occasional vertical diplopia: right eye image above left eye image with left head tilt or rightward gaze, and vice versa. Often, esotropia is seen in downgaze as well, because of loss of the abducting action of the superior obliques. They may adopt a chin-down head position without horizontal tilt.

A lesion interrupting both the predecussation trochlear fasciculus and the ipsilateral central tegmental (pupillary sympathetic) tract within the tectum produces an ipsilateral Horner syndrome with crossed CN-IV palsy. CN-IV palsy has occurred in the setting of idiopathic intracranial hypertension and after lumbar puncture—presumably because of tractional mechanisms—both with CN-VI coinvolvement. It can also occur in conjunction with CN-III involvement in spontaneous intracranial hypotension.

Perhaps because of their relatively fixed location within the lateral wall of the cavernous sinus, the trochlear and trigeminal nerves can be injured concomitantly. Patients with a posteriorly draining carotid–cavernous fistula may present with painful superior oblique dysfunction along with oculomotor nerve palsy, presumably due to local cavernous distention.

Differential Diagnosis

Other entities that produce vertical binocular diplopia with hypertropia may be initially confused with CN-IV palsy; myasthenia gravis is one such mimic. However, the pattern of changing misalignment in different directions of gaze will usually serve to distinguish true trochlear palsies from its simulators.

Restrictive diseases affecting the inferior rectus muscle (such as thyroid-related orbitopathy, orbital floor fracture with entrapment of the muscle, or injury from local anesthetic for cataract surgery) produce vertical diplopia; such diplopia, however, worsens in upgaze. Restrictive disease of the inferior oblique is a far better mimic, as patients would have ipsilateral hyperopia with excyclotorsion and worsening on attempted downgaze.

Injury to the orbital trochlea (through which the superior oblique tendon passes) typically produces *Brown tendon sheath syndrome*, with the eye shooting into downgaze on adduction because the tendon remains tight even when the muscle relaxes; however, on occasion, the injured trochlea will not allow the tendon to retract in response to superior oblique retraction, perfectly simulating CN-IV palsy. History of orbital trauma and trochlear abnormality on orbital imaging will serve to clarify the diagnosis.

Skew deviation due to imbalance of the otolithic inputs to the vestibulo-ocular system can also produce vertical misalignment. In such cases, reclining the patient to a supine position may eliminate the hypertropia.

Diagnostic Approach

Diagnosis of unilateral CN-IV palsy is made when ipsilateral hypertropia is demonstrated to worsen in downward gaze, contralateral gaze, and ipsilateral head tilt. Cases of bilateral trochlear palsies may present the seeming paradox of no hypertropia in primary gaze when the head is straight. However, these patients demonstrate a left hypertropia on right gaze and left head tilt, and right hypertropia on left gaze with a right head tilt.

Blood testing for infection, abnormal clotting, and systemic inflammation is usually done in nontraumatic cases. Patients with isolated CN-IV palsies may be observed for spontaneous improvement over 3–4 months if the history indicates a likely etiology (e.g., trauma or known diabetes); otherwise, neuroimaging is done upon diagnosis. Even in cases with a presumed etiology, nonresolution over time usually prompts imaging unless congenital CN-IV palsy is strongly suggested by history and examination findings (e.g., vertical fusional amplitude greater than 4 diopters and photographic evidence of life-long compensating head tilt).

Management and Therapy

Therapy directed at the cause of CN-IV palsy (when a cause other than trauma can be identified) will be dependent on the pathologic entity encountered. Symptomatic diplopia in nonhealing trochlear palsies may be reduced by the use of prismatic glasses to shift "second images" to line up with primary images. However, the utility of prismatic glasses in CN-IV palsy may be limited because such spectacles do not correct image tilt and because only one prismatic strength can be ground into the spectacles, but different strengths are needed for different gaze directions. Many patients prefer strabismic surgical treatment of nonresolving palsies; it offers correction of excyclotorsion and greater range of gaze without diplopia.

CRANIAL NERVE VI: ABDUCENS

CLINICAL VIGNETTE *A 68-year-old hypertensive, diabetic patient presented with isolated sixth cranial nerve (CN-VI) palsy, manifesting as inability to abduct the involved eye. No imaging was initially requested, given the presumed microvascular etiology. Four days later, the patient developed severe headache, and 2 days after that presented to the emergency room where computed tomographic scan revealed a hemorrhagic pituitary fossa mass.*

Two days later the patient expired due to hyperthermia from hypothalamic compression. It is argued that the sellar hemorrhage was in fact present at the time of the patient's initial symptoms and that this patient represents a case of pituitary apoplexy presenting with painless, isolated CN-VI palsy.

The sixth cranial nerve (CN-VI) innervates a single extraocular muscle, the lateral rectus, which is the primary abductor for the eyes.

The CN-VI nucleus, located just beneath the facial colliculi in the inferior pons, is enveloped by the turning CN-VII fascicular fibers of the facial genu and contains two physiologically—but not topographically—distinct groups of neurons (Fig. 6.5). One group innervates the ipsilateral lateral rectus; the other sends axons across the midline to the contralateral MLF. These latter axons ascend in the MLF to the ventral nucleus of the contralateral CN-III nuclear complex. These internuclear neurons connect the nuclei of CN-VI and -III, producing the almost simultaneous stimulation of the contralateral medial rectus during ipsilateral abducens nerve stimulation to produce lateral horizontal gaze.

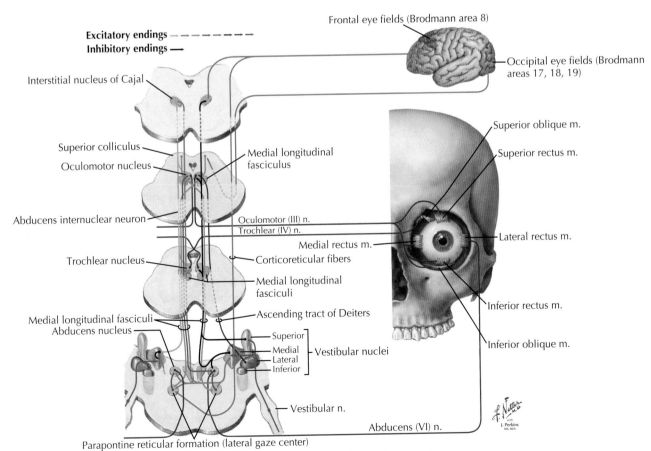

Fig. 6.5 Central Control of Eye Movements.

From its position laterally abutting the paramedian pontine reticular formation, the CN-VI fasciculus first travels medially (toward the MLF, temporarily with the interneuron axons) and then turns ventrally, passing through the paramedian pontine reticular formation and the undecussated corticospinal tract to reach the ventral surface of the brainstem at the inferior lip of the pons.

On exiting the ventral pons, the abducens nerve ascends between the pons and the clivus within the subarachnoid pontine cistern. After it enters the dura, CN-VI continues up the clivus to the posterior clinoid. It travels over the petrous ridge to lie beneath the inferior petrosal sinus and then enters the cavernous sinus via the Dorello canal just medial to the Meckel cave, which houses the gasserian ganglion.

After CN-VI traverses the cavernous sinus, it passes forward, adjacent to the lateral aspect of the ICA. Here, it likely carries the majority of the tertiary sympathetic pupillary axons the short distance from the carotid artery to the ophthalmic branch of the trigeminal nerve. The sympathetics then follow the ophthalmic nerve via its nasociliary branch to the ciliary ganglion; the sympathetic fibers pass through the ganglion without synapsing, entering the eye via the short ciliary nerves. Additional sympathetic fibers bypass the ciliary ganglion, entering the eye as the long ciliary nerves.

Etiology and Pathogenesis

Microvascular palsy, associated with risk factors such as hypertension or diabetes, is the most common cause of acquired, isolated CN-VI palsy. In some cases, advanced age is the only identifiable risk factor and the palsy is considered idiopathic. However, occasionally sixth-nerve palsy will be the presenting sign of other vasculitides such as *temporal arteritis* or treponematosis.

Within the brainstem, cranial nerve palsies can be caused by tumor, stroke, and demyelination. Often, other neurologic signs localizing to the pons will be present, but isolated abducens palsies can be seen.

The sixth nerve has the longest intracranial course of all the cranial nerves. It may suffer compression along this path from tumors at a number of locations, including at the cerebello-pontine angle, the clivus, the petrous bone, and the cavernous sinus. Tumors include acoustic neuroma, meningioma, hemangioma, lymphoma, chondrosarcoma, eosinophilic granuloma, and nasopharyngeal carcinoma, as well as various other carcinomas, both local and metastatic. Midline tumors of the skull base, such as chordoma, can cause bilateral CN-VI palsies by compressing both nerves as they ascend the clivus. Isolated unilateral palsy is, in rare cases, due to abducens schwannoma.

Within the cavernous sinus, the sixth nerve is often involved by disease of the carotid artery, including aneurysm, dissection, dolichoectasia, and carotid–cavernous fistula. The cavernous sinus is also a frequent location of hemangiomas, septic thrombosis, idiopathic inflammation *(Tolosa-Hunt syndrome)*, and metastatic carcinoma that can affect the sixth nerve. Pituitary apoplexy can cause CN-VI palsy by compressing against the cavernous sinus. Often, the other cranial nerves of the cavernous sinus will also be involved, along with the tertiary pupillary sympathetic neurons.

Traumatic CN-VI palsy is seen in the setting of a significant impact, severe enough to cause change of consciousness or bone fracture. CN-VI can also be injured during skull-based neurosurgery and can be seen after percutaneous radiofrequency ablation of CN-V for trigeminal neuralgia.

Vincristine produces CN-VI palsies, presumably from direct neurotoxicity of the nerve. Reports of CN-VI in patients using vitamin A and its analogs probably relate to increased ICP secondary to retinoid-induced pseudotumor cerebri.

Raised ICP alone, whether due to medication, tumor, obstructive hydrocephalus, meningitis, or idiopathic intracranial hypertension, can produce unilateral or bilateral CN-VI palsies. Such abducens palsy is a *falsely localizing sign,* suggesting impinging upon the sixth nerve, when in fact the causative tumor may be remote from the CN-VI territory, or there may be no tumor at all. The course of CN-VI between the internal auditory artery and the anterior inferior cerebellar artery makes it vulnerable to such palsy. As ICP begins to rise, downward brainstem herniation causes stretching of CN-VI, and perhaps compression against either artery. Similarly, downward shift of the pons in relation to the petrous ridge is thought to account for CN-VI palsies sometimes seen in spontaneous or postlumbar puncture intracranial hypotension.

Clinical Presentations

Patients with CN-VI paresis have an inward deviation of the affected eye and a noncomitant esotropia. Temporal eye movement beyond midline is lost or reduced. Patients with partial or mild abducens palsies adopt a posture with the head turned toward the affected side to minimize diplopia by keeping the eye adducted. In more severe palsies, this strategy often fails or is uncomfortable, so patients present with one eye shut, or covered.

The typical patient with microvascular CN-VI palsy will report painless, sudden-onset, horizontal binocular diplopia. Such patients typically show complete, spontaneous resolution within 2–4 months of onset.

Patients with unilateral or bilateral CN-VI palsy from high ICP will present with the symptoms of headache, worsening with recumbency, and visual symptoms ranging from mild dimming to 1–2 seconds of bilateral visual obscurations to profound visual field loss. In cases of *normal pressure hydrocephalus,* gait instability, urinary incontinence, and change in mental status are present. Primary nuclear CN-VI lesions typically have concomitant ipsilateral facial nerve involvement, because of the contact between the abducens nucleus and the genu of the facial fasciculus. For example, stroke of the inferior medial pons produces both ipsilateral gaze palsy and CN-VII as part of *Foville syndrome.* These deficits are accompanied by contralateral hemiplegia from more extensive involvement of the corticospinal tract prior to its decussation.

As Foville syndrome demonstrates, lesions of the CN-VI nucleus do not, in fact, result in clinical CN-VI palsy but rather ipsilateral *gaze palsy* with inability to move both eyes to the affected side. This gaze palsy occurs because the CN-VI nucleus contains both the motor neurons headed for the lateral rectus muscle and the interneurons going to the contralateral third-nerve nucleus via the MLF. The pontine localization of the gaze palsy can be inferred from the finding that such "lower" gaze palsies, in contradistinction to "higher" gaze palsies from frontal lobe disease, cannot be overcome with vestibulo-ocular reflex (e.g., doll's-eyes maneuver), caloric labyrinthine stimulation, or optokinetic stimulation.

Larger lesions affecting the CN-VI nucleus and extending rostrally into the ipsilateral MLF interrupt the crossed internuclear neurons from the opposite CN-VI nucleus coursing up toward the CN-III nucleus, with consequent inability to adduct the ipsilateral eye in horizontal gaze. This combined lesion of ipsilateral gaze palsy and internuclear ophthalmoplegia is known as the *Fisher "one-and-a-half" syndrome:* as with other internuclear ophthalmoplegia variants, convergence (the ability to adduct both eyes simultaneously for near vision) is spared as neither the upper midbrain pathways producing convergence nor the CN-III nuclei are affected.

Paramedian basilar artery branch occlusion causes infarction of the medial and ventral structures of the inferior pons, producing ipsilateral gaze palsy (paramedian pontine reticular formation involvement), hemifacial paralysis (CN-VII), limb ataxia and nystagmus (involvement of middle cerebellar peduncle and possibly vestibular nuclei efferents), crossed paralysis (corticospinal tract), and crossed tactile hypesthesia (medial lemniscus). More focal lesions may produce *Raymond syndrome* (abduction palsy and crossed hemiplegia) from abducens fascicular injury at the corticospinal tract in the basis pontis, whereas similar lesions with some lateral extension also involve the facial fasciculus, adding ipsilateral facial palsy to the presentation (*Millard-Gubler syndrome*).

Anterior inferior cerebellar artery occlusion typically produces more lateral damage characteristically to the vestibular nuclei, the auditory nerve, CN-VII, the paramedian pontine reticular formation, the spinothalamic tract, and the middle cerebellar peduncle and possibly extending dorsally to the cerebellar hemisphere and rostrally to the CN-V nucleus. The combined deficits produce a lateral inferior pontine syndrome of nystagmus (with beats or fast phase directed ipsilaterally), vertigo, gaze palsy, facial paralysis and hypesthesia, deafness, and ataxia, all with crossed body analgesia.

CN-VI, the carotid artery, and sympathetic pupil fibers are situated closely within the cavernous sinus, and an expanding *intracavernous carotid dissection or aneurysm* can compress these structures, producing painful abducens palsy with an ipsilateral Horner syndrome. Other pathologic processes, such as carotid cavernous fistula (CCF) and granulomas within this region sometimes produce a similar clinical picture. Patients with CCF may have additional features of headache, enlarged conjunctival vessels, proptosis, and an audible bruit over the orbit.

Processes that affect the anterior midline brainstem also deserve consideration in the differential diagnosis, including various posterior fossa tumors or inflammatory processes that affect the abducens nerve during its ascent of the clivus. Chordomas, slowly growing tumors that favor the midline skull base, occasionally present as isolated or bilateral CN-VI palsy as do durally based meningiomas.

Gradenigo syndrome is characterized by a painful abducens palsy resulting from mastoiditis and petrositis complicating chronic otitis media. The infectious process erodes the bone, affecting the abducens nerve and the gasserian ganglion and, at times, the CN-VII as it passes through the mastoid bone en route to the stylomastoid foramen. A combined trigeminal-abducens-facial nerve syndrome can be produced by other entities, particularly tumors that affect this region.

Differential Diagnosis

Möbius syndrome is a congenital, bilateral CN-VI and CN-VII palsy. MRI typically shows pontine hypoplasia in the region of the affected CN nuclei. The characteristic elongated, expressionless lower facies of these patients is usually sufficient to suggest the diagnosis, and such patients usually do not have symptomatic diplopia. However, Chiari malformation with syringomyelia can produce a similar, acquired picture.

Duane syndrome, a congenital condition of misdirected CN-III innervation of the lateral rectus, can also simulate abducens palsy. In patients with type I Duane syndrome, attempted lateral gaze reveals lack of abduction. Again, the chief clues to this diagnosis are life-long history and absence of symptomatic diplopia in lateral gaze despite the presence of noncomitant strabismus.

Inability to abduct the eyes, a seeming bilateral CN-VI palsy, can be seen in Wernicke encephalopathy resulting from thiamine depletion. Confusion, confabulation, ataxia, and history of alcoholism suggest the diagnosis, which is confirmed by low serum thiamine levels. Occasionally, sudden onset of esotropia simulating bilateral CN-VI palsy occurs because of divergence palsy, probably due to microvascular ischemia at the putative mesencephalic "divergence center." Spontaneous improvement in 2–3 months is expected. Divergence palsy can be differentiated from the more common, frequently psychogenic, convergence spasm by the miosis that accompanies convergence spasm as in normal close vision.

Myasthenia gravis may simulate CN-VI palsy but can be diagnosed by history of diurnal variation, variable ocular misalignment, presence of serum antibodies to acetylcholine receptors or striated muscle, and positive response to intravenous edrophonium chloride.

Traumatic fracture of the medial orbital wall (the lamina papyracea of the ethmoid sinus) with entrapment of the medial rectus muscle produces a restrictive esotropia that may at first suggest traumatic CN-VI palsy. Similarly, thyroid-related ophthalmopathy, which often preferentially restricts the medial rectus muscle or orbital tumor, may lead to restrictive esotropia and consideration of abducens palsy. *Force duction testing* (see below) will be normal in myasthenia, but positive—the eye resists the attempted movement—in cases of restrictive strabismus. Orbital imaging will confirm restrictive esotropia.

Diagnostic Approach

Complete palsy of CN-VI is usually evident, with examination revealing esotropia that lessens with gaze away from the affected side (direction in which the lateral rectus is usually least active). Abduction of the affected eye past midline is not possible, and the movement from adducted to midline position is slow.

Partial abducens palsies can be subtler, especially as only one muscle, and one plane of eye movement, is affected. Having the patient describe the diplopia will usually clarify that it is the binocular diplopia of ocular misalignment, and not the monocular diplopia or "ghosting" experienced when problems of the eye's optical system (e.g., cataracts) are present. The history should seek to uncover symptoms of myasthenia gravis, thyroid disease, or temporal arteritis, as well as any chronic or ongoing medical conditions that may suggest etiology (e.g., diabetes in microvascular palsies, cancer in compressive or infiltrative ones).

Alternately covering each eye with the patient refixating on a distant object each time will reveal the amplitude of the corrective saccade needed to compensate for the misalignment. This "alternate cover test," repeated in different directions of gaze, will confirm an incomitant (different in different gaze directions) esotropia, worse with ipsilateral horizontal gaze, in the case of abducens nerve palsy. This test will also serve to detect other directions of ophthalmoplegia in cases of multiple nerve involvement.

Forced-duction and *force-generation* testing are used clinically to differentiate paralytic abduction deficit from that due to restriction of the medial rectus muscle. The forced duction test is the passive movement of the eye into the apparently paralytic field of gaze; if the eye moves easily, there is no restriction and the diagnosis of palsy is supported. In the force-generation test for CN-VI palsy, the affected eye is passively adducted, and then the patient is instructed to shift gaze to attempt to abduct the eye. If no significant abducting force can be felt by the examiner, palsy is again suggested.

A screening examination of the other cranial nerves is then made, as structural lesions affecting CN-VI can also affect (depending on location and size of the responsible lesion) CN-II, -III, -IV, -V, -VII, and -VIII. Fundus examination to exclude papilledema is particularly important.

At this point, for patients for whom the history of present illness, past medical history, review of systems, or examination has suggested a specific diagnosis, directed diagnostic tests will be recommended. Chief among these tests is often an MRI of the brain and orbits with gadolinium contrast, and attention to the entire course of CN-VI.

However, for sudden-onset, painless, isolated CN-VI palsy in a patient with known vascular risk factors, a presumptive diagnosis of microvascular CN-VI palsy can be made. If the patient has no obvious risk factors for microvascular cranial mononeuropathy except age, blood pressure testing as well as screening blood tests—complete blood count, hemoglobin A1C, erythrocyte sedimentation rate, angiotensin-converting enzyme titer, and serologies for syphilis and Lyme disease—may be performed. In young patients, imaging will often be added to the initial workup, because of the relative rarity of microvascular disease in this population. Isolated CN-VI palsy with negative neuroimaging that improves spontaneously over 2–3 months is seen in children and can be presumed "viral" in origin.

Traditionally, patients with vasculopathic risk factors who present with a painless CN-VI palsy are given a presumptive microvascular CN-VI diagnosis and are followed expectantly for 2–4 months without imaging. If spontaneous resolution does not occur in that time frame, neuroimaging (MRI, as described above) typically is performed.

Management and Therapy

As with other ocular motor palsies, management of the cause of CN-VI palsy, when one can be identified, will depend on the specific etiology. Therapies may range from strategies to mitigate vasculopathic risk factors in microvascular cases, to neurosurgical interventions for those cases due to tumor, aneurysm, or high ICP.

Therapy for nonhealing CN-VI palsies can include the use of prismatic spectacles or strabismus surgery, both of which are most effective in cases with some preserved abducens function. In cases of persistent total sixth-nerve palsy, muscle-splitting surgery (dissecting out portions of the superior and inferior rectus muscles to fabricate a new abducting extraocular muscle) or vertical muscle transposition surgery can be attempted and frequently result in a good cosmetic and acceptable functional result. At times, however, cases of complete CN-VI palsy will be at last managed by use of a patch or obscuring lens in front of one eye to eliminate binocular diplopia in a dependable, if inelegant, fashion.

THE PUPILS

Examination

The pupillomotor examination is an assessment of two of the three internal motor functions of the eye, pupil constriction and dilation (the third is lens accommodation). The motor assessment is often supplemented by slit-lamp observation of the iris, which may reveal abnormalities of iris structure. Such iris defects can cause abnormalities of pupillary function that are unrelated to any neuropathy.

To examine pupillomotor functions, seat the patient comfortably with his or her gaze directed at a distance (12–20 ft forward). The examiner should position in front, and slightly to one side, so that the pupils may be observed without interrupting the patient's fixation. For examination of the light reflex, the room should be dim, and the examination light bright. The traditional stimulus is the ophthalmologic Finoff scleral transilluminator ("muscle light"), which features a shielded, directed beam of variable brightness, making it ideal for isolated illumination of one eye with minimal "scatter" illumination to the fellow eye. Any nonmedical light source with similar features will do as well.

In dim illumination, the pupil's shape (degree of roundness) is noted, its size is measured, and both are recorded. A "pupil gauge" (a printed card with full- or half-circles of given sizes, usually in 1-mm increments) is helpful, but a simple ruler may also be used. A dimmest-visible slit-beam directed from 45 degrees temporally can also be used to measure the pupil at the slit-lamp biomicroscope, if care is taken to avoid patient fixation on the slit-lamp or examiner. Alternatively, the pupil can be measured in dark conditions using a quantitative (scaled) infrared pupillometer; this device has become much more readily available in recent years because of the need to assess maximum pupil dilation at night in patients considering refractive corneal surgery.

Bright-light stimulus is then applied to one eye, and the pupil response of that eye (*direct response*) is observed. The final size of the pupil in response to light and the speed or briskness of that response is recorded. The normal pupillary light reaction is a brisk, uniform concentric constriction; when the light stimulus is removed, an equally brisk redilation is seen.

When light stimulation is prolonged, normal constriction is followed after about a second by minimal redilation. In some patients, cycles of small-amplitude redilation and reconstriction are seen and are termed *hippus*. Hippus can be quantified clinically: it can often be induced or emphasized with special lighting conditions ("edge lighting" at the slit-lamp), so that the frequency of the redilation/reconstriction cycles can be measured to give a "pupil cycle time" value. A prolonged pupil cycle time may suggest disease of the optic nerve or the pupilloconstrictive neural efferents.

Light stimulus is then applied to one eye while assessing the *indirect pupillary response* in the fellow eye. In healthy individuals, the indirect pupillary response should be clinically equivalent to the direct response. However, in many clinical settings, actual observation of an unilluminated pupil in a dim room is impractical. Instead, the *swinging flashlight test* is generally utilized to better document the indirect response by comparing it to the same eye's direct response.

The swinging flashlight test begins with the light directed to one eye; the direct response is observed. The flashlight is then quickly swung over to the other eye. Normally, the second pupil begins to dilate during the short time that neither is illuminated, but once it is directly stimulated a slight, brisk contraction is seen. If a large contraction or a continued dilation is seen after the flashlight has been swung, a relative afferent pupillary defect (RAPD) is suggested (see below).

Next, the reaction to near is checked; often in the clinical setting, the near reaction is only checked if the light reaction is found to be abnormal. The patient is asked to shift visual attention from the far fixation target to a minimally illuminated near fixation target, perhaps 6–10 inches away. The normal reaction of the pupil to near stimulus is a brisk, uniform constriction that may be of slightly greater amplitude than the light response. When gaze is redirected to the distant target, brisk redilation is normally observed. It should be noted that although the light reaction is involuntary, the near reaction requires voluntary triggering of the near triad and so is dependent on patient alertness, attention, and cooperation.

Notation of the complete clinical pupillary exam then consists of a description of the shape and measurement of the size of the pupil in dim lighting with distance fixation; speed of the reaction (both constriction and redilation) and final size of the light-stimulated pupil; presence (and severity) or absence of a RAPD; and reaction speed and final size of the near-stimulated pupil, especially if the light reaction is abnormal in any way.

Abnormalities of Pupil Function
Iris-Based Abnormalities

Iris abnormality will typically result in abnormal pupillary response. The cause may be a structural one (due to trauma or intrinsic iris degeneration), producing permanent pupil dysfunction, or pharmacologic, producing temporary motor abnormality. When the cause of pupillary dysfunction is an abnormal iris, the examiner will generally find several indications of that cause: irregular anatomic appearance of the iris and pupil, similar dysfunction to light and near stimuli, and inability of pharmacologic agents to produce full function of the iris.

Light Reflex Abnormalities, Afferent Limb

Light is detected at the retina, and the signal is sent via the optic nerve to the brain. Although the majority of visual information is transmitted to the lateral geniculate nucleus, the pupillary afferent fibers reach the pretectal nucleus via an extrageniculate pathway. The input from each eye reaches both the left and right nuclei, so that stimulation of one retina results in both the ipsilateral and contralateral pupillary

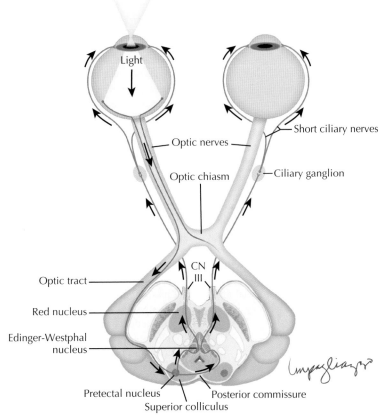

Fig. 6.6 Parasympathetic Pupillary Innervation and the Light Reflex Pathway.

constriction, producing a direct and consensual pupillary response, respectively (Fig. 6.6). Because of this anatomic property, disease of the pupillary afferents, even if unilateral, does not produce pupils that are unequal in size (*anisocoria*).

When the light-stimulated neural signal sent to the pretectal nucleus by one eye is significantly different from the other, an RAPD will result. Clinically, a RAPD is seen during the swinging flashlight test when, rather than "constricting" the affected pupil continues to dilate when the light is swung to that eye, the lack of "constriction" demonstrates that the (abnormal) direct pupillary response in the affected eye is not as strong as the (normal) indirect response produced by stimulating the fellow eye. When the flashlight is swung back to the normal eye, a larger-than-usual constriction is seen, as the direct response in that eye is greater than its consensual response.

It should be noted that a RAPD will only be detected if one eye's afferent system is appreciably more abnormal than that of the fellow eye. When, for example, both eyes have suffered extensive optic atrophy, the eyes will display *light-near dissociation* (absent light response with preserved near response; see below) as well as severe visual loss—but no RAPD.

The reasons for a detectable RAPD are legion. Although mild optical and cataract problems cannot cause a RAPD, a unilateral dark cataract may cause it, especially if the fellow eye has had its cataract removed. Retinal and optic nerve disease are the usual causes and typically can be correlated to defects in central and peripheral vision and to objective structural changes in the funduscopic examination. With complete optic tract lesions causing contralateral complete homonymous hemianopia, the contralateral eye (with temporal visual field loss and "bow-tie" optic atrophy) shows a RAPD, likely because that eye has lost more peripheral field (i.e., the temporal field of each eye is greater than the nasal) and a corresponding greater percentage of optic nerve fibers (53% loss in the contralateral optic nerve vs. 47% loss ipsilaterally).

Rarely, one encounters disease that has affected the extrageniculate pupillary afferent fibers only, after they separate from the geniculate-bound vision fibers. In those cases, the patient will show a clear afferent pupillary defect without any visual defect.

Efferent Limb Abnormalities: Parasympathetic

The pretectal nuclei receive input from both optic nerves, and in turn send efferents to both Edinger-Westphal nuclei. These nuclei send efferent pupilloconstrictive fibers via the oculomotor nerve (CN-III) to the ciliary ganglion, where they synapse with the short ciliary nerves carrying motor efferents to the pupillary sphincter (see Fig. 6.6).

Typically located on the exterior of the nerve, the pupilloconstrictive fibers of CN-III are particularly vulnerable to compression, but relatively resistant to microvascular ischemia (e.g., from diabetes mellitus). Hence, this leads to the classic (but occasionally inaccurate) clinical observation that ischemic CN-III palsies spare the pupil, whereas those due to compression palsies add pupillary dilation to the external oculomotor abnormalities.

Idiopathic, painless loss of pupillary constriction (and lens accommodation) is occasionally seen as an "acute *Adie pupil.*" Over weeks, such patients experience partial recovery of pupillary constriction, but with persistent abnormalities due to incomplete healing and aberrant regeneration. A typical (chronic) *Adie tonic pupil* will be mid-dilated, irregular, with areas of atonic iris sphincter, and showing asynchronous, segmental sphincter contraction (vermiform movement). The pupil shows *light-near dissociation,* with absent light reflex, and slow, strong constriction to near stimulus that persists for many seconds after gaze is redirected to distance (tonic constriction or dilation lag). Similar aberrant regeneration features can also be seen when a compressive, pupil-involving CN-III palsy recovers but absent in the few rare cases of ischemic CN-III palsy with pupillary involvement.

Efferent Limb Abnormalities: Sympathetic

The sympathetic innervation of the pupillary dilator muscle involves a three-chain pathway. The primary neuron runs from the hypothalamus to the ciliospinal center of Budge Waller at the junction of the thoracic and cervical spinal cord; the secondary neuron starts there, crosses over the lung apex and synapses in the superior cervical ganglion; and the tertiary neuron follows the ICA to the cavernous sinus, eventually reaching the eye after passing through the ciliary ganglion without synapsing (Fig. 6.7).

A pupil that has lost its sympathetic innervation will sluggishly redilate when light stimulus is removed (dilation lag), and will not open past mid-dilation even in darkness; in mesopic lighting, it is miotic compared to a normal pupil. The sympathetics innervating the facial arteries, sweat glands, and the Mueller muscle of the lid travel with the pupillary sympathetic; therefore sympathetic-denervation leads to miosis often accompanied by ipsilateral ptosis and hemifacial anhidrosis (Horner syndrome). Hemifacial flushing can also be present (harlequin syndrome).

Light-Near Dissociation

As has already been mentioned, light-near dissociation is the blunting or absence of the pupils' light response while the near response is preserved. Afferent pupil defect and the aberrant regeneration of Adie tonic pupil have already been given as two examples.

Two additional well-known examples will be discussed. The *Argyll Robertson pupil* was at one time a renowned feature of tertiary syphilis. In this condition, the pupils are miotic, irregular, and show absent or minimal reaction to light, but a brisk reaction to near-stimulus, however without the tonicity seen in Adie pupil. It has been proposed that Argyll Robertson pupil is due to a specific lesion of the pathway between the pretectal nucleus and the Edinger-Westphal nucleus, but the exact mechanism remains unknown.

Finally, in *Parinaud dorsal midbrain syndrome,* there is loss of pupillary light reflex, likely due to direct injury to the pretectal nuclei but with sparing of the presumably more ventral structures producing the near-response.

Pupil Abnormalities in Coma

Patients who have suffered intracranial catastrophe can also display characteristic pupillary syndromes. In patients with severe supratentorial edema or hemorrhage, the uncus is forced down upon the tentorial edge, compressing CN-III and producing mydriasis. It is often referred to as a "blown pupil," or *Hutchinson pupil.* The laterality of the mydriasis usually, but not invariably, indicates an ipsilateral location of the responsible mass.

In patients with pontine hemorrhagic stroke, "pontine pinpoint pupils" are encountered. Although very small, close examination, sometimes with a magnifying glass, shows that they do react to light stimulus. However, it should be kept in mind that the findings of miosis with stupor or coma may also suggest opiate poisoning.

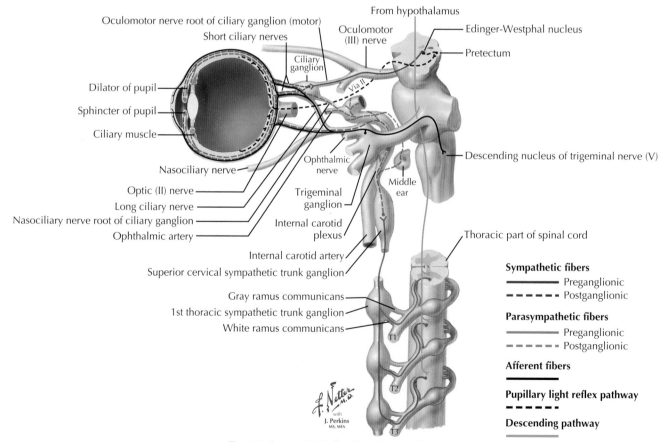

Fig. 6.7 Sympathetic Pupillary Innervation.

Laterality

Systemic disease, toxic exposure, and bilateral ocular or neuropathic conditions will cause bilateral pupillary dysfunction, but the pupils remain equal or show only minimal *anisocoria*. By contrast, obvious anisocoria suggests focal trauma, inflammation, ischemia, or compression (or perhaps topical pharmacologic exposure) as the likely etiology.

When anisocoria is present, the question arises: is the smaller or the larger pupil abnormal? When accompanying external signs are present (i.e., mydriasis with ipsilateral ptosis and loss of medial and vertical external movements such as in CN-III palsy), the answer may be obvious. Otherwise, the abnormal pupil can be determined by comparing the relative anisocoria in dark and light conditions. Anisocoria that is worse in dark conditions suggests a defect of dilation and that the smaller pupil is abnormal; conversely, anisocoria that is worse in bright light suggests the larger pupil is abnormal.

Physiological anisocoria is the term used to describe neurally based anisocoria which is not due to disease. The difference between the pupils is most often 0.5 mm or less, and very rarely exceeds 1 mm. It may vary from day to day. The anisocoria remains fairly constant in differing illumination levels and is eliminated by bilateral administration of topical pharmacologic miotic or mydriatic agents (confirming neural origin—see below).

Unilateral Adie tonic pupil is a fairly common idiopathic cause of anisocoria. When bilateral, it may (with tendon areflexia) form the *Holmes-Adie syndrome,* and investigation for signs of a more generalized dysautonomia, perhaps due to paraneoplastic autoantibodies or spirochetal infection, may be indicated. Bilateral tonic pupil, or even total pupillary areflexia, can be seen in the Miller Fisher variant of Guillain-Barré syndrome.

Pharmacologic Diagnosis of Pupillary Dysfunction

The diagnosis of anisocoria or of bilateral pupillomotor abnormality can be sharpened by the use of topical pharmacologic agents.

Incomplete (or asymmetric) response to standard pharmacologic dilation (phenylephrine 2.5%–10% with tropicamide 1%) suggests an iris structural abnormality, which may be more easily detected at slit-lamp after attempted dilatation. Conversely, incomplete miotic response to pilocarpine 1%–2% may suggest previous pupillary sphincter trauma, or recent exposure to an anticholinergic agent (topically to the eye if unilateral, and perhaps systemically if bilateral).

In contrast, weak mydriatic or miotic agents can be used to highlight denervation supersensitivity when it exists. Within days of sympathetic denervation of the iris, the dilator muscle will exhibit supersensitivity to weak alpha-1 adrenergic agonists (epinephrine 0.1%, phenylephrine 1%, or most recently apraclonidine 0.5%–1%); such agents (or cocaine, below) are often used to distinguish Horner pupil from physiological anisocoria. Similarly, a weak cholinergic agonist (pilocarpine 0.06%–0.12%) can demonstrate the cholinergic supersensitivity found in Adie tonic pupil.

Two additional agents are employed in the diagnosis of Horner pupil. Cocaine 10% solution has the unique property of preventing presynaptic norepinephrine reuptake; because of the steady baseline release of small amounts of norepinephrine into the neuromuscular cleft of the pupillary dilator muscle, the normal response to topical cocaine is pupillary dilatation. When baseline norepinephrine release is absent (because of either absence of the tertiary neuron or its neurochemical silence), cocaine will fail to dilate the Horner pupil.

Topical hydroxyamphetamine 1% causes release of stored presynaptic norepinephrine at the dilator's neuromuscular junction. Therefore lack of dilation in response to hydroxyamphetamine suggests absence of the tertiary neuron, helping to "localize" the lesion in the pupillary sympathetic chain.

FUTURE DIRECTIONS

Current discussions are focused upon developing better paradigms and practice pathways for proper and timely diagnosis of the many varied causes of ocular motor palsies and their mimics. The goal is a balance between exhaustiveness on one hand and cost-efficiency.

ACKNOWLEDGMENT

I am grateful and indebted for the suggestions of Professor Thomas R. Hedges III, MD, on modifying the form and content of this chapter.

ADDITIONAL RESOURCES

Oculomotor

Arle JE, Abrahams JM, Zager EL, et al. Pupil-sparing third nerve palsy with preoperative improvement from a posterior communicating artery aneurysm. Surg Neurol 2002;57:423–6.
Reports pupil-sparing in aneurysmal incomplete CN-III palsy.

Eyster EF, Hoyt WF, Wilson CB. Oculomotor palsy from minor head trauma. An initial sign of basal intracranial tumor. JAMA 1972;220(8):1083–6.
Notes frequent association of CN-III palsy after low-force head trauma with skull-base meningiomas.

Hamilton SR. Neuro-ophthalmology of eye-movement disorders. Curr Opin Ophthalmol 1999;10(6):405–10.
Discusses attempts to reach a best-practices approach to diagnosis of CN-III palsy.

Heinze J. Cranial nerve avulsion and other neural injuries in road accidents. Med J Aust 1969;2(25):1246–9.
Describes avulsion of CN-III and CN-IV nerve roots in trauma.

Lustbader JM, Miller NR. Painless, pupil-sparing but otherwise complete oculomotor nerve paresis caused by basilar artery aneurysm. Case report. Arch Ophthalmol 1988;106(5):583–4.
Presents the only clear case of pupil-sparing in aneurysmal complete CN-III palsy.

Trobe JD. Isolated pupil-sparing third nerve palsy. Ophthalmology 1985;92(1):58–61.
Articulates standard at that time regarding which third-nerve palsies need imaging.

Trochlear

Hara N, Kan S, Simizu K. Localization of post-traumatic trochlear nerve palsy associated with hemorrhage at the subarachnoid space by magnetic resonance imaging. Am J Ophthalmol 2001;132(3):443–5.
Offers MRI evidence regarding the probable locus minoris resistentiae in traumatic CN-IV palsy.

Moster ML, Bosley TM, Slavin ML, et al. Thyroid ophthalmopathy presenting as superior oblique paresis. J Clin Neuroophthalmol 1992;12(2):94–7.
Presents worsening in upgaze as the distinguishing feature of this diagnosis.

Parulekar MV, Dai S, Buncic JR, et al. Head position-dependent changes in ocular torsion and vertical misalignment in skew deviation. Arch Ophthalmol 2008;126(7):899–905.
Suggests that a decreased vertical misalignment with face-up head position in skew deviation can distinguish it from CN-IV palsy.

Abducens

Cushing H. Strangulation of the nervi abducentes by lateral branches of the basilar artery in cases of brain tumour. Brain 1910;33:204–35.
Classic reference regarding the possible mechanism of nonlocalizing CN-VI palsy.

Flanders M, Qahtani F, Gans M, et al. Vertical rectus muscle transposition and botulinum toxin for complete sixth nerve palsy. Can J Ophthalmol 2001;36(1):18–25.
Presents a treatment option for nonhealing CN-VI palsies.

Miller RW, Lee AG, Schiffman JS, et al. A practice pathway for the initial diagnostic evaluation of isolated sixth cranial nerve palsies. Med Decis Making 1999;19(1):42–8.

Articulation of the traditional standard of not initially imaging patients with presumptive vasculopathic CN-VI palsy, based on review of 407 cases.

Ouanounou S, Saigal G, Birchansky S. Möbius syndrome. AJNR Am J Neuroradiol 2005;26(2):430–2.

MRI finding of pontine hypoplasia in Möbius syndrome.

Pilon A, Rhee P, Newman T, et al. Bilateral abducens palsies and facial weakness as initial manifestations of a chiari 1 malformation. Optom Vis Sci 2007;84(10):936–40.

Syringomyelia producing "acquired" Möbius syndrome.

Warwar RE, Bhullar SS, Pelstring RJ, et al. Sudden death from pituitary apoplexy in a patient presenting with an isolated sixth cranial nerve palsy. J Neuroophthalmol 2006;26(2):95–7.

Report of the case used in this section's clinical vignette.

Pupils

Girkin CA, Perry JD, Miller NR. A relative afferent pupillary defect without any visual sensory deficit. Arch Ophthalmol 1998;116(11):1544–5.

Clinical description of a lesion of the extrageniculate pupillary afferent pathway.

Miller SD, Thompson HS. Pupil cycle time in optic neuritis. Am J Ophthalmol 1978;85:635–42.

Description of this clinical test.

Morales J, Brown SM, Abdul-Rahim AS, et al. Ocular effects of apraclonidine in horner syndrome. Arch Ophthalmol 2000;118(7):951–4.

First description of the usefulness of this agent in the diagnosis of Horner pupil.

Thompson HS, Kardon RH. The Argyll Robertson pupil. J Neuroophthalmol 2006;26(2):134–8.

Modern neuro-anatomic review of a classic pupillary syndrome.

Thompson S, Pilley SF. Unequal pupils (a flow chart for sorting out the anisocorias). Surv Ophthalmol 1976;21:45–8.

The diagnostic paradigm that has become a classic.

7

Cranial Nerve V: Trigeminal

Michal Vytopil

CLINICAL VIGNETTE *A 58-year-old retired town clerk presented with a 2-week history of numbness over her left chin and adjacent lower lip as well as vague pain in the left jaw. She explained that the area feels "Novacaine-like," exactly like the sensation she had experienced numerous times recently because of extensive "dental work" requiring mandibular blocks. She reported a 5-year history of lichen planus of her left mandibular gingival mucosa, which was biopsied two or three times over the preceding several years. Two months earlier, she noted swelling and bleeding in the vicinity of one of the left lower molars. She was referred to an endodontist, who extracted the seemingly involved tooth. Because the bleeding and uncomfortable sensation in the area persisted, a biopsy was performed by an oral surgeon; this revealed a well-differentiated squamous cell carcinoma. Computed tomography (CT) of head and neck was requested by the surgeon, but the patient missed her appointments because of her husband's health issues. She otherwise enjoys good health.*

Her exam revealed a 2-cm exophytic, ulcerated lesion in the left lower jaw area where the molar had been extracted. Examination of the cranial nerves demonstrated a quarter-sized area of numbness in the left chin and adjacent left lower lip. CT revealed a gingival mass invading the left mandible. Avid uptake in the mandible was noted on the positron emission tomography (PET) and bone scan images, which were obtained for staging purposes (Fig. 7.1).

Comment: Although seemingly harmless, the complaint of numb chin requires careful evaluation as it is often a harbinger of malignancy. In a patient with known cancer of the facial skin or oral mucosa, as in this vignette, one has to consider invasion of the tumor into the mandible, causing bone destruction and involving the mental or inferior alveolar nerves. Naturally other branches of the trigeminal nerve can be affected by the same locally destructive process, causing numbness in the distribution of the implicated nerves. CT of the facial bones is usually diagnostic.

ANATOMY

The trigeminal cranial nerve (CN V) is a mixed sensory and motor nerve (Fig. 7.2). The sensory component conveys general sensation from the facial skin and scalp to the top of the head, tragus of the ear, and anterior wall of the external auditory meatus (Fig. 7.3). It also provides general sensation from the mouth, including the tongue and teeth, nasal and paranasal sinuses, and meninges lining the anterior and middle cranial fossae. The motor portion of the trigeminal nerve supplies motor fibers to the muscles of mastication.

Sensory Nucleus

The **sensory nucleus** of the CN V is a large complex that begins rostrally within the midbrain and extends caudally through the pons and medulla into the second segment of the cervical spinal cord (Fig. 7.4). It is subdivided into three portions: (1) the *spinal tract nucleus,* primarily dedicated to pain and temperature fibers; (2) the *principal sensory nucleus*—the pontine trigeminal portion—which primarily receives tactile stimuli and therefore principally subserves light touch; and (3) the *mesencephalic sensory nucleus,* which contains cell bodies of sensory fibers carrying proprioceptive information from the masticatory muscles.

Trigeminal (Gasserian, Semilunar) Ganglion

The cell bodies of sensory CN V fibers are located within the trigeminal ganglion. This is contained within a skull-base depression, the *Meckel cave,* located near the apex of petrosal bone in the middle cranial fossa. Central processes of the neuronal cell bodies constitute the large sensory root that enters the pons and projects into the trigeminal sensory nucleus. Peripheral processes of the sensory neurons leave the trigeminal ganglion to form three sensory divisions (ophthalmic, maxillary, and mandibular) that, respectively, exit the skull through the superior orbital fissure, the foramen rotundum, and the foramen ovale (Fig. 7.5).

Sensory Divisions

The **ophthalmic division** collects touch, pain, temperature, and proprioceptive information from the upper third of the face, including the top of the nose, adjacent sinuses, and scalp regions. These nerve branches course posteriorly in the orbit toward the superior orbital fissure, where they enter the skull.

The **maxillary division** carries sensory information from the skin overlying the maxilla, side of the forehead, medial cheek and side of the nose, upper lip, palate, upper teeth, nasopharynx, and meninges of the anterior and middle cranial fossae.

The **mandibular division** primarily provides sensory innervation for the skin overlying the lower jaw (with the exception of the angle of the jaw innervated by both the second and third cervical nerves), cheeks, chin and lower lip, mucous membrane of the mouth, gums, inferior teeth, anterior two-thirds of the tongue, side of the head, anterior wall of the external auditory meatus, external wall of the tympanic membrane, and temporomandibular joint.

Motor Component

The *motor nucleus,* originating within the mid-pons, receives its major input from primary proprioceptive neurons in the mesencephalic subnucleus, creating a monosynaptic reflex arch similar to spinal reflexes; it can be assessed by eliciting the jaw jerk. Motor nucleus axons exit the pons as the motor root passing through the trigeminal ganglion and exiting the skull via the foramen ovale. Extracranially, motor fibers join the sensory mandibular division and provide innervation to the muscles of mastication: the masseter, temporalis, medial and lateral pterygoid, mylohyoid, and anterior digastric muscles.

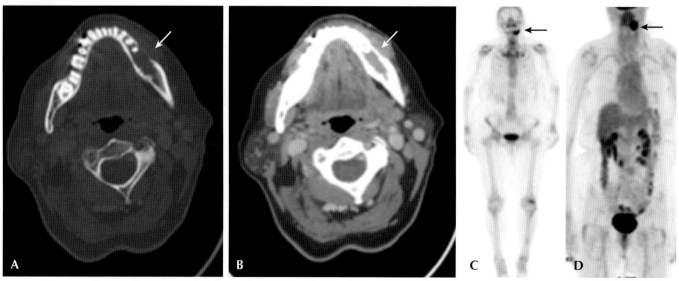

Fig. 7.1 Numb Chin Syndrome. Images of axial bone windows (A) and soft tissue windows (B) reveal a gingival squamous cell carcinoma invading the mandible *(arrows)*. Avid uptake is noted on positron emission tomography (C) and bone scan (D).

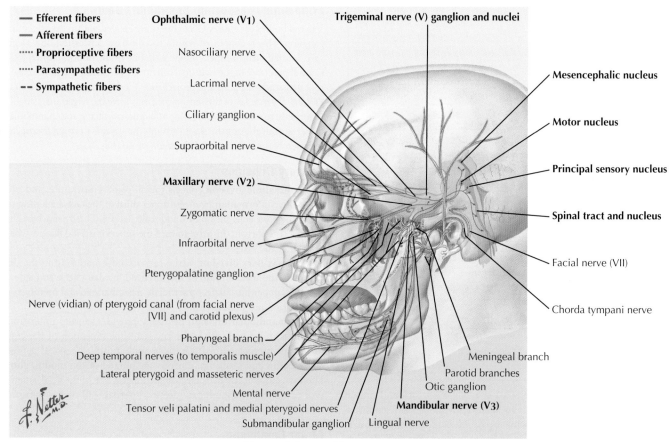

— Efferent fibers
— Afferent fibers
····· Proprioceptive fibers
····· Parasympathetic fibers
-- Sympathetic fibers

Ophthalmic nerve (V1)
Nasociliary nerve
Lacrimal nerve
Ciliary ganglion
Supraorbital nerve
Maxillary nerve (V2)
Zygomatic nerve
Infraorbital nerve
Pterygopalatine ganglion
Nerve (vidian) of pterygoid canal (from facial nerve [VII] and carotid plexus)
Pharyngeal branch
Deep temporal nerves (to temporalis muscle)
Lateral pterygoid and masseteric nerves
Mental nerve
Tensor veli palatini and medial pterygoid nerves
Submandibular ganglion

Trigeminal nerve (V) ganglion and nuclei
Mesencephalic nucleus
Motor nucleus
Principal sensory nucleus
Spinal tract and nucleus
Facial nerve (VII)
Chorda tympani nerve
Meningeal branch
Parotid branches
Otic ganglion
Mandibular nerve (V3)
Lingual nerve

Fig. 7.2 Schema of Trigeminal Nerve.

CN V LESIONS

Clinical Presentation and Diagnostic Approach

Trigeminal neuralgia is the most common disorder affecting the fifth cranial nerve, as discussed in Chapter 21.

Most trigeminal neuropathies are sensory, manifesting with facial numbness with or without pain. Patients with this complaint may have a lesion at any site along the trigeminal nerve's sensory pathway. To determine precisely which portion of the trigeminal nerve complex is affected, the examiner must initially test sensation within the distribution of each of the three major divisions. The cutaneous area over mandibular angle is supplied by upper cervical roots and not by the trigeminal nerve; this is a useful anatomic detail if one seeks to distinguish between trigeminal neuropathy and other (i.e., central or

Sensory distribution of trigeminal (V) nerve

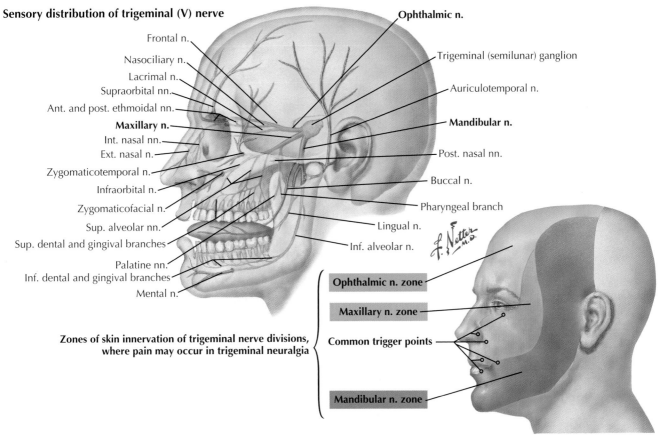

Ophthalmic n.
Frontal n.
Nasociliary n.
Lacrimal n.
Supraorbital nn.
Ant. and post. ethmoidal nn.
Maxillary n.
Int. nasal nn.
Ext. nasal n.
Zygomaticotemporal n.
Infraorbital n.
Zygomaticofacial n.
Sup. alveolar nn.
Sup. dental and gingival branches
Palatine nn.
Inf. dental and gingival branches
Mental n.

Trigeminal (semilunar) ganglion
Auriculotemporal n.
Mandibular n.
Post. nasal nn.
Buccal n.
Pharyngeal branch
Lingual n.
Inf. alveolar n.

Ophthalmic n. zone
Maxillary n. zone
Common trigger points
Mandibular n. zone

Zones of skin innervation of trigeminal nerve divisions, where pain may occur in trigeminal neuralgia

Fig. 7.3 Trigeminal Sensory Components.

Posterior phantom view

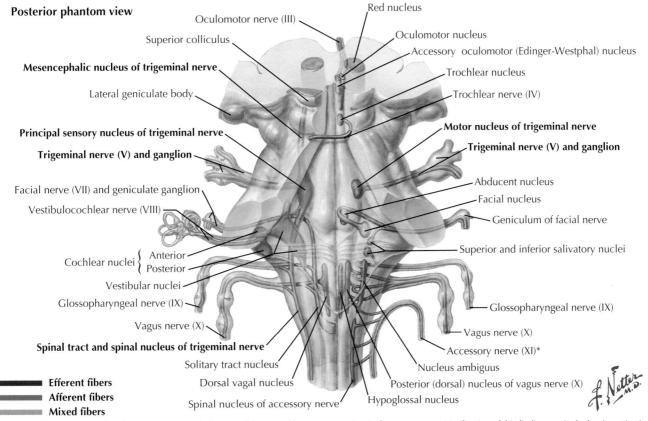

Oculomotor nerve (III)
Superior colliculus
Mesencephalic nucleus of trigeminal nerve
Lateral geniculate body
Principal sensory nucleus of trigeminal nerve
Trigeminal nerve (V) and ganglion
Facial nerve (VII) and geniculate ganglion
Vestibulocochlear nerve (VIII)
Cochlear nuclei { Anterior / Posterior
Vestibular nuclei
Glossopharyngeal nerve (IX)
Vagus nerve (X)
Spinal tract and spinal nucleus of trigeminal nerve
Solitary tract nucleus
Dorsal vagal nucleus
Spinal nucleus of accessory nerve

Red nucleus
Oculomotor nucleus
Accessory oculomotor (Edinger-Westphal) nucleus
Trochlear nucleus
Trochlear nerve (IV)
Motor nucleus of trigeminal nerve
Trigeminal nerve (V) and ganglion
Abducent nucleus
Facial nucleus
Geniculum of facial nerve
Superior and inferior salivatory nuclei
Glossopharyngeal nerve (IX)
Vagus nerve (X)
Accessory nerve (XI)*
Nucleus ambiguus
Posterior (dorsal) nucleus of vagus nerve (X)
Hypoglossal nucleus

███ **Efferent fibers**
███ **Afferent fibers**
███ **Mixed fibers**

*Recent evidence suggests that the accessory nerve lacks a cranial root and has no connection to the vagus nerve. Verification of this finding awaits further investigation.

Fig. 7.4 Schema of Cranial Nerve Nuclei in Brainstem.

Ophthalmic (V₁) and Maxillary (V₂) Nerves, Sensory

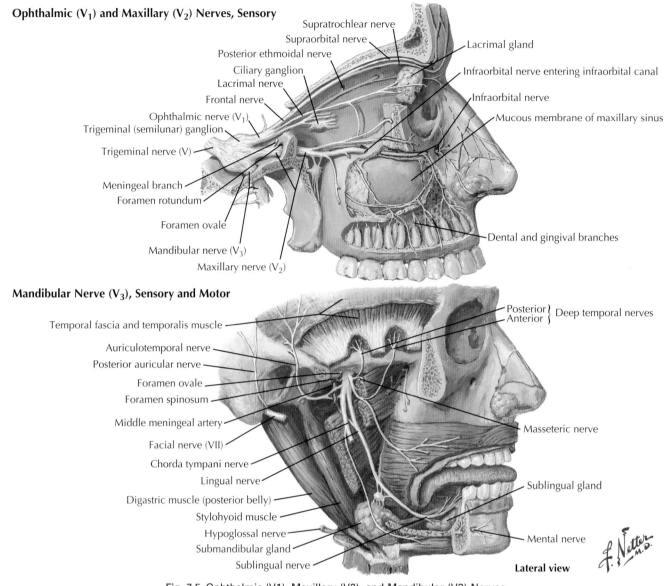

Ophthalmic (V₁) and Maxillary (V₂) Nerves, Sensory

Supratrochlear nerve
Supraorbital nerve
Posterior ethmoidal nerve
Ciliary ganglion
Lacrimal nerve
Frontal nerve
Ophthalmic nerve (V₁)
Trigeminal (semilunar) ganglion
Trigeminal nerve (V)
Meningeal branch
Foramen rotundum
Foramen ovale
Mandibular nerve (V₃)
Maxillary nerve (V₂)

Lacrimal gland
Infraorbital nerve entering infraorbital canal
Infraorbital nerve
Mucous membrane of maxillary sinus
Dental and gingival branches

Mandibular Nerve (V₃), Sensory and Motor

Temporal fascia and temporalis muscle
Auriculotemporal nerve
Posterior auricular nerve
Foramen ovale
Foramen spinosum
Middle meningeal artery
Facial nerve (VII)
Chorda tympani nerve
Lingual nerve
Digastric muscle (posterior belly)
Stylohyoid muscle
Hypoglossal nerve
Submandibular gland
Sublingual nerve

Posterior } Deep temporal nerves
Anterior }
Masseteric nerve
Sublingual gland
Mental nerve

Lateral view

Fig. 7.5 Ophthalmic (V1), Maxillary (V2), and Mandibular (V3) Nerves.

factitious) causes of facial numbness. Rarely, involvement of the spinal trigeminal nucleus within the rostral cervical cord can lead to facial numbness. The somatotopic organization of the nucleus explains why perioral areas are represented more rostrally within the nucleus and areas more removed from the mouth more caudally. Both general and special sensation to the tongue and palate are necessary for fully functional taste. Impairment of general sensation from the tongue and palate carried by CN V may cause taste disturbances, even though the special sensory fibers providing primary taste sensation are supplied by the facial and glossopharyngeal nerves. Motor trigeminal neuropathy causing masticatory weakness is often very difficult to test when the change is subtle. Normally both lateral pterygoid muscles pull the jaw forward. When there is a unilateral motor fifth nerve lesion, the healthy unopposed pterygoid pushes the jaw across the midline, thus leading to a deviation of the jaw to the side of the paretic motor fifth. In a case of more chronic motor trigeminal neuropathy, one can, after asking the patient to bite down forcefully, look for visible neuron atrophy of temporalis and masseter muscles on the affected side.

Examination of the *corneal reflex* and *jaw jerk* provides useful clinical tools. Application of a wisp of cotton to the cornea normally leads to

an eye blink provided that the facial nerve is intact. Asymmetric corneal responses or unilateral loss of this reflex provides objective evidence of a lesion involving the afferent sensory arc of the blink reflex, which is constituted by the ophthalmic division of CN V. The jaw reflex consists of contraction of the masseter and temporalis muscles in response to a gentle tap on the chin. In contrast to the corneal reflex, in which the efferent arm is subserved by the facial nerve, both afferent and efferent arms of the jaw reflex are supplied by trigeminal nerve fibers traveling in the mandibular division; the mesencephalic nucleus processing the proprioceptive information is where the two arms relay. A lesion anywhere along this pathway may depress the jaw jerk. A brisk jaw reflex, on the other hand, points to upper motor neuron dysfunction; in a patient with an atrophic tongue, brisk jaw jerk is often an ominous sign raising the specter of motor neuron disease.

Differential Diagnosis

Facial trauma, or rarely invasive **dental treatments,** accounts for the majority of trigeminal nerve injuries. CN V divisions and branches are exposed to **trauma** especially from **fractures of facial bones** within the face and neck. Dental pathology such as tooth abscesses as well as invasive dental procedures including wisdom tooth extraction and dental anesthetic injections may injure the lingual or inferior alveolar nerves. Typically these injuries lead to anesthesia and neuropathic pain within the specific distribution of whichever trigeminal branch is compromised.

In the Western world, *Herpes zoster* is the most common infectious cause of a trigeminal neuropathy, almost always affecting the ophthalmic division. *Herpes zoster ophthalmicus* occurs when latent varicella zoster virus infection within the trigeminal ganglion becomes reactivated. Most patients present with a characteristic periorbital vesicular rash and severe neuralgic pain within the ophthalmic division. Similar to other herpes zoster syndromes, the pain may precede the eruption of cutaneous lesions. Keratitis with subsequent scarring may lead to permanent visual impairment, the most serious outcome of ophthalmic zoster infection. Antiviral agents such as acyclovir, ideally started within 72 hours of onset, are the main therapy. Corticosteroid eye drops have been shown to decrease pain and hasten corneal healing and are sometimes considered by ophthalmologists. Postherpetic neuralgia (PHN), defined as persistence of pain for months after the rash has healed, develops in 10%–15% of patients. Patients over the age of 70 and those with severe rash and pain during the initial infection are at a higher risk of PHN. Early administration of antivirals reduces the risk of this intractable pain syndrome. Vaccination against herpes zoster is an effective means of decreasing the risk of both shingles and PHN. Rarely, infarction of the ipsilateral middle cerebral artery may be seen in these patients as a manifestation of central nervous system (CNS) vasculitis. The virus travels within the trigeminal nucleus and the adjacent intracavernous portion of the carotid artery or its branches, with resulting development of an inflammatory granulomatous angiitis of the brain. Cerebrospinal fluid (CSF) varicella zoster virus antibodies and a positive polymerase chain reaction (PCR) for viral antigen are frequently seen in this condition.

Worldwide, leprosy, or *Hansen disease,* is a more common cause of CN V neuropathy. This occurs primarily in economically depressed countries and generally affects the coolest areas of the skin. Thus, if sensory loss is confined to the tip of the nose or the pinna of the ear, Hansen disease is a primary consideration (Box 7.1).

The ophthalmic division may be involved within the wall of the *cavernous sinus* by a variety of processes, most often thrombosis of the sinus. Resultant numbness in the distribution of the first division of the trigeminal nerve is typically accompanied by various combinations of CN III, IV, and VI involvement as well as proptosis and conjunctival chemosis.

Middle ear infection leading to osteomyelitis of the petrous bone apex may present with a combination of otorrhea as well as trigeminal and abducens neuropathies (**Gradenigo syndrome**).

Trigeminal sensory neuropathy occurs when the trigeminal ganglion cell bodies are the primary pathologic target. Although the pathogenesis of this ganglionopathy is frequently unknown, an association with connective tissue disorders—particularly scleroderma, mixed connective tissue, and Sjögren syndrome—is recognized (Fig. 7.6). It is presumed that circulating autoantibodies attack the ganglion cells, as the blood-brain barrier here is more permeable to large molecules than is the blood-nerve barrier elsewhere in the nervous system. Numbness typically begins around the mouth and spreads slowly to involve other CN V divisions; the maxillary division is most frequently involved. The numbness may precede symptoms of systemic rheumatologic diseases. In Sjögren syndrome, trigeminal neuropathy is usually part of a more widespread sensory ganglionopathy. Other causes of unilateral or bilateral trigeminal neuropathy are sarcoidosis and rarely amyloidosis. The latter has been described to induce neuralgic pain mimicking tic doloreux.

BOX 7.1 Differential Diagnosis of CN V Lesion Origin

Brainstem: stroke, brainstem gliomas, multiple sclerosis, or syringobulbia

Intracranial: trigeminal neuroma, acoustic neuroma, meningioma, granuloma, amyloidoma, metastasis, herpes zoster, carotid or basilar aneurysms, trigeminal sensory neuropathy

Skull base lesions: metastasis, nasopharyngeal carcinoma, lymphoma, basilar meningitis

Trigeminal divisions and nerve branches: trauma, metastasis, spreading skin tumor, salivary tumor, vasculitis, leprosy (Hansen disease)

The possibility of *metastatic neoplasm* infiltrating a branch of CN V must always be considered in the differential diagnosis of persistent facial numbness or pain. Tumors involving the face and oral mucosa—such as *squamous cell carcinoma, melanoma, and microcystic adnexal (sweat gland) carcinoma*—have a proclivity for invading cutaneous nerves because of their innate neurotropism. Skull base tumors, such as **nasopharyngeal carcinoma** or **metastatic disease,** may directly invade various trigeminal divisions.

Primary trigeminal neuromas are rare, usually benign, well-demarcated, and slowly growing neoplasms. Most frequently these tumors arise near the trigeminal ganglion, usually extending into the middle and posterior cranial fossae. Rarely, they arise exclusively from one of the sensory divisions and spread extracranially. Rare instances of malignant schwannomas originating within the trigeminal ganglion also occur. Most neuromas have very slow growth, presenting with gradually developing numbness and paresthesias. Rarely, these sensory findings are accompanied by other neurologic symptoms resulting from damage to adjacent structures. For example, tumors growing downward into the posterior fossa may lead to cerebellar ataxia and lesions of CN VII and CN VIII, manifesting with facial palsy, tinnitus, or hearing loss. In contrast, neuromas exert pressure upward on the lateral wall of the cavernous sinus, leading to CN II, III, IV, and VI lesions.

Cerebellopontine angle tumors, typically vestibular schwannomas (acoustic neuromas) arising from CN VIII (Fig. 7.7), may enlarge and compress the trigeminal sensory root and lead to facial numbness or pain with subsequent ipsilateral loss of the corneal reflex. Other neoplasms include meningiomas, epidermoids, lymphomas, hemangioblastomas, gangliocytomas, chondromas, and sarcomas.

The **numb chin syndrome (NCS)** consists of unilateral and less often bilateral numbness of the chin and adjacent lower lip. Although NCS can be due to noncancerous causes—including dental procedure, dental abscess, connective tissue disease, and trauma—it is more often an ominous sign of primary or metastatic cancer involving the mandible, skull base, or meninges. Breast cancer and lymphoma, followed by prostate carcinoma and leukemia, are the malignancies most often associated with NCS. Direct invasion of the mandible by a local tumor, as described in the earlier vignette, can be seen with squamous cell carcinoma, melanoma, or myeloma. Indolently expanding numbness caused by perineural extension of a neurotropic tumor, most often squamous cell carcinoma, is an infrequent but important consideration in patients with a known history of facial skin or oral cancer. Of the benign etiologies, one of the more interesting causes of numb chin is salivary gland biopsy, typically utilized for the confirmation of Sjögren disease. Some primary trigeminal neuropathies defy specific definition and thus are labeled *idiopathic.* However, it is important to emphasize the need for a vigilant approach with frequent follow-up, especially in patients with prior known facial malignancies such as squamous cell cancer or melanoma.

Varicella-zoster with probable keratitis

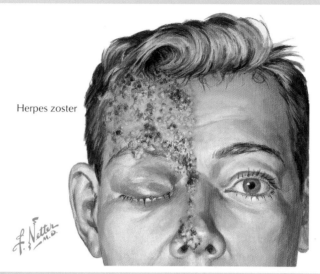

Herpes zoster

Progressive systemic sclerosis (scleroderma)

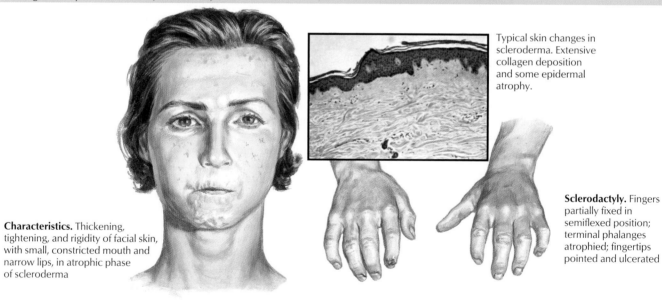

Typical skin changes in scleroderma. Extensive collagen deposition and some epidermal atrophy.

Characteristics. Thickening, tightening, and rigidity of facial skin, with small, constricted mouth and narrow lips, in atrophic phase of scleroderma

Sclerodactyly. Fingers partially fixed in semiflexed position; terminal phalanges atrophied; fingertips pointed and ulcerated

Fig. 7.6 Trigeminal Nerve Disorders.

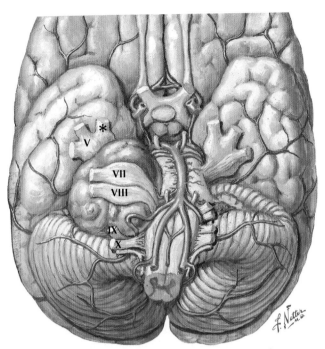

Large acoustic neurinoma filling cerebellopontine angle, distorting brainstem and cranial nerves V, VII, VIII, IX, X

Fig. 7.7 Acoustic Neuroma Compressing Trigeminal Nerve.

ADDITIONAL RESOURCES

Hughes RAC. Diseases of the fifth cranial nerve. In: Dyck PJ, Thomas PK, Griffin JW, et al, editors. Peripheral neuropathy. 3rd ed. Philadelphia, PA: WB Saunders Co; 1993. p. 801–17.

Oxman MN, Levin MJ, Johnson GR, et al. A vaccine to prevent herpes zoster and postherpetic neuralgia in older adults. N Engl J Med 2005;352: 2271–84.

The placebo arm of this randomized trial demonstrated that 18.5% of patients older than 70 developed PHN, in contrast to only 6.9% of those between 60 and 69.

Gonella MC, Fischbein NJ, So YT. Disorders of trigeminal system. Semin Neurol 2009;29, Number 1.

Comprehensive review of disorders of trigeminal nerve.

Smith RM, Hassan A, Robertson CE. Numb chin syndrome. Curr Pain Headache Rep 2015;19:44.

Practical and clinically oriented review of numb chin syndrome.

Gwathmey KG. Sensory neuronopathies. Muscle Nerve 2016;53(1):8–19.

8

Cranial Nerve VII: Facial

David P. Lerner, Michal Vytopil

CLINICAL VIGNETTE *A 62-year-old judge became aware of subtle weakness of his left lower face that he first noted while shaving. Two months later, he noted that he could no longer close his left eyelid fully and was having increasing weakness of the remainder of his left face. He was referred to a neurologist, who reassured him that he had a "benign" Bell palsy. He sought a second opinion when his facial weakness continued to worsen over another month with an inability to close the eye and to form a symmetric smile.*

Neurologic examination demonstrated weakness in all divisions of the left CN VII with total inability to close his eye or form a left-sided smile. Palpation of the cheek demonstrated some fullness in the left parotid gland, with the remainder of his head and neck examination being normal. Complete neurologic and otoscopic examinations were unremarkable. Audiologic test results were normal, including the left acoustic/stapedius reflex. A corneal reflex was sluggish on the left but present bilaterally.

A left parotid gland biopsy demonstrated a malignant adenocarcinoma with extension beyond the capsule at surgery. He died of metastatic cancer 20 months later.

Comment: Fortunately, this case represents a relatively rare occurrence. However, it emphasizes that what may initially look routine and benign indeed may have a much more serious pathophysiologic mechanism. The issue in this case is to appreciate the history of a gradual evolution of the neurologic deficits in contrast to the relatively acute onset of idiopathic Bell palsy. Furthermore, Bell palsy is typically preceded by retroauricular pain and often associated with hyperacusis and loss of taste on the anterior two-thirds of the tongue. When these symptoms are lacking, as in this instance, the pathoanatomic site is distal to the styloid foramen and potentially within the parotid gland as the facial nerve passes through its body. In addition, the gradual progression of this patient's symptoms provided a strong suspicion of a neoplasm.

Facial nerve (CN VII) lesions are the most common cranial mononeuropathy. This is one of the most complex cranial nerves with multiple functions (Fig. 8.1). It has a long and somewhat circuitous course with four primary components: (1) *motor fibers,* which constitute the major division and serve the primary function of CN VII: innervating the muscles of facial expression (unilateral, complete facial weakness is the hallmark of almost all facial neuropathies); (2) *autonomic fibers,* which are responsible for lacrimal, salivary, and mucous secretions; (3) *special sensory fibers,* which provide taste from the anterior two-thirds of the tongue; and (4) *general sensory fibers,* which innervate the external auditory canal and a small area behind the ear.

When a patient presents with facial weakness, differentiation should be made between peripheral facial nerve lesions and central nervous system (CNS) processes. With the latter, when the patient is relaxed, subtle suggestions of a facial nerve lesion may be appreciated by nasolabial fold flattening on the affected side. Brain lesions—such as cerebral infarction, tumor, inflammation, or demyelination—are often associated with other findings that can help with localization. For example, a small lesion near the Broca area may result in motor aphasia and facial weakness. Larger lesions affecting a significant portion of a hemisphere, as with large hemispheric strokes, cause a constellation of symptoms, including face, arm, and leg weakness and sensory loss; gaze deviation; and neglect or aphasia. Disruption of the posterior limb of the internal capsule results in face, arm, and leg weakness without sensory, visual, or cognitive changes. Although peripheral facial weakness involves the upper and lower part of the face to the same degree, **upper motor neuron lesions** typically present with a gradient of weakness (Fig. 8.2), with relative preservation of movement in the brow and forehead (orbicularis oculi and frontalis muscles, respectively). This is due to presumed dual hemispheric innervation of the forehead muscles. In addition, corticobulbar tract involvement, as in various suprabulbar palsies, leads to absence of *voluntary* facial movement but retained reflexive movements, as in response to emotional stimuli.

ANATOMY

Intrapontine Portion

CN VII consists of two primary roots (see Fig. 8.1). The larger division carries **somatic motor fibers** and has its origin within the facial nucleus in the caudal pons, where it lies adjacent to the spinal tract of the trigeminal nerve (CN V). It then passes dorsally and rostrally to curve around the abducens nerve (CN VI) nucleus (internal genu) and exits the brainstem at the bulbopontine angle between CN VI and CN VIII. Its smaller component, the **nervus intermedius** (intermediate nerve of Wrisberg), contains a combination of **autonomic, special sensory (taste),** and **general sensory** fibers. Its preganglionic parasympathetic fibers arise from the superior salivatory nucleus, relay through the pterygopalatine and submandibular ganglions, and eventually provide efferent function for lacrimation and salivation. The remaining intermediate nerve fibers carry taste and general somatic sensation and have their primary cell bodies in the geniculate ganglion and ultimately terminate within the nucleus solitarius and the spinal tract of CN V, respectively.

Peripheral CN VII

Both roots of CN VII leave the brainstem to enter the temporal bone via the internal auditory meatus, where they accompany the auditory nerve (CN VIII) passing through the internal auditory canal (see Fig. 8.1, *bottom*). CN VII continues to the periphery through the facial canal; this segment has five parts, based on their relation to surrounding anatomic structures. (1) The **labyrinthine segment** passes above the labyrinth and leads anterolaterally to the **geniculate ganglions,** which contain the cell bodies of CN VII afferents. (2) At this site, the canal

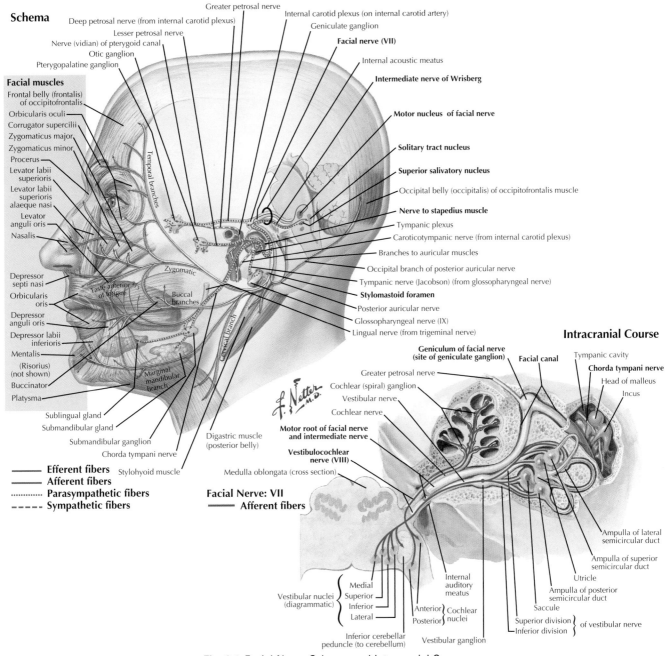

Schema

Greater petrosal nerve
Deep petrosal nerve (from internal carotid plexus)
Internal carotid plexus (on internal carotid artery)
Lesser petrosal nerve
Geniculate ganglion
Nerve (vidian) of pterygoid canal
Facial nerve (VII)
Otic ganglion
Internal acoustic meatus
Pterygopalatine ganglion
Intermediate nerve of Wrisberg

Facial muscles
Frontal belly (frontalis) of occipitofrontalis
Motor nucleus of facial nerve
Orbicularis oculi
Corrugator supercilii
Solitary tract nucleus
Zygomaticus major
Zygomaticus minor
Superior salivatory nucleus
Procerus
Levator labii superioris
Occipital belly (occipitalis) of occipitofrontalis muscle
Levator labii superioris alaeque nasi
Nerve to stapedius muscle
Levator anguli oris
Tympanic plexus
Nasalis
Caroticotympanic nerve (from internal carotid plexus)
Branches to auricular muscles
Zygomatic
Occipital branch of posterior auricular nerve
Depressor septi nasi
Taste anterior ⅔ of tongue
Tympanic nerve (Jacobson) (from glossopharyngeal nerve)
Orbicularis oris
Buccal branches
Stylomastoid foramen
Depressor anguli oris
Posterior auricular nerve
Depressor labii inferioris
Glossopharyngeal nerve (IX)
Mentalis
Lingual nerve (from trigeminal nerve)
(Risorius) (not shown)
Cervical branch
Buccinator
Platysma
Marginal mandibular branch

Sublingual gland
Submandibular gland
Submandibular ganglion
Digastric muscle (posterior belly)
Chorda tympani nerve

——— **Efferent fibers**
——— **Afferent fibers**
Stylohyoid muscle
·········· **Parasympathetic fibers**
– – – **Sympathetic fibers**

Intracranial Course

Geniculum of facial nerve (site of geniculate ganglion)
Facial canal
Tympanic cavity
Greater petrosal nerve
Chorda tympani nerve
Cochlear (spiral) ganglion
Head of malleus
Vestibular nerve
Incus
Cochlear nerve
Motor root of facial nerve and intermediate nerve
Vestibulocochlear nerve (VIII)
Medulla oblongata (cross section)

Facial Nerve: VII
——— **Afferent fibers**

Ampulla of lateral semicircular duct
Ampulla of superior semicircular duct
Utricle
Ampulla of posterior semicircular duct
Internal auditory meatus
Saccule
Medial
Vestibular nuclei (diagrammatic)
Superior
Inferior
Lateral
Anterior } Cochlear
Posterior } nuclei
Superior division } of vestibular nerve
Inferior division
Inferior cerebellar peduncle (to cerebellum)
Vestibular ganglion

Fig. 8.1 Facial Nerve Schema and Intracranial Course.

abruptly turns posteriorly and forms the ***external genu of CN VII.*** (3) The ***greater petrosal nerve*** originates here; it carries preganglionic parasympathetic fibers to the pterygopalatine ganglion, where they synapse and subsequently direct postganglionic fibers to the lacrimal gland. (4) The ***tympanic segment*** of CN VII travels posteriorly and laterally along the medial wall of the middle ear. At the posterior wall of the middle ear, the facial canal changes its course and travels inferiorly toward its exit at the stylomastoid foramen. (5) The vertical portion is named the ***mastoid segment*** and has two important branches: proximally, the *stapedius nerve* arises to innervate the stapedius muscle; more distally, the *chorda tympani* branches and exits the facial canal and, after traversing the middle ear, joins the lingual nerve belonging to the third division of CN V. The chorda tympani contains preganglionic parasympathetic fibers that synapse within the submandibular ganglion to innervate the submandibular and sublingual glands. The chorda

tympani also carries taste fibers. Their cell bodies originate within the geniculate ganglion, mediating taste sensation from the anterior two-thirds of the tongue.

Soon after leaving the skull at the stylomastoid foramen, the distal CN VII gives rise to several small motor branches innervating the posterior auricular, occipital, digastric, and stylohyoid muscles (see Fig. 8.1, *top*). The ***main motor trunk of CN VII*** then passes through the parotid gland to terminate as the temporal, zygomatic, buccal, mandibular, and cervical branches. The first two innervate the muscles involved in moving the forehead, closing the eyes, and wrinkling the nose. Muscles of the lower face and neck are primarily innervated by the latter two branches. CN VII subserves all muscles of facial expression except the levator palpebrae superioris; therefore, CN VII impairment, with a resultant asymmetric facies, is a major social and cosmetic impediment.

Hyperacusis

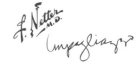

Left Peripheral VII Facial Weakness

Attempt to close eye results in eyeball rolling superiorly exposing sclera (Bell phenomenon) but no closure of the lid per se.

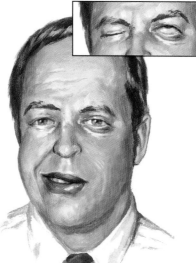

Left Central VII Facial Weakness

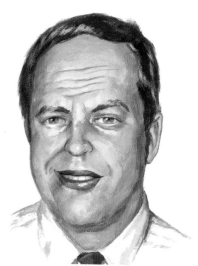

This may be early or initial symptom of a peripheral VII nerve palsy: patient holds phone away from ear because of painful sensitivity to sound. Loss of taste also may occur on affected side.

Patient unable to wrinkle forehead; eyelid droops very slightly; cannot show teeth at all on affected side in attempt to smile; and lower lip droops slightly.

Incomplete smile with very subtle flattening of affected nasolabial fold; relative preservation of brow and forehead movement.

Fig. 8.2 Central Versus Peripheral Facial Paralysis.

CLINICAL CORRELATIONS AND ENTITIES

The facial nerve can be damaged at any level along its complex course. Paralysis of the facial musculature is the hallmark of CN VII lesions regardless of the lesion's anatomic site. The clinical presence or absence of symptoms related to the various other components of the facial nerve is very important in identifying the lesion site.

The patient with a *peripheral CN VII* palsy, in most instances with the exception of an early very distal branch lesion within the parotid gland, loses function of the entire ipsilateral side of their face and cannot smile, close the eyelid (orbicularis oculi), or wrinkle (frontalis) the forehead on that side.

When *intrapontine* (Fig. 8.3, #1) lesions affect the facial motor nucleus per se as well as its exiting fibers, involvement of neighboring brainstem structures is typically seen. The association of peripheral facial paralysis with ipsilateral conjugate gaze palsy (paramedian pontine reticular formation lesion), ipsilateral lateral rectus palsy (CN VI lesion), or paresis of the opposite arm and leg (corticospinal tract lesion) usually indicates a pontine localization.

Extramedullary lesions (see Fig. 8.3, #2) affecting CN VII as it enters its intracranial course primarily occur within the cerebellopontine (CP) angle. Most commonly, these are benign, relatively large acoustic neuromas that initially involve CN VIII and later extend to produce a CN VII dysfunction. Thus, diminished hearing, sometimes initially presenting with tinnitus, usually precedes the onset of this type of peripheral facial paresis (Fig. 8.4). Occasionally, with very large CP angle tumors, there is concomitant involvement of the ipsilateral CN V (the trigeminal nerve) with unilateral facial numbness or initially only loss of the corneal reflex due to afferent dysfunction.

A relatively *proximal pregeniculate, intracanicular facial nerve* lesion (see Fig. 8.3, #3) characteristically leads to diminished lacrimation from greater petrosal nerve involvement as well as hyperacusis (an increased sensitivity to sound that is particularly noticeable while using a telephone); these effects are due to associated stapedius muscle paresis. Such lesions also lead to diminished salivation, absent or altered taste sensation for the anterior two-thirds of the tongue, and affected somatic sensation for the external auditory canal.

When a facial nerve lesion is more distally situated, *between the geniculate ganglion and the stapedius nerve,* all the previously noted findings occur but lacrimation is spared, as the greater petrosal nerve has already exited the geniculate ganglion. If damage occurs in the *facial canal,* involvement of the *stapedius nerve and the chorda tympani* (see Fig. 8.3, #4) leads to hyperacusis and impaired salivation and taste but no change in lacrimation. When the CN VII lesion is *distal to the chorda tympani,* it is characterized by a pure ipsilateral facial weakness (see Fig. 8.3, # 5). Very rarely, a lesion of this type occurs after the facial nerve exits the skull through the stylomastoid foramen. On occasion, this can cause diagnostic difficulty early on as it may initially involve just individual motor branches, with limited weakness of individual facial muscles before a complete palsy develops. Facial trauma is the most common cause of acute pure motor CN VII lesions; however, an insidious progressive course suggests that a parotid adenocarcinoma, as illustrated in the clinical vignette on p. 92 is the most likely cause.

CLINICAL VIGNETTE *A vigorous 18-year-old woman awakened with a mild dull ache behind her left ear. While washing her face she noted an inability to smile on that side and that her left eyelid could not close. As her grandparent had recently had a stroke presenting with facial weakness, she rushed to the local emergency room for immediate physician evaluation. Her clinical examination demonstrated that she was unable to smile, close her eyelid, or wrinkle the forehead on the left. Her left eye was slightly injected*

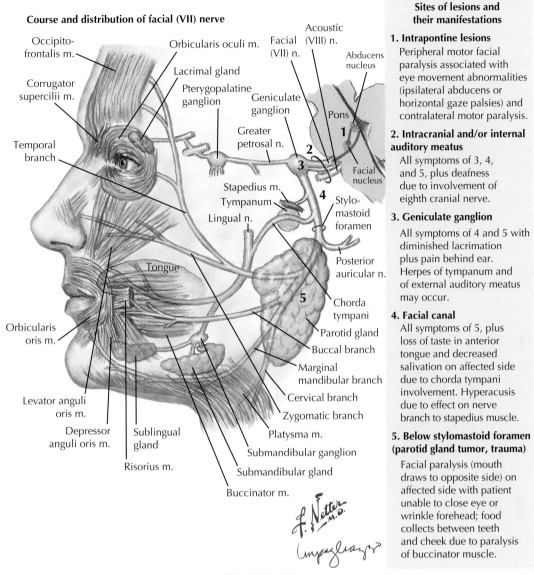

Course and distribution of facial (VII) nerve

Occipito-frontalis m.

Corrugator supercilii m.

Temporal branch

Orbicularis oculi m.

Lacrimal gland

Pterygopalatine ganglion

Geniculate ganglion

Greater petrosal n.

Facial (VII) n.

Acoustic (VIII) n.

Abducens nucleus

Pons

Facial nucleus

Stapedius m.

Tympanum

Lingual n.

Tongue

Orbicularis oris m.

Levator anguli oris m.

Depressor anguli oris m.

Sublingual gland

Risorius m.

Buccinator m.

Submandibular gland

Submandibular ganglion

Platysma m.

Cervical branch

Zygomatic branch

Marginal mandibular branch

Buccal branch

Parotid gland

Chorda tympani

Posterior auricular n.

Stylo-mastoid foramen

Sites of lesions and their manifestations

1. Intrapontine lesions
Peripheral motor facial paralysis associated with eye movement abnormalities (ipsilateral abducens or horizontal gaze palsies) and contralateral motor paralysis.

2. Intracranial and/or internal auditory meatus
All symptoms of 3, 4, and 5, plus deafness due to involvement of eighth cranial nerve.

3. Geniculate ganglion
All symptoms of 4 and 5 with diminished lacrimation plus pain behind ear. Herpes of tympanum and of external auditory meatus may occur.

4. Facial canal
All symptoms of 5, plus loss of taste in anterior tongue and decreased salivation on affected side due to chorda tympani involvement. Hyperacusis due to effect on nerve branch to stapedius muscle.

5. Below stylomastoid foramen (parotid gland tumor, trauma)
Facial paralysis (mouth draws to opposite side) on affected side with patient unable to close eye or wrinkle forehead; food collects between teeth and cheek due to paralysis of buccinator muscle.

Fig. 8.3 Bell Palsy.

and dry secondary to diminished tearing. She had no taste sensation on the anterior of the left tongue. The remainder of her neurologic examination was normal. No imaging studies were indicated.

A diagnosis of idiopathic Bell palsy was made; this patient was most relieved not to have had a stroke. As she lived in an endemic area for Lyme disease, specific antibodies were obtained before she was discharged on oral prednisone treatment. Over the next 2 months, she experienced a gradual and total return of her facial muscle function.

Comment: This is a classic case of idiopathic Bell palsy with no associated neurologic dysfunction or any specific evidence of systemic disorders predisposing to a facial nerve lesion. However, when the patient lives in an endemic Lyme disease region, it is reasonable to check Lyme-specific antibodies before corticosteroids are prescribed.

Idiopathic Facial Palsy (Bell Palsy)

The preceding vignette describes a benign, idiopathic facial palsy. The lesion had a proximal location, denoted by the loss of total motor function on one side of the patient's face involving the frontalis, orbicularis oculi, and the lower facial muscles, as well as loss of stapedius muscle action, taste, and lacrimal gland function.

Bell palsy is one of the most common and distinctive entities in clinical neurology. Typically, patients present with an acute unilateral partial weakness of all mimetic muscles that evolves over several hours to no more than a few days, at times leading to complete facial paralysis. Although Bell palsy is usually benign, its dramatic appearance initially creates in many individuals a major concern that they may have had a stroke and that permanent facial disfigurement will result.

Rare instances of direct examination of the facial nerve in the setting of Bell palsy have shown signs of edema with subsequent nerve compression within the facial canal and resultant ischemia and nerve fiber degeneration. There is evidence to support reactivation of latent herpes simplex or varicella-zoster virus (VZV) infection arising within the geniculate ganglion as the cause in a large proportion of common idiopathic cases of Bell palsy.

Clinical Presentation

In retrospect, a preceding dull ache behind the ipsilateral ear is a common initial sign. Patients usually first become aware of weakness per se when

Preoperative tumor compressing CN VII, VIII (not visualized)

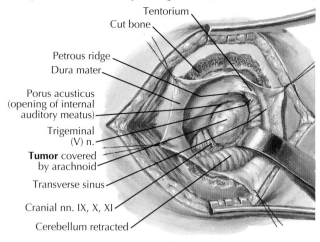

Tentorium
Cut bone
Petrous ridge
Dura mater
Porus acusticus
(opening of internal
auditory meatus)
Trigeminal
(V) n.
Tumor covered
by arachnoid
Transverse sinus
Cranial nn. IX, X, XI
Cerebellum retracted

Postoperative tumor bed revealing CN VI, VIII

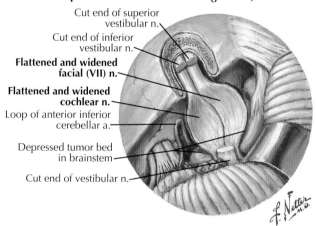

Cut end of superior
vestibular n.
Cut end of inferior
vestibular n.
**Flattened and widened
facial (VII) n.**
**Flattened and widened
cochlear n.**
Loop of anterior inferior
cerebellar a.
Depressed tumor bed
in brainstem
Cut end of vestibular n.

Fig. 8.4 Cerebellopontine Angle Tumor.

a family member points out facial asymmetry or when the individual personally notes an inability to close an eye or experiences difficulty holding saliva, food, and fluids in the affected side of the mouth. Less commonly, decreased taste or hyperacusis is the first symptom.

Facial asymmetry is unequivocally present; the affected frontalis is smooth and cannot be normally corrugated, whereas the angle of the mouth appears depressed even in repose. Inability to completely close the eyelids (lagophthalmos) results from orbicularis oculi weakness. The Bell phenomenon refers to the eyeball turning up without eyelid closure despite attempted contraction of the orbicularis oculi (see Fig. 8.2). Facial palsy accompanied by taste disturbances may help to distinguish whether the lesion is proximal or distal to the chorda tympani branch. For example, a pure motor lesion suggests a lesion at the distal part of the facial canal or within the parotid gland, whereas when all four primary functions are affected, an unusually proximal lesion is deduced.

Differential Diagnosis

The examiner must first differentiate between an upper or a lower motor neuron facial paralysis. Patients with upper motor neuron paralysis primarily have lower facial weakness with an asymmetric smile or unilateral drooling, whereas the upper face is relatively spared. In peripheral facial palsy, all musculature innervated by CN VII is affected.

Lyme disease is the primary identifiable infectious etiology that may present with an acute facial palsy; subsequently, a contralateral lesion

may develop. Typically, there are other neurologic signs such as headache or radiculitis and cerebrospinal fluid (CSF) pleocytosis. In the uncommon circumstance of a Bell palsy associated with VZV infection (Ramsay-Hunt syndrome), facial paralysis often precedes the appearance of typical herpetic vesicles within the external auditory canal. Middle ear infection can rarely damage the facial nerve as it travels through the petrous bone. In regions endemic to tuberculosis, facial nerve palsies in association with petrous bone or mastoid process infections have been described.

Bilateral sequential Bell palsies are the most common neurologic manifestation of sarcoidosis. Frequently associated hypothalamic–pituitary axis dysfunction (particularly impotence in men) and other cranial neuropathies are also present. Simultaneous bilateral facial weakness is an initial presentation of Guillain-Barré syndrome, which is soon followed by the more classic rapidly progressive polyradiculoneuropathy. Leprosy may lead to bilateral facial nerve lesions but with a unique patchy distribution.

A slowly progressive evolution of a unilateral facial palsy most typically suggests the presence of a neoplasm. Pontine lesions, especially **brainstem gliomas** (Chapter 49), are the most proximal cause for a peripheral facial weakness. These tumors usually present in conjunction with other signs, such as a lateral rectus palsy. Extramedullary tumors originating near the brainstem are often associated with facial nerve lesions and other cranial neuropathies, as with CN VIII acoustic neuromas or other **CP angle tumors** (see Fig. 8.4). When there is diffuse **leptomeningeal** involvement, as with metastatic carcinoma or lymphoma, the facial nerves may be part of the initial clinical profile of infiltration with these malignancies. Eventually other and often multiple cranial nerves become involved, particularly the trigeminal, oculomotor, and optic nerves. As noted in vignette on p. 92, evolving, progressive, and purely motor facial palsies presenting with varying degrees of individual facial muscle involvement are classic for a **parotid malignancy** (Fig. 8.5).

Treatment

Corticosteroids reduce the duration of paralysis and risk of permanent impairment. The typical regimen is 1 mg/kg of oral prednisone (or equivalent corticosteroid) up to 60 mg/day, but only if it can be initiated within the first 3 days. Treatment is continued for 5 days and then tapered by 10-mg decrements over each of the next 5 days. This leads to much earlier recovery, presumably by decreasing nerve swelling within the tight facial canal and thus diminishing nerve injury. There is no consistent evidence that antiviral medications, such as acyclovir or valacyclovir, shorten the course or improve outcome in Bell palsy when used alone. However, it is possible that combined therapy with steroids may be beneficial, and valacyclovir 1000 mg, three times a day for 1 week is used for severe idiopathic facial palsy. Although occasionally advocated, there is insufficient evidence to suggest that surgical CN VII decompression is effective.

During the period of facial paralysis with incomplete eye closure, great care is required to protect the exposed cornea, which is subject to trauma from simple things such as turning over in bed and dryness. Eye patching and artificial tears during the day and a lubricant eye gel at night are usually sufficient to prevent corneal abrasions.

Prognosis

The severity of the underlying facial nerve injury determines how quickly and completely recovery from Bell palsy occurs. The degree of injury ranges from mild, with pure demyelinating conduction block, to severe, with axonal loss and resulting wallerian degeneration. Up to 90% of Bell palsy cases are caused by a demyelinating conduction block with little or no associated axonal loss; therefore, recovery is prompt, complete, and without synkinesis. The remaining patients have axonal damage

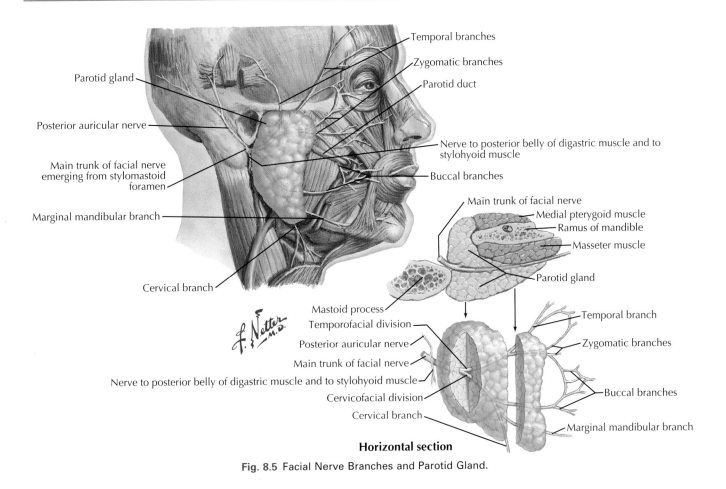

Labels: Parotid gland — Posterior auricular nerve — Main trunk of facial nerve emerging from stylomastoid foramen — Marginal mandibular branch — Cervical branch — Temporal branches — Zygomatic branches — Parotid duct — Nerve to posterior belly of digastric muscle and to stylohyoid muscle — Buccal branches — Main trunk of facial nerve — Medial pterygoid muscle — Ramus of mandible — Masseter muscle — Parotid gland — Mastoid process — Temporofacial division — Posterior auricular nerve — Main trunk of facial nerve — Nerve to posterior belly of digastric muscle and to stylohyoid muscle — Cervicofacial division — Cervical branch — Temporal branch — Zygomatic branches — Buccal branches — Marginal mandibular branch

Horizontal section

Fig. 8.5 Facial Nerve Branches and Parotid Gland.

with wallerian degeneration, and improvement requires regenerating axons to reinnervate paralyzed muscles, resulting in a slow and incomplete recovery.

The recovery rate from Bell palsy follows two patterns: most patients begin to regain facial strength within 3 weeks after onset, but in some patients, the initiation of recovery is delayed for at least 3–6 months. The overall prognosis is good; most patients (80%–85%) recover completely, but the rest may have various residual effects. These include synkinesis, residual weakness, tearing, or contracture. Synkinesis, the most frequent permanent sequela, clinically manifests as synchronized movement of different muscles that normally do not contract together. Typically, there is subtle eye closure with smiling or a lip or chin twitch with blinking. Synkinesis occurs when there is a misdirection of regenerating axons into muscles that they originally did not innervate. This is rarely disabling but can be disfiguring and cause involuntary eye closure at inopportune times. Botulinum toxin injections have emerged as a symptomatic treatment of these abnormal movements. Another rare phenomenon following recovery of facial nerve injury is excessive lacrimation while eating ("crocodile tears") and results from aberrant regeneration of salivatory fibers to the lacrimal glands.

Electromyography (EMG) provides valuable prognostic information, especially in those individuals not beginning to demonstrate improvement within the first few months after onset of Bell palsy. It should never be performed until approximately 3 weeks after onset. By then, it is possible to distinguish between nerve fibers that have undergone wallerian degeneration and those that are only temporarily blocked. A significantly reduced amplitude of the facial nerve compound muscle action potential and abundant fibrillation potentials in facial muscles indicate severe axonal damage, whereas a demyelinating conduction block is typically partially resolved by that time, evidenced by absent or scarce fibrillation potentials.

Infectious Facial Palsies
Varicella-Zoster Virus

The Ramsay-Hunt syndrome, caused by reactivation of the VZV within the geniculate ganglion, is the second most common cause of atraumatic facial palsy. Clinically, it is characterized by the triad of acute facial palsy, neuralgic pain, and the eruption of herpetic vesicles within the external auditory canal, ipsilateral palate, and anterior two-thirds of the tongue. The areas of pain and rash are appropriate to the general sensory innervation of the afferent facial nerve branches. The geniculate ganglion cell bodies host the latent VZV infection. The close proximity of the geniculate ganglion to the vestibulocochlear nerve in the bony facial canal explains the concomitant otologic symptoms, such as tinnitus, vertigo, and hearing loss in some patients. The detection of VZV immunoglobulin M (IgM) antibody in blood and CSF, or VZV DNA in CSF, saliva, or blood, is often helpful in assigning a viral etiology.

The prognosis for Ramsay-Hunt syndrome is worse than that of idiopathic Bell palsy, with frequent complete paralysis, incomplete recovery, and residual synkinesis. Therefore aggressive treatment with acyclovir (30 mg/kg IV daily or 4000 mg PO daily in divided doses) or valacyclovir 1000 mg three times daily is indicated. A course of prednisone similar to the one used for Bell palsy is probably reasonable, although no evidence-based data exist to support this treatment. The best long-term results are obtained when treatment is started within 3 days of onset.

Lyme Disease

> **CLINICAL VIGNETTE** *Five weeks after returning from her family's summer home in Old Lyme, Connecticut, this 32-year-old woman presented with left facial drooping and arm pain. Three days prior, she had woken up with severe pain behind the neck shooting down her right arm to the thumb. She noted difficulty holding a coffee mug to her lips.*
>
> *Her temperature was 38°C (100.6°F). There was a 10-cm circular rash on the medial aspect of her right thigh. Her neck was slightly rigid; no intra-auricular vesicles were noted. Neurologic examination results demonstrated severe left facial weakness associated with loss of taste. On attempted eye closure, her left eyelids remained 6 mm apart. Her right biceps, brachioradialis, and pronator teres were weak. The right brachioradialis reflex was absent.*
>
> *Brain computed tomography (CT) results were unremarkable. Lumbar puncture revealed a white blood cell count of 23/mm³, primarily lymphocytes, with a normal protein level and a slightly decreased glucose level. CSF and serum Lyme antibody test results were positive.*
>
> *Comment: This vignette is typical of facial palsy secondary to Lyme disease (neuroborreliosis). At times, as in this case, facial weakness occurs with concomitant, often very painful, nerve root lesions. Although relatively uncommon, this classic syndrome of Lyme meningoradiculitis should always be considered, particularly in endemic areas.*

Facial paralysis is the most common focal manifestation of neuroborreliosis; 40% of these patients have cranial neuropathies, and approximately 80% have CN VII involvement. Multiple cranial nerves are affected in one-fifth of those with a cranial neuropathy; two-thirds with multiple cranial neuropathies primarily have bilateral facial palsy. Patients with an acute facial palsy in the presence of systemic signs, such as erythema migrans, or a history of possible exposure to disease-transmitting ticks warrant further studies for neuroborreliosis.

Standard CSF analysis usually demonstrates a pleocytosis with lymphocytic predominance. Confirmatory studies include titers of anti–*Borrelia burgdorferi* antibodies and polymerase chain reaction detection of bacterial DNA in blood and CSF. Western blot improves sensitivity of serologic studies by identifying the specific antigens against which the patient generates antibodies. Facial paralysis may also occur before seroconversion (i.e., early in the disease before antibody testing results become positive). When clinical suspicion of Lyme disease is high, follow-up serologic tests are indicated.

Optimal treatment is still debated; the use of intravenous antibiotics is appropriate in severe cases with manifestations such as headache or radiculitis, in the presence of CSF pleocytosis, or when parenchymal brain or cord involvement is suspected. The typical regimen consists of ceftriaxone (2 g/day) or cefotaxime (6 g/day) for 2 weeks. In mild cases with an isolated facial neuropathy, oral doxycycline (200 mg/day) for 2 weeks is felt to be an acceptable option. Once this condition has been treated, the prognosis of facial palsy in Lyme disease is excellent, with most patients recovering completely.

Other Infections

Peripheral facial paralysis may occur with infectious mononucleosis caused by Epstein-Barr virus and poliomyelitis caused by an enterovirus.

Infectious conditions involving the temporal bone can cause peripheral facial paralysis, such as acute and chronic otitis media and osteomyelitis of diverse etiologies, including tuberculosis and syphilis. Acute bacterial and particularly tuberculous meningitis may affect multiple cranial nerves including CN VII. Leprosy is a common cause of facial palsy in endemic areas.

Granulomatous Disorders

Sarcoidosis is a disease of unknown etiology characterized by histopathologic findings of non-necrotizing granulomas within multiple organs. Unilateral or bilateral CN VII palsy with hyperacusis and dysgeusia, thought to result from granulomatous meningitis, is the most frequent neurologic manifestation. The prognosis is favorable, and most patients recover completely after steroid treatment.

Wegener granulomatosis is a systemic disease characterized by necrotizing granulomatous lesions of the upper and lower respiratory tract, glomerulonephritis, and systemic necrotizing vasculitis. Of the primary systemic vasculitides, only Wegener granulomatosis is associated with a significant frequency of cranial neuropathies. CN VII involvement, usually occurring in conjunction with other cranial neuropathies, may reflect granulomatous invasion of the temporal bone or granulomatous basilar meningitis. The 2-year fatality rate of untreated Wegener granulomatosis is greater than 90%, and aggressive immunotherapy is warranted immediately upon diagnosis.

Traumatic Facial Palsy

> **CLINICAL VIGNETTE** *A 40-year-old man was brought to emergency room after being hit by a motorcycle while crossing a busy street. He received a blow to the forehead as he fell to the pavement and was knocked unconscious for 2 minutes. In the emergency room, he complained of headache and decreased hearing on the right side. Urgent ear-nose-throat evaluation found fresh blood in the right meatus and a ruptured tympanic membrane. Neurologic exam demonstrated incomplete right peripheral facial weakness and loss of taste over the right anterior two-thirds of the tongue. High-resolution CT of the skull base revealed a transversely oriented fracture through the petrous bone as well as right hemotympanum, pneumocephalus, and occipital soft tissue swelling. The patient was treated conservatively, with complete resolution of the hearing loss and facial weakness within 3 months.*
>
> *Comment: This is a rather typical case of traumatic incomplete facial paralysis and thus has a good prognosis, in contrast to those who present with complete loss of facial nerve function.*

Nearly all patients with facial palsy after blunt head trauma have a temporal bone fracture. Concomitant damage to CN VIII, cochlea, labyrinth, or middle ear structures may produce hearing loss and vestibular dysfunction. Contusion, compression, and edema of CN VII have all been proposed as possible mechanisms of traumatic facial paralysis. Some of these processes can evolve gradually and lead to delayed facial palsy after several days. Immediate and complete facial palsy often indicates that the nerve has been transected and portends a poor prognosis for functional recovery. In such cases surgical exploration should be considered. Conversely, patients with incomplete weakness and with early signs of improvement, similar to the one in this vignette, usually achieve good recovery within months with conservative management alone.

Neoplasms

Several primary and metastatic malignancies may cause a facial palsy. Carcinomatous meningitis usually affects multiple cranial nerves; the most common sources are the lung, the breast, gastrointestinal cancers, and lymphomas. Typically these tumors have an aggressive clinical course; those that present with an isolated CN VII lesion soon demonstrate signs of multiple cranial or spinal nerve root involvement or both.

Certain benign tumors may exert chronic extrinsic pressure on the facial nerve. Schwannomas from the vestibular portion of CN VIII, typically occurring within the acoustic meatus at the CP angle, or less commonly meningiomas at similar sites, affect CN VII very gradually over time. When they eventually do so, they tend to predominantly and subtly affect sensory fibers over the motor fibers, which are more resilient to chronic deformation. Therefore, the only sign of early CN VII involvement may be relatively minor numbness behind the ear, on the floor of the ear canal, in the posteroinferior quadrant of the eardrum (Hitzelberger sign), or a combination of these. The change in hearing, however, usually leads to the diagnosis. Signs of a motor CN VII lesion do not occur until these lesions become large.

Malignant distal infiltration of CN VII is seen with parotid tumors (see Fig. 8.5).

Uncommon Mass Lesions

Cholesteatomas are rare mass lesions at the CP angle that deserve consideration in patients with slowly evolving facial paralysis. Other uncommon entities include pontine gliomas, arachnoid cysts, lipomas, and hemangiomas (Fig. 8.6).

Neuromuscular Disorders With Facial Weakness

The motor portion of the CN VII nucleus as well as the respective brainstem nuclei of CN V, IX, X, XI, and XII may be involved in various motor neuron diseases, particularly amyotrophic lateral sclerosis and bulbospinal muscular atrophy (Kennedy disease).

CN VII is affected in 33%–50% of cases of Guillain-Barré syndrome and often bilaterally. Although usually evident when limb weakness is severe, CN VII lesions may develop at any stage, including as the presenting sign. The Miller-Fisher syndrome, a variant of Guillain-Barré syndrome, is characterized by ophthalmoplegia, ataxia, and areflexia. However, involvement of cranial nerves other than CN III, IV, and VI occurs in many cases. Facial weakness has been reported in nearly half the cases of Miller-Fisher syndrome, underscoring the important clinical overlap between classic ascending Guillain-Barré syndrome and Miller-Fisher syndrome.

Neuromuscular junction disorders (NMJDs), particularly myasthenia gravis (MG), often lead to bifacial weakness. This is a common finding in the majority of MG patients where there is associated ptosis and extraocular muscle involvement. Interestingly, although some patients with the less common Lambert-Eaton myasthenic syndrome have diplopia, ptosis, dysphagia, and dysarthria, facial nerve weakness is not found in this presynaptic NMJD.

Some primary myopathies may cause bilateral facial weakness, typically accompanied by wasting. In adult-onset myotonic dystrophy, muscles innervated by CN III and CN V, such as the levator palpebrae superioris and the temporalis, are also involved. Therefore, ptosis and jaw weakness often also occur. Congenital myotonic dystrophy may present with bilateral facial diplegia and is sometimes associated with severe neonatal hypotonia. Facial weakness occurs in 95% of patients with facioscapulohumeral (FSH) dystrophy who are younger than 30 years. It affects predominantly the orbicularis oris and is often asymmetric. Although facial weakness is rarely the presenting problem, most patients with FSH dystrophy reveal long histories of difficulties in whistling or blowing balloons. Therefore, facial involvement is likely to be an early, slowly progressing sign.

An additional neurodegenerative disease that can present with bilateral lower motor neuron facial weakness is gelsolin amyloidosis. This is a progressive neurocutaneous disorder that results in gelsolin amyloid deposition in the cornea, skin, and the cranial nerves. It commonly presents with paresis of the area innervated by the upper branch of the facial nerve followed by progression to the area innervated by the lower branches. Although initially reported in families of Finnish descent, the disease is recognized throughout the world and is the result of point mutations in the gelsolin gene, resulting in misfolding, abnormal cleavage, and ultimately deposition of the protein.

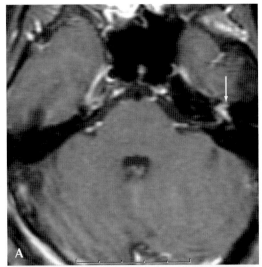

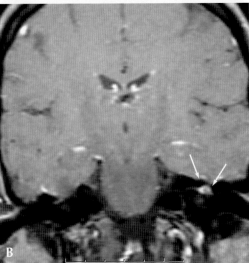

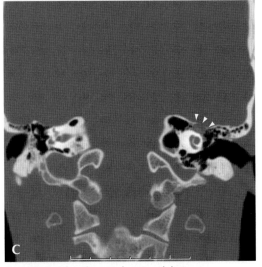

A and **B,** Axial and coronal post-gadolinium-enhanced, T1-weighted, fat-saturated MR images demonstrate enlargement and enhancement of the geniculate ganglion (thin arrows). **C,** Coronal thin section CT of petrous bone shows smooth enlargement of the geniculate region (arrowheads).

Fig. 8.6 Seventh Nerve Hemangioma.

Facial onset sensory motor neuropathy (FOSMN) syndrome is a rare progressive neuromuscular disease that presents with sensory loss with upper and lower motor neuron impairment that begins in the face and spreads to include the scalp, neck, and upper arms. With the combination of upper and lower motor neuron dysfunction, FOSMN may share pathophysiology with other neurodegenerative disorders such as amyotrophic lateral sclerosis.

Recurrent CN VII Palsy

Recurrence occurs in approximately 10% of Bell palsy cases, a circumstance necessitating careful diagnostic evaluation to exclude underlying causes, especially neoplasms and basilar meningeal involvement.

Melkersson-Rosenthal syndrome, an autosomal dominant hereditary disorder, is characterized by a triad of facial palsy, facial edema, and a furrowed tongue (lingua plicata). This often exhibits an incomplete penetrance. Each component may occur independently or in combination. The patient's history is characterized by recurrent attacks of facial paralysis, often beginning during childhood. Attacks can also include facial swelling, particularly affecting the upper lip. The tendency to recur is the only feature of facial paralysis that distinguishes it from most cases of Bell palsy.

Hereditary liability to pressure palsies is an allelic disorder with the Charcot-Marie-Tooth IA neuropathy, caused by deletion of the region containing the peripheral-myelin-protein 22 gene. It manifests with recurrent acute painless palsies from nerve lesions at sites of compression or increased exposure. Although the typical presentation is of peroneal or ulnar neuropathy, recurrent facial paralysis occasionally occurs.

CN VII Hyperactivity

Several positive symptoms occur from excessive reactivity of CN VII; synkinesis, facial myokymia, and hemifacial spasm are the most frequent.

Synkinesis is frequently observed subsequent to aberrant reinnervation in patients with antecedent severe Bell palsy; an inappropriate facial movement results, for example, concomitant blinking while smiling. Ephaptic transmission, or "artificial synapse," may arise at a lesion site where depolarization of the injured fibers acts as a stimulus to the intact portion of the nerve.

Facial myokymia is characterized by subtle, continuous, undulating movement of facial muscles. The movements are usually unilateral, subtle, often confined to one to two facial muscles, and sometimes accompanied by facial contracture or weakness. Observed mainly in multiple sclerosis, it much less commonly reflects an intrinsic brainstem tumor, particularly pontine gliomas. In the former it is usually self-limited and abates after several weeks. Some cases of facial myokymia are thought to be caused by antibody to a specific subtype of voltage-gated potassium channels. The specific antibody identified in some patients with facial myokymia also occurs with Isaac syndrome.

Hemifacial spasm consists of intermittent paroxysms of rapid, irregular, clonic twitching facial movements. The attack typically starts around the eyes and spreads to other ipsilateral facial muscles, especially in the perioral region. It is strictly confined to muscles innervated by CN VII; preceding CN VII lesions are rare. Paroxysms are often induced by voluntary or reflex facial movements, stress, and fatigue and may persist during sleep. The most common pathogenic mechanism for hemifacial spasm seems to be vascular compression of CN VII by an aberrant arterial loop near the brainstem. Therefore, detailed imaging studies including magnetic resonance angiography are essential for the diagnosis of hemifacial spasm. Less frequent pathophysiologic mechanisms include tumors and localized infectious processes. Botulinum toxin injections are an effective symptomatic treatment. Surgical decompression is an alternative sometimes leading to remission.

DIAGNOSTIC MODALITIES

Diagnostic modalities include imaging studies that may define direct involvement of CN VII or the presence of contiguous lesions. Other specialized testing modalities are used to study the various functions of CN VII. CSF analysis is important in infections, Guillain-Barré syndrome, and if meningeal infiltration (usually cancerous) is suspected. The use of EMG in Bell palsy is discussed earlier in this chapter.

Imaging Studies

The two primary imaging options are magnetic resonance imaging (MRI) and CT. MRI is best at imaging the intracranial facial nerve, CP angle, and parotid gland (Fig. 8.7). CT is the choice to image the temporal

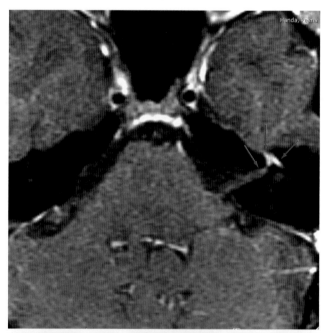

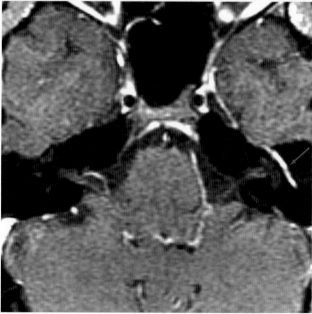

Axial T1-weighted, post-gadolinium MR image showing marked enhancement of fundal, geniculate, and tympanic segments of cranial nerve VII (arrows).

Fig. 8.7 Imaging of Bell Palsy.

bone and its facial (fallopian) canal. MRI must include primary and gadolinium-enhanced images. There may be unexpected relatively diffuse leptomeningeal enhancement when a facial neuropathy is the inciting lesion, leading to a diagnosis of metastatic carcinoma or lymphoma.

The very rare primary facial neuromas also strongly enhance with contrast. It is crucial that the ordering physician indicate a diagnosis of facial palsy and request an evaluation of CN VII along its entire course, not just the intracranial portion.

Extracranial lesions must also be considered in the imaging evaluation of facial weakness/palsy. If the neoplasm appears to be distal to the stylomastoid foramen, as with a highly malignant adenocarcinoma of parotid gland, MRI of the face may identify this tumor. Bone erosion or destruction versus remodeling is another important distinction that can be evaluated only on a bone window CT. Slow-growing benign lesions remodel bone, whereas bone erosion is more indicative of an aggressive or malignant process.

Intrinsic CN VII Topognostic Testing Studies

Intrinsic CN VII topognostic testing studies are based on the presence or absence of specific anatomic branch-point functions. With modern imaging studies, these are used less often but are occasionally valuable.

The Schirmer test of lacrimal flow depends on an intact geniculate ganglion, the site of the most proximal anatomic branch point along the course of CN VII, giving rise to the greater superficial petrosal nerve. The greater superficial petrosal nerve carries autonomic fibers to the lacrimal gland. Decreased lacrimation based on Schirmer testing suggests involvement of the greater superficial petrosal nerve or CN VII proximal to the ganglion. An associated facial palsy eliminates the former two possibilities.

EVIDENCE

Allen D, Dunn L. Aciclovir or valacyclovir for Bell's palsy (idiopathic facial paralysis). Cochrane Database Syst Rev 2004;(3):CD001869.
Review of data from three randomized studies including 246 patients found inconclusive evidence in regard to antiviral use in Bell palsy.
Engström M, Berg T, Stjernquist-Desatnik A, et al. Prednisolone and valacyclovir in Bell's palsy: a randomised, double-blind, placebo-controlled, multicentre trial. Lancet Neurol 2008;976-977:993–1000.

A randomized, double-blind, placebo-controlled, multicenter trial of patients aged 18–75 years who sought care directly or were referred from emergency departments or general practitioners within 72 hours of onset of acute Bell palsy. Prednisone was effective but acyclovir was of no value.
Grogan PM, Gronseth GS. Practice parameter: steroids, acyclovir, and surgery for Bell's palsy (an evidence-based review): report of the Quality Standards Subcommittee of the American Academy of Neurology. Neurology 2001;56:830–6.
This review summarizes available evidence for the treatment of Bell palsy.
Halperin JJ, Shapiro ED, Logigian E, et al. Practice parameter: treatment of nervous system Lyme disease (evidence-based review). Report of the Quality Standards Subcommittee of the American Academy of Neurology. Neurology 2007;69:91–102.
This review summarizes available evidence on treatment of neuroborreliosis and issues evidence-based recommendations. Some of the controversies are also discussed.
Sullivan FM, Swan IRC, Donnan PT, et al. Early treatment with prednisolone or acyclovir in Bell's palsy. N Engl J Med 2007;357:1598–607.
This well-conducted randomized, multicenter, placebo-controlled trial compares effectiveness of early treatment with corticosteroids, acyclovir, or both on outcome of patients with Bell palsy.

ADDITIONAL RESOURCES

Ang KL, Jones NS. Melkersson-Rosenthal syndrome. J Laryngol Otol 2002;116:386–8.
The differential diagnosis of MRS is discussed.
Finsterer J. Management of peripheral facial palsy. Eur Arch Otorhinolaryngol 2008;265:743–52.
This paper provides an excellent up-to-date review of idiopathic peripheral facial paralysis.
Grose C, Bonthius D, Afifi AK. Chickenpox and the geniculate ganglion: facial nerve palsy, Ramsay Hunt syndrome and acyclovir treatment. Pediatr Infect Dis J 2002;21:615–17.
This review suggests that facial palsy associated with VZV infection has a poorer outcome than Bell palsy and recommends the use of acyclovir.
Keane JR. Bilateral seventh nerve palsy: analysis of 43 cases and review of the literature. Neurology 1994;44:1198–202.
The differential diagnosis of facial diplegia is discussed.
Yanagihara N, Hato N, Murakami S, et al. Transmastoid decompression as a treatment of Bell's palsy. Otolaryngol Head Neck Surg 2001;124(3):282–6.
In this study, 58 patients with severe palsy underwent transmastoid decompression after steroid treatment and had better outcomes than 43 patients treated conservatively.

9

Cranial Nerve VIII: Auditory and Vestibular

Elizabeth Toh

AUDITORY NERVE

> **CLINICAL VIGNETTE** *A 68-year-old man presented with sudden onset of unilateral right-sided hearing loss. He stated that this was preceded by several months of constant ringing in his right ear. He had a history of hypertension and type 2 diabetes mellitus that was well controlled with oral hypoglycemic agents. He had no recent head trauma or previous head or neck surgeries. His only medications were atenolol and glyburide. There was no family history of hearing loss. He did not have a history of excess noise exposure or recent travel. No other otolaryngologic symptoms were reported.*
>
> *On examination, his external ears and tympanic membranes were normal. No middle ear effusions or masses were noted. The Weber tuning fork test lateralized to the left ear. Rinne test was positive in both ears confirming air conduction being louder than bone conduction in both ears. The rest of the head and neck examination including the remainder of his cranial nerve exam was unremarkable.*
>
> *Complete blood count was normal, and a fluorescent treponemal antibody absorption blood test was negative. The patient received a baseline audiogram demonstrating a high-frequency sensorineural hearing loss (SNHL) in the right ear. Gadolinium-enhanced brain MRI failed to demonstrate any retrocochlear tumor in the internal auditory canal or cerebellopontine angle.*
>
> *Sudden unilateral SNHL, such as in this vignette, in the absence of a tumor or lesion involving the vestibular nerve, can be attributed to a viral infection in the inner ear. In patients with diabetes or other microvascular risk factors, sudden unilateral sensorineural hearing loss may be attributed to microvascular infarction of the auditory nerve.*

Anatomy

The eighth cranial nerve (CN-VIII) is composed of two separate portions: the vestibular and cochlear nerves (vestibulocochlear nerve). The vestibular nerve has efferent and afferent fibers that control balance and equilibrium (see next section). The cochlear nerve, also called the auditory nerve, carries efferent and afferent fibers for hearing. To understand dysfunction of the auditory nerve, a brief description of the human hearing mechanism is required.

Sound waves travel through the external auditory canal and vibrate the tympanic membrane, which in turn produces motion of the middle ear ossicles (malleus, incus, and stapes). The vibrations are transmitted through the oval window at the stapes footplate, causing a fluid wave to travel through the cochlear perilymph. This in turn vibrates the basilar membrane and organ of Corti, stimulating inner and outer hair cells (Fig. 9.1). Hair cells, receptors of the sensorineural system, transmit action potentials to bipolar neurons, the bodies of which are in the spiral ganglion.

Afferent fibers projecting toward the central nervous system (CNS) constitute the auditory nerve (Fig. 9.2). They travel to the dorsal and ventral cochlear nuclei located in the caudolateral pons. Most of the secondary neurons project contralaterally across the midline to the superior olivary nucleus and then travel up the lateral lemniscus into the inferior colliculus of the midbrain. Decussating fibers from the cochlear nucleus to the superior olivary nucleus are located in the trapezoid bodies and also in the base of the pons. Fibers from the inferior colliculus continue to travel rostrally to the medial geniculate body of the thalamus and then terminate in the auditory cortex located in the transverse temporal gyri of Heschl.

Clinical Presentation

History

Hearing loss can result from pathologic conditions anywhere along the anatomic pathway for hearing. It may spare the auditory nerve, such as in middle ear pathology (e.g., serous otitis media), or involve the auditory nerve (e.g., acoustic tumors). SNHL is a hearing deficit from dysfunction of the cochlea (sensory), the auditory nerve (neural), or any part of the central auditory pathway. Auditory nerve dysfunction usually results in tinnitus, SNHL, or both. A targeted history and physical examination narrow the diagnosis. The temporal profile of symptom onset (i.e., sudden, progressive, fluctuating, or stable) is critical.

Tinnitus presents with or without concomitant SNHL and is classified into two groups. *Subjective tinnitus,* the most common, is heard solely by the patient. It can range from soft fluctuating ringing noise to loud constant debilitating roar. The cause of subjective tinnitus is usually unknown but is most often associated with SNHL or it can often be associated with exposure to loud noise, ototoxic drugs (such as aspirin, cisplatinum, and aminoglycosides), acoustic tumors, Meniere disease, and cochlear otosclerosis. *Objective tinnitus* is heard by the patient and the examiner and is usually not a sign of auditory nerve dysfunction. Pulsatile tinnitus is usually secondary to vascular causes, such as arteriovenous malformations or glomus tumors. Middle ear effusions, as in serous otitis media, can magnify vascular pulsations from the nearby internal carotid artery and produce vascular tinnitus. Pulsatile tinnitus may also occur with exposure to CNS pulsations or bone density changes allowing easier transmission of vascular flow sounds through the temporal bone to the cochlea. Clicking tinnitus is secondary to temporomandibular joint disease, palatal myoclonus, or spontaneous contraction of the middle ear muscles.

Determining the laterality of hearing loss is essential. Bilateral deficits occur in processes such as ototoxicity, noise exposure, and hearing loss related to aging (presbycusis). Unilateral hearing loss raises the concern of neoplastic, vascular, neurologic, or infectious etiologies. Fluctuation of hearing is seen in Meniere disease, autoimmune inner ear disease.

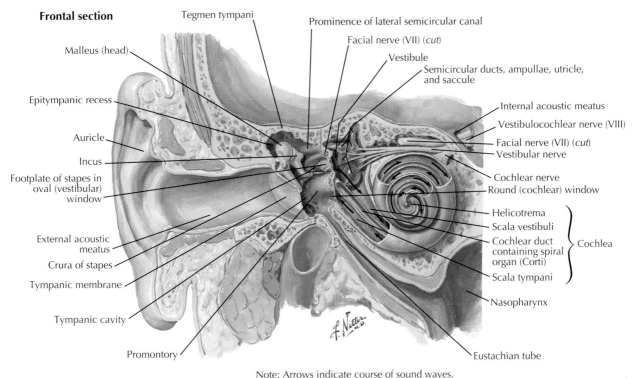

Frontal section

Tegmen tympani

Prominence of lateral semicircular canal

Facial nerve (VII) (*cut*)

Vestibule

Semicircular ducts, ampullae, utricle, and saccule

Malleus (head)

Epitympanic recess

Internal acoustic meatus

Vestibulocochlear nerve (VIII)

Auricle

Facial nerve (VII) (*cut*)

Vestibular nerve

Incus

Footplate of stapes in oval (vestibular) window

Cochlear nerve

Round (cochlear) window

Helicotrema

Scala vestibuli

Cochlear duct containing spiral organ (Corti)

Scala tympani

Cochlea

External acoustic meatus

Crura of stapes

Tympanic membrane

Tympanic cavity

Nasopharynx

Promontory

Eustachian tube

Note: Arrows indicate course of sound waves.

Fig. 9.1 Pathway of Sound Reception.

Progressive SNHL is usually seen with aging or tumors, whereas sudden SNHL occurs with viral neuritis or vascular processes.

Whether the hearing loss involves a process in the external or middle ear versus the inner ear must be determined. An audiogram should be performed on any patient with a complaint of a hearing disorder. The audiogram along with the history and physical examination will then lead to next steps of evaluation or diagnosis by the physician.

Only a few processes, such as otosclerosis and otitic meningitis, involve both the middle ear and the inner ear. Typically, tinnitus and vertigo are inner ear symptoms and indicate involvement of the cochlea, vestibular labyrinth, auditory nerve, or a combination of these structures. However, tinnitus, associated with SNHL, is now known to be a central event, based upon functional MRI studies, much like phantom limb syndrome.

Hearing loss associated with otalgia, otorrhea, headache, and aural fullness is most likely inflammatory and can be confirmed by physical examination. Concomitant tinnitus, vertigo, or both suggest the ominous extension of the inflammatory process to the inner ear or beyond. In this setting, a formal audiogram is indicated to determine whether the perceived hearing loss is secondary to a middle ear effusion or an additional sensorineural component. The latter is an otolaryngologic emergency.

With ototoxicity (aminoglycosides, salicylates, or loop diuretics), migraine headache disorders, and Meniere disease, vestibular symptoms, tinnitus, aural fullness, or a combination of these symptoms may accompany hearing loss. In conditions such as presbycusis and noise-induced hearing loss, vestibular symptoms are less likely to be part of the presentation.

Neurologic or ophthalmologic manifestations accompanying primary otologic symptoms occur with diseases such as multiple sclerosis or expanding neoplastic lesions, which may lead to combined facial nerve, trigeminal nerve, or ophthalmologic symptoms.

Trauma to the temporal bone, resulting in labyrinthine or auditory nerve injury, can result in auditory nerve dysfunction. Diving and flying may cause barotrauma, leading to rupture of the cochlear membranes, with subsequent SNHL. Occupational and recreational noise exposure damages the cochlea's outer hair cells, creating high-frequency SNHL. A family history of hearing loss is important to establish because this can be an important mechanism or predisposing factor for SNHL.

Physical Examination

Cerumen impaction or foreign bodies are easily identified *on inspection of the external auditory canal*. Otoscopic examination allows the physician to inspect the ear canal, tympanic membrane, and middle ear. This is important for identifying various conditions that can contribute to conductive hearing loss. It allows for the identification of fluid in the middle ear, cholesteatoma, or masses. Pneumatic *otoscopy* is used to assess the mobility of the tympanic membrane.

Tuning fork tests assess whether the hearing loss is conductive or sensorineural (Fig. 9.3). During the head and neck examination, a complete *cranial nerve examination* must also be performed to assess other potential cranial nerve abnormalities. Facial nerve weakness may be attributed to viral infections, such as herpes zoster oticus, or expanding neoplasms in the internal auditory canal or cerebellopontine angle, such as acoustic neuromas, meningiomas, or facial neuromas. *Auscultation* of the areas around the orbit and ear may detect objective pulsatile tinnitus. The pattern of SNHL can sometimes assist in the diagnosis of the etiology of hearing loss. The typical pattern for noise-induced SNHL is a drop in the 3–6 kHz frequency range which then improves in higher frequencies. Noise-induced SNHL may also be unilateral if the affected ear is closer to the noise source. Meniere disease and migraine disorders typically manifest with a low-frequency SNHL. Acoustic neuromas typically cause a unilateral SNHL. Speech discrimination significantly worse than would be expected on audiogram results may

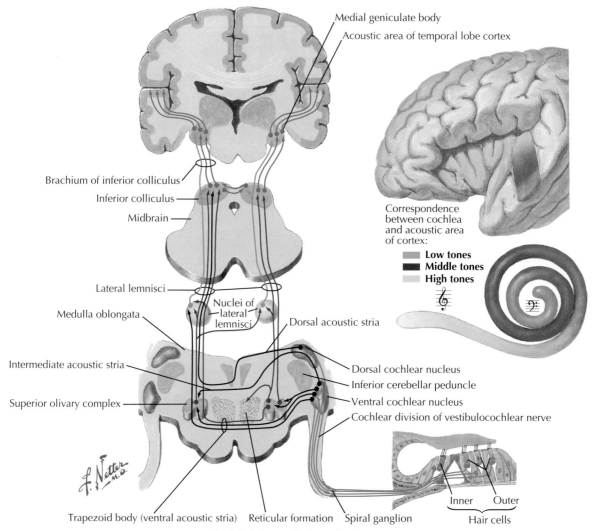

Brachium of inferior colliculus

Inferior colliculus

Midbrain

Lateral lemnisci

Medulla oblongata

Intermediate acoustic stria

Superior olivary complex

Medial geniculate body

Acoustic area of temporal lobe cortex

Correspondence between cochlea and acoustic area of cortex:

Low tones
Middle tones
High tones

Nuclei of lateral lemnisci

Dorsal acoustic stria

Dorsal cochlear nucleus

Inferior cerebellar peduncle

Ventral cochlear nucleus

Cochlear division of vestibulocochlear nerve

Inner   Outer

Hair cells

Trapezoid body (ventral acoustic stria)   Reticular formation   Spiral ganglion

Fig. 9.2 Afferent Auditory Pathways.

point to a central auditory processing disorder. Finally, a condition known as auditory neuropathy is manifested by normal auditory brainstem response testing and absence of otoacoustic emissions.

Diagnostic Approach

Standard laboratory blood tests are not routinely obtained for hearing loss unless a particular cause is suspected by history and physical examination.

A basic *audiogram* with pure tones and speech testing determines the type and amount of hearing loss. Unilateral decrease or asymmetries in speech discrimination, SNHL, or acoustic reflex abnormalities suggest a retrocochlear lesion, warranting further investigation.

Gadolinium-enhanced MRI scan of the brain (with particular attention to the internal auditory canals) is specifically indicated when history, symptoms, and audiometric tests strongly suggest retrocochlear disease. MRI is the diagnostic "gold standard" for tumors causing hearing loss. For patients presenting with asymmetric SNHL—especially if sudden—MRI is warranted to exclude acoustic neuromas or other cerebellopontine tumors. MRI may also detect acute and chronic vascular disease or infarction as well as demyelinating lesions.

Brainstem auditory evoked response (BAER) may be a useful objective and quantitative test when a retrocochlear deficit is suspected. It can suggest the site of lesions from the cochlea to the inferior colliculus at the pontine mesencephalic junction. BAER studies were initially considered highly sensitive for retrocochlear causes; however, as with most tests, false-negative and false-positive results are possible. For the purpose of screening for retrocochlear tumors, BAER is not as sensitive as gadolinium-enhanced MRI scans of the brain. The BAER uses electrodes attached to the patient's head and clicking sounds emitted through earphones. The sounds elicit action potentials through the peripheral and central auditory pathways, and the EEG activity is measured and averaged by a computer. Right and left ear waveform morphologic appearance and latencies are compared. Interaural differences suggest pathologic conditions. Five wave peaks characterize the BAER, corresponding to specific anatomic points within the auditory pathway: (1) CN-VIII action potential; (2) cochlear nucleus; (3) olivary complex; (4) lateral lemniscus; and (5) inferior colliculus. A change in peak morphology and latency helps localize the pathologic condition.

Differential Diagnosis

This section will briefly discuss some of the more common etiologies of SNHL, such as idiopathic sudden SNHL which is generally defined as greater than 30 dB decline in thresholds over at least three contiguous frequencies, occurring over a period of 72 hours or less.

Meniere Disease

Meniere disease is an idiopathic condition characterized by a combination of episodic vertigo, fluctuating SNHL, tinnitus, and aural fullness.

Weber Test

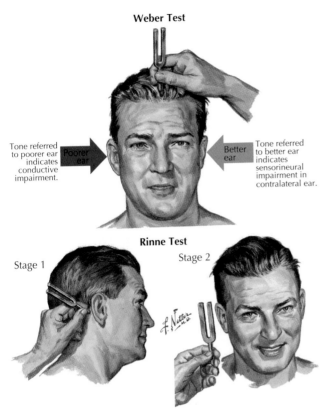

Tone referred to poorer ear indicates conductive impairment.

Poorer ear

Better ear

Tone referred to better ear indicates sensorineural impairment in contralateral ear.

Rinne Test

Stage 1

Stage 2

Normal: air conduction is twice as long as bone conduction.
Conductive loss: Bone conduction longer or equal to air conduction.
SNHL: Air conduction longer than bone conductions but both variably shortened.

Fig. 9.3 Hearing Tests: Weber and Rinne.

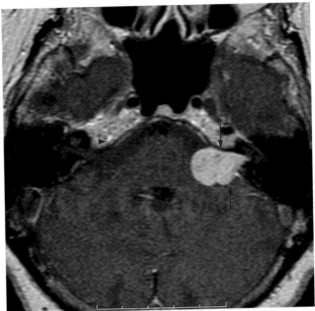

Axial T1-weighted, post-gadolinium-enhanced fat-saturated MR image shows an enhanced mass (arrows) widening the medial left internal auditory canal and extending into the cerebellopontine angle with indentation of the pons. The right side is normal (arrowhead).

Fig. 9.4 Vestibular Schwannoma.

These episodes typically last hours, and once the episode subsides the symptoms resolve. Over the course of time the hearing loss may become permanent, typically starting in the low-frequency tones before involving the mid- and high-frequency tones. A condition known as "cochlear Meniere disease" typically has the fluctuating hearing loss (maybe tinnitus and fullness) but no vertigo. Meniere disease is often a diagnosis of exclusion, so a full evaluation including MRI scan of the brain with contrast is warranted.

Neoplasms

In any case of sudden, unilateral SNHL, neoplastic lesions, although rare, should be considered in the differential until excluded by diagnostic and radiologic testing. Vestibular schwannomas (also known as acoustic neuromas) are benign tumors arising from the Schwann cells of CN-VIII and account for 6% of all intracranial tumors (Fig. 9.4). These occur on the vestibular portion of CN-VIII and involve the adjacent cochlear division by compression against the bony walls of the internal auditory canal. Less commonly, neuromas can also arise directly from the cochlear nerve.

Hearing loss is unilateral and is the most commonly reported symptom, occurring at some point in approximately 95% of patients with vestibular schwannoma. Progressive SNHL generally results from stretching or compression of the cochlear nerve as the tumor grows. In contrast, when hearing loss is precipitous, it is thought to be secondary to occlusion of the internal auditory artery supplying the cochlea. Tinnitus with acoustic neuromas is typically high pitched, continuous, and unilateral. Paradoxically, vestibular symptoms are less frequently reported with vestibular nerve schwannomas because as these lesions grow, the central vestibular system gradually compensates, often limiting any significant or longstanding vestibular symptomatology. Larger tumors occasionally lead to facial or trigeminal nerve involvement with symptoms of facial paralysis or paresthesias, respectively.

Before MRI, BAERs were the diagnostic test of choice for acoustic neuromas, with a sensitivity of 93%–98%. The sensitivity is significantly lower with tumors less than 1 cm (58%). Gadolinium-enhanced MRI scan of the brain (with particular attention to the internal auditory canals) will detect smaller tumors in patients who have had normal BAERs.

Vascular Etiologies

Vertebrobasilar stroke is another cause of sudden, unilateral SNHL with potentially devastating effects. Distinguishing whether hearing loss results from microvascular disease or a brainstem infarct is vital. The anterior inferior cerebellar artery supplies blood to the inferolateral portion of the pons, CN-VII, the spinal trigeminal tract, and the inferior cerebellum. A stroke from occlusion of this artery causes an infarct of the ipsilateral pons, creating a myriad of symptoms: ipsilateral hearing loss and vestibular symptoms, gait ataxia, conjugate gaze palsy, ipsilateral facial paralysis, and often contralateral loss of pain and temperature sensation in the extremities (see Chapter 54).

Computed tomography is usually the initial imaging study and excludes hemorrhagic infarction within the cerebellum and brainstem. MRI and MR angiography, however, provides better definition when available and concomitant imaging of the major vessels of the circle of Willis.

Unilateral SNHL also occurs secondary to occlusion of the cochlear blood supply from the internal auditory artery, a terminal branch of the anterior inferior cerebellar artery, or the basilar artery. This usually occurs secondary to compression by an acoustic neuroma in the internal auditory canal, but a thrombotic, vasculitis, or rarely embolic event can also be the cause.

Microvascular disease due to diabetes and hypertension is linked to sudden, unilateral SNHL, and the mechanism is thought to be similar to other diabetic cranial neuropathies with involvement of the vaso nervosum and nerve microinfarction.

Multiple Sclerosis

SNHL appears as a retrocochlear manifestation in approximately 4%–10% of patients with multiple sclerosis. However, it is rare for SNHL to be the initial or sole presentation. Usually, hearing loss is sudden but resolves within weeks of treatment. If multiple sclerosis is suspected, cerebrospinal fluid evaluation may be helpful; increased IgG index and oligoclonal bands in gel electrophoresis suggest multiple sclerosis. Audiometric testing can show normal or decreased speech discrimination in proportion to pure-tone threshold. MRI with and without gadolinium is the radiologic study of choice and can show periventricular white matter lesions on T2-weighted images within the inferior colliculus or cochlear nucleus in those who develop SNHL.

Infections

Various viral and bacterial infections can cause sudden SNHL. Herpes zoster oticus usually affects the sensory portion of the facial nerve, creating herpetic skin eruption around the auricle and in the external auditory canal with secondary inflammation and edema. Measles and mumps, previously a relatively common cause of hearing loss in children, have now been largely eliminated as a result of widespread vaccination in economically privileged countries.

Sudden deafness following a flulike illness or nonspecific viral processes is considered a common cause of sudden SNHL, especially when no vestibular symptoms coexist. The mechanism of action is unknown and it, therefore, should be considered a "diagnosis of exclusion."

Otosyphilis is defined as a positive syphilis serologic result in the setting of unexplained SNHL. The hearing loss, usually a late manifestation of the disease, begins at higher frequencies and can progress to bilateral cochlear and vestibular dysfunction. The exact causal mechanism is unknown; however, proposed theories include microvascular disease, direct spirochetal infiltration of the perilymph, and temporal bone osteitis. Diagnostic tests for syphilis, a treatable cause of SNHL, include the fluorescent treponemal antibody absorption blood test.

Lyme disease is another latent infection which can cause SNHL and patients with reasonable exposure risk should get appropriate testing to rule this out. Sudden SNHL is an otologic emergency, in that the sooner the patient is seen and evaluated by an ENT specialist, the sooner treatment can be initiated, preferably within 2–4 weeks of onset. Early treatment greatly enhances the chance of restoring hearing if the loss is due to a virus/infection.

Hematologic Disorders

Leukemia, sickle cell anemia, polycythemia, and macroglobulinemia can cause sudden SNHL, usually from sludging, hemorrhage into the inner ear, or microthrombi. A careful history, a complete blood count, and coagulation studies can exclude hematologic causes.

Presbycusis

This is the most common cause of slowly progressive, bilateral, symmetric, high-frequency SNHL with increasing age. Presbycusis originates from a pathologic condition that decreases the number of hair cells within the organ of Corti. It has an almost universal incidence in the elderly. Multiple factors determine its progression rate. Three of the most common are genetic predisposition, nerve toxins (particularly medications), and history of long exposure to loud noises.

Otosclerosis

Otosclerosis is the most common cause of conductive hearing loss in young adults and often affects both ears. It occurs as a result of foci of sclerosis within the endochondral temporal bone. The most common location for this is at the fissula ante fenestram just anterior to the oval window, causing fixation of the stapes footplate, which in turn dampens the transfer of sound vibrations to the inner ear. Rare cases of associated cochlear sclerosis and SNHL have been described. Hearing loss is usually gradual but may be accelerated during pregnancy. Some patients may have tinnitus and dizziness. The condition is hereditary but with variable expression, and middle-aged women are most at risk. An audiogram and tympanogram help in making the diagnosis, and hearing may be rehabilitated with a hearing aid or stapedectomy surgery.

Treatment

When the primary cause of hearing loss is determined, in some cases, such as a sudden SNHL or syphilis, treatment is available and hearing loss is potentially reversible depending on when the treatment is initiated in the course of the illness. There is no treatment for vascular lesions with infarction of the auditory nerve. However, for common disorders such as presbycusis, a variety of high-technology hearing-enhancing modalities can be designed, with the aid of an otologist and audiologist, to meet the patient's needs.

VESTIBULAR NERVE

CLINICAL VIGNETTE *A 65-year-old woman came to the emergency department with a chief complaint of "dizziness." At 3:00 AM, she had awoken to an odd feeling in her head, which was accompanied by nausea. As she turned to her right to ask her husband for help, she experienced a severe spinning sensation with increased nausea followed by vomiting. The symptoms lasted for a minutes or so. However, in the car and subsequently in the emergency department, any head movement in the supine position precipitated recurrent symptoms. Her medical history included diabetes mellitus, hypertension, and a remote transient ischemic attack (TIA) manifested by right-sided weakness.*

Her blood pressure was 180/90 mm Hg. She appeared pale and uncomfortable and refused to open her eyes or move her head during the examination. The findings of her neurologic examination were normal, with the exception that she was hesitant to get off the exam table to allow gait testing. Brain MRI results were normal. Dix-Hallpike testing elicited typical nystagmus for posterior semicircular canal benign paroxysmal positional vertigo (BPPV). Subsequently, otolith particle-repositioning (Epley) maneuver successfully alleviated her symptoms.

This vignette describes a classic case of an individual with acute BPPV. In most patients, this annoying disorder can be successfully treated by a simple maneuver. However, the possibility of a stroke, especially in those with cerebrovascular risk factors, or other cerebellar lesions must be considered before making this diagnosis.

Dizziness is a common nonspecific symptom. In patients older than 75 years, it is one of the more common medical complaints that bring individuals to a physician; dizziness is the third most common symptom among all age groups. In the United States, there are 8 million visits annually for dizziness; chronic dizziness affects 16% of the self-reported population.

When patients report dizziness, one of the primary challenges is to define its precise character. Feeling lightheaded, experiencing loss of equilibrium, vertigo, unsteady gait, and fainting can all be grouped under a patient's ill-defined description of "dizziness," although these symptoms often suggest different etiologies. Clarification of the precise historical details—onset, duration, positional and other exacerbating factors, and associated symptomatology—is essential to determine the likely cause.

Vertigo is the illusory perception of motion. Patients describe it as a sensation similar to that experienced on a merry-go-round. An inquiry as to whether things actually move in front of the patient's eyes or a sense that they themselves are moving helps the patient define this symptom. Typical associated clinical findings include sudden precipitous onset, nausea, vomiting, and nystagmus during the vertiginous symptoms.

Typically, in the acute setting, horizontal direction-fixed nystagmus is suggestive of a peripheral etiology (vestibular labyrinth) with the fast component of the nystagmus beating toward the affected ear. However, there are some forms of nystagmus that are more typical of a central etiology. **Gaze-dependent nystagmus** occurs in processes that affect the ipsilateral cerebellum. **Vertical nystagmus** seen **with upward gaze** is often the result of disease in the cerebellum or tegmentum. **Downward gaze vertical nystagmus** is most often found in processes at the foramen magnum level, especially Chiari malformations. *Optokinetic* nystagmus refers to a normal phenomenon of reflexive slow movement of the eye in **pursuit** followed by a cortically driven corrective fast movement or **saccade.** Patients with parietal lobe lesions lose the fast, saccadic elements of the optokinetic response when the strip is moved in the direction of the abnormal hemisphere.

Anatomy

The vestibulocochlear nerve, CN-VIII, is actually composed of two nerves: the vestibular and cochlear nerves. The vestibular nerve is responsible for efferent and afferent fibers that control balance and equilibrium. The cochlear nerve, also called the *auditory nerve,* carries the efferent and afferent fibers for hearing. The vestibular system provides specific sensory input that influences motor function in reference to postural control (Figs. 9.1 and 9.5); the latter depends on interrelated mechanisms,

including perception of position and motion in relation to gravity and orientation of the head and body in relation to the vertical axis during quiet stance. Other vestibular functions include integrating selected postural and orientation sensory cues in various environments; this aids in controlling the center of gravity when the body is static or moving and stabilizes the head during bodily movements. Because the vestibular system primarily provides sensory information about the head on the body, the CNS must rely on other sensory modalities to determine overall body position and movement.

The visual system provides multiple information modes about head position and movement with respect to the environment, the direction of the vertical axis, and low-frequency information regarding slow or static tilts. Joint position and muscle stretch contribute somatosensory information about the relative alignment of body segments with each other and the supporting surface. Postural control involves the combination of the complex organization of this sensory information, a "central set" based on previous experience and biomechanical constraints. Normally, to maintain proper body alignment over the support base, the individual generates a motor output via the vestibulospinal and corticospinal systems.

There are numerous central as well as peripheral processes that cause symptoms of vertigo (Fig. 9.6). During the patient's initial evaluation it is important to differentiate a CNS lesion from a peripheral lesion by determining whether any associated neurologic deficits are present and their exact characteristics.

CNS Disorders

Brainstem dysfunction typically includes prominent dysmetria, diplopia, dysphagia, dysarthria, perioral numbness, or weakness. Twenty-five

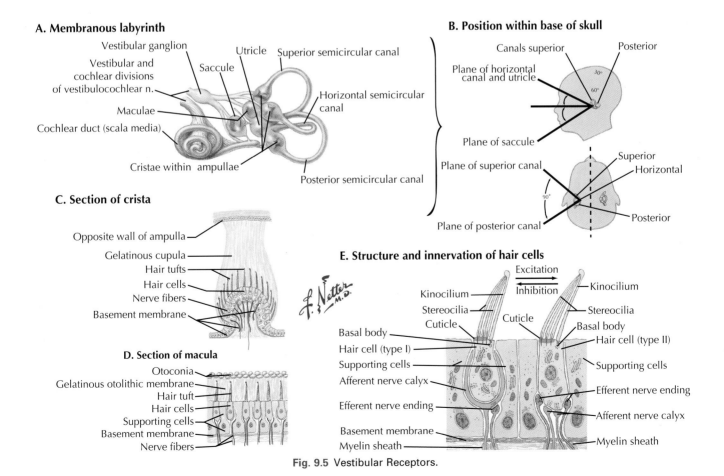

Fig. 9.5 Vestibular Receptors.

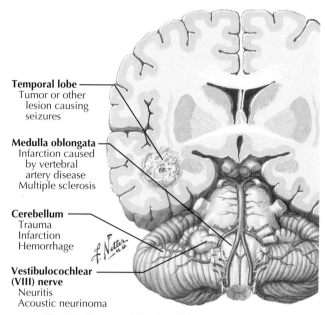

Temporal lobe
Tumor or other
lesion causing
seizures

Medulla oblongata
Infarction caused
by vertebral
artery disease
Multiple sclerosis

Cerebellum
Trauma
Infarction
Hemorrhage

**Vestibulocochlear
(VIII) nerve**
Neuritis
Acoustic neurinoma

Fig. 9.6 Causes of Vertigo (Classified by Region).

percent of patients with stroke risk factors who present to emergency medical settings with isolated vertigo, nystagmus, and postural instability have an infarction within the territory of the posterior inferior cerebellar artery (PICA). The acute postural instability with a PICA infarction is usually so severe that independent ambulation is not possible. Other than difficulty walking, there may be no cerebellar or central findings with a PICA infarction. This diagnosis is particularly important because acute postinfarction swelling or hemorrhage within the cerebellar hemisphere may cause brainstem compression and death (see Chapter 54).

Similarly, multiple sclerosis patients with demyelinating lesions in the brainstem may present with acute vertigo and gait dysfunction.

In contrast, patients with peripheral vestibular disorders have preserved ambulation, although they may have feelings of disequilibrium and be frightened to move, as noted in the vignette. If carefully brought into the upright posture, most of these individuals can ambulate well and do not exhibit cerebellar ataxia or limb dysmetria.

Therefore, for patients presenting with vertigo who cannot ambulate independently, and particularly those with vascular risk factors, brain imaging is mandatory to rule out cerebellar infarction or multiple sclerosis.

Peripheral Nervous System Disorders

The matched tonic input of both vestibular end organs is processed centrally to mediate head stability. Unilateral reduction or differential in vestibular input is interpreted as turning. Acute peripheral vestibular dysfunction causes vertigo by interrupting the normal tonic discharge of one labyrinth. In the intact vestibular system, upright head rotation causes a reduction in horizontal semicircular canal firing rate on one side, paired with an increased firing rate on the other side. With acute unilateral vestibular loss, the reduced firing rate simulates the normal response to turning, generating fast phase nystagmus away from the affected ear. The nystagmus is usually more pronounced in gaze toward the affected side and reduced in gaze away from the affected side (law of Alexander). Veering or tilting toward the side of lesion may be present, through effects on the vestibular–spinal, vestibular–ocular, and vestibular–cerebellar pathways.

Etiologic Classification of Peripheral Vestibulopathies

Etiologic classification of peripheral vestibulopathies is initially based on symptoms, duration, episodic nature, and other associated auditory dysfunctions.

Meniere disease is characterized by recurrent vertigo, fluctuating SNHL, tinnitus, and aural fullness, as discussed above. The prevalence of the disease ranges from 500 to 1000 per million, with no difference in regard to gender. Patients often present in their fourth decade, usually with unilateral symptoms, although some will develop bilateral symptoms within a few years. The vertigo spells typically last hours during which time the patient is incapacitated and the vertigo symptoms are continuous and nonpositional. Patients can have multiple attacks per month or only one every few years. In the early stages of the disease, symptoms often appear in isolation, and the hearing deficit is not always initially noticeable, rendering diagnosis difficult. As the disease progresses, prominent low-frequency SNHL appears, and the symptoms are more prolonged and recur more frequently. Some patients are left with a chronic sense of imbalance as a permanent weakness of the peripheral vestibular system occurs.

The underlying pathophysiology of Meniere disease is presumably related to either excessive production or decreased absorption of endolymph. An autoimmune etiology has been proposed, but the exact mechanism remains unclear. Diagnostic tests such as glycerol dehydration test and audiometry have high sensitivity for Meniere disease, especially if performed during an attack. Other tests such as electrocochleography are useful for the diagnosis of the disease. Serologic tests to exclude comorbid conditions, including thyroid function test, antinuclear antibody, rheumatoid factor, complement antibodies, serum immunoglobulin levels, anticardiolipin antibodies, C-reactive protein, syphilis, and Lyme treponemal, titer may be indicated in some patients. Symptomatic treatment includes antiemetics, benzodiazepines, and steroids (administered orally, intratympanically, or both). Preventative treatment for the episodic attacks may include diuretics, a low-salt diet, and avoidance of alcohol, caffeine, nicotine, and stress. Intratympanic instillation of drugs such as dexamethasone may be helpful to control vertigo for months/years and may be helpful for recovery of any associated acute SNHL. Intratympanic gentamicin and streptomycin, strong vestibular toxins, are used as a last resort to eliminate vestibular function in cases of intractable vertigo and poor hearing in the affected ear. Endolymphatic sac decompression and shunting, as well as surgical labyrinthectomy and vestibular neurectomy, have also been used in cases with refractory vertigo.

Vestibular neuritis is characterized by prolonged vertigo with or without hearing loss. Unlike Meniere disease this vertigo typically lasts days and then as it subsides, patients experience imbalance which persists for weeks to months. It is not episodic and typically is thought to be caused by a virus.

Initially, it is important to exclude vertebrobasilar TIAs, particularly in those with vascular risk factors or in young persons with associated recent neck injury and possible vertebral artery dissection. However, it is rare for vertigo to be the sole manifestation of a TIA, emphasizing the importance of a careful history, as patients may overlook seemingly less important symptoms that could lead to a central diagnosis and may focus on the vertigo.

Types of Vertigo and Disorders

Benign paroxysmal positional vertigo (BPPV) is the most common cause of vertigo in the elderly, although this condition may occur at all ages. The typical presentation is that of recurrent bouts of positionally triggered vertigo with either a transient spinning sensation or an illusion of side-to-side movement. Spells are brief, lasting seconds to minutes, and often associated with nausea and sometimes vomiting. Symptoms occur with sudden shift in position, when turning in bed, or with neck extension, as while looking up or while in a dentist or hairdresser chair. Often patients become anxious and guard against fast movements. Episodes become gradually shorter and symptoms improve over 72 hours but can occasionally linger for many days or even months. BPPV results from otolith debris errantly entering the semicircular canals, usually the posterior semicircular canal, rendering them gravitationally sensitive with the solid material acting as a plunger or weight within the fluid-filled system. Symptoms become less defined when the horizontal or superior canal is involved or bilateral vestibular disruptions are present. Although many cases can be diagnosed in the emergency department or outpatient clinic, BPPV patients are often referred either to neurology or otolaryngology specialists. When the presentation is not typical, tests such as brain MR and electronystagmograms are done to exclude other pathology. Recurrent symptoms can lead to vascular evaluations to rule out possible vertebral artery compromise. Although unusual, vertigo as the sole manifestation of vertebrobasilar disease has been reported, especially with posterior inferior cerebellar artery ischemia, and caution is advised when vascular risk factors are present in those with atypical presentations. However, distinct positionally inducible isolated short-lived vertigo remains more a feature of a peripheral vestibulopathy than of cerebral ischemia.

The diagnosis of BPPV in large part depends on the clinical history and bedside testing. The Dix-Hallpike maneuver, when performed and interpreted properly, is diagnostic. Studies suggest that the Dix-Hallpike maneuver has a sensitivity and specificity of approximately 75% but higher when using video goggles. In our experience the ability to perform the maneuver properly in anxious patients fearful of provocative maneuvers is a major limiting factor for accurate evaluation. Head Impulse test is another maneuver that is useful to differentiate peripheral from central vertigo (Fig. 9.7). This is a bedside test that has higher specificity in patients with peripheral vertigo and assesses the function of the horizontal semicircular canal. The patient is seated and asked to fixate on a target (e.g., the examiner's nose). The examiner turns the patient's head laterally by about 15–30 degrees. Normal response is for the patient's eyes to stay fixated on the target. If the eyes move with the head turn, that is they are dragged off the target followed by a corrective saccade back to the target, it suggests impairment of the vestibulocochlear reflex on the side ipsilateral to the head turn. In patients with cerebellar lesions causing vertigo, the head impulse test is usually normal.

Risk factors for BPPV include recent head trauma (which can be relatively minor); otologic surgery or disease; habitual unusual positioning such as is a daily occurrence for plumbers, mechanics, and yoga enthusiasts; or advanced age. Particle repositioning maneuvers or canalith repositioning maneuvers are the main treatment for BPPV (Fig. 9.8). Another maneuver known as the liberatory maneuver, developed by Dr. Alain Semont, relies on rapidly swinging the patient from lying initially on the involved side through 180 degrees to the opposite, uninvolved side. Unfortunately, any repositioning maneuver can be limited by the inability of the patient to physically participate (musculoskeletal and orthopedic limitations, especially of the head and neck) or when induced symptoms are intolerable. In 5% of patients, symptoms may worsen with repositioning maneuvers in part due to conversion from posterior to horizontal semicircular canal involvement. Outcome studies regarding the effectiveness of the canalith repositioning maneuver provide

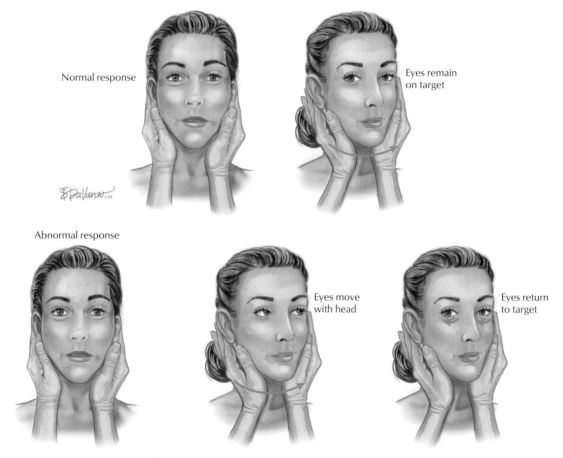

Fig. 9.7 Head Impulse Test.

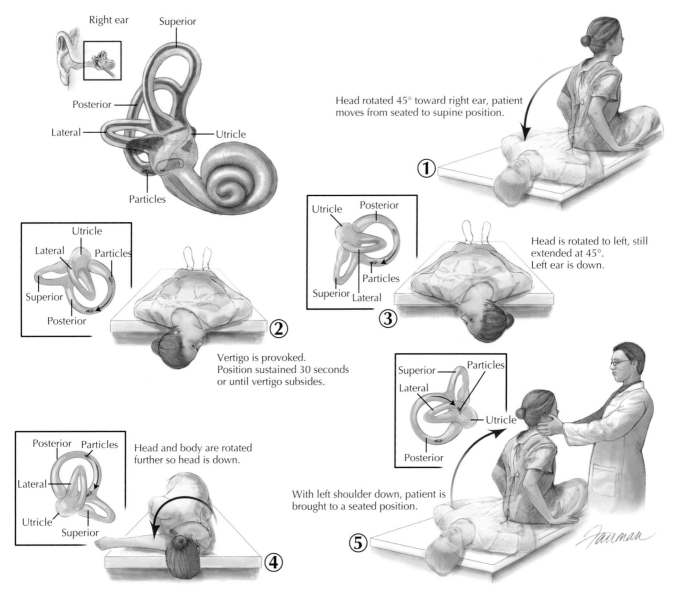

Right ear

Superior

Posterior

Lateral

Utricle

Particles

Utricle

Lateral

Particles

Superior

Posterior

Vertigo is provoked.
Position sustained 30 seconds
or until vertigo subsides.

Head rotated 45° toward right ear, patient
moves from seated to supine position.

①

Utricle   Posterior

Particles

Superior   Lateral

③

Head is rotated to left, still
extended at 45°.
Left ear is down.

Posterior   Particles

Lateral

Utricle

Superior

Head and body are rotated
further so head is down.

④

Superior   Particles

Lateral

Utricle

Posterior

With left shoulder down, patient is
brought to a seated position.

⑤

Fig. 9.8 Canalith Repositioning (Epley) Maneuver.

a range of reported success, as most studies rely on subjective reporting, which is inherently unreliable because patients quickly develop adaptive behavior spontaneously. Overall, however, there is evidence to favor repositioning maneuvers, with some studies demonstrating resolution of symptoms in 90% of patients after only one treatment. Self-administered maneuvers in combination with guided treatments can often help expedite improvement in the remaining patients. Successful treatment with the repositioning maneuvers does not influence recurrence rate, which averages around 20% over a 20-month period. Persistent vertigo or frequent recurrences of BPPV is uncommon, but under such circumstances surgical occlusion of the posterior semicircular canal with bone grafts and fibrin glue is an effective treatment. Medications can provide temporary relief by controlling nausea and suppressing the vestibular responses. Meclizine and benzodiazepines are the most frequently prescribed medications but can be sedating and should be used only for a few days. In general, definitive treatment with particle repositioning is favored over symptomatic control with central vestibular suppressants for BPPV.

Chronic vestibulopathies are less likely to cause vertigo because their duration allows for CNS compensation. Acoustic neuromas and other slow-growing neoplasms affecting CN-VIII may cause unilateral tinnitus, hearing loss, and abnormal hypoactive caloric responses on electronystagmogram. However, these tumors rarely present with vertigo. These conditions are typically noted to be associated with disequilibrium complaints.

Bilateral vestibulopathy typically do not cause vertigo or a sensation of turning. However, bilateral vestibular disruption does affect the vestibular–ocular reflex, which stabilizes visual perception during head motion. The main symptoms in these cases are a sense of imbalance, especially when visual cues are altered (unequal surface, dim illumination, and quick head movements), and oscillopsia (see below). Vestibulotoxic agents, such as aminoglycosides, alcohol, and heavy metals, can lead to transient or permanent vestibular damage, but bilateral vestibular hypofunction can also occur in otherwise healthy adults (idiopathic) or can result from a genetic predisposition.

Oscillopsia, or failure to stabilize vision during head movement, can cause bobbing visual perception and loss of dynamic visual acuity while walking. Because some patients call this "dizziness," a close history is needed to help differentiate it from true vertigo. In addition to bilateral peripheral vestibulopathies, oscillopsia can be seen with central lesions involving the brainstem and cerebellar, particularly mass lesion around the foramen magnum. It is typically seen in patients with the Arnold–Chiari syndrome, a developmental condition often associated with syringomyelia and syringobulbia, and is rarely observed in patients with multiple sclerosis. This phenomenon is usually binocular, and monocular symptoms raise the possibility of ocular muscle myokymia instead.

Canal dehiscence syndrome, first described in 1998 by Lloyd B. Minor, is caused by thinning or developmental absence of part of the temporal bone overlying the superior semicircular canal leading to an extra direct conduit for impulses into the inner ear in addition to normal conduction through the oval window. Canal dehiscence presents with a variety of symptoms in the affected ear including a sensation of ear blockage that is relieved with Valsalva maneuver, hyperacusis, sound distortion, conductive hearing loss, and chronic imbalance. Abrupt vertigo, disequilibrium, nystagmus, oscillopsia, and nausea induced by external sounds and even one's own voice or pulsations occur in some cases and is known as the Tullio phenomenon. These symptoms may also be induced by tragal pressure on the affected ear. Clinical diagnosis, however, can be difficult, as symptoms may often be nonspecific or occur in isolation. Some seemingly bizarre complaints, such as hearing louder than usual gastric noises and being aware of the eyeballs moving in the socket, are reported. Pulsatile tinnitus is also common and often leads to a suspicion of vascular causes.

A combination of tests helps establish the diagnosis of canal dehiscence and differentiates it from conditions such as Meniere disease or perilymphatic fistulas. An abnormally reduced vestibular-evoked myogenic threshold in the affected ear in the presence of a dehiscent superior semicircular canal seen on high-resolution CT scan has more than 90% diagnostic sensitivity and specificity. Low-frequency conductive hearing with normal tympanometry and an intact acoustic reflex provide further support. A variety of surgical techniques to repair or plug the superior semicircular are effective for eliminating clinical symptoms.

Diagnostic Approach

A **complete neurologic examination** is of the utmost importance in the evaluation of dizziness or vertigo. When one sensory vestibular mechanism is absent, the remaining sensory inputs are used to elicit corrective postural reactions. Superimposed neurologic disorders, including stroke, Parkinson disease, cerebellar pathology, or peripheral neuropathy, may affect the potential of the nervous system to compensate, and symptoms are amplified significantly.

Video electronystagmogram (VNG): This test is intended to evaluate the effects of vestibular input on the ocular system. Disorders of both the otoliths and the vestibular nerve can cause abnormalities on the VNG. The basic elements of the VNG include the bithermal caloric testing, smooth pursuit, optokinetic, saccade, and positional testing. Vestibular nerve abnormalities can manifest as a delay in conduction of the vestibular–ocular reflex via the medial longitudinal fasciculus. Additionally, rotatory chair testing may be used by some testers. Rotatory chair testing may elicit abnormal responses in patients with otolith dysfunction as well as in those with vestibular nerve dysfunction. Other tests include the VHIT and ocular and cervical VEMPs. The tests are affected by medications and patient cooperation and depend on comparison to standard tables or to the normal side. The results should be interpreted with the clinical presentation and potential confounding variables taken into account.

Dynamic posturography is a complex testing modality that defines the extent to which a patient is able to use visual, somatosensory, and vestibular input for postural control. The patient stands on a shifting platform in front of a simulated visual field. The postural response to various shifts can be assessed and quantitated. This test is useful for diagnosis and it is sometimes used for designing rehabilitation strategies.

The clinical test of sensory interaction and balance (foam posturography) uses a combination of two visual (eyes open or closed) and two support surface (soft unstable, firm stable) conditions to clinically measure a patient's sensory interaction for postural stability. The **Romberg (stationary) and sharpened Romberg (tandem stance) test** with eyes open and eyes closed, and unilateral standing with eyes open and eyes closed are not specific for postural deficits secondary to vestibular pathologic conditions. However, patients with vestibular damage may demonstrate increased sway or falling during these tests.

Dynamic tests, such as floor walking with the eyes closed, measure tandem walking for up to 10 steps. Persons with acute or chronic vestibular disorders may fail this test based on established age-related norms.

Several performance tests may be used to establish a baseline functional analysis and measure outcome in individuals with impairments of static and dynamic postural control. These include the Timed Up and Go Test, the Dynamic Gait Index, the Fukuda stepping test, and the Berg Balance Scale.

The **Timed Up and Go** test measures the time required to rise from a standard chair, walk 10 feet, return to that chair, and sit. The norm for neurologically intact older adults is 10–12 seconds. The results may be a predictor for falls in community-dwelling elders. There is a maximum of 14 seconds for elders at minimal risk for falls and less than 30 seconds for elders who are dependent on assistance for ambulation in the community. There is no threshold established for patients with vestibular disorders.

The **Dynamic Gait Index** measures the ability to modify gait in response to eight different tasks during ambulation. Each task is given a score of 0 to −3. A score of 11 ± 4 is found in older adults with a history of falls but no neurologic disorders.

The **Berg Balance Scale** uses 14 test-specific items rated 0–4 that measure postural control during functionally related tasks. These require anticipatory abilities and are performed only while sitting and standing. Test scores are a good predictor of elderly fall risk. Scores less than 45 were associated with an increased risk for falls; scores less than 36 were associated with a 100% risk of falls.

General Treatment Considerations
Rehabilitation

Many vestibular rehabilitation programs provide a range of treatment modalities aimed to facilitate acute recovery and ongoing compensation programs for patients with varying degrees of residual vestibular deficit. Some are useful for acute or chronic vestibular lesions and are equally applicable to vertigo, dizziness, and disequilibrium in general.

Pharmacologic Therapy

Recent studies suggest that high-dose steroid therapy (orally, intratympanic, or both) significantly improves the recovery of peripheral vestibular neuritis. Antiviral therapy is generally not indicated. Vestibular suppressant medications such as meclizine, scopolamine, and benzodiazepines are useful for relief of acute symptoms of vertigo and dizziness from any vestibular process. However, long-term use interferes with central vestibular compensation mechanisms and should preferably be avoided.

Nonpharmacologic Therapy

Vestibular compensation results from active neuronal changes in the cerebellum and the brainstem in response to sensory conflicts created by vestibular pathology. Despite spontaneous "recovery," patients still experience disequilibrium, motion-provoked vertigo, or both because the vestibular system, inhibited to a certain degree by the cerebellum, is unable to respond appropriately to labyrinthine input produced by normal head movements.

Because movement provokes a sense of disequilibrium and vertigo, patients with vestibular disorders may restrict their activity level and trunk and head movements to avoid these symptoms. This provides for greater short-term compensatory stability but interferes with long-term recovery if patients are not challenged to increase movement to facilitate vestibular compensation. Educating patients about vestibular function encourages and reassures them to safely increase their activity level even though early recovery movement provokes symptoms.

Initially, an assistive device such as a cane or walker may be recommended. Sensory input through the upper extremity from a cane or light touch through fingertips can reduce postural sway in patients without proper vestibular function.

Motor organization exercises help to improve standing, ambulation, and functional activities such as moving at various speeds, changing directions, and maneuvering around obstacles.

Weekly therapy visits for 4–12 weeks help to monitor the effectiveness of assigned home exercise programs. Treatment success depends on the nature of the primary underlying neurologic dysfunction. Peripheral vestibular disorders such as BPPV and stable vestibular hypofunction are most amenable to treatment. In contrast, individuals with primary CNS disorders have poorer outcomes but still demonstrate reduced symptomatology with treatment.

Other factors influencing treatment effectiveness include the degree of initial disability and a more recent time of onset. Comorbidities, such as underlying musculoskeletal dysfunction and other neurologic impairments and patient compliance also affect outcomes. Elderly patients often require longer treatment times to reach maximum benefit.

ADDITIONAL RESOURCES

Auditory

Calabresi P. Multiple sclerosis and demyelinating conditions of the central nervous system. In: Goldman L, Schafer AI, editors. Cecil textbook of medicine. 25th ed. Philadelphia, PA: Elsevier Saunders; 2016. pp. 2471–9.

Horikawa C, Kodama S, Tanaka S, et al. Diabetes and risk of hearing impairment in adults: a meta-analysis. J Clin Endocrinol Metab 2013;98:51–8.

Metselaar M, Demirtas G, van Immerzeel T, et al. Evaluation of magnetic resonance imaging diagnostic approaches for vestibular schwannoma based on hearing threshold differences between ears: added value of auditory brainstem responses. Otol Neurotol 2015;36:1610–15.

Sheth SA, Kwon CS, Barker FG 2nd. The art of management decision making: from intuition to evidence-based medicine. Otolaryngol Clin North Am 2012;45:333–51.

Sismanis A. Pulsatile tinnitus: contemporary assessment and management. Curr Opin Otolaryngol Head Neck Surg 2011;19:348–57.

Vestibular

Chien WW, Carey JP, Minor LB. Canal dehiscence. Curr Opin Neurol 2011;24:25–31.

Furman J, Cass S. Benign paroxysmal positional vertigo. N Engl J Med 1999;341:1590–6.

Furman J, Whitney S. Central causes of dizziness. Phys Ther 2000;80: 179–87.

Hall CD, Herdman SJ, Whitney SL, et al. Vestibular rehabilitation for peripheral vestibular hypofunction: an evidence-based clinical practice guideline: from the American Physical Therapy Association Neurology Section. J Neurol Phys Ther 2016;40:124–55.

Harris JP, Nguyen QT. Meniere's disease. Otolaryngol Clin North Am 2010.

Lauritsen CG, Marmura MJ. Current treatment options: vestibular migraine. Curr Treat Options Neurol 2017;19:38.

Nguyen-Huynh AT. Evidence-based practice: management of vertigo. Otolaryngol Clin North Am 2012;45:925–40.

Strupp M, Zingler VC, Arbusow V, et al. Methylprednisolone, valacyclovir, or the combination for vestibular neuritis. N Engl J Med 2004;351: 354–61.

Venhovens J, Meulstee J, Verhagen WI. Acute vestibular syndrome: a critical review and diagnostic algorithm concerning the clinical differentiation of peripheral versus central aetiologies in the emergency department. J Neurol 2016;263:2151–7.

10

Cranial Nerves IX and X: Glossopharyngeal and Vagus

Timothy D. Anderson

CRANIAL NERVE IX: GLOSSOPHARYNGEAL NERVE AND SWALLOWING

The glossopharyngeal nerve is a mixed nerve, containing both sensory and motor fibers along with parasympathetic, special sensory, and visceral sensory components. The motor component is fibers to the stylopharyngeus muscle, as well as the superior pharyngeal constrictors, and the sensory component has a similar distribution over the upper pharynx and posterior $\frac{1}{3}$ of the tongue, as well as the sensation of taste from the posterior $\frac{1}{3}$ of the tongue (bitter and sour). The visceral sensory afferents are from the carotid body and sinus. Dysfunction of the glossopharyngeal nerve can cause some disturbance in taste, but the primary disability with glossopharyngeal injury is in swallowing.

Swallowing dysfunction (dysphagia) is a serious and debilitating problem, with potential for inadequate nutrition, aspiration, and potentially life-threatening aspiration pneumonia. Normal swallow is very complex, with multiple cranial nerves (CNs) required for sensory feedback and motor control in a very precise and ordered process. Dysphagia can be a result of a multitude of central and peripheral neurologic disorders and sometimes is the first and most prominent sign of neuromuscular disorders.

Swallowing Physiology

Swallowing is a complex process involving motor control and sensory feedback from anatomic structures within the oral cavity, pharynx, larynx, and esophagus (Fig. 10.1). The trigeminal (CN V), facial (CN VII), glossopharyngeal (CN IX; Fig. 10.2), vagus (CN X; Fig. 10.3), and hypoglossal (CN XII) CNs are involved. A "normal swallow" comprises two major components, bolus transport and airway protection. The swallowing process is typically classified into four phases: oral preparatory, oral swallowing, pharyngeal, and esophageal (Fig. 10.4). The pharyngeal phase of swallow is the most complex, and problems in this phase are most likely to cause aspiration.

1. The **oral preparatory phase** involves voluntary motor function during which food or liquid is taken into the mouth, masticated, and mixed with saliva to form a cohesive bolus (see Fig. 10.4A). This phase requires tension in the labial and buccal musculature (CN VII) while rotary mandible motion produces chewing (CN V_3). Tongue mobility is the most important neuromuscular function involved in this first phase.

2. The **oral swallowing phase** is initiated when the tongue (CN XII) sequentially squeezes the bolus posteriorly against the hard palate and initiates propulsion into the oropharynx (see Fig. 10.4B). The soft palate (CN IX), critical to containing the bolus within the oral cavity during the oral preparatory phase, now moves posteriorly to allow the bolus to pass through the faucial arches and simultaneously prevents the bolus from entering the nasopharynx. The swallowing reflex is triggered as the bolus passes the anterior tonsillar pillars, which initiates the pharyngeal phase.

3. The **pharyngeal phase** begins with the bolus passing into the throat, triggering the swallowing reflex and causing several pharyngeal physiologic actions to occur simultaneously, allowing food to pass into the esophagus (see Fig. 10.4C). Intrinsic laryngeal muscles close the larynx, creating a seal that separates the airway from the digestive tract. The tongue is the major force pushing the bolus through the pharynx. Synergistic actions with CN X produce pharyngeal peristalsis as it innervates the pharyngeal constrictors. The food bolus moves around the closed airway and into the piriform sinuses, then is squeezed through the open upper esophageal sphincter and into the esophagus. The motion of the bolus is aided by forward and upward motion of the larynx, widening the esophageal inlet. Once the bolus passes into the esophagus, the larynx returns to its former position and the vocal folds open and respiration resumes. CN IX mediates the sensory portion of the pharyngeal gag but innervates just one muscle, the stylopharyngeus. The gag reflex is the best direct test of glossopharyngeal function, although it requires both CNs IX and X to be functioning. When swallowing is inefficient and aspiration occurs, a reflexive cough needs to occur as a respiratory defense against foreign matter. The cough reflex is induced by irritation of afferent CN IX and CN X sensory fibers in the larynx, trachea, and larger bronchi (see Figs. 10.2 and 10.3).

4. The **esophageal phase** starts with the passage of the bolus through the upper esophageal sphincter (also called the cricopharyngeus) (see Fig. 10.4D). CN X mediates the action of the cricopharyngeus, which relaxes to allow food to pass from the hypopharynx into the esophagus. Once the bolus enters the esophagus, serial contractions of the esophageal muscle push the bolus down to the lower esophageal sphincter (LES) and into the stomach.

Clinical Presentation

There are myriad presentations of dysphagia; although some complaints are more concerning than others, it is frequently difficult to determine the severity of a patient's dysphagia based solely on symptoms. Less concerning symptoms are a sensation of something being stuck in the throat (globus) or difficulty swallowing one's own saliva, and the most concerning presentation is recurrent aspiration pneumonia. In swallowing evaluations, two terms are commonly used to identify events that increase the risk of aspiration pneumonia: penetration and aspiration. **Penetration** is defined as the entry of material into the laryngeal introitus, where it is more likely to be aspirated. **Aspiration** is the entry of an inappropriate substance below the level of the vocal folds. If the aspirated material is not quickly and completely cleared, aspiration pneumonia can occur.

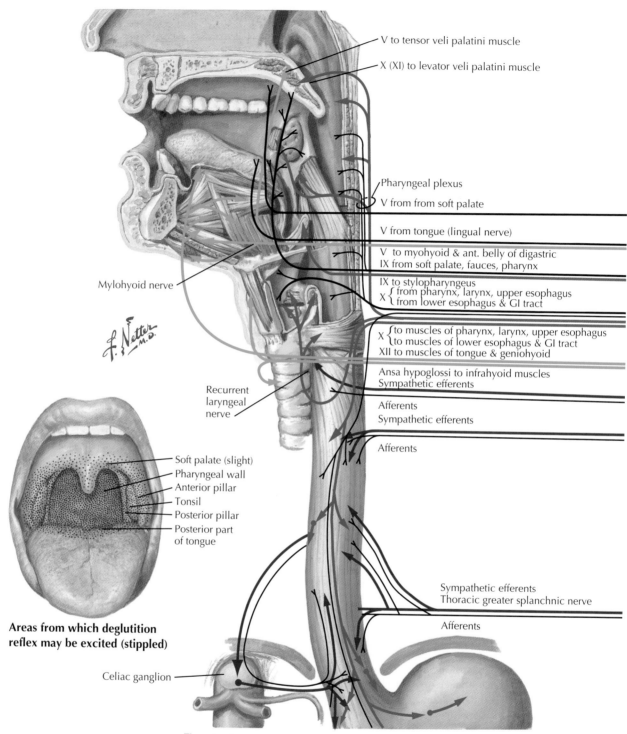

V to tensor veli palatini muscle

X (XI) to levator veli palatini muscle

Pharyngeal plexus

V from from soft palate

V from tongue (lingual nerve)

V to myohyoid & ant. belly of digastric
IX from soft palate, fauces, pharynx

IX to stylopharyngeus
X { from pharynx, larynx, upper esophagus
{ from lower esophagus & GI tract

X { to muscles of pharynx, larynx, upper esophagus
{ to muscles of lower esophagus & GI tract
XII to muscles of tongue & geniohyoid

Ansa hypoglossi to infrahyoid muscles
Sympathetic efferents

Afferents
Sympathetic efferents

Afferents

Mylohyoid nerve

Recurrent
laryngeal
nerve

Sympathetic efferents
Thoracic greater splanchnic nerve

Afferents

Soft palate (slight)
Pharyngeal wall
Anterior pillar
Tonsil
Posterior pillar
Posterior part
of tongue

**Areas from which deglutition
reflex may be excited (stippled)**

Celiac ganglion

Fig. 10.1 Neuroregulation of Deglutition.

Odynophagia, or pain on swallowing, occurs most frequently due to infectious or neoplastic causes. The mechanism of swallowing is generally preserved, and aspiration is rare. If the symptoms are acute, bacterial and viral pathogens are more likely, and prompt evaluation is warranted because serious conditions such as epiglottis or neck abscess could be the cause. More chronic, indolent presentations tend to occur with fungal infections; these are more likely in patients with diabetes, patients using inhaled steroids, or in immunocompromised patients. Cancers of the base of tongue, supraglottis, or hypopharynx generally present with progressive odynophagia and, in the later stages, may cause swallowing dysfunction and malnutrition. Esophageal cancers are asymptomatic in the early stages but can cause symptoms of food sticking in the throat or chest in later stages.

Dysphagia, or difficulty swallowing, is usefully divided by the consistency of the swallowed bolus. Dysphagia to saliva but not to other consistencies is the least concerning. This symptom frequently occurs with globus sensation. This seems to occur due to minor sensory changes in the hypopharynx or due to mild edema of the larynx and is most

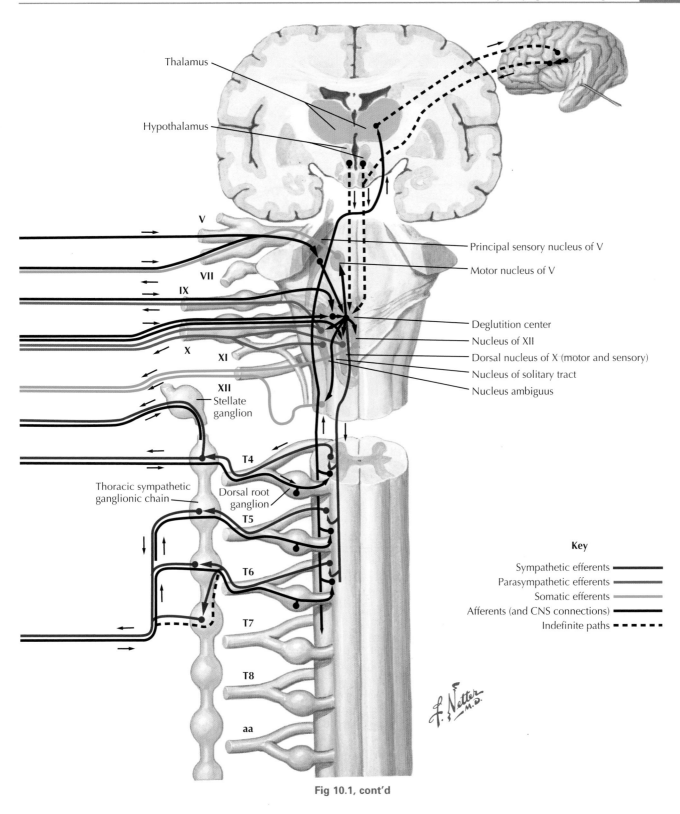

Thalamus

Hypothalamus

V

VII

IX

X

XI

XII
Stellate
ganglion

Thoracic sympathetic
ganglionic chain

Dorsal root
ganglion

T4

T5

T6

T7

T8

aa

Principal sensory nucleus of V

Motor nucleus of V

Deglutition center
Nucleus of XII
Dorsal nucleus of X (motor and sensory)
Nucleus of solitary tract
Nucleus ambiguus

Key

Sympathetic efferents
Parasympathetic efferents
Somatic efferents
Afferents (and CNS connections)
Indefinite paths

Fig 10.1, cont'd

often ascribed to laryngopharyngeal reflux. Some of these patients have anxiety about swallowing, which leads to oral aversive behaviors; they may refuse to eat specific foods or consistencies. Dysphagia to solids is often localizable to a narrow, specific area in the swallowing system. In this case, dysphagia starts with the largest and firmest boluses, such as large pills or meats, then progresses to smaller and less solid boluses. Some patients can point to a specific spot where the food becomes stuck. Patients may also develop dysphagia to solids due to loss of pharyngeal muscle strength. In these cases, all solids will be equally difficult, and they have frequent coughing or regurgitation of the bolus. Speech is frequently affected and may be wet and gurgly sounding due to accumulation of secretions in the larynx. Patients with dry mouth or throat may have difficulty with bread and crackers, which are inadequately moisturized and remain very sticky.

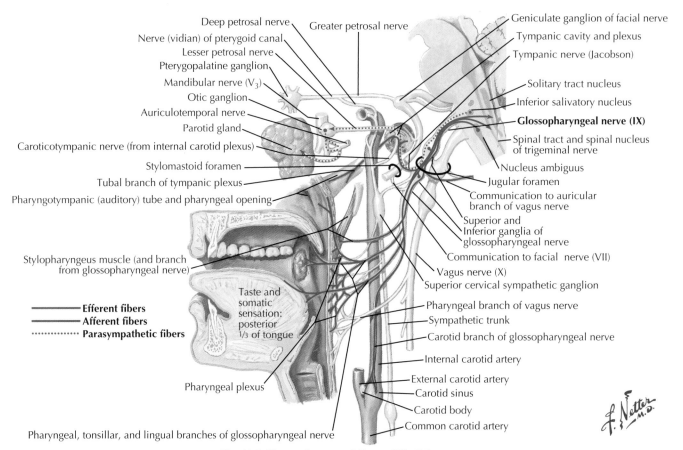

Deep petrosal nerve
Nerve (vidian) of pterygoid canal
Lesser petrosal nerve
Pterygopalatine ganglion
Mandibular nerve (V₃)
Otic ganglion
Auriculotemporal nerve
Parotid gland
Caroticotympanic nerve (from internal carotid plexus)
Stylomastoid foramen
Tubal branch of tympanic plexus
Pharyngotympanic (auditory) tube and pharyngeal opening

Greater petrosal nerve

Geniculate ganglion of facial nerve
Tympanic cavity and plexus
Tympanic nerve (Jacobson)
Solitary tract nucleus
Inferior salivatory nucleus
Glossopharyngeal nerve (IX)
Spinal tract and spinal nucleus of trigeminal nerve
Nucleus ambiguus
Jugular foramen
Communication to auricular branch of vagus nerve
Superior and Inferior ganglia of glossopharyngeal nerve
Communication to facial nerve (VII)
Vagus nerve (X)
Superior cervical sympathetic ganglion

Stylopharyngeus muscle (and branch from glossopharyngeal nerve)

Taste and somatic sensation: posterior ⅓ of tongue

——— **Efferent fibers**
——— **Afferent fibers**
·········· **Parasympathetic fibers**

Pharyngeal plexus

Pharyngeal branch of vagus nerve
Sympathetic trunk
Carotid branch of glossopharyngeal nerve
Internal carotid artery
External carotid artery
Carotid sinus
Carotid body
Common carotid artery

Pharyngeal, tonsillar, and lingual branches of glossopharyngeal nerve

Fig. 10.2 Glossopharyngeal Nerve (IX): Schema.

Dysphagia to liquids is the best indicator of a neurologic cause of dysphagia. Liquids do not form a cohesive bolus, and dysphagia can occur during any phase of the swallow. If oral control and sensation are lacking, the liquids can leak into the pharynx before the swallow is initiated. Sometimes they will trigger the swallow when they reach the larynx (secondary trigger of swallow), and the patient will protect the airway and successfully manage the swallow. In more concerning cases the liquids will enter the laryngeal introitus (penetration) and even make it to the trachea or beyond before a cough is triggered. Other patients can hold the liquids in the oral cavity without difficulty but have problems once the swallow is initiated. If the larynx does not close fully due to vocal fold paralysis or structural abnormality, the sphincteric effect is impaired and liquids may penetrate below the vocal folds during the swallow. In these cases the cough is also generally impaired, and it may be very difficult to clear any aspirated material. Finally, in some patients the coordination of swallowing is abnormal. One of the most common problems in coordination is early closure of the upper esophageal sphincter, leading to a portion of the bolus being trapped in the hypopharynx. The larynx then opens, and secondary aspiration of the residual material can occur.

Silent aspiration is the combination of swallowing dysfunction, leading to aspiration, and sensory loss, causing a lack of reflexive actions to clear the aspirated material. In patients with aspiration events, but normal sensation, reflexive coughing can efficiently clear the airway and prevent aspirated material from reaching the lung. These patients are at higher risk of aspiration pneumonia but can go years between episodes. Patients with abnormal sensation but normal swallow cannot sense aspiration but rarely or never have aspiration events that would normally trigger the cough reflex. Many of these patients have only

rare aspiration pneumonias. The patients with silent aspiration are the ones at highest risk of pneumonia and are the least able to modify the swallow to increase safety. Many of these patients are maintained on no-oral feeding due to the frequency and severity of their aspiration pneumonias.

Diagnostic Approach

Occult swallowing problems are common in hospitalized patients, and failure to recognize the presence of dysphagia increases the risk of aspiration pneumonia, prolonged hospitalization, and death. Techniques for rapid universal dysphagia screening have been developed and are increasingly being implemented in the hospital setting. For patients who fail the dysphagia screening, formal assessment of swallowing function serves to confirm the severity of dysphagia and to identify therapeutic strategies to minimize the risk of aspiration.

Dysphagia screening begins with a simple evaluation of the patient's mental status and ability to follow commands. Hospitalized patients who are not oriented to person, place, and time or who cannot follow simple commands ("stick your tongue out") should be kept NPO (nothing by mouth) unless evaluated and cleared for oral intake by a speech-language pathologist. Other patients can be screened with the **3-ounce swallow test:** the patient is asked to drink a 3-oz cup of water continuously until empty. If they stop between swallows, cough or choke, or have a wet, gurgly vocal quality after drinking the water, the test is considered a failure. In a large study of 3000 patients, the 3-ounce swallow test was found to be highly sensitive but had a 51% false-positive rate. Some institutions have developed different screening protocols with better specificity; the 3-ounce swallow test has the advantage of being simple and quick to administer.

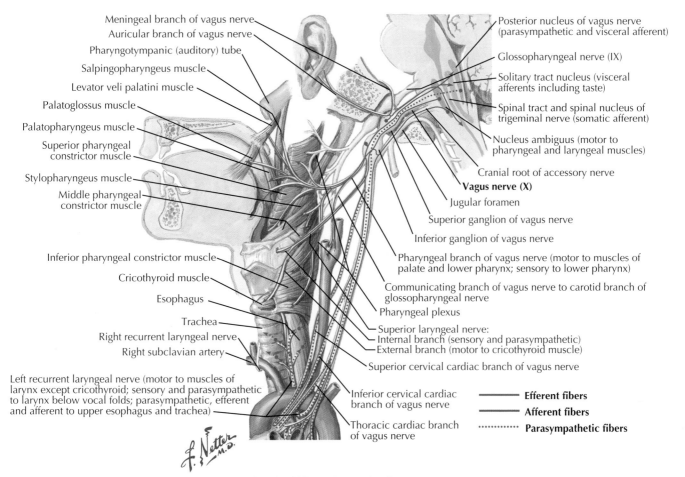

Meningeal branch of vagus nerve
Auricular branch of vagus nerve
Pharyngotympanic (auditory) tube
Salpingopharyngeus muscle
Levator veli palatini muscle
Palatoglossus muscle
Palatopharyngeus muscle
Superior pharyngeal constrictor muscle
Stylopharyngeus muscle
Middle pharyngeal constrictor muscle

Inferior pharyngeal constrictor muscle
Cricothyroid muscle
Esophagus
Trachea
Right recurrent laryngeal nerve
Right subclavian artery
Left recurrent laryngeal nerve (motor to muscles of larynx except cricothyroid; sensory and parasympathetic to larynx below vocal folds; parasympathetic, efferent and afferent to upper esophagus and trachea)

Posterior nucleus of vagus nerve (parasympathetic and visceral afferent)
Glossopharyngeal nerve (IX)
Solitary tract nucleus (visceral afferents including taste)
Spinal tract and spinal nucleus of trigeminal nerve (somatic afferent)
Nucleus ambiguus (motor to pharyngeal and laryngeal muscles)
Cranial root of accessory nerve
Vagus nerve (X)
Jugular foramen
Superior ganglion of vagus nerve
Inferior ganglion of vagus nerve
Pharyngeal branch of vagus nerve (motor to muscles of palate and lower pharynx; sensory to lower pharynx)
Communicating branch of vagus nerve to carotid branch of glossopharyngeal nerve
Pharyngeal plexus
Superior laryngeal nerve:
Internal branch (sensory and parasympathetic)
External branch (motor to cricothyroid muscle)
Superior cervical cardiac branch of vagus nerve
Inferior cervical cardiac branch of vagus nerve
Thoracic cardiac branch of vagus nerve

—— **Efferent fibers**
—— **Afferent fibers**
·········· **Parasympathetic fibers**

Fig. 10.3 Vagus Nerve (X): Schema.

Flexible endoscopic evaluation of swallowing (FEES) allows direct evaluation of motor and sensory aspects of the pharyngeal swallow. It requires transnasal passage of a fiberoptic laryngoscope to view the larynx and surrounding structures. Laryngeal airway protection and the integrity of the oropharyngeal swallow are assessed by giving various foods tinted with coloring to enhance visualization. Velopharyngeal closure, abduction and adduction of the vocal folds, pharyngeal contraction, and the patient's ability to manage secretions are assessed. If abnormalities are detected, compensatory strategies and postures are also assessed.

Modified barium swallow (MBS), also called **videofluoroscopy,** is a functional radiologic evaluation intended to determine appropriate therapeutic intervention strategies to facilitate safe and efficient swallowing function.

FEES and MBS are complementary modalities; MBS provides better views of the upper esophageal sphincter and esophagus, whereas FEES can be performed by the bedside and uses real food. Sometimes one of these modalities will identify a problem missed by the other due to these differences. Both FEES and MBS have been validated as objective swallowing tests able to accurately evaluate dysphagia and identify patients at risk of aspiration.

Clinical Considerations and Outlook

There are three major considerations for resumption of oral intake in dysphagic patients: safety of swallow, ability to maintain oral nutritional support, and quality of life. In patients with central neurologic compromise, safety of swallow is often grossly impaired and the risk of aspiration pneumonia significantly increased. In addition, many of these patients are bedridden and have cognitive impairment or decreased levels of alertness. In this setting, even small amounts of aspiration are likely to progress to serious aspiration pneumonia. Although the majority of stroke patients improve over time and resume oral intake, other neurodegenerative disorders such as amyotrophic lateral sclerosis (ALS) have an unrelenting course with progressive dysphagia and increasing risk of aspiration. Patients with neuromuscular disorders, such as myasthenia gravis, may begin with a strong swallow but fatigue over the course of a meal and cannot safely complete a meal. For many patients, eating becomes progressively time consuming and effortful, making consumption of enough calories difficult. Elucidating the exact etiology and pathophysiology for dysphagia in each case helps to direct the treatment approach and predict outcome.

Interventions for dysphagia are individually determined based on the location and type of dysphagia, the patient's desires, and the risks of oral intake. There is no "one-size-fits-all" approach. Patients with oral-motor abnormalities can frequently use assistive devices such as long-handled spoons to bypass their problem, and oral motor exercises can restore function. Abnormalities of the pharyngeal swallow are most common, and there are many potential interventions: specific exercises can strengthen weak pharyngeal or base of tongue muscles, a preswallow breath-hold can help to close the larynx before the swallow, and a planned cough after the swallow can clear material that penetrates the larynx. For upper esophageal sphincter abnormalities, surgical intervention can

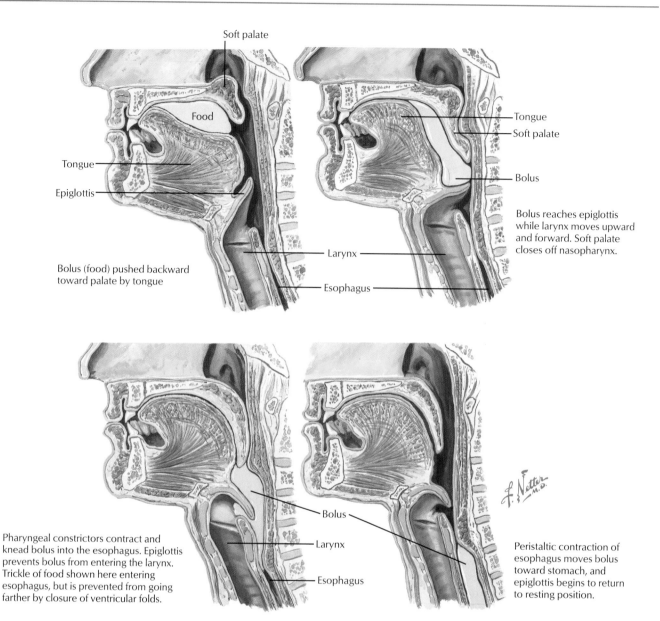

Bolus (food) pushed backward toward palate by tongue

Bolus reaches epiglottis while larynx moves upward and forward. Soft palate closes off nasopharynx.

Pharyngeal constrictors contract and knead bolus into the esophagus. Epiglottis prevents bolus from entering the larynx. Trickle of food shown here entering esophagus, but is prevented from going farther by closure of ventricular folds.

Peristaltic contraction of esophagus moves bolus toward stomach, and epiglottis begins to return to resting position.

Fig. 10.4 Deglutition.

be helpful. Surgery in this area should start with esophageal dilation and injections of botulinum toxin into the upper esophageal sphincter. If these temporary measures improve the swallow, permanent surgical division of the upper esophageal sphincter can be performed endoscopically or via an open approach. In patients with severe swallowing dysfunction, nonoral feeding (gastrostomy or jejunostomy) can be life-saving. In some patients, a gastrostomy tube maintains nutrition while the patient recovers. In others, a gastrostomy tube maintains hydration or nutrition while they continue to take small amounts of food by mouth for social reasons, as well as to continue having the pleasure of eating. Some patients accept the risk of deadly aspiration pneumonia in order to maintain a normal life, whereas others undergo early gastrostomy because maintaining nutrition is time consuming and not enjoyable. Optimal management of dysphagia requires a multidisciplinary approach and awareness of the natural history of the underlying disorder, as well as taking the patient's desires, fears, and social situation into account.

CRANIAL NERVE X, VAGUS: VOICE DISORDERS

CLINICAL VIGNETTE *A 33-year-old female computer programmer with no prior medical problems presented with abrupt onset of a weak, breathy voice and coughing and choking when drinking thin liquids. Physical examination revealed a healthy female with a very breathy and weak voice. Otolaryngologica examination found a complete left vocal fold paralysis, with the vocal fold in the paramedian position. Chest x-ray and computed tomography (CT) of the neck revealed no lesions or masses along the course of the left vagus nerve. Idiopathic vocal fold paralysis was diagnosed, and the patient deferred temporary injection of the vocal fold to improve voice and swallowing. Over the next 12 weeks, the patient noted a slow but steady return of her voice, and reexamination of the larynx 4 months after symptom onset showed near-normal function of the left vocal fold.*

Although the larynx is usually considered the source of speech, speech production requires precise coordination of multiple organ systems. Contraction of the abdominal musculature, diaphragm, and chest wall provides a power source for the voice. The larynx acts as a pressure regulator and vibratory source. The pharynx, tongue, nose, and mouth shape these vibrations into recognizable speech and singing. However, the larynx is the most easily injured of these systems, and most vocal problems originate within it.

Anatomy/Pathophysiology

The motor supply of the laryngeal muscles begins in the nucleus ambiguus (see Fig. 10.3). These fibers travel within the vagus nerve (CN X) as it exits the cranium via the jugular foramen, traveling through the neck within the carotid sheath (Fig. 10.5). High in the neck, the superior laryngeal nerve (SLN) splits away from CN X. It then divides into internal and external branches. The internal branch pierces the thyrohyoid membrane and provides sensory innervation to the pharynx and larynx. The external branch travels lower in the neck past the superior pole of the thyroid gland to innervate the cricothyroid muscle.

The recurrent laryngeal nerve (RLN) takes a more tortuous path. It separates from CN X, loops around the aortic arch on the left and the brachiocephalic artery on the right, and travels back toward the larynx in the tracheoesophageal groove bilaterally. It passes under the thyroid gland and inserts into the larynx under the thyroid cartilage, innervating all other intrinsic laryngeal muscles. Both these nerves are vulnerable to injury and have distinct symptoms when injured.

Clinical Presentation: Disorders of Voice
Recurrent Laryngeal Nerve

RLN damage usually causes vocal fold immobility on the side of injury. Depending on the position of the vocal fold, symptom severity varies greatly. If the vocal fold is lateral, the larynx cannot close and symptoms include breathy, hoarse voice, dysphagia to liquids, and ineffective cough. If the paralyzed vocal fold is in the midline, the vocal folds will close better, and the only symptoms may be vocal fatigue and slight breathiness. Most patients eventually compensate somewhat.

Surgical injuries remain the most common cause of unilateral vocal fold paralysis. In nonsurgical injuries, more frequent underlying causes

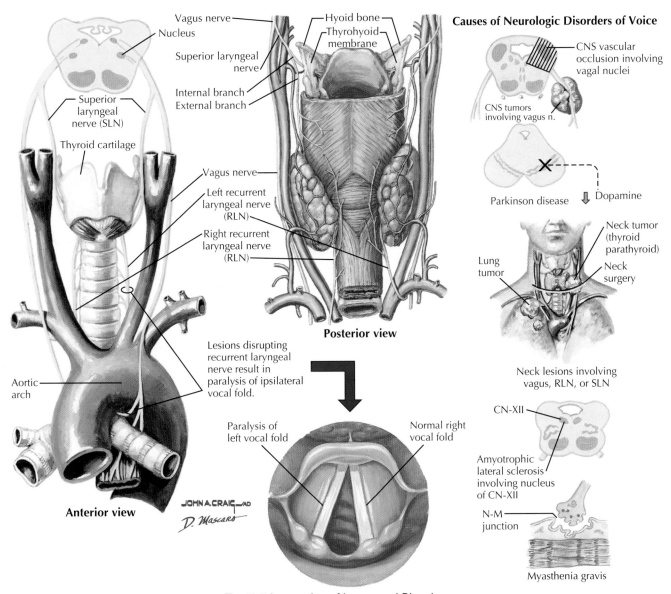

Fig. 10.5 Innervation of Larynx and Disorders.

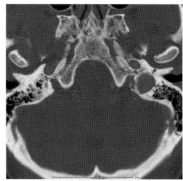

Axial skull base brain CT: Smoothly marginated left jugular fossa expansion (arrowheads).

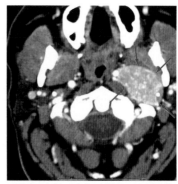

Postcontrast axial neck CT: Markedly enhancing, well marinated, posterior left carotid space mass lesion (arrows).

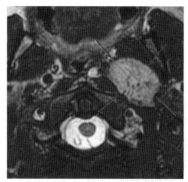

Axial T2 neck MR: Discrete, left posterior carotid space mass with "salt and pepper" signal pattern (arrows).

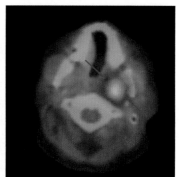

Axial octreotide scan of the neck: Markedly avid uptake left carotid space mass lesion (arrows).

Fig. 10.6 Glomus Tumor of Vagal Nerve.

include thyroid, lung, or neck tumors; cerebrovascular accidents; and CN X tumors (paragangliomas or glomus vagale [Fig. 10.6]). Many patients have no identifiable cause of their paralysis, although a viral/inflammatory cause is posited, no proof is yet available, and treatment with steroids or antivirals has not been shown to be helpful.

Superior Laryngeal Nerve

The classic symptom of SLN dysfunction is the inability to raise the vocal pitch. Patients also frequently have weak voices that tire easily. High CN X lesions and cerebrovascular accidents cause combined SLN and RLN injuries. These patients are at high risk for aspiration because they can neither close the larynx nor sense when they are about to aspirate. Most cases of isolated SLN paresis are from thyroid surgery or are idiopathic.

Other Neurologic Disorders of the Larynx

Spasmodic dysphonia is a task-specific dystonia affecting the larynx. Patients have irregular voice breaks when trying to speak, but many can sing normally. Its cause is unknown. Treatment involves identifying the involved muscles and paralyzing them with injections of botulinum toxin.

Patients with laryngeal tremor have regular voice breaks and a tremulous voice. Laryngeal examination reveals regular contractions of the laryngeal muscles at rest and during phonation. Singing is not spared. It can be difficult to distinguish spasmodic dysphonia from tremor.

Vocal fold bowing occurs due to a loss of vibratory material and muscle mass in the larynx. Although it can be a natural consequence of aging, it is a prominent feature of Parkinson disease and can occur

in several other neurologic disorders. The voice is weak and breathy, and accessory muscle compensation is common, causing neck pain and vocal fatigue. Speech therapy significantly reduces symptoms in 85% of patients with idiopathic bowing, and an intensive form of speech therapy (Lee Silverman Voice Technique) has been shown to be very successful in patients with Parkinson disease. For those who have inadequate response to speech therapy, surgery is available to straighten and bulk the bowed vocal folds.

Diagnostic Approach

Diagnosis of laryngeal motion abnormalities is primarily done via direct visualization of the larynx. Mirror examination (Fig. 10.7) is technically difficult and limited by the gag reflex. Fiberoptic laryngoscopy is a simple, fast, well-tolerated procedure that allows determination of the cause of hoarseness in most cases. For patients with hoarseness that is not easily diagnosed by flexible laryngoscopy, more advanced investigations including laryngeal stroboscopy and laryngeal electromyography can be helpful. In patients with vocal paralysis without obvious cause, imaging of the vagus nerve course can help to find an underlying diagnosis.

Treatment: Vocal Fold Paralysis

Although many patients will have spontaneous recovery of vocal fold function, some patients do not want to wait to regain their voice and some do not recover spontaneously. Treatment is usually directed at moving the paralyzed vocal fold to the midline with an injection into the paralyzed side, or placement of implant below the vocal fold via an external approach. Reinnervation procedures have been described but are not widely used because of inconsistent results.

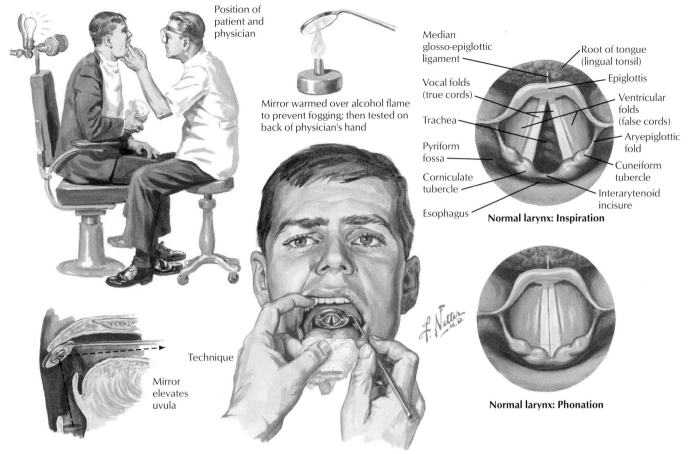

Position of patient and physician

Mirror warmed over alcohol flame to prevent fogging; then tested on back of physician's hand

Median glosso-epiglottic ligament

Vocal folds (true cords)

Trachea

Pyriform fossa

Corniculate tubercle

Esophagus

Root of tongue (lingual tonsil)

Epiglottis

Ventricular folds (false cords)

Aryepiglottic fold

Cuneiform tubercle

Interarytenoid incisure

Normal larynx: Inspiration

Technique

Mirror elevates uvula

Normal larynx: Phonation

Fig. 10.7 Mirror Examination of the Larynx.

ADDITIONAL RESOURCES

Suiter DM, Leder SB. Clinical utility of the 3-ounce water swallow test. Dysphagia 2008;23(3):244–50.

Study of 3000 patients demonstrating the high sensitivity of the 3-oz water test in a wide variety of patients.

Rosenthal LH, Benninger MS, Deeb RH. Vocal fold immobility: a longitudinal analysis of etiology over 20 years. Laryngoscope 2007;117(10):1864–70.

A large study of patients with vocal fold paralysis showing the changing trends in etiology over two decades of study.

Langmore SE, Skarupski KA, Park PS, et al. Predictors of aspiration pneumonia in nursing home residents. Dysphagia 2002;17:298–307.

Risks and results of aspiration pneumonia in a high-risk cohort.

Paniello RC, Barlow J, Serna JS. Longitudinal follow-up of adductor spasmodic dysphonia patients after botulinum toxin injection: quality of life results. Laryngoscope 2008;118(3):564–8.

Quality of life improvements in patients with spasmodic dysphonia treated with botulinum toxin injections.

Rosen CA, Gartner-Schmidt J, Casiano R, et al. Vocal fold augmentation with calcium hydroxylapatite: twelve-month report. Laryngoscope 2009;119(5):1033–41.

One of the largest multiinstitutional studies of the treatment of vocal fold paralysis.

11

Cranial Nerves XI and XII: Accessory and Hypoglossal

David P. Lerner, Michal Vytopil

CRANIAL NERVE XI: THE SPINAL ACCESSORY NERVE

Cranial nerve (CN) XI, or the spinal accessory nerve (SAN), serves primarily as the motor nerve for the sternocleidomastoid (SCM) and trapezius muscles in the neck and shoulder. It has an intriguing functional array with one of the two major muscles it innervates, the SCM, inserting on the ipsilateral occiput. When one side contracts, it turns the head in the opposite direction; for example, a right SCM contraction turns the head to the left and vice versa. Both SCM muscles contracting simultaneously results in neck flexion.

The seemingly paradoxical function of the SCM is also of interest and used in rare circumstance of a *hysterical pseudohemiparesis* or *functional somatization*. Patients feigning a right hemiparesis will give way when asked to turn their head against resistance to the right, not realizing that it is the left SCM that turns the head contralaterally; also when asked to turn their head to the asymptomatic left, they use the right SCM without difficulty.

Anatomy

The SAN is primarily a motor nerve innervating the SCM and trapezius muscles in the neck and back (Fig. 11.1). In contrast to the other CNs, its lower motor neuron cell bodies are located primarily within the spinal cord. The accessory nucleus is a cell column within the lateral anterior gray column of the upper five or six cervical spinal cord segments. Proximally it lies nearly in line with the nucleus ambiguus and caudally within the dorsolateral ventral horn. Originating from the accessory nucleus, the rootlets emerge from the cord and unite to form the trunk of CN XI. This extends rostrally through the foramen magnum into the posterior cranial fossa. Intracranially, it accompanies the caudal fibers of the vagus nerve (CN X) exiting the skull through the jugular foramen. The SAN then descends in close proximity to the internal carotid artery and internal jugular vein (Fig. 11.2).

Once the SAN is extracranial, it is joined by fibers derived from the third and fourth upper cervical ventral rami. Some of these cervical fibers may innervate the caudal trapezius, whereas the proximal trapezius and the entire SCM muscle are primarily innervated by CN XI. The SAN then emerges from the midpoint of the posterior border of the SCM, to cross the posterior triangle of the neck superficial to the levator scapulae. It is here that this CN is in close proximity to the superficial cervical lymph nodes. Further caudally, approximately 5 cm above the clavicle, it passes into the anterior border of the trapezius muscle, which it also innervates.

There is a minor afferent component to the SAN that carries primary proprioceptive function for the two muscles it innervates. In addition, a minor cranial root contribution to the spinal accessory consists of a few fibers originating in the caudal portion of the nucleus ambiguus. These fibers traverse with the intracranial SAN and exit through the jugular foramen.

The supranuclear innervation of the CN XI nuclei is still a matter of debate. Although the trapezius muscle is innervated from the opposite hemisphere, there is some question as to whether the supranuclear innervation of the SCM is also contralateral. One standard neuroanatomy text (Brodal, 1998) states that with clinical corticobulbar lesions there is paresis of the contralateral SCM as well as the trapezius. Others note, based on intracarotid sodium amytal injections, that the SCM is innervated predominantly from the ipsilateral hemisphere. Suffice it to say that the most proximal and midline musculature can be activated bilaterally. Therefore one needs to be circumspect when attempting to lateralize the source of unilateral SCM weakness.

Clinical Presentation and Diagnostic Approach

SAN lesions located intracranially or proximally to the innervation of the SCM cause weakness of both the SCM and the trapezius. If the SCM is weak, the patient experiences weakness when turning the head to the opposite side. Damage to the nerve within the posterior triangle of the neck spares the SCM and results in weakness of the trapezius only. Involvement of the trapezius manifests as drooping of the shoulder and mild scapular winging away from the chest wall with slight lateral displacement. Weakness in shoulder elevation and arm abduction above horizontal is typical. Winging is apparent with arms hanging along the trunk and becomes accentuated when patients abduct the arms. In contrast, scapular winging from serratus anterior weakness due to long thoracic nerve palsy is most prominent on forward elevation of the arms (Fig. 11.3).

Most individuals with CN XI palsies present with shoulder or neck pain or both. The painful paresis can be sudden because of direct injury during procedures such as excision biopsies of lymph nodes in the posterior triangle of the neck, radical dissection of lymph nodes in the neck, or with trauma, or the paresis can be subacute such as with entrapment of the nerve within scar tissue or structural lesions such as tumors. As in all patients with neck and shoulder pain, careful exam and history are necessary to exclude lesions at the level of the cervical nerve roots or brachial plexus.

Electromyography is important for confirming that the lesion is confined to the distribution of CN XI. In addition, a gadolinium-enhanced magnetic resonance imaging (MRI) is appropriate if any question exists of a more widespread lesion other than a simple CN XI neuropathy.

Differential Diagnosis

The most common site of isolated CN XI neuropathy is within the neck. The close association of CN XI with superficial cervical lymph nodes renders it vulnerable to iatrogenic damage during lymph node biopsy or a radical neck surgical dissection. The SAN can also be directly compressed by swollen lymph nodes or other solid tumors. Rarely, CN XI neuropathy occurs after blunt or penetrating **neck trauma** or due to **radiation injury** with treatment of adjacent tumors. Although it is

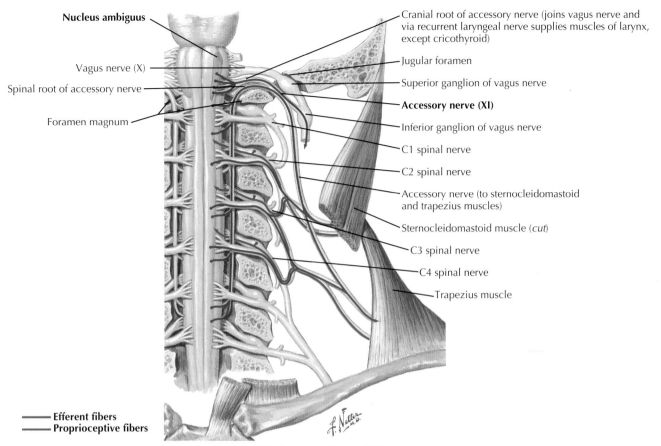

Fig. 11.1 Accessory Nerve (XI): Schema.

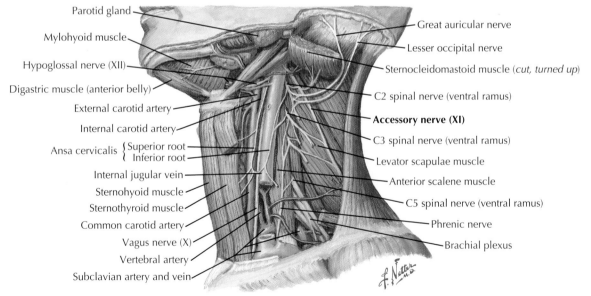

Fig. 11.2 Cervical Plexu in Situ.

not part of the brachial plexuus, CN XI can be involved in patients with **brachial plexitis** (neuralgic amyotrophy). Damage also rarely occurs after carotid endarterectomy or jugular vein cannulation because of the nerve's proximity to large neck vessels.

Intraspinal and intracranial portions of CN XI may be affected by **intrinsic spinal cord lesions,** posterior fossa **meningiomas,** or **metastases.** Benign tumors such as an en plaque meningioma at the base of the

brain or **metastatic tumors** at the jugular foramen or foramen magnum may impinge on the SAN; however, these various lesions usually affect concomitantly the glossopharyngeal, vagal, and sometimes even the hypoglossal nerve exiting through the adjacent hypoglossal foramen. Very rarely, varied pathologic lesions of the SAN occur just after it leaves the skull and courses through the space behind the parotid gland and pharynx. CNs IX, X, XI, and XII and adjacent sympathetic chain

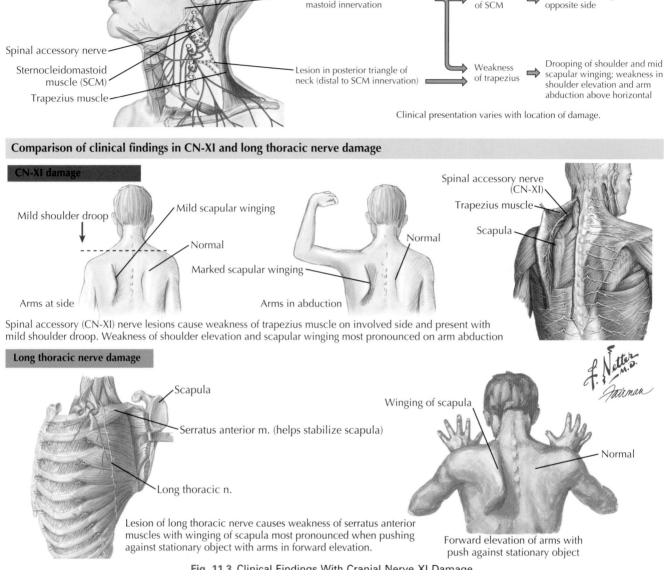

Clinical presentation varies with location of damage.

Comparison of clinical findings in CN-XI and long thoracic nerve damage

Fig. 11.3 Clinical Findings With Cranial Nerve XI Damage.

fibers (causing Horner syndrome) are potentially involved in variable combinations with primary or metastatic tumors.

Various disorders at the anatomic level of the anterior horn cell are within the differential of CN XI neuropathy, including **motor neuron disease, syringomyelia,** and **poliomyelitis.** In these cases, one finds prominent atrophy and fasciculations affecting both the SCM and trapezius muscles.

Prognosis

For patients with benign traumatic lesions, the likelihood of reinnervation is good unless the proximal and distal SAN segments are widely separated. Sometimes surgical exploration is helpful. The time frame for reinnervation is similar to that for any peripheral nerve: 1 mm/day or 3 cm/month.

CRANIAL NERVE XII: HYPOGLOSSAL

Despite being the most distal of the 12 paired CNs, the hypoglossal nerve (CN XII) controls what is teleologically an important human function: the final common pathway for verbal language implementation. Phylogenetically, the hypoglossal nerve also has major significance

in its role in food intake. As with any cranial nerve, CN XII is susceptible to numerous pathologic processes.

Anatomy

CN XII carries motor fibers that supply all intrinsic and most extrinsic tongue muscles (i.e., the hyoglossus, styloglossus, genioglossus, and geniohyoid) (Fig. 11.4). Its fibers originate from the hypoglossal nucleus beneath the floor of the fourth ventricle (Fig. 11.5). In its intramedullary course, CN XII axons pass ventrally and lateral to the medial lemniscus emerging from the medulla in the ventrolateral sulcus between the olive and the pyramid. The rootlets unite to form CN XII, which exits the skull through the hypoglossal foramen adjacent to the foramen magnum within the posterior cranial fossa (Fig. 11.6).

After exiting the skull, CN XII runs medial to CN IX, X, and XI. It continues between the internal carotid artery and internal jugular vein, and deep into the posterior belly of the digastric muscle. It then loops anteriorly, coursing on the lateral surface of the hyoglossus muscle, and later, it divides to supply the intrinsic and extrinsic muscles of the ipsilateral tongue (see Fig. 11.4).

The anterior primary ramus of the spinal nerve C1 sends fibers to accompany CN XII for a short distance; these fibers later connect with

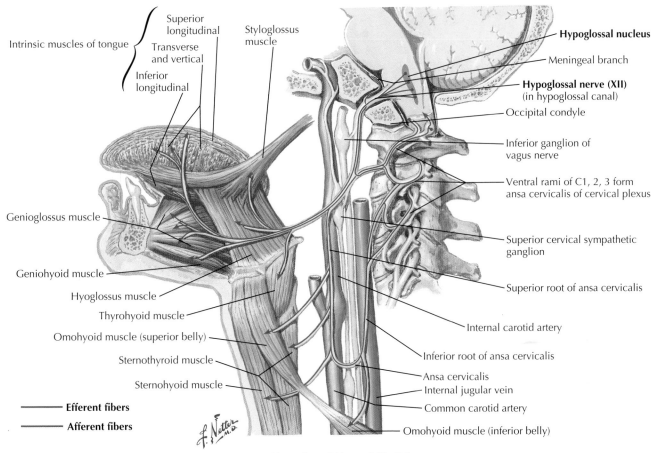

Superior longitudinal

Styloglossus muscle

Intrinsic muscles of tongue

Transverse and vertical

Inferior longitudinal

Hypoglossal nucleus

Meningeal branch

Hypoglossal nerve (XII) (in hypoglossal canal)

Occipital condyle

Inferior ganglion of vagus nerve

Ventral rami of C1, 2, 3 form ansa cervicalis of cervical plexus

Genioglossus muscle

Geniohyoid muscle

Hyoglossus muscle

Thyrohyoid muscle

Superior cervical sympathetic ganglion

Superior root of ansa cervicalis

Omohyoid muscle (superior belly)

Sternothyroid muscle

Sternohyoid muscle

Internal carotid artery

Inferior root of ansa cervicalis

Ansa cervicalis

Internal jugular vein

Common carotid artery

—— **Efferent fibers**

—— **Afferent fibers**

Omohyoid muscle (inferior belly)

Fig. 11.4 Hypoglossal Nerve (XII): Schema.

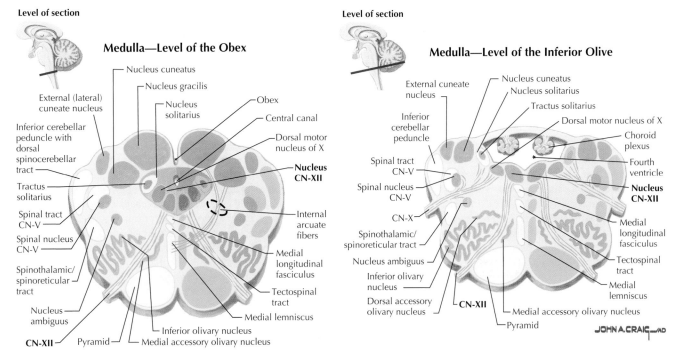

Level of section

Medulla—Level of the Obex

Nucleus cuneatus

Nucleus gracilis

External (lateral) cuneate nucleus

Nucleus solitarius

Obex

Central canal

Inferior cerebellar peduncle with dorsal spinocerebellar tract

Dorsal motor nucleus of X

Nucleus CN-XII

Tractus solitarius

Spinal tract CN-V

Internal arcuate fibers

Spinal nucleus CN-V

Spinothalamic/ spinoreticular tract

Medial longitudinal fasciculus

Nucleus ambiguus

Tectospinal tract

CN-XII

Pyramid

Inferior olivary nucleus

Medial lemniscus

Medial accessory olivary nucleus

Level of section

Medulla—Level of the Inferior Olive

External cuneate nucleus

Nucleus cuneatus

Nucleus solitarius

Tractus solitarius

Inferior cerebellar peduncle

Dorsal motor nucleus of X

Choroid plexus

Spinal tract CN-V

Fourth ventricle

Spinal nucleus CN-V

Nucleus CN-XII

CN-X

Medial longitudinal fasciculus

Spinothalamic/ spinoreticular tract

Nucleus ambiguus

Tectospinal tract

Inferior olivary nucleus

Medial lemniscus

Dorsal accessory olivary nucleus

CN-XII

Medial accessory olivary nucleus

Pyramid

Fig. 11.5 Hypoglossal Nerve Intramedullary Course.

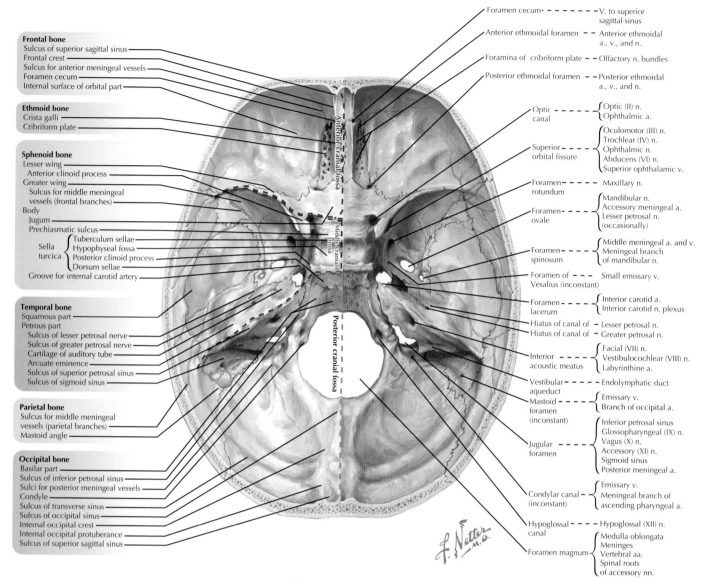

Fig. 11.6 Base of Skull.

the fibers of C2 and C3 anterior primary rami, forming a loop called the *ansa cervicalis*. This innervates the infrahyoid muscles (i.e., sternohyoid, omohyoid, sternothyroid, thyrohyoid, and geniohyoid). These small muscles aid in head flexion.

CLINICAL VIGNETTE *This 64-year-old lady presented with a 2-month history of unrelenting, increasingly disconcerting left occipital headache. This occasionally radiated with brief jabs toward her left ear. Whenever she bent her head forward, the pain became unbearable. Although she was initially diagnosed with occipital neuralgia, two local nerve blocks were ineffective. She admitted that her tongue also felt "leathery" and "numb." One year earlier she was treated for adenocarcinoma of the breast with a partial mastectomy and axillary node dissection. Sampled lymph nodes were negative for cancer.*

Neurologic exam demonstrated atrophy and fasciculations of the left half of the tongue. This was best observed with the tongue at rest inside the mouth. Upon protrusion, the tongue deviated to the left. The head pain was aggravated by neck flexion and suboccipital palpation.

Contrast-enhanced computed tomography (CT) of the skull base revealed an infiltrating lesion eroding the left occipital condyle. Further imaging showed

multiple metastases in the ribs and thoracic vertebrae, as well as liver and lungs. The lesions were assumed to represent metastatic carcinoma. Radiation therapy led to resolution of her headache; however, her hypoglossal neuropathy persisted. Subsequently, she was placed on systemic chemotherapy for disseminated cancer.

*A unilateral hypoglossal neuropathy must always lead to consideration of the presence of a neoplasm, particularly in a patient with history of cancer. In this case, the nerve was damaged by a destructive metastasis as it exited the skull through the hypoglossal foramen at the occipital condyle. Bony metastases at this location, also called **occipital condyle syndrome,** are typically accompanied by occipital pain and neck stiffness. Breast, lung, and prostate cancer account for most of these metastatic lesions.*

Patients with a unilateral hypoglossal neuropathy rarely present with complaints related to tongue function. They may comment that their tongue feels "numb" or "clumsy" but not necessarily weak, yet when asked they are unaware of any intraoral sensory loss per se. This vignette illustrates the value of a careful clinical evaluation and its unique potential to lead to the diagnosis of a unilateral hypoglossal palsy, in this instance a most sinister etiology for this woman's headache.

Clinical Presentation

Clinical evaluation of the hypoglossal nerve requires careful observation of the tongue at rest and during activation by attempting to protrude it directly forward.

Straight protrusion of the tongue is accomplished by balanced action of both genioglossus muscles. Therefore bilateral CN XII lesions impair tongue protrusion, as well as up, down, and side-to-side movements. This in turn causes dysarthria and swallowing difficulties. A *unilateral lower motor neuron hypoglossal nerve lesion* causes the tongue to *deviate toward the side of the lesion* when the patient attempts to protrude the tongue forward. Typically, these lesions are also associated with atrophy, fasciculations, and increased furrowing of the ipsilateral side of the tongue (Fig. 11.7). Swallowing and/or speech dysfunction may not be present early on. Fine quivering or flickering movements are normally seen in healthy patients asked to hold the tongue protruded for more than a few seconds, and these may occasionally be confused with true fasciculations. The most reliable way to evaluate for fasciculations is to keep the tongue at rest on the floor of the mouth. Sometimes, fasciculations may be enhanced by stroking the lateral aspect of the resting tongue with a standard wooden tongue blade. A *unilateral upper motor neuron lesion* may on occasion result in deviation of the tongue; however, this is contralateral to the central lesion, and there is never any accompanying atrophy or fasciculations. In certain disorders, particularly amyotrophic lateral sclerosis, both upper and lower motor neuron components may be present, with the combination leading to some initial diagnostic confusion if this area is the first to become clinically affected.

Differential Diagnosis

Anterior horn cell disorders frequently affect the hypoglossal nucleus, particularly with **motor neuron disease,** spinal muscular atrophy, or **poliomyelitis.** Other intramedullary processes such as **syringobulbia, intramedullary tumors, cavernomas,** or **multiple sclerosis** may also lead to tongue paresis. Because of the close midline proximity of the two hypoglossal nuclei, these structural intramedullary lesions often lead to bilateral tongue paralysis.

When there is a precipitous onset of tongue weakness, this is usually caused by rare atherosclerotic occlusion within a midline penetrating branch of the vertebral basilar system and stroke. This leads to damage of the hypoglossal nucleus and its emerging fibers, the corticospinal tract, and the medial lemniscus. This **medial medullary syndrome** is clinically characterized by an ipsilateral lower motor tongue weakness accompanied by a contralateral hemiparesis and loss of proprioception and vibration. The more proximally innervated face is spared.

The intracranial course of the 12th CN can also be damaged by lesions, typically neoplasms, at the basal meninges and skull base. **Metastatic** lung or breast cancer, lymphomas, or benign lesions such as **meningiomas, chordomas,** or **cholesteatomas** occasionally affect the hypoglossal nerve. The proximity of hypoglossal and jugular foramina explains frequent concomitant involvement of other lower CNs (CN IX, X, and XI) in these cases. Both neoplastic and infectious-inflammatory lesions may lead to a basal meningitis affecting multiple CNs, including the hypoglossal. Rarely, other nonneoplastic, primary bony processes, such as platybasia and Paget disease, may be implicated.

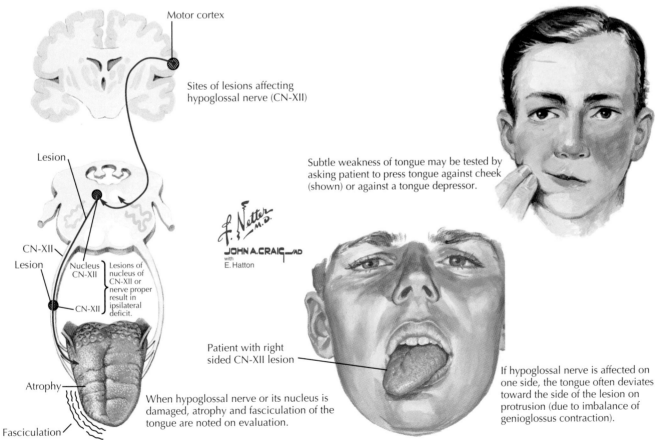

Motor cortex

Sites of lesions affecting hypoglossal nerve (CN-XII)

Lesion

CN-XII

Lesion

Nucleus CN-XII

Lesions of nucleus of CN-XII or nerve proper result in ipsilateral deficit.

CN-XII

Atrophy

Fasciculation

When hypoglossal nerve or its nucleus is damaged, atrophy and fasciculation of the tongue are noted on evaluation.

Subtle weakness of tongue may be tested by asking patient to press tongue against cheek (shown) or against a tongue depressor.

Patient with right sided CN-XII lesion

If hypoglossal nerve is affected on one side, the tongue often deviates toward the side of the lesion on protrusion (due to imbalance of genioglossus contraction).

Fig. 11.7 Hypoglossal Nerve (XII).

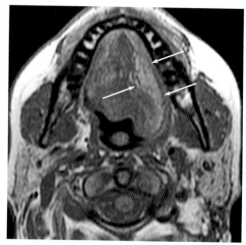

A. Axial neck MR: Denervation atrophy left hemitongue (arrows).

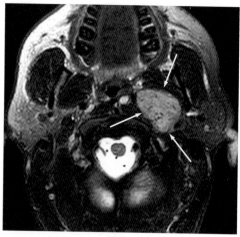

B. Axial T2 neck MR: Discrete, large, left carotid space mass with distinctive "salt and pepper" signal pattern (arrows).

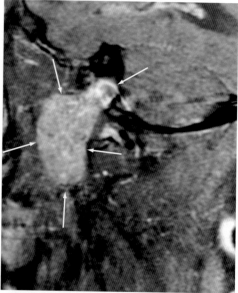

C. Sagittal T2 neck MR: large jugular fossa and carotid space mass with "salt and pepper" signal pattern (arrows).

Fig. 11.8 Glomus Jugulare With Hypoglossal Palsy.

The close spatial relation between the hypoglossal nerve and the carotid artery makes this nerve vulnerable to primary carotid pathology within the neck. Very rarely, *dissection of the internal carotid artery* is accompanied by a CN XII neuropathy, most likely related to nerve compression by the increased circumference of the dissected vessel. Occasionally, an iatrogenic hypoglossal neuropathy occurs subsequent to a *carotid endarterectomy* or other types of neck surgery. A **naso-pharyngeal cancer** may damage CN XII along its intracranial course or within the neck; this is usually in conjunction with involvement of other CNs. **Glomus jugulare tumor** is a rare hypervascular malignancy that arises from the paraganglionic tissue at the jugular foramen and can compress CN XII either at the base of the brain or within the neck (Fig. 11.8A to C). Similar to other CNs, the CN XII may also be affected by **radiation therapy** and **neck trauma.** Most uncommonly, the hypoglossal nerve is affected as part of two primary demyelinating peripheral nerve syndromes, namely, **hereditary neuropathy with liability to pressure palsies (HNPP)** or a variant of chronic inflammatory demyelinating polyneuropathy (CIDP), the **Lewis-Sumner syndrome.**

Glossodynia is a controversial syndrome with no specific etiology as yet defined and can be a feature of the burning mouth syndrome. This is characterized by an uncomfortable burning pain within the tongue, unassociated with any tongue weakness or atrophy. The condition occurs more frequently in women. Vitamin B_1, or B_{12}, deficiency, as well as Sjögren syndrome, have been suggested as pathophysiologic mechanisms. Unfortunately, many of these patients with idiopathic tongue pain are subsequently suspected of having a psychogenic basis, but this may simply reflect our lack of full understanding of this often-distressing complaint.

Diagnostic Approach

MRI of the brain, skull base, and neck are the diagnostic tests of choice. If these imaging studies do not define evidence of a specific mass lesion, a careful search for leptomeningeal enhancement is in order. This is typically seen with metastatic tumors, sarcoidosis, or other rare leptomeningeal infiltrating lesions such as tuberculosis. Contrast-enhanced CT with thin slices through the skull base may also be useful to identify very discrete bony lesions.

Cerebrospinal fluid (CSF) analysis is indicated if an infiltrative process is clinically suspected or suggested from MRI. CSF analysis must include routine studies and cytologic analysis for malignant cells.

Electromyography of the genioglossus and anatomically adjacent muscles is indicated when the previously mentioned studies are unremarkable. Unfortunately, an asymmetrically atrophied tongue is commonly the presenting sign of motor neuron disease.

ADDITIONAL RESOURCES

Berger PS, Bataini JP. Radiation-induced cranial nerve palsy. Cancer 1977;40:152–5.
This classic paper describes 25 patients with cranial nerve palsies following radiation therapy for head and neck cancer; the spinal accessory nerve was involved in 5 patients.

Brodal P. The central nervous system, structure and function. 2nd ed. Oxford: Oxford University Press; 1998. pp. 452–3.

Brown H. Anatomy of the spinal accessory nerve plexus: relevance to head and neck cancer and atherosclerosis. Exp Biol Med (Maywood) 2002;227:570–8.
This article provides a detailed review of surgical anatomy of spinal accessory nerve and its relationship to cervical and brachial plexus, as well as other neck structures. Special attention is given to the nerve's vascular supply.

DeToledo JC, Dow R. Sternomastoid function during hemispheric suppression by amytal: insights into inputs to the spinal accessory nerve nucleus. Mov Disord 1998;13:809–12.

Weakness of the SCM ipsilateral to the Amytal carotid injection argues that ipsilateral hemisphere is the one more involved in supranuclear innervation of the SCM.

Friedenberg SM, Zimprich T, Harper CM. The natural history of long thoracic and spinal accessory neuropathies. Muscle Nerve 2002;25:535–9.

This retrospective review of 56 cases seen at the Mayo Clinic over 22 years provides insight into the natural history, outcome predictors, and role of electrophysiology in spinal accessory nerve lesions.

Greenberg HS, Deck MD, Vikram B, et al. Metastasis to the base of the skull: clinical findings in 43 patients. Neurology 1981;31(5):530–7.

In this classic paper, the combination of occipital headache and unilateral hypoglossal palsy due to a skull base metastasis was first described as the occipital condyle syndrome.

Gutrecht JA, Jones HR. Bilateral hypoglossal nerve injury after bilateral carotid endarterectomy. Stroke 1988;19:261–2.

This instructive case points out the often-dramatic difference between the clinical presentation of bilateral versus unilateral hypoglossal neuropathy.

Keane JR. Twelfth-nerve palsy. Analysis of 100 cases. Arch Neurol 1996;53:561–6.

In this large series, nearly half of the cases of hypoglossal neuropathy were due to a neoplasm.

Kim DH, Cho YJ, Tiel RL, et al. Surgical outcomes of 111 spinal accessory nerve injuries. Neurosurgery 2003;53:1106–12.

This is a retrospective review of injury mechanisms, operative techniques, and surgical outcomes of 111 cases of spinal accessory neuropathy that underwent surgical repair.

Wesselmann U, Reich SG. The dynias. Semin Neurol 1996;16:63–74.

In this review of "dynias," authors discuss the controversial syndrome of glossodynia.

Neurologic Emergencies and Critical Care

Brian J. Scott

12

Neurologic Emergencies and Neurocritical Care

David P. Lerner, Anil Ramineni, Joseph D. Burns

CLINICAL VIGNETTE *A 62-year-old man with hypertension and diabetes mellitus type 2 was brought to the emergency department via Emergency Medical Services for evaluation of acute onset of obtundation. Over the course of approximately 1 minute, he changed from being fully alert and talking normally to minimally responsive. En route, his vital signs were blood pressure 156/82 mm Hg, pulse 92 beats/minute, oxygen saturation 95% on 2 L via nasal cannula. A finger stick glucose was 197 mg/dL.*

He is stuporous on initial examination. His Glasgow Coma Score is 8 (verbal 2, eyes 1, motor 5). There is anisocoria (right pupil 6 mm and unreactive to direct and indirect light, left pupil 3 mm and briskly responsive to direct and indirect light). At primary gaze, the right eye is inferior and lateral relative to the position of the left eye (Fig. 12.1). There is decreased tone in all extremities but more so on the left. To noxious stimulation, his right arm localizes, the left arm withdraws minimally, and his legs withdraw equally to a painful stimulus.

The differential diagnosis for abrupt onset stupor/coma is quite broad. Rapid assessment of reversible and treatable causes is paramount. Although multiple metabolic derangements can present with coma, rarely do they result in focal neurologic deficits as seen in this patient. Right cranial nerve III (oculomotor) dysfunction and asymmetric motor responses to pain in the upper extremities should prompt concern for a structural central nervous system etiology. The examination suggests midbrain dysfunction potentially consistent with vertebrobasilar ischemia or a transtentorial herniation syndrome. Rapid symptom onset fits best with either seizure or cerebrovascular etiology. Consideration of intracranial hemorrhage within any compartment (epidural, subdural, subarachnoid, intraparenchymal), and large vessel occlusion with ischemia or infarction are most likely. An immediate noncontrast head computed tomography (CT) is indicated and can assist with diagnosis.

The patient underwent a noncontrast head CT (Fig. 12.2), which demonstrated an acute-on-subacute large right subdural hematoma. There is associated compression of the right hemisphere with subfalcine and uncal herniation. Neurosurgery completed an emergent craniotomy and subdural evacuation with limited radiographic improvement but excellent clinical improvement. Additional investigation revealed an acquired von Willebrand factor deficiency, which was likely to be the primary contributor to his spontaneous subdural hemorrhage.

INTRODUCTION

Nearly all subspecialties of neurology can have patients present with a life-threatening emergency. Over the past 15 years, many healthcare systems have created dedicated neurocritical care units and/or teams of neurocritical care providers who are specifically trained to care for this complex group of patients. With the ever-growing field of neurointensive care, the emphasis on early diagnosis and management to limit secondary injury is vital because there are still limitations in curative therapies.

Many of the other chapters in this work address specific disease processes in more detail. Diseases commonly managed in neurocritical care include severe traumatic brain injury (TBI), which is the leading cause of death between the ages of 1 and 45 (Chapter 19), large vessel ischemic stroke, which constitutes approximately 3% of all ischemic stroke in the United States (Chapter 15), status epilepticus occurring with an incidence of 41 cases per 100,000 (Chapter 23), and subarachnoid hemorrhage (Chapter 17). Together, they comprise a substantial portion of emergency and acute neurologic care.

PRINCIPLES OF EMERGENCY NEUROLOGY AND NEUROCRITICAL CARE

The principles that guide management of any life-threatening emergency also hold true for care of acute neurologically injured patients. The dogged approach of A-B-Cs (airway-breathing-circulation) remains:

- **Airway:** ensure a patent airway via oropharyngeal suctioning, and assess the potential need for intubation. If needed, ensure adequate cervical spine stabilization
- **Breathing:** evaluate oxygenation and ventilation. Augment as needed to maintain normal oxygenation and ventilation
- **Circulation:** evaluate end organ perfusion via blood pressure monitoring and organ function. Administer intravenous crystalloid and blood products as needed to ensure adequate perfusion.

After addressing the A-B-Cs as noted previously, there is additional focus on D (disability) in the management of potential acute neurologic injury:

- **Disability:** although a rapid Glasgow Coma Scale (Fig. 12.3) and brief cranial nerve examination are adequate for an initial rapid assessment, there needs to be a more thorough neurologic examination completed once the patient is stabilized. This may be a full neurologic examination or a thorough coma examination, depending on the patient's level of consciousness.

Clinical history may be limited in the very early stages of care, but prodromal symptoms (fever, behavioral change, headache, neurologic dysfunction), past medical history, and environmental factors (ingestion, trauma) are important and may substantially impact clinical decision making, diagnostic testing, and early treatment. High clinical suspicion for neurologic injury in those presenting with encephalopathy and/or coma is appropriate and may lead to early identification of cerebrovascular disease, structural brain lesion(s), or central nervous system (CNS) infection. The rapid neurologic assessment begins the goal of lesion localization.

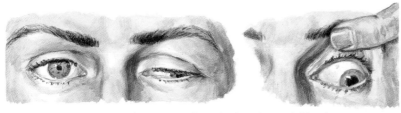

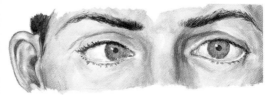

Oculomotor palsy: Ptosis, eye turns laterally and inferiorly, pupil dilated; common finding with cerebral aneurysms, especially carotid-posterior communicating aneurysms

Abducens palsy: Affected eye turns medially. May be first manifestation of intracavernous carotid aneurysm. Pain above eye or on side of face may be secondary to trigeminal (V) nerve involvement.

Retinal changes

Superior cerebellar artery aneurysm with CN III and IV compression

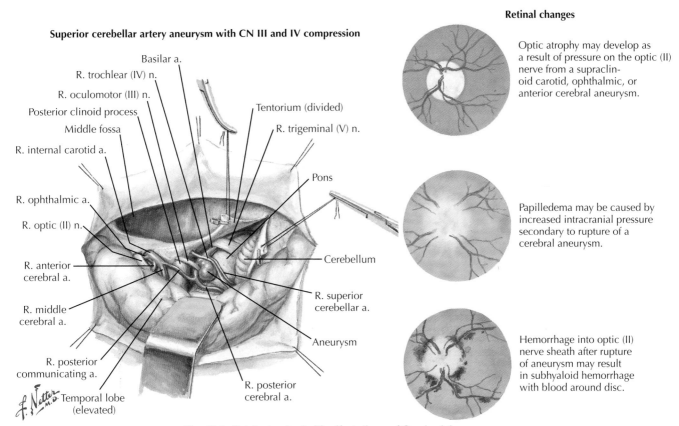

Optic atrophy may develop as a result of pressure on the optic (II) nerve from a supraclinoid carotid, ophthalmic, or anterior cerebral aneurysm.

Papilledema may be caused by increased intracranial pressure secondary to rupture of a cerebral aneurysm.

Hemorrhage into optic (II) nerve sheath after rupture of aneurysm may result in subhyaloid hemorrhage with blood around disc.

Fig. 12.1 Ophthalmologic Manifestations of Cerebral Aneurysms.

PRESERVATION OF NORMAL NEUROLOGIC FUNCTION

Although the early restoration of normal neurologic function is ideal, commonly neurologic injuries are not fully reversible. Much of the focus in the management of neurologic emergencies and neurocritical care is the maintenance of normal neurologic physiology—ensuring adequate delivery of glucose and oxygen, removal of carbon dioxide, cessation of seizure activity, and maintenance of normal intracranial pressure (ICP)—to prevent secondary brain injury.

As noted previously, the neurologic assessment follows cardiopulmonary stabilization. This emphasizes the dynamic physiologic interplay between the cardiac, pulmonary, and nervous system. Injured brain/spinal cord has a reduced physiologic reserve compared with uninjured tissue. Normal cerebral autoregulation allows for maintenance of blood flow over a broad range of mean arterial pressure (MAP = ⅓ systolic blood pressure + ⅔ diastolic blood pressure), but injured brain can lose this autoregulatory feature. As a result, hypotension will cause oligemia or ischemia, whereas hypertension results in hyperperfusion.

Although management of global hypoperfusion is addressed by standard resuscitation efforts, focal hypoperfusion as seen in ischemic stroke may be effectively reversed or reduced with prompt diagnosis and intervention as appropriate (intravenous tissue plasminogen activator [tPA] or mechanical thrombectomy). Normal brain perfusion is 25–50 mL blood/g brain tissue/min. If perfusion drops to 5 mL blood/g brain tissue/min, there is electrical quiescence (essentially brain function cessation given lack of oxygen, blood, and nutrients), and at less than 2 mL/g brain tissue/min, there is neuronal cell death.

Although maintenance of normotension is ideal, this may not be adequate to ensure normal brain perfusion. As there is normal intraarterial and venous pressure, so too is there a normal physiologic range for ICP. The cranial vault is a fixed volume encased by the calvarium with different compartments established by the dura. The ICP results from the volume of brain, blood, and cerebrospinal fluid within the cranial vault (Fig. 12.4). In a normal physiologic state, the ICP is the same throughout the compartments (typically <20 mm H_2O). However, in brain injury, there can be global elevation in the ICP, compartmental increase in ICP, or a combination of global and regional intracranial

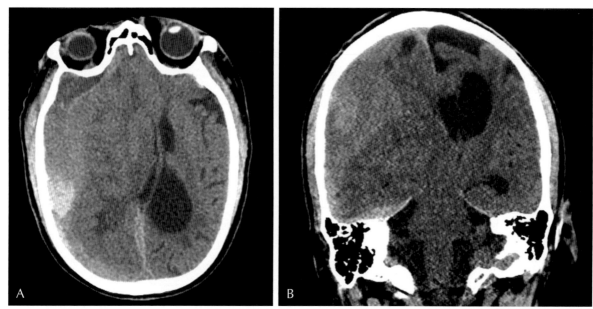

Fig. 12.2 Noncontrast Head Computed Tomography. (A) Axial image cranial to the thalami demonstrating a large right-sided subdural hematoma with mainly subacute (isodense) but also an acute (hyperdense) component with right-to-left subfalcine midline shift and entrapment of the left lateral ventricle resulting in ventriculomegaly. (B) Coronal image at the mid-uncus demonstrating the subdural hematoma with right-to-left subfalcine shift and right uncal herniation, as well as compression of the right midbrain.

hypertension. Maintenance of normal ICP may require medical or surgical treatments, as discussed later, and is critical to survival and the preservation of neurologic function.

SPECIFIC DISEASE PROCESSES

Coma/Stupor

Coma is the loss of awareness of external stimuli and voluntary reaction to these stimuli. There are varying degrees of coma, discussed in detail in Chapter 13. The differential diagnosis for coma is broad and is not limited to central nervous system etiology.

The initial evaluation of comatose patients includes early treatment of reversible causes—typically considered toxic or metabolic—such as hypoglycemia, drug intoxication, uremia, and hyperammonemia. A thorough general physical examination may give clues to the underlying etiology. A neurologic examination will be limited, but abnormal findings indicative of focal or regional brain dysfunction can assist with determining central nervous system localization and potential causes. Most patients presenting in coma will undergo central nervous system imaging with noncontrast head computed tomography (CT). Many of the findings that would result in coma—intracerebral hemorrhage, hydrocephalus, brainstem compression—will be obvious, but subtle findings of anoxic brain injury or diffuse TBI may not be present on noncontrast head CT.

An important point of care in the comatose patient is to not prognosticate very early in the hospital course. While still determining the etiology of coma, in the presence of severe organ dysfunction or recent exposure to drugs or medications, it may be impossible to accurately predict an individual's clinical outcome. Providers tend to have a bias toward negative outcomes in the earliest points of critical neurologic illness, yet some comas are partially or fully reversible.

Intracranial Hypertension/Herniation

As touched on earlier in the chapter, intracranial hypertension and herniation is a feared complication of many neurologic diseases. There are multiple causes of increased ICP, including both central nervous system etiologies and systemic causes, such as fulminant cirrhosis. Patients with increased ICP can present with headache, papilledema, nausea, and vomiting that may progress to stupor/coma. If herniation occurs, focal weakness, pupillary changes, posturing, and cardiopulmonary arrest may occur (Fig. 12.5).

The initial evaluation of patients presenting with signs/symptoms of increased ICP are rapid treatment followed by determining the cause. It may be appropriate to treat these patients with hyperosmolar therapy prior to obtaining CNS imaging, because herniation is a life-threatening illness that can result in irreversible neurologic injury. Early treatment consists of maneuvers to decrease ICP—elevation of the head of bed, maintaining the head in midline, and ensuring adequate pain control and sedation if intubated. Inducing hyperventilation in intubated patients with elevated ICP can provide a transient reduction in ICP by causing vasoconstriction of intracerebral vessels. However, the effect of hyperventilation lasts only a few minutes and carries the risk of ischemic brain injury. It should therefore only be used as a bridge to more definitive therapy such as hyperosmolar therapy or neurosurgical intervention.

There are two primary etiologies of cerebral edema: vasogenic and cytotoxic. Vasogenic edema results from an inflammatory process resulting in flow from the vasculature into the interstitial space. This is commonly seen with brain tumors and responds to treatment with high-dose steroids. Cytotoxic edema results from cellular death, such as following an ischemic stroke, and can respond to hyperosmolar therapy like mannitol and/or hypertonic saline.

The cranial vault is divided into different compartments by the dura—cerebral falx (left and right hemisphere) and the cerebellar tentorium (supratentorial and infratentorial fossa). When there is a pressure gradient different from one compartment to another, there is shift of brain tissue and resultant neuronal dysfunction. Subfalcine herniation results in a lateral hemisphere moving under the cerebral falx and compressing the anterior cerebral arteries, causing potential lower extremity paraparesis. Uncal herniation is movement of the medial temporal lobe

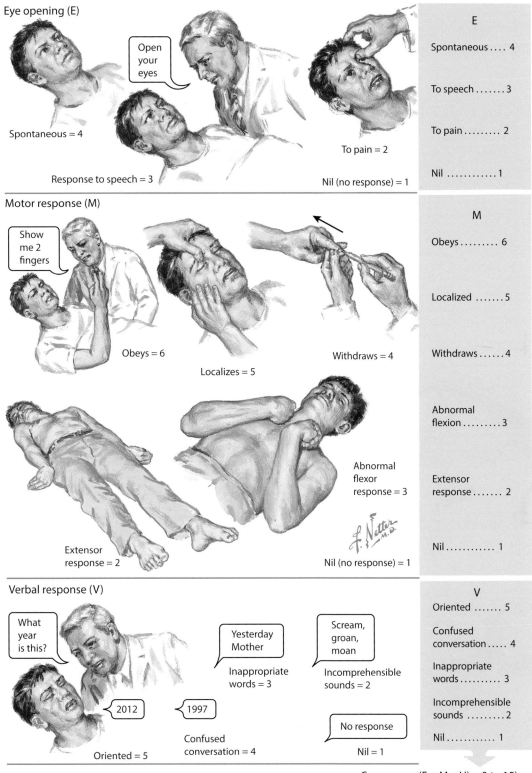

Eye opening (E)

Open your eyes

Spontaneous = 4

Response to speech = 3

To pain = 2

Nil (no response) = 1

E
Spontaneous 4
To speech 3
To pain 2
Nil 1

Motor response (M)

Show me 2 fingers

Obeys = 6

Localizes = 5

Withdraws = 4

Abnormal flexor response = 3

Extensor response = 2

Nil (no response) = 1

M
Obeys 6
Localized 5
Withdraws 4
Abnormal flexion 3
Extensor response 2
Nil 1

Verbal response (V)

What year is this?

Yesterday Mother

Inappropriate words = 3

Scream, groan, moan

Incomprehensible sounds = 2

2012   1997

No response

Oriented = 5

Confused conversation = 4

Nil = 1

V
Oriented 5
Confused conversation 4
Inappropriate words 3
Incomprehensible sounds 2
Nil 1

Coma score (E + M + V) = 3 to 15

Fig. 12.3 Glasgow Coma Scale.

(the uncus) across the cerebral tentorium and compressing the midbrain. Upward herniation results from posterior fossa lesion causing herniation of the cerebellum upward and causing compression of the midbrain. Additional herniation from the posterior fossa can cause the cerebellar tonsils to move into the foramen magnum and result in medulla and spinal cord compression. Lastly, if there is a breach in the cranial vault

(from a hemicraniectomy), brain tissue can herniate out of the vault, termed fungating herniation.

Acute Ischemic Stroke

Nearly 800,000 strokes occur every year in the United States and result in more than 100,000 deaths and is a leading cause of disability. Advances

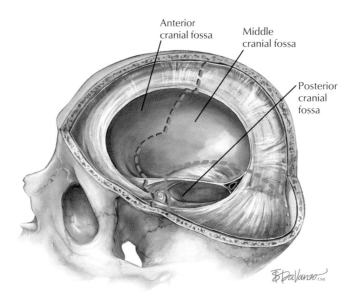

Fig. 12.4 Brain in a Box Model.

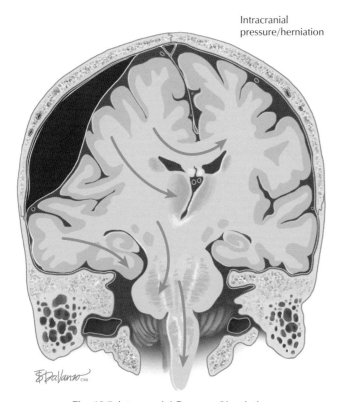

Intracranial
pressure/herniation

Fig. 12.5 Intracranial Pressure/Herniation.

in endovascular interventions have changed the acute stroke treatment paradigm. Despite these advances, there are still many ischemic strokes that are either unsuccessfully treated or cannot be treated.

Chapter 15 contains much more detail than what is presented here. Rapid evaluation for eligibility for intravenous tissue plasminogen activator (tPA) and/or endovascular therapy are still paramount in acute ischemic stroke evaluation. There are specific stroke processes that may require intensive care management. Large vessel occlusion that does or does not undergo endovascular therapy should have close neurologic

monitoring given the potential for reperfusion injury or malignant cerebral edema.

Commonly, postintraarterial therapy uses blood pressure augmentation in attempts to maintain perfusion to at-risk tissue. For those with large-vessel occlusion, resultant cytotoxic edema can result in herniation, and the potentially life-saving hemicraniectomy may need to be offered (Fig. 12.6). Another feared complication is hemorrhagic conversion of a stroke following intravenous (IV) tPA or endovascular therapy (Fig. 12.7). This may require reversal of tPA and strict blood pressure augmentation. There is no true reversal agent for tPA, but given that it degrades fibrin administration of fibrin-rich products such as fresh frozen plasma, cryoprecipitate and fibrinogen concentrate can promote thrombus formation. Lastly, posterior circulation ischemic strokes require frequent neurologic examinations because obstructive hydrocephalus in the days following ictus may require acute neurosurgical intervention such as placement of an external ventricular drain (EVD) and/or suboccipital craniectomy.

Prognosis from large vessel ischemic stroke has drastically improved within the past several years, mainly as a result of the advances in endovascular therapy. Individuals with large vessel ischemic strokes are more likely to have a good neurologic functional outcome if there is a small area of core infarct and if the team is able to achieve reperfusion of the at-risk brain tissue as quickly as possible from the onset of stroke symptoms.

Intracerebral Hemorrhage

Intracerebral hemorrhage accounts for approximately 10% of all strokes in the United States (Fig. 12.8). Although less common than ischemic stroke, hemorrhagic stroke has higher acute mortality and higher rate of decompensation and is more likely than ischemic stroke to cause disability.

Intraparenchymal hemorrhage presents similarly to ischemic stroke—acute onset of focal neurologic symptoms that can be ascribed to a single vascular territory. Those with an alteration in consciousness out of proportion to their examination, headache, and nausea with emesis are more likely to have hemorrhage rather than ischemic stroke. Initial evaluation with a noncontrast head CT must be completed quickly because there is no definitive way to determine ischemic versus

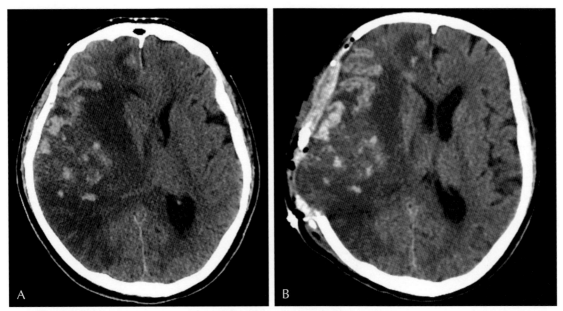

Fig. 12.6 Malignant Middle Cerebral Artery Ischemic Stroke. Noncontrast head computed tomography. (A) Axial image through thalami demonstrating a large right-sided middle cerebral artery ischemic stroke (hypodense tissue) with hemorrhagic conversion (hyperdense material) with compression of the right lateral ventricle and entrapment of the left lateral ventricle resulting in ventriculomegaly. (B) The same axial image following a right-sided hemicraniectomy. Resultant improvement in the compression of the right lateral ventricle and herniation of the infarcted brain outside the normal confines of the cranial vault at the posterior portion of the hemicraniectomy.

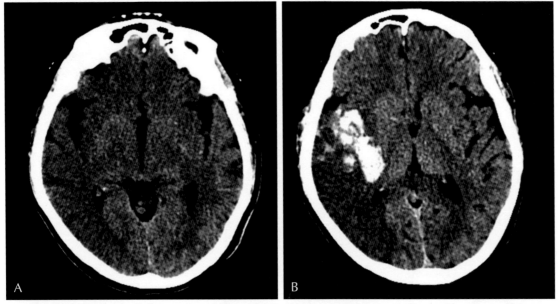

Fig. 12.7 Hemorrhagic Conversion of Right Middle Cerebral Artery Ischemic Stroke After Tissue Plasminogen Activator. Noncontrast head computed tomography: (A) Axial image at the level of the thalami demonstrating subtle early ischemic changes in the right frontal and temporal lobes with hypodensity and loss of gray-white differentiation. (B) Axial image at the level of the thalami 12 hours after the initial image (A). There is hemorrhage (hyperdensity) within the right frontal and temporal lobe and evolution of the ischemic stroke of the right fontal and temporal lobes.

hemorrhagic stroke without imaging. A CT angiogram of the intracerebral vessels is often appropriate as well to evaluate for underlying vascular lesions because these are a common cause for hemorrhage.

Initial assessment should include an assessment of hemorrhage location, size, and clinical presentation. Early interventions include blood pressure management to avoid hypertension (leading to extension of the hemorrhage) or hypotension (which may cause regional brain ischemia), reversal of any coagulopathy, and specific management of any causative underlying vascular lesion. Neurosurgical intervention may be appropriate for hematoma evacuation or for placement of an external ventricular drain (EVD) if there is intraventricular hemorrhage or hydrocephalus (see Chapter 16 for additional details).

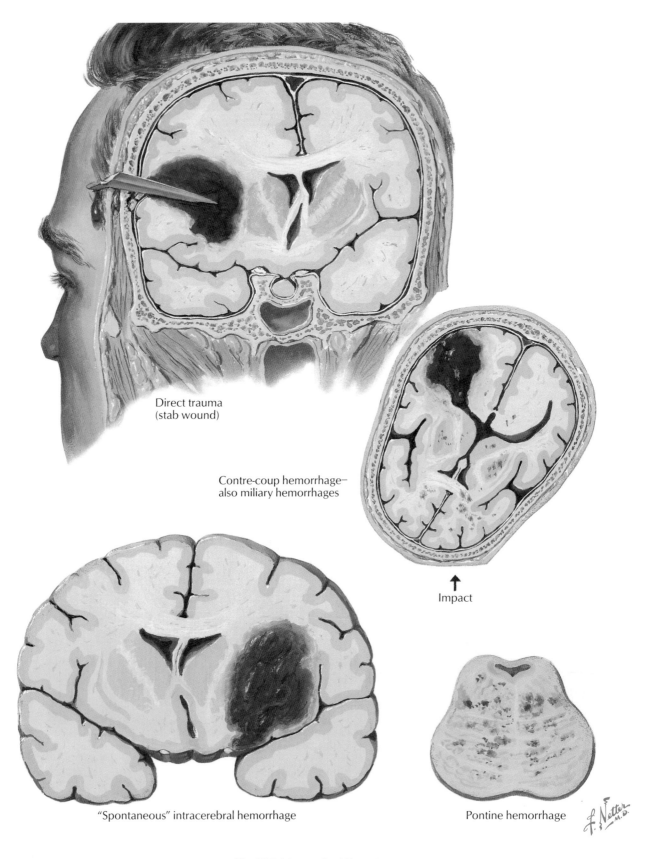

Direct trauma
(stab wound)

Contre-coup hemorrhage–
also miliary hemorrhages

Impact

"Spontaneous" intracerebral hemorrhage

Pontine hemorrhage

Fig. 12.8 Intracerebral Hematoma.

Subarachnoid Hemorrhage

Subarachnoid hemorrhage, as stated in the name, is venous or arterial blood that enters the subarachnoid space, including the ventricles, via multiple mechanisms with the most common being trauma or aneurysmal rupture (Fig. 12.9). It accounts for approximately 3% of stroke within the United States. Approximately 10% of those with aneurysmal subarachnoid hemorrhage die prior to emergency department arrival. For those who do receive medical care, the in-hospital mortality ranges widely from 8% to 67%. Among posthospital survivors, approximately 50% have significant chronic reduction in health-related quality of life.

Subarachnoid hemorrhage typically presents with abrupt/"thunderclap" onset of a severe headache ("worst headache of life") and can be accompanied by nausea, emesis, photophobia, meningismus, loss of consciousness/alteration in mental status, and focal neurologic deficits. To confirm the diagnosis of subarachnoid hemorrhage, noncontrast

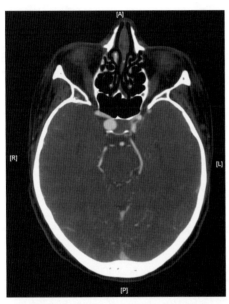

CT Angio source image showing an aneurysm.

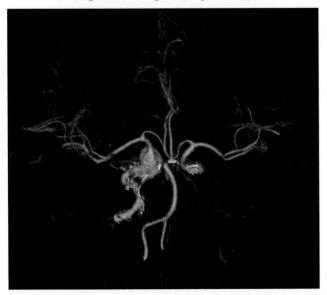

CTA 3-D reconstruction showing detailed anatomy of the aneurysm.

Fig. 12.9 Subarachnoid Hemorrhage.

head CT is highly sensitive (98%–100%) within the first 12 hours of symptom onset. The sensitivity of head CT drops over the course of a week to approximately 50% at 7 days after symptom onset. If there is high suspicion for subarachnoid hemorrhage but a normal head CT, lumbar puncture should be completed to assess for the presence of red blood cells and cerebrospinal fluid (CSF) xanthochromia. Digital subtraction catheter angiography is the "gold standard" for detecting an intracerebral aneurysm; however, most investigations start with a CT angiogram because it is less invasive than conventional angiography yet still quite sensitive in detecting aneurysms in the large cerebral vessels around the circle of Willis.

Initial assessments should be focused on both radiographic and clinical findings that can be used to assist with risk stratification of potential complications and prognostication. Early interventions that may include placement of an EVD if there are findings of hydrocephalus, initiation of an antiepileptic medication, treatment of hypertension, management of pain, and surgical or interventional treatment to secure the aneurysm (see Chapter 17).

Traumatic Brain Injury

TBI (Fig. 12.10) can occur in isolation or in conjunction with other systemic injuries, but in either case, it is important to complete a full trauma evaluation at presentation to ensure there are no missed injuries. Management of these patients will occur in a multidisciplinary team. The "A-B-C" paradigm for management is paramount for trauma management, and this is the followed by a thorough neurologic examination to determine disability, "D." Other important components of the history include the mechanism of injury, others injured at the scene, initial Glasgow Coma Scale, and potential medication or drug ingestion prior to arrival in the emergency department.

Although the grading of TBI based on presenting Glasgow Coma Scale (mild 13 to 15/moderate 9 to 12/severe 3 to 8) is useful and easy to ascertain, it may not give a full description of the neurologic injuries sustained. Patients with focal neurologic findings, worsening mental status or failure of mental status to improve, loss of consciousness for more than 5 minutes, seizures, penetrating head trauma, or signs of basal or depressed skull fracture should undergo imaging with a noncontrast head CT. There is a broad array of findings that may be present: epidural, subdural, subarachnoid, and intraparenchymal hemorrhage, skull fracture, diffuse axonal injury (DAI), venous sinus injury, nasal sinus injury, globe/orbit injury. Those injuries that require surgical management need to be determined quickly and the appropriate surgical team contacted. Although rarely seen with isolated head injury, coagulopathy may occur as a result of trauma and needs to be identified and treated appropriately.

The complications that can occur with TBI vary depending on the mechanism and extent of injury found on initial workup. The most common imaging finding is DAI which results from shear injury to axons typically during rapid acceleration-deceleration of the cranium or torsional injury. DAI is best evaluated by MRI, specifically susceptibility-weighted imaging (SWI), and graded based on findings of hemorrhage within particular brain locations including the corpus collosum and brainstem. A rapid elevation in ICP (ICP crisis) may occur in TBI, and therefore extremely close monitoring for clinical neurologic deterioration is critical. ICP monitors are indicated for those with Glasgow Coma Scale (GCS) less than 8 and an abnormal admission head CT. Monitoring is also recommended for those with two of the following: older than 40 years, unilateral or bilateral motor posturing, or an episode of systolic blood pressure less than 90 mm Hg. Other issues that may arise in the intensive care unit (ICU) include sympathetic storming, traumatic intracranial vasospasm, and systemic complications associated with critical illness such as deep vein thrombosis or nosocomial infections.

Intracerebral Hematoma

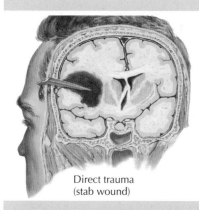
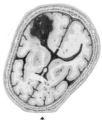

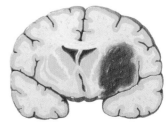

Direct trauma
(stab wound)

Impact
Contre-coup hemorrhage–
also miliary hemorrhages

Pontine hemorrhage

"Spontaneous" intracerebral hemorrhage

Acute Subdural Hematoma

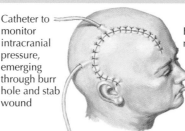
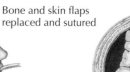

"Question mark"
skin incision
(black); outline
of free bone
flap and burr
holes (red)

Skin flap reflected (Raney clips control
bleeding); free bone flap removed and
dura opened; clot evacuated by
irrigation, suction, and forceps.

Catheter to
monitor
intracranial
pressure,
emerging
through burr
hole and stab
wound

Bone and skin flaps
replaced and sutured

Jackson-Pratt drain,
emerging from
subdural space
via burr hole
and stab wound

Section showing acute
subdural hematoma on
right side and subdural
hematoma associated with
temporal lobe intracerebral
hematoma ("burst" temporal
lobe) on left

Temporal Fossa Hematoma

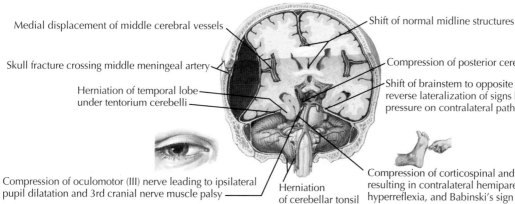
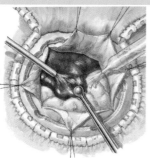
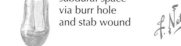
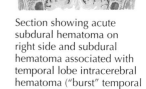

Medial displacement of middle cerebral vessels

Skull fracture crossing middle meningeal artery

Herniation of temporal lobe
under tentorium cerebelli

Compression of oculomotor (III) nerve leading to ipsilateral
pupil dilatation and 3rd cranial nerve muscle palsy

Herniation
of cerebellar tonsil

Shift of normal midline structures

Compression of posterior cerebral artery

Shift of brainstem to opposite side may
reverse lateralization of signs by tentorial
pressure on contralateral pathways.

Compression of corticospinal and associated pathways,
resulting in contralateral hemiparesis, deep tendon
hyperreflexia, and Babinski's sign

Fig. 12.10 Acute Traumatic Brain Injury.

Clinical outcome in TBI is quite variable and depends on the extent of systemic injuries, mechanism of injury, region of brain injury, extent of DAI, and complications within the intensive care unit. Advances in imaging with tractography have shed light into recovery from severe TBI, but this remains investigational (Chapter 19).

Spinal Cord Injury

Spinal cord dysfunction is rare, but a neurologic emergency as early recognition and treatment can preserve or improve functional outcomes (Fig. 12.11). The common findings in spinal cord disease can include pain, a spinal sensory level, weakness, and/or autonomic dysfunction.

Early evaluation should include a thorough neurologic examination in an attempt to localize the lesion within a region of the spinal cord. Stabilization of the spinal column and limitation of additional cord injury are the primary goals. Imaging with CT scan, although adequate to evaluate the thoracoabdominal structures and bone injury, has limitations evaluating the spinal cord and epidural space, making CT imaging an inadequate imaging modality. Patients with concern for spinal cord injury should be transferred to facilities with immediate capability for MRI imaging and an available spine surgery team for prompt surgical management if needed. If there is a suspicion for cord compression due to malignancy, initiation of high-dose steroids (dexamethasone)

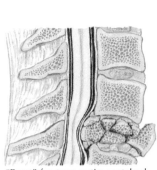

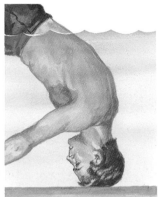

"Burst" fracture: entire vertebral body crushed, with intraspinal bone fragments

Mechanism: vertical blow on the head as in diving or surfing accident, being thrown from car, or football injury

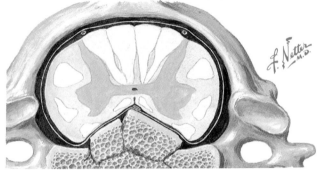

Dislocated bone fragments compressing spinal cord and spinal artery: blood supply to anterior two thirds of spinal cord is impaired

Fig. 12.11 Trauma of the Spinal Cord.

"… a condition resulting either from the failure of the mechanisms responsible for seizure termination or from the initiation of mechanisms, which lead to abnormally, prolonged seizures (after time point t1). It is a condition, which can have long-term consequences (after time point t2), including neuronal death, neuronal injury, and alteration of neuronal networks, depending on the type and duration of seizures."

(Trinka et al., Epilepsia, 2015)

For convulsive status epilepticus, t1 = 5 minutes (the time point at which treatment should be considered or started), and t2 = 30 minutes (the time beyond which there is permanent neurologic injury). These times are longer for focal and nonconvulsive status epilepticus. Although this is an all-encompassing definition, the operational definition of ongoing seizure activity for greater than 5 minutes or recurrent seizures without complete recovery of consciousness is more practical to guide treatment decisions. Although status epilepticus constitutes a neurologic emergency, the timing and aggressiveness of treatment depend on the type—nonconvulsive versus focal without changes in consciousness versus generalized convulsive status epilepticus.

Early evaluation of status epilepticus should be completed in parallel with early management (Fig. 12.12). Clinical evaluation of patients in status epilepticus will be limited given ongoing seizure activity or stupor/coma. Seizures and status epilepticus are typically symptoms of an underlying disease process, and the search for the underlying etiology is important. An extensive metabolic evaluation and toxicology screen should be completed. Central nervous system imaging with a noncontrast head CT can be helpful to evaluate for structural lesions that may result in status epilepticus. Early consideration of lumbar puncture and empiric treatment for meningitis in new-onset status epilepticus or status epilepticus accompanied by fever or other signs or symptoms suggestive of infection is appropriate.

Early management of status epilepticus is to abort seizure activity because persistence of seizure can result in permanent neuronal dysfunction and is more difficult to treat. The first-line treatment of status epilepticus is benzodiazepines followed by an antiepileptic medication, and, although there is an ever-expanding list of anticonvulsant medications, those with an approved indication for status epilepticus include only valproic acid, phenytoin, and phenobarbital. If there is ongoing seizure activity despite benzodiazepine and primary antiepileptic medication administration, intubation and sedation with an anesthetic medication should be completed. Typically, patients treated with any combination of these medications will have an alteration in the level of consciousness, and it can be difficult to determine if this is due to medications or ongoing subclinical seizures. Continuous video EEG monitoring is more sensitive than short-duration (30–60 minutes) studies in detecting subtle or nonclinical seizure activity. While treating with antiepileptic medications, it is also important to investigate and treat any underlying metabolic derangements such as hypoglycemia or metabolic acidosis.

is appropriate. If there is concern for an infectious etiology, empiric treatment with antibiotics that will cover gram-positive skin flora is appropriate and should include treatment for methicillin-resistant *Staphylococcus aureus* (MRSA).

Cervical spinal cord injury can result in neurogenic shock due to loss of descending sympathetic fibers from the lateral cord. Treatment of neurogenic shock starts with adequate volume resuscitation but may also require vasopressor medications to compensate for the loss of both alpha- and beta-adrenergic tone (epinephrine and norepinephrine are the medications of choice). Attempts to maintain autonomic function with Foley catheter placement and an aggressive bowel regimen are important. The paralysis following spinal cord injury places patients at high risk for deep vein thrombosis, and therefore prevention with sequential compression devices or medication prophylaxis is an important component of care.

Prognosis in spinal cord injury depends on the extent of weakness and sensory loss, as well as the underlying mechanism of injury. The American Spinal Injury Assessment (ASIA) grading system uses a 5-point grading scale to describe the severity of spinal cord injury. Functional outcome tools such as the Spinal Cord Independence Measure (SCIM III) can provide some insight into recovery (Chapter 20).

Status Epilepticus

Status epilepticus has undergone multiple definition changes, especially with the increased use of electroencephalography (EEG) monitoring in the intensive care unit. The International League Against Epilepsy defines status epilepticus as:

Encephalitis/Meningitis

Although both encephalitis and meningitis are uncommon diseases with a combined annual incidence rate of 4–6 cases per 100,000 person/year, they can cause profound disability (Fig. 12.13). The complete classic triad of fever, meningismus, and altered mental status is encountered in only 44% of patients, but one or more of these signs is characteristic. Other common signs and symptoms include headache, rash, new seizure, or a focal neurologic deficit. Clinical exam findings of a positive Kernig sign (passive knee and hip flexion resulting in neck flexion) and/or Brudzinski sign (passive neck flexion resulting in knee flexion) are strongly supportive, but their absence does not exclude the diagnosis of meningitis.

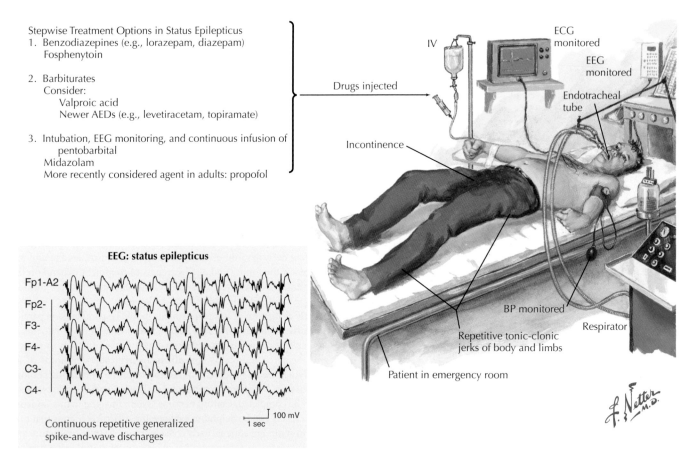

Stepwise Treatment Options in Status Epilepticus
1. Benzodiazepines (e.g., lorazepam, diazepam)
   Fosphenytoin

2. Barbiturates
   Consider:
       Valproic acid
       Newer AEDs (e.g., levetiracetam, topiramate)

3. Intubation, EEG monitoring, and continuous infusion of
       pentobarbital
   Midazolam
   More recently considered agent in adults: propofol

Drugs injected

IV

ECG monitored

EEG monitored

Endotracheal tube

Incontinence

BP monitored

Respirator

Repetitive tonic-clonic jerks of body and limbs

Patient in emergency room

EEG: status epilepticus

Fp1-A2
Fp2-
F3-
F4-
C3-
C4-

100 mV
1 sec

Continuous repetitive generalized
spike-and-wave discharges

Fig. 12.12 Status Epilepticus.

Early clinical suspicion for infection is the key to management of these diseases. Early empiric antibiotic treatment with broad-spectrum antibiotics, antivirals, and potentially dexamethasone can be life-saving (Section XIII). Administration of these medications should not be delayed for lumbar puncture or imaging. Strictly speaking, not all patients with suspected meningitis or encephalitis require imaging, but those with fever, encephalopathy, focal deficit, papilledema, new-onset seizure, or chronic immunosuppression must have a noncontrast head CT prior to lumbar puncture. In practice, a noncontrast head CT is almost always performed prior to lumbar puncture in cases of suspected meningitis or encephalitis.

The prognosis varies greatly depending on the causative organism and clinical severity, but it is well established that delays in antibiotic initiation are associated with worse outcomes for those with sepsis of all causes, including those with CNS infections.

Severe Neuromuscular Weakness/Neuromuscular Respiratory Failure

Although rare, severe Guillain-Barré syndrome and myasthenia gravis are two neuromuscular disease processes that may require ICU care. Severe respiratory muscle weakness can result in hypoventilation and acute respiratory failure, whereas bulbar dysfunction can result in the inability to protect the upper airway. Both may require intubation and mechanical ventilation.

The physiology of neuromuscular respiratory failure is fundamentally different than respiratory failure from lung disease. The initial evaluation includes concomitant neurologic examination and a thorough systemic evaluation of other disease processes that may result in or contribute to weakness. Bedside respiratory mechanics to assess

vital capacity and negative inspiratory force can measure the severity of neuromuscular respiratory failure as both a single assessment and to track trends in respiratory function over the course of the hospital stay.

In those with neuromuscular respiratory weakness, the 20-30-40 rule can help to determine who needs intubation. A vital capacity less than 20 mL/kg (ideal body weight), negative inspiratory force greater than −30 cm H_2O, or maximal expiratory pressure less than 40 cm H_2O or decline of greater than 30% from previous measurements is indicative of severe respiratory muscle weakness. Respiratory compromise and failure can occur quite rapidly in neuromuscular patients, and measures used to assess respiratory distress for intrinsic lung disease such as respiratory rate, accessory muscle, use and pulse oximetry have limited value because hypoxia is a very late feature of respiratory failure in neuromuscular weakness. The single-breath count test is a bedside maneuver that can be helpful to assess respiratory muscle weakness in which a patient takes a deep breath and counts out loud to the highest number possible.

Monitoring in the Intensive Care Unit

Neuromonitoring devices in critical care are tools to help understand pathophysiologic states, guide treatment decisions, and assess an individual's response to therapeutic interventions. As with all of neurology and medicine, information from monitoring devices cannot be interpreted in isolation and must be closely correlated with careful observation of the patient's neurologic exam whenever possible. In cases where the neurologic exam is not able to be performed safely (such as severe trauma in which removing sedation would risk further injury to the patient) or is extremely limited (such as hepatic coma),

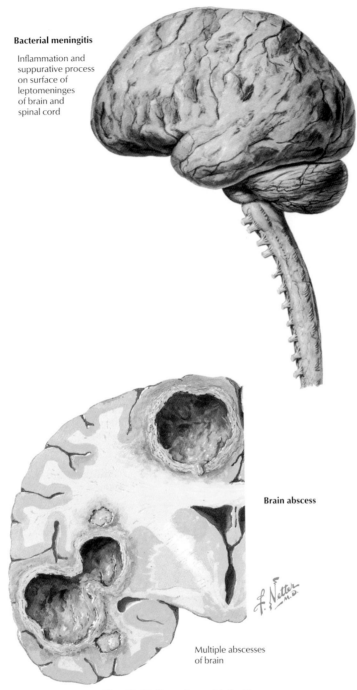

Bacterial meningitis

Inflammation and suppurative process on surface of leptomeninges of brain and spinal cord

Brain abscess

Multiple abscesses of brain

Fig. 12.13 Overview of Infections.

neuromonitoring devices can provide information about ICP or cerebral blood flow that can help to guide management.

VENOUS ACCESS AND MONITORING

First, in critically ill patients and those with life-threatening illness, adequate venous access is key to ongoing management of the patient. There may be a need for multiple medication administrations (as is the case in status epilepticus), close monitoring of blood pressure and continuous augmentation with intravenous medications (as is the case with intracerebral hemorrhage), additional information for volume assessment and need for use of vasopressor medications (as is the case in meningitis), or rapid administration of medications that are caustic

to peripheral vasculature (such as 23% sodium chloride for elevated ICP). Central access typically via the subclavian, internal jugular, or common femoral vein allows reliable long-term access for these needs (Fig. 12.14).

ELECTROENCEPHALOGRAPHY (EEG) MONITORING

Injured brain, no matter the mechanism, has a high potential for seizures. Commonly, patients will have encephalopathy in the neurointensive care unit, and it is difficult to ascertain the etiology. Therefore EEG can be helpful in determining if there are subclinical seizures contributing to the patient's mental status. EEG leads in the intensive care unit are placed in the standard 10-20 international standard placement with

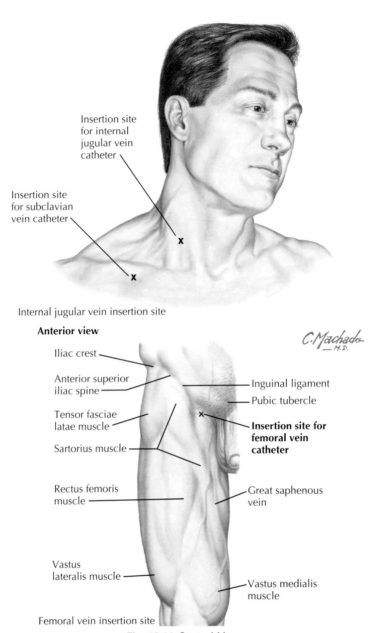

Insertion site
for internal
jugular vein
catheter

Insertion site
for subclavian
vein catheter

Internal jugular vein insertion site

Anterior view

C. Machado
M.D.

Iliac crest

Anterior superior
iliac spine

Tensor fasciae
latae muscle

Sartorius muscle

Rectus femoris
muscle

Inguinal ligament

Pubic tubercle

**Insertion site for
femoral vein
catheter**

Great saphenous
vein

Vastus
lateralis muscle

Vastus medialis
muscle

Femoral vein insertion site

Fig. 12.14 Central Lines.

the understanding that there may be limited lead placement in patients with recent neurosurgical interventions, intracranial monitors, or wounds (Fig. 12.15).

EEG monitoring in the ICU commonly is not straightforward with clear electrographic seizures but rather will have abnormal EEG discharges or rhythms (e.g., periodic lateralized discharge, generalized periodic discharges, and rhythmic activity). These findings, although abnormal, fall on a spectrum between ictal (clearly seizure) and nonictal (clearly not seizure) brain activity. Not all abnormal findings require treatment with anticonvulsant medications, but monitoring for changes in the EEG pattern over time or in response to anticonvulsant medications is useful.

Quantitative EEG (qEEG) is an additional tool used within the intensive care unit. qEEG uses digital signal analysis to generate condensed graphical displays of multiple EEG parameters including power, wave variability, rhythmicity, and symmetry. By condensing hours of EEG into graphical representation, there are multiple trends that may

be better assessed including the percentage of slow waves present during the recording, seizure frequency, and asymmetry (Fig. 12.16).

INTRACRANIAL PRESSURE MONITORING

ICP monitoring (Fig. 12.17) can be done using various devices, most commonly EVD, intraparenchymal monitors, and subdural pressure monitors. Each monitoring system has benefits and drawbacks. EVDs are inserted into the third ventricle using cranial surface landmarks, so placement may be difficult with small ventricles or distorted cranial anatomy. The catheter is then attached to a pressure monitoring and drainage system. One advantage of EVDs over other intracranial monitoring devices is that the catheter can remove CSF if there is elevated ICP or hemorrhage within the ventricular system. An intraparenchymal monitor is placed directly into the brain tissue through a burr hole (approximate size 2 cm diameter) in the skull. The monitor measures the ICP near the brain surface in the surrounding region. Although

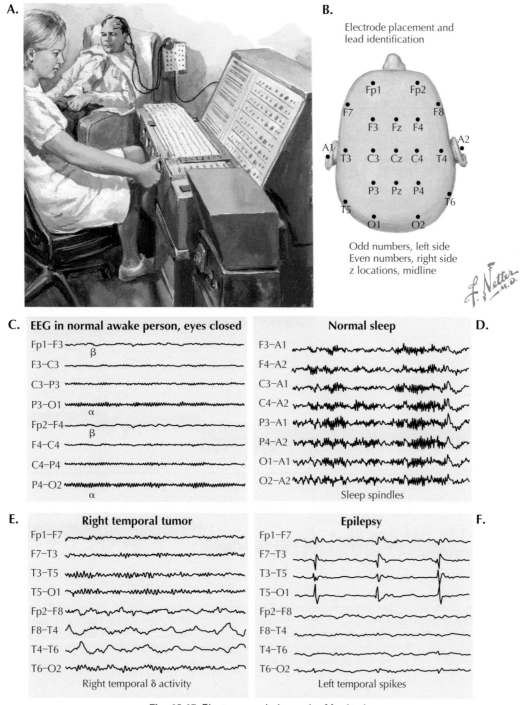

Fig. 12.15 Electroencephalography Monitoring.

placement is easier than an EVD, it is not possible to drain CSF or make central ICP measurements with an intraparenchymal monitor. Intraparenchymal monitors also tend to become inaccurate after 48–72 hours. Subdural ICP monitors are placed in similar fashion to intraparenchymal monitors with similar drawbacks.

Normal ICP is less than 20 mm H_2O. The waveform tracing generated from the EVD reflects the ICP, which can be monitored over time and treated as appropriate (Fig. 12.18). The waveform generated from an EVD provides dynamic ICP measurements throughout the cardiac cycle, which appear different in physiologic versus disease states. There are three peaks (or waves) seen within each ICP wave—percussion waves 1, 2, and 3, respectively. P_1 is formed by the flow of arterial blood into

the capillary beds of the brain. P_2 is known as the dicrotic wave, which corresponds to the flow of blood in the early venous phase. Lastly, P_3 is the tidal wave, the physiology of which is not fully elucidated, but thought to be due to flow of blood into the large venous structures.

In normal brain, $P_1 > P_2 > P_3$, but in injured brain there may be a shift with $P_1 < P_2 > P_3$, suggestive of poor brain compliance. Compliance reflects the ability of brain tissue to accommodate additional blood volume, measured as the change in volume over the change in pressure ($C = \Delta V / \Delta P$). Normally the additional or normal fluctuation in blood flow during the cardiac cycle produces minimal change in the ICP, and the brain demonstrates a state of normal compliance. However, when the intracranial volume increases (i.e., from cerebral edema), the

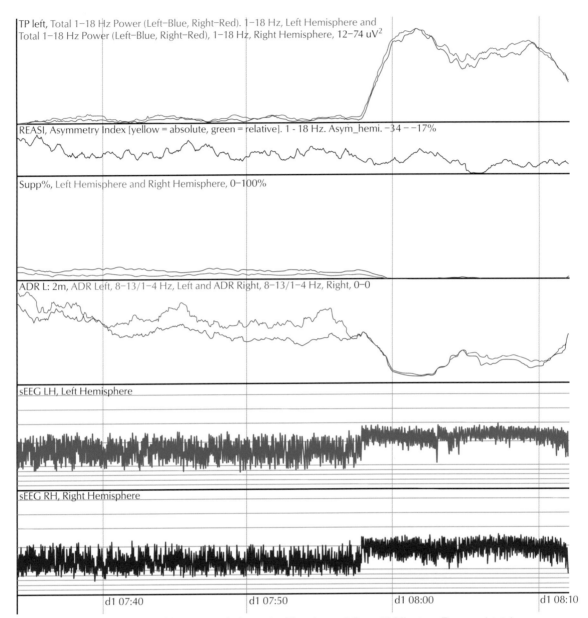

TP left, Total 1–18 Hz Power (Left–Blue, Right–Red). 1–18 Hz, Left Hemisphere and Total 1–18 Hz Power (Left–Blue, Right–Red), 1–18 Hz, Right Hemisphere, 12–74 uV²

REASI, Asymmetry Index [yellow = absolute, green = relative]. 1 - 18 Hz. Asym_hemi. –34 – –17%

Supp%, Left Hemisphere and Right Hemisphere, 0–100%

ADR L: 2m, ADR Left, 8–13/1–4 Hz, Left and ADR Right, 8–13/1–4 Hz, Right, 0–0

sEEG LH, Left Hemisphere

sEEG RH, Right Hemisphere

d1 07:40   d1 07:50   d1 08:00   d1 08:10

Fig. 12.16 Quantitative Electroencephalography Time Lapsed Over 45 Minutes. *Top panel:* total power (total voltage of electroencephalography [EEG]). *Second panel:* asymmetric index right-left balance of power in EEG. *Third panel:* suppression percentage (amount of time with suppression). *Fourth panel:* alpha-delta ratio is ratio of time with alpha frequency compared with the delta frequency. *Fifth and sixth panels:* amplitude = integrated EEG (left and right hemispheres, respectively).

edematous brain has reduced compliance and small changes in volume result in large changes in the ICP. At times when there is low compliance, extra vigilance is needed because small changes in intracranial volume can lead to ICP crisis (ICP > 60 mm H_2O). When ICP is sustained above a determined threshold, treatment to reduce ICP should proceed. If an EVD is in place, drainage of CSF may result in ICP reduction, but treatment with hyperosmolar therapy, such as mannitol or hypertonic saline, or in some cases surgical intervention may be needed to effectively reduce ICP to normal levels.

INVASIVE NEUROMONITORING

Although there are multiple noninvasive monitoring tools, these have limitations in that they indirectly measure the physiology of the brain. There are additional monitoring devices that more directly measure

physiologic parameters within the brain tissue itself. These types of monitors include parenchymal microcatheters placed much like an intraparenchymal pressure monitor. There are a number of physiologic data points that can be recorded with microcatheters: brain tissue oxygen level, brain temperature, cerebral conductance, and microdialysis are the most common.

Although invasive monitoring is not standard of care, many neurointensive care units use these tools to help guide patient management. For example, microdialysis provides important physiologic data. The brain uses solely carbohydrates as a fuel source via complete aerobic oxidative phosphorylation and metabolizes glucose into pyruvate and ultimately CO_2. When the brain is underperfused, there is a shift from oxidative phosphorylation to anaerobic glycolysis and formation of lactate. Microdialysis can monitor the concentrations of both pyruvate and lactate, and the ratio thereof, to best understand the metabolic

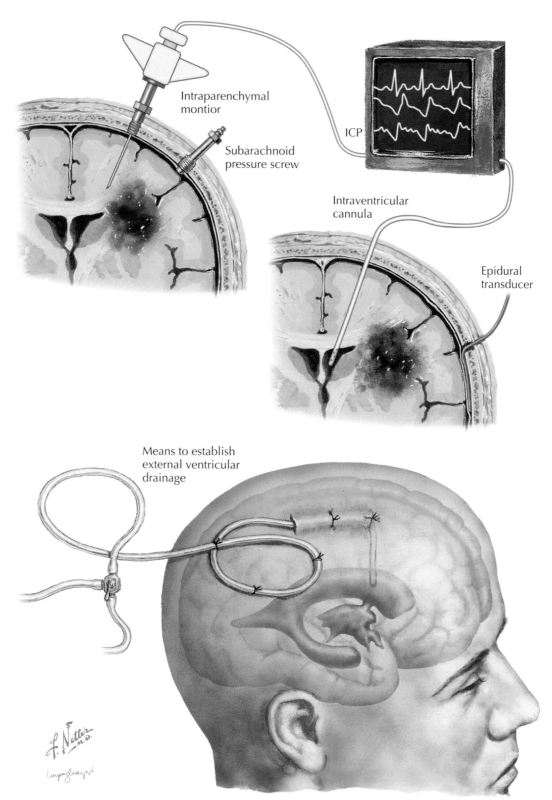

Fig. 12.17 Monitoring Intracranial Pressure.

state of brain tissue at a regional level. If the lactate to pyruvate ratio is high, suggesting anaerobic glycolysis, adjustment to increase blood pressure (increase cerebral perfusion), hemoglobin (oxygen carrying capacity), decrease ICP (perfusion), and temperature may improve this ratio, suggesting improvement in carbohydrate use and return to a more normal physiologic state.

The brain functions via electrical impulses among cells. The principle of conductance is the ability of an electrical impulse generated by one cell to be transmitted to another. In the normal brain, this occurs quite easily given the high concentrations of sodium, potassium, and chloride. In a diseased brain where there is increased fluid, there is a decrease in the concentration of the interstitial solute, which impairs the ability of

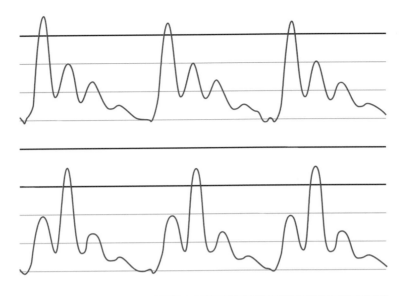

Fig. 12.18 Intracranial Pressure (ICP) Waveform. ICP waveform tracings from the same patient taken at different times during their hospital course. *Top* is hospital day 1 following a large intraparenchymal and intraventricular hemorrhage. This is a normal wave form with the first wave (P_1) larger than the second wave (P_2), which is larger than the third wave (P_3). *Bottom* is the tracing at hospital day 4 when the patient was experiencing ICP elevations and the edema from the intraparenchymal hemorrhage was near peak. The waveform has characteristic findings of noncompliance, with the second wave (P_2) larger than the first or third wave.

neurons to transfer electrical impulses, or a decrease in the conductance. The decrease in cerebral conductance marks vasogenic and/or cytotoxic edema. Treatment for these conditions with either hyperosmolar therapy or steroids can reverse the abnormality. Conductance can normalize if the cerebral edema improves or is treated.

TRANSCRANIAL DOPPLER ULTRASOUND

Transcranial Doppler ultrasound (TCD) is a noninvasive imaging technique used most commonly for evaluation of vasospasm associated with aneurysmal subarachnoid hemorrhage. Using the B-mode of an ultrasound probe, the evaluation of flow within vessels can occur. There are two primary monitoring sites—over the temporalis muscle for the anterior circulation and over the posterolateral neck into the foramen magnum for vertebrobasilar arteries. From these two positions, the large intracranial arteries can be evaluated.

Vasospasm associated with subarachnoid hemorrhage results in blood vessel narrowing through a complex mechanism of actions that can result in cerebral infarction. TCDs are completed daily on patients at risk, and blood flow velocities are measured to monitor for vasospasm but not necessarily brain ischemia. Most neurovascular laboratories have established protocols and normal values, but the most common value monitored is the mean arterial velocity (cm/s). Other points of interest are the **pulsatility index,** which is an indirect evaluation of cerebral blood flow dynamics, and the **Lindegaard ratio,** which relates to the severity of arterial vasospasm.

$$\text{Pulsatility Index (PI)} = \frac{\begin{array}{c}(\text{peak systolic velocity (cm/s)}\\ -\text{ end diastolic velocity (cm/s)})\end{array}}{\text{Mean flow velocity (cm/s)}}$$

Lindegaard Ratio = peak systolic velocities (cm/s) of ipsilateral:

$$\frac{\text{middle cerebral artery} - \text{extracranial internal carotid artery}}{\text{extracranial internal carotid artery}}$$

Although TCD is a noninvasive and inexpensive test, it has limited sensitivity and specificity in the detection of cerebral vasospasm (approximately 50% for both) and has limitations related to the level of experience of the ultrasound technician.

FUTURE DIRECTIONS

Although neurocritical care has been a subspecialty for the past 15 years, the field continues to grow. There are more fellowship training programs and more neurointensive care units opening throughout the United States and worldwide. As advances in surgical techniques push the boundaries on which interventions can be performed in the cranial vault (e.g., minimally invasive surgery for intraparenchymal hematoma evacuation), we will have more effective therapies to offer patients and families, as well as better information about the disease processes. The ongoing advances in neuromonitoring continue to provide insight into the primary and secondary brain injuries that occur following life-threating diseases. Although studies using invasive monitoring have yet to demonstrate clinical benefit, neurosurgeons and neurointensivists remain early adopters of this technology and will be leaders in determining how to best use these devices and the clinical information they provide.

ADDITIONAL RESOURCES

Emergency Neurological Life Support (ENLS). Available from: http://www.neurocriticalcare.org/enls.

Frontera JA, editor. Decision making in neurocritical care. 1st ed. New York, NY: Thieme Medical Publishers; 2009.

Lee K, editor. The neuroICU book. 2nd ed. New York, NY: McGraw-Hill Education; 2017.

Lewis SL. CONTINUUM: lifelong learning in neurology. Neurocrit Care 2015;21(5).

Wijdicks EFM, Rabinstein AA, editors. Neurocritical care (what do I do now). 2nd ed. Oxford, UK: Oxford University Press; 2016.

13

Coma, Vegetative State, and Brain Death

Anil Ramineni, Gregory J. Allam, David P. Lerner, Joseph D. Burns

COMA

> **CLINICAL VIGNETTE** *A 57-year-old man with coronary artery disease develops severe chest pain and heaviness on exertion, then loses consciousness while working in the garden with his wife. Emergency Medical Services is called immediately and arrives at the scene within minutes. The man is found pale, unresponsive, and flaccid. The systolic blood pressure is low, approximately 70–85 mm Hg, and he is found to be in ventricular tachycardia, but he promptly reverts to sinus rhythm with cardiac defibrillation. In the hospital, he is found to have roving eye movements and does not open his eyes even to noxious stimulus. He makes incomprehensible sounds but does not clearly produce or understand language, and he grimaces and withdraws his limbs to painful stimuli. Over a 3-day period, he becomes awake and conversant but has poor short-term memory and ataxia. These symptoms gradually resolve over a 3-week period.*

> **CLINICAL VIGNETTE** *A 76-year-old man is found unconscious in bed at home. His wife informs the emergency physician that he has a history of prostate cancer but no risk factors for vascular disease. She denies knowledge of any recent head injury. He is totally unresponsive to verbal and painful stimuli. Neurologic examination shows he is comatose with pinpoint pupils. Eye movements to doll's-eyes maneuvers are full and conjugate, and cold caloric stimulation of the ear canals produces ipsilateral tonic deviation of the eyes without nystagmus. There are bilateral withdrawal responses of his extremities to noxious stimuli and bilateral Babinski signs.*
>
> *Intravenous administration of 0.4 mg naloxone produces dramatic change, with full awakening within a few minutes. Results of a brain computed tomography (CT) are normal, confirming that there is no evidence of intracerebral, subarachnoid, or subdural hemorrhage, cerebral infarction, or mass lesions. When asked about narcotic use, the patient states that he was no longer able to tolerate the pain of metastatic prostate cancer; he had taken an overdose of an opioid analgesic.*

The first vignette reflects a common clinical presentation for anoxic-ischemic brain injury secondary to cardiac arrest. The chance of good neurologic recovery depends on a number of factors that include age, extent or duration of brain ischemia, effective targeted temperature management (when appropriate), and the severity of coexisting medical conditions. A detailed history, review of in-field records, and serial neurologic examinations are the essential first steps in understanding the extent and mechanism of brain injury, identifying potential ingestions or exposures, and determining the need for further workup.

The second vignette illustrates the classic case of a "toxic-metabolic" coma. Despite profound unresponsiveness and miotic pupils, the patient's neurologic examination demonstrates retained brainstem reflexes, and CT results are normal. Although pontine hemorrhage is often suspected in a comatose septuagenarian with pinpoint pupils, intact reflexive eye movement strongly indicates a metabolic cause. Reversal of an opiate overdose with an antagonist such as naloxone can result in rapid neurologic recovery. However, more severe overdoses may be associated with respiratory suppression leading to anoxic brain injury or death.

Consciousness is the state of awareness of internal and external stimuli and is manifested by the ability to react to these stimuli through thought or by directed physical movement. Coma is a lack of consciousness characterized by the absence of wakefulness and awareness of surroundings. Full consciousness can be disrupted without total loss of arousal or wakefulness. Varying degrees of consciousness can be approximately delineated by the response to a particular stimulus, and terms such as *drowsiness, obtundation,* or *stupor* are sometimes used as a reflection of severity. However, the most useful means to communicate a state of altered level of consciousness remains the accurate description of patient behavior and reactions to specific stimuli. For example, it is preferable to indicate that a patient opens his or her eyes to voice but does not maintain eye opening and responds only after repeated questioning than to say that the patient is obtunded. Nevertheless, defining terms are often used as descriptors of a patient's level of consciousness, even though they tend to be imprecise. *Lethargy* consists of significant drowsiness in which a mild to moderate stimulus is required to arouse a patient's response to questions or commands. *Obtundation* describes a condition in which repeated stimuli are needed to draw the patients' attention back to a task. *Stupor* is a state of more severely depressed level of consciousness in which wakefulness and minimal interaction with the examiner can be achieved only for brief intervals by repeated and/or noxious stimulation.

Delirium is a term used to describe a disorder of attention and orientation that may occur in association with an altered level of consciousness. It is an acute confusional state with a disturbance in attention, awareness, and cognition (see Chapter 26). This state develops over a short period of time, typically hours to days, and most often fluctuates in severity throughout the day. Delirium may be divided into hyperactive, hypoactive, or mixed subtypes depending on the clinical features. Hyperactive delirium is characterized by sympathetic nervous system overactivity with attention marred by hyperexcitability, tachycardia, perspiration, hypertension, hallucinations, and disturbance of the normal sleep-wake cycle. Hypoactive delirium manifests with decreased responsiveness and apathy. Mixed delirium involves a combination of features that are both hyperactive and hypoactive. Delirium is common in hospitalized individuals and is associated with prolonged hospitalization, increased healthcare costs, and mortality.

Because the examining physician can only infer thought from patients' actions (e.g., speech or movement), a reliable and reproducible physical examination is essential in evaluating the patient with altered consciousness. The neurologist must make every effort to establish the presence or absence of a directed nonreflexive response and judge its quality. Discerning whether there is a disorder of consciousness or an inability to respond is sometimes challenging. For example, in basilar occlusion with infarction of the posterior circulation but preserved bihemispheric function, a "locked-in" syndrome occurs (Fig. 13.1). In this condition, the patient will seemingly have no directed response to stimuli because disruption of the corticospinal and corticobulbar tracts results in severe quadriplegia and facial weakness. Yet on close examination, blinks or vertical eye movements may be preserved, and this patient may blink or move his or her eyes in an exact fashion to instructions, demonstrating full awareness and intact cognition. Similarly, in patients with severe acute polyneuropathies such as Guillain-Barré syndrome, consciousness is preserved but difficult to assess and quantify secondary to profound generalized weakness.

The Glasgow Coma Scale assesses and quantifies the degree of consciousness across three measures: eye opening, verbal response, and motor response. It is the most common scoring system used in prehospital and acute care settings as a fast and reliable way to describe level of consciousness and prognosticate, particularly in traumatic brain injury. Those with a Glasgow Coma Scale score of 3–8 are defined as having a severe injury (Fig. 13.2).

The prevalence of the different etiologies for coma varies depending on the age and demographics of a patient. Overall, trauma, stroke, diffuse anoxic-ischemic brain insult (secondary to cardiorespiratory arrest), and intoxicants are the leading mechanisms. Infections, seizures, and metabolic-endocrine disorders account for many of the remaining cases of coma (Fig. 13.3).

States that affect cognition and attention without affecting wakefulness such as the dementias (characterized by progressive cognitive deterioration) and structural brain lesions such as strokes or tumors when they cause focal or regional cerebral dysfunction do not fit within the designation of coma. Sleep is also distinct from coma because it is a normal patterned physiologic disconnection of the cortex from external stimuli (see Chapter 24).

Evaluation and Treatment of the Comatose Patient

The initial evaluation of a patient in coma must occur simultaneously with its management. Any delay in treatment while waiting to determine the exact cause should be avoided. Clearing the airway and ensuring adequate ventilation and oxygenation with a bag-valve mask or intubation, if needed, must be addressed immediately. Management of severe hypotension must be prompt, especially in suspected cases of increased intracranial pressure (ICP). Hemodynamic collapse should never be attributed to an intracranial process, without rapid and thorough evaluation and treatment of cardiac or circulatory causes. These form the "ABCs of coma management": airway, breathing, and circulation (Fig. 13.4). Immobilizing the neck until a cervical spine injury is excluded and performing a focused assessment with sonography for trauma (FAST) and CT scan of the cervical spine is also important in cases of suspected head or neck trauma (see Chapter 20).

Emergent evaluation of patients in coma of indeterminate etiology requires the following blood studies: a complete blood count, fingerstick glucose level, serum chemistry, urine and serum toxicology screens, ethanol level, liver profile, thyroid function tests, arterial blood gas, and blood cultures. Creatine kinase and troponin measurements, in conjunction with electrocardiography, are important for excluding myocardial infarction and transient cardiac arrest. Drug levels may be crucial in cases of suspected ingestion or overdose, including acetaminophen, lithium, or anticonvulsants based on available clinical history. Electroencephalography (EEG) can help to identify patients with nonconvulsive status epilepticus. Suspicion should be high for alternative causes of coma such as carbon monoxide poisoning in the proper clinical context, which may require additional laboratory tests.

Among the most common immediately treatable causes of coma are hypoglycemia and narcotic intoxication. These should be considered early and managed promptly, once oxygenation and hemodynamic status are stable. Infusion of 100 mg thiamine must precede the infusion of 50 mL of 50% dextrose in water as a precaution against Wernicke encephalopathy. This is postulated to be due to osmotic or metabolic damage to periventricular structures, such as the mammillary bodies and the medial thalamus (Fig. 13.5). When a narcotics overdose is suspected, such as in comatose patients with miotic pupils, intravenous (IV) naloxone, a

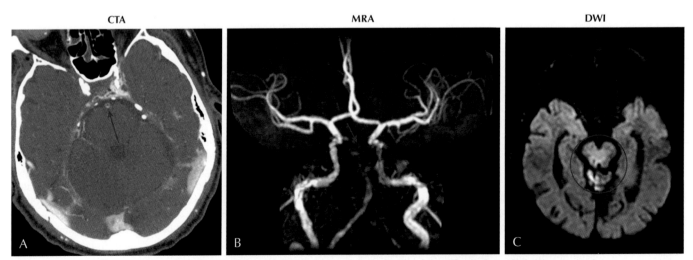

CTA **MRA** **DWI**

Fig. 13.1 Neuroimaging in "Locked-in" Syndrome Due to Basilar Artery Occlusion. (A) Axial computed tomography angiography *(CTA)* demonstrating occlusion of the basilar artery *(red arrow)*. (B) Magnetic resonance (MR) angiogram *(MRA)* of the intracranial circulation demonstrating absent flow in the distal basilar artery as well as bilateral posterior cerebral arteries *(red arrow)*. (C) MR axial diffusion-weighted image *(DWI)* showing bright signal in the midbrain consistent with recent infarct.

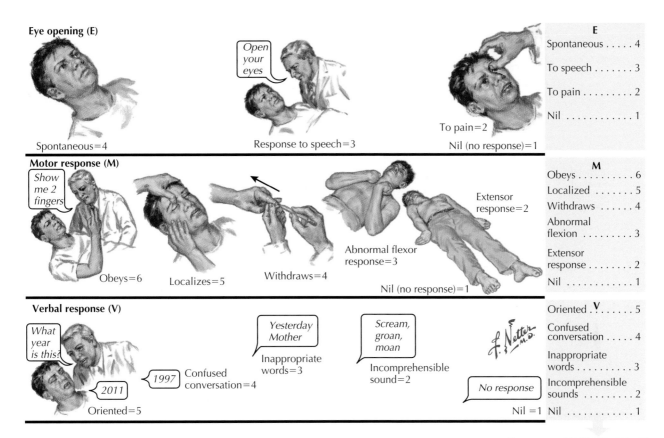

Eye opening (E)

Spontaneous=4

Open your eyes

Response to speech=3

To pain=2

Nil (no response)=1

E
Spontaneous 4
To speech 3
To pain 2
Nil 1

Motor response (M)

Show me 2 fingers

Obeys=6

Localizes=5

Withdraws=4

Abnormal flexor response=3

Extensor response=2

Nil (no response)=1

M
Obeys 6
Localized 5
Withdraws 4
Abnormal flexion 3
Extensor response 2
Nil 1

Verbal response (V)

What year is this?

2011

1997 Confused conversation=4

Yesterday Mother

Inappropriate words=3

Scream, groan, moan

Incomprehensible sound=2

No response

Oriented=5

Nil =1

f. Netter M.D.

V
Oriented 5
Confused conversation 4
Inappropriate words 3
Incomprehensible sounds 2
Nil 1

Coma score (E+M+V)=3 to 15

Fig. 13.2 Glasgow Coma Scale.

central opioid antagonist, can improve the level of consciousness within minutes. Repeated doses may be needed to maintain wakefulness and reverse respiratory depression. Caution should be exercised in those with long-standing known or suspected opioid dependency because abrupt or complete reversal of opioid effects by repeated doses may precipitate an acute withdrawal state.

Administration of flumazenil, a pure benzodiazepine antagonist (0.2 mg IV), given one to five times, can improve the mental state and reverse respiratory depression in benzodiazepine overdose. It must be used cautiously in those with a history of long-term benzodiazepine use or dependency because it can precipitate seizures. It should generally be avoided in patients with epilepsy and those at risk for seizures.

Urgent IV broad-spectrum antimicrobial coverage is indicated for patients presenting with coma and fever because early empiric treatment is crucial to improve clinical outcomes for meningitis and septicemia (see Chapter 44). In patients with altered consciousness, lumbar puncture should be performed only after brain imaging has excluded lesions that could lead to herniation, but imaging must not delay antibiotic administration.

Assessment of the comatose patient should include examination of the skin. Rashes may indicate streptococcal or staphylococcal meningitis, bacterial endocarditis, or systemic lupus erythematosus. Purpura may indicate meningococcal meningitis, a bleeding diathesis, or aspirin intoxication. Skin dryness suggests anticholinergic or barbiturate overdose, whereas excessive perspiration indicates cholinergic poisoning, hypoglycemia, or other causes of sympathetic overactivity. Dark pigmentary changes in the axillary and genital areas suggest adrenal insufficiency, whereas doughy pale skin is typical of myxedema. Renal failure may present with urea salt crystal skin condensations or "urea frost." Facial or basal skull fractures often cause ecchymosis around the eyes

(raccoon eyes or panda bear sign) or in the mastoid area (Battle sign), respectively. Extremities must be examined for needle and track marks that indicate IV drug use or subcutaneous self-injection.

The patient's breath may be uremic, fruity as in ketoacidosis, or have the musty fishy odor of hepatic failure. Fever may indicate meningitis or encephalitis but also occurs with sympathomimetic or tricyclic (anticholinergic) overdose or drug or alcohol withdrawal. Occasionally a low-grade fever can occur with subarachnoid hemorrhage or brainstem lesions. Cardiovascular examination in a febrile comatose patient should include investigation for stigmata of endocarditis such as a heart murmur.

A cautious and thorough neurologic assessment should be performed in any patient with coma. Particular attention should be paid to pupillary responses and other brainstem reflexes. Fundoscopic examination or ocular ultrasound may suggest papilledema indicative of intracranial hypertension. Motor examination (including noxious stimulation) may elicit signs of decorticate (flexor) or decerebrate (extensor) posturing and assist further in localization. In addition, it is important to assess for meningismus.

Focal neurologic signs on initial examination may implicate a structural lesion as the cause of coma and should be followed closely for signs of evolving herniation concurrently as urgent brain imaging is being obtained. Other causes of focal presentation are compensated old brain injuries clinically reemerging as a result of seizures, toxins, or metabolic derangements. However, metabolic disorders including nonketotic hyperosmolar hyperglycemia, hypoglycemia, and hepatic coma may cause focal seizures or lateralizing neurologic signs without focal brain lesions. Evolving signs of increased ICP or herniation must be treated promptly regardless of cause; additional neurologic injury may occur in waiting for brain CT results or other tests.

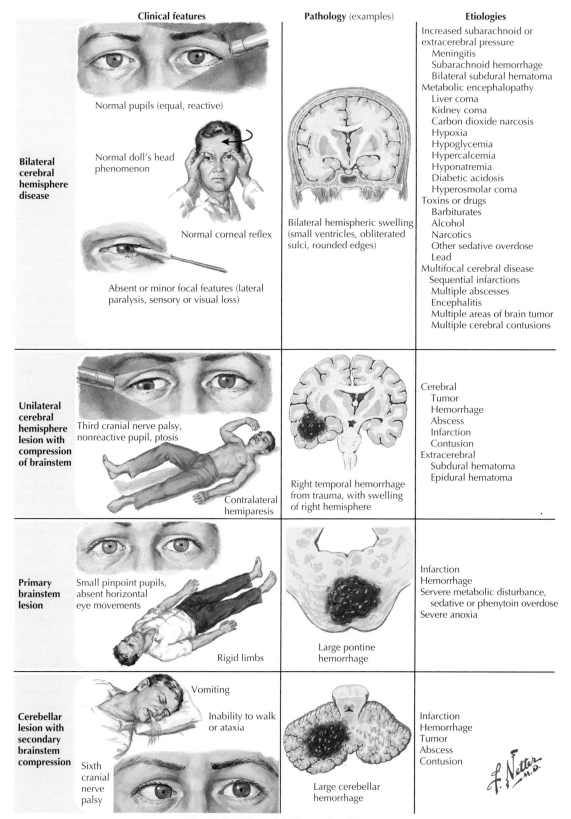

Clinical features	Pathology (examples)	Etiologies

Bilateral cerebral hemisphere disease

Normal pupils (equal, reactive)

Normal doll's head phenomenon

Normal corneal reflex

Absent or minor focal features (lateral paralysis, sensory or visual loss)

Bilateral hemispheric swelling (small ventricles, obliterated sulci, rounded edges)

Increased subarachnoid or extracerebral pressure
  Meningitis
  Subarachnoid hemorrhage
  Bilateral subdural hematoma
Metabolic encephalopathy
  Liver coma
  Kidney coma
  Carbon dioxide narcosis
  Hypoxia
  Hypoglycemia
  Hypercalcemia
  Hyponatremia
  Diabetic acidosis
  Hyperosmolar coma
Toxins or drugs
  Barbiturates
  Alcohol
  Narcotics
  Other sedative overdose
  Lead
Multifocal cerebral disease
  Sequential infarctions
  Multiple abscesses
  Encephalitis
  Multiple areas of brain tumor
  Multiple cerebral contusions

Unilateral cerebral hemisphere lesion with compression of brainstem

Third cranial nerve palsy, nonreactive pupil, ptosis

Contralateral hemiparesis

Right temporal hemorrhage from trauma, with swelling of right hemisphere

Cerebral
  Tumor
  Hemorrhage
  Abscess
  Infarction
  Contusion
Extracerebral
  Subdural hematoma
  Epidural hematoma

Primary brainstem lesion

Small pinpoint pupils, absent horizontal eye movements

Rigid limbs

Large pontine hemorrhage

Infarction
Hemorrhage
Servere metabolic disturbance, sedative or phenytoin overdose
Severe anoxia

Cerebellar lesion with secondary brainstem compression

Vomiting

Inability to walk or ataxia

Sixth cranial nerve palsy

Large cerebellar hemorrhage

Infarction
Hemorrhage
Tumor
Abscess
Contusion

Fig. 13.3 Differential Diagnosis of Coma.

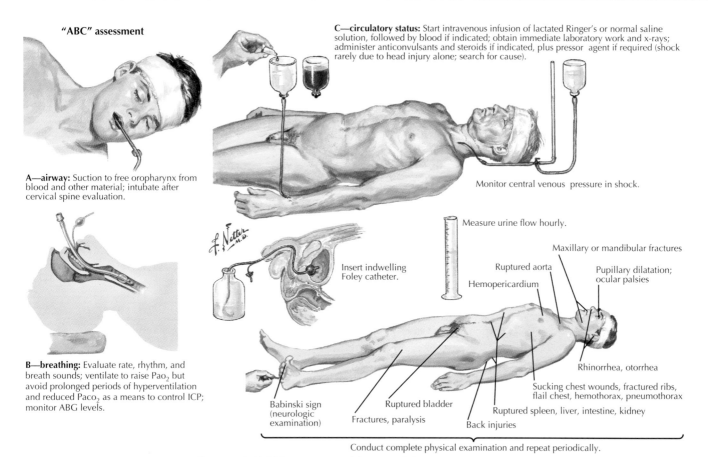

"ABC" assessment

A—airway: Suction to free oropharynx from blood and other material; intubate after cervical spine evaluation.

B—breathing: Evaluate rate, rhythm, and breath sounds; ventilate to raise Pao_2 but avoid prolonged periods of hyperventilation and reduced $Paco_2$ as a means to control ICP; monitor ABG levels.

C—circulatory status: Start intravenous infusion of lactated Ringer's or normal saline solution, followed by blood if indicated; obtain immediate laboratory work and x-rays; administer anticonvulsants and steroids if indicated, plus pressor agent if required (shock rarely due to head injury alone; search for cause).

Monitor central venous pressure in shock.

Measure urine flow hourly.

Insert indwelling Foley catheter.

Maxillary or mandibular fractures

Pupillary dilatation; ocular palsies

Ruptured aorta

Hemopericardium

Rhinorrhea, otorrhea

Sucking chest wounds, fractured ribs, flail chest, hemothorax, pneumothorax

Ruptured spleen, liver, intestine, kidney

Back injuries

Babinski sign (neurologic examination)

Ruptured bladder

Fractures, paralysis

Conduct complete physical examination and repeat periodically.

Fig. 13.4 Initial Management of Coma and Severe Head Injuries.

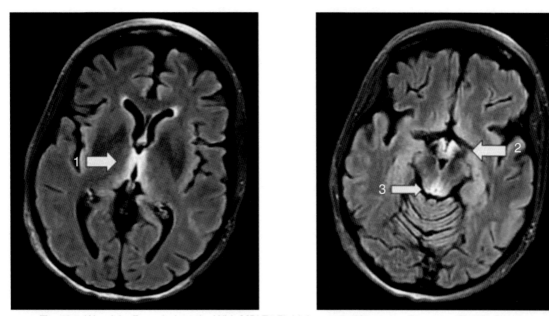

Fig. 13.5 Wernicke Encephalopathy With MRI T2 Fluid-Attenuated Inversion Recovery (FLAIR) Changes Involving Medial Thalamus (1), Mammillary Bodies (2), and Periaqueductal Gray (3).

EEG is often helpful in evaluating patients with altered consciousness or coma. An abnormal EEG tracing makes psychogenic coma unlikely. EEG detects nonconvulsive status epilepticus, which can present without a history of epilepsy. Although nonspecific, diffuse EEG background slowing correlates with metabolic derangements and focal slowing with localized structural brain disease. Hepatic and other metabolic encephalopathies may show triphasic waves (Fig. 13.6). In herpes simplex encephalitis, periodic lateralized epileptiform temporal lobe discharges are often seen and support the clinical diagnosis. In addition, when a basis pontis lesion with the "locked-in syndrome" is suspected, a normal EEG background rhythm shows that the patient is alert despite limited or no obvious response to stimuli (alpha coma pattern).

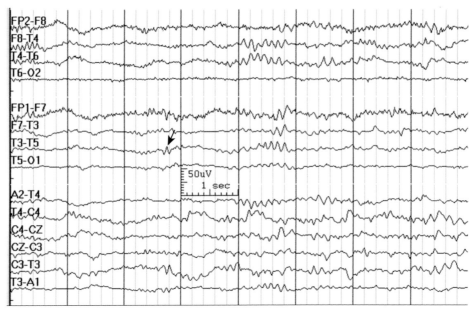

Fig. 13.6 Triphasic Waves on EEG as Seen in Metabolic and Hepatic Coma.

Neurologic Assessment

> **CLINICAL VIGNETTE** *A 76-year-old man is found lying on the floor at home. Examination in the emergency department demonstrates a left hemiplegia, with conjugate eye deviation to the right. He is awake, calm, and able to answer questions but with a left homonymous visual field deficit, dysarthria, and a left facial droop. He has no movement in the left arm or leg, and when his left hand is placed in his right visual field, he does not recognize it as his own. In spite of his hemiplegia, he denies having any difficulties with his limbs. Brain CT demonstrates a large right middle cerebral artery and anterior cerebral artery territory stroke. In the next hour, the patient becomes obtunded and progressively less responsive to external stimulation. Repeat brain CT scan shows a large intraparenchymal hemorrhage within the infarct territory and a right cerebral shift across the falx cerebri and downward through the cerebellar tentorium, with compression of the midbrain.*
>
> *The patient undergoes endotracheal intubation due to his depressed level of consciousness and inability to protect his airway. Soon afterward, he cannot be aroused. On exam, he has right-sided flexed arm posturing and left-sided extension, with tonic leg extension and plantar flexion. His pupils are irregular and sluggishly reactive to light. Vestibuloocular reflex is absent. His examination does not improve with administration of hypertonic saline, mannitol, or hyperventilation. An emergency, right decompressive hemicraniectomy is performed; however, he remains comatose and the family choses to transition to comfort care. He dies hours after mechanical ventilation is discontinued.*

Rostrocaudal Signs of Brain Compromise

As pressure from a hemispheric lesion increases, patients gradually move from being easily roused, but inattentive, to sleepy and unable to maintain wakefulness, then to coma. The ascending reticular formation, stimulated by sensory input, mediates arousal and consciousness to the cortex via the thalamic nuclei. Lesions that cause coma are at one of three levels along the neuraxis: bilateral cerebral cortex, the thalami, or the upper brainstem. The classic concept of coma stages produced by brain mass lesions pertains to a hemispheric process that worsens until it ultimately causes "rostrocaudal" deterioration of function from the hemispheres into the medulla. Although these stages rarely manifest symmetrically or in a strict and clearly delineated sequential pattern, this paradigm remains useful for evaluating patients with hemispheric lesions and deterioration of their neurologic examination (such as the patient in the vignette) and to conceptualize the associated functional brainstem neuroanatomy. In addition to the level of consciousness, important physical examination elements include pupillary size and reactivity, reflexive eye movements, limb posturing, and breathing pattern (Fig. 13.7).

Pupillary Reactivity and Eye Movements

When pressure onto or across the diencephalon exists, loss of wakefulness results, but patients may transiently continue to withdraw appropriately from uncomfortable stimuli and to resist passive limb movements. Pupils are small and reactive, although at times reactivity is blunted and subtle to detect. Although there is no visual fixation, eye movements are conjugate and full. As pressure mounts across the thalami onto the mesencephalon, pupillary and eye movement abnormalities appear. Involvement of cranial nerve (CN) III or its nucleus initially causes irregular, dilated, and poorly reactive pupils. Eventually, eye movements are disrupted by CN III or CN VI lesions or from involvement of the medial longitudinal fasciculus (MLF).

The MLF, a paracentral dorsally located tract coursing up the vestibular nuclei to the CN III nucleus, maintains conjugate eye movements either initiated voluntarily in the waking state or induced reflexively from cervical or vestibular inputs in comatose patients. This pathway provides the basis of doll's-eyes testing (aka vestibuloocular reflex) or caloric stimulation testing of the semicircular canals. An intact MLF system keeps the eyes from moving passively when the examiner moves the head to one side or the other. The eyes remain in their primary position in relation to the examiner or seem to move to the opposite side in relation to the head turning. With unilateral caloric stimulation of the ears, an intact MLF causes the eyes to deviate conjugately to one side or another, depending on the water temperature used for irrigation. The direction of the convection current induced in the semicircular canals by different temperatures determines the direction of eye movement. With the head maintained in the neutral position, cold water causes the eyes to deviate to the side of the stimulated ear, with horizontal nystagmus beating away from the ear tested. Warm water causes the eyes to move away from the stimulated ear, with nystagmus toward

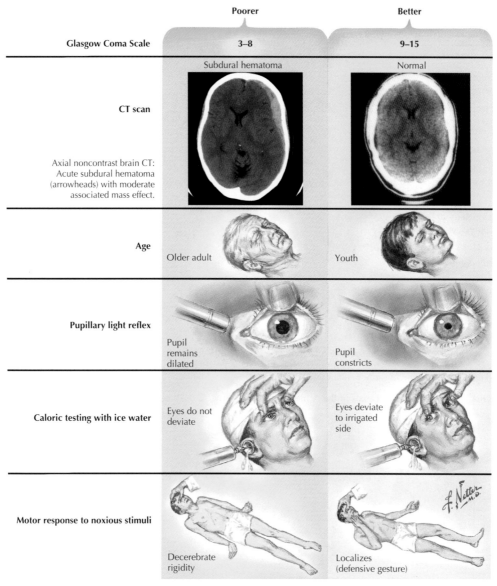

Fig. 13.7 Prognosis in Coma Related to Severe Head Injuries.

the ear being tested. Disruption of the MLF system results in abnormal or absent responses to caloric stimulation (Fig. 13.8). Therefore oculocephalic testing checks the integrity of a large portion of the brainstem from the vestibular nuclei to the mesencephalic third-nerve nucleus.

Movement

If the motor pathways of the brainstem are disconnected from corticothalamic input, certain primitive tonic postures may be observed that reflect the level of central nervous system (CNS) damage. With supratentorial injury, depending on the area of frontal cortex involved, patients may show unilateral signs of upper motor neuron dysfunction, with the typical triad of increased flexor tone, hyperreflexia, and paralysis. The opposite side may still show semivoluntary or directed movements, such as withdrawing from noxious stimuli or breaking the fall of a limb held against gravity. When damage progresses below the diencephalon or to the upper reticular activating system, a decorticate posture appears, characterized by rigid arm adduction, forearm pronation with flexion of the elbow and wrist, and leg extension at the hips and knees. With involvement of the brainstem below the diencephalon (classically below the level of the red nucleus), decerebrate rigidity evolves, with arm

extension at the elbows, hyperextension of the trunk and legs, and prominent plantar flexion of the feet. Arm adduction, wrist flexion, and forearm pronation persist. Animal models suggest that decerebrate rigidity corresponds to mesencephalic lesions at the level of the red nucleus. With ischemia to the lower pons and medulla, the body becomes flaccid, with no reactivity except for occasional bilateral toe extensor responses with knee and hip flexion that are mediated by spinal motor and sensory reflex pathways.

Breathing

Respiratory patterns also change with worsening levels of consciousness in coma (Fig. 13.9). The earliest breathing alterations are Cheyne-Stokes respirations. Hemispheric forebrain structures serve to regulate breathing by mechanisms independent of CO_2 accumulation. With bilateral cerebral cortex damage, this breathing control is lost and CO_2-driven breathing is accentuated with only modest CO_2 accumulations, thus inducing an increased rate and depth of respiration. This reactive hyperpnea leads to an increased minute ventilation and decreased arterial CO_2. Low arterial CO_2 without intact forebrain control causes a loss of respiratory drive. The ensuing apnea leads to CO_2 reaccumulation. This

Doll's eye phenomenon

Direction of maintained
head acceleration

Horizontal semicircular
canal excited

Horizontal semicircular
canal depressed

Medial rectus motor
neurons excited

Medial rectus motor
neurons depressed

Medial and lateral vestibular
nuclei excited

Inhibitory interneurons

Abducens nucleus excited

Abducens nucleus
depressed

Abducens (VI) nerve

Oculomotor (III) nerve

Pontine reticular formation

Lateral rectus
muscle

Lateral rectus muscle

Medial
rectus
muscles

Eyes move in opposite direction from head;
tend to preserve visual fixation: rate determined by degree of horizontal canal
excitation

Medial longitudinal fasciculus (MLF) maintains conjugate eye movements initiated voluntarily in waking
state or induced reflexively from cervical or vestibular inputs in comatose patients. MLF provides basis for
doll's eye testing and caloric stimulation of semicircular canals.

JOHN A. CRAIG—AD

Testing for doll's head conjugate eye movement

Head rotated and observed for
presence and direction of eye
movement; intact MLF prevents
passive eye movement; with
head rotation.

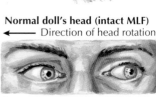

Normal doll's head (intact MLF)
← Direction of head rotation

Apparent eye movement ——→
Eyes remain in primary position in
relation to examiner or appear to
"move opposite" to direction of
head rotation.

**Abnormal doll's head
(disrupted MLF)**
← Direction of head rotation

← Direction of eye movement
Eyes remain centered following
same direction as rotation of head.

Ice water caloric testing of the semicircular canals in the comatose patient

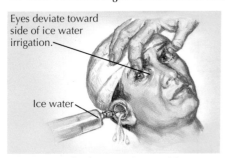

Eyes deviate toward
side of ice water
irrigation.

Ice water

Normal caloric test (intact MLF)

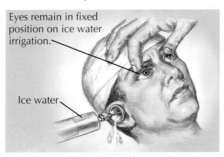

Eyes remain in fixed
position on ice water
irrigation.

Ice water

Abnormal caloric test (disrupted MLF)

One ear irrigated with ice water solution and
patient observed for presence and direction of
eye movement relative to side of irrigation

Fig. 13.8 Eye Movements in Coma.

cycle repeats itself, resulting in hyperpnea of a crescendo-decrescendo pattern, alternating with intervening episodes of brief apnea.

Midbrain and upper pons lesions cause hyperventilation with a constant rate and amplitude, without periods of apnea. The reasons for the so-called central neurogenic hyperventilation are unclear but are unlikely to be of purely neuronal origin. Lung congestion caused by immobility and poor airway protection likely play a major role. Hypothalamic and midbrain lesions engender increased sympathetic activity, which in turn promotes capillary fluid seepage, worsening lung congestion, and, in extreme cases, pulmonary edema.

Injury to the lower half of the pons damages the respiratory control system, possibly generating apneustic breathing; a pattern of prolonged end-inspiratory pauses alternating with end-expiratory pauses of several seconds, without the crescendo-decrescendo pattern of Cheyne-Stokes breathing. Further damage causes this pattern to fragment into an irregular, unpredictable rhythm of varying amplitude, intermixed with pauses of variable length. Ultimately, destruction of the centrally located dorsomedial medullary respiratory center causes total cessation of breathing, even before circulatory collapse occurs.

Coma from metabolic disease rarely conforms to the typical rostrocaudal stages and often shows concurrent findings that implicate multiple nervous system levels. For example, hypoglycemia can cause

unconsciousness with decerebrate posturing but preserved oculocephalic responses and pupillary reactivity. In metabolic coma from opioid overdose, pupils are tiny but reactive to light, even though respiratory drive may be obliterated. In addition, oculocephalic responses are commonly intact, despite drug-induced pinpoint pupillary changes mimicking the exam findings found with pontine hemorrhage, as the vignette at the beginning of this chapter illustrates. Finally, pupillary reactivity remains relatively resistant to metabolic effects; when other brainstem signs are absent, the presence of brisk pupillary reactivity suggests a nonstructural metabolic or toxic cause.

Prognosis

Determining the degree of neurologic recovery for an individual comatose patient is a difficult task. Although many families ask, it is often not accurate or practical to apply statistics in framing an individual's chances for recovery or good neurologic outcome except at the best and worst ends of the prognostic spectrum. The focus usually shifts to the chances of recovery, no matter how limited, rather than the likelihood of severe disability. For each individual case, numerous factors, including age, the cause of the coma, the evolution of the neurologic examination, and medical comorbidities, factor into an assessment of prognosis. All of these, as well as the religious or philosophical beliefs

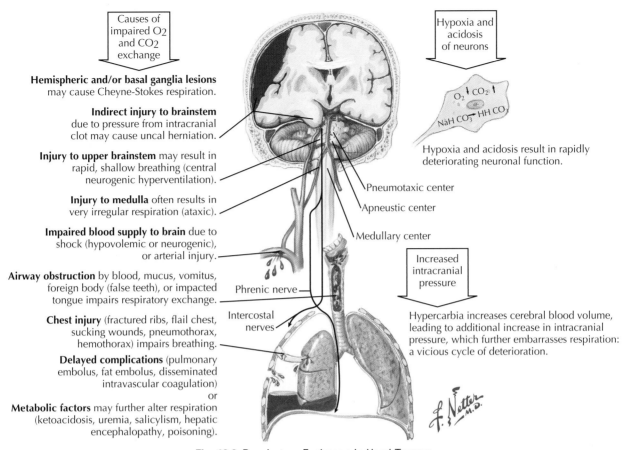

Causes of impaired O₂ and CO₂ exchange

Hemispheric and/or basal ganglia lesions may cause Cheyne-Stokes respiration.

Indirect injury to brainstem due to pressure from intracranial clot may cause uncal herniation.

Injury to upper brainstem may result in rapid, shallow breathing (central neurogenic hyperventilation).

Injury to medulla often results in very irregular respiration (ataxic).

Impaired blood supply to brain due to shock (hypovolemic or neurogenic), or arterial injury.

Airway obstruction by blood, mucus, vomitus, foreign body (false teeth), or impacted tongue impairs respiratory exchange.

Chest injury (fractured ribs, flail chest, sucking wounds, pneumothorax, hemothorax) impairs breathing.

Delayed complications (pulmonary embolus, fat embolus, disseminated intravascular coagulation) or **Metabolic factors** may further alter respiration (ketoacidosis, uremia, salicylism, hepatic encephalopathy, poisoning).

Hypoxia and acidosis of neurons

Hypoxia and acidosis result in rapidly deteriorating neuronal function.

Pneumotaxic center
Apneustic center
Medullary center

Phrenic nerve
Intercostal nerves

Increased intracranial pressure

Hypercarbia increases cerebral blood volume, leading to additional increase in intracranial pressure, which further embarrasses respiration: a vicious cycle of deterioration.

Fig. 13.9 Respiratory Exchange in Head Trauma.

of the patient and family, help with communication in the process of surrogate medical decision making and goals of care conversations.

Recovery from drug intoxication in individuals without associated ischemic brain injury from secondary hypoxemia or circulatory collapse is usually good. In hepatic and other metabolic comas, brainstem dysfunction with disruption of oculocephalic reflexes and/or loss of pupillary reactivity is a marker of severity and increases the likelihood of poor prognosis or death. A long duration of coma or absent localizing motor responses does not exclude the possibility of a good recovery in hepatic coma and probably reflects prolonged metabolic derangement.

Numerous theories have been proposed as to the cause of hepatic encephalopathy in patients with cirrhosis. The predominant mechanism relates to neurotoxic substances, such as ammonia, which enter the brain due to liver failure. These substances may cause dysfunction of astrocytes and neurons, as well as cerebral inflammation, in addition to other deleterious effects. Many precipitants for hepatic encephalopathy in those with hepatic failure have been identified (anemia, constipation, dehydration, gastrointestinal bleeding, metabolic alkalosis, hypoglycemia, hypothyroidism, hypoxia, infection, medications), and aggressive treatment is necessary to reverse the encephalopathy. Removal of intestinal ammonia with nonabsorbable disaccharides (lactulose) and antibiotics such as neomycin or rifaximin are commonly used and are effective, although it may take several days for the encephalopathy to improve.

Acute fulminant liver failure often leads to altered consciousness, via similar mechanisms to those described for chronic liver failure. However, patients with acute liver failure may develop cerebral edema and intracranial hypertension that can rapidly progress to death. Treatment consists of the previously outlined measures and the preservation of cerebral perfusion pressure (CPP) by close monitoring and aggressive control of ICP by clinical examination or invasive neuromonitoring in select cases for those with a Glasgow Coma Scale (GCS) less than or equal to 8. With severe acute liver failure, liver transplantation remains the most effective and immediate treatment to control brain edema and to reverse coma.

Coma after cardiac arrest has a mortality rate of up to 60%–70%, with generally only 10%–15% of patients returning to a good functional status. Randomized controlled trials of therapeutic hypothermia and targeted temperature management (i.e., 24 hours of induced hypothermia—goal temperature 32°C–34°C) followed by passive rewarming following out of hospital cardiac arrest in those with an initial cardiac rhythm of ventricular fibrillation or pulseless ventricular tachycardia has resulted in improved neurologic outcomes and has been widely adopted in critical care. More recent data suggest that targeting milder hypothermia to 36°C may be equally effective to 33°C. The lack of bilateral pupillary responses, absent corneal responses, or absent/extensor motor responses at 3 days postarrest has been associated with a poor neurologic prognosis following cardiac arrest. Myoclonus status epilepticus (generalized multifocal unrelenting myoclonus) within the first day postarrest correlates with severe ischemic damage to the cortex, brainstem, and spinal cord and is strongly associated with poor neurologic recovery. These findings must be interpreted cautiously following the use of targeted temperature management as data suggest that they may not be as reliable.

Other laboratory and electrophysiologic findings have been associated with a poor neurologic prognosis and can be used to help understand the severity of brain injury. Elevation of serum neuron specific enolase greater than 33 µg/L (measured 1–3 days postarrest) suggests significant neurocellular injury. The absence of bilateral cortical N20 somatosensory evoked potentials (SSEPs) is strongly indicative of a poor prognosis, although is not definitive. Burst suppression or malignant patterns on EEG are associated with poor prognosis. Neuroimaging must be interpreted cautiously after cardiac arrest; however, severe diffuse anoxic brain injury on CT scan is likely associated with poor prognosis.

Ultimately, a multimodal approach utilizing all of these tests together to increase their predictive ability is the most judicious approach.

These observations can guide families and staff toward the best course of action for each patient. Evolution of the neurologic examination and assessment with as many confounding or sedating factors removed helps to clarify whether there are signs of neurologic improvement or not. Consequently, further waiting and repeated coma examination, although potentially stressful for the family, result in more certainty regarding the appropriateness of the eventual decisions taken. Those showing unfavorable prognostic signs early and no improvement or evolution in their neurologic examination over time are less likely to have a favorable neurologic recovery. However, for individuals who exhibit even subtly improving neurologic function, it may be reasonable to extend the duration of observation to give a more accurate determination of their neurologic outcome.

PERSISTENT VEGETATIVE STATE

CLINICAL VIGNETTE *A 23-year-old woman is an unrestrained driver in a "head-on" automobile accident. She is ejected 30 feet through the windshield and sustains major head trauma. On arrival in the emergency department, she is totally unresponsive, hypotensive, and tachycardic. Brain CT demonstrates generalized cerebral edema and diffuse subarachnoid hemorrhage. Neurologic examination shows her to be unresponsive even to painful stimuli, other than some rare nonpurposeful right leg movements. Pupils are minimally and inconsistently reactive, and she has a dense left hemiplegia. Subsequent magnetic resonance imaging (MRI) demonstrates bilateral focal contusions of the cerebral hemispheres, shear injury to the splenium of the corpus callosum, and brainstem edema. Four months later, after no improvement in her clinical state, she is diagnosed with persistent vegetative state (PVS).*

Condition is called *persistent* when it lasts without change for more than 1 month.

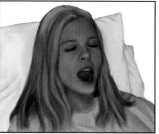 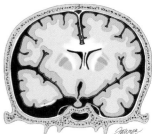

Patients may startle, look about, or yawn, but none of these actions are in conscious response to a specific stimulus.

Subarachnoid hemorrhage

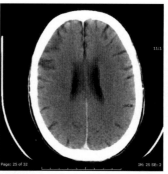 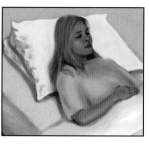

Non-contrast brain CT demonstrating ominous sign of diffuse brain injury and possible prelude to a persistent vegetative state: sulcal effacement (diffuse edema) and subtle disappearance of normal differentiation between gray and white matter.

Fig. 13.10 Persistent Vegetative State.

PVS most frequently occurs in young individuals with healthy cardiovascular and pulmonary systems. PVS, or unresponsive wakefulness syndrome, is a state of preserved brainstem and hypothalamic function with absent or insufficient cortical function to sustain awareness of environment and self. Wakefulness is the requisite feature distinguishing vegetative state from coma, and patients in a vegetative state may cycle through sleep stages. There is no behavioral evidence of even the simplest reproducible response. Patients may startle, look about, occasionally move a limb, shift position, or yawn, but none of these actions are in response to an environmental stimulus (Fig. 13.10). Even the most basic voluntary actions, such as chewing and swallowing, are lost. With reversible metabolic or exogenous causes eliminated, the condition is called persistent when it lasts without change for more than 1 month. For adults, a vegetative state lasting more than 12 months may be referred to as permanent. If the mechanism of brain injury is nontraumatic, some may refer to a vegetative state as permanent after only 3 months. In permanent vegetative state, the chance of recovery is exceedingly low and the condition is generally associated with long-term completely dependent care.

As with coma, individuals in a posttraumatic PVS have better chances of recovery than cases due to medical causes. Nevertheless, one-third of all these patients die within the first year. Of patients with head trauma, one-third regain consciousness after 3 months and approximately one-half in a year. Overall, one-fourth of all patients with traumatic PVS recover to a level of moderate disability, mostly those who regain awareness within 3 months.

Of patients with nontraumatic PVS, more than 50% die within a year and only approximately 10%–15% regain consciousness by the third month. Most remain severely disabled. If the condition persists longer, there is minimal chance of significant functional recovery. For a patient in a vegetative state, discontinuation of nutritional support and hydration is ethically acceptable and may be discussed with the patient's surrogate medical decision maker(s). Any decisions regarding continuation versus discontinuation of medical intervention are undoubtedly complex and require detailed counseling, as well as clear communication regarding the best assessment of prognosis and the patient's wishes.

DEATH BY NEUROLOGIC CRITERIA/BRAIN DEATH

CLINICAL VIGNETTE *A 56-year-old man suddenly collapses at home after experiencing severe chest pain. His wife calls Emergency Medical Services, who find him pulseless and cyanotic. ECG demonstrates ventricular fibrillation, and he is successfully defibrillated. After an airway is established and 100% oxygen is given, he is transported to the emergency department (ED). There, neurologic evaluation shows that he is unresponsive to any form of communication. His pupils are large and not reactive to light stimulation. Decerebrate posturing is noted to suctioning and to noxious stimulation. Bilateral Babinski signs are present. Over hours, his tone becomes flaccid, and cold caloric stimulation testing shows no response on either side. The next day, he develops generalized myoclonus and continued hemodynamic instability, requiring cardiac and ventilatory support. Three days later, there is no change in his neurologic status. An apnea test following the institutional protocol shows no spontaneous respirations. He is declared brain dead at the conclusion of the apnea test.*

This vignette is a characteristic example of a patient with prolonged cardiorespiratory arrest resulting in devastating diffuse cerebral ischemic damage. Until a precise determination of brain death is established, aggressive medical care continues, although there are many medical, ethical, and legal considerations in caring for individuals who have no clinical evidence of brain function despite artificial maintenance of cardiopulmonary function with modern intensive care.

In most medical communities, a person is considered dead once there is irreversible and total cessation of all brain function, regardless of a continuing functional circulatory system. The cause of brain death must be clearly elucidated by history, examination, or medical tests before pursuing clinical brain death testing to exclude reversible causes or confounders. Intoxicants, sedatives, and hypothermia may present similarly to brain death but are potentially reversible and must always be considered and eliminated as a potential cause for absent brainstem responses. In many countries, including the United States, "brain death" or death by neurologic criteria (DNC) constitutes a legal definition of death. Once a DNC determination is made, all life support measures should be halted.

It is appropriate to respect the patient's and family's wishes, religious or personal, regarding the diagnosis of brain death and discontinuation of life support. There is considerable cultural and religious variability in beliefs and attitudes toward medical care at the end of life and noncardiac death. It is important to explain the difference between brain death and other conditions such as coma or vegetative state. It is also essential to meet with the family and communicate throughout the clinical assessment process. The team needs to explain and reinforce that once a brain death determination is made, the condition is irreversible and regarded legally and medically in the same way as cardiac death. It is expected that upon discontinuation of the ventilator and other critical care interventions, circulatory collapse will invariably occur within minutes to hours.

Honoring the wishes of registered organ donors and realizing the potential to bring something positive out of tragedy for an ever-growing list of patients awaiting transplant procedures make it requisite for the team to contact local organ donation services as soon as a patient is identified as potentially meeting DNC criteria. It is critical from an ethical standpoint that the primary caregivers for the patient perform their duties and make all medical decisions independently from the organ donation representatives. Organ donation nurses, social workers, and coordinators are trained in these conversations and, with the care team's permission, will approach family members at the appropriate time to discuss organ donation.

Brain Death Criteria

The criteria for brain death vary among states and countries. The determination is based on clinical examination findings including apnea testing, with other testing used only as an ancillary or confirmatory measure. The following are generally accepted principles of brain death determination:

1. A preceding coma of known irreversible cause must **not** be due to, or influenced by, CNS depressants, intoxicants, paralytic agents, hypothermia (<32°C/90°F), endocrine, or metabolic disturbances.
2. Cessation of all brain function must be documented as follows:
   a. There must be **no response to stimuli** in any way **other than** spinal cord–mediated **reflexive movements** in the legs and arms. Muscle stretch reflexes or extensor responses of the toes (Babinski signs) can be seen, but there must be no other spontaneous limb movements or posturing to painful stimuli, including decerebrate rigidity.
   b. **Brainstem reflexes must be absent,** including pupillary response to light (without mydriatic agents), oculocephalic reflexes by caloric stimulation, corneal reflexes, oropharyngeal reflexes (gag

or swallowing), respiratory activation (spontaneous breaths or cough), and snout or jaw jerk reflex (Fig. 13.11).
   c. **Apnea test must be positive,** wherein the patient exhibits no evidence of respiratory effort with induced hypercapnia. In this instance, the patient is ventilated with 100% O_2 for 15 minutes and then disconnected while an endotracheal catheter provides passive supplemental oxygen. Apneic oxygenation is maintained while serial blood gas measurements are taken at approximately 5-minute intervals. The apnea test is confirmatory of DNC if the partial pressure of arterial carbon dioxide ($Paco_2$) increases by 20 points or is greater than 60 mm Hg. Institutional protocols may vary slightly in the requirements to successfully complete the apnea test.
3. When the clinical evaluation, apnea test, or both are unclear or unfeasible, confirmatory tests to document the absence of electrical or metabolic cerebral activity are conducted at the discretion of the physician making the brain death determination. CT or MRI scan may clarify the etiology of neurologic injury but in themselves do not add to a determination of death by neurologic criteria.
   a. A high-quality 30-minute or longer EEG isoelectric tracing meeting strict technical standards (including a maximum 2 μV/mm sensitivity, interelectrode impedances between 100 and 10,000 Ohms, and "double" interelectrode distance bipolar montage) is sought. If there is uncertainty after an initial EEG recording, a second recording 6 or more hours after the first in adults (>24 hours in neonates and children) to document electrocerebral inactivity is indicated (2016 American Neurophysiology Society Guideline Recommendations).
   b. Documentation of cessation of cerebral circulation by conventional angiography, technetium (99mTc hexamethylpropyleneamine oxime [HMPAO]) brain single-photon emission computerized tomography (SPECT) study, or transcranial Doppler ultrasonography.

Confounding Factors

When a severe cerebral insult is suspected but brain death determination cannot be confirmed because of confounding issues, everything possible should be done to correct for these specific factors before a brain death assessment can proceed. For example, hypothermia must be treated to bring and maintain core body temperature to greater than 36.5°C, fluid and at times vasopressor agents must be administered for patients to maintain systolic blood pressures above 90 mm Hg, and acute kidney injury must be reversed to the extent possible.

A Pco_2 of approximately 60 mm Hg or greater (as seen in chronic obstructive lung disease) may not necessarily stimulate chemoreceptors in the brainstem to initiate respiration, even with a functioning brainstem. In such cases, the CO_2 level may be allowed to climb to approximately 80 mm Hg during the apnea test, but such levels risk direct cardiodepressant effects, as well as arrhythmias and hypotension due to acidemia. Therefore it is preferable in these instances to forgo apnea testing and obtain ancillary tests to confirm the diagnosis without risking iatrogenic complications.

Although most centers in the United States uphold the general outline of the principles mentioned previously and in the American Academy of Neurology (AAN) guideline on determining brain death in adults, there are numerous variations and differences concerning how best to ensure diagnostic certainty. Most medical centers do not require confirmatory tests when all clinical criteria are met. The number of evaluations and the time span between them may also differ between institutions. The specific brain death criteria and protocol for each medical center must be consulted before the evaluation is begun and a diagnosis is substantiated.

Border zone ischemia (shock, circulatory insufficiency)

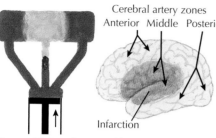

Cerebral artery zones
Anterior Middle Posterior

Infarction

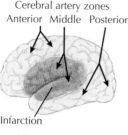

Diffuse cortical necrosis; persistent vegetative state

Border zone
between artery zones

Infarction

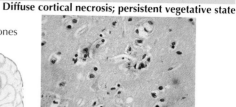

Few anoxic neurons in early anoxia

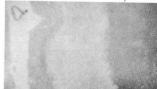

Extensive laminar necrosis

Pump with 3 outflows, one outflow blocked. Deficit occurs in zone supplied by it.

If brain artery is blocked, infarction occurs in zone supplied by that vessel.

If pump is weak, deficit is between zones supplied by 3 outflows.

If total blood flow is inadequate, deficit is mostly at border zone between supply zones.

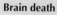 **Brain death**

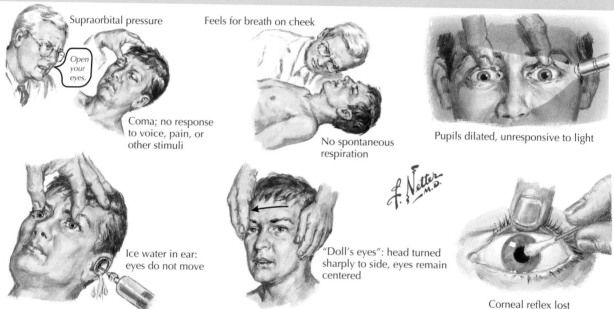

Supraorbital pressure

Open your eyes.

Coma; no response to voice, pain, or other stimuli

Feels for breath on cheek

No spontaneous respiration

Pupils dilated, unresponsive to light

Ice water in ear: eyes do not move

"Doll's eyes": head turned sharply to side, eyes remain centered

Corneal reflex lost

F. Netter M.D.

Fig. 13.11 Hypoxic Brain Damage and Brain Death.

ADDITIONAL RESOURCES

Posner JB, Saper CB, Schiff ND, et al. The diagnosis of stupor and coma. 4th ed. Contemporary Neurology Series. 71. New York: Oxford University Press; 2007.

An expanded and exhaustive edition of the classic monogram on the pathophysiology of coma and its various etiologies. Detailed description of the associated vascular and anatomic pathology. It ends with a small section on the approach to the unconscious patient and treatment.

Conrad GR, Sinha P. Scintigraphy as a confirmatory test of brain death. Semin Nucl Med 2003;33:312–23.

Stecker MM, Sabau D, Sullivan L, et al. American Clinical Neurophysiology Society guideline 6: minimum technical standards for EEG recording in suspected cerebral death. J Clin Neurophysiol 2016;33:324–7.

Wijdicks EFM, Hijdra A, Young GB, et al. Practice parameter: prediction of outcome in comatose survivors after cardiopulmonary resuscitation (an evidence-based review): report of the quality standards subcommittee of the American Academy of Neurology. Neurology 2006;67:203–10.

A systematic review of the outcomes in coma after cardiopulmonary arrest identifying the factors that most reliably predict a poor prognosis.

Geocadin RG, Wijdicks E, Armstrong MJ, et al. Practice guideline summary: reducing brain injury following cardiopulmonary resuscitation. Neurology 2017;88:2141–9.

Levy DE, Bates D, Corona JJ, et al. Prognosis in non-traumatic coma. Ann Intern Med 1981;94:293–301.

Landmark paper that details the examination of postanoxic coma and the various findings that predict outcomes.

Sazbon L, Zagreba F, Ronen J, et al. Course and outcome of patients in vegetative state of non-traumatic aetiology. J Neurol Neurosurg Psychiatry 1993;56:407–9.

Teasdale G, Jennet B. Assessment of coma and impaired consciousness: a practical scale. Lancet 1974;ii:81–4.

The first description of the Glasgow Coma Scale that has acquired widespread use and has subsequently been shown to be a reliable tool in predicting outcome in head trauma.

The Multi-Society Task Force on PVS. Medical aspects of the persistent vegetative state: parts I and II. N Engl J Med 1994;330:1499–508, 1572–9.

American Psychiatric Association. Diagnostic and statistical manual of mental disorders: DSM-5. 5th ed. Arlington: American Psychiatric Association; 2013. pp. 372–8.

Vahedi K, Hofmeijer J, Juettler E, et al; for the DECIMAL, DESTINY, and HAMLET investigators. Early decompressive surgery in malignant infarction of the middle cerebral artery: a pooled analysis of three randomized controlled trials. Lancet Neurol 2007;6: 315–22.

Data pooled from three different studies showing that decompressive hemicraniectomy more than doubles the chance of survival from "malignant" middle cerebral artery stroke, and likely improves outcomes regardless of the side affected. However, most survivors are left with significant disability.

Cerebrovascular Diseases

Claudia J. Chaves

Anatomic Aspects of Cerebral Circulation

Claudia J. Chaves

The brain and meninges are supplied by arteries derived from the common carotid artery (CCA) and vertebrobasilar system (Fig. 14.1). The right CCA usually originates from the brachiocephalic trunk, whereas the left CCA originates directly from the aortic arch. Both vertebral arteries (VAs) originate from the subclavian arteries. The morphologic variants of the CCA and VAs usually are not clinically significant.

The CCA bifurcates at approximately the level of the sixth cervical vertebrae into the external and internal carotid arteries. The external carotid artery (ECA) supplies the neck, face, and scalp. The internal carotid artery (ICA) and its branches are mostly responsible for the arterial supply of the anterior two-thirds of the cerebral hemispheres (anterior circulation).

The vertebrobasilar and posterior cerebral arteries (PCAs) supply blood to the brainstem, cerebellum, occipital lobes, and posterior portions of the temporal and parietal lobes (posterior circulation).

THE CAROTID ARTERY SYSTEM

External Carotid Artery

At its origin, the ECA deviates anteriorly and medially in relation to the ICA in the neck and provides many branches to the neck (superior thyroid, ascending pharyngeal arteries) and face (lingual and facial arteries). As the artery ascends, occipital and posterior auricular branches supply the scalp in their named areas. However, the occipital artery also has several meningeal branches that supply the posterior fossa and dura. Within the substance of the parotid gland, the ECA divides into its two terminal branches: the superficial temporal and maxillary arteries. The superficial temporal artery is the main supply to the scalp over the frontoparietal convexity and its underlying muscles. The more proximal branches also supply the masseter muscle. The superficial temporal artery is commonly involved in giant cell arteritis, an important consideration in the elderly with headaches, and can be palpated anterior to the tragus and in the temporal area (see Chapter 21).

The maxillary artery supplies the face and, through its middle meningeal branch, provides most of the blood supply to the dura mater covering the brain. The middle meningeal artery is often implicated in the formation of epidural hematomas in patients with temporal or parietal bone skull fractures (see Chapter 19).

The ECA occasionally has an important role in supplying collateral flow for ICA occlusive disease through anastomoses between its facial, maxillary, and superficial temporal branches and the ophthalmic artery.

Internal Carotid Artery

There are four ICA segments: cervical, petrous, cavernous, and supraclinoid. The cervical segment ascends vertically in the neck, posterior and slightly medial to the ECA. Significant atherosclerotic disease is usually located at the ICA origin, with potential for artery-to-artery embolism, stenosis with eventual occlusion, or both (see Chapter 15). Unlike the ECA, this segment does not have branches, allowing differentiation between the two vessels on imaging scans.

The ICA enters the skull through the carotid canal within the petrous bone. This petrous segment has two small branches, the caroticotympanic and pterygoid branches, which are usually clinically irrelevant.

The cavernous segment, usually called the carotid siphon because of its shape, is the portion of the ICA within the cavernous sinus and provides minor branches supplying the posterior pituitary (meningohypophyseal artery) and the abducens nerve. Of its many branches, the ophthalmic artery is the most significant. The ophthalmic artery arises from the ICA just as it pierces the dura and emerges from the cavernous sinus to pass through the optic canal into the orbit just below and lateral to the optic nerve. It supplies the globe and orbital contents through its three major branches: the ocular (central retinal and ciliary arteries), orbital, and extraorbital branches. The ophthalmic artery forms extensive anastomoses with branches of the ECA.

The supraclinoid segment is the last portion of the ICA. It begins when this segment penetrates the dura. The *posterior communicating artery* (P-com) and the *anterior choroidal artery* are the two important branches originating at this level. The ICA then bifurcates into *the anterior cerebral artery* (ACA) and *middle cerebral artery* (MCA).

The P-com is often hypoplastic. When present, it travels posteriorly to communicate with the posterior circulation at the level of the PCA. The P-com also provides thalamoperforate branches that supply the anteromedial thalamus and parts of the cerebral peduncles. Its presence and size are variable but often serves as an important collateral pathway in extensive cerebrovascular disease allowing flow from the anterior to the posterior circulation or vice versa.

The anterior choroidal artery arises from the posterior surface of the ICA just above the P-com origin. This artery supplies an extensive cerebral area, including the visual system (optic tract, anterior portion of the lateral geniculate body, and optic radiations), genu and posterior limb of the internal capsule, basal ganglia (medial globus pallidus and tail of the caudate), the diencephalon (portions of the lateral thalamus and the subthalamic nuclei), the midbrain (substantia nigra and portions of the cerebral peduncle), the medial temporal lobe (uncus, pyriform cortex, amygdala), and the choroidal plexus of the temporal horn and atrium.

The ACA travels medially and anteriorly toward the interhemispheric fissure. It supplies the anterior portions of the basal ganglia and internal capsule and most of the mesial portion of the frontal and parietal lobes. The first segment of the ACA, the A1 segment, begins at the carotid bifurcation and terminates at the level of the anterior communicating artery, which connects opposite A1 segments and

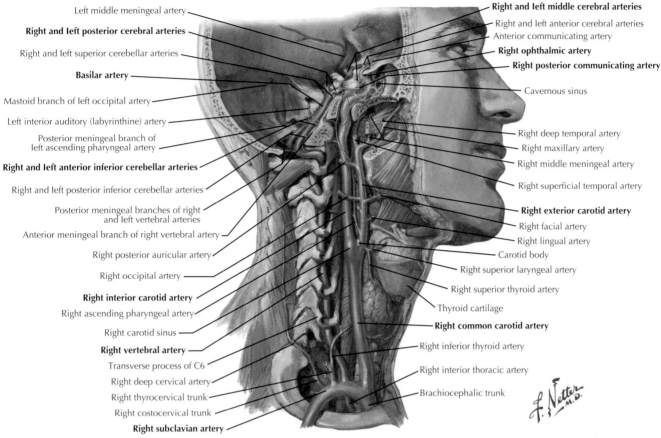

Left middle meningeal artery

Right and left posterior cerebral arteries

Right and left superior cerebellar arteries

Basilar artery

Mastoid branch of left occipital artery

Left interior auditory (labyrinthine) artery

Posterior meningeal branch of
left ascending pharyngeal artery

Right and left anterior inferior cerebellar arteries

Right and left posterior inferior cerebellar arteries

Posterior meningeal branches of right
and left vertebral arteries

Anterior meningeal branch of right vertebral artery

Right posterior auricular artery

Right occipital artery

Right interior carotid artery

Right ascending pharyngeal artery

Right carotid sinus

Right vertebral artery

Transverse process of C6

Right deep cervical artery

Right thyrocervical trunk

Right costocervical trunk

Right subclavian artery

Right and left middle cerebral arteries

Right and left anterior cerebral arteries

Anterior communicating artery

Right ophthalmic artery

Right posterior communicating artery

Cavernous sinus

Right deep temporal artery

Right maxillary artery

Right middle meningeal artery

Right superficial temporal artery

Right exterior carotid artery

Right facial artery

Right lingual artery

Carotid body

Right superior laryngeal artery

Right superior thyroid artery

Thyroid cartilage

Right common carotid artery

Right inferior thyroid artery

Right interior thoracic artery

Brachiocephalic trunk

Fig. 14.1 Arteries to Brain and Meninges.

constitutes an important collateral pathway in carotid artery occlusive disease. Occasionally, a single A1 exists supplying both medial frontal hemispheres from a single side and is termed an azygous ACA. The recurrent artery of Heubner is the most important branch of the A1 segment and supplies the anteroinferior portion of the head of the caudate, the putamen, and the anterior limb of the internal capsule. The ACA continues as the A2 segment, where the orbitofrontal branch arises and travels around the genu of the corpus callosum to the orbital and medial surface of the frontal lobe, whereas the frontopolar branch supplies the rest of the medial surface of the frontal lobe. The ACA then gives off its two major branches, the pericallosal artery that runs just above the corpus callosum and the callosomarginal artery paralleling the cingulate gyrus. These two arteries supply the mesial portions of the frontal and parietal lobes.

One of the major fail-safe systems within the cerebral circulation is the circle of Willis, formed by the connections between the ACAs, the anterior communicating arteries, the supraclinoid carotid, the P-coms, and the PCAs. This vascular network often provides alternative conduits for perfusion avoiding the development of cerebral infarction when a major vessel becomes significantly diseased or occluded, as with cervical ICA atherosclerotic disease. The respective junctions of each of these vessels in the circle of Willis is the primary site of berry aneurysm formation, which is the major cause of subarachnoid hemorrhages (see Chapter 17).

The MCA originates from the supraclinoid carotid stem and, subsequently, travels laterally to the Sylvian fissure as the main-stem M1 segment, giving off lenticulostriate branches to the basal ganglia. As the MCA approaches the Sylvian fissure, it usually divides into two large trunks: the superior and inferior divisions. Occasionally, the MCA

trifurcates, and a middle trunk is also present. Different branches supply the frontal (orbitofrontal, ascending frontal, precentral, and central branches), parietal (anterior and posterior parietal and angular branches), and temporal (anterior and posterior temporal) lobes. The orbitofrontal, ascending frontal, precentral, and central branches usually arise from the superior division of the MCA, whereas the angular, anterior, and posterior temporal branches arise from the inferior division. The anterior and posterior parietal branches can arise from either division (Fig. 14.2). The MCA stem or its distal bifurcation point are classic sites where large cerebral artery emboli lodge and are sometimes amenable to emergent intraarterial thrombolytic therapy (see Chapter 15).

VERTEBROBASILAR ARTERIES

The VAs usually originate from the subclavian arteries on either side (see Fig. 14.1). They have four portions: three extracranial and one intracranial. From their origin, the VAs travel posteriorly (prevertebral segment) and enter the transverse foramen of the sixth cervical vertebrae. They then extend superiorly to exist at C2 (cervical segment), sharply turning posteriorly around the auricular process of the atlas (atlantic segment), then proceeding rostrally, piercing the posterior atlanto-occipital membrane and the dura mater to enter the intracranial cavity through the foramen magnum (intracranial or intradural segment). The VAs are prone to dissection at their entry and exit sites through the vertebra and are prone to temporal arteritis right at the dural junction.

The intracranial segments course anteriorly lateral to the medulla, then ascend medially to the pontomedullary junction, where they unite at the pontine midline to from the *basilar artery* (Fig. 14.3).

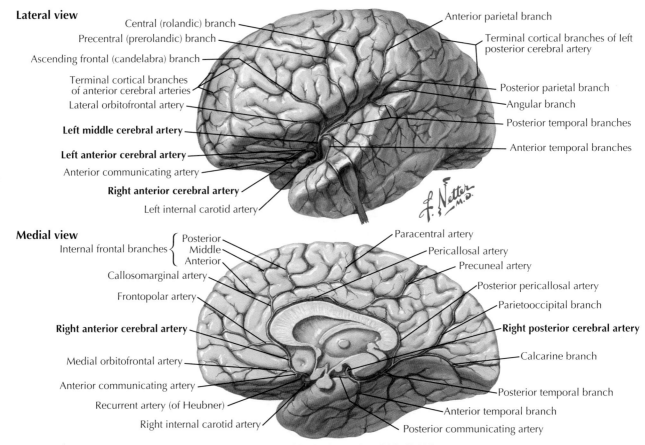

Lateral view

Central (rolandic) branch
Precentral (prerolandic) branch
Ascending frontal (candelabra) branch
Terminal cortical branches of anterior cerebral arteries
Lateral orbitofrontal artery
Left middle cerebral artery
Left anterior cerebral artery
Anterior communicating artery
Right anterior cerebral artery
Left internal carotid artery

Anterior parietal branch
Terminal cortical branches of left posterior cerebral artery
Posterior parietal branch
Angular branch
Posterior temporal branches
Anterior temporal branches

Medial view

Internal frontal branches { Posterior, Middle, Anterior
Callosomarginal artery
Frontopolar artery
Right anterior cerebral artery
Medial orbitofrontal artery
Anterior communicating artery
Recurrent artery (of Heubner)
Right internal carotid artery

Paracentral artery
Pericallosal artery
Precuneal artery
Posterior pericallosal artery
Parietooccipital branch
Right posterior cerebral artery
Calcarine branch
Posterior temporal branch
Anterior temporal branch
Posterior communicating artery

Fig. 14.2 Arteries of Brain: Lateral and Medial Views.

The cervical branches of the VAs give muscular, vertebral body and radicular branches and may serve as collateral conduits in cases of cervical artery compromise or occlusion. The intracranial branches are neurologically more significant and, if diseased, often give definite neurologic syndromes. The first of these are the lateral medullary branches supplying the lateral portions of the medulla. Distally the *posterior-inferior cerebellar arteries* (PICAs) primarily supply the posterior and inferior regions of the cerebellum but also the dorsum of the medulla oblongata. Classic Wallenberg syndrome results from occlusion of medullary arteries of the PICA or penetrator branches of the VAs.

The anterior spinal artery arises from paired medial VA branches just before the basilar junction unites in the midline to form a single vessel running the full length of the spinal cord caudally in the antero-medial sulcus. It also supplies the medial portions of the medulla; however, adequate collateral circulation in this location makes the medial medullary syndrome rare. In contrast, the anterior spinal artery within the cord is crucial to spinal cord function, and its occlusion leads to an anterior spinal artery syndrome (see Chapter 55). The posterior spinal arteries arise from the PICAs or intracranial VAs and run caudally, supplying the posterior and lateral aspects of the spinal cord.

The basilar artery courses rostrally on the anterior surface of the pons and along the clivus to end at the pontomesencephalic junction, providing a number of important branches on its way.

The *anterior-inferior cerebellar arteries* (AICAs) usually arise from the midportion of the basilar artery and supply the brachium pontis, lateral pontine tegmentum, flocculus, and anteroinferior portions of the cerebellum. The internal auditory artery may arise from the AICAs or the basilar itself, and supplies the vestibular and cochlear structures.

The *superior cerebellar arteries* (SCAs) arise from the distal portion of the basilar artery before it bifurcates into the *PCAs*. During their course around the midbrain, the SCAs provide branches to the superior lateral pontine tegmentum and the tectum of the mesencephalon. The SCAs then travel toward the cerebellum, supplying the superior vermis, the lateral portion of the cerebellar hemispheres, and most of the cerebellar nuclei and the cerebellar white matter. When the basilar artery reaches the level of the cerebral peduncles, it divides into opposite PCAs that loop laterally and posteriorly around the midbrain supplying the medial temporal lobe, portions of the parietal lobe, and the occipital lobes. Perforator branches are given off to the thalamus. Distal to the posterior communicating artery, medial and lateral posterior choroidal branches off the PCA supply the posterior portion of the lateral geniculate body, optic tract, pulvinar, hippocampus, and parahippocampal gyrus, as well as the choroid plexus of the lateral and third ventricles.

The basilar artery is particularly prone to atherosclerotic deposition throughout its length, and at its extremes can cause either severe stenosis or occlusion, or formation of a fusiform aneurysm by weakening the vessel wall. The rostral end of the basilar, just before bifurcating into the PCAs, is the site most likely to be occluded by an embolus leading to the classic "top of the basilar" syndrome (see Chapter 15). Similarly, this is one of the most common sites for berry aneurysms within the vertebrobasilar system (see Chapter 17).

CEREBRAL SINUSES AND VEINS

Surrounded by dura, cerebral sinuses and veins are the venous structures of the brain. They have neither valves nor tunica muscularis, but

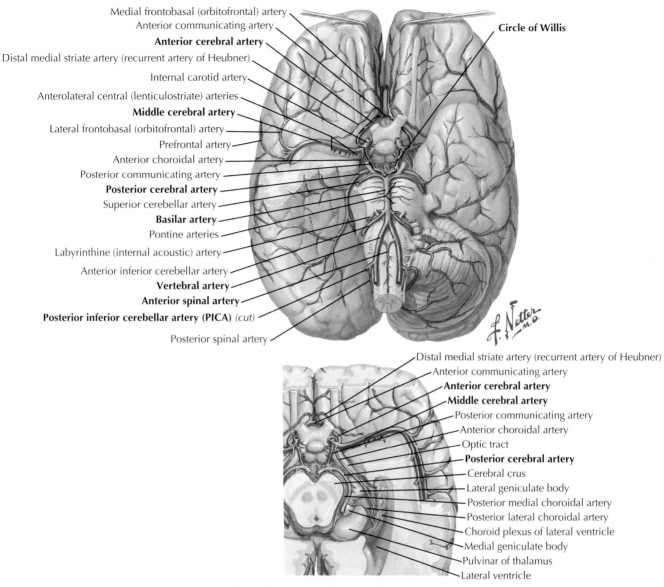

Medial frontobasal (orbitofrontal) artery
Anterior communicating artery
Anterior cerebral artery
Distal medial striate artery (recurrent artery of Heubner)
Internal carotid artery
Anterolateral central (lenticulostriate) arteries
Middle cerebral artery
Lateral frontobasal (orbitofrontal) artery
Prefrontal artery
Anterior choroidal artery
Posterior communicating artery
Posterior cerebral artery
Superior cerebellar artery
Basilar artery
Pontine arteries
Labyrinthine (internal acoustic) artery
Anterior inferior cerebellar artery
Vertebral artery
Anterior spinal artery
Posterior inferior cerebellar artery (PICA) *(cut)*
Posterior spinal artery

Circle of Willis

Distal medial striate artery (recurrent artery of Heubner)
Anterior communicating artery
Anterior cerebral artery
Middle cerebral artery
Posterior communicating artery
Anterior choroidal artery
Optic tract
Posterior cerebral artery
Cerebral crus
Lateral geniculate body
Posterior medial choroidal artery
Posterior lateral choroidal artery
Choroid plexus of lateral ventricle
Medial geniculate body
Pulvinar of thalamus
Lateral ventricle

Fig. 14.3 Arteries of Brain: Inferior Views.

typically contain inpouchings of arachnoid cells, called arachnoid granulations, which allow cerebrospinal fluid drainage. These granulations function as one-way valves and are pressure dependent. Malfunction of these valves can occur in subarachnoid hemorrhage or meningitis, leading to normal pressure hydrocephalus (see Chapter 38).

The main venous sinuses include the superior and inferior sagittal sinuses, the straight sinus, the transverse sinuses, the sigmoid sinuses, the occipital sinus, the cavernous sinuses, the superior and inferior petrosal sinuses, and the sphenoparietal sinuses. Acute or subacute cerebral venous thrombosis can be the cause of a wide range of neurologic pathology from isolated chronic headache to venous infarction with seizures to obtundation and coma. Anatomic images and a full discussion of this subject are provided in Chapter 18.

The *superior sagittal sinus* is located within the midline of the cerebral hemispheres running posteriorly from the foramen cecum to the occipitocerebellar junction. This sinus drains the venous flow of both the frontal and parietal lobes most often into the right transverse sinus. Occasionally its anterior portion can be hypoplastic and that is usually

associated with dominance of the cavernous sinuses draining the frontal lobes.

The *inferior sagittal sinus* is smaller and inconstant. When present, the inferior sagittal sinus parallels the corpus callosum, traveling in the inferior portion of the falx cerebri, and drains the region of the medial hemispheres and cingulate gyrus, flowing into the straight sinus.

The *straight sinus* is formed by the intersection of the inferior sagittal sinus and the great vein of Galen (see Cerebral Veins). The straight sinus often drains into the left transverse sinus.

The *transverse sinuses* are often asymmetric, the left being more frequently hypoplastic than the right. In those cases, the ipsilateral jugular foramen is correspondingly small, helping distinguish between developmental hypoplasia and local thrombosis. The transverse sinuses lie in the grooves of the occipital bone and run laterally and forward for a short distance before diving down to become the sigmoid sinuses. In addition to receiving blood flow from the superior sagittal and straight sinuses, each transverse sinus also receives blood from the superior petrosal sinuses, mastoid and condyloid emissary veins, inferior cerebral and cerebellar veins, and diploic veins. The *sigmoid sinuses* are the continuation of the transverse sinuses and end at the jugular foramina, becoming the internal jugular veins. At times, the sigmoid sinus can be larger than its transverse tributary, usually secondary to the presence of an ipsilateral large vein of Labbé emptying into its proximal segment.

The *cavernous sinus* is an intricate venous channel interconnecting with its contralateral partner via intercavernous channels around the infundibulum. The cavernous sinus is important for the structures that it drains and for the structures that run through it. Laterally in the cavernous sinus wall are CN III, IV, and V (V1 and V2 segments), and through its center runs the intracavernous portion of the ICA, the sympathetic plexus, and CN VI. The cavernous sinuses drain into paired superior and inferior petrosal sinuses that, in turn, drain into the transverse sinus and internal jugular veins, respectively.

The *superior petrosal sinus* connects the cavernous with the transverse sinus. It drains the tympanic cavity, cerebellum, and inferior portions of the cerebrum. The *inferior petrosal sinus* connects the cavernous sinus with the internal jugular vein and drains the inner ear, medulla, pons, and cerebellum. The *sphenoparietal sinuses* lie below the lesser wings of the sphenoid bone and drain the dura mater into the cavernous sinuses.

CEREBRAL VEINS

The cerebral veins are classified into three groups: superficial, deep, and posterior fossa veins.

The superficial group drains the cerebral cortex through the superior, middle, and inferior cerebral veins and flows to nearby sinuses, including the superior sagittal, inferior sagittal, cavernous, superior petrosal, and transverse sinuses. This group also has two important anastomotic veins connecting the superficial middle cerebral vein on each hemisphere to the superior sagittal sinus (vein of Trollard) and with the ipsilateral transverse sinus (vein of Labbé).

The deep veins drain the corpus callosum, basal ganglia, thalamus, and posterior portions of the limbic system. The two more important veins of this group are the internal cerebral vein and the basal vein of Rosenthal. The intersection of them both forms the great cerebral vein—also called the vein of Galen—a 2-cm long U-shaped vein that courses under the splenium of the corpus callous in the quadrigeminal cistern draining into the straight sinus.

The posterior fossa veins include both the brainstem and cerebellar venous systems and they can be quite variable. However, in general, the midbrain veins drain into the vein of Galen and the basal vein of Rosenthal while the pons and medulla tend to drain into the transverse, occipital, superior, and inferior petrosal sinuses. Regarding the cerebellum, its most important veins are the superior and inferior cerebellar veins. The superior cerebellar vein drains into the straight, transverse, or superior petrosal venous sinuses, while the inferior cerebellar vein drains into the sigmoid, inferior petrous, or straight sinuses.

ADDITIONAL RESOURCES

Damasio H. A computed tomographic guide to the identification of cerebrovascular territories. Arch Neurol 1983;40(3):138–42.
This article depicts computed tomography templates of the different cerebrovascular arterial territories.
Netter FM. The Netter collection of medical illustrations, vol. 7. Parts I and II: Nervous System. Philadelphia, PA: Elsevier; 2013.
Tatu L, Moulin T, Bogousslavsky J. Arterial territories of the human brain. Neurology 1998;50:1699–708.
This article presents a system of 12 axial sections of the cerebral hemispheres showing its arterial territories, most important anatomic structures, and Brodmann's areas.
Salamon G, Huang YP. Radiologic anatomy of the brain. Berlin Heidelberg: Springer-Verlag; 1976.
Extensive review of the cerebral vascular supply.
Rhoton AL Jr. The cerebral vessels. Neurosurgery 2002;S1(4 Suppl.):S159–205.
Review of the anatomy of cerebral sinuses and veins.
Nowinski WL. Proposition of a new classification of the cerebral veins based on their termination. Surg Radiol Anat 2012;34(2):107–14.
Detailed review of prior classifications of the cerebral veins and the proposition of a new one.

15

Ischemic Stroke

Barbara Voetsch, Matthew E. Tilem, Michael Adix II, Ian Kaminsky

While in recent years ischemic stroke has dropped to the fifth most frequent cause of death in the United States, it remains a leading cause of morbidity, mortality, and long-term disability worldwide with a devastating impact on patients, families, and communities. It is well understood that ischemic stroke represents a constellation of etiologies and mechanisms that often present with similar signs and symptoms. Advances in technology have improved understanding of stroke pathophysiology that promises to translate into more specific treatments and better outcomes.

The distinction between transient ischemic attacks (TIAs) and strokes based on the duration of ischemic symptoms has become less clinically relevant over the past couple decades. With the more widespread use of magnetic resonance imaging (MRI), it has become evident that about a third of patients with transient ischemic symptoms actually have evidence of diffusion restriction on MRI. Therefore vascular neurologists have advocated for a new, tissue-based definition of TIA that implies the absence of acute imaging abnormalities. More importantly, strokes and TIAs share pathophysiologic mechanisms, and the same preventative measures may apply to both. Therefore, the diagnostic approach to patients with transient or persistent ischemic symptoms should be the same, and treatment should be guided toward the underlying cause of the brain ischemia.

ETIOLOGY AND PATHOPHYSIOLOGY

The most common ischemic stroke etiologies are large artery occlusive disease, cardioembolism, and small vessel disease.

Large Artery Occlusive Disease

Atherosclerosis causes stenosis or occlusion of extracranial and intracranial arteries and is directly responsible for a significant percentage of cerebral ischemic events. Atheroma formation involves the progressive deposition of circulating lipids and ultimately fibrous tissue in the subintimal layer of the large and medium arteries, occurring most frequently at branching points (Fig. 15.1). Plaque formation is enhanced by blood-associated inflammatory factors as well as increased shear injury from uncontrolled blood pressure (BP). Intraplaque hemorrhage, subintimal necrosis with ulcer formation, and calcium deposition can cause enlargement of the atherosclerotic plaque with consequent worsening of the degree of arterial narrowing.

Disruption of the endothelial surface triggers thrombus formation within the arterial lumen through activation of nearby platelets by the subendothelial matrix. When platelets become activated, they release thromboxane A_2, causing further platelet aggregation. The development of a fibrin network stabilizes the platelet aggregate, forming a "white thrombus." In areas of slowed or turbulent flow within or around the plaque the thrombus develops further, enmeshing red blood cells (RBCs) in the platelet–fibrin aggregate to form a "red thrombus" (Fig. 15.2). This remains poorly organized and friable for up to 2 weeks and presents a significant risk of propagation or embolization. Either the white or red thrombus, however, can dislodge and embolize to distal arterial branches. Large artery disease can cause ischemic strokes by either intraarterial embolism, as described previously and, less commonly, hemodynamic ischemia or hypoperfusion through a significantly narrowed vessel.

Frequent sites for carotid system or anterior circulation atherosclerosis are the origin of the internal carotid artery (ICA), the carotid siphon at the base of the brain (Fig. 15.3), and the main stem of the middle cerebral artery (MCA) and the anterior cerebral artery (ACA). The ICA at or around the bifurcation is usually affected in Caucasians, whereas in Asian, Hispanic, and African American populations, intracranial atherosclerosis may be more common than cervical carotid disease. In the vertebrobasilar system, the origins of the vertebral arteries in the neck and the distal portion of the intracranial vertebral arteries are the most commonly affected areas. The basilar artery and origins of the posterior cerebral arteries (PCAs) are other sites.

The main modifiable risk factors for large artery disease are arterial hypertension (HTN), diabetes, hypercholesterolemia, and smoking. The most important nonmodifiable risk factors are age and family history.

Cardiac Embolism

Several types of cardiac disease lead to cerebral embolism: atrial fibrillation (AF), ischemic heart disease, valvular disease, dilated cardiomyopathies, atrial septal abnormalities, and intracardiac tumors (Fig. 15.4).

Chronic or paroxysmal AF is the rhythm most associated with cardioembolic events, with stroke often being their first manifestation. Atrial flutter is also implicated as a cardioembolic risk due to its tendency to convert back and forth with AF. Because such arrhythmias are often intermittent, careful, and at times repeated, monitoring is needed to identify their presence, as they pose a significant risk for recurrent stroke.

Within the first 4 weeks of myocardial infarction (MI), particularly with ischemia of the anterior wall, there is a higher risk of embolic stroke. More remote MIs can be a potential embolic source, particularly in patients who develop akinetic segments or left ventricular aneurysms. Mural thrombi are common in patients with dilated cardiomyopathies. Brain embolism is estimated to occur in approximately 10%–15% of these patients.

Rheumatic valvular disease, mechanical prosthetic heart valves, and infective endocarditis are well-known cardiac sources of embolism. Other relatively common abnormalities, such as mitral valve prolapse,

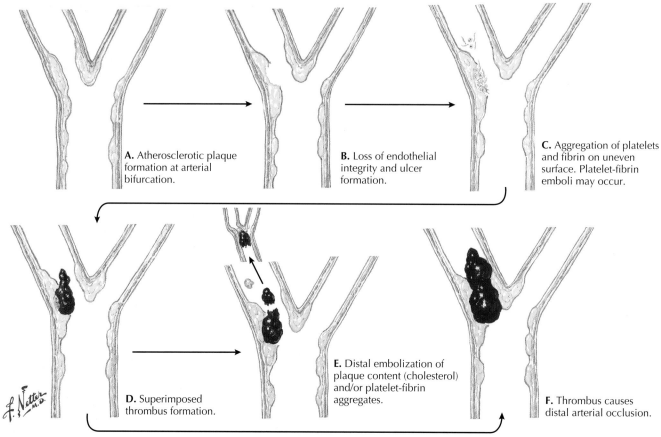

A. Atherosclerotic plaque formation at arterial bifurcation.

B. Loss of endothelial integrity and ulcer formation.

C. Aggregation of platelets and fibrin on uneven surface. Platelet-fibrin emboli may occur.

D. Superimposed thrombus formation.

E. Distal embolization of plaque content (cholesterol) and/or platelet-fibrin aggregates.

F. Thrombus causes distal arterial occlusion.

Fig. 15.1 Atherosclerosis, Thrombosis, and Embolism.

mitral annulus calcification, and bicuspid aortic valve, have suspected embolic potential. However, these should be considered as a potential cause of stroke only after other etiologies have been excluded.

Patent foramen ovale (PFO) and atrial septal aneurysm are risk factors for stroke. A meta-analysis of case-control studies comparing patients younger than 55 years with ischemic stroke to nonstroke controls showed an odds ratio for stroke of 3:1 for PFO alone and of 6:1 for PFO with an associated atrial septal aneurysm. Potential or presumed mechanisms of stroke included venous "paradoxical embolism," direct embolization from thrombi formed within the PFO or atrial septal aneurysm, and thrombus from atrial arrhythmias thought to be more prevalent in this population.

Intracardiac tumors are a rare but important cause of embolic stroke. Atrial myxoma and papillary fibroelastoma are the two most common and relevant neoplasms in the provocation of cardioembolism.

Small Vessel Disease (Lacunes)

The capillary vessel and the end penetrating arteries that supply the basal ganglia, thalamus, internal capsule, and white matter tracts are not prone to atherosclerosis, as in the large-caliber cerebral circulation, but undergo a characteristic pathologic degeneration in response to endothelial damage. Fibrinoid degeneration with focal enlargement of the vessel wall, foam cell invasion of the lumen, and hemorrhagic rupture through the vessel wall characterize this process known as fibrinoid degeneration or lipohyalinosis. Occlusion of these arteries causes small (1–20 mm), discrete, and often irregular lesions called *lacunes*. As previously alluded to, lacunes do not involve the cortical ribbon and occur most often in the basal ganglia, thalamus, pons, internal capsule, and

cerebral white matter, and may cause discrete clinical syndromes but often go clinically unnoticed. Arterial HTN and diabetes are the main risk factors (Fig. 15.5).

Arterial Dissection

Dissection of the cervical ICA tends to occur several centimeters distal to the bifurcation or at the skull base. The cervical vertebral artery (VA) is most frequently dissected where it engages the spine, coursing through transverse foramina from C6 to C2 (V2) and then through the transverse foramen of V1 before entering foramen magnum (V3). Dissection occurring between the intima and media usually causes stenosis or occlusion of the affected artery, whereas dissection between the media and adventitia is associated with aneurysmal dilatation. Congenital abnormalities in the media or elastica of the arteries, as seen in Marfan syndrome, fibromuscular dysplasia, and type IV Ehlers-Danlos, can predispose patients to arterial dissection. Although often associated with acute trauma, arterial dissection may result from seemingly innocuous incidents, such as a fall; sports activities, particularly wrestling or diving into a wave; and paroxysms of coughing or vomiting. Dissection causes stroke by one of two mechanisms. Clot may accumulate at the intimal tear and subsequently embolize to the distal cerebral circulation. Alternatively, expanding thrombus within the media may cause some dissections to progress to severe stenosis or complete occlusion of the true lumen resulting in cerebral hypoperfusion (Fig. 15.6).

Less Common Stroke Etiologies

Although frequently considered in the differential diagnosis of ischemic stroke, arteritis is a rare stroke etiology. Usually, central nervous

Platelets circulating in blood contain thromboxane A$_2$, a substance that promotes their aggregation, while vascular endothelium secretes prostacyclin, an aggregation inhibitor that balances this effect. These products are synthesized after conversion of arachidonic acid into intermediate endoperoxides by cyclooxygenase enzymes.

If endothelial continuity is interrupted by trauma, atherosclerosis, etc., subsurface collagen is exposed to blood and stimulates adhesion of platelets to vessel wall. Platelets then discharge thromboxane A$_2$, causing aggregation of adjacent platelets.

As more platelets aggregate, fibrin network develops and stabilizes mass into "white thrombus," which then retracts into vascular wall. In some cases, endothelium may later heal over with or without narrowing of lumen.

If thrombus develops further, red blood cells become enmeshed in platelet-fibrin aggregate to form "red thrombus," which may grow and block vessel lumen. Either platelet-fibrin aggregates or more fully formed clots may break off, with embolization into distal arterial branches.

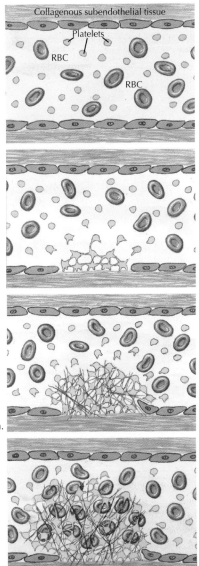

Fig. 15.2 Role of Platelets in Arterial Thrombosis. *RBCs,* Red blood cells.

system vasculitis presents as an encephalopathy with multifocal signs.

Cocaine and amphetamine are the most frequent drugs associated with ischemic strokes. Vasoconstriction and vasculitis are the proposed mechanisms. Other illicit drugs, in particular marijuana, as well as a growing list of medications (classically antidepressants) can trigger reversible cerebral vasoconstriction syndrome, which typically presents with a thunderclap headache sometimes accompanied by focal neurologic deficits.

Hematologic disorders such as polycythemia, sickle cell disease, and thrombocytosis (usually platelets >1,000,000/dL) can cause ischemic strokes by increasing blood viscosity, hypercoagulability, or both. Antithrombin III, protein S, protein C deficiencies, factor V Leiden, and prothrombin gene mutation are usually associated with venous and not arterial thrombosis but may take on importance in cases of stroke associated with PFO due to the passage of venous clots through an intraatrial defect (paradoxical embolization). Moderate to severe hyperhomocysteinemia and antiphospholipid syndrome are causes of arterial ischemic stroke, even in the absence of PFO.

CLINICAL PRESENTATION

Large Artery Occlusive Disease
Carotid Artery Disease

CLINICAL VIGNETTE *A 54-year-old man presented to his optometrist after experiencing a 2-minute episode of painless transient monocular vision loss in the left eye. Two weeks earlier he had been seen in the emergency room for a 1-hour episode of transient right-hand tingling which was attributed to carpal tunnel syndrome. His past medical history was notable for 40 pack-years of smoking, poorly controlled type 2 diabetes, and untreated obstructive sleep apnea. He had two younger siblings with coronary stents. On exam, he had bilateral carotid bruits and a delayed left radial pulse. His speech was mildly dysfluent, and he made subtle naming errors for low frequency words. He was referred for an emergent carotid ultrasound, which demonstrated greater than 70% bilateral carotid stenosis with an ICA/CCA ratio of 9.0 on the left and 5.5 on the right. A contrast-enhanced MRI demonstrated small, scattered, acute, and subacute embolic ischemic strokes in the left MCA and ACA territories. He was admitted to the hospital and placed on aspirin 325 mg daily and a statin. A left carotid endarterectomy was performed with no subsequent neurologic events.*

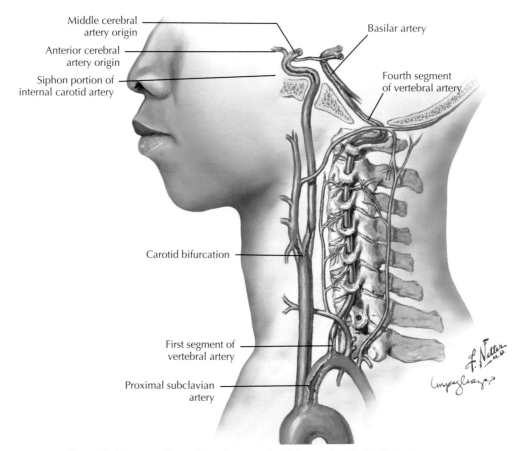

Fig. 15.3 Common Sites of Cerebrovascular Atherosclerotic Occlusive Disease.

Middle cerebral artery origin

Anterior cerebral artery origin

Siphon portion of internal carotid artery

Basilar artery

Fourth segment of vertebral artery

Carotid bifurcation

First segment of vertebral artery

Proximal subclavian artery

CLINICAL VIGNETTE *A 70-year-old white man with arterial hypertension and high cholesterol presented with 1 month of recurrent 1- to 2-minute episodes of left extremities shaking that occurred only on standing. His blood pressure was 110/80 mm Hg, and neurologic examination showed a left pronator drift, but was otherwise normal.*

Head computed tomography (CT) showed small strokes in the arterial border zone between the right MCA and ACA, and right MCA and PCA distributions. Head and neck computed tomography angiography (CTA) demonstrated a right ICA occlusion. CT perfusion showed hypoperfusion in the right MCA territory, worse in the border zone areas. Collateral flow through the right ophthalmic, anterior communicating, and posterior communicating arteries was detected by transcranial Doppler and conventional angiogram. Patient was started on antiplatelet treatment as well as a statin drug, and his antihypertensive medication dose was decreased, with a subsequent increase in the systolic BP to 140–150 mm Hg. No further episodes occurred.

The previous vignettes illustrate the two mechanisms of stroke or TIA in large artery atherosclerotic disease, intraarterial embolism (the first vignette), and hypoperfusion (the second vignette). Identification of the exact mechanism has important therapeutic implications.

TIAs are common in patients with carotid artery disease and usually precede stroke onset by a few days or months. TIAs caused by intraarterial embolism from a carotid source may not be stereotypical. TIA symptoms vary, depending on which ICA branch is involved. For example, patients can have a first episode of a transient right leg weakness and weeks later have another spell characterized by expressive aphasia, right facial droop, and weakness of the right hand. This depends on the destination of the emboli. In the first example, the ACA territory is the

destination, and in the later example, the MCA territory. In contrast, hemodynamic "limb-shaking" TIAs, as in the second vignette presented previously, are often stereotypical and posturally related and are usually seen in patients with high-grade ICA stenosis or occlusion. In this classic example of a hemodynamic ischemia, patients present with recurrent, irregular, and involuntary movements of the contralateral arm, leg, or both, usually triggered by postural changes and lasting a few minutes. These spells likely represent intermittent loss of cortical control and paralysis and differ from a focal seizure, in which the movements are more regular and rhythmic and usually correlate with focal repetitive cortical hyperexcitability seen on electroencephalogram.

Another important clue to ICA disease is episodes of transient monocular blindness (TMB). *TMB* refers to the occurrence of temporary unilateral visual loss or obscuration that is classically described by careful observers as a horizontal or vertical "shade being drawn over one eye," but most frequently as a "fog" or "blurring" in the eye, lasting 1–5 minutes. It often occurs spontaneously but at times is triggered by position changes. Positive phenomena such as sparkles, lights, or colors evolving over minutes are more typical of migrainous phenomena and help differentiate such benign visual changes from the more serious TMB, a frequent harbinger of cerebral infarct within the carotid artery vasculature. Rarely, with critical ipsilateral internal carotid stenosis, gradual dimming or loss of vision when exposed to bright light, such as glare of snow on a sunlit background, can be reported and is due to limited vascular flow in the face of increased retinal metabolic demand. Besides carotid atherosclerosis, other etiologies of TMB include cardiac embolism and intrinsic ophthalmic artery disease due to processes such as atherosclerosis or arteritis (see "Giant Cell or Temporal Arteritis" in Chapter 21), as well as decreased retinal perfusion from glaucoma or increased intraocular pressure. It is not uncommon that homonymous

Cardiac Sources of Cerebral Emboli

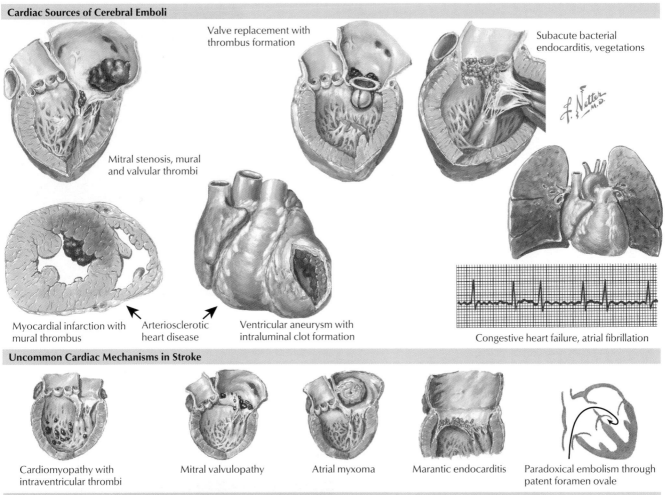

Mitral stenosis, mural and valvular thrombi

Valve replacement with thrombus formation

Subacute bacterial endocarditis, vegetations

Myocardial infarction with mural thrombus

Arteriosclerotic heart disease

Ventricular aneurysm with intraluminal clot formation

Congestive heart failure, atrial fibrillation

Uncommon Cardiac Mechanisms in Stroke

Cardiomyopathy with intraventricular thrombi

Mitral valvulopathy

Atrial myxoma

Marantic endocarditis

Paradoxical embolism through patent foramen ovale

MRI Showing Scattered Areas of Diffusion Restriction in Multiple Vascular Territories

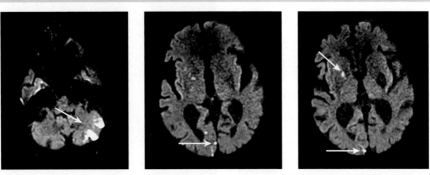

Fig. 15.4 Cardiac Embolism. *White arrows* demonstrate areas of acute infarction. *MRI,* Magnetic resonance imaging.

field deficits are reported by patients as monocular visual loss off to the affected side, and careful questioning as to whether each eye was checked independently and whether the visual difficulty involved the perception of a quadrant or one-half of the visual world is essential. For example, patients with left occipital infarctions or transient ischemia may report right-sided vision loss, but further questioning reveals that they were unable to read the right side of street signs or a license plate, and while covering the "unaffected" left eye, the seemingly abnormal right eye had retained vision within the distribution of the unaffected left homonymous field (Fig. 15.7).

As in the first vignette, strokes from intraarterial embolism from ICA disease are usually cortically based. Symptoms depend on whether branches of the MCA, ACA, or both are involved. The PCA territory may rarely be affected by intraarterial emboli from ipsilateral ICA stenosis or occlusion in patients with anomalous normal vascular variants, as in a persistent fetal PCA.

Neurologic findings vary by the location of the occlusion and presence of collateral circulation (Fig. 15.8). A large MCA stroke is usually seen in patients with MCA main stem occlusion without good collateral flow, whereas deep or perisylvian strokes are the most common presentation when enough collateral flow is present over the convexities.

Contralateral motor weakness involving the foot more than the thigh and shoulder, with relative sparing of the hand and face, is the typical presentation of distal ACA branch occlusion. Conversely, prominent cognitive and behavioral changes associated with contralateral hemiparesis predominate in patients with proximal ACA occlusions and the

Lacunar infarcts in base of pons interrupting some corticospinal (pyramidal) fibers. Such lesions cause mild hemiparesis.

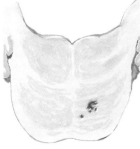

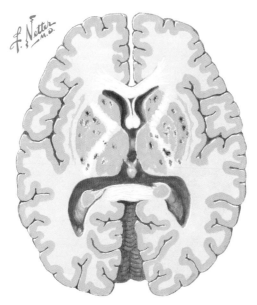

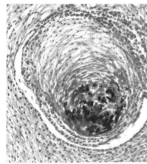

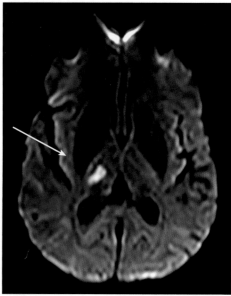

Multiple bilateral lacunes and scars of healed lacunar infarcts in thalamus, putamen, globus pallidus, caudate nucleus, and internal capsule. Such infarcts produce diverse symptoms.

Acute thalamic lacunar stroke on MRI.

Small (100-μm) artery within brain parenchyma showing typical pathologic changes secondary to hypertension. Vessel lumen almost completely obstructed by thickened media and enlarged to about 3 times normal size. Pink-staining fibrinoid material within walls.

Fig. 15.5 Lacunar Infarction. *MRI,* Magnetic resonance imaging.

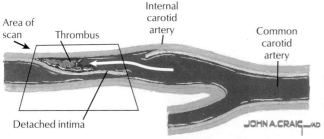

Intimal tear allows blood flow to dissect beneath intimal layer, detaching it from arterial wall. Large dissection may occlude vessel lumen.

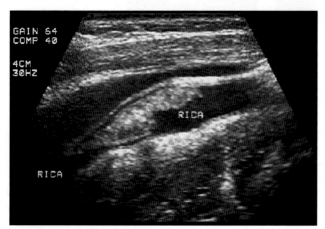

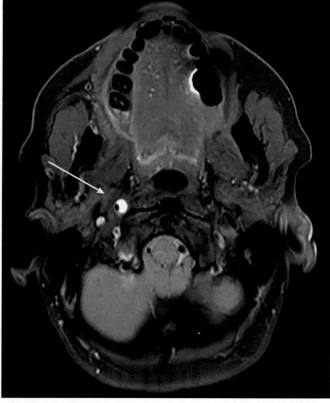

Carotid dissection: Ultrasound of the carotid artery with clot formed between layers of the artery (near the upper RICA label).

MRI with fat saturation showing carotid dissection with large false lumen.

Fig. 15.6 Arterial Dissection. *MRI,* Magnetic resonance imaging; *RICA,* right internal carotid artery.

Ocular Signs of Carotid Artery Ischemia (Transient Monocular Blindness [TMB])

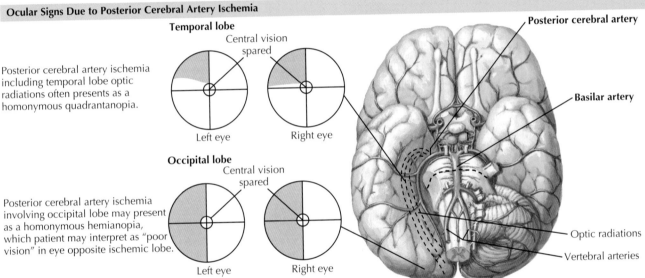

Internal carotid artery

Ophthalmic artery

Central retinal artery

Covering one eye may reveal unsuspected monocular vision loss

Left eye   Right eye

Episodes generally transient (3-5 min). Visual fields during episode show monocular decreased vision.

Other Causes of Transient Monocular Blindness

Typical scintillating scotoma helps to diagnose TMB due to migraine.

Erythrocyte sedimentation rate should be obtained to rule out TMB due to temporal arteritis.

⇧ESR

Fundus examination may reveal signs of retinal ischema, hemorrhages, and anterior ischemic optic neuritis.

Ocular Signs Due to Posterior Cerebral Artery Ischemia

Temporal lobe

Central vision spared

Posterior cerebral artery ischemia including temporal lobe optic radiations often presents as a homonymous quadrantanopia.

Left eye   Right eye

Occipital lobe

Central vision spared

Posterior cerebral artery ischemia involving occipital lobe may present as a homonymous hemianopia, which patient may interpret as "poor vision" in eye opposite ischemic lobe.

Left eye   Right eye

Posterior cerebral artery

Basilar artery

Optic radiations

Vertebral arteries

Fig. 15.7 Ocular Signs of Large Vessel Disease.

involvement of the recurrent artery of Huebner (caudate and anterior limb of internal capsule infarct).

Hemodynamic strokes usually involve the border zone territory between ACA and MCA (anterior border zone), MCA and PCA (posterior border zone), or between deep and superficial perforators (subcortical border zone), and cause the typical clinical symptoms outlined in Table 15.1.

Intracranial Middle Cerebral Artery and Anterior Cerebral Artery Disease

CLINICAL VIGNETTE *A 70-year-old woman with history of diabetes mellitus (DM) and hypercholesterolemia presented to the ED reporting mild right-sided weakness, first noticed on awakening 2 days previously. The hemiparesis progressed to a right hemiplegia with dysarthria within 48 hours without change in the patient's level of consciousness. Head CT demonstrated a stroke involving the left centrum semiovale. Head CTA showed a distal M1 segment stenosis. The patient was started on an antiplatelet treatment and a statin. Pharmacologic treatment for her diabetes was maximized. Once stable, the patient was transferred to a rehabilitation facility with partial recovery of her motor deficits.*

TABLE 15.1   Clinical Symptoms in Patients With Border Zone Strokes

Stroke Location	Clinical Symptoms
Anterior border zone	Contralateral weakness (proximal > distal limbs and sparing face), transcortical motor aphasia (left-sided infarcts), and mood disturbances (right-sided infarcts)
Posterior border zone	Homonymous hemianopsia, lower-quadrant-anopsia, transcortical sensory aphasia (left-sided infarcts), hemineglect, and anosognosia (right-sided infarcts)
Subcortical border zone	Brachiofacial hemiparesis with or without sensory loss, subcortical aphasia (left-sided infarcts)

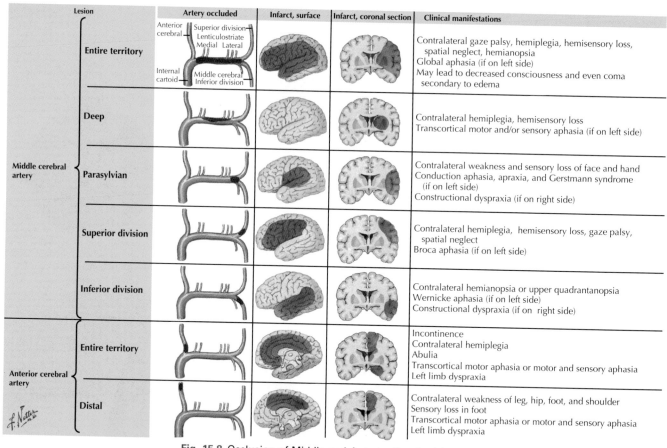

Lesion		Artery occluded	Infarct, surface	Infarct, coronal section	Clinical manifestations
Middle cerebral artery	Entire territory	Anterior cerebral — Superior division Lenticulostriate Medial Lateral Internal cartoid — Middle cerebral Inferior division			Contralateral gaze palsy, hemiplegia, hemisensory loss, spatial neglect, hemianopsia Global aphasia (if on left side) May lead to decreased consciousness and even coma secondary to edema
	Deep				Contralateral hemiplegia, hemisensory loss Transcortical motor and/or sensory aphasia (if on left side)
	Parasylvian				Contralateral weakness and sensory loss of face and hand Conduction aphasia, apraxia, and Gerstmann syndrome (if on left side) Constructional dyspraxia (if on right side)
	Superior division				Contralateral hemiplegia, hemisensory loss, gaze palsy, spatial neglect Broca aphasia (if on left side)
	Inferior division				Contralateral hemianopsia or upper quadrantanopsia Wernicke aphasia (if on left side) Constructional dyspraxia (if on right side)
Anterior cerebral artery	Entire territory				Incontinence Contralateral hemiplegia Abulia Transcortical motor aphasia or motor and sensory aphasia Left limb dyspraxia
	Distal				Contralateral weakness of leg, hip, foot, and shoulder Sensory loss in foot Transcortical motor aphasia or motor and sensory aphasia Left limb dyspraxia

Fig. 15.8 Occlusion of Middle and Anterior Cerebral Arteries.

This vignette describes a classic course of subcortical infarct from poor perfusion of the lenticulostriate vessels secondary to a fixed lesion in the ipsilateral MCA. The patient's symptoms evolved from relatively mild hemiparesis to complete paralysis within 2 days. Unlike large MCA infarctions, there was no impairment of the patient's level of consciousness despite the progressive nature of the neurologic deficit. In contrast, large cortical MCA lesions may also evolve over 2–4 days, but due to development of cerebral edema and increased intracranial pressure, altered levels of consciousness and even coma are commonly seen.

Intrinsic occlusive disease of the MCA and ACA are more common in Asians, Hispanics, and African Americans than in Caucasians. Arterial HTN, diabetes, and smoking are the most common risk factors, with a lower incidence of high cholesterol, coronary artery disease, and peripheral vascular disease. Although TIAs can occur, they are not as common as in patients with ICA disease and usually occur over a shorter period of hours or days. When strokes occur, initial symptoms are typically noticed on awakening and often fluctuate during the day, supporting a hemodynamic mechanism.

Vertebrobasilar Disease

CLINICAL VIGNETTE *A 76-year-old white man with a history of hypercholesterolemia and a previous myocardial infarction had acute onset of vertigo associated with vomiting and gait difficulties 2 days before presentation. On admission, he had sudden onset of slurred speech and lack of right arm coordination. Head CT demonstrated an old right posterior-inferior cerebellar artery (PICA) stroke and a subacute left PICA stroke. Head MRI with diffusion-weighted imaging showed a new right superior cerebellar artery stroke. Head and neck CTA showed occlusion of the left vertebral artery (VA) origin, a hypoplastic right VA, and an embolus in the middistal portion of the basilar artery. He was started on a statin and on antiplatelet therapy. Clinically the patient improved significantly.*

The vertebral arteries originate from the subclavian arteries in the neck. Stenosis or occlusion of the proximal subclavian arteries and the vertebral arteries at their origin rarely causes symptoms because of the concomitant development of adequate collateral circulation within the neck through the thyrocervical and costocervical trunks and other subclavian artery branches eventually flowing into the distal VA (see Fig. 15.3). More often, patients with subclavian and concomitant vertebral-origin stenosis have symptoms related only to upper extremity ischemia. They report pain, coolness, and weakness of the ipsilateral arm. Rarely does chronic atherosclerotic disease at the vertebral origins, even when bilateral, cause significant vertebrobasilar system flow reduction symptoms. When stenosis or occlusion of the VA origin leads to TIAs or stroke, intraarterial embolism is the commonly recognized mechanism. The embolus usually lodges in the distal VA, causing a PICA stroke, or passes through, leading to a "top of the basilar syndrome" (Table 15.2).

Distal intracranial VA atherosclerotic disease most often occurs at the level of the penetrators to the lateral medulla and at the takeoff to the PICA. Occlusion at this site presents as Wallenberg syndrome (lateral medullary syndrome), cerebellar PICA stroke, or both. Lateral medullary syndrome progressing into coma and herniation due to an associated large PICA cerebellar infarction is not uncommon and emphasizes the need to investigate and closely observe those with Wallenberg syndromes for unfolding signs of wider neurologic involvement.

TABLE 15.2 Clinical Manifestations of Ischemia in the Vertebrobasilar System According to the Artery Involved

Involved Artery	Ischemic Manifestations
Vertebral or PICA penetrator arteries (lateral medullary or Wallenberg syndrome)	Ipsilateral limb ataxia and Horner syndrome, crossed sensory loss, vertigo, dysphagia, and hoarseness
PICA	Vertigo, nausea, vomiting, and gait ataxia
AICA	Gait and limb ataxia, dysfunction of ipsilateral CN-V, -VII, and -VIII
SCA	Dysarthria and limb ataxia
PCA right	Contralateral visual field cut and sensory loss, visual neglect, and prosopagnosia (inability to recognize faces)
Left	Contralateral visual field cut and sensory loss, alexia without agraphia, anomic or transcortical sensory aphasia, impaired memory, and visual agnosia
Top of the basilar syndrome	Rostral brainstem—somnolence, vivid hallucinations, dreamlike behavior, and oculomotor dysfunction. Temporal + occipital regions—hemianopsia, fragments of Balint syndrome, agitated behavior, and amnestic dysfunction

AICA, Anterior inferior cerebellar artery; *PCA,* posterior cerebral artery; *PICA,* posterior–inferior cerebellar artery; *SCA,* superior cerebellar artery.

Atherosclerosis of the basilar artery most often affects its proximal and mid portions. Patients experience TIAs characterized by transient diplopia, dizziness, incoordination, and weakness affecting both sides at once or alternating between sides over minutes and even hours or days (Fig. 15.9). When stroke occurs, the most commonly affected area is the basis pons, with bilateral, often asymmetric, hemiparesis, pseudobulbar syndrome, abnormalities of eye movements (sixth nerve palsy, unilateral or bilateral internuclear ophthalmoplegia, ipsilateral conjugate gaze palsy, "one and one-half syndrome"), nystagmus, and if the reticular activating system is involved, coma (Fig. 15.10). Presence of coma or altered level of consciousness is dependent on collateral flow to the tegmentum from other vessels. If the pontine and midbrain tegmentum is spared, bilateral motor and sensory signs as well as varying degrees of ophthalmoplegia may be present without altered consciousness, such as in the "locked in" syndrome.

Embolus to the distal basilar artery leads to the classic top of the basilar syndrome (Fig. 15.11). Affected areas are the rostral brainstem (penetrator branches from distal basilar artery), the thalamus (penetrators of the proximal PCAs), and the medial temporal and occipital lobes. Clinical presentation includes bilateral homonymous hemianopsias or cortical blindness, confusion, and inability to form new memories. Cortical blindness may be accompanied by anosognosia and visual confabulations (Anton-Babinski syndrome). Patients with this syndrome are unaware of their blindness and may fabricate responses to questions about what they can see. In contrast, emboli moving past the basilar

tip cause only unilateral PCA occlusions, with isolated homonymous hemianopsia.

Most PCA infarcts are either cardioembolic or from intraarterial embolism. Intrinsic PCA stenosis is a less common cause of infarction. Clinical symptoms consist of transient episodes of hemivisual loss with, at times, associated contralateral sensory symptoms. Headache is a common associated symptom. In addition to visual and sensory abnormalities, patients with left PCA strokes often have concurrent anomic or transcortical sensory aphasia, impaired memory, and when involving the splenium of the corpus callosum, alexia without agraphia (inability to read with preserved writing). Patients with right PCA stroke often have associated visual neglect. The prominent neglect results in delayed presentation, as patients tend not to identify the presence of stroke symptoms. Patients with a right PCA stroke may present after a motor vehicle accident involving the left side of the car. Less frequently, there is an inability to recognize familiar faces (prosopagnosia). Bilateral parieto-occipital damage (Balint syndrome) leads to an inability to view a grouped visual stimulus as a whole (simultanagnosia), loss of accurate visual fixation and ocular tracking (optic apraxia), and impaired precision pointing to a visual target ("optic ataxia").

Cardioembolic Disease

> **CLINICAL VIGNETTE** *An 80-year-old woman was brought to the emergency room by ambulance after her husband heard her fall while walking to the bathroom. He immediately attended to her but found her to be unarousable. She had a history of mechanical aortic valve replacement 25 years earlier and took warfarin with a target INR of 2.0–3.0. On arrival she was found to be comatose. Her blood pressure was 190/110 mm Hg, and her pulse was 110 beats/min. Her pupils were 4 mm and reactive to light. Corneal reflexes were intact. She had dysconjugate gaze. There was no blink to visual threat. There was no response to sternal rub or nail bed pressure, with the exception of Babinski signs. However, she consistently demonstrated volitional upgaze on command. Her electrocardiogram revealed atrial fibrillation. INR was found to be 1.6. A noncontrast brain CT demonstrated a subtle hyperdensity of the basilar artery, and a CT angiogram confirmed occlusion of the basilar artery. She received intravenous tPA within the 3 hours of symptom onset and was referred for emergent mechanical thrombectomy with a stent retriever.*

AF, paroxysmal or chronic, is one of the most common sources of cardiac brain embolism and accounts for up to 15%–20% of all ischemic strokes. The incidence of AF in the population older than age 65 years is estimated at around 6%, but most patients do not experience embolic events. Risk factors that predispose to stroke or embolization from nonvalvular AF include age older than 75 years, female gender, atherosclerotic disease, HTN, DM, reduced cardiac ejection fraction, and congestive heart failure. Multiple risk factors increase the likelihood of major stroke up to sevenfold and should be strongly considered for anticoagulation. Those who present with TIA or stroke hold the highest risk of recurrence around 12% a year for the first year, then 5%–6% yearly thereafter. Atrial flutter, although a more organized cardiac arrhythmia, still predisposes to emboli formation and has a high risk of conversion to AF. Atrial flutter should be approached in the same fashion as AF.

Strokes secondary to cardiac sources typically present with acute onset of focal neurologic deficits, such as sudden loss of hand control or drooping of the mouth, often associated with language dysfunction, if involving the dominant hemisphere, or neglect if involving the nondominant hemisphere. Cerebral emboli are most clinically apparent during the day, and patients often provide a precise time of stroke or TIA onset. The anterior carotid circulation receives 80% of cerebral blood flow and is four times more likely than the posterior vertebrobasilar

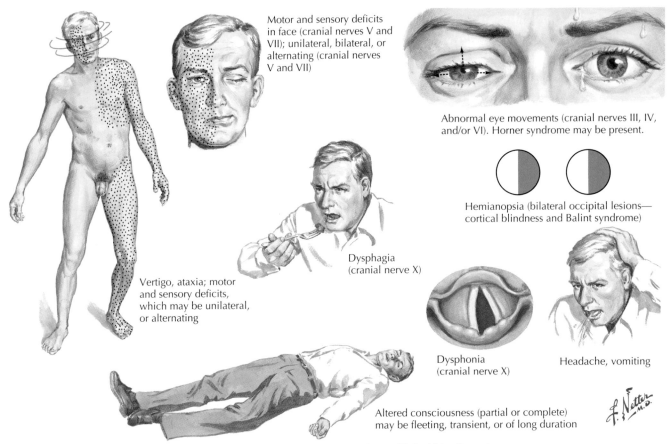

Motor and sensory deficits in face (cranial nerves V and VII); unilateral, bilateral, or alternating (cranial nerves V and VII)

Abnormal eye movements (cranial nerves III, IV, and/or VI). Horner syndrome may be present.

Hemianopsia (bilateral occipital lesions—cortical blindness and Balint syndrome)

Dysphagia (cranial nerve X)

Vertigo, ataxia; motor and sensory deficits, which may be unilateral, or alternating

Dysphonia (cranial nerve X)

Headache, vomiting

Altered consciousness (partial or complete) may be fleeting, transient, or of long duration

Fig. 15.9 Ischemia in Vertebrobasilar Territory: Clinical Manifestations.

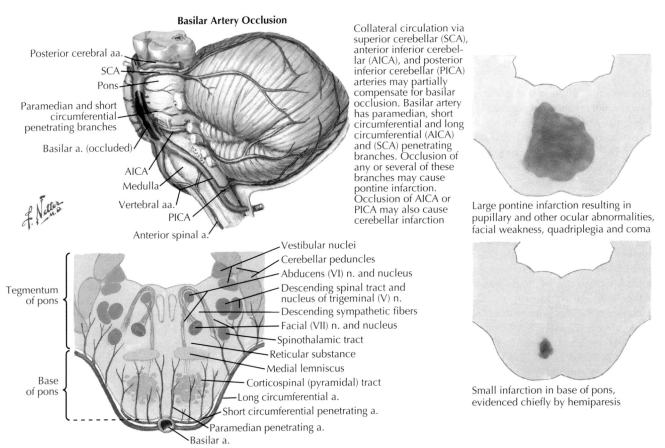

Basilar Artery Occlusion

Posterior cerebral aa.
SCA
Pons
Paramedian and short circumferential penetrating branches
Basilar a. (occluded)
AICA
Medulla
Vertebral aa.
PICA
Anterior spinal a.

Collateral circulation via superior cerebellar (SCA), anterior inferior cerebellar (AICA), and posterior inferior cerebellar (PICA) arteries may partially compensate for basilar occlusion. Basilar artery has paramedian, short circumferential and long circumferential (AICA) and (SCA) penetrating branches. Occlusion of any or several of these branches may cause pontine infarction. Occlusion of AICA or PICA may also cause cerebellar infarction

Large pontine infarction resulting in pupillary and other ocular abnormalities, facial weakness, quadriplegia and coma

Tegmentum of pons

Vestibular nuclei
Cerebellar peduncles
Abducens (VI) n. and nucleus
Descending spinal tract and nucleus of trigeminal (V) n.
Descending sympathetic fibers
Facial (VII) n. and nucleus
Spinothalamic tract
Reticular substance
Medial lemniscus

Base of pons

Corticospinal (pyramidal) tract
Long circumferential a.
Short circumferential penetrating a.
Paramedian penetrating a.
Basilar a.

Small infarction in base of pons, evidenced chiefly by hemiparesis

Fig. 15.10 Basilar Artery Occlusion.

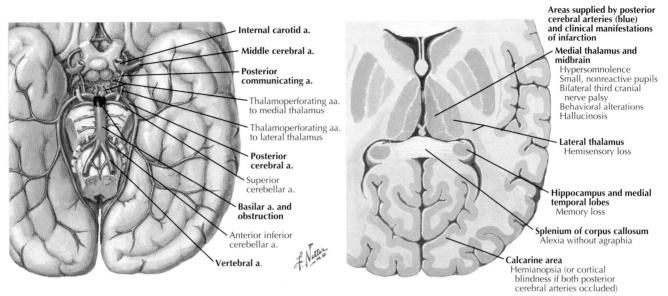

Fig. 15.11 Occlusion of "Top Basilar" and Posterior Cerebral Arteries.

circulation to be affected with emboli. Furthermore, a history of TIAs or strokes affecting both carotid territories or affecting both carotid and vertebrobasilar territories increases the suspicion of cardiac embolism. The vessels more often affected by cardiac emboli are the MCA and its branches, followed by the distal portion of the intracranial VA, distal basilar (top of the basilar syndrome), and PCA territory.

Embolism as a complication of acute MI is more likely to occur within the first 2 weeks of the acute event. Patients with anterior wall MIs may develop segmental hypokinetic myocardial wall defects or even aneurysms. Such lesions provide a potential nidus for platelet aggregation with subsequent embolus formation.

Infective endocarditis presents with TIA or stroke in approximately 15% of cases, but eventually 30% of patients are likely to experience a major neurologic complication throughout the course of the illness. Individuals with valvular heart disease are particularly at risk for developing endocarditis after any procedure that leads to transient bacteremia, even those as innocuous as dental cleaning, and should be treated beforehand with prophylactic antibiotics. Intravenously illicit drug use is also a major risk for infective endocarditis because of the reuse of nonsterilized needles. Endocarditis commonly presents with systemic symptoms, such as fever, weight loss, and malaise, as well as signs of a new-onset or changing cardiac murmur and petechial rash. Microemboli may manifest in the nail beds and conjunctiva as splinter hemorrhages, in the palms and finger pads as tender nodules or erythematous lesions (Osler nodes and Janeway lesions), and as hemorrhagic, edematous retinal exudates (Roth spots). Microemboli affecting the brain diffusely often present as an encephalopathy rather than with focal neurologic findings, and may be hard to diagnose in the setting of chronic medical illness.

Despite a clinically normal initial cardiac examination, the TEE confirmed a congenital intraatrial heart defect. The symptom complex acuity was consistent with a cardioembolic source, justifying a careful heart evaluation. In patients of this age group, PFO is the most likely associated condition with embolic stroke.

PFO is common, occurring in up to one-fourth of the population, and usually asymptomatic. This intraarterial connection is a remnant of the intrauterine fetal circulation that allows placental oxygenated blood to bypass the fetal lung vasculature directly to the left atrium and fetal systemic circulation. This conduit, which usually closes within a few months of birth, remains partially patent in a large proportion of the population. The usual left to right intraatrial gradient may become transiently reversed by any activity that increases pulmonary arterial and right atrial pressure (Valsalva, squatting, straining, lifting, coughing, etc.). Passing venous thromboemboli that might normally be dissolved or filtered by the pulmonary circulation have the potential to cross from pulmonary to systemic and cerebral arterial circulation by this mechanism, which is called paradoxical embolism.

Another presumed mechanism is turbulent or stagnant flow in and around the defect itself, with subsequent clot formation and propagation. PFOs are usually detected by Doppler echocardiography. After a brief delay, intravenous agitated saline injection is seen as echo-dense air bubbles crossing the intraatrial septum from right to left. This is often aided by a Valsalva maneuver that transiently increases right-sided atrial pressure with respect to the left. TEE holds a higher sensitivity as compared with a transthoracic approach and is considered the test of choice. PFO has been shown to be more common in young adults with cryptogenic stroke, as compared with the general population and as compared with those with identifiable sources of stroke. Being a common finding, the presence of a PFO as a cause of paradoxical embolism in cryptogenic stroke remains, however, presumptive, and other situational, hematologic, and anatomic factors likely come into play that make the PFO clinically relevant. For example, a paradoxical embolism becomes more suspicious in a young patient with a prior history of deep venous thrombosis who presents with a stroke after a bout of coughing from an upper respiratory tract infection during a period of relative immobility. As illustrated in the vignette, patients at risk include those who are nonambulatory from prolonged illness or even seemingly inconsequential settings, such as during prolonged transoceanic flights or car trips where venous flow in the legs is diminished or stagnant.

CLINICAL VIGNETTE *A previously healthy 41-year-old woman had a right facial droop and difficulty speaking 1 day after she had made a continuous 10-hour car trip. At the ED, neurologic examination confirmed right central facial weakness and a mild mixed expressive and receptive aphasia. Cardiac examination and an electrocardiograph were normal. Brain MRI with diffusion-weighted imaging showed a small left insular stroke. Head and neck MRA results were normal. Transesophageal echocardiography (TEE) showed a patent foramen ovale (PFO), and her hypercoagulable screen was remarkable for protein S deficiency. Symptoms gradually improved, clearing completely within 72 hours.*

Those with coagulation disorders, either hereditary or acquired, such as with hormone replacement therapy or pregnancy, are also at a higher risk. Studies show that the incidence of an associated hypercoagulable hematologic abnormality is higher in patients with cryptogenic stroke and PFO than the general population. Coagulation studies and a search for deep vein thrombosis should be included in the workup for all young patients with cryptogenic stroke and an associated PFO. Anatomic considerations also come into play. A PFO with an associated atrial septal aneurysm (>10 mm protrusion into either atrium) holds a much higher risk of recurrence of up to 19.2% over 4 years, even when treated with antiplatelets. A large-size PFO (>1 cm) with many microbubbles crossing the intraarterial septum, especially without the aid of a Valsalva maneuver, likely represents a high risk of recurrence.

Lacunar Small Vessel Disease

> **CLINICAL VIGNETTE** *A 68-year-old woman developed sudden right hemiplegia while watering her lawn. She had not seen a physician in years and did not take any medications. Her neighbors called 911, and she was brought to the emergency room by ambulance. On arrival, her blood pressure was 220/112 and pulse was 68 beats/min. She was severely dysarthric, but there was no aphasia. She had right facial weakness and complete paralysis of the right arm and leg. The remainder of her neurologic examination was normal. A noncontrast brain CT demonstrated multiple, bilateral but chronic lacunar infarcts of the brainstem, thalami, and basal ganglia. There was also advanced calcification of the carotid siphons and distal vertebral arteries. Immediately following the CT scan, her symptoms completely resolved. A carotid ultrasound showed no hemodynamically significant carotid artery stenosis. LDL was 166; HgA1c was 7.2. She was admitted to the hospital for blood pressure control and an MRI scan. Aspirin 325 mg and atorvastatin 80 mg were started. Several hours later the dysarthria and right hemiplegia recurred. She was treated emergently with intravenous tPA within the 3-hour window. The following day, a brain MRI demonstrated an acute lacunar stroke in the left basis pontis.*

TABLE 15.3 Most Frequent Lacunar Syndromes and Their Locations

Clinical Syndrome	Location
Pure motor stroke: weakness equally involving face, arm, and leg	Internal capsule (posterior limb) or basis pontis
Pure sensory stroke: numbness or paresthesia equally involving face, arm, leg, and usually trunk	Lateral thalamus (posteroventral nucleus)
Ataxic hemiparesis: weakness and incoordination in the arm and/or leg	Basis pontis or internal capsule
Dysarthria—clumsy hand syndrome: facial weakness, severe dysarthria, dysphagia, mild hemiparesis inconsistently present and clumsiness of the hand	Basis pontis
Sensorimotor stroke: combination of pure motor/pure sensory symptoms and findings	Thalamus or internal capsule

> *while watching television, he developed abrupt onset of vertigo with profuse vomiting. His wife brought him to the emergency room, where a brain CT was done. The CT was read as normal, and he was discharged with a diagnosis of labyrinthitis. The following morning he awoke with a hoarse voice, right facial pain, and pins-and-needles sensation of the left arm. He returned to the emergency room and was found to have direction-changing nystagmus. There was sensory loss of the right side of his face and the left side of his body. He had right hemiataxia on finger-to-nose and heel-to-shin testing. His uvula deviated to the left with elevation of the palate. A repeat brain CT showed a large acute right posterior inferior cerebellar artery infarct without hemorrhage. CT angiography of the head and neck demonstrated a right vertebral artery dissection. He was admitted to the neurologic intensive care unit for close observation. He was kept NPO to prevent aspiration, and 300 mg of aspirin was administered per the rectum.*

Lacunar strokes affecting the internal capsule, thalamus, striatum, or brainstem (see Fig. 15.5) can often be clinically distinguished from embolic disease by the tendency toward a more fluctuating course, with deficits progressing or "stuttering" over 2–4 days. In addition, lacunar deficits have a relatively typical distribution; they affect the entire side of the body with motor and/or sensory symptoms without cortically based findings or visual changes. This is in contrast with MCA cortical branch occlusions that tend to have a brachiofacial distribution often associated with other cognitive and/or visual signs.

Patients experiencing lacunar strokes can present with TIA in up to 15%–20% of instances. TIAs are stereotypical, and tend to cluster over 2–5 days, at times occurring frequently over a 24-hour period and in a crescendo fashion. Signs and symptoms vary according to the location of the ischemia (Table 15.3).

HTN and diabetes are the most important risk factors, and proper treatment of these conditions is essential to prevent further strokes.

Arterial Dissection

> **CLINICAL VIGNETTE** *A 48-year-old male carpenter developed sudden onset right-sided neck pain and occipital headache while carrying lumber on his shoulders. With the exception of longstanding cigarette smoking, he had no significant past medical history. He presented to an urgent care center where he was diagnosed with cervical muscle spasm. He was given a prescription for cyclobenzaprine and referred for physical therapy. Two days later,*

Extracranial carotid artery dissection occurs predominantly in patients aged 20–50 years. The characteristic clinical presentation is unilateral neck or face pain, sometimes followed a few days later by acute onset of neurologic signs. In patients with carotid dissection, pain is usually referred to the eye, temple, or forehead. Ipsilateral Horner syndrome occurs in 40%–50% of patients and is due to distension or pressure against the oculosympathetic fibers running along the ICA to the eye. Pulsatile tinnitus is common. Often, a history of minor trauma exists (violent coughing, cervical manipulation, whiplash injury, etc.) in the days preceding symptom onset. As in the preceding vignette, benign traumatic events can cause a slight intima tear in the carotid or vertebral arteries, leading to platelet fibrin aggregation with potential for developing artery-to-artery emboli.

Similar to the carotid artery within the neck, the extracranial VA has a significant potential for sustaining traumatic dissection. Dissection usually occurs in the distal extracranial portion at C1–C2, also called the *third segment*, just before it penetrates the dura at the skull base. In those patients, pain is referred to the neck or back of the head and usually precedes the onset of neurologic signs by days and rarely weeks.

TIAs are more common in ICA than in VA dissections. In ICA dissection, TIAs usually involve the ipsilateral eye and cerebral hemisphere. Ischemic symptoms of VA dissection are of dizziness, diplopia, gait unsteadiness, and dysarthria. In extracranial ICA and VA dissections, strokes usually affect the MCA and distal VA (PICA and lateral medullary) territories.

Both carotid and VA dissection may be asymptomatic or present with subtle symptoms that are not always recognized. The incidence of spontaneous dissection according to different studies is approximately 2.6/100,000. However, this is likely an underestimation, considering that many dissections may escape detection, as subtle symptoms can easily be dismissed. It is not uncommon to discover a previously unknown, chronic cervical artery dissection on MRA or CTA.

DIAGNOSTIC APPROACH

For every patient evaluated with ischemic stroke or TIA, the location of the lesion and mechanism should be investigated thoroughly to most effectively direct treatment and to better predict potential complications. CT and MRI brain scanning have greatly enhanced our ability to diagnose and follow neurologic disease, as well as guide treatment.

Noninvasive arterial imaging with CTA and MRA has largely replaced catheter angiography in the initial evaluation of cerebrovascular disease and shows great promise in advancing acute stroke care (Fig. 15.12).

Anatomic Site

Although the precise anatomic location of an acute TIA or stroke can frequently be deduced by the history and neurologic examination, confirmation with an imaging study is needed and often provides more specific etiologic information that can direct potential treatment. In addition, intracerebral hemorrhages, subdural hematomas, or other structural lesions, including benign and malignant tumors, are occasionally found on brain CT and MRI in patients presenting with seemingly typical cerebrovascular events.

Brain CT examination, with its immediate availability in most hospitals and short scanning time, is usually the initial study performed

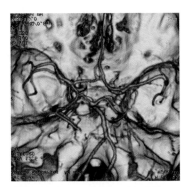

A. 3-D reconstructed image of the Circle of Willis on computed tomography angiography (CTA).

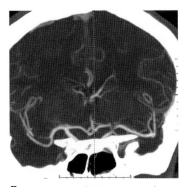

B. Reconstructed CTA images of coronal intracerebral vessels.

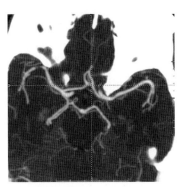

C. Reconstructed CTA images of axial intracerebral vessels.

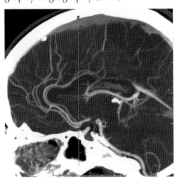

D. Reconstructed CTA images of sagittal intracerebral vessels.

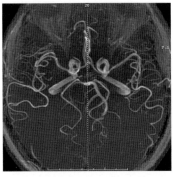

E. Reconstructed magnetic resonance angiography (MRA) composite of all proximal vessels.

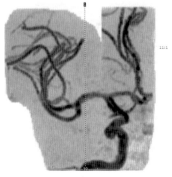

F. Reconstructed magnetic resonance angiography (MRA) of the right internal carotid circulation.

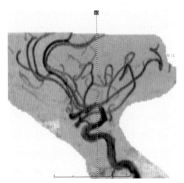

G. Reconstructed magnetic resonance angiography (MRA) of the right internal carotid circulation.

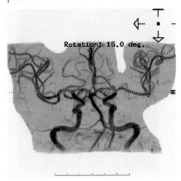

H. Reconstructed magnetic resonance angiography (MRA) composite of all proximal vessels.

Fig. 15.12 Intracranial Arterial Imaging With CT and MRI.

in individuals presenting with an acute focal neurologic deficit. Its sensitivity to detect the presence of a primary cerebral hemorrhage or a hemorrhagic infarct is a crucial starting point in determining the future course of action such as the use of thrombolytics, the need for surgical intervention, and the degree of BP control. The head CT is often normal in the first few hours of an ischemic stroke. However, in some cases, the presence of an acute arterial occlusion can be detected by the presence of a localized intraluminal hyperdense signal, often seen in patients with MCA occlusion (Fig. 15.13A), even when the brain parenchyma shows no evolving processes. Head CT may also show early infarct changes characterized by sulcal effacement or loss of gray-white matter differentiation (see Fig. 15.13B). Such findings have important therapeutic implications. A CT angiogram can confirm the presence of a thrombus (see Fig. 15.13C) and help guide further intervention concerning intravenous thrombolysis, endovascular mechanical thrombectomy, anticoagulation, and management of BP. CT perfusion has evolved into a valuable tool to screen acute stroke patients for consideration of urgent endovascular thrombectomy by defining core infarct volume and the potentially salvageable ischemic penumbra. This approach has allowed for the expansion of the previously narrow treatment window for ischemic stroke.

Diffusion-weighted MRI is the most sensitive and specific test for acute ischemia, and abnormalities have been demonstrated as early as 1 hour after symptom onset. Other MRI sequences, such as FLAIR and T2-weighted imaging, can show the area of stroke, often 6–12 hours after onset of symptoms (see Fig. 15.13D and E).

Etiologic Mechanism

To define the specific pathophysiologic mechanism for a TIA or stroke, patency of the extracranial and intracranial arteries, the character of

their endothelial surface, and the adequacy of cerebral perfusion are required.

Complete assessment of cardiac function is essential and includes the electrical stability of the cardiac rhythm, myocardial contractility, valvular status, and whether a PFO is present. TEE provides more sensitivity and anatomic details and is preferred over the transthoracic approach for valvular lesions, intraatrial abnormalities (PFO and ASD), and aortic arch disease. Ultrasound of the carotid arteries at their bifurcation in the neck and transcranial Doppler of the intracranial vessels can functionally assess cerebral flow and determine the presence of critically stenotic extracranial or circle of Willis arteries, respectively. Carotid ultrasound helps characterize the carotid plaque as "soft," consisting of cholesterol deposits and clot, which is more prone to ulceration and artery-to-artery embolization, or "hard," where the vessel wall has fibrosed and calcified over time, making it a less likely source of distal embolization. MRA or CTA of the head and neck is appropriate to assess patency of intracranial and extracranial arteries. The more recent addition of perfusion scanning helps define the effect of any stenotic or occlusive lesion upon regional blood flow and now plays an integral role in identification of patients for late window mechanical thrombectomy (Table 15.4)

Information gathered from imaging studies allows differentiation of three primary carotid or vertebrobasilar stroke mechanisms: large artery disease with intraarterial embolism, small vessel disease, and large artery disease with hemodynamic ischemia.

Renal failure or pacemaker devices limit the imaging studies that can be performed in patients with TIAs and strokes. Gadolinium-based contrast agents have been linked to the development of nephrogenic systemic fibrosis and nephrogenic fibrosing dermopathy, often with serious and irreversible skin or organ pathology in patients with

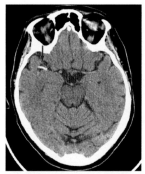

A. Axial CT scan demonstrates increased density in distal right M1 segment (arrow); a hyperdense MCA sign.

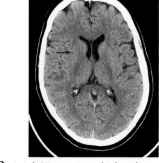

B. Axial CT scan 2 cm higher demonstrates normal insular ribbon and imperceptible change in right basal ganglia (arrow).

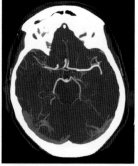

C. Computed tomography angiography (CTA) shows opacification of a few branches proximal to the previously demonstrated clot and expected obstruction of distal right M1 segment (arrow).

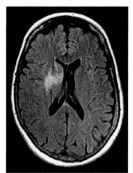

D. Axial FLAIR image 11 hours later demonstrates edema in the ischemic basal ganglia (arrows) where restricted diffusion was also noted.

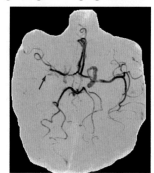

E. MR angiography shows obstruction of distal right M1 segment similar to CTA (arrow).

Fig. 15.13 Acute Ischemic Infarct With a Right Middle Cerebral Artery Clot.

TABLE 15.4 Comparison of Neurologic Imaging Techniques

Imaging Method	Advantages	Disadvantages
MRI/MRA	DWI and PWI demonstrate the area of stroke and the area at risk (penumbra), respectively.	Prolonged test (30–60 min); patient must cooperate or sedation is required. Cannot be performed in patients with PCM. MRA can overestimate tight stenosis as an occluded vessel.
CTA/CTP	Images can be obtained rapidly (<5 min).	Patient must have normal renal function because CTA and CTP require high doses of contrast, 100 and 50 mL, respectively.
Ultrasonography of the neck	Easy to perform, can be done at the bedside	No detailed information about the vertebral arteries or the intracranial vessels.
TCD	Easy to perform, even at the bedside	Poor transtemporal windows limit the information about the intracranial vessels.

CTA, Computed tomography angiography; *CTP,* computed tomography perfusion; *DWI,* diffusion-weighted imaging; *MRA,* magnetic resonance angiography; *MRI,* magnetic resonance imaging; *PCM,* pacemaker; *PWI,* perfusion-weighted imaging; *TCD,* transcranial Doppler.

moderate to end-stage renal disease. The mechanism is unclear but thought to be due to stimulation of tissue fibrosis similar to that seen in scleroderma.

A hypercoagulable screen is part of the evaluation of patients younger than 50 years and in patients of any age without identifiable risk factors. It should be kept in mind that most inherited coagulopathies are more associated with systemic and cerebral venous thrombosis rather than arterial stroke, and a direct relation cannot be made. Other factors such as the presence of PFO or other intraatrial shunt may make them more relevant in cases of ischemic stroke without any other clear source. Antiphospholipid syndrome and homocysteinemia may predispose to arterial ischemic stroke, even in the absence of PFO.

TREATMENT

The treatment of TIAs and arterial ischemic strokes consists of acute reperfusion therapies including thrombolysis with IV recombinant tPA and mechanical thrombectomy, general supportive measures, identification and control of vascular risk factors, secondary stroke prevention, carotid revascularization in selected patients, and rehabilitation.

Acute Reperfusion Therapy

Acute stroke care begins in the prehospital setting and depends on public awareness of stroke signs and symptoms, and recognition that immediate medical management is necessary. Emergency medical services should initiate care in the field, use standardized scales for stroke screening (e.g., FAST scale—Face, Arm, Speech, Time), and transport patients rapidly to the nearest primary or comprehensive stroke center after providing prehospital notification that a potential stroke patient is en route. The receiving hospital should ideally have a designated stroke team and, if not available, telestroke consultation can be implemented to improve and expedite care.

Once a safe airway and hemodynamic stability are established, patients are submitted to brain imaging with the main purpose of ruling out acute intracranial hemorrhage. This can be achieved with a noncontrast head CT, which is widely available in most emergency rooms. If there is suspicion for large vessel occlusion (LVO), noninvasive vascular imaging is optimally obtained as part of the initial imaging evaluation, as long as this does not delay the administration of IV tPA. A systematic review evaluating the accuracy of prediction instruments for diagnosing LVO determined that the National Institutes of Health Stroke Scale (NIHSS) is the most reliable predictor. Specifically, NIHSS of 6 or higher was found to have 87% sensitivity and 52% specificity, and while LVO can be present in patients with lower NIHSS, this is accepted as the threshold above which vascular imaging should routinely be obtained.

Timely restoration of cerebral blood flow using reperfusion therapy is the most effective strategy for salvaging ischemic brain tissue that is not already infarcted. There is a narrow window during which this can be accomplished, since the benefit of reperfusion decreases over time. This can be achieved pharmacologically with the use of recombinant tPA to lyse the thrombus or via mechanical thrombectomy.

Thrombolysis With IV Recombinant Tissue Plasminogen Activator

Recombinant tPA was first approved by the US Food and Drug Administration (FDA) in 1996 after the pivotal NINDS trial (National Institute of Neurological Disorders and Stroke), a randomized double-blind trial of IV tPA in patients with ischemic stroke treated within the first 3 hours of symptom onset. As compared with patients given placebo, those receiving tPA were at least 30% more likely to have minimal or no disability at 3 months. Importantly, the benefit was present for all stroke subtypes analyzed. Similar results of early treatment with tPA within a 3-hour window were found in a subpopulation analysis of patients in the ATLANTIS (Alteplase Thrombolysis for Acute Noninterventional Therapy in Ischemic Stroke) trial. In 2008, with the release of the ECASS III trial (European Cooperative Acute Stroke Study), the window for thrombolysis was then safely expanded to 4.5 hours. The safety and efficacy of thrombolysis with IV tPA have since been well established, and this remains the standard of care for acute stroke treatment within 4.5 hours. The eligibility criteria for IV tPA have evolved over time to become more inclusive, and a recent meta-analysis of tPA trials demonstrated that the benefit of IV tPA is well established for adult patients with disabling stroke symptoms, regardless of age and stroke severity. An American Heart Association/American Stroke Association (AHA/ASA) statement published in 2016 provides a detailed discussion of the inclusion and exclusion criteria for tPA, and these are again summarized in the 2018 AHA/ASA acute stroke management guidelines. The main exclusion criteria are listed in Box 15.1.

Despite the longer window, however, it is critical to continue to treat patients as quickly as possible as the benefit of tPA is strictly time-dependent. At the time of this publication, the door-to-needle time of 60 minutes recommended by the AHA/ASA is being reduced to 45 minutes. Recombinant tPA protocols are being made leaner by eliminating unnecessary steps and testing. The only laboratory test that must precede the initiation of IV tPA is the assessment of blood glucose, as both hypoglycemia and hyperglycemia can mimic acute stroke presentations. Given the extremely low risk of unsuspected thrombocytopenia or coagulation studies in a population, it is reasonable that thrombolysis not be delayed while waiting for platelet and coagulation studies if there is no reason to suspect an abnormal test. Many centers are initiating tPA infusion in the CT scanner to save time. ECG and chest radiographs can be obtained after tPA, unless there is concern for an acute cardiac or pulmonary condition.

BOX 15.1 Contraindications for IV Recombinant Tissue Plasminogen Activator

Strong Contraindications for IV rt-PA
1. Unclear time of onset
2. CT evidence of acute intracranial hemorrhage
3. CT evidence of suspected large infarct (more than ⅓ MCA territory or mass effect)
4. Signs or symptoms suggestive of subarachnoid hemorrhage
5. Known history of intracranial hemorrhage
6. Previous stroke or serious head trauma within the past 3 months
7. Intracranial or intraspinal surgery within the past 3 months
8. Acute aortic arch dissection
9. Infective endocarditis
10. Administration of DOACs within previous 48 hours unless appropriate lab tests are normal
11. Administration of therapeutic dose of LMWH within previous 24 hours
12. Platelet count < 100,000/mm³, INR > 1.7, PTT > 40s

Relative Contraindications
1. Seizure at onset of stroke
2. Serum glucose <50 mg/dL or >400 mg/dL
3. Myocardial infarction in the previous 6 weeks
4. Intracranial vascular malformations

DOAC, Direct oral anticoagulant; *INR,* international normalized ratio; *LMWH,* low molecular weight heparin; *PTT,* partial thromboplastin time; *rt-PA,* recombinant tissue plasminogen activator.

Mechanical Thrombectomy

The approach to treatment of acute ischemic stroke has undergone major advancements over the past several years, particularly with respect to the role of endovascular therapy. Early endovascular trials, including IMS III (Interventional Management of Stroke), MR Rescue (Mechanical Retrieval and Recanalization of Stroke Clots Using Embolectomy), and Synthesis Expansion, failed to show a benefit of mechanical thrombectomy in acute stroke patients with LVO. In fact, the IMS III trial was stopped prematurely due to futility. In retrospect, these negative results can be attributed to a number of factors, including prolonged times to groin puncture and reperfusion, poor rates of recanalization, and treatment of a large percentage of patients with old thrombectomy devices or intraarterial tPA only. In addition, and perhaps more importantly, patient selection was inadequate, and the following requirements necessary to demonstrate the benefit of endovascular therapy were not met: (1) presence of a target vascular occlusion, (2) presence of target salvageable tissue, and (3) fast and effective reperfusion.

Taking these aspects into account, a flood of more strictly designed randomized controlled trials, starting with MR CLEAN (Multicenter Randomized Clinical Trial of Endovascular Treatment for Acute Ischemic Stroke in the Netherlands) and followed by ESCAPE, SWIFT-PRIME, REVASCAT, and EXTEND-IA, compared best medical therapy alone to medical therapy combined with intervention using more modern devices and techniques and more stringent patient selection criteria. A meta-analysis of these trials, with pooled data from 1287 subjects, showed that the rate of functional independence (90-day modified Rankin scale score of 0–2) was significantly better for the intervention group compared with the control group (46% vs. 27%, OR 2.35, 95% CI 1.85–2.98). The number needed to treat (NNT) for one additional person to achieve functional independence ranged from approximately 3 to 7.5. Mechanical thrombectomy was beneficial across a wide range of patient subgroups, including age 80 years or older, high initial stroke severity, and those not treated with IV rtPA. In addition, there was no significant difference between the mechanical thrombectomy and control groups for rates of symptomatic intracranial hemorrhage or 90-day mortality. These trials erased the skepticism surrounding mechanical thrombectomy and established this interventional treatment strategy as the standard of care in the management of acute LVOs (Fig. 15.14).

Until recently, neurointerventionalists performed mechanical thrombectomy up to 6 hours from symptom onset based on time windows extrapolated from rtPA trials. This changed rather drastically with the recent publication of the DAWN and DEFUSE 3 trials, which showed that endovascular therapy can be effective and safe for selected patients beyond 6 hours from symptom onset who have a clinical deficit and area of hypoperfusion that is disproportionally severe when compared with the volume of infarction on imaging studies.

The DEFUSE 3 trial enrolled patients with ischemic stroke due to occlusion of the proximal MCA or ICA who were last known to be well 6 to 16 hours earlier. Patients were required to have an infarct size of less than 70 mL and a ratio of ischemic tissue volume to infarct volume of 1.8 or more, as measured by automated software processing of diffusion-weighted MRI or CT perfusion imaging. Patients were treated with medical therapy alone or with mechanical thrombectomy using the Trevo, Solitaire, or MindFrame devices or the Penumbra thrombectomy system. The DAWN trial was similar in its methodology but enrolled patients up to 24 hours from onset of stroke symptoms. About half of the patients in both trials were "wake-up strokes." The results of both trials were overwhelmingly positive with significantly better outcomes in the thrombectomy group at 90 days and low NNT, to the point that they were stopped early for efficacy. Based on these promising results, the AHA/ASA updated the 2018 guidelines for the early management of patients with acute stroke to reflect the extended time windows for mechanical thrombectomy. A Class I recommendation with Level A evidence was assigned to performing mechanical thrombectomy in patients 6–16 hours since onset of acute stroke symptoms who meet either DEFUSE 3 or DAWN trial criteria, and a Class IIa recommendation with Level B-R evidence to performing mechanical thrombectomy in patients 6–24 hours since symptom onset who meet DAWN trial requirements. The most commonly used endovascular techniques currently include aspiration of clot by an aspiration catheter and removal of clot using a stent retriever with or without concomitant aspiration. These trials represent a landmark in the endovascular treatment of stroke and will allow neurointerventionalists to positively impact the lives of many more patients suffering from ischemic strokes.

When selecting patients for mechanical thrombectomy, NIHSS is commonly used to assess the severity of a patient's neurologic deficit and to identify patients suffering from an LVO. A common cutoff below which patients are considered unlikely to have an LVO is an NIHSS less than 6. However, this is not absolute, and it is very important to consider which patient deficits are relative to their baseline quality of life and functional ability. An NIHSS less than 6 can still be devastating to someone who was previously high-functioning, particularly if the deficits include aphasia.

ASPECTS scoring is a commonly used radiologic method for evaluating a noncontrast head CT in a patient having an acute stroke affecting the MCA territory. It divides the MCA territory into 10 regions. A point is lost for every region exhibiting loss of gray-white matter differentiation. ASPECTS scores of 7 or less are associated with worse functional outcomes at 90 days. Clinicians often use 6 as a minimum score for performing mechanical thrombectomy.

While each of these criteria is important to consider, it has become increasingly apparent that every patient with an acute LVO needs to be evaluated individually. Not every patient with a high NIHSS or high ASPECTS score should be treated, even if they present shortly after the onset of the stroke. Similarly, not every patient with a low NIHSS or a

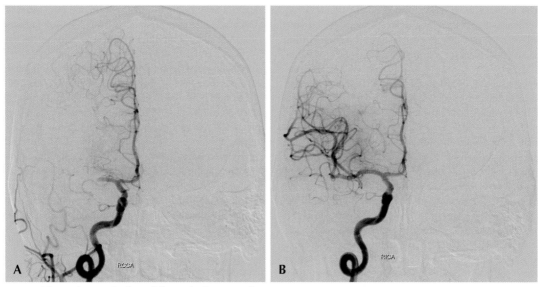

Successful reperfusion of right middle cerebral artery with stent retriever (A, Pre; B, Post).

Fig. 15.14 Mechanical Thrombectomy of Large Vessel Occlusion.

relatively long time since the onset of the stroke should be excluded. In addition to the easily quantifiable criteria described previously, a patient's premorbid function and his or her personal and family goals of care need to be considered. Advanced imaging techniques such as multiphase computed tomography angiography (CTA), CT, MR perfusion, and diffusion-weighted imaging (DWI) can also be helpful when trying to determine whether a patient may benefit from intervention in challenging cases.

General Supportive Measures

The care of a stroke patient is multifaceted and early key general medical management issues that often arise include BP control, fluid management, treatment of abnormal blood glucose levels, treatment of fever and infection, swallowing assessment, and prophylaxis of venous thromboembolism. Because of the complexity of the care, treatment in a dedicated stroke unit has been shown to be associated with better outcomes.

Systemic BP is often elevated in patients with acute ischemic stroke. Possible etiologies include chronic HTN, an acute sympathetic response, and other stroke-mediated mechanisms that occur to maintain perfusion in borderline ischemic areas. While elevated BP can increase the risk of hemorrhagic transformation, cerebral edema, and further vascular damage, aggressive BP reduction can compromise cerebral blood flow surrounding the area of ischemia, further increasing the infarct size. Despite these considerations, optimal BP management in the acute phase of a stroke has not been well established.

According to the latest guidelines, when thrombolysis is not being considered, BP levels as high as 220/120 mm Hg are permissible assuming patients have no comorbid conditions that require stricter levels (e.g., concomitant acute coronary syndrome). In patients receiving rt-PA BP should be strictly maintained below 180/105 mm Hg for at least 24 hours postthrombolysis. Post-tPA BP protocol violations have been independently associated with higher likelihood of symptomatic intracranial hemorrhage and worse outcome. When BP lowering is indicated, reversible and titratable agents are favored, and intravenous calcium channel blockers and beta blockers such as nicardipine and labetalol tend to be first-line agents.

Intravascular volume depletion is frequent in the setting of acute stroke and may worsen cerebral blood flow. For most patients, isotonic saline is the best choice for volume repletion and maintenance fluid therapy. Fluids containing dextrose or glucose should be avoided, as they may lead to hyperglycemia. Hypotonic fluids and free water should also be avoided, as they may exacerbate cerebral edema. If significant cerebral edema is present, hyperosmolar therapy with 3% hypertonic saline or mannitol may need to be considered in an intensive care setting.

Hypoglycemia and hyperglycemia can mimic stroke symptoms, delay recovery, and worsen outcomes. Hypoglycemia less than 60 mg/dL should be aggressively corrected. Hyperglycemia should be treated to a goal blood glucose level of 140 to 180 mg/dL. If glucose levels are difficult to control, patient has newly diagnosed DM or hemoglobin A1c is significantly elevated, an endocrinology consultation could be considered.

Hyperthermia has been shown to cause direct neuronal injury in animal models of stroke and is associated with unfavorable outcomes in human studies. Sources of hyperthermia (temperature >38°C) should be investigated and treated accordingly. This is particularly important in the first days after a stroke. Induced hypothermia is not currently recommended for patients with ischemic stroke, outside of clinical trials.

Dysphagia is common after stroke and is a major risk factor for developing aspiration pneumonia. It is important to assess swallowing function prior to administration of any oral medications or food. Patients should be kept nil per os (NPO) until they have bedside dysphagia screening or a formal evaluation with a swallow therapist. Once swallowing permits or, if that's not the case, once a nasogastric tube is placed, nutrition should be started.

Other simple yet important measures include maintaining head of bed at 30 degrees for most patients, prevention of venous thromboembolism, and screening for depression.

Identification and Treatment of Vascular Risk Factors

The most important nonmodifiable stroke risk factors are advanced age, gender, ethnicity, and family history, and while these cannot be altered, their recognition is useful in identifying patients at increased risk. While the incidence of stroke rapidly increases with age, doubling for each decade after age 55, strokes can occur as early as infancy and childhood. The list of traditional modifiable risk factors includes HTN, DM, hyperlipidemia, obesity, cigarette smoking, alcohol abuse, and the more recent recognition of obstructive sleep apnea. Regular screening for modifiable risk factors should be performed in all patients, along with aggressive management, including pharmacologic treatment, increased physical activity, and dietary changes introduced according to the 2014 AHA/ASA guidelines for the prevention of stroke in patients with stroke and TIA.

Stroke risk is consistently linked to elevated BP independently of other risk factors, and there is overwhelming evidence that treatment of **HTN** is possibly the single most important intervention for secondary stroke prevention. Meta-analyses of randomized controlled trials have shown that BP management is associated with a 35%–45% stroke risk reduction among hypertensive subjects. Initiation of BP therapy is indicated for previously untreated patients with ischemic stroke or TIA who, after the first several days, have an established BP 140 mm Hg or higher systolic or 90 mm Hg or higher diastolic. Resumption of BP therapy is indicated for previously treated patients with known HTN. It appears that the choice of antihypertensive agent is not as relevant as the degree of BP reduction achieved. In addition, several lifestyle modifications associated with BP reductions should be included as part of a comprehensive approach to antihypertensive therapy, including salt restriction, weight loss, consumption of a fruit- and vegetable-rich diet, and low-fat dairy products, regular aerobic physical activity, and limited alcohol consumption.

Patients with **DM** and impaired glucose tolerance have approximately twice the risk of ischemic stroke compared with those without diabetes, mediated by endothelial dysfunction, dyslipidemia, and platelet and coagulation abnormalities. A major concern is that the burden of obesity and consequently DM is rapidly rising in both developed and developing countries. The 2014 AHA/ASA guidelines recommend screening for DM with testing of fasting plasma glucose, hemoglobin A1c, or an oral glucose tolerance test and the use of guidelines from the American Diabetes Association for glycemic control and cardiovascular risk factor management. A reasonable goal of therapy is hemoglobin A1c of 7% or less and glucose control to near normoglycemic levels, based on evidence that tight glucose control reduces microvascular complications. Diet, exercise, oral hypoglycemic drugs, and insulin are proven methods to achieve glycemic control.

Statins have been approved for prevention of ischemic strokes or TIAs in patients with **hyperlipidemia,** comorbid coronary artery disease, or evidence of an atherosclerotic origin. Treatment should aim for a target low-density lipoprotein cholesterol (LDL-C) level of less than 100 mg/dL. For high-risk patients with multiple risk factors, an LDL-C less than 70 mg/dL is usually recommended.

Since the publication of the Stroke Prevention by Aggressive Reduction in Cholesterol Levels (SPARCL) trial, statins have been recommended for patients with atherosclerotic ischemic stroke or TIA even without known coronary heart disease to reduce the risk of both subsequent stroke and cardiovascular events. This trial showed a 5-year absolute risk reduction of 2.2% for the combination fatal and nonfatal stroke and of 3.5% absolute risk reduction for major cardiovascular events in patients receiving 80 mg of atorvastatin as compared with placebo. The two treatment groups have no significant differences in the incidence of serious adverse events; however, there were slightly more hemorrhagic strokes in the atorvastatin group as compared with placebo (55 vs. 33). Hemorrhagic strokes were more frequent in male, older patients, with hemorrhagic stroke as an entry event, and in patients with stage 2 HTN (systolic BP ≥160 mm Hg, diastolic BP ≥100 mm Hg) at the last visit just prior to the hemorrhagic stroke. There was no relationship between the hemorrhagic risk and the LDL cholesterol levels.

Cigarette smoking is associated with an increased risk of all stroke subtypes and has a strong, dose-response relationship for both ischemic stroke and subarachnoid hemorrhage. While there are no randomized controlled trials of smoking cessation for stroke prevention, observational studies have shown that the elevated risk of stroke due to smoking declines after quitting and is eliminated by 5 years. Therefore AHA/ASA guidelines recommend smoking cessation for patients with stroke or TIA who have smoked in the year prior to the event and suggest avoidance of environmental tobacco smoke.

Obstructive sleep apnea as defined by an apnea-hypopnea index of 5 or more events/hour is present in approximately half to three-quarters of patients with stroke or TIA. Despite being highly prevalent, as many as 70% to 80% of stroke patients with sleep apnea are neither diagnosed nor treated. A few small randomized controlled trials have shown improved outcome with treatment of obstructive sleep apnea; however, no large trials have been completed. Continuous positive airway pressure therapy and behavioral modifications are the mainstays of treatment for patients diagnosed with sleep-related breathing disorders.

Additional behavioral and lifestyle modifications that may be beneficial for reducing the risk of ischemic stroke include limited alcohol consumption, weight control, regular aerobic physical activity, salt restriction, and a low-fat or Mediterranean diet.

Secondary Prevention
Antiplatelet Therapy

The benefit of antiplatelet therapy for secondary stroke prevention and reduction of risk of other cardiovascular events in patients with a history of noncardioembolic stroke or TIA is well established. The most common antiplatelet agents used are aspirin, clopidogrel, and a combination of dipyridamole and low-dose aspirin.

Aspirin is the oldest and systematically best studied antiplatelet agent. It is available worldwide and inexpensive. It inhibits cyclooxygenase preventing production of thromboxane A_2, a stimulator of platelet aggregation. A meta-analysis published in 2002 by the Antithrombotic Trialists' Collaboration established that patients at high risk for cardiovascular disease treated with antiplatelet agents (primarily aspirin) have a 25% relative risk reduction in nonfatal stroke when compared with placebo. The International Stroke Trial (IST) and Chinese Acute Stroke Trial (CAST) each included ~20,000 subjects and showed that the introduction of aspirin within 48 hours of symptom onset is both safe and effective. This was recently confirmed by a large Cochrane review of aspirin trials. A caveat is patients treated with IV thrombolysis, in which aspirin administration is generally delayed until 24 hours post-tPA. The dose of aspirin used in the different trials varied from 20 to 1300 mg, but most studies have found that 50–325 mg of aspirin daily is as effective as higher doses, with less bleeding complications. In patients unsafe or unable to swallow, rectal or nasogastric administration is appropriate.

Clopidogrel is a thienopyridine that inhibits ADP-dependent platelet aggregation. In the CAPRIE trial (Clopidogrel versus Aspirin in Patients at Risk of Ischemic Events), patients with recent stroke, MI, or peripheral vascular disease were randomly assigned to 75 mg/day of clopidogrel or 325 mg/day of aspirin. The primary endpoint (composite outcome of stroke, MI, or vascular death) was significantly reduced with clopidogrel as compared with aspirin, with a relative risk reduction of 8.7%. However, most of the benefit was observed in the subgroup of patients with peripheral vascular disease. Clopidogrel had a favorable gastric side effect profile when compared with aspirin, but this was offset by an increased risk of rash and diarrhea.

Interestingly, two trials comparing the effect of long-term therapy with **combination of aspirin and clopidogrel** versus either agent alone did not show greater benefit for stroke prevention but rather significantly increased the risk of life-threatening bleeding complications. The MATCH (Management of Atherothrombosis with Clopidogrel in High-Risk Patients) trial compared dual antiplatelet therapy with aspirin and clopidogrel versus clopidogrel alone, while in the CHARISMA (Clopidogrel for High Atherothrombotic Risk and Ischemic Stabilization, Management, and Avoidance) trial, combination therapy was compared with aspirin alone. Finally, in a randomized trial evaluating more 3000 patients with subcortical stroke confirmed by MRI, the Secondary Prevention of Small Subcortical Strokes (SPS3) trial, the arm testing the combination of aspirin plus clopidogrel versus aspirin alone was terminated early because of a higher frequency of hemorrhagic events (mostly gastrointestinal) and a higher all-cause mortality rate.

Dual antiplatelet therapy with aspirin and clopidogrel for secondary stroke prevention therefore fell into disfavor until the recent CHANCE (Clopidogrel in High-Risk Patients with Acute Nondisabling Cerebrovascular Events) trial, which focused on acute secondary prevention. This was a randomized, double-blind, placebo-controlled trial conducted in China to study the efficacy of short-term dual antiplatelet therapy begun within 24 hours of symptom onset in patients with minor stroke (NIHSS score ≤3) or high-risk TIA (ABCD^2 [Age, Blood Pressure, Clinical Features, Duration, Diabetes] score ≥4). Patients received clopidogrel plus aspirin for 21 days followed by clopidogrel alone for 90 days. The primary outcome of recurrent stroke at 90 days (ischemic or hemorrhagic) significantly favored dual antiplatelet therapy over aspirin alone with a hazard ratio of 0.68. A subsequent report of 1-year outcomes found a durable treatment effect, but the HR for secondary stroke prevention was only significantly beneficial in the first 90 days. The recently published POINT trial (Platelet-Oriented Inhibition in New TIA and Minor Ischemic Stroke), which used a higher loading dose of clopidogrel and extended the combination of aspirin and clopidogrel to 90 days (rather than 21 days in the CHANCE trial), broadened the findings of the CHANCE trial of reducing early major ischemic events to more diverse, non-Asian populations, but did again show an increased risk of hemorrhage that remained relatively constant throughout the 90-day trial period.

Despite its benefits on stroke prevention, ticlopidine, another thienopyridine, is rarely used because of its potentially serious side effects of severe neutropenia, which occurs in approximately 1% of patients, and its mandated weekly monitoring of complete blood count for the first months of therapy.

Dipyridamole inhibits platelet aggregation induced by the phosphodiesterase. The combination of low-dose aspirin (50 mg/day) and sustained-release dipyridamole (400 mg/day) for secondary stroke prevention has been shown to be more effective than either drug alone. The relative risk reduction of stroke compared with placebo in the European Stroke Prevention Study (ESPS-2) was 37% for the combination of aspirin and dipyridamole, 18.1% for aspirin monotherapy, and 16.3% for dipyridamole monotherapy when compared with placebo. Bleeding was not significantly increased by dipyridamole, but headache and gastrointestinal symptoms were more common among the combination group. Similar benefits were later reported in the European/Australasian Stroke Prevention in Reversible Ischemia Trial (ESPRIT). The Prevention Regimen for Effectively Avoiding Second Strokes (PROFESS) trial compared clopidogrel with the combination of aspirin and dipyridamole in more than 20,000 patients with recent noncardioembolic ischemic stroke and showed no statistical difference between the groups in the primary outcome of recurrent stroke or the secondary composite endpoint of stroke, MI, or vascular death. Adverse events that led to drug discontinuation were more common among patients assigned to aspirin plus extended-release dipyridamole (16.4% compared with 10.6%) and were mostly on account of headache. Taken together, these trials indicate that the combination is at least as effective as aspirin or clopidogrel alone for secondary stroke prevention but less well tolerated by patients.

Anticoagulants

Warfarin inhibits vitamin K–dependent coagulation factor synthesis (II, VII, IX, X, proteins C and S). Warfarin has a significant benefit compared with placebo for secondary stroke prevention in patients with AF, with an annual stroke rate of 4% in patients receiving warfarin compared with approximately 12% in patients receiving placebo.

According to the WARSS trial, warfarin was not superior to aspirin for prevention of recurrent ischemic strokes or death in patients with prior noncardioembolic ischemic strokes. Most patients in this trial had small vessel disease (56%) or stroke of unclear etiology (26.1%). Warfarin also showed no advantage over aspirin for prevention of ischemic stroke or vascular death in patients with symptomatic intracranial artery stenosis (WASID trial) and was associated with significantly higher rates of adverse events. Anticoagulation with warfarin is indicated for stroke prevention in patients with AF who have valvular heart disease, particularly mechanical valve or moderate-to-severe mitral stenosis. For patients with nonvalvular AF, stratification according to stroke risk following the CHA$_2$DS$_2$-VASc score (congestive heart failure, hypertension, age ≥ 75 years [doubled], diabetes mellitus, prior stroke or TIA or thromboembolism [doubled], vascular disease, age 65–74 years, sex category) is recommended. This risk stratification score assigns 1 point for each risk factor and 2 points for strokes or TIAs and for age 75 or older. Nonvalvular AF patients with CHA$_2$DS$_2$-VASc score of 0–1 have an annual stroke risk of approximately 1%, and aspirin treatment is generally recommended. Among patients with AF at moderate to high risk of thromboembolic events (CHA$_2$DS$_2$-VASc ≥2), warfarin significantly reduces the incidence of stroke at an acceptable risk of bleeding compared with placebo, assuming there are no contraindications. It is generally recommended that the target international normalized ratio (INR) be in the range of 2.0–3.0. Aspirin treatment alone holds modest benefit for stroke prevention in AF and should be considered only in patients who cannot take warfarin or any of the novel anticoagulants.

While warfarin is effective for the prevention of cardioembolic stroke in patients with AF, it has several unique drawbacks. Numerous drug interactions and intrinsic variability from patient to patient result in fluctuating levels of anticoagulation as measured by the INR. Supratherapeutic and subtherapeutic levels are common, leading to an increased risk of bleeding or ischemic stroke, respectively. Patients must submit to regular blood testing and individualized dosing. Dietary restrictions require patients to avoid healthy, leafy vegetables, which may counter the effect of warfarin's vitamin K antagonism.

Several non–vitamin K antagonist oral anticoagulants have therefore been developed in an attempt to provide comparable stroke protection without the limitations that accompany warfarin therapy. These medications directly target the enzymatic activity of thrombin and factor Xa, and are collectively referred to as direct oral anticoagulants (DOACs) or novel oral anticoagulants (NOACs). Twice daily dabigatran is a direct thrombin inhibitor, while once daily rivaroxaban and twice daily apixaban inhibit factor Xa. All three of these medications are FDA approved for the prevention of stroke in patients with nonvalvular AF.

Therapy with a DOAC has a number of advantages, as it requires neither INR monitoring nor vitamin K restriction, substantially increasing convenience and ease of compliance for patients. These drugs have rapid onset and offset of action, so that bridging with parenteral anticoagulant therapy is not needed during initiation or in patients who require interruption of anticoagulation for invasive procedures. All three drugs do, however, require dosage adjustment on the basis of renal function.

Overall, all-cause mortality from DOACs appears to be lower than that from *warfarin*, driven primarily by a decrease in fatal intracranial bleeding. While there is not enough evidence to support the use of DOACs in the acute phase of stroke treatment, these medications are now becoming the preferred choice for most AF patients in whom long-term oral anticoagulant therapy is indicated, as endorsed by the AHA and European Society of Cardiology. As no blinded head-to-head trial comparisons between individual DOACs have been carried out, it is unclear which is superior, if any. One consideration is that intravenous idarucizumab has recently become available as a reversal agent for dabigatran.

Specific Scenarios

The best treatment for stroke prevention in patients with extracranial dissections remains unclear. The 2018 AHA/ASA guidelines recommend the use of either warfarin or antiplatelets for 3–6 months in patients with extracranial vessel dissections. Beyond 3–6 months, long-term antiplatelet is reasonable for most patients, but anticoagulation may be considered for those with recurrent ischemic events.

For patients with ischemic strokes or TIAs and a PFO, antiplatelet therapy is reasonable to prevent recurrent events, but warfarin may be preferable for patients with an underlying hypercoagulable state and for those with high-risk anatomic features such as large PFOs associated with atrial septal aneurysms or a spontaneous right-to-left atrial shunt. Five randomized clinical trials have evaluated mechanical closure of PFO in patients without an obvious stroke etiology, yet they employed variable eligibility criteria, used different closure devices, and had different guidelines for antithrombotic therapy, rendering comparisons difficult. While there is suggestion that patients 60 years or younger with a cryptogenic, nonlacunar ischemic stroke who have a PFO with high-risk features may be reasonable candidates for percutaneous PFO closure, it remains unclear for which subset of patients this procedure provides the most benefit over medical therapy alone. It is strongly recommended that these cases be reviewed by both cardiologists and vascular neurologists prior to any decision in favor of closure.

Surgical Treatment

Carotid endarterectomy (CEA) for prevention of ischemic stroke has been performed since the early 1950s, but it was only in the 1990s that several large-scale trials were completed, comparing this surgery against best medical treatment in patients with ICA stenosis.

For symptomatic patients, evidence from the North American Symptomatic Carotid Endarterectomy Trial (NASCET) and the European Carotid Surgery Trial (ECST) support CEA for severe (70%–99%) symptomatic stenosis over best medical treatment, with a 17% absolute risk reduction and a 65% relative risk reduction of ipsilateral stroke at 2 years. CEA was not indicated for patients with stenosis less than 50%. For the symptomatic patients with stenosis between 50% and 69%, CEA is moderately useful and can be considered in selected patients. There is increasing evidence that specific plaque morphologic features, such as "soft" noncalcific plaque with intraplaque hemorrhage and ulceration, increase the risk of stroke, and CEA may be a treatment option in symptomatic patients with only moderate degrees of ICA stenosis. NASCET showed that in symptomatic patients with stenosis of 50%–69%, the 5-year rate of ipsilateral stroke in the surgical group was 15.7% compared with 22.2% among those treated medically.

For patients with asymptomatic ICA stenosis from 60% to 99%, evidence from the Asymptomatic Carotid Atherosclerosis Study (ACAS) and Asymptomatic Carotid Surgery Trial (ACST) showed a modest benefit favoring CEA, with an absolute risk reduction at 5 years of 5.9% and 5.4%, respectively. The stroke risk reduction was more prominent in men and independent of the degree of stenosis or contralateral disease. Therefore, it is reasonable to consider CEA for asymptomatic stenosis of 60%–99% if the patient has a life expectancy of at least 5 years and if the rate of perioperative stroke or death for the institution or particular surgeon can be reliably kept to less than 3%.

CEA is one of the more common vascular procedures, with rates of perioperative mortality or stroke below 1% being achieved in many centers (Fig. 15.15). A complication rate of less than 3%–5% is thought to ensure overall patient benefit, and most go home 1 or 2 days following

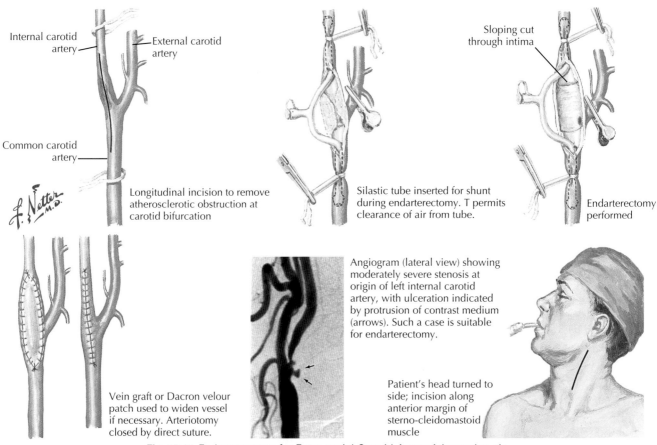

Internal carotid artery

External carotid artery

Common carotid artery

F. Netter M.D.

Longitudinal incision to remove atherosclerotic obstruction at carotid bifurcation

Silastic tube inserted for shunt during endarterectomy. T permits clearance of air from tube.

Sloping cut through intima

Endarterectomy performed

Vein graft or Dacron velour patch used to widen vessel if necessary. Arteriotomy closed by direct suture.

Angiogram (lateral view) showing moderately severe stenosis at origin of left internal carotid artery, with ulceration indicated by protrusion of contrast medium (arrows). Such a case is suitable for endarterectomy.

Patient's head turned to side; incision along anterior margin of sterno-cleidomastoid muscle

Fig. 15.15 Endarterectomy for Extracranial Carotid Artery Atherosclerosis.

surgery. Postoperative cranial neuropathies, cardiac complications, and hyperperfusion syndrome manifested by intracranial hemorrhage and seizures are uncommon complications.

Carotid angioplasty and stenting have emerged as attractive alternatives for patients with symptomatic carotid disease who cannot undergo CEA. Accumulating data suggest that stenting and CEA achieve similar long-term outcomes; however, the periprocedural 30-day stroke and death rates are greater with stenting. Therefore, CEA remains the preferred method assuming patients meet the following conditions: a life expectancy of at least 5 years, a surgically accessible carotid lesion, no prior ipsilateral endarterectomy, and absence of clinically significant cardiac, pulmonary, or other disease that would greatly increase the risk of anesthesia and surgery.

Rehabilitation

Advances in basic and clinical research have shown that the human brain is capable of significant recovery after stroke, provided appropriate rehabilitation treatment is applied. Several new techniques have become available in the past decade, such as task-specific therapy, robotic-assisted rehabilitation, and constraint-induced movement therapy with ongoing studies about their short- and long-term efficacy.

Task-specific therapy is designed to deal with loss of particular abilities and seems to be more efficacious than traditional approaches for patients with motor deficits. Robotic-assisted rehabilitation, especially for the upper extremities, has been shown to reduce even severe motor impairment in stroke patients. Constraint-induced movement therapy, where the unaffected arm is restrained while the paralyzed limb is left to perform intense exercises over 2 consecutive weeks, has shown a statistically and clinically significant improvement in motor arm function as compared with traditional therapy. Persistent benefits up to 2 years have been reported.

ADDITIONAL RESOURCES

Demaerschalk BM, Kleindorfer DO, Adeoye OM, et al. Scientific rationale for the inclusion and exclusion criteria for intravenous alteplase in acute ischemic stroke. A statement for healthcare professionals from the American Heart Association/American Stroke Association. Stroke 2016;47:581–641.

Goyal M, Menon BK, van Zwam WH, et al. Endovascular thrombectomy after large-vessel ischaemic stroke: a meta-analysis of individual patient data from five randomised trials. Lancet 2016;387:1723–31.

Heart Association task force on practice guidelines and the heart rhythm society. Circulation 2014;130:e199–267.

January CT, Wann LS, Alpert JS, et al. 2014 AHA/ACC/HRS guideline for the management of patients with atrial fibrillation. A report of the American College of Cardiology/American Heart Association Task Force on Practice Guidelines and the Heart Rhythm Society. J Am Coll Cardiol 2014;64:e1–76.

Kernan WN, Ovbiagele B, Black HR, et al. Guidelines for the prevention of stroke in patients with stroke and transient ischemic attack. A guideline for healthcare professionals from the American Heart Association/American Stroke Association. Stroke 2014;45:2160–236.

National Institute of Neurological Disorders and Stroke rt-PA Stroke Study Group. Tissue plasminogen activator for acute ischemic stroke. N Engl J Med 1995;333:1581–7.

Powers WJ, Rabinstein AA, Ackerson T, et al. 2018 guidelines for the early management of patients with acute ischemic stroke. A guideline for healthcare professionals from the American Heart Association/American Stroke Association. Stroke 2018;49:e46–110.

16

Intracerebral Hemorrhage

Joseph D. Burns, David P. Lerner, Anil Ramineni

> **CLINICAL VIGNETTE** *A 40-year-old right-handed man with a past medical history significant for hypertension presented to the emergency department (ED) via ambulance with sudden-onset right hemiparesis. He did not take antithrombotic medications. His initial blood pressure was 184/93 mm Hg. The neurologic exam was notable for normal alertness, preserved ability to follow commands with the left limbs, anarthria, normal brainstem reflexes, leftward gaze deviation, and right hemiplegia. Glasgow Coma Scale (GCS) 14, National Institutes of Health Stroke Scale (NIHSS) 19, ICH score 0. The platelet count and INR were normal, and serum and urine toxicology screens were negative. CT (Fig. 16.1) showed a 25 mL left putaminal ICH with no intraventricular hemorrhage and minimal local mass effect and no evidence of culprit macrovascular lesion on computed tomography angiography (CTA). He was treated with a nicardipine infusion to a target systolic blood pressure of 140–160 mm Hg and admitted to the intensive care unit. His 7-day hospitalization was uncomplicated, and on discharge to acute inpatient rehabilitation, his right hemiparesis and aphasia had improved to an NIHSS of 5, although the modified Rankin scale was still 4.*

Intracerebral hemorrhage (ICH) is a type of stroke caused by bleeding directly into brain parenchyma owing to rupture of small arteries and arterioles. It is classified as primary (due to hypertensive or cerebral amyloid angiopathy [CAA]) or secondary (directly related to congenital or acquired microvascular abnormalities, tumors, and other identifiable etiologies). Brain hemorrhages caused by trauma are a distinct entity. ICH is the second most common type of stroke, is often devastating, and no specific treatment for it exists. Although it has been recognized (initially as "apoplexy") phenomenologically since the time of Hippocrates and clinicopathologically since the mid-15th century, more refined understanding of ICH is a much more recent development. Clinically meaningful understanding of ICH began in the mid-20th century with the recognition, based on clinicopathologic correlation and epidemiologic work, of hypertension as a major risk factor. Beginning in the mid-1970s, the introduction of computed tomography (CT) and magnetic resonance imaging (MRI) (and, more recently, CT- and MRI-based angiography) to routine clinical practice allowed for accurate premortem distinction between ischemic stroke and ICH as the cause of stroke syndromes in individual patients, differentiation of primary ICH from secondary etiologies, correlation between hemorrhage size and location and clinical presentation and prognosis, and better understanding of the dynamic nature of hematoma and perihematomal edema (PHE) formation and growth. Deeper understanding of the pathophysiology of ICH at the physiologic, cellular, and molecular levels is advancing, but remains an ongoing endeavor. The recent proliferation of clinical trials of treatments for ICH provides reason for optimism about the future of this condition despite the fact that a "magic bullet" specific treatment remains elusive.

This chapter will focus on the epidemiology, pathophysiology, diagnosis, management, and prognosis of primary ICH. Secondary causes of ICH are discussed elsewhere in this book. Despite the lack of an effective specific treatment, a solid understanding of primary ICH can allow the clinician to limit its negative impact. Prompt diagnosis and skillful care of ICH patients based on knowledge about clinical presentation and diagnosis, pathophysiology, natural history, and empiric data regarding the utility or harm of supportive treatments can have an important influence on outcome. Finally, confident prognostication, including an appreciation of its often uncertain nature, is crucial for optimal care of ICH patients and their loved ones.

ETIOLOGY

Primary Intracerebral Hemorrhage

Primary ICH is the end result of chronic damage to cerebral small arteries and arterioles caused by either chronic hypertension (hypertensive arteriopathy, Figs. 16.1 and 16.2) or β-amyloid deposition (CAA, Fig. 16.3). The location of the hemorrhage is largely determined by the underlying vascular pathology: hypertensive arteriopathy typically causes deep hemorrhages, while CAA more typically causes superficial hemorrhages.

Cerebral arterioles are important resistance vessels, playing a crucial role in reducing blood pressure and pulse pressure in the microvasculature of the brain. The perforating arterioles at the base of the brain that arise directly from the major cerebral arteries (in the basal ganglia, internal capsule, deep lobar white matter, thalamus, cerebellum, and pons) are therefore selectively vulnerable to the stress of chronic hypertension. This hemodynamic stress leads initially to smooth muscle hyperplasia, followed by smooth muscle cell death, and culminates in arteriolar lipohyalinosis, in which the media of the affected arterioles is devoid of smooth muscle cells and consists largely of fibrotic material. Such changes render these vessels noncompliant, fragile, and thus susceptible to rupture. While microaneurysms (Charcot-Bouchard) are a typical feature of this disease, they have not clearly been established as the proximate cause of rupture.

The central feature of the pathophysiology of CAA is deposition of β-amyloid in the media and adventitia of superficial capillaries and arterioles of the cortex and leptomeninges, particularly but not exclusively in the occipital lobes. There are multiple mechanisms by which β-amyloid, likely derived from neurons, is cleared from the interstitial fluid of the brain: active transport into the circulation through capillaries, degradation by enzymes in the interstitium as well as within astrocytes and microglia, and bulk flow along the perivascular pathways that drain fluid from the brain. With age, bulk flow becomes the predominant clearance route and amounts of β-amyloid in the perivascular space increase, leading to accumulation within the walls of capillaries and small arterioles. This accumulated mural β-amyloid causes impaired vascular

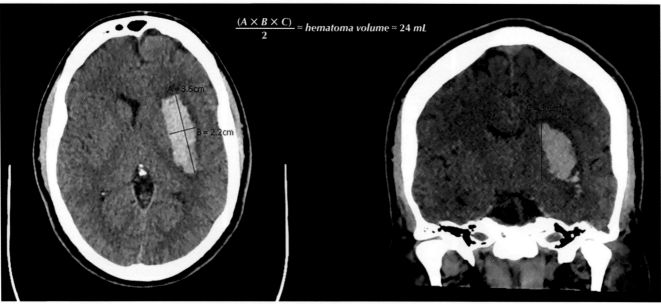

$$\frac{(A \times B \times C)}{2} \approx hematoma\ volume \approx 24\ mL$$

Fig. 16.1 CT Images of a Typical Hypertensive Putaminal Intracerebral Hemorrhage. The ABC/2 method of estimating the hematoma volume is shown. First, the axial slice in which the hematoma area is largest is identified. *A* is defined as the longest dimension of the hematoma in this slice. *B* is the longest line through the hematoma that is perpendicular to *A*. *C* is the rostrocaudal extent of the hematoma and can be determined by multiplying the number of axial slices on which the hematoma appears by the slice thickness or, as shown here, directly on the coronal reconstruction.

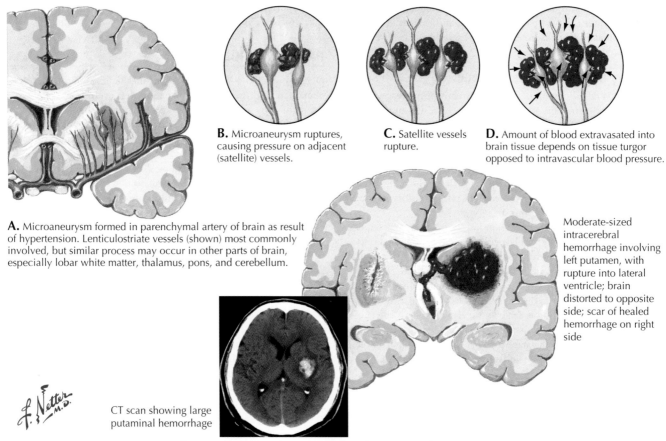

B. Microaneurysm ruptures, causing pressure on adjacent (satellite) vessels.

C. Satellite vessels rupture.

D. Amount of blood extravasated into brain tissue depends on tissue turgor opposed to intravascular blood pressure.

A. Microaneurysm formed in parenchymal artery of brain as result of hypertension. Lenticulostriate vessels (shown) most commonly involved, but similar process may occur in other parts of brain, especially lobar white matter, thalamus, pons, and cerebellum.

Moderate-sized intracerebral hemorrhage involving left putamen, with rupture into lateral ventricle; brain distorted to opposite side; scar of healed hemorrhage on right side

CT scan showing large putaminal hemorrhage

Fig. 16.2 Hypertensive Intracerebral Hemorrhage: Pathogenesis.

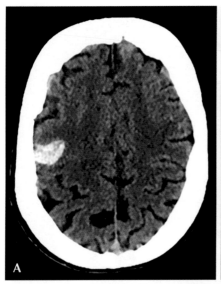
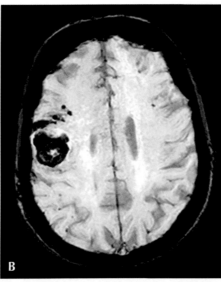
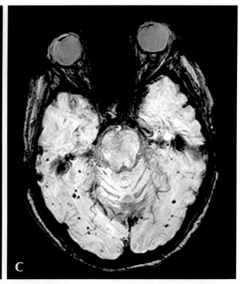

Fig. 16.3 Typical CT (A) and susceptibility-weighted MR imaging (B and C) of intracerebral hemorrhage (ICH) due to probable cerebral amyloid angiopathy. There is a right frontal cortico-subcortical hematoma with overlying subarachnoid hemorrhage (A and B), as well as numerous, predominantly cortico-subcortical micro-hemorrhages (hypointense dots) in both the region of the ICH (B) and the posterior regions of the cerebral hemispheres (C).

reactivity and inflammation, which in turn cause microvascular injury consisting of loss of smooth muscle cells, wall thickening, concentric splitting of the vessel wall, wall weakening, and ultimately hemorrhage.

In both hypertensive vasculopathy and CAA, the pathologic changes in the vessel walls not only make hemorrhage more likely to occur, but they also impair vessels' response to hemorrhage. Loss of smooth muscle in the media in both conditions leaves the affected arterioles less able to mount the vasospastic response that forms an important part of the initial hemostatic process, thereby exacerbating hemorrhages once they occur.

Secondary Intracerebral Hemorrhage

Secondary ICH refers to nontraumatic intracerebral hemorrhage caused by an identifiable etiology other than hypertensive vasculopathy or CAA. A number of macrovascular lesions (those discernable on brain or vessel imaging), detailed in other chapters, can lead to ICH, as can multiple other conditions (Box 16.1, Fig. 16.4). Although such hemorrhages may have distinctive clinical and radiographic features, there is often little to distinguish them from primary ICH in the initial evaluation, and the cause is only uncovered by a proper history, physical examination, lab, and imaging investigation.

The roles played by acute hypertension and coagulopathy are complex and deserve special consideration. Hypertension most commonly causes ICH through its chronic deleterious effects on deep cerebral arterioles, as detailed previously. And although many patients with ICH present with acute, severe hypertension, this is thought to be more of an effect of the hemorrhage's injury to the brain than a cause of the hemorrhage. However, when hypertension is acute and severe enough, it can cause ICH in the absence of other causes. It is possible, therefore, that while chronic hypertension sets the stage for ICH by weakening arterioles, acute hypertension can be a more proximate cause of ICH by exploiting underlying arteriolar weakness from any cause. Coagulopathy probably contributes to ICH by making any bleeding that occurs worse. There is normally no spontaneous bleeding in the brain despite the fact that, as in other organs, the endothelium of the microcirculation is disrupted from time to time because such disruptions are normally promptly repaired by an intact coagulation system. However, such breaches can become symptomatic hemorrhages in the presence of a coagulopathy, and breaches are more likely to occur when there is an underlying vasculopathy. Accordingly, the likelihood that symptomatic cerebral bleeding will occur in the setting of coagulopathy depends on the combined severity of the coagulopathy and vasculopathy. Whereas a young, healthy person may not sustain ICH, even in the setting of severe DIC, comparatively much milder therapeutic anticoagulation with warfarin may provoke symptomatic hemorrhage in a patient with CAA.

PATHOPHYSIOLOGY

Once considered a simple process of mechanical brain injury due to hematoma and then edema formation that evolved over a few days, the manner by which ICH causes brain injury has more recently been shown to be more complex, consisting of numerous biologic processes that develop over at least a week (Fig. 16.5). Accordingly, from both mechanistic and temporal perspectives, contemporary knowledge of ICH pathophysiology has revealed multiple distinct potential treatment targets.

ICH first injures the brain due to dissection of the hemorrhage along white matter tissue planes, creating a mixture of blood and isolated regions of intact brain tissue. Importantly, bleeding is typically not a monophasic process. Hematoma expansion occurs to some extent in more than 70% of patients in the first 24 hours after symptom onset, with about one-third of patients experiencing significant hematoma growth of at least 33% of the initial volume. The likelihood of hematoma growth declines rapidly with time elapsed after symptom onset such that most expansion occurs within the first 6 hours, and expansion is rare after 24 hours in noncoagulopathic patients. Expansion is highly consequential, with just a 10% increase in hematoma volume over baseline conferring significant increase in the risk of death and worse disability. Although hematoma expansion has been shown to be more likely in patients with untreated coagulopathy, more severe acute hypertension, and higher initial hematoma volume, the mechanism by which it occurs is unknown. Specifically, whether expansion occurs due to continued bleeding from the vessel that ruptured initially, an "avalanche" of progressive rupture of neighboring vessels due to mechanical disruption from the mass effect of the growing hematoma (as initially

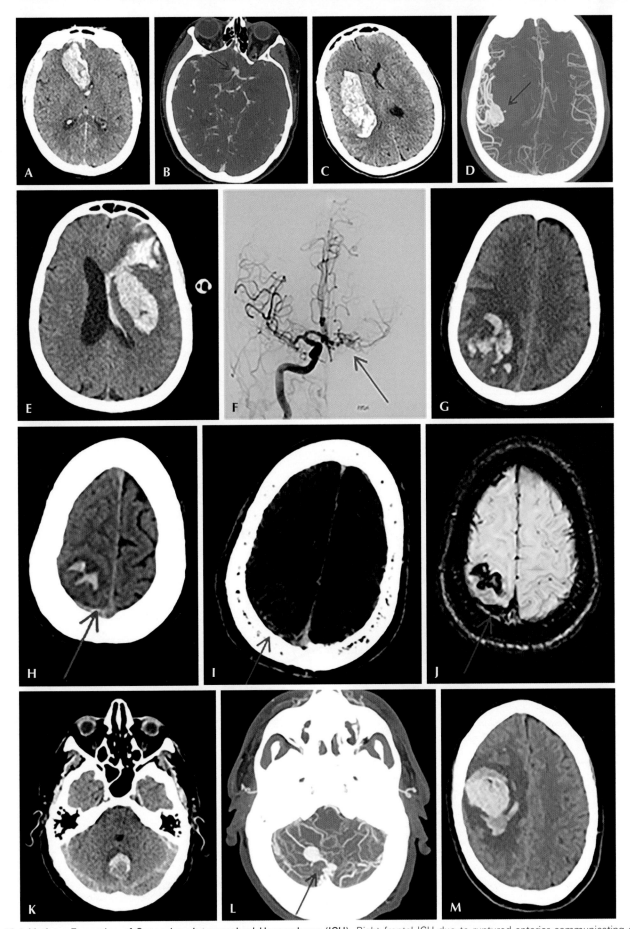

Fig. 16.4 Various Examples of Secondary Intracerebral Hemorrhage (ICH). Right frontal ICH due to ruptured anterior communicating artery aneurysm (A and B; *arrow* is showing the anterior communicating aneurysm). Right deep insular/putaminal ICH due to ruptured AVM (C and D; *arrow* is showing the AVM). L basal ganglia ICH with intraventricular hemorrhage caused by left internal carotid artery (ICA) moyamoya syndrome (E and F; *arrow* is showing the LICA Moyamoya syndrome). Right frontoparietal ICH (G) due to right vein of Trolard thrombosis visible as hyperdense vein on CT (H), filling defect in vein (I), and susceptibility artifact on susceptibility-weighted MRI (J; *arrow* is showing the right vein of Trolard thrombosis). Vermian ICH due to dural arteriovenous (AV) fistula (K and L; *arrow* is showing the dural AV fistula). R frontal ICH due to hemorrhagic metastasis from renal cell carcinoma (M). Note the significant perihematomal edema apparent just 1 hour after symptom onset.

BOX 16.1   Causes of Secondary Intracerebral Hemorrhage[a]

Macrovascular lesions
- Arteriovenous malformation
- Saccular aneurysm
- Cavernous malformation
- Dural arteriovenous fistula
- Intracranial artery dissection +/− pseudoaneurysm
- Moyamoya syndrome and disease

Hemorrhagic transformation of infarct
- Bland
- Septic embolic (endocarditis)
- Posterior reversible encephalopathy syndrome
- Reversible cerebral vasoconstriction syndrome

Intracranial neoplasm
- Primary
  - Glioblastoma multiforme
  - Oligodendroglioma
  - Meningioma
- Metastatic
  - Lung
  - Melanoma
  - Breast
  - Renal cell

Intracranial venous thrombosis
- Cerebral venous sinus thrombosis
- Cortical vein thrombosis

Sudden severe hypertension[b]
- Sympathomimetic drugs (cocaine, amphetamines)
- Pheochromocytoma

Coagulopathy[b]
- Anticoagulant therapy
- Liver disease
- Diffuse intravascular coagulation (DIC)
- Immune thrombocytopenic purpura
- Thrombotic thrombocytopenic purpura
- Congenital bleeding diatheses

Vasculitis
- Infectious
- Primary central nervous system
- Systemic vasculitis

Intravascular lymphoma

[a]Major categories are presented in approximate order of decreasing frequency.
[b]Hypertension and coagulopathy are rarely the sole cause of intracerebral hemorrhage and most often contribute by exacerbating other, more common etiologies.

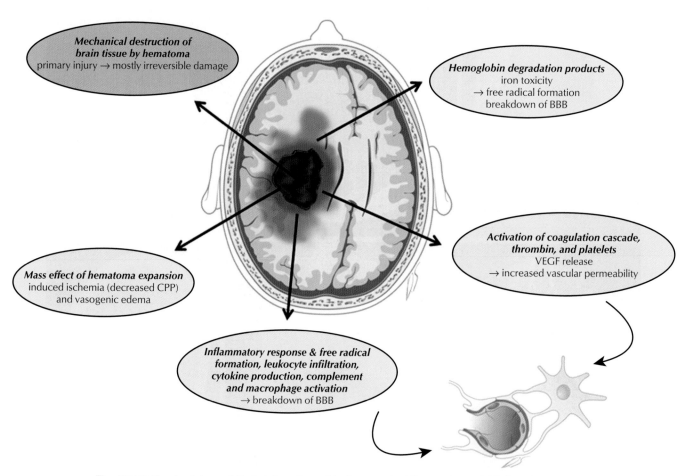

Fig. 16.5 Pathophysiology of Brain Injury Caused by Intracerebral Hemorrhage. *BBB,* Brain blood barrier; *CPP,* cerebral perfusion pressure; *VEGF,* vascular endothelial growth factor. (Reused with permission from Kim H, Edwards NJ, Choi HA, Chang TR, Jo KW, Lee K. Treatment strategies to attenuate perihematomal edema in patients with intracerebral hemorrhage. *World Neurosurg.* 2016;94:32-41. Fig. 1, p. 33.)

proposed by Fisher), some other mechanism, or a combination of these is unknown.

PHE begins to form within minutes after a hemorrhage occurs and expands most rapidly in the first 48 hours, thereafter growing more slowly until reaching its peak 7–14 days after symptom onset, and rarely may continue to progress in a delayed manner. PHE that develops over the first few hours is largely the result of clot organization and retraction—the center of the hematoma contracts and becomes concentrated clot. This leads to accumulation of serum proteins in the interstitium of the brain surrounding the hematoma, which serve as effective osmoles drawing water across the still intact blood-brain barrier (BBB). Thereafter, PHE forms because of disruption of the BBB caused by inflammation. In the first few days, this inflammation is primarily driven by thrombin and complement. Hemoglobin and the products of its degradation (heme, iron, and bilirubin), derived from the lysis of red blood cells within the clot that typically occurs several days after the initial bleeding, probably cause the latest phases of edema formation. Matrix metalloproteinases play a key role in increasing BBB permeability. Glutamate-mediated excitotoxicity, mitochondrial dysfunction, and neuronal apoptosis also contribute to secondary injury in the PHE region. Higher absolute amounts and faster rates of PHE growth in the first 24–72 hours are associated with delayed neurologic deterioration, increased mortality, and worse functional outcomes. The clinical significance of delayed PHE growth is uncertain overall, but a subset of patients, not identifiable *a priori,* can have late delayed deterioration from this process many days after the hemorrhage began.

Perihematomal ischemia is not as important in the pathophysiology of ICH-induced brain injury as once thought. Cerebral blood flow (CBF) is reduced in the perihematomal region, as well as diffusely in the hemisphere ipsilateral to an ICH in the acute setting, and normalizes over 3–7 days. However, studies using PET CT and CT perfusion have shown that despite reduced blood flow, these areas of oligemia are not ischemic due to decreased metabolic rate and therefore decreased oxygen extraction that occurs in perihematomal brain regions.

EPIDEMIOLOGY

ICH is a common and devastating disease. In the United States and other high income countries ICH composes approximately 10% of all strokes, whereas this figure is 20% in low-middle income countries. Worldwide, the incidence rate of ICH has been estimated to be approximately 25 per 100,000 person-years. Thus approximately 1.9 million incident ICHs occur worldwide each year, 80,000 of them in the United States. While the worldwide incidence rate for ICH has not significantly changed since early estimates from the 1980s, some studies indicate a modest decrease in high income countries.

Box 16.2 lists the most important risk factors for ICH. Interestingly, despite the fact that warfarin anticoagulation nearly triples the risk of ICH, antiplatelet therapy (including dual antiplatelet therapy) confers only a very small risk, if any. Also of note is that while hypertension remains the most important risk factor associated with ICH, due to effective treatment across populations its primacy as an etiology is waning. This, combined with an aging population and increasing use of anticoagulants, has led to CAA and anticoagulation assuming more prominence as risk factors. Although some data suggest a small increased risk of ICH conferred by statin therapy, contradicting data exist, making the effect of statins on ICH risk uncertain.

ICH is frequently fatal, and survivors often have poor functional outcomes. One-month case fatality worldwide has been estimated to be 40%, nearly twice that of ischemic stroke. At 1 year after ICH, mortality is approximately 55%, and at 5 years it is 70%. Importantly, these rates have not changed since they were first measured in the 1980s. The

---

BOX 16.2   Risk Factors for Intracerebral Hemorrhage

Modifiable
- Hypertension
- Coagulopathy
  - Therapeutic anticoagulation
  - Liver disease
  - Antiplatelet therapy
- Smoking
- Heavy alcohol use

Nonmodifiable
- Cerebral amyloid angiopathy
- Increasing age
- Asian race
- Male sex
- Lower socioeconomic status
- History of stroke

---

probability of functional independence (modified Rankin Scale 0–2) at 1 year has been estimated to be only 17%–25% for all ICH patients, or approximately 55% when considering only survivors.

CLINICAL PRESENTATION

ICH is a type of stroke, and its clinical presentation holds true to this definition. The most prominent and invariable feature of the presentation of ICH is the sudden onset of neurologic deficits referable to the location of the hemorrhage. Unlike ischemic stroke, however, the early pathophysiology involves more than just focal brain injury. Globally increased intracranial pressure, tissue shifts, and meningeal and ependymal irritation due to hematoma dissection into (respectively) the subarachnoid and intraventricular spaces lead to somewhat distinctive general features of the presentation of ICH beyond focal neurologic dysfunction.

General Signs and Symptoms

Headache is a frequent feature of the early course of ICH, occurring in about a third of patients soon after presentation. It may be more common in patients with cerebellar and lobar hematomas compared with deep hematoma locations. Few features specific to ICH-related headache have been found, although putaminal hemorrhages tend to cause ipsilateral frontal headaches, cerebellar hemorrhages typically cause occipital headaches, and occipital lobar ICH has been associated with ipsilateral occipital and periorbital headache. About 5% of ICH patients experience *seizures* within 24 hours of presentation, with lobar hematoma location serving as a strong risk factor. *Vomiting* is a common feature of both hemorrhage and ischemia in the brainstem and cerebellum. However, when the lesion is supratentorial, vomiting is far more common in ICH than in ischemic stroke. *Depressed level of consciousness* is more common in all-comers with ICH than with acute ischemic stroke and results from globally increased ICP (large hemorrhages, intraventricular hemorrhage [IVH] with hydrocephalus), direct involvement of the reticular activating system in the brainstem or thalamus by the hemorrhage, or indirect involvement of these structures by way of tissue shifts caused by hematomas in the cerebellum or deep supratentorial regions. Finally, ICH is more likely to present with *deficits that gradually progress after onset,* typically over the course of minutes to an hour, than ischemic stroke. Importantly, while these general signs and symptoms are more common in ICH than in ischemic stroke, they are not, neither alone nor in combination, nearly sufficient enough to truly distinguish between these two very different conditions—brain imaging is required for this.

Deep Supratentorial Hemorrhages

Hemorrhages of the deep gray nuclei and surrounding white matter tracts in the supratentorial region compose about 50% of all primary ICHs. Located in regions of the brain where structures subserving many functions lie close together, these hemorrhages frequently cause clinical syndromes with severity disproportionate to their size. Furthermore, deep hemorrhages occur close to the ventricles, making IVH a frequent complication and introducing its clinical features to the presenting syndrome, which often dominate the initial clinical picture. Detailed comparison of the clinical presentation of ICH in each of the major deep supratentorial locations is presented in Fig. 16.6.

Location	Pathology (ruptured arteries)	CT scan	LOC	Pupils	Eye movements	Motor	Sensory	Other
Putamen	Lenticulostriates, medial and/or lateral	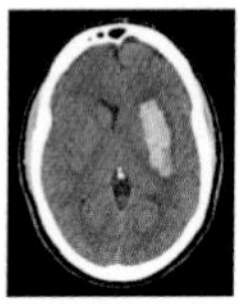	Normal (small-medium hematoma) Decreased (large hematoma, IVH)	Normal (small-medium hematoma) Ipsilateral dilated and poorly reactive (if associated transtentorial herniation) Ipsilateral midposition and reactive (if extension into thalamus/mid brain extension)	Normal (most often) Contralateral conjugate supranuclear gaze palsy (severity proportionate to size of hematoma)	Contralateral hemiparesis (severity proportionate to size of hematoma and degree of involvement of internal capsule)	Contralateral hemi-sensory loss sparing the trunk, typically milder than motor deficits (severity proportionate to size of hematoma)	Aphasia (dominant) Contralateral hemineglect (nondominant) Contralateral homonymous hemianopia (large hematomas only)
Thalamus	Posteromedial = Thalamoperforator Posterolateral = Thalamogeniculate Dorsal = posterior choroidal branches Anterior = tuberothalamic branches	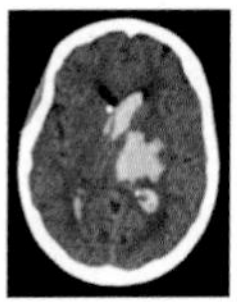	Normal (small-medium hematoma) Decreased (large hematoma, IVH, extension to midbrain)	Normal Ipsilateral > contralateral miosis and poorly reactive	Contralateral conjugate supranuclear gaze palsy Paresis of upgaze Bilateral esotropia ("pseudo-sixth nerve palsy") Ipsilateral conjugate supranuclear gaze palsy ("wrong-way eyes") Skew deviation	Contralateral hemiparesis Contralateral hemiasterixis Contralateral ataxic hemiparesis (small posterolateral hematomas)	Contralateral hemihypesthesia involving face, limbs, and trunk	Aphasia (dominant, especially posterolateral, posterior dorsal) Contralateral hemineglect (nondominant, especially posterolateral) Abulia (anterior) Amnesia (anterior, posteromedial, posterior dorsal)
Caudate	(Lenticulostriates, medial; branches of Heubner's artery)	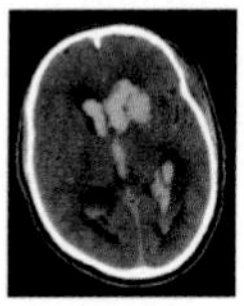	Normal to mildly decreased Decreased (IVH)	Normal	Normal (most often). Occasional contralateral conjugate supranuclear gaze palsy	Normal (most often) Occasional contralateral hemiparesis (if extension into internal capsule)	Normal (most often) Occasional sensory symptoms without abnormality on exam	Prominent neuropsychological abnormalities: abulia, confusion, disorientation, amnesia Aphasia (dominant, infrequent) Hemi-inattention (nondominant, infrequent)

Fig. 16.6 Clinical Presentation of Deep Supratentorial Intracerebral Hemorrhage by Anatomic Location.
IVH, Intraventricular hemorrhage; *LOC,* loss of consciousness.

Hemorrhages into the *putamen,* caused by rupture of the lenticulostriate arteries, are the most common type of deep supratentorial hemorrhage. Depending upon their size and precise location, they cause a syndrome of hemispheric dysfunction in which motor findings are more apparent than sensory abnormalities. Other abnormalities such as aphasia (dominant hemisphere), hemineglect (nondominant hemisphere), supranuclear horizontal gaze palsy, and visual field defects may be present in various degrees of severity.

Thalamic hemorrhages adjusted for volume are the most devastating of all supratentorial hemorrhages due to the centrality of the thalamus in consciousness and the major functions of the overlying hemisphere. As with putaminal hemorrhages, the clinical syndrome depends on the size and precise location within the thalamus. However, certain clinical features are fairly consistently shared among most thalamic hemorrhages, especially contralateral hemiparesis (due to involvement of the adjacent posterior limb of the internal capsule). Hemisensory loss is also frequently present, with a characteristic pattern that is highly specific to thalamic lesions: hypesthesia for pinprick and temperature more than touch involving the contralateral *trunk,* as well as the face and limbs. Ophthalmologic abnormalities, while less consistent than the sensory and motor findings, are also frequently present. Small to mid-position, poorly reactive pupils, either ipsilateral to the hemorrhage or bilateral, are common. The most common eye movement abnormality is a contralateral supranuclear gaze palsy producing conjugate deviation of the eyes toward the side of the hemorrhage. The opposite abnormality infrequently occurs, called "wrong-way eyes," in which dysfunction of already-crossed descending tracts connecting cortical and pontine centers of horizontal gaze cause conjugate horizontal gaze deviation *away* from the side of the hemorrhage. A combination of convergence and gaze depression is also characteristic.

Hemorrhage into the head of the *caudate* nucleus is the least common of the deep supratentorial hemorrhages. Because IVH occurs so frequently with hemorrhages in this location and the associated focal neurologic abnormalities can be subtle, general features such as headache, vomiting, and decreased level of consciousness tend to dominate the clinical syndrome. The most prominent and consistent focal features of caudate hemorrhage are neuropsychological abnormalities, including abulia, confusion, disorientation, and amnesia. Abulia must be parsed carefully from depressed consciousness, as the latter is indicative of concerning complications such as acute hydrocephalus due to IVH. Features more typical of putaminal and thalamic hemorrhages, such as hemiparesis, hemisensory dysfunction (typically subjective without corresponding abnormalities on exam), contralateral supranuclear gaze palsy, aphasia, and hemi-inattention, may variably be present but tend to be less severe.

Lobar Hemorrhages

Lobar hemorrhage is the second most common location for ICH. Headache, vomiting, and seizures are common, while depressed level of consciousness is seen only in patients with hemorrhages of size and location sufficient to cause displacement of the mesencephalic-diencephalic junction. Focal neurologic dysfunction depends on the precise location of the hemorrhage and is detailed in Fig. 16.7.

Cerebellar Hemorrhages

Hemorrhage into the cerebellum (Fig. 16.8C and D) usually begins and is centered in the region of the *dentate nucleus* and has a hypertensive etiology. Patients typically complain of ataxia and vertigo that lead to an inability to stand or walk. Headache (typically occipital), vomiting, and dysarthria are common. The neurologic examination usually reveals limb ataxia without true weakness ipsilateral to the hemorrhage. If the hematoma is large enough to compress the anteriorly adjacent pontine

tegmentum, ipsilateral abducens and facial nerve palsies and Horner syndrome may occur as very worrisome signs. IVH into the adjacent fourth ventricle is another common and serious complication that can cause hydrocephalus that occurs either very early or in delayed fashion up to days after ictus. In such cases, patients will have a depressed level of consciousness. ICH can also infrequently occur in the *vermis.* These hemorrhages typically extend into the fourth ventricle and pontine tegmentum, and their clinical presentation is very similar to that of a primary pontine hemorrhage (as discussed later).

Brainstem Hemorrhages

Hemorrhages into the brainstem compose only about 5% of all ICHs, but they are very frequently devastating. As in the thalamus, multiple critical neural structures subserving numerous crucial functions are contained within a very small space in the brainstem, making the precise anatomy of a patient's hemorrhage crucial for determination of the presenting clinical syndrome and prognosis.

Pontine hemorrhages compose at least 75% of all brainstem ICHs and are typically divided into paramedian, basal/basotegmental, and lateral tegmental subtypes based on anatomy and functional significance. *Paramedian pontine hemorrhages* (Fig. 16.9A) tend to be the largest pontine ICHs and, adjusted for volume, are the most devastating form of ICH. They occur due to rupture of the distal-most portion of a basilar artery-derived paramedian perforating artery near the junction of the basis pontis and tegmentum, and expand in both the anterior-posterior plane and often more extensively along white matter tracts in the rostrocaudal plane. The clinical presentation typically begins with occipital headache, vomiting, numbness, or weakness involving the face and limbs on one or both sides of the body, dysarthria, or diplopia, but frequently evolves rapidly to coma with pinpoint pupils, complete horizontal ophthalmoplegia (including absent vestibulo-ocular reflex movements), and extensor posturing. Convulsive movements, as seen in the "brainstem fits" of acute basilar artery occlusions, as well as shivering can occur and may be mistaken for seizure. Finally, autonomic dysregulation can be prominent and severe, with hyperthermia being the most common manifestation. *Basal and basotegmental pontine hemorrhages* (see Fig. 16.9B) are similar in location to paramedian hemorrhages, but are smaller and frequently unilateral. As such, their clinical manifestations tend to be more focal, the most common of which is ataxic hemiparesis. *Lateral tegmental pontine hemorrhages* are caused by rupture of penetrating arteries derived from the long circumferential arteries. These hemorrhages are typically small and confined to one side of the lateral tegmentum, producing predominantly oculomotor abnormalities such as abducens palsy, complete ipsilateral horizontal gaze palsy, or ipsilateral "one-and-a-half syndrome." Ataxia, dysarthria, contralateral face and body sensory loss, and ipsilateral miosis are also common. When these hemorrhages uncommonly expand to involve the tegmentum bilaterally, including the reticular activating system, the results can be devastating with coma dominating the clinical picture.

Midbrain ICH (see Fig. 16.9C) is uncommon and, when present, usually occurs as an extension of far more common primary thalamic or pontine primary ICH. ICH confined to the midbrain is often caused by an underlying arteriovenous malformation (AVM), cavernous malformation, or a related to bleeding diathesis. Primary hypertensive midbrain ICH is uncommon. Typical clinical manifestations include dysfunction of the ipsilateral oculomotor nerve (partial or complete), ipsilateral ataxia, and contralateral hemiparesis. When the dorsal portion of the midbrain is involved, various features of the dorsal midbrain syndrome (vertical gaze palsy, light-near dissociation of pupillary reactivity, and convergence-retraction nystagmus) are present.

The *medulla* is the least common location for ICH (see Fig. 16.9D) and, like hemorrhages into the midbrain, are more often secondary to

Location	CT scan	Aphasia/ Hemi-neglect	Motor	Sensory	Visual	Eye Movements	Headache	Other
Frontal	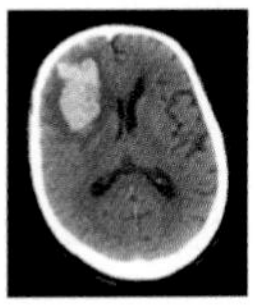	Less frequent, relatively mild	Prominent Superior: leg > face, arm weakness Inferior: face, arm > leg paresis	Variable cortical sensory loss, more prominent with inferior and posterior hemorrhages	None	Contralateral supranuclear gaze palsy	Bifrontal, worse ipsilateral to hemorrhage	Abulia, frontal release signs with anterior hemorrhages
Temporal	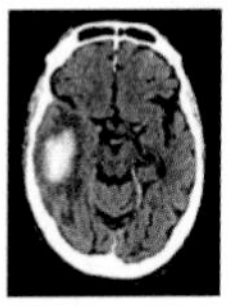	Prominent Dominant hemisphere: Wernicke aphasia prominent Non-dominant: confusion, often with agitated delirium; hemi-neglect uncommon	Infrequent hemiparesis	Infrequent pinprick hypesthesia in the limbs	Common Hemianopia or superior quadrantanopia	Normal	Ipsilateral temporal, periorbital	Transtentorial herniation more common than in other lobar hemorrhage locations due to proximity to the mesencephalic -diencephalic junction
Parietal	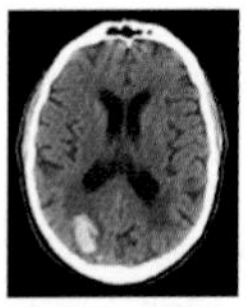	Common Dominant: aphasia Non-dominant: hemi-neglect	Common Hemiparesis of variable severity	Prominent Hypesthesia of limbs and trunk in all modalities	Common Hemianopia or inferior quadrantanopia	Contralateral supranuclear gaze palsy	Ipsilateral temporal	Depressed level of consciousness and other signs of Transtentorial herniation possible with inferomedial hemorrhages
Occipital	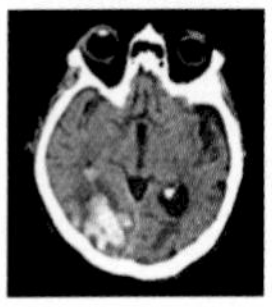	Infrequent Dominant: dyslexia, dysgraphia, alexia without agraphia Non-dominant: anosognosia for visual deficits	None	Infrequent tactile extinction	Prominent "Blurred' vision Homonymous hemianopia	Normal	Prominent Ipsilateral periorbital	Lateral hematomas can present with headache without focal abnormalities

Fig. 16.7 Clinical Features of Lobar Intracerebral Hemorrhage. *IVH,* Intraventricular hemorrhage.

local AVM, cavernous malformation, or a bleeding diathesis. Clinically, medullary ICH can be differentiated from medullary infarction on the basis of having clinical features of both medial and lateral medullary infarct syndromes: hypoglossal nerve palsy, limb weakness (ipsilateral, contralateral, or both, depending on the extent and location of the hemorrhage in relation to the decussation of the corticospinal tract), vertigo, nystagmus, ataxia, dysphonia, dysphagia, dysarthria, and ipsilateral Horner syndrome.

Intraventricular Hemorrhage

IVH that occurs without ICH is relatively uncommon, comprising 3%–9% of all cases of spontaneous intracerebral hemorrhage. While such *"primary"* IVH can be due to hypertensive arteriopathy, bleeding due to an underlying macrovascular lesion is more likely, and its occurrence should prompt a search for lesions such as aneurysm, AVM, or moyamoya disease/syndrome. *Secondary IVH* occurs when a hematoma that begins in the brain parenchyma ruptures into the relatively

low-pressure ventricular system. This is common, occurring in 35%–45% of patients with primary ICH. It is more common when the site of bleeding is adjacent to the ventricles or when the hematoma is large. Once in the ventricles, blood causes inflammation, fibrosis, hydrocephalus, and increased intracranial pressure, and these effects are directly proportional to the amount of intraventricular blood. Through these mechanisms, IVH substantially increases the mortality and decreases the likelihood of a good functional outcome.

DIAGNOSTIC EVALUATION

CLINICAL VIGNETTE *A 64-year-old right-handed woman with a past medical history of hypertension presented to the ED via EMS due to an acute headache and decrease in level of alertness that began 45 minutes prior to arrival while she was eating dinner. According to her dining companion, she*

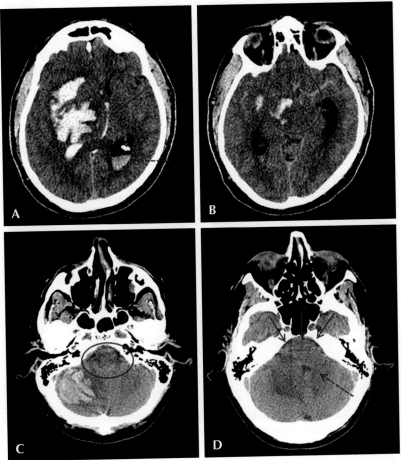

Fig. 16.8 Structural complications from thalamic (A and B) and cerebellar (C and D) intracerebral hemorrhages on CT. Panel A shows a large right thalamic hemorrhage with significant leftward shift of the third ventricle and IVH *(solid arrow)*, as well as trapping with hydrocephalus of the left lateral ventricle *(dashed arrow)*. Panel B shows severe effacement of the perimesencephalic cisterns and significant compression of the rostral midbrain *(Circle is showing the effacement of the perimesencephalic cisterns and compression of rostral midbrain.)*. Panel C demonstrates a large hematoma in the inferior R cerebellar hemisphere with effacement of the perimedullary cisterns *(Oval shape is showing the effacement of the perimedullary cisterns.)*. Slightly more rostrally there is compression and shift of the fourth ventricle (Panel D, *dashed arrow*) and effacement of the prepontine cistern (Panel D, *solid arrows*).

suddenly complained of a very severe headache and then became confused and poorly responsive. EMS arrived 10 minutes later and found the patient to be having a seizure: she was turning her head to the left and her right arm was rigidly extended for about 90 seconds, after which she vomited. She did not take antithrombotic medications. The blood pressure was 175/100 mm Hg. On arrival to the ED, the blood pressure was 170/95 and the neurologic exam showed that she only momentarily opened her eyes in response to a loud voice, followed simple axial and right limb commands inconsistently, normal brainstem reflexes, and severe left arm and leg weakness without facial weakness. GCS 8, NIHSS 20. Labs were notable for normal platelet count and INR, and negative serum and urine toxicology screens. CT head (image) showed a 60 mL right parasagittal inferior frontal ICH with significant IVH. Due to the history of thunderclap headache and characteristic hemorrhage appearance, a ruptured aneurysm of the anterior communicating artery was strongly suspected. CTA was immediately performed (image) and confirmed this diagnosis.

The diagnostic evaluation in patients with ICH (Box 16.3) has four main aims:

1. Identification of immediately life-threatening complications
2. Identification of ICH, as opposed to some other disease process, as the cause of the patient's clinical syndrome
3. Evaluation for the presence or risk of the development of complications, such as hematoma expansion, hydrocephalus, and brainstem compression
4. Determination of the hemorrhage's underlying etiology

The most common life-threatening complication in ICH in the acute setting is respiratory failure due to insufficient airway control. This is caused by some combination of depressed level of consciousness and direct lesioning brain regions responsible for sensorimotor function of the facial, oral, and pharyngeal regions (i.e., frontal operculum, insula, internal capsule, lower cranial nerve nuclei). The relatively high risk of vomiting—and therefore aspiration—makes the presence of insufficient airway control especially problematic in ICH. Accordingly, all ICH patients should immediately be assessed for adequacy of airway

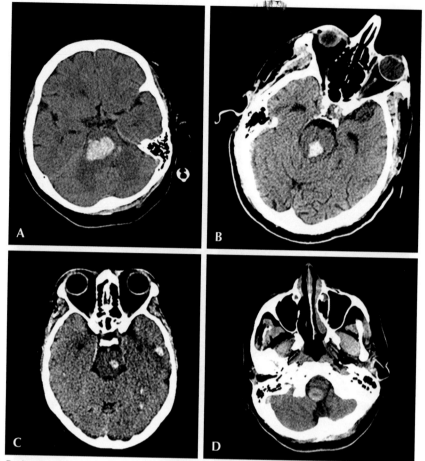

Fig. 16.9 Brainstem Intracerebral Hemorrhage. (A) Paramedian pons (hypertensive). (B) Pontine basotegmental (hypertensive). (C) Midbrain (disseminated intravascular coagulation). (D) Medulla (cavernous malformation).

BOX 16.3 Initial Diagnostic Evaluation of Intracerebral Hemorrhage Patients

History
- Time of symptom onset or time last seen well
- Specifics of the presenting stroke syndrome
- Elapsed time from initial manifestations to the peak stroke syndrome
- Headache: presence, evolution over time, location, and quality
- Recent trauma
- Medications, especially antithrombotic drugs and antihypertensives
- Detailed past medical history focusing on presence or absence of hypertension, malignancy
- Personal or family history of stroke and/or abnormal bleeding or clotting.
- Use of illicit drugs

Physical Examination
- Vital signs
- Detailed neurologic examination
- NIHSS
- GCS or FOUR score
- General medical examination to detect signs of cardiorespiratory dysfunction
- Examination for signs of possibly associated conditions
  - Head lacerations or contusions, Battle sign, raccoon eyes (recent head trauma)
  - Meningismus (infectious vasculitis, septic venous thrombosis, aneurysmal SAH)
  - Cutaneous embolic lesions (endocarditis)
  - Jaundice, chest spider angiomata, palmar erythema (cirrhosis)

Laboratory
- PT, INR, PTT
- CBC (platelets)
- Serum or capillary glucose
- Electrolytes and renal function
- Serum troponin concentration
- Serum and urine screening tests for drugs of abuse
- β–HCG (women of childbearing age)
- EKG (LVH)

Imaging
- NCCT for all patients
- Strongly consider CT or MR angiography and venography for patients with any of the following features
  - Age < 60 years
  - No significant known history of hypertension or coagulopathy
  - Pregnant, ≤6 months postpartum, or on oral contraceptives
  - Known thrombophilia
  - History of DVT or PE
  - Lobar, infratentorial, parasagittal, or bithalamic location
  - Multiple acute/subacute hemorrhages
  - Associated intraventricular or subarachnoid hemorrhage
  - Multiple acute hemorrhages

β-HCG, Beta human chorionic gonadotropin; *CBC,* complete blood count; *CT,* computed tomography; *DVT,* deep venous thrombosis; *EKG,* electrocardiogram; *FOUR score,* full outline of unresponsiveness; *GCS,* Glasgow Coma Scale; *INR,* international normalized ratio; *LVH,* left ventricular hypertrophy; *MRI,* magnetic resonance imaging; *NCCT,* noncontrast CT; *NIHSS,* National Institutes of Health Stroke Scale; *PE,* pulmonary embolism; *PT,* prothombin time; *PTT,* partial thromboplastin time; *SAH,* subarachnoid hemorrhage.

control, as indicated by level of consciousness and oropharyngeal dysfunction.

Patients with large hemorrhages, IVH, and/or hydrocephalus may show signs of intracranial hypertension and/or brainstem compression. Therefore, signs indicating the presence of these complications, such as coma, cranial nerve dysfunction, and extensor posturing, should be promptly identified.

The diagnostic evaluation begins with defining the precise manifestations and temporal course of the presenting stroke syndrome. Despite the fact that certain clinical features such as headache, vomiting, seizures, depressed level of consciousness, and gradually evolving deficits are more common in ICH than ischemic stroke, historical and physical exam features are not adequate for reliable differentiation between the conditions. Neuroimaging is therefore the next and most important step in the diagnostic pathway and should occur as soon as the patient is safe to travel to the CT scanner.

CT is the preferred imaging modality for ICH diagnosis. It is nearly 100% sensitive and specific while being faster, more readily available, and less expensive than MRI. The precise location and volume of the hematoma should be noted (see Fig. 16.1). Infrequent potential pitfalls in the diagnosis of ICH with CT include difficulty in differentiating small subacute ICHs from infarcts with hemorrhagic transformation and the rare "CT negative" ICH. Both problems occur almost exclusively in patients who present in the subacute phase because (1) the density of an ICH decreases with time and (2) hemorrhagic infarct transformation is rare before 24 hours after symptom onset.

Identification of the risk for complications from ICH begins with an assessment of the blood pressure, because systolic blood pressure (SBP) above about 160 mm Hg probably represents a modifiable risk for hematoma expansion. Next, the patient should be assessed for the presence of a correctable coagulopathy or thrombocytopenia with a detailed history focusing on a history of liver, kidney, or hematologic disease, recent ingestion of anticoagulants or antiplatelet agents, and personal or family history of excessive bleeding; and laboratory assessment of the complete blood count, activated partial thromboplastin time, and prothrombin time with international normalized ratio. The CT should be examined for the presence of IVH, hydrocephalus, and mass effect (see Fig. 16.8A and B). In supratentorial hemorrhages, concerning mass effect is generally considered to be present when the perimesencephalic cisterns are crowded or the third ventricle is horizontally displaced by 5 mm or more. For cerebellar hemorrhages, mass effect is assessed by determining the degree of compression and horizontal displacement of the fourth ventricle and the degree of effacement of the prepontine cistern.

The last step in the diagnostic process is determination of the hemorrhage etiology. Although most ICHs are primary and caused by hypertensive angiopathy or CAA, identifying secondary etiologies, especially macrovascular lesions and cerebral venous thrombosis, is crucial, as these necessitate the urgent application of unique treatments. This assessment begins with a thorough history and physical examination (see Box 16.3) and select laboratory studies. The results of this evaluation will then inform interpretation of the initial noncontrast CT scan and help determine the need for additional imaging. CT or MR angiography and venography should be strongly considered in patients whose clinical, laboratory, and noncontrast CT assessment suggests an increased risk for macrovascular lesion as the etiology of the hemorrhage (see Box 16.3). Depending upon the index of suspicion for an underlying lesion, conventional angiography and/or delayed (4–8 weeks) MRI may be appropriate if the CT or MR angiography is unrevealing. MRI evidence of asymptomatic lobar microhemorrhages is also central in making the diagnosis of CAA (Box 16.4, see Fig. 16.3).

BOX 16.4   Modified Boston Criteria for the Diagnosis of Cerebral Amyloid Angiopathy

Definite:
- Full postmortem examination demonstrating:
  - Lobar, cortical, or cortico-subcortical hemorrhage
  - Severe CAA with vasculopathy
  - Absence of other diagnostic lesion

Probable With Supporting Pathology:
- Clinical data and pathologic tissue (evacuated hematoma or cortical biopsy) demonstrating:
  - Lobar, cortical, or cortico-subcortical hemorrhage
  - Some degree of CAA in specimen
  - Absence of other diagnostic lesion

Probable:
- Clinical data and MRI or CT demonstrating:
  - Multiple hemorrhages restricted to lobar, cortical, or cortico-subcortical regions (cerebellar hemorrhage allowed), or
  - Single lobar, cortical, or cortico-subcortical hemorrhage and focal or disseminated superficial siderosis
  - Age ≥ 55 years
  - Absence of other cause of hemorrhage or superficial siderosis

Possible:
- Clinical data and MRI or CT demonstrating:
  - Single lobar, cortical, or cortico-subcortical hemorrhage, or
  - Focal or disseminated superficial siderosis
  - Age ≥ 55 years
  - Absence of other cause of hemorrhage or superficial siderosis

CAA, Cerebral amyloid angiopathy.
Modified from Linn J, Halpin A, Demaerel P, et al. Prevalence of superficial siderosis in patients with cerebral amyloid angiopathy. *Neurology.* 2010;74:1346-1350.

MANAGEMENT (Box 16.5)

CLINICAL VIGNETTE *A 67-year-old right-handed man with a history of coronary artery disease and atrial fibrillation for which he took aspirin and warfarin was found by his wife on the floor next to their bed one hour after he had gone to sleep. He was alert, slurring his speech, and could not move his left limbs. Paramedic assessment in the field revealed a blood pressure of 250/115 mm Hg, normal alertness, dysarthria, left hemineglect, and left hemiparesis. He was taken to a community hospital emergency department where his initial evaluation did not differ from that of the paramedics. GCS 15, NIHSS 14, ICH score 1. His INR was 2.0; platelet count was 169 k/μL. CT (Fig. 16.10A) showed a 20 mL R putaminal ICH with mild shift of the third ventricle and small intraventricular hemorrhage. He was given vitamin K 10 mg IV, and arrangements were made for transfer to a tertiary hospital. No acute coagulopathy reversal or blood pressure management was undertaken. Three hours after ED arrival, with the systolic blood pressure remaining 180–220 mm Hg, he suddenly developed vomiting and coma. He was intubated and promptly transferred. On arrival to the tertiary hospital ICU, 4 hours after his initial ED presentation, his blood pressure was 202/130 mm Hg, GCS 3T, NIHSS 35, ICH score 4. His neurologic exam was notable for coma; 6 mm fixed pupils; absent corneal, oculocephalic, and cough reflexes; and absent motor responses in all limbs. The INR was 2.3. CT head (Fig. 16.10B) showed that the hematoma volume had increased 5-fold to 105 mL and that it was now causing more intraventricular hemorrhage along with transtentorial herniation. The patient was declared brain dead 2 days later.*

BOX 16.5   Basic Management of Intracerebral Hemorrhage

Acute Phase

- Assess and stabilize airway, breathing, and circulation
  - Head of bed ≥30 degrees
  - Suction secretions, vomitus from oropharynx
  - Goal oxygen saturation ≥94%
  - Tracheal intubation for inadequate airway control (or other causes of respiratory failure)
- Treat ongoing or impending herniation syndromes and/or intracranial hypertension
  - Sedation
  - Hyperventilation to goal $PaCO_2$ 30–35 mm Hg
  - Osmotherapy
    - Mannitol or hypertonic saline bolus
  - Consider EVD, surgical decompression
- Minimize hematoma expansion
  - Control hypertension
    - Use nicardipine or labetalol to keep SBP 140–160 mm Hg
    - Maintain MAP > 65 mm Hg
  - Treat coagulopathy
    - Warfarin
      - Four-factor PCC
      - Vitamin K IV
    - Dabigatran
      - Idarucizumab if dTT prolonged
    - Oral FXa inhibitors
      - Consider andexanet alfa or four-factor PCC
    - Heparins (unfractionated, low molecular weight)
      - Protamine

- Oral antiplatelet drugs
  - Getting surgery
    - 1 apheresis unit platelet transfusion
  - Not getting surgery
    - Single agent: no platelet transfusion
    - ≥2 agents: can consider platelet transfusion

Detect and Treat Complications

- Admit to neuro-ICU at a designated stroke center
- Hourly neurologic examinations
- Minimal necessary sedation
- Seizures
  - Treat if they occur
  - Avoid primary prophylactic treatment
- Fever control with acetaminophen
- Normoxia, normocapnia
- Maintain blood pressure as above
- Maintain sodium homeostasis
  - Avoid hypotonic fluids
  - Avoid drops in serum sodium concentration >4–5 mEq/L/24 hr
- Dysphagia management
  - Avoid oral medications or nutrition unless a formal dysphagia screen is passed
  - NG or OG tube as needed
- VTE prophylaxis
  - IPC devices on admission

SC UFH or LMWH at prophylactic doses at 48 hr after ictus if hematoma stable and no ongoing coagulopathy.

dTT, Diluted thrombin time; *EVD,* external ventricular drain; *FXa,* factor Xa; *ICU,* intensive care unit; *IPC,* intermittent pneumatic compression; *IV,* intravenous; *LMWH,* low molecular weight heparin; *MAP,* mean arterial pressure; *NG,* nasogastric; *OG,* orogastric; *PCC,* prothrombin complex concentrate; *SBP,* systolic blood pressure; *SC,* subcutaneous; *UFH,* unfractionated heparin; *VTE,* venous thromboembolism.

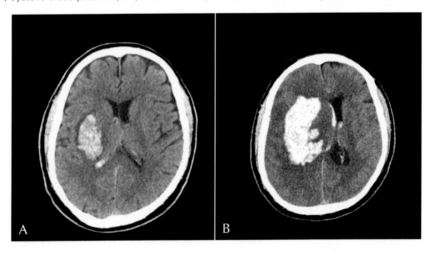

Fig. 16.10 Axial Noncontrast Head CT. A, Initial image completed at time of presentation with approximately 15 mL intraparenchymal hemorrhage with small amount of intraventricular extension and associated cytotoxic edema. B, Repeat head CT following neurologic worsening. Significant expansion of the intraparenchymal hemorrhage, now with volume of approximately 80 mL and increased mass effect with right to left midline shift.

Rapid stabilization of respiratory, hemodynamic, and neurologic function is the first step in the care of the patient with ICH. Compromised airway control with or without pulmonary dysfunction from aspiration is common and should be managed by keeping the head of the patient's bed elevated to at least 30 degrees, clearing the oropharynx of secretions and vomitus by suctioning, providing supplemental oxygen to keep the oxygen saturation 94% or more, and tracheal intubation if needed. Shock is unusual in patients with ICH and should be assessed and managed as in any other patient. In addition, cardiogenic shock from neurogenic stress cardiomyopathy should be considered in the differential diagnosis, especially in patients with large hemorrhages. Finally, patients with clinical and radiographic signs of ongoing or impending herniation syndromes and/or intracranial hypertension should be treated with intubation, sedation, hyperventilation, and bolus-dose osmotherapy (mannitol or hypertonic saline) before neurosurgical treatment, if appropriate, can be undertaken.

Minimizing hematoma expansion is the next priority and is achieved through rapid control of hypertension and reversal of coagulopathy. The consequences of not doing this effectively in what began as a non-severe hypertensive putaminal ICH in a patient anticoagulated with warfarin are illustrated by Vignette 3. The management of hypertension in patients with ICH has recently been investigated in two large randomized control trials. Compared with no goal-directed antihypertensive treatment, blood pressure control in the acute stages of ICH seems to be associated with less hematoma expansion. INTERACT 2 and ATACH 2, however, showed that aggressive lowering of the SBP to 110–140 mm Hg did not lead to better outcomes and might have been associated with more renal complications than more moderate control to the range of 140–160 mm Hg. To maximize the benefits of hypertension control, the goal SBP range of 140–160 mm Hg should be reached within an hour of patient presentation. Intravenous nicardipine or labetalol given as a continuous infusion or intermittent boluses, respectively, work well for this purpose. Warfarin coagulopathy is best reversed using four-factor prothrombin complex concentrate (PCC), which, as a lyophilized concentrate of vitamin K–dependent coagulation factors, is essentially a specific antidote to warfarin that can be infused much faster and in much smaller volumes than the traditionally used fresh frozen plasma (FFP). The INCH trial, in which PCC was compared with FFP in patients with acute vitamin K–antagonist-associated ICH demonstrated much faster normalization of the INR with PCC (40 vs. 1482 minutes) and less extensive hematoma expansion. The trial was not adequately powered to detect a difference in the rate of thromboembolic events, but no increased risk was found in the small number of patients studied ($n = 50$). Importantly, PCC (or, if used, FFP) should always be immediately followed by 10 mg of intravenous vitamin K to prevent a rebound rise in the INR that can otherwise occur hours later due to the short half-lives of the coagulation factors that they supply. Patients taking dabigatran should have a dilute thrombin time checked immediately. If prolonged, reversal of dabigatran coagulopathy with the specific antidote idarucizumab should be considered. If this laboratory test is unable to be obtained in a timely manner, and there is suspicion that a patient ingested dabigatran recently, consider empiric administration of idarucizumab. A single dose of IV desmopressin (DDAVP) should be considered in all ICH patients taking oral antiplatelet medications. Evidence of reasonable quality indicates that patients taking oral antiplatelet drugs who are planned to undergo surgery, including external ventricular drain (EVD) placement, benefit from transfusion of one apheresis unit of platelets prior to surgery. For patients taking a single antiplatelet drug who are not undergoing operation, platelet transfusion was shown not to be beneficial but instead possibly harmful in the recent PATCH trial. The safety and efficacy of platelet transfusion in nonsurgical patients on combination oral antiplatelet therapy are not known. Oral factor Xa inhibitors recently had a reversal agent FDA approved, andexanet alfa. However, data regarding its use is limited. An alternative to this agent is PCC, which may partially reverse their anticoagulant effects. Protamine can reverse the effects of unfractionated heparin and may have some effect in bleeding patients anticoagulated with low molecular weight heparin.

Early involvement of the neurosurgery team is necessary in patients with IVH and patients with or at risk for developing significant mass effect from the hematoma and anticipated hematoma expansion and/or PHE. EVD placement should be strongly considered in patients with hydrocephalus and/or IVH, particularly if the level of alertness is depressed. Ventricular irrigation via an EVD with alteplase used in the manner investigated in the CLEAR-III trial is probably safe and can be considered in patients with significant IVH and small (<30 mL) ICH. However, this was not shown to clearly improve functional outcomes in the trial. Cerebellar ICH is a neurosurgical emergency, with emergent hematoma evacuation being clearly indicated for potentially salvageable patients who demonstrate clinical and radiographic signs of brainstem compression and/or hydrocephalus from fourth ventricle compression. Such signs include decreased levels of consciousness and cranial neuropathies, especially involving the third, sixth, and seventh cranial nerves. Patients with cerebellar hematomas of greater than 3 cm diameter are at particularly high risk for this. Decompression with EVD alone for mass effect from cerebellar hemorrhages is generally not recommended because of the risk of treatment failure and worsening due to upward cerebellar herniation. Surgical evacuation of brainstem hematomas due to primary ICH is not useful.

Despite the strong biologic plausibility that hematoma removal in supratentorial ICH should be beneficial by limiting secondary injury due to both mass effect and the downstream inflammatory/cytotoxic injury incited by the presence of extravasated blood, how, when, and in whom (if anybody) to effectively use surgery in this group remain uncertain. The STICH trials, in which hematoma evacuation was achieved with traditional craniotomy and corticotomy in the vast majority of patients, showed that early surgery led to equivalent outcomes when compared with a strategy of early conservative treatment with delayed surgery in salvageable patients who experienced delayed neurologic deterioration. At present, therefore, it is reasonable to consider surgical hematoma evacuation and/or decompressive craniectomy as a life-saving measure in patients deteriorating due to mass effect from a supratentorial ICH, especially those with superficial hematomas. Minimally invasive, image-guided surgical (MIS) techniques for hematoma evacuation are current areas of clinical investigation. The hope for these techniques is that they will allow the theoretical benefits of hematoma evacuation on not just mortality but also ultimate neurologic function to be realized by minimizing the injury to salvageable perihematomal brain that is inherent to traditional techniques. Thus far a variety of MIS techniques have been shown to be safe and effective in hematoma evacuation for even deep basal ganglia hemorrhages. Advanced phase trials are ongoing to assess for functional outcome benefits.

Once through the first few hours, management is focused on preventing, detecting, and treating neurologic deterioration and secondary dysfunction of other organ systems. Hourly neurologic examinations by the nurse coupled with frequent reassessments by the physician and/or advanced practitioner for detecting the earliest signs of deterioration, judicious and conservative use of sedation and analgesia to prevent clouding the neurologic assessment, and elevation of the head of the bed to at least 30 degrees to optimize cerebral venous drainage and prevent aspiration are simple yet essential. While seizures should be treated with benzodiazepines (as necessary) and antiepileptic drugs, the utility of seizure prophylaxis is less clear. Coupled with the fact that at least phenytoin for seizure prophylaxis has been associated with higher mortality and worse neurologic outcomes, prophylactic AED treatment is not recommended. Because both hyper- and hypoglycemia exacerbate neurologic injury, the serum glucose concentration should be maintained in the range of 100–180 mg/dL. Fever can also exacerbate neurologic injury, and treatment with acetaminophen should be considered. More aggressive measures of induced normothermia using external and intravascular cooling devices have not been sufficiently studied, and existing data have not demonstrated effectiveness and indicate the possibility of harm. Thus these methods cannot be recommended as routine clinical practice at present. Mechanically ventilated patients should be kept meticulously normocapnic and normoxic. Hypertension is treated as described previously, with enteral agents typically being added in hemodynamically stable patients on the second hospital day. Hypotonic IV fluids and serum sodium reductions of more than 4–5 mEq/L over 24 hours should be avoided and, if needed, treated with hypertonic saline to avoid exacerbation of PHE.

All ICH patients should be formally assessed for dysphagia prior to any oral intake to reduce the risk of pneumonia; oral medications and enteral nutrition should be provided by oro- or nasogastric tube in patients deemed unsafe to swallow. Finally, ICH patients are at very high risk for venous thromboembolic complications. Prophylaxis with lower extremity intermittent pneumatic compression devices should be started immediately upon admission, and pharmacoprophylaxis with subcutaneous unfractionated or low molecular weight heparin should begin 48 hours after ictus in patients with no ongoing coagulopathy and a stable hematoma.

Managing ICH patients within the appropriate systems of care is crucial for optimizing outcomes. Neurologic, neurosurgical, nursing, and allied health expertise in caring for patients with stroke are clearly beneficial and are most consistently achieved by admitting ICH patients to formally designated stroke centers. Except for patients with very small supratentorial hematomas at minimal risk for hematoma expansion or hydrocephalus, most ICH patients should initially be admitted to an intensive care unit. Admission to a dedicated neuro-ICU as compared with general medical, surgical, or mixed ICUs has been shown to be associated with significantly lower mortality.

PROGNOSTICATION

Despite the inherent difficulty and uncertainty, patients and families need accurate prognostic information as the basis on which to make decisions about critical matters such as continuation or discontinuation of life-sustaining measures. In general, prognosis depends on relatively few data points, including age, premorbid cognitive and functional status, severity of the clinical syndrome, size and location of the hemorrhage, and the presence of IVH. Multiple scoring systems have been devised that combine these elements to predict the probability of mortality and poor functional outcomes, the most useful of which are the ICH (Fig. 16.11, best for mortality) and FUNC (Fig. 16.12, best for functional outcome) scores. Although the use of these scores adds some objectivity

	Component	ICH Score points
GCS Score	3–4	2
	5–12	1
	13–15	0
ICH volume, mL	≥30	1
	<30	0
IVH	Yes	1
	No	0
Infratentorial origin of ICH	Yes	1
	No	0
Age, years	≥80	1
	<80	0

A. ICH Score.

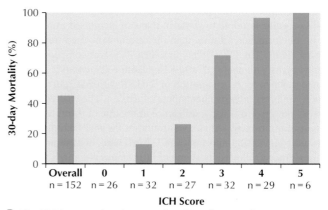

B. The ICH Score and 30-day mortality. Thirty-day mortality increases as ICH Score increases. No patient with an ICH Score of 0 died. All patients with an ICH Score of 5 died. No patient in the UCSF ICH cohort had an ICH Score of 6, although this would be expected to be associated with mortality.

Fig. 16.11 Intracerebral hemorrhage (ICH) Score. *IVH,* Intraventricular hemorrhage. ([B], Reused with permission from Hemphill JC, Bonovich DC, Besmertis L, Manley GT, Johnston SC. The ICH score: a simple, reliable grading scale for intracerebral hemorrhage. *Stroke.* 2001;32:891-897, Fig. 1, p. 894).

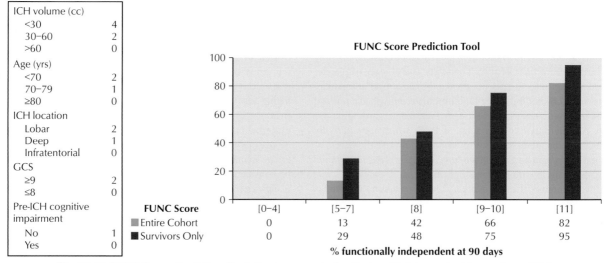

Fig. 16.12 FUNC Score Prediction Tool. Y-axis: percent of patients with intracerebral hemorrhage (ICH) who reach functional independence at 90 days. X-axis: FUNC score categories. Data table: percent of functionally independent patients among the entire cohort and survivors only (per FUNC score category). Inset: FUNC score determinants provided to facilitate clinical use of this ICH outcome prediction tool. (Reused with permission from Rost NS, Smith EE, Chang Y, et al. Prediction of functional outcome in patients with primary intracerebral hemorrhage: the FUNC score. *Stroke.* 2008;39:2304-2309. Fig. 1, p. 2307.)

to prognostication that may counterbalance the biases of the prognosticating physician, *they should not be relied upon as the primary basis of prognostication at the level of the individual patient.* These scales themselves are inevitably affected by the biases of the physicians who cared for the patients from which they were derived, do not provide precise enough information on which to base decisions about the level of aggression of care, and do not consider the eloquence of the brain region injured by the hematoma. Furthermore, it was recently demonstrated that the subjective prognosis of experienced clinicians may more accurately predict actual outcome than either the ICH or FUNC score. Taken together, this information indicates that prognostication in ICH is best performed by an experienced clinician who combines more objective data from the ICH and FUNC scores with his or her subjective, "gestalt" prognosis to reach a final formulation. This final prognosis should be determined and delivered to the family not earlier than 24 hours after the onset of symptoms to avoid premature withdrawal of life-sustaining therapy, except in the most obviously devastating cases. The degree of uncertainty in the prognosis should be openly discussed with the family.

ADDITIONAL RESOURCES

Carhuapoma JR, Mayer SA, Hanley DF, editors. Intracerebral hemorrhage. Cambridge: Cambridge University Press; 2010.
A comprehensive, modern textbook that reviews all aspects of basic and clinical science concerning ICH.
Frontera JA, Lewin JJ 3rd, Rabinstein AA, et al. Guideline for reversal of antithrombotics in intracranial hemorrhage: a statement for healthcare professionals from the Neurocritical Care Society and Society of Critical Care Medicine. Neurocrit Care 2016;24:6–46.
Detailed yet practical review and guidelines for the reversal of antithrombotics of all types in patients with intracranial bleeding.
Hemphill JC 3rd, Greenberg SM, Anderson CS, et al. Guidelines for the management of spontaneous intracerebral hemorrhage: a guideline for healthcare professionals from the American Heart Association/American Stroke Association. Stroke 2015;46:2032–60.
The most recent edition of the comprehensive, evidenced-based ICH management guidelines from the AHA/ASA.
Chu SY, Hwang DY. Predicting outcome for intracerebral hemorrhage patients: current tools and their limitations. Semin Neurol 2016;36:254–60.
Useful, comprehensive review of prognostication in ICH.
Kase CS, Caplan LR. Intracerebral hemorrhage. Boston: Butterworth-Heinemann; 1994.
The definitive textbook on ICH, especially for history concerning the evolution of thought on the condition and clinico-anatomic correlation.
Kim H, Edwards NJ, Choi HA, et al. Treatment strategies to attenuate perihematomal edema in patients with intracerebral hemorrhage. World Neurosurg 2016;94:32–41.
Up-to-date review of the pathophysiology of secondary injury and perihematomal edema as well as possible treatment strategies.
Qureshi AI, Qureshi MH. Acute hypertensive response in patients with intracerebral hemorrhage pathophysiology and treatment. J Cereb Blood Flow Metab 2018;38:1551–63.
Up-to-date review and synthesis of the large, important recent trials on blood pressure management in acute ICH.
Ziai W, Nyquist P, Hanley DF. Surgical strategies for spontaneous intracerebral hemorrhage. Semin Neurol 2016;36:261–8.
Contemporary review of surgery for ICH with an emphasis on clinical studies of minimally invasive surgery.

17

Subarachnoid Hemorrhage

David P. Lerner, Anil Ramineni, Michael Adix II, Ian Kaminsky, Joseph D. Burns

---

CLINICAL VIGNETTE *A 66-year-old woman experienced the near immediate onset of a terrible temporal pain that radiated into her forehead. She almost lost consciousness. She became nauseated, vomited, and felt disoriented. Her family called emergency medical services, who brought her to the emergency department. There, she was noted to be arousable but sleepy and confused, with no focal motor deficit. She had nuchal rigidity and photophobia. An unenhanced head computed tomography (CT) showed subarachnoid hemorrhage centered in the right sylvian fissure but no brain parenchymal abnormalities. Angiography demonstrated a ruptured middle cerebral artery aneurysm that was successfully clipped the next morning. The patient's postoperative course was uneventful (Figs. 17.1 and 17.2).*

Subarachnoid hemorrhage (SAH) refers to bleeding into the subarachnoid space, which is located between the arachnoid mater and the pia mater. The pia mater is tightly adherent to the brain parenchyma, and the subarachnoid space lies atop it. This space is occupied by connective tissue, blood vessels, and intercommunicating channels that contain cerebrospinal fluid (CSF) (Fig. 17.3). In addition, there are larger openings at the base of the brain referred to as subarachnoid cisterns. Nontraumatic SAH is the smallest subset of stroke, composing approximately 5%. However, it has a disproportionately high associated mortality and morbidity. While there are many causes, the most common is a rupture of an intracranial aneurysm. Early recognition and diagnosis, coupled with timely treatment by a multidisciplinary team of neurosurgeons, neurointerventionalists, and neurointensivists in an institution with significant experience caring for patients with aneurysmal SAH (aSAH) is essential to optimize the likelihood of a favorable outcome.

EPIDEMIOLOGY

Subarachnoid hemorrhage is a catastrophic neurologic event having a precipitous onset, frequently without any premonitory warning. Approximately 50% of patients die secondary to aneurysmal SAH. 10%–15% of these patients die prior to reaching the hospital, and 25% die within 24 hours of aneurysmal rupture. In patients who survive, less than half will have a favorable outcome and reach functional independence. aSAH, although catastrophic, can be treated successfully.

The incidence of nontraumatic SAH varies around the world, with rates of 2–4 per 100,000 persons in China and Central America, 5–15 per 100,000 persons in the United States and most other Western populations, 20 per 100,000 persons in Japan, and 35 per 100,000 persons in Finland. A total of 80% of these are due to ruptured intracranial aneurysms. Accordingly, there are approximately 20,000 incident aSAH cases per year in the United States. The mean age of aneurysm rupture is 55 years; however, patients may be significantly younger or older. Only 20% of aneurysm ruptures occur in patients aged between 15 and 45 years. The incidence is higher in women compared with men, with a ratio of about 1.5:1.

There are both modifiable and nonmodifiable risk factors for intracranial aneurysm formation and rupture. Nonmodifiable risk factors include prior SAH, polycystic kidney disease, connective tissue disease, family history of intracranial aneurysms, and female sex. In the United States, SAH is more common in African American and Hispanic populations. Despite lack of a specific gene, there appears to be some genetic component to aneurysm formation and aSAH. Those with more than one first-degree relative should be screened for intracranial aneurysms. The strongest modifiable risk factor for both aneurysm formation and rupture is smoking. Heavy smoking (greater than one pack per day) is associated with a higher risk of SAH, and smoking cessation reduces the risk of SAH. Hypertension is also consistently associated with SAH. Other modifiable risk factors include drug abuse, particularly cocaine, and heavy alcohol abuse. A list of risk factors for aSAH can be found in Box 17.1.

While no predisposing activity has been identified, some literature suggests that patients with rupture of aneurysm are more likely to engage in moderate to strenuous exertion in the 2 hours preceding SAH. Nevertheless, aSAH may also occur in sleep or during routine daily activities.

ETIOLOGY

Approximately 20% of nontraumatic SAH cases have causes other than a ruptured intracranial aneurysm. This nonaneurysmal SAH group has a wide spectrum of etiologies as detailed in Box 17.2 (in approximate order of frequency).

Nonaneurysmal Perimesencephalic Subarachnoid Hemorrhage

CLINICAL VIGNETTE *A 48-year-old male with no past medical history was lifting weights at the gym when he felt a "pop" in the back of his head immediately followed by a 10/10 holocephalic headache. Associated with his headache was nausea with one episode of emesis, but he retained normal consciousness. EMS brought him to the emergency department, and on arrival his vitals were: heart rate 82 beats/min, blood pressure 124/74, temp 96.6°F, oxygen saturation 96% in room air. His neurologic examination was normal with the exception of nuchal rigidity. A head CT was completed shortly after arrival and is shown as follows. A CTA was completed, which was negative for an aneurysm or vascular malformation. The following morning, a digital subtraction angiogram was completed and did not demonstrate any vascular abnormality. The patient was diagnosed with perimesencephalic subarachnoid hemorrhage and was discharged from the hospital 7 days after his initial presentation and had no hospital complications and returned to his normal activities (Fig. 17.4).*

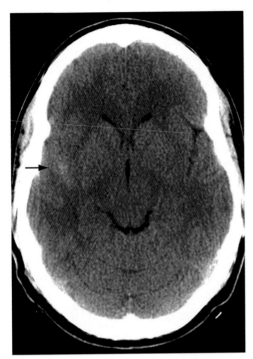

A. Axial CT exam shows subarachnoid hemorrhage lateralized to the right extending into the right sylvian fissure (arrow).

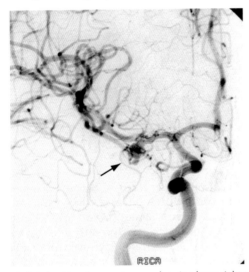

B. Frontal digital subtraction angiogram showing large right middle cerebral artery aneurysm (arrow).

Fig. 17.1 Right Middle Cerebral Artery Aneurysm.

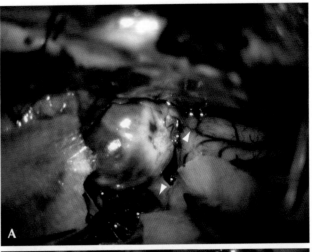

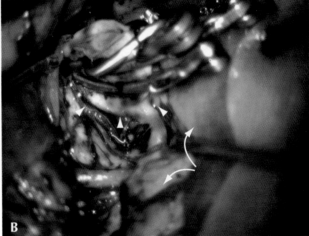

Right-sided pterional approach depicting large bulging MCA aneurysm (arrowheads) before (**A**) and after (**B**) surgical clipping. Aneurysm has been decompressed with surgical clips at its base with preservation of the parent artery (arrowheads).

Fig. 17.2 Middle Cerebral Artery Aneurysm Clipping.

Of the approximately 20% of SAH patients who have negative initial angiograms, repeated angiography may demonstrate the culprit in another 7% of patients. However, a specific subset of patients with definitively negative imaging for aneurysms displays SAH with a specific CT distribution of blood over the anterior aspect of the brainstem or perimesencephalic regions. Termed *nonaneurysmal perimesencephalic SAH*, it is typically associated with a more benign clinical course. Specifically, the risk for recurrent hemorrhage is extremely low, and the risks of hydrocephalus or cerebral vasospasm/delayed cerebral ischemia (DCI) are much lower than in patients with aSAH. Although the presentation is similar to that of an aSAH, symptom onset may be more gradual, and patients often appear less ill. In patients who have a characteristic presentation and CT findings, alongside a high-quality angiogram that is negative, a follow-up angiogram is not always needed. The cause of nonaneurysmal perimesencephalic SAH is unknown. Current theories include the rupture of small perforating vessels across the perimesencephalic cistern or a venous source of bleeding.

CLINICAL PRESENTATION

The classic symptom of aSAH is the "thunderclap headache" (TCHA), occurring in at least 50% of cases. TCHA is sudden in onset and often described as severe, excruciating, and unbearable. The headache peaks rapidly, within 1 minute, and is frequently associated with pain extending across the head and toward the neck. Although the headache of aSAH is typically severe, it is not always the worst headache that the patient has ever experienced. The pain is usually holocephalic and constant with occasional throbbing. However, in some patients the headache may be lateralized to the side of the aneurysm. Retroorbital stabbing pain raises suspicion for an ipsilateral posterior communicating artery aneurysm. The headache's character and quality is due to the rapid upsurge in intracranial pressure and rapid spread of blood through the subarachnoid space. Sentinel hemorrhage, also known as a "warning

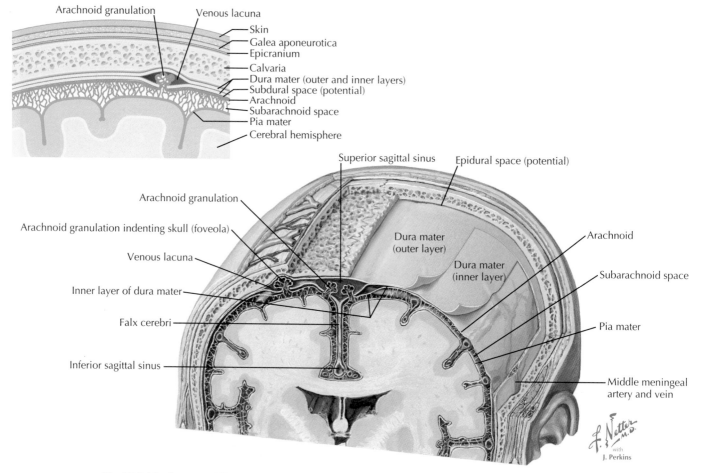

Fig. 17.3 Meninges and Their Relationship to the Brain Parenchyma. Top: Layers of the scalp, bone, and meninges in relation to the brain parenchyma. Bottom: Blown-up image of the meninges in relation to the brain. Green: pia mater, Pink: subarachnoid space.

BOX 17.1 Risk Factors for Aneurysmal Subarachnoid Hemorrhage

- Advancing age
- Female sex
- Ethnicity
  - African American
  - Hispanic American
  - Japanese
  - Finnish
- Family history
- Hypertension
- Cigarette smoking
- Polycystic kidney disease
- Connective tissue disease
- Substance abuse
  - Cocaine
  - Alcohol

---

leak," is a fleeting but severe headache within 3 weeks of the major ictus that occurs in 15%–60% of aSAH patients. This headache may be somewhat milder and usually is not associated with meningismus. It is often ignored until a catastrophic major aneurysmal rupture highlights its significance in retrospect.

Alteration in consciousness, nausea and/or vomiting, and meningismus are often associated with the headache. Approximately 30% of patients are found to be confused and lethargic after the ictus. During the moment of rupture, one-fourth patients become comatose and greater than 50% have transient loss of consciousness.

Seizurelike activity may be observed. The incidence of true seizure activity in patients with aSAH is estimated to be less than 10%, although this is difficult to ascertain accurately. Seizures in aSAH are most commonly associated with middle cerebral artery (MCA) and anterior communicating artery (AComm) aneurysm rupture causing intracerebral hematomas.

When evaluating patients with suspected aneurysm rupture, special attention should be focused on the level of consciousness, focal neurologic signs such as hemiparesis or cranial nerve palsies, and signs of meningismus (Fig. 17.5). Brudzinski's maneuver is a useful means of evaluating meningismus; the examiner flexes the patient's neck, precipitating hip flexion, knee flexion, and hamstring pain. Diplopia (due to abducens or oculomotor nerve palsies) and visual loss (chiasmal or optic nerve involvement) may be caused by cranial nerve compression from the aneurysmal dome or aneurysmal rupture and resultant increased intracranial pressure (Fig. 17.6).

Examination of the optic fundi may disclose retinal, preretinal, or subhyaloid hemorrhages and occasional papilledema. The combination of vitreous hemorrhage with SAH is referred to as Terson syndrome, which is a potential cause of visual loss and often goes unnoticed until the patient regains consciousness 1–2 weeks later. The overall prognosis for patients with Terson syndrome is worse, and it is found more in severe subarachnoid bleeds. Vision may recover without intervention; however, a vitrectomy is occasionally required.

BOX 17.2 Differential Diagnosis of Nontraumatic, Nonaneurysmal Subarachnoid Hemorrhage

- Vascular
  - Nonaneurysmal perimesencephalic subarachnoid hemorrhage
  - Reversible cerebral vasoconstriction syndrome
  - Cerebral amyloid angiopathy
  - Brain arteriovenous malformation
  - Intracranial dural arteriovenous fistula
  - Cerebral venous and venous sinus thrombosis
  - Intracranial artery dissection
  - Moyamoya disease/syndrome
  - Other vascular malformations (cavernous malformation, angioma, spinal arteriovenous fistula)
- Tumor
  - Pituitary apoplexy
  - Spinal ependymoma
- Infectious
  - Bacterial endocarditis with or without mycotic aneurysm
  - Infectious vasculitis
- Inflammatory
  - Primary angiitis of the central nervous system
  - Polyarteritis nodosa
  - Churg-Strauss syndrome
  - Wegner granulomatosis
  - Bechet disease
- Sympathomimetic drug abuse
- Severe coagulopathy

DIFFERENTIAL DIAGNOSIS

Patients presenting with a TCHA, especially those with associated meningismus or altered mental status, should be considered to have aSAH until proven otherwise because of (1) the importance of making this diagnosis as early as possible, and (2) approximately 25% of patients with TCHA have aSAH. However, this clinical picture may be associated with other disorders (Box 17.3).

Reversible cerebral vasoconstriction syndrome (RCVS) accounts for approximately 25% of TCHA cases. RCVS consists of multifocal narrowing of cerebral arteries that is typically reversible and of uncertain etiology, which, by definition, presents with TCHA (Fig. 17.7). It is more common in women and may be related to pregnancy, oral contraceptive use, drug abuse (especially marijuana and sympathomimetics), and the use of various prescription medications (especially triptans, selective serotonin reuptake inhibitors [SSRIs], and serotonin and norepinephrine reuptake inhibitors [SNRIs]). RCVS can also result in subarachnoid hemorrhage. While RCVS and aSAH can initially be difficult to distinguish, certain clues are helpful. Recurrent TCHAs without major neurologic abnormalities on examination, as well as subarachnoid blood on the cortical surface rather than the basal cisterns, argue strongly for RCVS.

Although migraines are often characterized by the patient as sudden, a careful history reveals that they typically have a gradual onset, with progression over minutes to hours. Many are preceded by a classic visual aura of fortification spectra or scintillating scotoma that gradually grows and then regresses over 5–30 minutes before the headache occurs. A personal or family history of migraines is helpful in making this diagnosis, especially when a headache is a characteristic of a patient's typical migraine syndrome.

Cluster headache is another benign but severe headache syndrome with a well-defined clinical presentation. These headaches typically affect

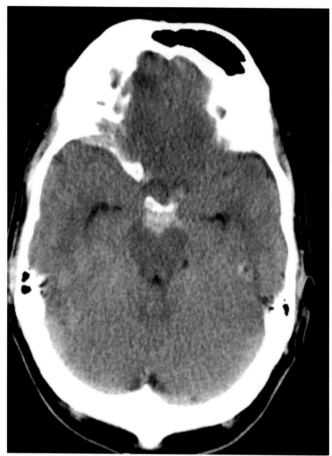

Fig. 17.4 Perimesencephalic Subarachnoid Hemorrhage. Axial non-contrast head computed tomography at the level of the midbrain. The intrapendicular cistern filled with hyperdensity, consistent with hemorrhage. The limitation of hemorrhage to this location is termed perimesencephalic subarachnoid hemorrhage.

men and consist of incredibly severe unilateral periorbital and frontal pain. Cluster headaches are almost always associated with unilateral conjunctival injection with excessive lacrimation and nasal congestion. They have a limited time course, usually lasting 45–60 minutes. They occur nightly in a temporal cluster for 6–8 weeks but may recur several times within a day. When this pattern is established, the diagnosis is secure. However, when the patient first experiences this headache in early midlife, a careful evaluation is indicated to exclude SAH. A therapeutic response to inhalation of 100% oxygen can be diagnostic. Paroxysmal hemicrania is a related disorder that is characterized by a robust response to indomethacin.

TCHA associated with cough, exercise, or sexual activity can be difficult to distinguish from aSAH, as these activities not infrequently also precede intracranial aneurysm rupture and mimic the rapidity of onset and severity of aSAH. Accordingly, patients with a first-time TCHA related to these activities should be thoroughly evaluated with a focus on excluding the diagnosis of aSAH.

DIAGNOSTIC APPROACH

Crucial points in the history of patients with a recent headache are the abruptness of pain onset and the severity of discomfort. Lack of abnormality on the neurologic examination does not exclude aSAH, and therefore a detailed history and careful evaluation of such patients are essential. Furthermore, a mild hemorrhage, as in the clinical vignette, may not be

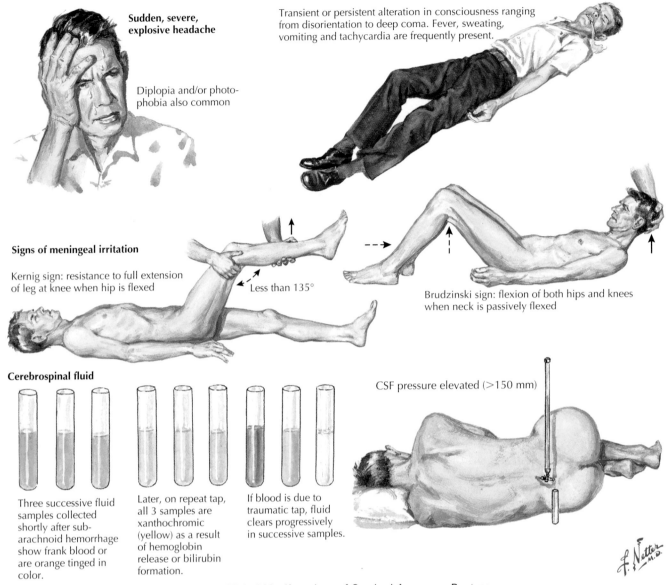

Sudden, severe, explosive headache

Transient or persistent alteration in consciousness ranging from disorientation to deep coma. Fever, sweating, vomiting and tachycardia are frequently present.

Diplopia and/or photophobia also common

Signs of meningeal irritation

Kernig sign: resistance to full extension of leg at knee when hip is flexed

Less than 135°

Brudzinski sign: flexion of both hips and knees when neck is passively flexed

Cerebrospinal fluid

CSF pressure elevated (>150 mm)

Three successive fluid samples collected shortly after subarachnoid hemorrhage show frank blood or are orange tinged in color.

Later, on repeat tap, all 3 samples are xanthochromic (yellow) as a result of hemoglobin release or bilirubin formation.

If blood is due to traumatic tap, fluid clears progressively in successive samples.

Fig. 17.5 Clinical Manifestations of Cerebral Aneurysm Rupture.

observed on CT, particularly if there is a delay in presentation. The clinical diagnosis of SAH is best confirmed with noncontrast brain CT (NCCT; Fig. 17.8), which can confirm the presence of SAH and frequently highlights associated issues such as hydrocephalus, intraparenchymal hematoma, or intraventricular hemorrhage. The sensitivity of NCCT declines as time passes after headache onset. For optimal scans performed on modern generation scanners with slice thickness less than 5 mm, the sensitivity for detecting aSAH is greater than 98% within 6 hours, 95% at 12 hours, 90% at 2 days, 75% at 3 days, and 50% after 5 days. A small hemorrhage may not be apparent after only 24 hours. Although MRI may be as sensitive as CT scan within the first 48–72 hours, it is rarely used due to more difficulty with completing and interpreting the imaging. Nonetheless, the use of hemosiderin-sensitive sequences (e.g., susceptibility-weighted imaging) may be more sensitive than CT scan.

Whenever the clinical suspicion of SAH exists but CT is negative, a lumbar puncture must be performed because of the imperfect sensitivity of CT for aSAH at even early time points and the essential nature of making this diagnosis before rerupture. A nontraumatic lumbar puncture is crucial. When the presence of blood in the CSF does not

clear between the first and fourth tubes, this is particularly suggestive of SAH (see Fig. 17.5). However, a more sensitive and specific indicator is CSF xanthochromia, or yellow discoloration of spun CSF. This results from lysis of erythrocytes with degradation of heme products into bilirubin within the CSF, which renders the CSF a yellowish color within 1–3 hours after an SAH and often persists for approximately 2–3 weeks. While the sensitivity of CSF analysis for xanthochromia is not maximal until 6–12 hours after ictus, one should not wait to perform LP in patients with suspected aSAH for this time to elapse, again because of the importance of making a timely diagnosis.

When SAH is confirmed by CT or lumbar puncture, the cause of the hemorrhage is best evaluated with a four-vessel cerebral angiogram. Although CT angiography is often used as a screening method to evaluate for aneurysms, catheter angiography remains the accepted standard for evaluating aneurysms in patients with aSAH: it is the gold standard for sensitivity, provides an increased level of anatomic detail often needed for aneurysm treatment planning, and allows for the option of simultaneous aneurysm treatment when appropriate. An aneurysmal source is found in 80%–85% of angiograms performed for suspected aSAH.

A. Cranial neuropathies

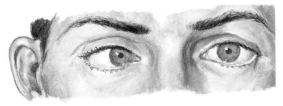 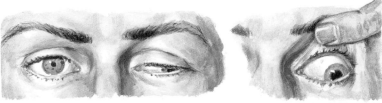

Abducens nerve palsy: affected eye turns medially. May be first manifestation of intracavernous carotid aneurysm. Pain above eye or on side of face may be secondary to trigeminal (V) nerve involvement.

Oculomotor nerve palsy: ptosis, eye turns laterally and inferiorly, pupil dilated. Common finding with cerebral aneurysms, especially carotid-posterior communicating aneurysms.

B. Visual field disturbances

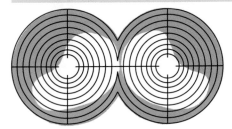 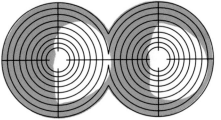 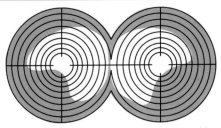

Superior bitemporal quadrantanopia caused by supraclinoid carotid aneurysm compressing optic chiasm from below

Right (or left) homonymous hemianopsia caused by compression of optic tract. Unilateral amaurosis may occur if optic (II) nerve is compressed.

Inferior bitemporal quadrantanopia caused by compression of optic chiasm from above

C. Retinal changes

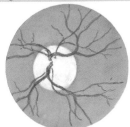 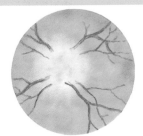 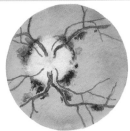

Optic atrophy may develop as result of pressure on optic (II) nerve from a supraclinoid carotid, ophthalmic, or anterior cerebral aneurysm.

Papilledema may be caused by increased intracranial pressure secondary to rupture of cerebral aneurysm.

Hemorrhage into optic (II) nerve sheath after rupture of aneurysm may result in subhyaloid hemorrhage, with blood around disc.

Fig. 17.6 Ophthalmologic Manifestations of Cerebral Aneurysms.

When the initial angiogram is negative in patients with suspected aSAH, a repeat angiogram is often performed within 5–10 days.

GRADING SCALES

To ensure proper communication, predict outcomes, and guide management, a clinical and radiographic grade for aSAH is needed. Several grading scales are available (Hunt and Hess, World Federation of Neurosurgeons, and modified Fisher scale); the most widely used is the Hunt–Hess scale—a quantifier from 1 (best) to 5 (worst) of the patient's state and an indicator of prognosis. The modified Fisher scale is a radiographic scale determined by the extent of subarachnoid hemorrhage and presence or absence of intraventricular hemorrhage and is related to the risk of DCI (Table 17.1).

PATHOPHYSIOLOGY

Intracranial Aneurysms

Subtypes of intracranial aneurysms include saccular, fusiform, dissecting, and infectious (mycotic) aneurysms. Saccular aneurysms are by far the most common type. They are spherical in shape but frequently have asymmetric outpouching and multilobulated characteristics that are felt to be potential rupture sites for the aneurysm. The aneurysm fundus or body is connected to the parent vessel via a small neck region, and as the aneurysm grows, this neck region may broaden and incorporate normal branching vessels.

Intracranial aneurysms characteristically occur at branch points of major cerebral arteries. Almost 85% of aneurysms are found in the anterior circulation and 15% within the posterior circulation (Fig. 17.9). Overall, the most common sites are the anterior communicating artery followed by the posterior communicating artery and the MCA bifurcation. Within the posterior circulation, the most frequent site is at the top of the basilar artery at the bifurcation into the posterior cerebral arteries.

Aneurysms are frequently classified according to size, with small being less than 10 mm, large 10–25 mm, and giant aneurysms larger than 25 mm. At presentation, most aneurysms are small, with only 2% found to be giant. Giant aneurysms are more likely to cause symptoms by compressing surrounding brain and/or cranial nerves. Rarely, involvement of tributary vessels, either due to aneurysm expansion or cavitary clot, may lead to ischemic symptoms as well. Controversy remains

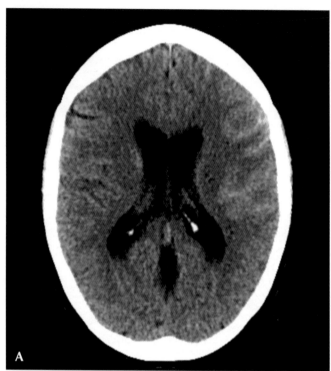

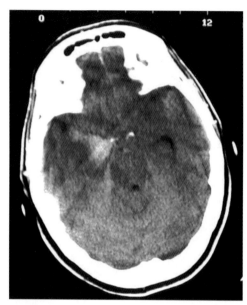

Unenhanced axial CT of the brain with SAH centered in the right sylvian fissure

Fig. 17.8 CT Brain With Subarachnoid Hemorrhage.

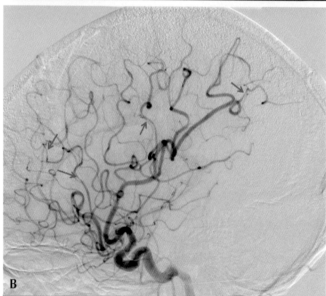

Fig. 17.7 (A) Reversible cerebral vasoconstriction syndrome subarachnoid hemorrhage. Axial noncontrast head CT with hyperdensity in the left frontal sulci consistent with cortical subarachnoid hemorrhage. (B) Reversible cerebral vasoconstriction syndrome—angiography. Left internal carotid artery injection with demonstration of multifocal narrowing of multiple distal branches in the left middle cerebral artery *(red arrows)* territory consistent with reversible cerebral vasoconstriction syndrome.

BOX 17.3 Differential Diagnosis for Thunderclap Headache

- Vascular
  - Ruptured intracranial aneurysm
  - Reversible cerebral vasoconstriction syndrome
  - Intracerebral hemorrhage
  - Cervical artery dissection
  - Cerebral venous sinus thrombosis
  - Subdural hematoma
  - Ischemic stroke (especially cerebellar)
  - Hypertensive crisis (with or without pheochromocytoma)
  - Giant cell arteritis
- Infectious
  - Meningitis/encephalitis
  - Subdural empyema
  - Severe sinusitis
- Neoplastic
  - Pituitary apoplexy
  - Brain tumor
- Disorders of cerebrospinal fluid hydrodynamics
  - Intracranial hypotension
  - Third ventricle colloid cyst with obstructive hydrocephalus
  - Aqueductal stenosis
- Primary headache syndromes
  - Primary thunderclap headache
  - Cough, exercise, or sexual activity associated thunderclap headache

---

regarding the precise relationship between aneurysm size and the risk of rupture. Overall, ruptured aneurysms tend to be larger than unruptured aneurysms, although many ruptured aneurysms are small.

MANAGEMENT

The first step in management of any neurologic emergency includes stabilization of the airway, breathing, and circulation and treatment of ongoing life-threatening neurologic complications. Once this is accomplished, the next, urgent goal of aSAH management should be to exclude the aneurysm from the circulation. This can be achieved via two approaches: endovascular with angiography and coiling or craniotomy with direct visualization and clipping. Treatment of unruptured intracranial aneurysms differs in some important ways from the treatment of ruptured aneurysms and will not be discussed in this chapter.

TABLE 17.1 Grading Systems for Aneurysmal Subarachnoid Hemorrhage

World Federation of Neurological Surgeons Grading System

Grade	Glasgow Coma Score	Motor Deficit
1	15	Absent
2	13–14	Absent
3	13–14	Present
4	7–12	Absent or Present
5	3–6	Absent or Present

Hunt and Hess Grade

Grade	Description	Mortality
1	Asymptomatic or minimally headache and slight nuchal rigidity	3%
2	Moderate or severe headache, nuchal rigidity, no neurologic deficit other than cranial nerve palsy	3%
3	Drowsiness, confusion, or mild focal deficit	9%
4	Stupor, moderate to severe hemiparesis, possibly early decerebrate rigidity and vegetative disturbance	24%
5	Deep coma, decerebrate posturing, moribund appearance	71%

Modified Fisher Grade

Grade	Criteria on CT	Incidence of Symptomatic Vasospasm
0	No SAH or IVH	0%
1	Focal of diffuse, thin SAH; no IVH	24%
2	Thin, focal or diffuse SAH; with IVH	33%
3	Thick, focal or diffuse SAH; no IVH	33%
4	Thick, focal or diffuse SAH; with IVH	40%

CT, Computed tomography; *IVH*, intraventricular hemorrhage; *SAH*, subarachnoid hemorrhage.

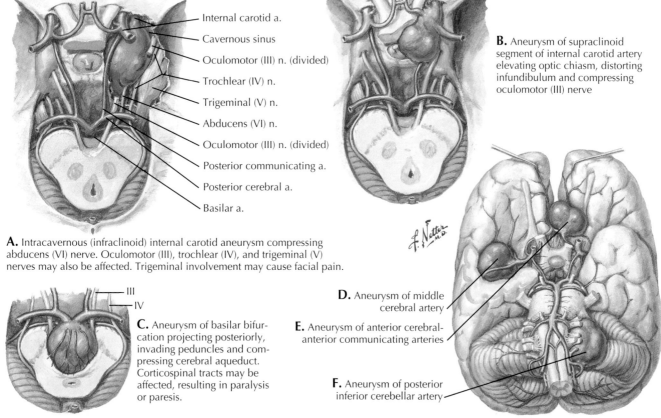

Internal carotid a.
Cavernous sinus
Oculomotor (III) n. (divided)
Trochlear (IV) n.
Trigeminal (V) n.
Abducens (VI) n.
Oculomotor (III) n. (divided)
Posterior communicating a.
Posterior cerebral a.
Basilar a.

B. Aneurysm of supraclinoid segment of internal carotid artery elevating optic chiasm, distorting infundibulum and compressing oculomotor (III) nerve

A. Intracavernous (infraclinoid) internal carotid aneurysm compressing abducens (VI) nerve. Oculomotor (III), trochlear (IV), and trigeminal (V) nerves may also be affected. Trigeminal involvement may cause facial pain.

III
IV

C. Aneurysm of basilar bifurcation projecting posteriorly, invading peduncles and compressing cerebral aqueduct. Corticospinal tracts may be affected, resulting in paralysis or paresis.

D. Aneurysm of middle cerebral artery

E. Aneurysm of anterior cerebral-anterior communicating arteries

F. Aneurysm of posterior inferior cerebellar artery

Fig. 17.9 Typical Sites of Cerebral Aneurysms.

Until the early 1990s, surgical clipping was the indisputable best treatment modality for ruptured intracranial aneurysms. This changed in 1991 when Gugliemi and colleagues published the first description of obliteration of an intracranial aneurysm by endovascular deployment of platinum coils into the aneurysm lumen. Introduced into the aneurysm using long, flexible catheters via femoral artery access, these coils subsequently **induce** rapid thrombosis of the aneurysm, thereby excluding it from the circulation. The coils stay in the aneurysm, as opposed to herniating into and embolizing the parent vessel, because they are held in initially by the relatively small neck of the aneurysm, and later by thrombosis and fibrosis (Fig. 17.10). Accordingly, aneurysms with a wide neck relative to the size of the dome are less favorable for coiling. As with the evolution of surgical clipping, several refinements of endovascular aneurysm treatment techniques and devices have over time led to greater success and less risk with this treatment. While simple coiling is the preferred method of treatment when possible, newer techniques such as balloon-assisted and stent-assisted coiling allow for successful endovascular treatment of otherwise uncoilable aneurysms.

Walter Dandy in 1937 described the first case of surgical clipping of an intracranial aneurysm, and this remains an essential treatment option for intracranial aneurysms today. The surgical approach to an aneurysm depends on its location, size, and shape. Most anterior circulation aneurysms are accessed via a pterional craniotomy, whereas posterior circulation aneurysms can be accessed by a variety of different skull base craniotomy approaches (Figs. 17.11 and 17.12). Once the craniotomy has been performed and the dura has been opened, a surgical microscope is used to facilitate operative dissection down to the aneurysm, followed by placement of one or more metallic clips across the neck of the aneurysm. Many additional advanced surgical techniques are available, including temporary clipping (allowing for temporary cessation of flow in the parent artery to facilitate safer aneurysm manipulation), cerebral arterial bypasses (to allow for parent vessel sacrifice in cases in which the aneurysm cannot be otherwise excluded from the circulation), aneurysmorrhaphy, and wrapping of dissecting aneurysms. Aneurysms that are difficult for the surgeon to access, especially posterior circulation aneurysms, are least favorable for this method.

DECIDING ON CLIPPING VERSUS COILING FOR RUPTURED SACCULAR ANEURYSMS

The relative superiority of clipping versus coiling for the treatment of ruptured intracranial aneurysms has been controversial since coiling first entered mainstream practice in the 1990s. Since then, two large clinical trials that have addressed this question and provide high-quality evidence now serve as a guide for this decision in individual patients: the International Subarachnoid Aneurysm Trial (ISAT), performed in the 1990s with up to 18 years of follow-up data published, and the Barrow Ruptured Aneurysm Trial (BRAT), performed in the 2000s with up to 6 years of follow-up data published.

At 1 year after aSAH, the risk of death or severe disability was significantly higher in the clipping groups in both trials (31% vs. 24% ISAT, 34% vs. 23% BRAT) despite a higher risk of aneurysm rerupture and need for retreatment in the coiled patients. The risk of posttreatment rerupture of the initially ruptured aneurysm was higher in the coiling group (2.6% vs. 1%) in ISAT, but higher in the clipping group in BRAT (0% vs. 0.08%). Finally, retreatment of the ruptured aneurysm in the first year was more frequent in the coiled group: 11% versus 3% (ISAT) and 11% versus 4.5% (BRAT). Additional advantages of coiling over clipping include a lower risk of DCI, epilepsy, and cognitive dysfunction. Taken together, these data indicate that the advantages conferred by clipping—avoiding a relatively small risk of rerupture and a larger risk of retreatment—are far outweighed, at least in the first year, but the much higher upfront risk conferred by surgery for mortality, functional disability, and complications. This conclusion is supported by long-term follow-up data from both trials.

Importantly, these trial results do not mean that coiling is the better treatment in all aSAH patients. Surgical aneurysm clipping remains an essential technique. In ISAT, patients were only randomized if a neurosurgeon and neurointerventionalist both agreed that the aneurysm was equally amenable to treatment by either modality. In BRAT, although patients were randomized regardless of the appearance and location of the aneurysm, there was significant crossover from one assigned group to the other based on what the treating physicians deemed the most appropriate treatment when equipoise did not exist. Therefore, patients with aneurysm or other characteristics that favored one treatment modality over the other (Box 17.4) were not included at all in ISAT and not randomly assigned treatment in BRAT. Although newer techniques and devices, as well as overall increased experience in the field, have expanded the indications for endovascular treatment, surgical clipping remains an important option, particularly in patients with space-occupying hematomas or aneurysms with anatomy not favorable for endovascular treatment (very small size, low dome:neck ratio, many MCA aneurysms). Young (<40–50 years old) patients with easily surgically accessible aneurysms (because of their lower risk with surgery and higher lifetime risk of rerupture) may also benefit more from clipping. Conversely, endovascular treatment is almost always the preferred method for treating posterior circulation aneurysms due to the high surgical risks.

Because of the complexity of the decision making involved in determining the optimal mode of treatment in any given aSAH patient, treatment of ruptured aneurysms should only be undertaken in a hospital with expertise in both surgical and endovascular techniques. Furthermore, the decision of clipping versus coiling should be made after careful review by physicians (or a single physician) experienced in the use of both modalities.

Ruptured Dissecting Aneurysms

The treatment of ruptured dissecting aneurysms is much more challenging than that of saccular aneurysms, and they are extremely dangerous regardless of the chosen treatment. Historically, the primary methods of treatment included surgical or endovascular sacrifice of the affected vessel, surgical wrapping of the dissecting aneurysm, and various other endovascular techniques involving the use of stents and/or coils. Unfortunately, all of those strategies are associated with high morbidity and mortality.

More recently, the use of flow diverters has become the favored approach at many institutions. The benefit of using flow diverters is that their placement is minimally invasive, the affected artery remains patent, and they allow for remodeling of the affected artery with a legitimate chance at a cure. The major downside is that they do not immediately secure the lesion while at the same time requiring the use of dual antiplatelet therapy, which might increase the risk of early rerupture. Regardless of the chosen treatment strategy, it is extremely important to communicate the gravity of the situation to the patient and their family prior to proceeding with treatment.

Ruptured Mycotic Aneurysm

Mycotic aneurysms are uncommon, infectious aneurysms caused by a number of infectious etiologies, most commonly bacterial endocarditis. In this disease, they are caused by embolization of infected thrombi from cardiac valvular vegetations. Because such emboli are typically small, they characteristically (although not exclusively) embolize to distal branches of intracranial vessels. Thus, as compared with typical saccular aneurysms which occur in the proximal intracranial arterial

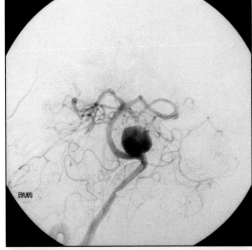

Large berry aneurysm at junction of vertebral and basilar artery

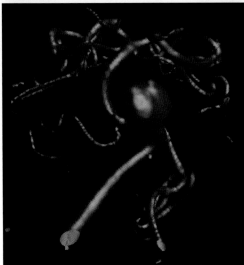

Three-dimensional reconstruction of a giant vertebrobasilar junction aneurysm

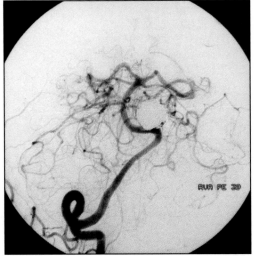

Total obliteration of the aneurysm with interventional radiology placement of coils within the aneurysm

Fig. 17.10 Interventional Radiologic Repair of Berry Aneurysm.

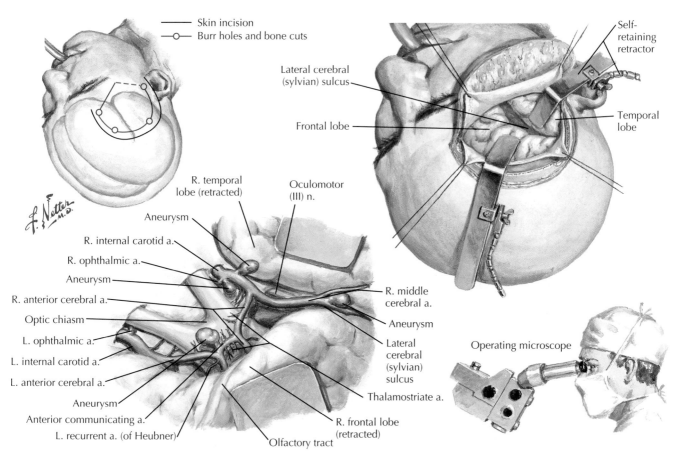

Fig. 17.11 Frontotemporal Approach for Internal Carotid, Ophthalmic, Anterior Communicating, and Middle Cerebral Aneurysms.

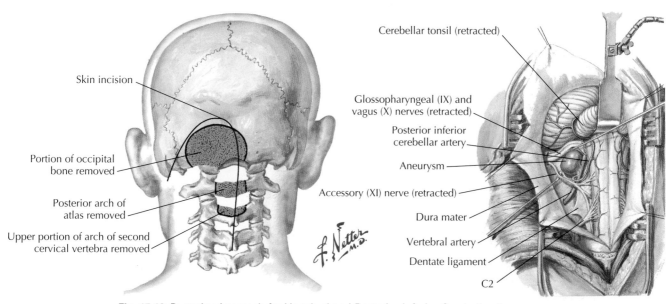

Fig. 17.12 Posterior Approach for Vertebral and Posterior Inferior Cerebellar Aneurysms.

branch points, mycotic aneurysms typically arise in more distal branches. The inflammatory response to the infected embolus results in vessel wall degradation, which in the presence of the physical stress of arterial blood flow results in aneurysm formation and possibly rupture. Medical management of ruptured mycotic aneurysms includes blood pressure control, maintenance of normal coagulation function, avoidance of

anticoagulants, and especially prolonged antibiotic therapy directed at the causative organism. There are no definitive guidelines on procedural management of ruptured mycotic aneurysms, but considerations include endovascular sacrifice of the vessel by polymer occlusion or open surgical approach with aneurysmal clipping, which is commonly reserved for those requiring hematoma evacuation/intracranial pressure

BOX 17.4 Clipping Versus Coiling of Ruptured Aneurysms: Effect of Patient and Aneurysm Characteristics

- Favors clipping
  - Wide aneurysm neck
  - Very small aneurysm
  - Middle cerebral artery bifurcation location
  - Associated intracranial hematoma with mass effect
  - Younger patient age
- Favors coiling
  - Posterior circulation and other locations with difficult surgical access
  - Small aneurysm neck
  - Elderly patients
  - Poor clinical grade patients

management. Endovascular therapy with coils and/or stents, while possible, is often avoided due to the possibility of infection seeding these devices.

Neurologic Complications of Aneurysmal Subarachnoid Hemorrhage

Rebleeding

If a ruptured aneurysm is not treated, the risk of subsequent rupture is very high: at least 4% (and possibly up to 15%–20%) in the first 24 hours and 1.5% per subsequent day, leading to approximately 27% incidence of subsequent aneurysmal rupture within the first 2 weeks of hemorrhage and 50% in the first 6 months. Thereafter the rebleeding rate decreases to 3%–5% per year. Crucially, rebleeding most often has catastrophic consequences, with a mortality rate of 70%. Therefore, an essential component of the early phase of aSAH treatment is to prevent rebleeding using surgical or endovascular methods to obliterate the aneurysm as soon as it is safe, ideally within 24–48 hours of ictus.

If aneurysm treatment is expected to be delayed by more than approximately 6–12 hours, a short (<72 hours) course of the antifibrinolytic agent tranexamic acid can be used up to 6 hours before the endovascular or surgical treatment to reduce rerupture risk without increasing the risk of thromboembolic complications or DCI. Maintaining a systolic blood pressure of less than 160–180 mm Hg, while being careful not to provoke cerebral hypoperfusion due to elevated ICP and/or early vasospasm, may also decreased the risk of pretreatment rerupture.

Hydrocephalus

About 25% of patients with aSAH develop acute hydrocephalus, independent of clinical grade, that worsens if left untreated. As common as it is, the etiology is not known. Factors associated with increased risk of hydrocephalus include intraventricular hemorrhage, low GCS, hypertension, older age, posterior circulation aneurysm, and increasing amounts of SAH. External ventricular drainage is recommended in patients if there is any suspicion that hydrocephalus might be contributing to more than mild neurologic impairment. Although most of these patients no longer require ventricular drainage after about 2–3 weeks, chronic hydrocephalus develops in 25% of aSAH patients who survive the acute period. These patients require permanent ventricular drainage with a ventriculoperitoneal shunt.

Cerebral Vasospasm and Delayed Cerebral Ischemia

Cerebral vasospasm, which may cause DCI, is a common complication after SAH, and contributes to significant morbidity and mortality. Vasospasm occurs in 30%–70% of aSAH patients, and DCI occurs in 20%–30%. Importantly, not all cerebral vasospasm causes DCI, and not all DCI can be explained by angiographically detectable cerebral vasospasm. Vasospasm and/or DCI can occur any time in the first 3 weeks after aneurysm rupture, although it is uncommon before the third to fourth day after SAH and usually peaks between days 7 and 14. The most potent risk factor is the volume of blood in the subarachnoid cisterns and ventricles. Beginning with C. Miller Fisher's score in 1980, several semiquantitative CT grading scales have been devised that correlate the amount to SAH to vasospasm and DCI risk. At present, the most clinically useful of these is the modified Fisher scale (see Table 17.1).

The mechanism underlying cerebral vasospasm and DCI is poorly understood, a fact emphasized by vasospasm and DCI, while commonly referred to synonymously, are actually clinically related but separable entities. The pathophysiology is likely quite complex, involving but not limited to macrovascular (angiographically detectable vasospasm) and microvascular components, inflammation driven primarily by oxyhemoglobin in the extravasated arterial subarachnoid blood, and cortical spreading depression/ischemia. To date there is no known preventative treatment. One study using oral nimodipine demonstrated improved functional outcome at 90 days, but no change in the rate of vasospasm. Based on this and multiple other studies with similar findings, nimodipine is used to improve functional outcome at a standard dose of 60 mg every 4 hours or 30 mg every 2 hours for a total of 21 days after the hemorrhage. Hypovolemia and hypotension can precipitate DCI. Therefore, euvolemia should be carefully maintained throughout the DCI window. Once the aneurysm has been secured, permissive hypertension is advisable, with cessation of all antihypertensive agents (with the exception of nimodipine) and treatment of hypertension only when severe (above systolic 200–220 mm Hg or lower if causing end-organ dysfunction) and there is no ongoing DCI.

Monitoring for and treating DCI and vasospasm is a central part of neurocritical care for aSAH patients. The neurologic examination remains the cornerstone for detection of DCI. However, there are three major limitations to this strategy: (1) changes in examination may be due to a multitude of factors unrelated to DCI, (2) changes in examination are reflective of brain ischemia and therefore do not allow for preemptive treatments, and (3) in comatose patients detectable changes in exam may not be appreciated until DCI is severe. Therefore, additional surveillance tools are used to augment the neurologic exam. Transcranial Doppler (TCD) ultrasound measures the velocity of blood within the major (internal carotid, middle, anterior, posterior cerebral, vertebral, and basilar arteries) intracranial and extracranial vessels. As the vessels become stenotic due to vasospasm, the velocity of blood increases. TCD has limitations with regard to sensitivity, specificity, and positive predictive value—90%, 71%, and 50%, respectively. Its noninvasive nature and ease of use make it probably the most widely used vasospasm monitoring method, but its diagnostic performance is less than ideal, and crucially, it can detect only vasospasm but not DCI. MR and CT angiography and perfusion imaging can be used to objectively detect both vasospasm and cerebral ischemia, and these are quite useful screening tools in comatose patients. Their utility is limited by the need to transfer the patient to the radiology suite, the fact that they assess only a single time point in a notoriously dynamic process, as well as exposure to radiation (CT) and contrast material. Continuous electroencephalography (EEG) can also be used for DCI monitoring. As blood flow decreases, the normal fast-wave activity of the brain decreases and the background rhythm slows. Quantitative EEG can determine the ratio of time with fast and slow frequencies, and this ratio will decrease as blood flow decreases and brain tissue becomes infarcted. Brain ischemia can also be detected using intraparenchymal monitors that can measure parameters such as brain tissue oxygen tension, cerebral interstitial fluid lactate/pyruvate ratio, and cerebral blood flow. Limitations of these techniques include their invasive nature, lack of validated diagnostic thresholds, and the fact that they monitor only a very small region of the brain.

Medical management of DCI has evolved in recent years. It is crucial to acknowledge that the target for treatment is DCI and not vasospasm. Triple H therapy, consisting of hypervolemia, hemodilution, and hypertension, has been replaced by euvolemic hypertensive therapy. The first objective is to optimize volume resuscitation, typically with isotonic crystalloid intravenous fluids. The target should be euvolemia rather than hypervolemia, as the latter may lead to additional complications (primarily pulmonary) without clear added benefit. Augmentation of the blood pressure with vasopressors, most commonly phenylephrine or norepinephrine, to allow for improved blood flow through or around (by collateral routes) stenotic vessels is the next step in management. Inotropic agents, especially milrinone, can be useful in patients with significantly reduced cardiac output as well as in patients refractory to euvolemic hypertension. The goal with all of these is to prevent development of permanent neurologic deficits by reversing DCI before it can lead to brain infarction without causing severe nonneurologic complications. If complications, such as pulmonary edema, myocardial dysfunction or ischemia, or arrhythmias, develop, the intensity of hemodynamic augmentation should be decreased. Occasionally, DCI continues despite aggressive medical therapy. If significant DCI persists for more than approximately 1–4 hours despite maximal safe hemodynamic augmentation, urgent cerebral angiography should be performed to assess the severity of vasospasm and provide direct intraarterial treatment, if indicated. The first-line endovascular treatment option is the direct intraarterial infusion of a vasodilatory agent such as verapamil, nicardipine, or milrinone. Unfortunately, while quite effective, intraarterial vasodilators' effects are transient, typically lasting a period of several hours. As such, this procedure may need to be performed multiple times in patients who develop recurrent clinical symptoms of vasospasm. Balloon angioplasty, which is a more durable treatment, also carries higher procedure-related risks. It is most useful in patients with severe, early vasospasm in proximal large vessels that are expected to be problematic for many days.

Nonneurologic Complications of aSAH

The nonneurologic complications of aSAH demonstrate the intimate interplay between the brain and body. It is not uncommon to see multisystem organ dysfunction in the setting of acute SAH.

At the moment of aneurysm rupture, experimental evidence suggests that a massive surge in ICP overcomes MAP, resulting in a momentary global arrest in cerebral circulation. As the increased ICP begins to wane, the circulation is reinstated, at which point a small fibrin plug is created at the site of rupture, sealing the aneurysm and preventing further bleeding. The sudden ICP increase affects the hypothalamus, and when combined with the associated global ischemia, there is a **massive neuroendocrine response** with a **catecholamine surge** consequently leading to systemic dysfunction, especially of the heart, lungs, and kidneys.

One consequence of this catecholamine surge is myocardial injury, known as **neurogenic stress cardiomyopathy.** Abnormalities may be identified on electrocardiogram (ECG) in up to 90% of patients at admission, including T-wave abnormalities, ST-segment alterations, prominent U waves, or prolongation of the QT interval (Fig. 17.13), and can be seen in up to 10%. Minor troponin elevations occur in the majority of aSAH patients. Transient regional systolic dysfunction of the left ventricle with regional wall motion abnormalities primarily of the cardiac base (so-called takotsubo cardiomyopathy) is characteristic. When severe, this can cause cardiogenic shock. It is essential to recognize these common consequences of aSAH and distinguish them from true myocardial ischemia, which is quite uncommon in aSAH, as treatments for MI and aSAH are often contradictory.

Neurogenic pulmonary edema is another important nonneurologic complication of aSAH. Interstitial and alveolar edema can occur within minutes to hours after aSAH, and resolution can take several days. Neurogenic pulmonary edema initially appears similar to acute

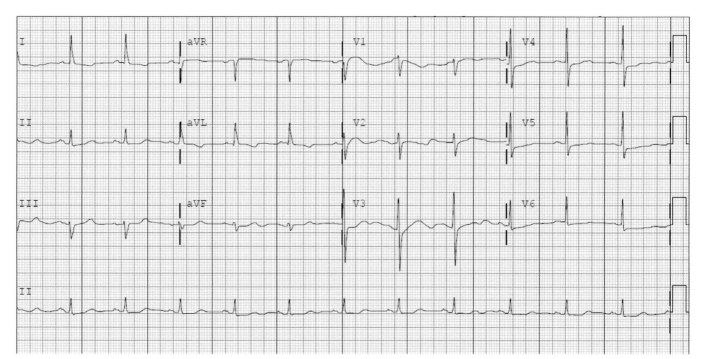

Fig. 17.13 ECG Changes Associated With Subarachnoid Hemorrhage. Electrocardiogram demonstrating QT prolongation and ST depressions in precordial leads. Another commonly encountered finding, not pictured here, is T-wave inversion in precordial leads.

respiratory distress syndrome (ARDS): bilateral opacities on x-ray and severely decreased arterial to inspired oxygen ratio ($PaO_2/FiO_2 < 200$). Although the pathophysiology is not fully understood, it appears to be related to the transient sympathetic surge, although how much of this is due to a direct effect on the pulmonary alveolar endothelium and how much is secondary cardiogenic pulmonary edema due to neurogenic stress cardiomyopathy has not been well worked out. Management of neurogenic pulmonary edema is mainly supportive and does not substantially alter the prognosis following SAH. Intubation and mechanical ventilation are typically required. Thereafter, supplemental oxygenation, increased levels of positive end expiratory pressure (PEEP), adjustment of tidal volumes, and optimization of fluid status all may be considered. Unlike ARDS, most cases of neurogenic pulmonary edema begin to resolve within 48–72 hours.

There is usually associated **acute hypertension,** sometimes as part of the Cushing response related to increased ICP. This reflexive mechanism may be protective, as it maintains mean arterial pressure and cerebral circulation in the face of a dramatic increase in ICP. Management of hypertension in this setting requires treatment of the increased ICP, such as ventricular drainage of the CSF. As discussed in a previous section, prior to aneurysm treatment, care should be taken to manage hypertension to reduce the risk of aneurysmal rebleeding while avoiding provocation of cerebral hypoperfusion.

Frequently, abnormalities of electrolytes occur, particularly hyponatremia. The two primary causes of hyponatremia in SAH are **cerebral salt wasting (CSW)** and **syndrome of inappropriate antidiuretic hormone (SIADH)** (Table 17.2). These two conditions typically present with mild to moderate hyponatremia (125–134 mEq/L), although rarely it may be severe (<125 mEq/L). The primary means of differentiating CSW from SIADH is the volume status of the patient, which can be quite difficult. In SIADH, the intravascular volume is normal to mildly elevated, whereas in CSW it is reduced. Commonly used volume status assessments include:

- Passive leg raise: placing patient flat and raising the legs to 45 degrees for 5 minutes. If there is an increase in mean arterial pressure, end-tidal CO_2, then the patient is likely fluid responsive (71% sensitive and 100% specific).
- IVC ultrasound: measurement of the inferior vena cava at the point just proximal to the right atrium is the ideal place for monitoring. If the diameter is less than 1.5 cm or there is collapse of the vein greater than 50% with the respiratory cycle, these point to a patient who is fluid response (78% sensitive and 86% specific).
- Arterial waveform-derived stroke volume variability: the beat-to-beat variation of the stroke volume as measured by area under the curve of an arterial waveform is associated with volume responsiveness. Stroke volume variability greater than 9% indicates hypovolemia with 81% sensitivity and 80% specificity.
- Pulmonary artery catheterization: this is a less commonly used volume assessment tool due to its invasiveness and potential complications.

CSW results in hypovolemia due to natriuresis, probably primarily driven by dysregulation of atrial natriuretic peptide secretion from the hypothalamus. The patient with CSW requires replacement of both volume and sodium, which can be achieved with hypertonic solutions (3% NaCl). The mineralocorticoid fludrocortisone can be used to partially counter the natriuretic process. SIADH is the result of hypothalamic–pituitary axis dysregulation and release of excessive ADH. This results in excessive free water resorption and resultant hyponatremia. Although fluid restriction is used in other patients with SIADH, given the great difficulty in distinguishing it from CSW and the risks of provoking DCI with hypovolemia, in aSAH patients SIADH is treated in the same manner as CSW, with provision of both sodium and volume with hypertonic saline solutions.

ADDITIONAL RESOURCES

Connolly ES, Rabinstein AA, Carhuapoma JR, et al. Guideline for the management of aneurysmal subarachnoid hemorrhage: a guideline for healthcare professionals from the American Heart Association/American Stroke Association. Stroke 2012;43:1711–37.

The American Heart Association/American Stroke Association have extensive published guidelines on treatment recommendations for those with aneurysmal subarachnoid hemorrhage. This is a broad review of the literature and basic treatment outline for aneurysmal subarachnoid hemorrhage.

Diringer MN, Bleck TP, Hemphill JC III, et al. Critical care management of patients following aneurysmal subarachnoid hemorrhage: recommendations from the Neurocritical Care Society's multidisciplinary consensus conference. Neurocrit Care 2011;15:211–40.

The Neurocritical Care Society guidelines for aneurysmal subarachnoid hemorrhage provide focused literature review of relevant treatments and management of the disease and complications thereof.

Molyneux AJ, Birks J, Clarke A, et al. The durability of endovascular coiling versus neurosurgical clipping of ruptured cerebral aneurysms: 18 year follow-up of the UK cohort of the International Subarachnoid Aneurysm Trial (ISAT). Lancet 2015;385:691–7.

The ISAT update from 2015 gives the longest follow-up for patients who have undergone endovascular coiling and open clipping of ruptured aneurysmal subarachnoid hemorrhage.

Spetzler RF, McDougall CG, Zabramski JM, et al. The Barrow Ruptured Aneurysm Trial: 6-year results. J Neurosurg. 2015;123:609–17.

The BRAT 6-year follow-up results are the single institution, Barrow Neurologic Institute, results on endovascular coiling and open clipping of ruptured aneurysms. This study, although smaller than ISAT, is only North American patients, making it potentially more relevant for those practicing in the United States.

TABLE 17.2 Differentiation of Cerebral Salt Wasting and Syndrome of Inappropriate Antidiuretic Hormone

Laboratory/Clinical Finding	CSW	SIADH
Urine osmolality	↑	↑
Urine Na concentration	↑	↑
Extracellular fluid volume	↓	↔ or ↑
Fluid balance	↓	↔ or ↑
Urine volume	↑	↔ or ↓
Serum bicarbonate	↑	↓
Blood urea nitrogen (BUN)	↑	↔ or ↓
Sodium balance	↓	↔ or ↑
Treatment in aSAH	Volume resuscitation Hypertonic saline Mineralocorticoids Salt tablets	Free water restriction Hypertonic saline Salt tablets Vaptans Demeclocycline

aSAH, Aneurysmal subarachnoid hemorrhage; *CSW,* cerebral salt wasting; *SIADH,* syndrome of inappropriate antidiuretic hormone.

18

Cerebral Venous Thrombosis

Gregory J. Allam

CLINICAL VIGNETTE *A 45-year-old man with a history of bipolar disorder and binges of alcohol abuse gradually developed global headaches that abruptly worsened over a 6-day period. He presented to the emergency room with excruciating headaches, especially while lying flat or after coughing. He described visual blurring and transient visual dimming with straining or getting up rapidly. He was slightly inattentive but had no focal weakness or numbness on examination. Ophthalmoscopy showed severe bilateral papilledema with peripapillary flame-shaped hemorrhages but no visual field loss. Computed tomography (CT) scan of the brain showed hyperdensity in the sagittal sinus and the left transverse sinus. Cerebrospinal fluid (CSF) fluid opening pressure was elevated but with a normal analysis. Magnetic resonance imaging (MRI) of the brain showed no acute stroke or hemorrhage, but magnetic resonance venography (MRV) showed partial occlusion of the sagittal sinus, left transverse sinus, and the left jugular vein. He later admitted to drinking and smoking heavily just before his headaches worsened. There was no evidence of malignancy, and initial coagulation studies were normal. He was treated with warfarin and acetazolamide with gradual resolution of the headaches. Serial MRVs showed partial recanalization of the occluded cerebral sinuses and he was eventually taken off warfarin. He was admitted about 6 months later with recurrent episodes of shortness of breath and palpitations and was found to have multiple small pulmonary emboli and deep vein thrombosis. A more extensive hypercoagulability screen now revealed a lupus anticoagulant, and the presence of a prothrombin (factor II) gene mutation. He was subsequently advised to stay on lifelong warfarin.*

CLINICAL VIGNETTE *A 34-year-old man presented to the hospital after 1 week of increasing occipital headache, stiff neck, and chills. Although brain CT scanning and CSF analysis were normal, the patient was admitted to the hospital for reported worsening confusion and behavioral changes. Soon after admission, he had a generalized tonic-clonic seizure and was intubated for airway protection.*

A brain MRI demonstrated bilateral frontal hemorrhagic infarctions with edema and a MRV showed a sagittal sinus thrombosis. Because of obtundation and signs of increased intracranial pressure (ICP), hyperosmolar therapy and an intravenous heparin infusion were started. A continuous intrasinus infusion of tissue plasminogen activator was given over 2 days. The thrombosis resolved, and he recovered consciousness.

Eventually, the patient was discharged from the hospital on warfarin and anticonvulsants, with only minor left-sided sensory changes and mild left leg weakness. Unfortunately, he did not continue the prescribed anticoagulants and was readmitted 20 days later with pleuritic chest pain and shortness of breath. Bilateral deep vein thrombosis and a pulmonary embolism were diagnosed. An infrarenal inferior vena cava filter was inserted, and anticoagulation was resumed. The patient had a positive test result for anticardiolipin antibodies. This led to the diagnosis of an anticardiolipin antibody syndrome, confirming the need for long-term systemic anticoagulation.

When venous drainage of the brain is compromised, back-pressure into the parenchymal tissue causes capillary congestion, interstitial edema, decreased tissue perfusion, and ultimately ischemia. Eventually capillary rupture causes hematoma formation. This process of cerebral venous congestion followed by hemorrhagic infarction, not conforming to strict arterial territories, is the hallmark of cerebral sinus thrombosis. The causes of cerebral venous thrombosis (CVT) vary (Box 18.1), but often relate to transient or permanent hypercoagulable states, with dehydration acting as a common precipitating event. A thorough investigation for such etiologies is crucial to directing long-term treatment and anticipating potential comorbidities.

Attention should be given to signs of meningitis, such as fever, stiff neck, and rash. Examining the ears, sinuses, and face for infection or discharge may provide clues to possible septic venous thrombosis. Physical evidence or a history of head or neck trauma is important. Ocular pain, proptosis, chemosis, and cranial neuropathies are significant signs that often indicate a venous occlusion along the skull base such as cavernous sinus, petrosal sinus, or jugular vein thrombosis.

ANATOMY

Although complex, cerebral venous system anatomy is best considered in three levels: the dural-based superior group, the dural inferior or basal skull group, and the deep veins of the brain.

The dura is formed of two layers, one abutting the inner calvarium and the other forming the outer meningeal covering. These layers separate in the midsagittal and transverse planes, forming dural venous sinuses that ultimately drain into the jugular veins. A single superior sagittal sinus joins the often asymmetric but paired transverse sinus at the confluence of sinuses or torcular herophili (Fig. 18.1). The transverse sinuses run laterally from the occipital bone to the middle cerebral fossa along the tentorium cerebelli. The right is often larger and is continuous with the superior sagittal sinus whereas the left curves out laterally as an extension of the single midline straight sinus. The straight sinus runs downward from near the splenium of the corpus callosum to the occipital protuberance. From the transverse sinus the sigmoid sinus curves down toward the skull base and joins the inferior petrosal sinus at the jugular foramen to form the jugular vein.

The straight sinus (Figs. 18.1–18.4) is formed by the splayed falx layered over the cerebellar tentorium. The inferior sagittal sinus runs in the fold of the lower arch of the falx cerebri and joins the cerebral vein of Galen in the proximity of the posterior horns of the lateral ventricles to form the straight sinus. The superior and inferior sagittal sinuses provide drainage for the cerebral hemispheres.

The great cerebral vein of Galen drains through paired internal cerebral veins, and the paired basal vein of Rosenthal drains the basal ganglia, thalamus, posterior portions of the limbic system, the hippocampus, and mesencephalon.

BOX 18.1 Causes of Venous Sinus Thrombosis

- Hypercoagulable states, anticardiolipin antibody syndrome, etc.
- Head trauma, jugular trauma, or canalization
- Parameningeal infection of the face, eye, ear, mastoids, or sinuses
- Meningitis, subdural empyema, brain abscess
- Hormonally related: pregnancy, postpartum period, oral contraceptives
- Dehydration
- Infiltrative malignancies
- Ulcerative colitis
- Systemic lupus erythematosus
- Human immunodeficiency virus infection
- Nephrotic syndrome
- Behçet disease

The cavernous sinus runs posteriorly at the skull base from the sphenoid bone in the area of the superior orbital fissure to the petrous temporal bone. Cavernous sinus tributaries include cerebral veins and the ophthalmic vein. The cavernous sinus drains along the medial upper layer of the tentorium and through the superior petrosal sinus, coursing posteriorly to the transverse sinus. The cavernous sinus houses the carotid artery and the oculomotor, trochlear, and abducens cranial nerves, as well as the ophthalmic division of the trigeminal nerve. The maxillary division of the trigeminal nerve also goes through the lower portion of the lateral wall (Fig. 18.5), but in some patients it can lie just outside the sinus. A mesh of venous sinuses around the pituitary and the anterior skull base connects the two cavernous sinuses across the midline. The superior petrosal sinus drains the anterior brainstem and the anterior superior and inferior cerebellar hemispheres. Below the tentorium, along the skull base, the inferior petrosal sinus links the cavernous sinus to the sigmoid sinus (see Fig. 18.1).

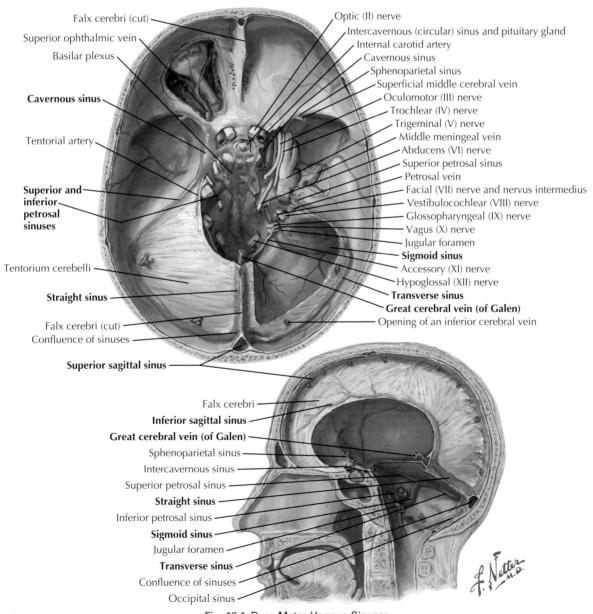

Fig. 18.1 Dura Mater Venous Sinuses.

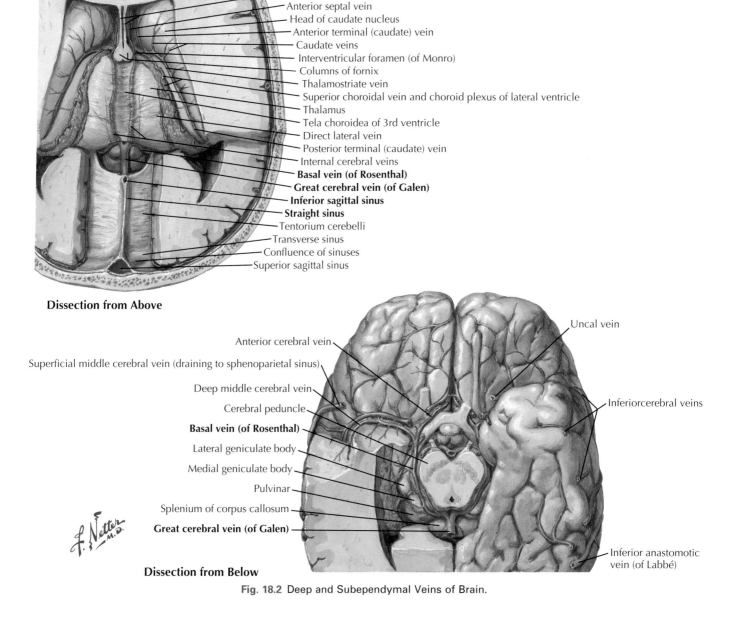

Dissection from Above

Longitudinal fissure
Anterior cerebral veins
Rostrum of corpus callosum
Septum pellucidum
Anterior septal vein
Head of caudate nucleus
Anterior terminal (caudate) vein
Caudate veins
Interventricular foramen (of Monro)
Columns of fornix
Thalamostriate vein
Superior choroidal vein and choroid plexus of lateral ventricle
Thalamus
Tela choroidea of 3rd ventricle
Direct lateral vein
Posterior terminal (caudate) vein
Internal cerebral veins
Basal vein (of Rosenthal)
Great cerebral vein (of Galen)
Inferior sagittal sinus
Straight sinus
Tentorium cerebelli
Transverse sinus
Confluence of sinuses
Superior sagittal sinus

Anterior cerebral vein
Superficial middle cerebral vein (draining to sphenoparietal sinus)
Deep middle cerebral vein
Cerebral peduncle
Basal vein (of Rosenthal)
Lateral geniculate body
Medial geniculate body
Pulvinar
Splenium of corpus callosum
Great cerebral vein (of Galen)

Uncal vein
Inferiorcerebral veins
Inferior anastomotic vein (of Labbé)

Dissection from Below

Fig. 18.2 Deep and Subependymal Veins of Brain.

CLINICAL PRESENTATION

General Aspects

The neurologic presentation of CVT is protean. General features depend on the location of venous thrombosis and the abruptness of occlusion. In most patients, the earliest sign is an evolving, constant, diffuse headache that worsens with recumbence. Blurred vision from papilledema is often present but, unless it persists for weeks, it rarely leads to significant or permanent visual loss. Sudden brief spells of visual obscuration can occur with abrupt positional changes and are thought to represent transiently decreased perfusion of swollen optic nerves. Slowed cognition or encephalopathy without localized brain lesions or focal neurologic signs may occur with long-standing cerebral thrombosis of gradual evolution, as seen in the first vignette presented above.

Patients who have a more abrupt onset of cortical vein or superficial venous sinus thrombosis develop cortically based, often hemorrhagic lesions with focal neurologic signs, and focal or generalized seizures. If the hemispheric lesion is large, increased ICP and coma with possible transtentorial brain herniation can occur. With involvement of the deep cerebral veins or extensive involvement of the superficial sinuses with more than two-thirds of the superior sagittal sinus and/or transverse and sigmoid sinuses, obtundation followed by coma with decorticate or decerebrate posturing are presenting signs reflecting bihemispheric, bithalamic basal ganglionic, or brainstem dysfunction. Combinations of painful cranial neuropathies with little involvement of consciousness occur with basal skull, jugular vein, cavernous, or petrosal sinus venous thrombosis.

Specific Clinical Presentations

In **superior sagittal sinus thrombosis** (SSST), increased venous pressure from decreased drainage initially causes generalized headaches with paroxysms of pain occurring with any Valsalva-like maneuver,

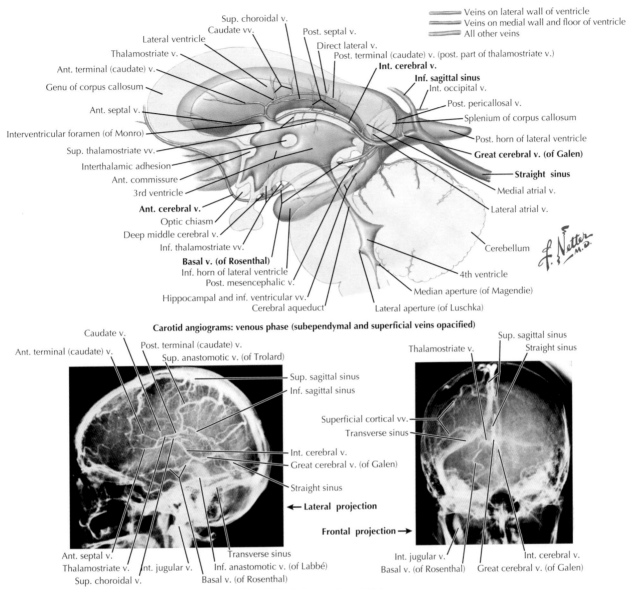

Fig. 18.3 Subependymal Veins.

such as coughing, sneezing, straining, lifting, or bending. Blurred vision may occur secondary to optic nerve head edema or associated exudates, particularly involving the macula. Permanent visual compromise is unusual and only happens when papilledema persists unaddressed for weeks. Light-headedness, transient blindness, and tinnitus can occur with sudden head elevation from a lying or bending position, similar to pseudotumor cerebri.

Intracerebral cortically based hemorrhages, which are common with SSST, are often associated with focal neurologic signs and seizures. Confusion, behavioral changes, somnolence, and coma may occur as thrombosis propagates within the sinus and ICP increases. These signs usually develop after the clot extends into the posterior third of the sinus toward the confluence of sinuses (torcula). In most cases of SSSTs, one of the lateral sinuses is concomitantly involved (Fig. 18.6).

Occasionally, **isolated cortical vein thrombosis** is seen without sagittal sinus involvement. The clinical picture is again one of headaches, focal neurologic dysfunction, and seizure—however, without increased ICP or papilledema. Underlying causes are similar to sagittal sinus

thrombosis, and treatment generally follows the same principles. Neuroimaging shows isolated, often hemorrhagic, ischemic lesions that are not confined to a cerebral artery territory.

Deep cerebral vein thrombosis is present in 40% of superior sagittal sinus cases and is more likely to produce coma, pupillary abnormalities, ophthalmoplegia, and increased ICP than SSST alone. Sole or predominant deep venous system involvement mostly occurs in children but is reported in adults with presentations ranging from isolated drowsiness or obtundation to coma with bilateral posturing and ocular abnormalities. Survivors experience bilateral weakness, rigidity, dystonia or athetosis, memory loss, personality changes, and various neuropsychological disturbances.

Base of the skull sinus thrombosis has a clinical presentation of painful cranial neuropathies. *Cavernous sinus thrombosis* is often septic from facial, orbital, or middle ear infections with eye pain, proptosis, and chemosis as frequent features (Fig. 18.7). Varying degrees of ophthalmoplegia are present secondary to involvement of CN III, IV, and VI running through the cavernous sinus. The ophthalmic division of the trigeminal nerve (V1) also courses through this sinus as well as in

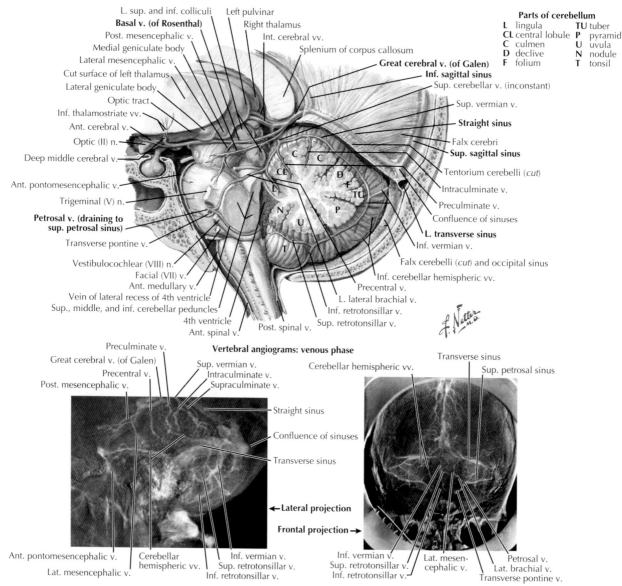

Parts of cerebellum
L	lingula	**TU**	tuber
CL	central lobule	**P**	pyramid
C	culmen	**U**	uvula
D	declive	**N**	nodule
F	folium	**T**	tonsil

Vertebral angiograms: venous phase

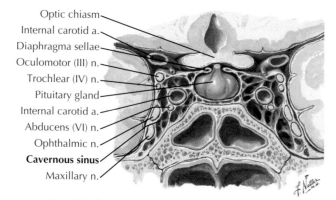

Fig. 18.4 Veins of Posterior Cranial Fossa.

Fig. 18.5 Cavernous Sinus and Its Cranial Nerves.

some patients its maxillary division (V2), and facial sensory changes are occasionally seen. Inferior petrosal sinus thrombosis, often septic, causes retro-orbital pain, trigeminal V1 sensory changes, and abducens nerve palsy (Gradenigo syndrome; CN V, CN VI). Localized thrombosis involving the internal jugular vein may be an extension of transverse or sigmoid sinus thrombosis or may result from catheterization or trauma. This often presents with CN IX, X, and XI dysfunction (jugular foramen or Vernet syndrome) and varying degrees of ipsilateral trapezius and sternocleidomastoid weakness, change in voice with vocal cord and palatal weakness, general sensory loss in the ipsilateral oropharynx as well as loss of special sensory taste sensation in the posterior third of the tongue.

DIAGNOSTIC APPROACH

Routine blood work including complete blood count, basic metabolic profile, prothrombin time, and activated partial thromboplastin time should be obtained in all patients with suspected CVT, according to the guidelines of the American Heart Association/American Stroke

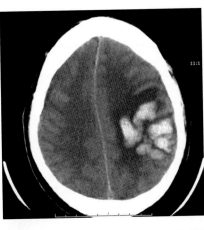

A. CT 2 days after admission showing left posterior frontal parietal patchy hemorrhage within the ischemic region.

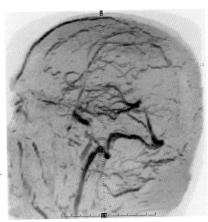

B. Magnetic resonance venography (MRV) demonstrates absence of flow in posterior sagittal sinus and some cortical veins.

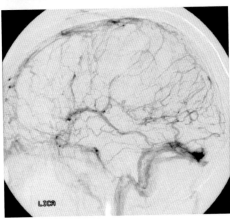

C. Digital angiogram, venous phase confirms the MRV findings.

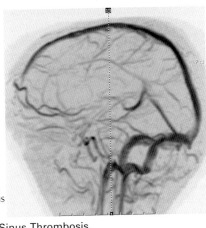

D. Normal MRV for comparison.

Fig. 18.6 Sagittal Sinus Thrombosis.

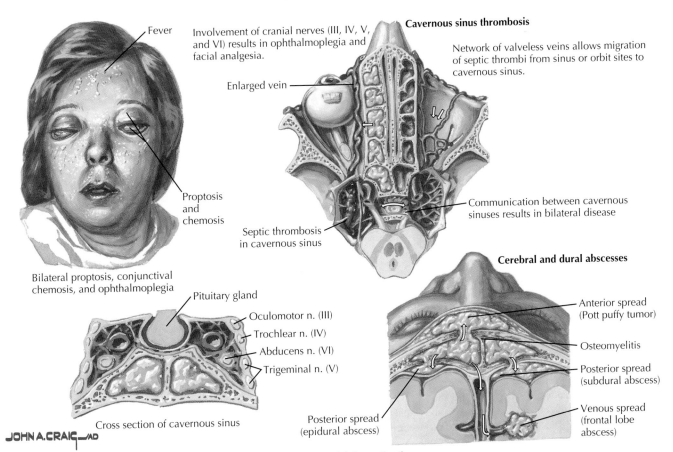

Fever

Involvement of cranial nerves (III, IV, V, and VI) results in ophthalmoplegia and facial analgesia.

Cavernous sinus thrombosis

Network of valveless veins allows migration of septic thrombi from sinus or orbit sites to cavernous sinus.

Enlarged vein

Proptosis and chemosis

Communication between cavernous sinuses results in bilateral disease

Septic thrombosis in cavernous sinus

Bilateral proptosis, conjunctival chemosis, and ophthalmoplegia

Cerebral and dural abscesses

Pituitary gland

Oculomotor n. (III)

Trochlear n. (IV)

Abducens n. (VI)

Trigeminal n. (V)

Anterior spread (Pott puffy tumor)

Osteomyelitis

Posterior spread (subdural abscess)

Venous spread (frontal lobe abscess)

Posterior spread (epidural abscess)

Cross section of cavernous sinus

JOHN A. CRAIG—AD

Fig. 18.7 Intracranial Complications.

Association, while evaluation for a thrombophilic state, either genetic or acquired, should be pursued in high probability patients, such as those with CVT at young age, personal or family history of venous thrombosis, and in patients without a CVT risk factor. The hypercoagulable screen commonly includes protein C and S quantification, lupus anticoagulant, anticardiolipin antibodies, homocysteine levels, and DNA testing for factor V (Leiden factor) and prothrombin gene mutation.

Lumbar puncture often shows an opening pressure greater than 200 mm H_2O. The CSF protein is increased but the glucose content, unless there is associated meningitis, is usually normal. CSF red blood cells, xanthochromia, and pleocytosis are commonly seen, especially in cases of septic sinus thrombosis and in cases associated with meningitis. Normal CSF analysis, although rare, does not exclude the diagnosis.

Acutely, brain CT without contrast is obtained to assess for intracranial hemorrhage. It may reveal irregularly shaped paramedian cortical venous infarctions that do not conform to defined arterial distributions. The "empty delta sign," where contrast partially fills the sinus, leaving an unenhanced island of clot within the occipital confluence, occurs in 50% of cases. Over the hemispheric convexities, thrombosed cortical vessels sometimes appear as hyperintense coiled or serpiginous signals. Diffuse edema and narrowed lateral ventricles may be apparent with or without hemorrhagic lesions.

MRI and MRV have largely replaced angiography as standard imaging techniques to confirm cerebral sinus thrombosis (see Fig. 18.6). Cerebral angiography with a prolonged venous phase is now reserved for cases not clearly diagnosed by MRI or CT and for patients requiring intrasinus thrombectomy/thrombolysis.

Cerebral sinus thrombosis is often a clinical diagnosis based on a detailed history and corroborating physical findings. However, imaging studies have become crucial in the management of these patients from confirming the diagnosis to guiding treatment and to help in predicting the clinical course and outcome.

TREATMENT

The management of sagittal sinus thrombosis consists of hydration, anticoagulation, and the treatment of any underlying cause. Because dehydration enhances clot propagation, early volume repletion is of utmost importance. Anticoagulation with either intravenous unfractionated heparin to achieve a partial thromboplastin time double the control value, or subcutaneous low molecular weight heparin (LMWH), is appropriate, although more recent evidence suggests somewhat better outcomes with LMWH treatment. Anticoagulation is indicated despite hemorrhagic infarctions because the overall outcome is improved and intracranial hemorrhage is rarely worsened. Close clinical follow-up and serial brain CT scanning to monitor hematomas remain necessary because expanding hemorrhagic infarcts may cause shift and herniation, necessitating acute treatment of increased ICP with osmotic agents or, rarely, decompressive surgical intervention. Warfarin is given for long-term anticoagulation and is started after 24 hours of intravenous heparin treatment or after the patient is stable. When indefinite anticoagulation is not needed, the duration of warfarin treatment remains unclear; accepted practice is 3–6 months knowing that 90% of patients recanalize, at least partially, by 6 months. A few case series and case reports suggest that the novel oral anticoagulants or factor Xa inhibitors can be used safely without major bleeding complications and with good recanalization rates, but more research and experience are needed before these agents can be recommended over warfarin. After the precipitating cause is resolved, it is best to confirm that headache and papilledema are controlled and that MRV shows, at least, partial recanalization of the sagittal sinus before discontinuing oral anticoagulants.

Seizures occur in the acute phase in up to 30% of patients and are usually focal but can be generalized. Recurrent seizures should be treated promptly because they can cause ICP, clinical deterioration, and increased mortality. The effectiveness of routine seizure prophylaxis treatment remains unclear but is a reasonable intervention in those with cortical lesions and suspected seizures on presentation. It has been estimated that 3%–4% of patients may experience pulmonary embolism. This is suspected when respiratory deterioration and increased oxygen needs suddenly occur.

If deterioration continues despite systemic anticoagulation, many advocate a more invasive endovascular approach with the combined use of rheolytic mechanical thrombectomy catheters and in situ clot thrombolysis. An initial attempt at partial thrombolysis is usually followed by a continuous 12-hour intrasinus infusion. Numerous case series have shown significant neurologic recovery, even in patients with several hemorrhagic infarcts and days of obtundation or coma, with only a minor increase in bleeding complications.

PROGNOSIS AND LONG-TERM COMPLICATIONS

With anticoagulation, about 80% of patients have good recovery with little or no residual disability. Poor outcomes correlate with rapid deterioration after admission, coma or obtundation on presentation, involvement of the deep venous system, older age, and multiple cerebral hemorrhages with focal deficits, especially if present for days. Before the advent of anticoagulation, the mortality rate was 30%–50%. A mortality rate of 3%–6% remains in the acute phase. Aggressive treatment with endovascular intrasinus thrombolysis and mechanical thrombectomy, especially in those with evolving venous infarctions and progressive obtundation in spite of medical management, may improve outcomes and decrease the rate of early mortality. However, to date, there are no randomized controlled studies to support its routine use.

Long-term complications with approximately 10% occurrence rate for each, include headaches, papilledema with progressive visual loss, and focal or generalized seizures. Headache usually resolves with increasing recanalization and better venous drainage, and often does not necessitate long-term therapy. In cases where the headaches persist, a lumbar puncture helps clarify if CSF pressure remains elevated despite recanalization and if lumboperitoneal shunting is an option. Recurrent or worsening headache as well as new bruits should prompt reimaging to exclude recurrent thrombosis or the rare occurrence of arteriovenous dural fistulas.

Papilledema, when present, should be followed by an ophthalmologist and with serial visual fields. If uncontrolled, progressive visual loss (arcuate midperipheral field constriction and central visual loss with widening blind spot) is dangerous secondary to gradual optic nerve atrophy. Treatment of papilledema involves decreasing CSF pressure with serial spinal taps, carbonic anhydrase inhibitors, and, in those not responding to medical management, lumboperitoneal shunting or optic nerve fenestration into the orbit. Optic nerve fenestration is generally safer than CSF shunting procedures and rarely reoccludes, but still holds a risk of ocular complications with rare worsening optic neuropathy and ocular vascular complications. It is done unilaterally with, at times, positive effects on both eyes. The exact mechanism of action is unknown but is thought to locally shunt or blunt transmission of increased subarachnoid CSF pressure on to the optic nerve head, and many cases still demonstrate high lumbar puncture pressures after fenestration.

Seizures, particularly in those presenting with recurrent seizures and cortically based lesions, may necessitate continued anticonvulsant therapy despite sinus recanalization and the resolution of all other symptoms. The recurrence rate of cerebral thrombosis and other thrombotic events, such as deep vein thrombosis or pulmonary embolism, is estimated around 2%–7% with those who are known to have specific thrombophilia disorders at a higher risk. The majority of these patients would likely require lifelong systemic anticoagulation.

ADDITIONAL RESOURCES

Coutinho JM, Zuurbier SM, Stam J. Declining mortality in cerebral venous thrombosis: a systematic review. Stroke 2014;45(5):1338.

de Freitas GR, Bogousslavsky J. Risk factors of cerebral vein and sinus thrombosis. Front Neurol Neurosci 2008;23:23–54.

Devasagayam S, Wyarr B, Levden J, et al. Cerebral venous sinus thrombosis incidence is higher than previously thought: a retrospective population-based study. Stroke 2016;47(9):2180–2.

Ferro JM, Bousser M-G, Canhão P, et al. European Stroke Organization guideline for the diagnosis and treatment of cerebral venous thrombosis—endorsed by the European Academy of Neurology. Eur J Neurol 2017;24:1203–13.

Misra UK, Kalita J, Chandra S, et al. Low molecular weight heparin versus unfractionated heparin in cerebral venous sinus thrombosis: a randomized controlled trial. Eur J Neurol 2012;19(7):1030–6.

Saponsnik G, Barinagarrementeria F, Brown RD Jr, et al. Diagnosis and management of cerebral venous thrombosis: a statement for healthcare professionals from the American Heart Association/American Stroke Association. Stroke 2011;42:1158.

Siddiqui FM, Dandapat S, Banerjee C, et al. Mechanical thrombectomy in cerebral venous thrombosis: systematic review of 185 cases. Stroke 2015;46(5):1263–8.

Trauma

Brian J. Scott

19

Trauma to the Brain

Khaled Eissa, Carlos A. David, Jeffrey E. Arle

Traumatic brain injury (TBI) is a worldwide major source of lifelong morbidity and mortality. It is the leading cause of death in North America for individuals between the ages of 1 and 45. The societal cost is substantial, with approximately 2.5 million emergency department visits per year and 3–5 million Americans living with a TBI-related disability. Many of these injuries involve young individuals; contact sports and motor vehicle accidents are the most common causes of TBI in individuals 15–19 years old. Of patients with severe TBI, about 40% die from their illness and 60% will have lifelong disability. Young men are overrepresented in this illness. Individuals over 75 have the highest rates of hospitalization and death among all age groups with TBI. Coexisting medical conditions and higher rates of anticoagulation contribute to the increased severity in this population.

Various head injury classification systems exist. These are based on (1) *severity* (mild, moderate, severe), (2) *mechanism* (closed vs. penetrating), (3) *skull fractures* (depressed vs. nondepressed), (4) presence of *intracranial lesions* (focal vs. diffuse), and (5) *hemorrhages* (extraaxillary epidural or subdural, subarachnoid, focal parenchymal/lobar, or brainstem Duret hemorrhage).

TBI is a sequence of two related processes: primary and secondary brain injury. Primary brain injury is a result of the initial event such as direct impact, penetrating injury, acceleration/deceleration injuries, and others. Secondary brain injury occurs as a result of a sequence of multiple cascades of molecular injuries that results in cell death and brain swelling.

> **CLINICAL VIGNETTE** *An emergency physician is requesting an emergent evaluation for a 26-year-old male who was transferred to your emergency room by ambulance after being hit by a speeding car. Eyewitnesses report that the patient lost consciousness for less than a minute after the accident but he then regains consciousness and is able to ambulate afterward. En route to the emergency room his mental status declines. On physical examination upon admission to the emergency room, his Glasgow Coma Scale (GCS) is 5. His right pupil is 11 mm and nonreactive. After emergency endotracheal intubation and application of a cervical collar application, computed tomography (CT) of the head is performed in addition to body imaging, and shows a lens-shaped density compressing the right parietal lobe and a small fracture of the right temporal bone consistent with an epidural hematoma. Body imaging shows multiple fractured ribs on the right side and a tension pneumothorax. A right-sided chest tube is emergently placed and the patient is emergently transferred to the operating room where he has a craniotomy and evacuation of the hematoma.*
>
> *Comment: This patient presents with a classic history of epidural hematoma (EH). He has an initial lucid interval but soon after his mental status deteriorates as the hematoma size expands and compresses his brain, resulting in transtentorial herniation.*

GENERAL PRINCIPLES OF HEAD INJURY CARE

The initial management of severe head injuries follows the Advanced Trauma Life Support guidelines by the American College of Surgeons. Most often, patients have other injuries warranting resuscitation and a primary and secondary trauma survey, which consists of:
- A—**Airway:** Assess airway patency and establish a patent airway and cervical immobilization with neck collar.
- B—**Breathing:** Evaluate rate, rhythm, and breath sounds. Provide ventilatory support if indicated.
- C—**Circulation:** Assess for external source of bleeding, heart rate, skin color, and blood pressure.
- D—**Disability—Neurologic:** Assess level of consciousness using Glasgow Coma Scale (Fig. 19.1), evaluate pupil size and reaction, assess for lateralizing neurologic signs or spinal cord injury.
- E—**Exposure/Environmental Control:** Expose the patient for comprehensive assessment and prevent hypothermia.
- **Secondary Survey & Management:** This includes head-to-toe evaluation and examination to assess for possible injuries and provide initial management.

Concomitantly, the patient's general level of responsiveness must be assessed using the GCS (Fig. 19.1). The lowest possible score of 3 means that individuals have no ability to open their eyes, no motor response to verbal command or direct stimuli, and no verbal response to the physician's questions, giving a score of 1 for each of the three components. The highest possible score is 15 in a fully alert and responsive individual. A complete examination of the exterior surface of the face and head is vital. Blood loss can be extensive given the location of blood vessels within the dense connective tissue of the scalp, which decreases retraction of cut vessels and promotes bleeding.

SKULL FRACTURES

Skull fractures can be located in the calvarium (vault) and/or the basal skull. Fractures of the cranial vault carry a 20 times greater incidence of intracranial hematoma in comatose patients and a 400 times greater incidence in conscious patients. Basal skull fractures, often difficult to identify on head CT, can present with pathognomonic signs, including raccoon or panda bear eyes, battle sign (ecchymosis over the mastoid process), and cerebrospinal fluid (CSF) leakage from the nose, throat, or ears (Fig. 19.2). Most leaks resolve spontaneously. Persistent leaks necessitate operative treatment (Fig. 19.3).

Depressed fractures and those along the temporal bone are more commonly associated with injury to the brain or blood vessels. A fracture across the middle meningeal artery may produce an epidural hematoma (EH). Open fractures with their communication between the intracranial

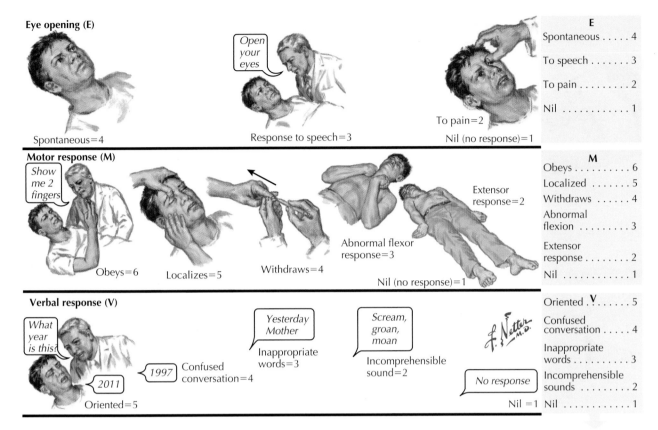

Eye opening (E)

Spontaneous=4

Open your eyes

Response to speech=3

To pain=2

Nil (no response)=1

E	
Spontaneous	4
To speech	3
To pain	2
Nil	1

Motor response (M)

Show me 2 fingers

Obeys=6   Localizes=5   Withdraws=4

Abnormal flexor response=3

Extensor response=2

Nil (no response)=1

M	
Obeys	6
Localized	5
Withdraws	4
Abnormal flexion	3
Extensor response	2
Nil	1

Verbal response (V)

What year is this?

2011

1997   Confused conversation=4

Oriented=5

Yesterday Mother

Inappropriate words=3

Scream, groan, moan

Incomprehensible sound=2

No response

Nil =1

V	
Oriented	5
Confused conversation	4
Inappropriate words	3
Incomprehensible sounds	2
Nil	1

Coma score (E+M+V)=3 to 15

Fig. 19.1 Glasgow Coma Scale.

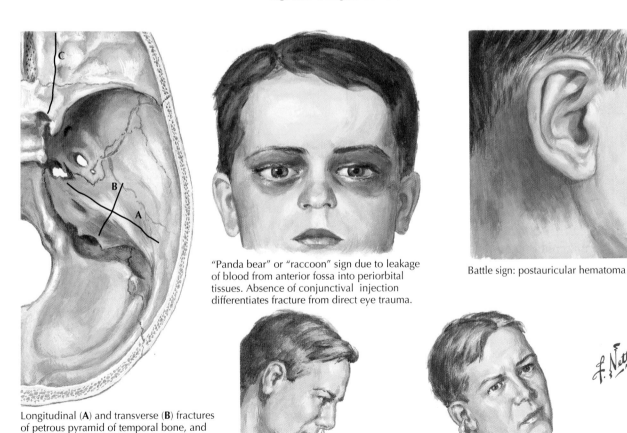

Longitudinal (**A**) and transverse (**B**) fractures of petrous pyramid of temporal bone, and anterior basal skull fracture (**C**)

"Panda bear" or "raccoon" sign due to leakage of blood from anterior fossa into periorbital tissues. Absence of conjunctival injection differentiates fracture from direct eye trauma.

Battle sign: postauricular hematoma

Rhinorrhea

Otorrhea or ear hemorrhage

Fig. 19.2 Basilar Skull Fractures.

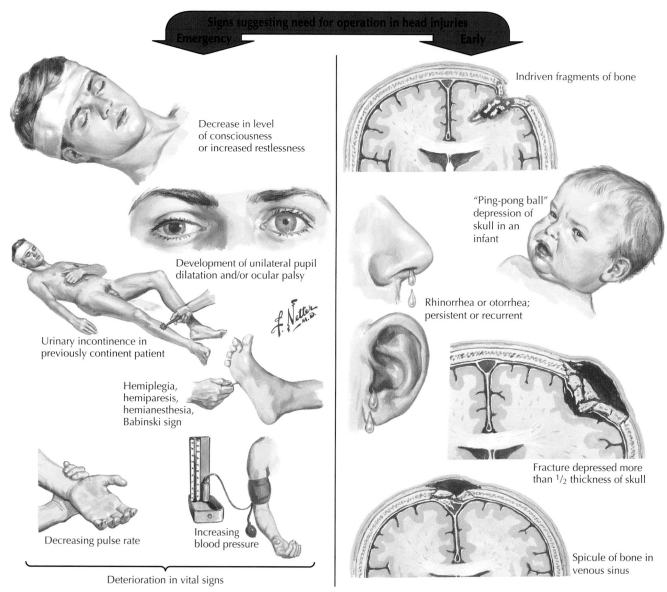

Signs suggesting need for operation in head injuries

Emergency — Early

Decrease in level of consciousness or increased restlessness

Development of unilateral pupil dilatation and/or ocular palsy

Urinary incontinence in previously continent patient

Hemiplegia, hemiparesis, hemianesthesia, Babinski sign

Decreasing pulse rate

Increasing blood pressure

Deterioration in vital signs

Indriven fragments of bone

"Ping-pong ball" depression of skull in an infant

Rhinorrhea or otorrhea; persistent or recurrent

Fracture depressed more than 1/2 thickness of skull

Spicule of bone in venous sinus

Fig. 19.3 Signs Suggesting Need for Operation.

vault and the external environment are associated with higher risks of spinal fluid leaks and infection (Fig. 19.4).

EXTRAAXIAL TRAUMATIC BRAIN INJURIES

Traumatic Subarachnoid Hemorrhage

Subarachnoid hemorrhage (SAH) is the most common sequela of TBI and is typically associated with additional intracranial lesions. SAH can range from clinically asymptomatic to fatal. These SAH blood products can obstruct CSF circulation or reabsorption, leading to increased intracranial pressure (ICP) with hydrocephalus. Depending on the severity of the hemorrhage, treatment of traumatic SAH may include placement of a ventricular drain or shunting system for secondary hydrocephalus.

Epidural Hematomas

EH represents an acute blood collection contained between the dura and inner table of the skull. These occur in approximately 2% of all TBIs (Fig. 19.5) and 5%–15% of fatal head injuries. EHs most commonly develop in the temporal and parietal regions; 90% of EH are associated with a skull fracture that results in lacerations of vascular

structures, more commonly the middle meningeal artery (Fig. 19.6) or, less commonly, venous injuries.

Immediately after the closed head injury, the patient classically experiences an initial but relatively brief loss of consciousness secondary to the primary concussive injury. This is then followed by a "lucid interval" with return of wakefulness, which can be reassuring. Subsequently, as the torn vessels leak and the EH expands, regional brain compression leads to a rapid lapse into coma (see Fig. 19.3). This presentation occurs in less than one-third of affected individuals. Most patients do not have a lucid interval. Cranial CT imaging usually demonstrates a hyperdense, biconvex collection between the skull and brain (Fig. 19.7). EHs do not cross cranial suture lines and they expand in thickness under the effect of high pressure arterial bleeding. On occasion, the initial CT is normal. Thus, when the patient is at high risk (i.e., moderate to severe TBI and/or skull fractures) it is essential to closely observe the patient's neurologic exam and level of consciousness and to repeat the CT scan at the slightest clinical change. Once the EH is identified, emergency surgical evacuation is indicated. EHs are one of the most serious sequelae of brain trauma and can be fatal without immediate recognition and surgical evacuation.

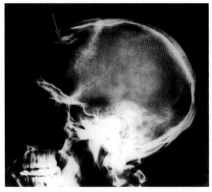

Left lateral skull film showing left frontal depressed skull fracture

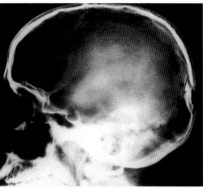

Left lateral skull film revealing occipital depressed skull fracture

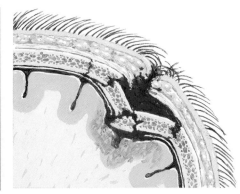

Compound depressed skull fracture. Note hair impacted into wound

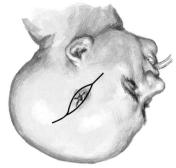

Elliptical incision with extensions to remove devitalized skin and pericranium

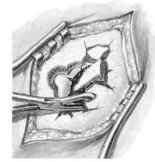

Burr hole placed at margin of fracture to facilitate elevation of depressed bone fragments. Bone edges, dura, and brain then debrided

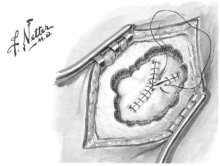

Watertight dural closure. Optionally, bone fragments may be cleaned and wired in place Skin is closed in one layer

Fig. 19.4 Compound Depressed Skull Fractures.

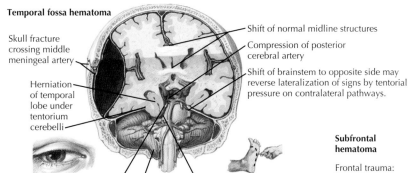

Temporal fossa hematoma

Skull fracture crossing middle meningeal artery

Herniation of temporal lobe under tentorium cerebelli

Compression of oculomotor (III) nerve leading to ipsilateral pupil dilatation and third cranial nerve palsy

Herniation of cerebellar tonsil

Shift of normal midline structures

Compression of posterior cerebral artery

Shift of brainstem to opposite side may reverse lateralization of signs by tentorial pressure on contralateral pathways.

Compression of corticospinal and associated pathways, resulting in contralateral hemiparesis, deep tendon hyperreflexia, and Babinski sign

Subfrontal hematoma

Frontal trauma: headache, poor cerebration, intermittent disorientation, anisocoria

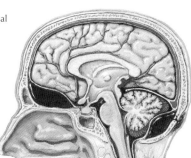

Posterior fossa hematoma

Occipital trauma and/or fracture: headache, meningismus, cerebellar and cranial nerve signs, Cushing triad

Fig. 19.5 Epidural Hematoma.

CLINICAL VIGNETTE *An 85-year-old man is being evaluated in the Emergency Department (ED) for weakness. He reports headache, dizziness, and weak legs for the past few days. On further questioning, he recalls that 7 weeks earlier he had slipped on the ice, striking his occiput, while helping to push a car out of a snow bank.*

His neurologic examination is significant only for tandem ataxia but is otherwise unremarkable. Head CT demonstrates large biparietal subdural hematomas. Bilateral craniotomies are performed, draining both hematomas. Postoperatively, he has a few focal motor and sensory seizures that stopped after he was started on phenytoin. His neurologic and functional recovery is otherwise excellent.

Acute Subdural Hematoma

Subdural hematomas (SDHs) are located between the arachnoid and the dural membranes and are classified by their temporal profile. *Acute SDHs* occur in 15% of TBI patients; these are seven to eight times more common than EHs. Advanced age is associated with greater risk because of atrophy of the cerebral cortex. With cerebral atrophy, an increasing space develops within the subdural compartment. In turn this leads to increased stretch on the bridging veins between the skull and the surface of the brain (Fig. 19.8). When any individual sustains direct head trauma, the brain parenchyma accelerates and decelerates in relation to fixed dural structures. This leads to a tearing of the now anatomically stretched veins that form a "bridge" between the cerebral cortex and the skull.

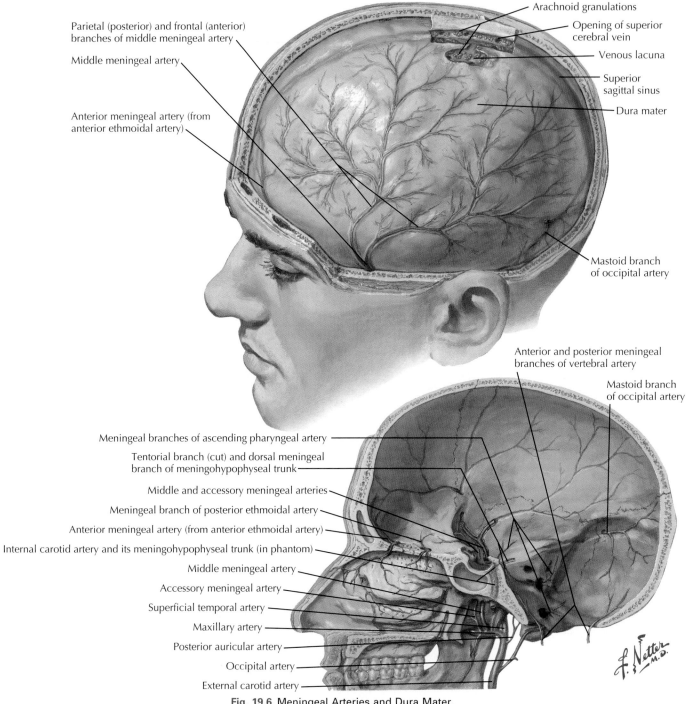

Parietal (posterior) and frontal (anterior) branches of middle meningeal artery

Middle meningeal artery

Anterior meningeal artery (from anterior ethmoidal artery)

Arachnoid granulations

Opening of superior cerebral vein

Venous lacuna

Superior sagittal sinus

Dura mater

Mastoid branch of occipital artery

Anterior and posterior meningeal branches of vertebral artery

Mastoid branch of occipital artery

Meningeal branches of ascending pharyngeal artery

Tentorial branch (cut) and dorsal meningeal branch of meningohypophyseal trunk

Middle and accessory meningeal arteries

Meningeal branch of posterior ethmoidal artery

Anterior meningeal artery (from anterior ethmoidal artery)

Internal carotid artery and its meningohypophyseal trunk (in phantom)

Middle meningeal artery

Accessory meningeal artery

Superficial temporal artery

Maxillary artery

Posterior auricular artery

Occipital artery

External carotid artery

Fig. 19.6 Meningeal Arteries and Dura Mater.

Concomitant injury to cortical arteries can also lead to bleeding into the subdural space (Fig. 19.9).

Clinical Presentation and Diagnosis

The initial severity and location of the injury determines the patient's clinical presentation; this varies from neurologically intact, to altered mental states, which are subsequently associated with pupillary inequality and motor weakness, with the patient eventually becoming comatose with signs of decorticate or decerebrate posturing. The lucid interval, a classical finding with EH, is also commonly seen with acute SDH. Brain CT is the initial test of choice for detecting SDH and other traumatic brain injuries. An acute SDH is recognized by its hyperdense crescent-shaped appearance between the brain and skull (see Fig. 19.7). Unlike EH, SDHs typically cross skull suture lines, and sometimes extend along the falx cerebri. Head CT sometimes underestimates the size of the SDH given the similar imaging density of the nearby bone.

Treatment and Prognosis

If the patient has evidence of increased ICP or compartmental herniation, medical management to decrease ICP, such as mannitol or hypertonic saline, may be considered. Surgical intervention with a craniotomy is indicated for thick SDH or if it is associated with shifting of the brain midline structures. Surgical evacuation of the clot must be expeditiously performed. A burr-hole trephine evacuation is inadequate because the

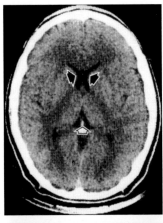

A. Normal brain. CT scan demonstrating normal anatomy at level of frontal horns of lateral ventricles (black arrows). Pineal gland (white arrow) is in normal midline location.

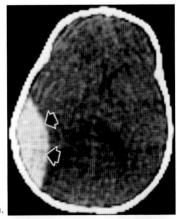

B. Epidural hematoma. CT scan demonstrating hyperdense right parietal epidural hematoma (black arrows), which has assumed classic biconvex lens configuration secondary to adherence of dura to inner table of skull. Other structures are compressed and shifted.

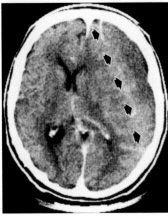

C. Subacute subdural hematoma. CT scan demonstrating large iso-dense mass over left cerebral convexity. Compressed cerebral cortex (black arrows) shows enhanced density delineating inner border of subacute subdural hematoma. Normal structures are shifted across midline.

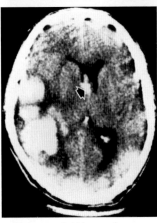

D. Acute intracerebral hematoma. CT scan demonstrating hyperdense mass in right parietotemporal area. Large acute intracerebral hematoma has shifted lateral ventricle toward midline. Blood is visualized within ventricular system (black arrow).

Fig. 19.7 CT and Angiogram of Intracranial Hemorrhage.

clot is often already more viscous than normal blood. Residual and recurrent hematomas are also postoperative concerns.

Chronic Subdural Hematoma

Subdural blood collections commonly appear 2–3 weeks after an often seemingly innocuous injury, as illustrated in the initial vignette. Their incidence is 1–2 per 100,000 persons each year. Most chronic SDH patients are over 50 years old. Chronic alcoholics or patients with coagulopathies (either innate or induced by medications such as antiplatelet or anticoagulants), are more prone to bleeding with relatively minor trauma such as striking one's head on the door frame on entering an automobile, or a minor fall with head strike.

Initially, relatively minor amounts of blood enter the subdural space after trauma or spontaneous hemorrhages. The collected blood may get reabsorbed without producing significant symptoms, or may proceed over a few weeks' interval to form a membrane at both the inner and outer aspects of the hematoma. Eventually, these membranes are prone to low-grade bleeding and thus lead to slow enlargement of the SDH. Concomitantly a higher osmotic pressure develops within the SDH leading to an osmotic gradient that promotes the passage of CSF into the initial SDH; consequently this mass lesion gradually enlarges. The clinical course is variable and not predictable. If the SDH reaches a critical size to compromise brain function, symptoms will develop.

Clinical Presentation and Diagnosis

The presentation may range from subtle focal signs of cerebral compromise as determined by the site of injury (e.g., such as aphasia, focal weakness or sensory loss, confusion, or seeming early dementia with bifrontal lesions) to symptoms of the various herniation syndromes.

A high clinical suspicion of SDH must always occur especially with the at-risk individual whenever there is a remote history of head trauma. CT is the study of choice (see Fig. 19.7), although SDH is also visible on brain magnetic resonance imaging (MRI) scans.

Treatment and Prognosis

Medical management and observation are recommended for individuals with mild clinical symptoms and signs: discontinuation of anticoagulant medications, close observation, and serial CT scans to confirm clinical and radiographic stability are reassuring. Surgical therapy is advisable for any chronic SDH that is causing significant mass effect or is associated with significant clinical impairment. As chronic SDH undergoes liquefaction, burr-hole trephine evacuation can be performed with the placement of a drainage catheter. Up to 45% of chronic SDHs reaccumulate. Craniotomy with membrane formation is required for SDHs that reaccumulate after drainage.

INTRAAXIAL TRAUMATIC INJURIES

Cerebral Contusions

These are the second most common TBI lesions. Usually the frontal and temporal lobes are affected. A contusion is a bruised area of brain tissue composed of hemorrhage, infarcted tissue, and necrosis. *Coup* lesions are those found under the sites of direct injury; *contrecoup* lesions are located at sides opposite to impact secondary to brain tissue necrosis and edema sites, where the brain decelerates against the skull (often the frontal and temporal poles). Cortical contusions are most common, but they also occur within the deep white matter.

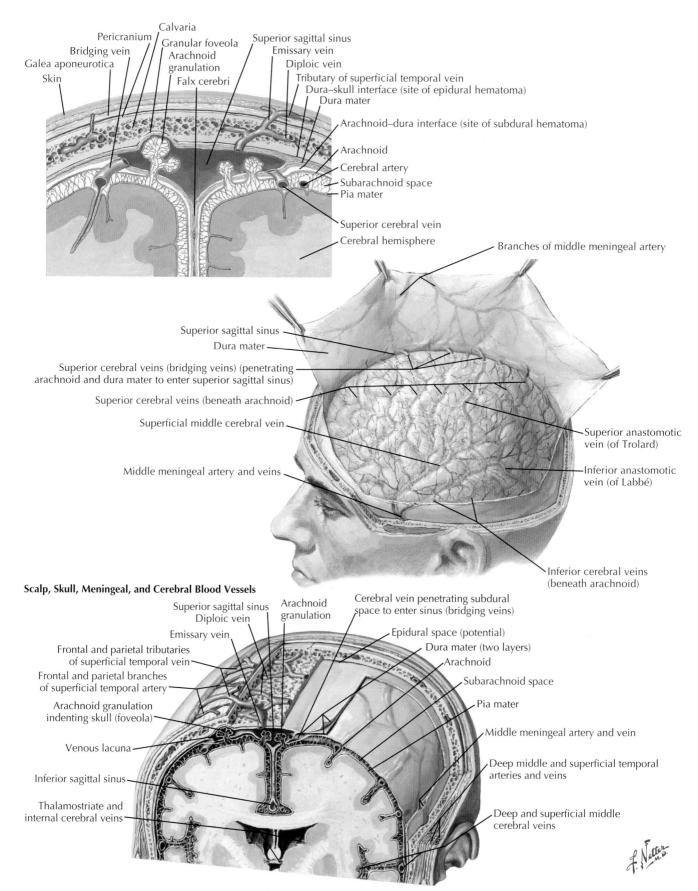

Calvaria
Pericranium
Bridging vein
Galea aponeurotica
Skin
Granular foveola
Arachnoid granulation
Falx cerebri
Superior sagittal sinus
Emissary vein
Diploic vein
Tributary of superficial temporal vein
Dura–skull interface (site of epidural hematoma)
Dura mater
Arachnoid–dura interface (site of subdural hematoma)
Arachnoid
Cerebral artery
Subarachnoid space
Pia mater
Superior cerebral vein
Cerebral hemisphere

Branches of middle meningeal artery
Superior sagittal sinus
Dura mater
Superior cerebral veins (bridging veins) (penetrating arachnoid and dura mater to enter superior sagittal sinus)
Superior cerebral veins (beneath arachnoid)
Superficial middle cerebral vein
Middle meningeal artery and veins
Superior anastomotic vein (of Trolard)
Inferior anastomotic vein (of Labbé)
Inferior cerebral veins (beneath arachnoid)

Scalp, Skull, Meningeal, and Cerebral Blood Vessels

Superior sagittal sinus
Diploic vein
Emissary vein
Frontal and parietal tributaries of superficial temporal vein
Frontal and parietal branches of superficial temporal artery
Arachnoid granulation indenting skull (foveola)
Venous lacuna
Inferior sagittal sinus
Thalamostriate and internal cerebral veins
Arachnoid granulation
Cerebral vein penetrating subdural space to enter sinus (bridging veins)
Epidural space (potential)
Dura mater (two layers)
Arachnoid
Subarachnoid space
Pia mater
Middle meningeal artery and vein
Deep middle and superficial temporal arteries and veins
Deep and superficial middle cerebral veins

Fig. 19.8 Superficial Cerebral Veins and Diploic Veins.

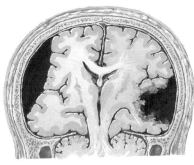

Section showing acute subdural hematoma on right side and subdural hematoma associated with temporal lobe intracerebral hematoma ("burst" temporal lobe) on left

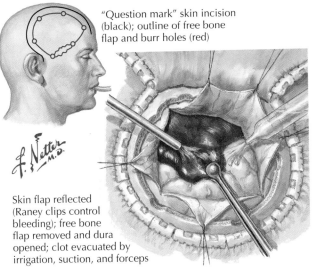

"Question mark" skin incision (black); outline of free bone flap and burr holes (red)

Skin flap reflected (Raney clips control bleeding); free bone flap removed and dura opened; clot evacuated by irrigation, suction, and forceps

Fig. 19.9 Acute Subdural Hematoma.

Clinical presentation varies widely and is predicated on the location and size of the lesion. Many brain contusions develop surrounding brain edema and regional brain compression within the first 1–3 days. This can become clinically significant in patients who sustain high-impact trauma. Surgical intervention is usually not required for intracerebral contusions, especially for small, deep subcortical contusions; these are generally observed or managed medically. However, large lobar contusions with associated mass effect sometimes require craniotomy and evacuation. Temporal lobe contusions are potentially the most dangerous given their location near the brainstem and the higher potential for uncal herniation and brainstem compression. Repeat CT scanning is essential to follow these lesions. Mortality due to cerebral contusions ranges from 25% to 60%.

Intraparenchymal Hematomas

Approximately one-quarter of head injury patients develop intraparenchymal hematomas; these are well-demarcated areas of acute hemorrhage. The basic pathophysiology is similar to contusions. Most (90%) occur within the frontal and temporal lobes. Shear injury leads to deep cerebral white matter hematomas. Two-thirds of intraparenchymal hematomas are associated with concomitant subdural or EHs (see Fig. 19.9). An intraventricular hemorrhage, often complicated by obstructive hydrocephalus, may also commonly develop.

Depending on the severity of the injury, almost half of these patients present with a loss of consciousness. Other signs and symptoms relate to the size and location of the hemorrhage.

Medical management is the treatment of choice for deep or small hemorrhages and in unstable patients. Surgical resection is indicated for large superficial lobar hematomas associated with clinical signs of mass effect (depressed level of consciousness and/or focal neurologic

deficits). Ventricular CSF drains may be placed to relieve obstructive hydrocephalus and to monitor ICP. These provide a means to follow neurologically severely compromised patients. Mortality rates vary from 25% to 75% in patients with an intraparenchymal hemorrhage.

Diffuse Axonal Shear Injury

The combination of rotational acceleration and deceleration of the brain during traumatic impact results in shearing of diffuse axonal pathways and small capillaries. High-speed motor vehicle accidents are the most common etiology in the civilian population. Microscopic penetrating blood vessels are damaged at multiple levels including the corticomedullary junction, corpus callosum, internal capsule, deep gray matter, and upper brainstem, leading to numerous small hemorrhagic foci. However, immediately following axonal shear injury, the initial brain CT is often unremarkable, especially when there are no concomitant areas of intraaxial or extraaxial hematoma or punctate contusion. During the first 48–72 hours after the injury (even with normal or minimal findings on initial CT), cerebral edema may become obvious on clinical examination and follow-up imaging. Pressure monitors are recommended in TBI patients with a GCS of 3–8 and an abnormal head CT. As the lateral ventricles are often small and/or compressed, ventricular catheter placement is technically difficult and intraparenchymal catheters are more commonly used (Fig. 19.10).

MRI is more sensitive in detecting axonal shear injury. Microhemorrhages may be seen on gradient echo T2-weighted sequences (Fig. 19.11). Later, nonspecific white matter T2 hyperintense lesions with atrophic changes are characteristic.

Shear injury is a major prognostic contributor to head injury morbidity. Survivors may have moderate to severe neurocognitive deficits, or may remain comatose or minimally conscious for extended periods. Another potential outcome is that of preserved wakefulness without any awareness of internal or external stimuli classified as a persistent vegetative state (see Chapter 13). This entity carries an extremely poor prognosis (Fig. 19.12).

POSTERIOR FOSSA LESIONS

Cerebellar and posterior fossa traumatic brain lesions account for only 5% of post-TBI sequela. EH, SDH, and intraparenchymal cerebellar hematomas are the most common traumatic lesions at this level. Because of the limited space within the posterior fossa, lesions can rapidly lead to early neurologic decline secondary to brainstem compression and/or acute obstructive hydrocephalus. Careful assessment of patients for these life-threatening injuries is critical, especially in high-risk individuals such as those with basal skull fractures. MRI is superior to CT to visualize nonosseous posterior fossa pathology. Normal bony architecture, as imaged with brain CT, frequently prevents identification of posterior fossa lesions in patients with TBI. Hematoma evacuation via posterior fossa craniectomy is the primary treatment modality when there is a critical mass lesion (Fig. 19.13).

TRAUMATIC BRAIN INJURY IN MILITARY COMBAT SETTINGS

Significant effort has gone into defining appropriate guidelines of care for TBI since 1990. In 2005, Guidelines for Field Management of Combat-Related Head Trauma was offered by the Brain Trauma Foundation; it also provides levels of evidence found in published literature supporting its conclusions. Nearly all of the relevant scientific literature is Class III evidence. Combat TBI tends to occur from high-velocity rifle rounds (as opposed to handguns) and penetrating shrapnel and debris, with or without blast injury. The differences between field combat and

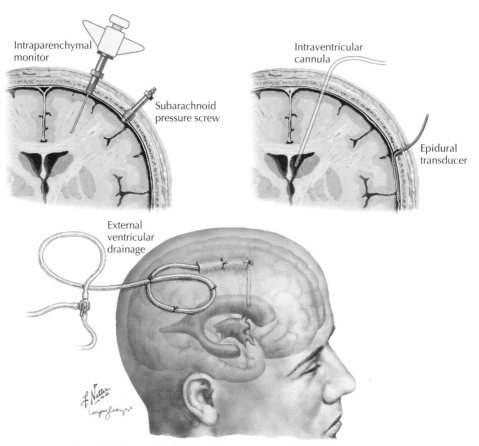

Fig. 19.10 Intensive Medical Management of Severe Head Injury.

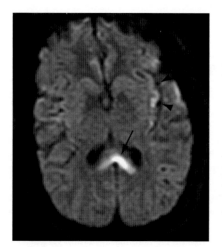

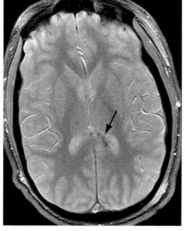

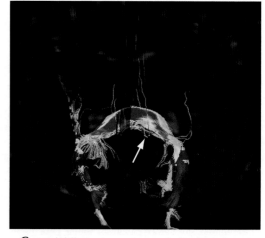

A. Restricted diffusion is quite prominent in left splenium of corpus callosum (arrow) and less so involving left insular white matter (arrowheads).

B. Paramagnetic signal within corpus callosum on gradient echo image confirms associated petechial hemorrhage (arrow).

C. Axial diffusion tensor image shows disruption of fibers (arrow).

Fig. 19.11 Shear Injury.

civilian care may include a limited ability to obtain an adequate exam or history, delay in transportation of patient, or no access to the patient. Inability to secure an area may require assessment of the casualty while under heavy fire. Chemical or radioactive contamination may require medical personnel to wear protective clothing that can severely limit assessment, and finally the tactical plans may hamper mobilization of appropriate resources. The supply of bandages, fluids, and medications alone for field medics who are under siege for days or even weeks at a time may be extremely difficult. Not all aspects of the care and assessment of neurologic injuries in a combat setting are negative relative to the civilian world. The dedication of medics for saving casualties and "leaving no one behind" is extraordinarily high and is an important foundation to support the confidence of combat soldiers. Soldiers are among the most physiologically robust and compliant of patients, and medics' acts of fearlessness to provide care in the battlefield setting are legendary.

Condition is called *persistent* when it lasts without change for more than 1 month.

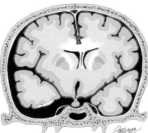

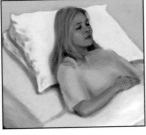

Subarachnoid hemorrhage

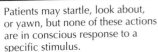

Patients may startle, look about, or yawn, but none of these actions are in conscious response to a specific stimulus.

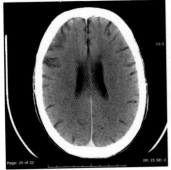

Noncontrast brain CT demonstrating ominous sign of diffuse brain injury and possible prelude to a persistent vegetative state: sulcal effacement (diffuse edema) and subtle disappearance of normal differentiation between gray and white matter.

Fig. 19.12 Persistent Vegetative State.

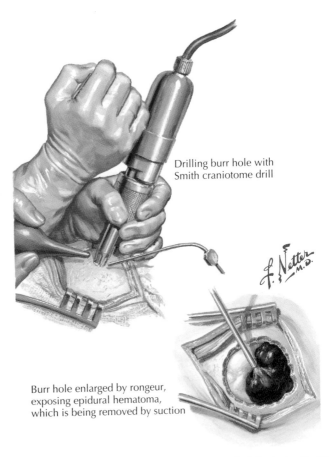

Drilling burr hole with Smith craniotome drill

Burr hole enlarged by rongeur, exposing epidural hematoma, which is being removed by suction

Fig. 19.13 Exploratory Burr Holes and Removal of Posterior Fossa Hematoma.

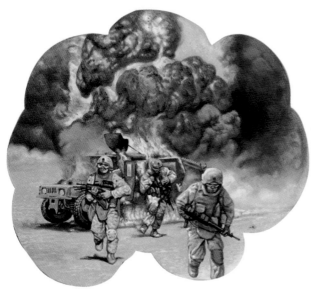

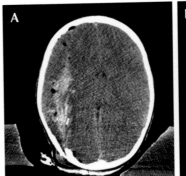

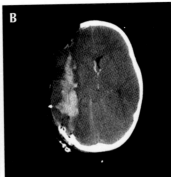

Infant hit by IED (improvised explosive device) with brain injury in the right hemisphere **(A). B** shows the hemicraniectomy performed to mitigate brain injury from swelling

Fig. 19.14 Brain Injury in Military Combat.

One main difference between the civilian and combat settings is the need for multicasualty triage in the field; this is one of the primary responsibilities of combat medics, who have limited ability, if any, to provide mechanical ventilation or ICP management. Measurement of GCS serves to assess the severity of TBI and the outcome, and may be a useful baseline measure for triage decisions. However, its use is only helpful once casualties reach a military hospital level of assessment.

Moreover, the reliability of combat medics, and even military physicians, in measuring GCS has been shown to be poor compared to civilian first-responders.

Experience in Afghanistan and Iraq by US neurosurgeons has led to a more aggressive surgical approach in handling brain trauma: aggressive cranial decompression (Fig. 19.14) to help manage brain edema, including bilateral hemicraniectomies to allow the brain to swell without

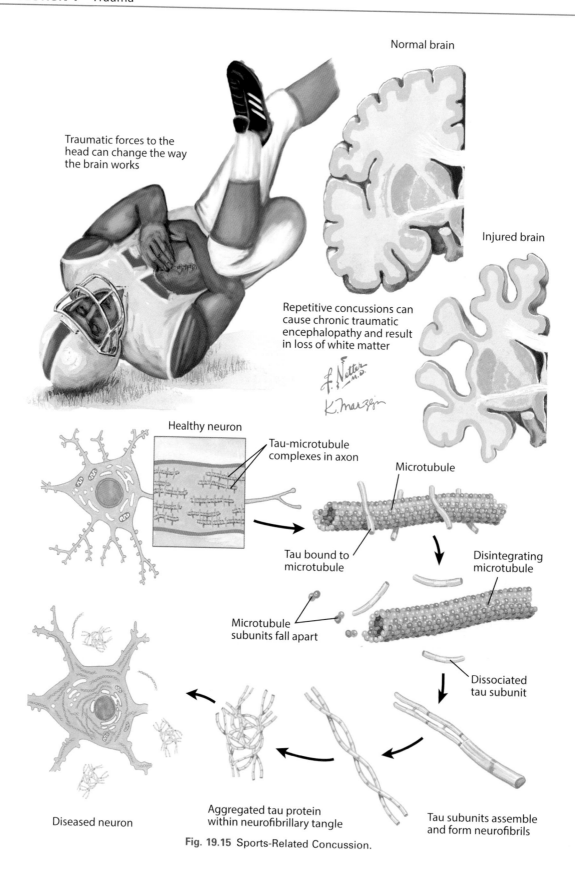

Normal brain

Traumatic forces to the head can change the way the brain works

Injured brain

Repetitive concussions can cause chronic traumatic encephalopathy and result in loss of white matter

Healthy neuron

Tau-microtubule complexes in axon

Microtubule

Tau bound to microtubule

Disintegrating microtubule

Microtubule subunits fall apart

Dissociated tau subunit

Aggregated tau protein within neurofibrillary tangle

Tau subunits assemble and form neurofibrils

Diseased neuron

Fig. 19.15 Sports-Related Concussion.

pressure from the fixed cranial volume (Personal communication, Brett Schlifka, MD, Maj, USA 2006). This minimizes the need for intensive ICP medical management in these initial combat hospital facilities. If patients survived this acute care, better and longer-term management and ultimately cranioplasty repair could be performed at better-equipped facilities in higher-level settings.

RECURRENT TRAUMATIC BRAIN INJURY

Recurrent concussion/mild TBI related to contact sports, military service, and domestic abuse has garnered increasing attention from the neuroscience community as well as the general public over the past decade. Repetitive mild brain injury, as can occur in competitive football, soccer, or boxing, can be associated with subsequent neurocognitive symptoms, including mood disorders (especially depression), memory loss, and parkinsonism—collectively termed chronic traumatic encephalopathy (CTE). Exposure to repetitive TBI early in life and prolonged duration of exposure both appear to increase the risk for symptoms. The imaging of individuals with CTE has demonstrated regional or global brain atrophy and thinning of the corpus callosum. Neuropathology characteristically shows degeneration of neurons with regional or widespread neurofibrillary tangles containing phosphorylated tau protein (Fig. 19.15).

Current research is actively seeking to more precisely characterize the pathologic changes that occur in repetitive mild TBI, which will hopefully lead to effective prevention of the neurocognitive sequelae. Major medical associations and competitive sports organizations have strict guidelines relating to head injury and concussion. Fundamental to these is the requirement that athletes who sustain a concussion are removed from all participation until symptoms have completely resolved to avoid more severe and, rarely, even life-threatening injury.

LONG-TERM PROGNOSIS OF TRAUMATIC BRAIN INJURY

It is often difficult to accurately determine a patient's long-term functional outcome despite the physician's desire to answer this very critical question for the patient's family. Although it is relatively easy to identify individuals at both ends of the trauma severity spectrum, it is more difficult in the gray middle-zone area. Useful factors include injury severity, the initial GCS, response to therapy, global (diffuse axonal/shear) versus focal injuries, associated injuries, age, medical comorbidities, and the ability to rapidly commence medical and surgical interventions. Rehabilitation that includes both physical and cognitive/behavioral therapies is an important component of post-TBI care that influences recovery and long-term prognosis.

ADDITIONAL RESOURCES

Aarabi B. Surgical outcome in 435 patients who sustained missile head wounds during the Iran-Iraq war. Neurosurgery 1990;27:692–5.

Chestnut R, Temkin N, et al. Trial of Intracranial-pressure monitoring in traumatic brain injury. N Engl J Med 2012;367:2471–81.

Cooper D, Rosenfeld J, et al. Decompressive craniectomy in diffuse traumatic brain injury. N Engl J Med 2011;364:1493–502.

Fakhry SM, Trask AL, Waller MA, et al. Management of brain-injured patients by an evidence-based medicine protocol improves outcomes and decreases hospital charges. J Trauma 2004;56:492–500.

Giza CC, Kutcher JS, Ashwal S, et al. Summary of evidence-based guideline update: evaluation and management of concussion in sports. Neurology 2010;80(24):2250–7.

McKee AC, Stein TD, Nowinski CJ, et al. The spectrum of disease in chronic traumatic encephalopathy. Brain 2013;136:43–64.

Riechers GR, Ramage A, Brown W, et al. Physician knowledge of the Glasgow Coma Scale. J Neurotrauma 2005;22(11):1327–34.

Stocchett N, Maas A. Traumatic intracranial hypertension. N Engl J Med 2014;370:2121–30.

20

Trauma to the Spine and Spinal Cord

Jian Guan, Subu N. Magge

CLINICAL VIGNETTE *After a day of skiing, six teenagers packed into a small hatchback on their way home. Conditions were icy, and the driver lost control of the vehicle near the base of the mountain, rear-ending another vehicle at approximately 30 miles/h. One of the passengers, an 18-year-old man, struck his head on the seat in front of him. When Emergency Medical Services arrived on scene, the patient's primary complaint was neck pain. He was subsequently placed in a hard cervical collar and transported to the nearest trauma center.*

On arrival, computed tomography (CT) of the patient's cervical spine demonstrated a fracture of the axis through the base of the odontoid process. The patient was neurologically intact, with no complaints apart from continued neck pain. After extensive discussions regarding possible options for management, the patient underwent odontoid screw fixation. The operation was uncomplicated, and the patient was released after a 2-day stay in the hospital.

At the 1-month follow-up, the patient was recovering well. His neck pain had completely resolved, and he had no new neurologic deficits. Imaging showed good positioning of the odontoid screw and reapproximation of the fractured odontoid with the body of the axis. The patient had no limitations in his cervical range of motion and had returned to school 2 weeks earlier to continue his senior year.

Comment: This patient represents a common spine fracture in an unusual demographic; odontoid fractures are most common in the elderly population. Although the majority of patients who present to the hospital with this fracture have no evidence of neurologic deficit, odontoid fractures are unstable and require stabilization—either externally with a brace or internally through surgical fixation. The morphology of the fracture and individual patient characteristics are the key factors to be weighed in making the treatment plan.

In this case, the patient's fracture anatomy made the success of external fixation unlikely; the majority of fractures through the base of the dens (so-called type II fractures) fail to resolve with bracing alone. On the basis of the patient's imaging findings, the decision was made to proceed with placement of an odontoid screw, using a ventral approach that places a single screw through the axis and the fractured fragment. Such an approach allows for the preservation of rotational motion at the atlantoaxial junction, an especially important consideration in a young, active patient.

This case illustrates many of the complexities of spine trauma management:
- *the need for appropriate evaluation and stabilization of patients from the arrival of emergency medical services to the patient's initial evaluation in the hospital*
- *the importance of accurate imaging and appropriate diagnosis*
- *numerous subtle but vital patient characteristics that determine the final course of management.*

Traumatic spine fractures and associated traumatic spinal cord injury (TSCI) are among the most devastating injuries that medical professionals encounter. Apart from the acute challenges represented by such patients (who frequently present with multiple life-threatening injuries and are in need of rapid and definitive treatment), TSCI invariably results in social, economic, and medical challenges, which, in many ways, are unparalleled. Early documented recognition of the seriousness of spinal cord injury is recorded on the Edwin Smith Surgical Papyrus, Egypt (17th century BC). Modern causes of spinal cord injury are diverse, ranging from motor vehicle accidents (Fig. 20.1) to sports-related injuries to trauma sustained in armed conflicts. Regardless of etiology, these patients require comprehensive multidisciplinary care to identify and address the long-term medical, social, and psychological issues following spinal cord injury.

Despite the multiple challenges faced by patients with TSCI, most of them are able to live active, productive lives that are substantially longer than could be achieved after TSCI 50 years ago. To watch paraplegic individuals in wheelchairs come to the finish line of the Boston Marathon or those competing in the Paralympic Games speaks to these triumphs. The future of TSCI treatment also holds great promise, with advances in stem cell technology and robotics progressing at a staggering rate.

Major trauma centers evaluate 2 to 3 TSCI individuals out of every 100 patients brought to their emergency departments. The very high mortality (50%) associated with TSCI occurs mainly at the initial accident or injury scene. In addition to TSCI, many of these patients have injuries to other body systems, including traumatic brain injuries, orthopedic injuries, cardiopulmonary injuries, and visceral injuries. Of the patients who make it to the hospital, mortality is approximately 16%.

Although young men sustain 85% of TSCIs, the increasing age of the overall population in many Western countries is shifting the demographics of TSCI. In the older population, individuals with significant cervical spinal spondylosis and/or stenosis are much more likely to develop TSCIs, such as a central cord injury (Fig. 20.2), from relatively simple ground-level falls.

In the United States alone, the annual cost of caring for TSCI patients is estimated to be over $9.7 billion. Furthermore, the patient with a spinal cord injury must adjust to limited mobility, psychiatric issues, urologic problems, pulmonary difficulty, skin breakdown, sexual dysfunction, and frequently the inability to perform his or her job. The higher the neurologic injury within the spinal cord, the more difficult the patient's adjustment to the injury and the higher the associated costs. The patient in the opening vignette of this chapter was fortunate to not experience any long-term sequelae from his injury, as a large proportion of patients presenting with spine trauma do have persistent neurologic dysfunction. Although we may have interventions in the near future that can ameliorate the effects of TSCI, prevention of such injuries remains the best way to reduce the burden of TSCI. *Think First,* a program sponsored by the American Association of Neurological

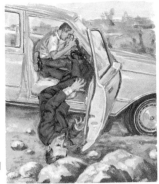
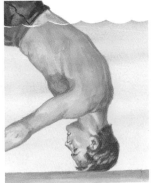

Use of seat belt could have prevented this injury.

Mechanism. Vertical blow on head as in diving or surfing accident, being thrown from car, or football injury

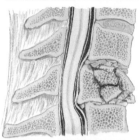
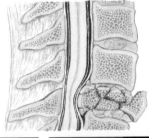

Burst fracture with characteristic vertical fracture through vertebral body

More severe trauma explodes vertebral body. Posteriorly displaced bone fragments frequently produce spinal cord injury.

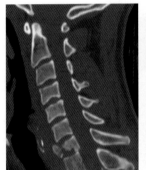
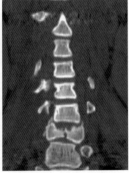
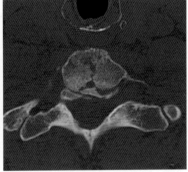

Sagittal CT reconstruction shows compressed comminuted fracture of C7 vertebral body with minimal posterior displacement into the spinal canal.

Coronal CT reconstruction showing disrupted C7 vertebral body.

Axial CT demonstrates comminuted fracture of the vertebral body with sparing of the posterior arch.

Fig. 20.1 Cervical Spine Injury: Compression.

Surgeons that reaches millions of students across the United States and in a number of foreign countries, seeks to educate school-aged children about TSCI prevention.

PATHOPHYSIOLOGY

Traumatic injuries of various types can result in TSCI. Among the most common, particularly among adolescents, are those related to diving accidents or vehicular trauma resulting in compression injury to the vertebrae and the spinal cord (see Fig. 20.1). TSCI in the elderly population is often the result of ground-level falls in the home (see Fig. 20.2); similarly, individuals with ambulatory instability are at significantly increased risk of spinal cord trauma due to falls (Fig. 20.3).

Vertebral fractures can result in damage to the spinal cord (Fig. 20.4), which may range in severity from a mild contusion to a total severing of the cord. In addition to the initial trauma during the event, there is often significant delayed intramedullary microvascular thrombosis within the spinal cord. This frequently leads to progressive secondary injury due to cord ischemia, microhemorrhages, and necrosis. Toxic excitatory amines produced by the trauma worsen the secondary injury.

INITIAL MANAGEMENT

As with any serious traumatic event, patients with TSCI often present with multiple concurrent injuries that may lead to issues such as hypotension, hypoxia, and infection. Some of these may require surgical intervention or stabilization before any TSCI may be addressed, and these patients frequently benefit from advanced multidisciplinary care. As with any trauma, the ABCs of Advanced Trauma Life Support (i.e., airway, breathing, and circulation) demand immediate medical attention. Because any degree of hypotension and hypoxia will further exacerbate the intrinsic spinal cord injury, it is absolutely essential that everything be done to minimize any subsequent injury to the contused spinal cord secondary to inadequate blood supply and/or oxygen (Fig. 20.5). Once the patient is stabilized, a detailed neurologic examination is undertaken. Any motor deficits, sensory changes, and deep tendon reflex abnormalities must be documented meticulously. Several classification schemes assist in describing findings. The American Spinal Injury Association (ASIA) scale is commonly used and stratifies injuries from A (no motor or sensory function) through E (normal sensory and motor function) (Table 20.1). Positive findings also guide further evaluation with diagnostic imaging.

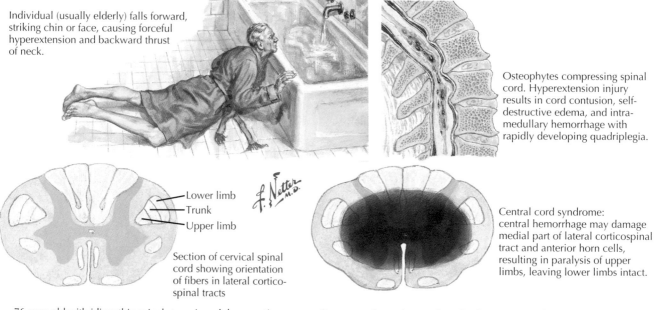

Individual (usually elderly) falls forward, striking chin or face, causing forceful hyperextension and backward thrust of neck.

Osteophytes compressing spinal cord. Hyperextension injury results in cord contusion, self-destructive edema, and intra-medullary hemorrhage with rapidly developing quadriplegia.

Lower limb
Trunk
Upper limb

Section of cervical spinal cord showing orientation of fibers in lateral cortico-spinal tracts

Central cord syndrome: central hemorrhage may damage medial part of lateral corticospinal tract and anterior horn cells, resulting in paralysis of upper limbs, leaving lower limbs intact.

76-year-old with idiopathic spinal stenosis and degenerative subluxation fell down 4 steps.

Posttraumatic cord contusion, disc herniation, and epidural hematoma.

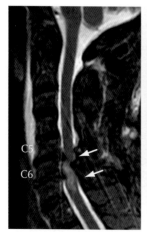
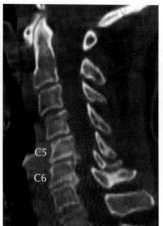
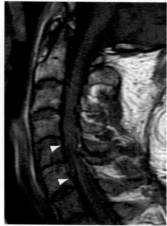
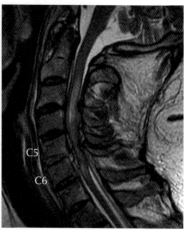

Sagittal T2-weighted cervical MRI shows degenerative bars indenting the spinal cord at C5-C6 and C6-C7 with thickening of ligamentum flavum posteriorly and edema within the spinal cord (arrows) indicating spinal cord injury.

Sagittal cervical CT reconstruction demonstrates multilevel subluxation and degenerative spurs at C5-C6 and C6-C7.

Sagittal T1-weighted cervical MRI demonstrates anterior epidural mass consisting of disc herniation and epidural hematoma between (arrowheads).

Sagittal T2-weighted cervical MRI demonstrates a similar epidural process in addition to showing edema anterior to a partially disrupted C5-C6 disc and probable disruption of posterior longitudinal ligament. Spinal cord edema extends from C2 to C7.

Fig. 20.2 Cervical Spine Injury: Hyperextension.

DIAGNOSTIC APPROACH

Cervical Spine

In any patient in whom cervical spinal injury is suspected, the neck should be immobilized in a rigid collar as soon as possible. Most trauma patients require spinal CT examination, and injuries may be detected even in patients who complain of neck pain and/or tenderness without obvious neurologic deficits. The advantages of CT scanning are the rapidity with which imaging can be obtained and its high sensitivity and specificity for bony spinal injury (see Figs. 20.1 and 20.2). CT also offers the ability to digitally reconstruct acquired images in sagittal, coronal, axial, and oblique views to better detect abnormalities. In settings lacking CT scan capabilities, plain x-ray remains a valuable screening resource, especially when making decisions about the escalation of care in patients with suspected spinal injury. This three-view cervical spine study must include lateral, anteroposterior, and open-mouth views of the odontoid. It is essential to visualize the entire cervical spine from the occiput through T1. Whenever this traditional imaging is inadequate or provides questionable findings, thin-cut CT scanning with reconstruction through the questionable areas must be obtained.

Whenever there is any neurologic deficit, magnetic resonance imaging (MRI) (see Fig. 20.2) is performed before removing the collar or instituting therapy. An MRI will provide evidence of any spinal cord injury, nerve root compression, disc herniation, or ligamentous/soft tissue injury. A normal examination provides evidence that it may be safe to remove the collar support and allow early mobilization. Formal MRI may not be necessary if the trauma patient is alert, has no neck pain

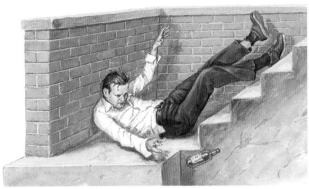

Blow to back of head from falling against hard surface when balance is compromised

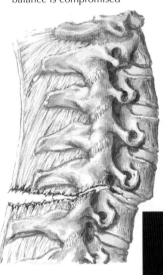

Anterior dislocation of C5-6 with tear of interspinal ligament, facet capsules, and posterior fibers of intervertbral disc

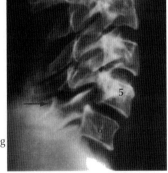

X-ray film (lateral view) showing bilateral interfacet dislocation at C5-6 (arrow)

Fig. 20.3 Cervical Spine Injury: Hyperextension Flexion-Rotation.

TABLE 20.1 American Spinal Injury Association Classification

ASIA Classification	Description
A (Complete)	No motor or sensory function below level of injury preserved including the sacral segments S4 or S5
B (Sensory Incomplete)	Sensory but no motor function is preserved below the level of injury, including the sacral segments S4 and S5
C (Motor Incomplete)	Motor function is preserved below the level of injury, with more than half of muscle groups having a muscle grade of <3/5
D (Motor Incomplete)	Motor function is preserved below the level of injury, with more than half of muscle groups having a muscle grade of ≥3/5
E (Normal)	No motor or sensory deficits

ASIA, American Spinal Injury Association.
From American Spinal Injury Association. *International Standards for Neurological Classifications of Spinal Cord Injury.* Revised edition. Chicago, IL: American Spinal Injury Association; 2000:1–23.

MRI is mandatory whenever there is any question of injury to the spinal cord or ligamentous structures or a potential of disc rupture. Plain radiographs may demonstrate a large proportion of bony injuries, but a CT scan allows for greater resolution and may detect subtle abnormalities that cannot be visualized on x-ray alone.

TREATMENT

Immediate

Treatment begins at the scene of the injury with immediate spine immobilization. The patient is placed on a backboard with his or her neck in a collar, taped to the board with the spine stabilized to prevent secondary injury (see Fig. 20.5). This position must be maintained until the entire spine is clinically, and usually radiographically, cleared by the appropriate physicians. Because of spinal instability, the condition of 4% of patients with TSCI deteriorates after initial attempts at treatment. Nonoperative spinal stabilizing techniques include a rigid collar, craniocervical traction, a halo, a rotating frame, or rocking bed (Fig. 20.6). Patients who are managed with nonoperative stabilization alone must be evaluated for healing of their fracture and for the possible development of progressive deformity over time, as they may require fusion at a later date should they experience decompensation.

Corticosteroids

The use of corticosteroids for treatment of spinal cord injury has undergone a number of profound changes over the past several decades and remains somewhat controversial even today. Following the positive results of the second National Acute Spinal Cord Injury Study (NASCIS II), a multicenter, double-blind, placebo-controlled trial of methylprednisolone therapy for acute spinal cord injury, corticosteroids were used in a high proportion of spinal cord injury cases. However, the results of NASCIS II were not without significant controversy, and many argued that the study was flawed methodologically and that benefits were only seen in posthoc analysis.

Subsequent studies have failed to demonstrate significant benefits with corticosteroid therapy in TSCI or have demonstrated higher rates of morbidity and mortality. These include a prospective, randomized, double-blinded study in 2000 by Pointillart et al.,

or tenderness, has full painless range of motion of the neck, demonstrates a normal neurologic examination, and shows no evidence of active intoxication.

In the case of the neurologically intact patient with definite posttraumatic neck pain whose cervical radiographic and/or CT findings are normal, it is still essential to evaluate for the possibility of a subtle but unstable fracture dislocation with potential for severe cord injury. Dynamic, lateral flexion/extension radiographs or fluoroscopy will indicate dislocation. The neck excursions required for these procedures can be performed only when the patient is lucid and cooperative. If the patient is uncooperative or obtunded, he or she must be kept in the rigid collar until flexion-extension films can be performed passively by a trained provider.

Thoracic, Thoracolumbar, and Lumbar Spine

For injuries to the thoracic, thoracolumbar, and lumbar spine, plain radiographs, CT, and MRI are all used. Similar to the cervical spine,

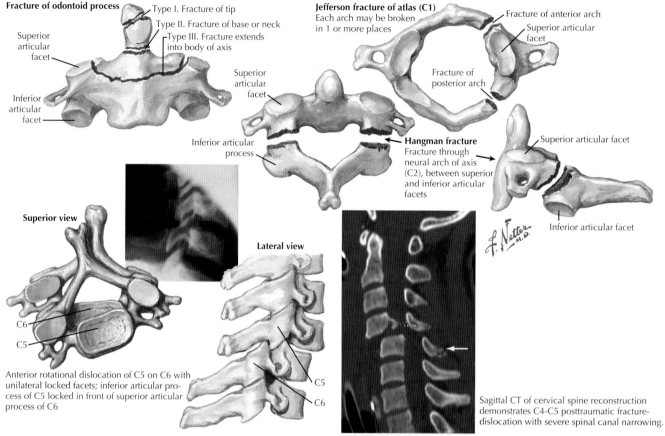

Fig. 20.4 Fracture and Dislocation of Cervical Vertebrae.

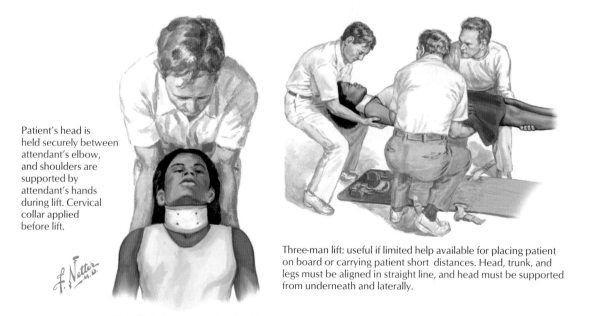

Fig. 20.5 Suspected Cervical Spine Injury: Treatment at Site of Accident.

which showed a significantly higher rate of transient hyperglycemia with corticosteroid therapy. In a prospective, randomized, double-blinded study evaluating adverse events specifically, Matsumoto et al. noted that complications seen more frequently with corticosteroid therapy included gastrointestinal bleeding, and respiratory compromise. The higher rate of adverse events, combined with the lack of definitive evidence for benefit, resulted in the most recently published consensus guidelines recommending against routine use of corticosteroids in TSCI.

Surgery

When spinal cord neural compression is documented or spinal misalignment is evident, surgical intervention must be considered immediately. The degree of neural compression is first assessed using CT and

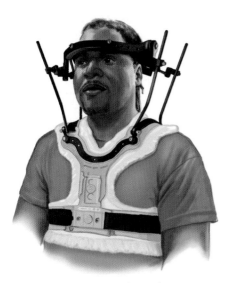

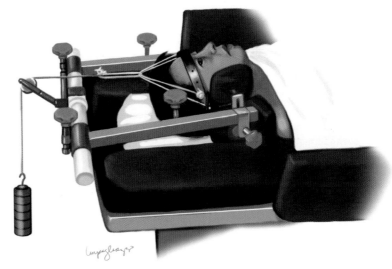

A halo vest is frequently used to treat many types of bony cervical spine injury

A halo ring can be used to stabilize cervical fractures that will require operative intervention or by applying traction that can reduce cervical spine subluxations

Fig. 20.6 Cervical Spine Injury: Traction and Bracing.

MRI. Significant spinal cord or nerve root compression requires surgical decompression and stabilization. Stability, which is the ability of the spine to withstand physiologic loads through normal ranges of motion, can be difficult to evaluate. One commonly used heuristic described by Denis involves dividing the spine into three columns: anterior (consisting of the anterior longitudinal ligament and anterior two-thirds of the vertebral body), middle (posterior one-third of the vertebral body and the posterior longitudinal ligament), and posterior (all structures posterior to the posterior longitudinal ligament). In this method, typically all injuries involving two or more columns are at high risk for instability.

There is also disagreement among neurosurgeons regarding the timing of surgery. Some champion earlier surgical decompression and stabilization when there is an incomplete injury, especially with residual autonomic function. This is thought by some to improve the potential for neurologic improvement. Early decompression is supported by studies, such as the Surgical Timing in Acute Spinal Cord Injury Study (STASCIS) by Fehlings et al. in 2012, where decompression within 24 hours for cervical TSCI was associated with better neurologic function at the 6-month follow-up. Although the outlook for improvement with a complete spinal cord lesion is poor, some neurosurgeons believe that early surgery and stabilization—even with complete lesions—allows for early mobilization and rehabilitation, possibly reducing the significant morbidity of prolonged bed rest. Other neurosurgeons are more conservative and wait until the patient is fully stabilized medically prior to surgical intervention. This is because a number of these patients can demonstrate profound autonomic instability, and anesthesia under such circumstances can precipitate profound hypotension, possibly precipitating devastating cord ischemia. It is generally thought that regardless of the timing, surgical decompression and fusion provide better overall outcomes than nonoperative treatment even after a long delay. This applies to spinal cord and/or nerve root injury. Controversy continues to exist as to whether early surgery with complete cord injury improves neurologic function compared with delayed surgery. Early surgical stabilization can be facilitated by new technologies, such as intraoperative imaging and navigation, which can help with instrumentation and localization even when normal anatomy is compromised by the injury itself (Fig. 20.7).

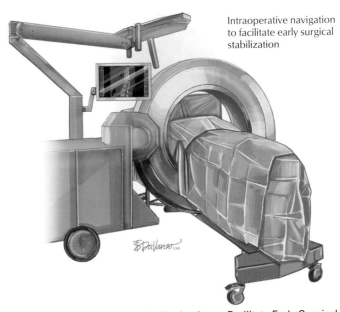

Intraoperative navigation to facilitate early surgical stabilization

Fig. 20.7 Use of Intraoperative Navigation to Facilitate Early Surgical Stabilization.

In summary, the goals of surgery are twofold: to decompress the neural elements and to stabilize the spine. This allows the best chance for early mobilization. There are also specific evaluation and therapeutic approaches that are necessary depending on the anatomical site of injury.

Atlanto-Axial (C1–C2)

In the cervical spine, open-mouth odontoid x-rays are used to demonstrate the relationship of the lateral masses of C1 with the articular pillars of C2. The "rule of Spence" states that if the sum of the overhang of both C1 lateral masses on C2 is greater than 7 mm, then the transverse ligament is likely disrupted, resulting in C1–C2 instability. Treatment typically involves halo vest immobilization or occipitocervical fusion (see Fig. 20.4).

Dens fractures are subclassified depending on fracture location and morphology (see Fig. 20.4). Type 1 fractures occur through the tip of the dens above the transverse ligament. They are quite rare and may be associated with atlantoaxial instability, although they commonly heal on their own with rigid external bracing alone. Type 2 fractures, the most common, occur through the base of the dens and are usually unstable (Figs. 20.4 and 20.6). Type 2 fractures show a higher risk for pseudoarthrosis with external bracing alone and often require surgical arthrodesis. Type 3 fractures involve the body of C2. These fractures often heal with immobilization in a hard collar or halo vest alone (see Fig. 20.6). Surgical options for treatment of dens fractures that fail or are not candidates for conservative management with rigid cervical bracing include posterior fusion of C1 and C2 using a variety of techniques or anterior fixation through an odontoid screw.

Prior to selection of a fixation technique, careful assessment of the patient and the fracture must be undertaken to avoid poor outcomes. For example, although placement of an odontoid screw (Fig. 20.8) allows for the preservation of rotation at the atlantoaxial junction, the technique has many contraindications including comminuted C2 fractures, transverse ligament disruption, and chronic nonunions (greater than 6–8 months). Relative contraindications for odontoid screw fixation include severe osteopenia, oblique fractures of the odontoid (where the fracture is parallel to the planned trajectory of the screw), and technically challenging anatomy such as a bull-neck or barrel chest.

Traumatic spondylolisthesis of the axis caused by bilateral fractures of the C2 pars interarticularis is known as a "hangman's fracture," as this is the mechanism of injury seen in individuals who are executed via hanging. The most common modern-day cause of this fracture is motor vehicle collisions; the striking of the chin on the steering wheel results in a combination of hyperextension and axial loading (Fig. 20.9).

Type 1 hangman's fractures have minimal angulation and less than 3 mm of subluxation. These are considered most likely to heal with external bracing alone. Treatment involves fracture reduction and stabilization in a hard collar or halo. *Type 2 hangman's fractures* have 4 mm or more subluxation. These are usually unstable and require reduction and stabilization in halo. *Type 3 hangman's fractures* involve marked disruption of C2–C3 posterior elements and wide subluxation. These injuries are often fatal, but survivors require open reduction and

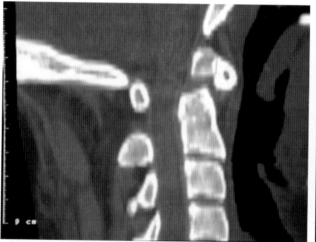 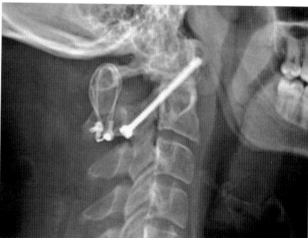

A. Reformatted sagittal CT scan of type 2 dens fracture.   **B.** Plain radiograph of post C1-2 transarticular fixation and fusion.

Fig. 20.8 Dens Fracture of Cervical Spine.

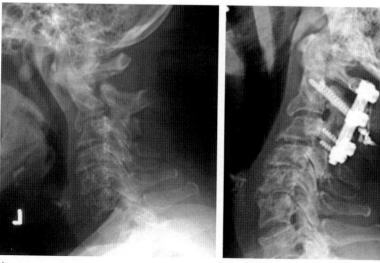

A. Hangman's fracture   **B.** Post repair

Fig. 20.9 Plain Radiograph of Hangman's Fracture: Cervical Spine.

stabilization via C2–C3 anterior discectomy and fusion, or posterior C1–C3 fusion.

Subaxial Cervical Spine

Subluxation is defined by neutral spinal radiographs demonstrating instability with greater than 3.5 mm or angulation greater than 11 degrees. Injuries resulting in stable fractures usually heal well with

immobilization in a hard collar or halo. Grossly unstable injuries require surgical stabilization (Figs. 20.9 and 20.10).

Thoracolumbar Spine

Approximately 64% of spine fractures occur at the thoracolumbar junction (Fig. 20.11). The degree of initial spinal cord injury usually determines the long-term prognosis. Most injuries that are relatively stable

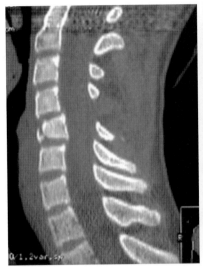
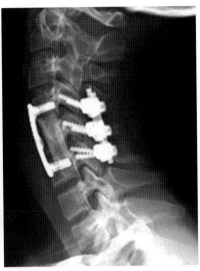

A. Reformatted sagittal CT of C5 "burst" fracture

B. Plain radiograph of C5 vertebrectomy/ fusion with posterior C4-6 lateral mass fixation/fusion

Fig. 20.10 Nonaxial Burst Fracture: Cervical Spine.

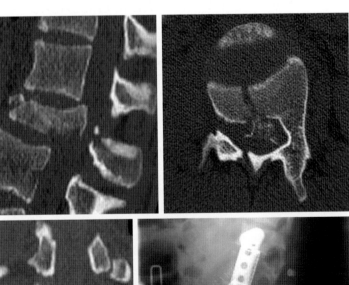
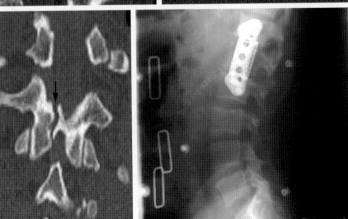

A. Midsagittal CT reconstruction showing markedly compressed and disrupted L1.

B. Axial CT demonstrates fracture in vertebral body, retropulsed fragment occupying the anterior aspect of the spinal canal, and disruption of the posterior arch.

C. Coronal CT reconstruction demonstrates fracture in posterior arch (arrow).

D. Reformatted sagittal CT scan of vertebrectomy and fusion using anterior titanium mesh cage and anterior plate.

Fig. 20.11 Burst Fracture: Lumbar Spine.

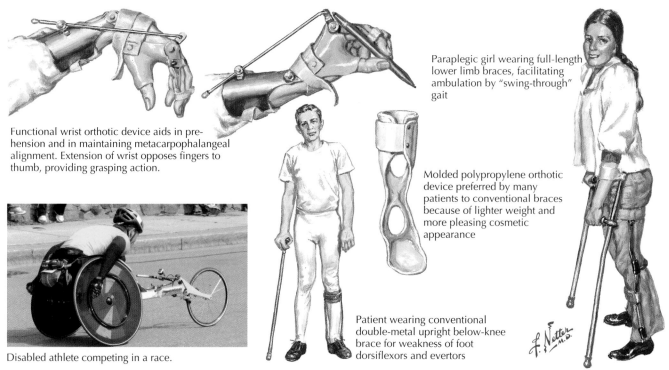

Functional wrist orthotic device aids in pre-hension and in maintaining metacarpophalangeal alignment. Extension of wrist opposes fingers to thumb, providing grasping action.

Disabled athlete competing in a race.

Paraplegic girl wearing full-length lower limb braces, facilitating ambulation by "swing-through" gait

Molded polypropylene orthotic device preferred by many patients to conventional braces because of lighter weight and more pleasing cosmetic appearance

Patient wearing conventional double-metal upright below-knee brace for weakness of foot dorsiflexors and evertors

Fig. 20.12 Cervical Spine Injury: Rehabilitation of Patient.

may be managed with external bracing and mobilization. The decision to operate on thoracolumbar spine fractures is often complex and relies on an assessment of a variety of factors including the presence of neurologic injury, ongoing compression of neurologic structures, the type and severity of bony injury, and the presence of damage to ligamentous elements of the spine. Although some instruments, such as the thoracolumbar injury classification and severity (TLICS) score, exist to assist in decision making, clinical acumen remains paramount when assessing individual cases.

PROGNOSIS

Spinal cord injury remains a devastating, life-altering injury. When there is complete loss of neurologic function, clinical improvements allowing return to activities of daily living are currently largely dependent on the availability of superior physiatric rehabilitation rather than anatomic spinal cord regeneration. Many patients with incomplete spinal cord injuries can recover some degree of neurologic function, although this frequently requires months of intensive therapy. Complete spinal cord injury remains an incredibly difficult condition to manage, and the majority of patients have fixed deficits that are unrecoverable.

In any case of TSCI, early patient mobilization is vital. Deconditioning and poor functional recovery are associated with any significant period of bed rest. Immobility also makes the patient more susceptible to major complications, including deep venous thrombosis, pneumonia, and skin breakdown.

Fortunately, many patients with TSCI are now able to return to a relatively normal life. Many hold full-time jobs (Fig. 20.12), and an ever-increasing number of athletic endeavors are also now accessible to patients with disabilities resulting from TSCI (see Fig. 20.12).

FUTURE DIRECTIONS

Given its immense individual and societal impact, it is unsurprising that TSCI remains an intense area of research. Although current therapeutic options for TSCI are extremely limited, there is reason to believe that significant advancements may be made in the next several years. A number of pharmacologic therapeutic options, predominantly aimed at reducing secondary injury, are currently in various stages of clinical trials. One promising agent, currently under evaluation in a phase 3 trial, is riluzole, a sodium channel blocker previously approved for amyotrophic lateral sclerosis.

Advances in stem cell technology—buoyed by improved methods of both stem cell derivation and an ever-increasing understanding of the factors promoting stem cell differentiation—raise the possibility of someday achieving the regeneration of injured cord cells. Actively recruiting trials include a study investigating Schwann cell transplantation for patients with long-term deficits from TSCI and another study examining transplantation of oligodendrocyte progenitor cells.

Pioneering efforts in biotechnology, specifically in the realm of mind–machine interfaces, have allowed for the development of devices that allow patients with spinal cord injury to regain function in impacted limbs by bypassing the injured cord segment and directly translating brain signals into muscle movement. Bouton et al. recently described their experience with a patient driving an arm-sleeve stimulator using signals derived from cortical electrical activity (Fig. 20.13). Although significant hurdles remain before these next-wave therapeutic options can be used in the average TSCI patient, the current trajectory of research gives hope to the millions of patients suffering from the effects of TSCI.

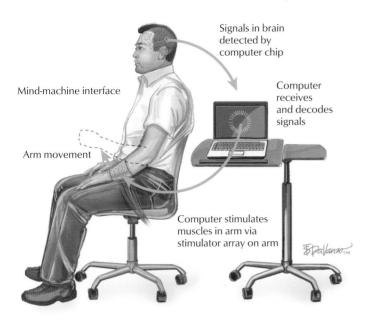

Signals in brain detected by computer chip

Mind-machine interface

Computer receives and decodes signals

Arm movement

Computer stimulates muscles in arm via stimulator array on arm

Fig. 20.13 Mind–Machine Interface.

ADDITIONAL RESOURCES

American Association of Neurological Surgeons/Congress of Neurological Surgeons. Guidelines for the management of acute cervical spine and spinal cord injuries. Neurosurgery 2013;72(Suppl. 3).

This supplemental volume of the journal Neurosurgery *represents the latest guidelines for the management of spinal cord injury. These recommendations are made based on the best available evidence and are derived from expert consensus.*

Guan J, Hawryluk GW. Advancements in the mind-machine interface: toward re-establishment of direct cortical limb movement in spinal cord injury. Neural Regen Res 2016;11(7):1060–1.

Brief review of the use of mind-machine interface to bypass spinal cord injury and reestablish direct control of limbs below the level of damage. Presents the latest research in the field and gives a mini-summary of progress to date.

National Spinal Cord Injury Statistical Center. Facts and figures at a glance. Birmingham, AL: University of Alabama at Birmingham; 2016. Available from: http://www.nscisc.uab.edu.

Clearinghouse for national statistics on spinal cord injury in the United States. Provides estimates of the national economic impact of spinal cord injury and acts as a longitudinal record of the impact of spinal cord injury year to year.

Sahni V, Kessler JA. Stem cell therapies for spinal cord injury. Nat Rev Neurol 2010;6:363–72.

Succinct review of recent progress in stem cell therapies for spinal cord injury. Discusses both the mechanisms and theory behind stem cell use for spinal cord injury and recent clinical trials.

Lee JY, Vaccaro AR, Lim MR, et al. Thoracolumbar injury classification and severity score: a new paradigm for the treatment of thoracolumbar spine trauma. J Orthop Sci 2005;10(6):671–5.

Paper detailing a decision-making support algorithm for determining the need for surgical intervention in thoracic and lumbar spine injuries. This is only one of many algorithms that have been developed for this purpose.

Guan J, Bisson EF. Treatment of odontoid fractures in the aging population. Neurosurg Clin N Am 2017;28(1):115–23.

Review of management of odontoid fractures, focusing on management in older patients. Includes a brief discussion of the changing demographics of spinal cord injury with the aging population.

Anwar MA, Al Shehabi TS, Eid AH. Inflammogenesis of secondary spinal cord injury. Front Cell Neurosci 2016;10:98.

Review of secondary injury mechanisms, with a focus on the inflammatory cascade. Also discusses possible avenues for future treatments that may target these pathways.

Pointillart V, Petitjean ME, Wiart L, et al. Pharmacologic therapy of spinal cord injury during the acute phase. Spinal Cord 2000;38:71–6.

Prospective, randomized trial of spinal trauma patients randomized to receive methylprednisolone and/or nimodipine in addition to early surgical decompression. There was a higher incidence of hyperglycemia in the steroid-treated group, and no difference in 1-year clinical outcomes.

Matsumoto T, Tamaki T, Kawakami M, et al. Early complications of high-dose methylprednisolone sodium succinate treatment in the follow-up of acute cervical spinal cord injury. Spine 2001;16(4):426–30.

Prospective, double-blinded study that randomized 46 patients to either high-dose steroid therapy or placebo. It found increased pulmonary and gastrointestinal side-effects in the steroid group and a trend toward worse steroid complications in those over 60.

Fehlings MG, Vaccaro A, Wilson JR, et al. Early versus delayed decompression for traumatic cervical spinal cord injury: Results of the surgical timing in acute spinal cord injury study (STASCIS). PLoS ONE 2012;7(2):e32037. doi:10.1371/journal.pone.0032037.

Multicentered prospective cohort study of early (<24 hrs after injury) versus late (≥ 24 hrs) surgical decompression showing better functional outcomes at 6 months with early surgical decompression.

Bouton CE, Shaikhouni A, Annetta NV, et al. Restoring cortical control of functional movement in a human with quadriplegia. Nature 2016;533(7602):247–50.

Report of muscle activation in a paralyzed human using an implanted cortical microelectrode system and neuromuscular electrical stimulation.

Headache and Pain

Jayashri Srinivasan

21

Primary and Secondary Headache

Carol L. Moheban, Daniel Vardeh

CLINICAL VIGNETTE *A 50-year-old woman is referred to a neurologist because of severe headaches. She first developed headaches during adolescence, and they worsened in the setting of menopause. A typical headache is unilateral and localized to the right frontotemporal and periorbital regions. The pain is described as throbbing and pulsating. When severe, her headaches are associated with nausea, vomiting, photophobia, phonophobia, and visual symptoms. Her headaches had increased in frequency and were occurring a few times a month, lasting for at least 12 hours, and causing her to miss work. Her examination was normal. Blood work and a magnetic resonance imaging (MRI) of the brain were normal.*

Headache is one of the most common symptoms in medicine and is often the primary complaint presented to the internist, neurologist, or emergency room physician. Despite this, like many pain syndromes, headaches are underdiagnosed and undertreated. Accurate headache diagnosis is important before specific treatment can be initiated. It can be the presenting symptom in many primary neurologic illnesses and in a number of serious systemic disorders. The preceding vignette is typical of migraines, one of the most common headache syndromes. Distinguishing features of more serious causes, such as brain tumors, ruptured aneurysms, low cerebrospinal pressure syndromes, subdural hematoma, meningitis, and temporal arteritis, should be deliberately inquired of and must not be overlooked. Assessment of a patient presenting with headache starts with a detailed history. Essential characteristics should be defined: any premonitory symptoms, manner of onset (e.g., precipitous or gradual), diurnal variation, provoking and alleviating factors, location, pain characteristics, duration, medical and psychiatric comorbidities, and degree of disability. Family and social history, current medications, drug allergies, and review of systems are also important. A detailed neurologic and general medical examination is essential to the evaluation, particularly with individuals having a recent or precipitous onset or experiencing changes in headache characteristics. Ancillary laboratory and neuroradiologic testing are often indicated.

Headache syndromes must first be classified as primary (without significant underlying neurologic pathology) or secondary (due to intracranial pathology). The differentiation between primary and secondary headache is critical; it dictates the diagnostic approach and guides treatment and prognosis.

PRIMARY HEADACHE DISORDERS

Migraine

Epidemiology

Migraine is the most common type of headache that makes patients seek medical care. Recent epidemiologic studies reveal a worldwide prevalence of 10%–15% with the highest prevalence in South and Central America. Females are affected twice as often as men, and prevalence is especially high in younger females and the urban population. According to the *Global Burden of Disease Survey 2010* conducted by the World Health Organization (WHO), migraine ranks as the third most common disease worldwide (after dental caries and tension type headaches), the seventh most disabling disease, and the third most expensive neurologic disease after dementia and stroke. The estimated heritability of migraine is 40%–60% based on family and twin studies; a child with a migraineur parent has about a 50% chance of developing a migraine, and this number rises to 75% if both parents are affected. First migraine attacks often manifest in the teens and early 20s, and 80% of patients have had their first migraine by age 30. Typically, migraines diminish or disappear in the older population and with menopause; one should be particularly cautious in making a new migraine diagnosis in the elderly.

Pathophysiology

Migraine pathophysiology is likely linked to cortical hyperexcitability in genetically susceptible patients, which subsequently activates trigeminal pathways and results in release of vasoactive neuropeptides and proinflammatory substances (including substance P and calcitonin gene-related peptide [CGRP]) in the trigeminal nociceptive nerve endings. These nociceptive nerve endings are located in pial, arachnoid, and dural blood vessels, as well as large cerebral arteries and sinuses; they are carried mostly by V1 and to lesser degree V2 and V3 nerve roots (Figs. 21.1 and 21.2). The release of vasoactive substances promotes meningeal blood vessel dilatation and release of inflammatory cytokines, leads to peripheral trigeminal nerve sensitization as well as central sensitization in the spinal trigeminal nucleus. Ultimately, these changes not only cause a throbbing headache, but via activation of the pulvinar, hypothalamus, and periaqueductal gray in the brainstem result in widespread symptoms of allodynia, malaise, and autonomic responses. The convergence of trigeminal sensory afferents and C1–C3 occipital afferents in the trigeminal nucleus spinalis likely allows for cross sensitization and referred pain in the occipital region and neck (see Fig. 21.1). The phenomenon of an aura (i.e., a transient focal neurologic symptom heralding or accompanying a migraine headache) represents a slowly propagating wave (2–6 mm/min) of neuronal and glial depolarization followed by a prolonged inhibition (15–30 min) of cortical activity, termed cortical spreading depression. Because this phenomenon can occur anywhere on the cortex, auras can produce a wide range of symptoms including visual, motor, sensory, and cognitive alterations.

Clinical Symptoms (Fig. 21.3)/Diagnostic Criteria

Migraine is a primary headache disorder; however it can and often does coexist with other either primary (e.g., tension type headache) or secondary (medication-overuse headache) headache disorders. Migraine

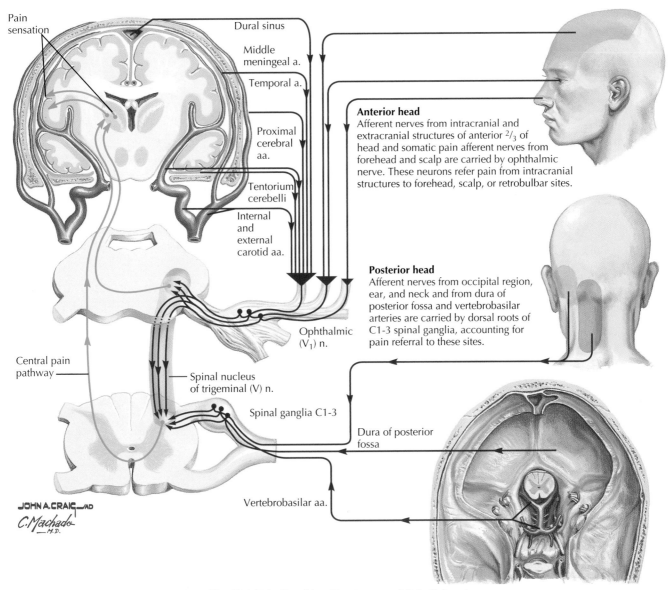

Fig. 21.1 Pain-Sensitive Structures and Pain Referral.

has two major subtypes, based on the presence or absence of an aura; furthermore, migraine frequency distinguishes between episodic and chronic migraines; the latter is characterized by greater than 15 headache days per month for 3 months.

According to the International Headache Society (IHS) classification, migraine headaches are characterized by
- Recurrent headache attacks lasting 4–72 hours AND
- Typical headache characteristics (2 out of 4): unilateral location, pulsating quality, moderate or severe intensity, aggravation by routine physical activity, AND
- Association with (1 out of 2) nausea/vomiting or photophobia and phonophobia.

The location of migraine headache is typically frontotemporal, but can involve the entire hemicranium and sometimes the face. Laterality can switch from attack to attack, however typically there is a strong side preference for most attacks. Migraine onset in children can often have a bilateral presentation, and lateralizes typically as they reach adolescence. Symptoms of cutaneous/scalp allodynia as well as more widespread neck muscle tenderness are not uncommon and are likely attributed to sensitization of the trigeminocervical complex.

Patients with migraine often have premonitory symptoms which occur up to 1–2 days before the actual migraine attack. These include fatigue, neck tenderness, thirst, anorexia, fluid retention, food cravings, gastrointestinal symptoms, and emotional or mood disturbances such as irritability, elation, or depression.

Approximately 15% of migraine patients have an aura, characterized by focal, transient neurologic symptoms which typically precede but also can accompany the headache phase. By far the most common aura symptoms (>90%) are of visual character, followed by sensory and speech/language disturbance. Rarer presentations include motor weakness (referred to as hemiplegic migraine) and brainstem symptoms (e.g., vertigo). Aura phenomena are diagnosed according to their time of onset, duration, and relation to the headaches (IHS criteria). Most auras typically spread over 5–20 minutes (e.g., spreading tingling sensation or flashing lights), last 5–60 minutes, are typically unilateral, and are followed by the headache phase within 1 hour of onset. Gradual spreading of symptoms within one modality (tingling starting in the face and gradually involving the arm) or even spreading to other modalities (e.g., flashing lights followed by tingling) is the result of continuous spreading across various cortical areas. Prolonged inhibition after the

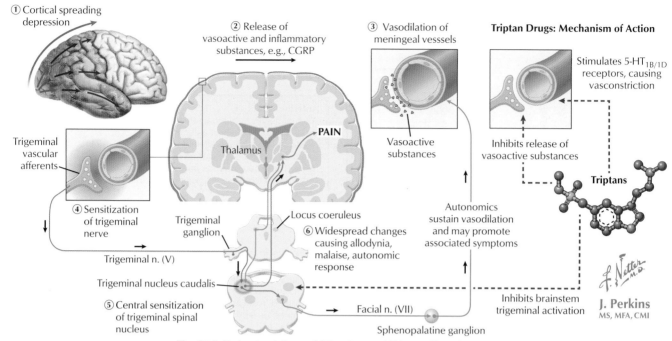

Fig. 21.2 Pathophysiology of Migraine and Triptan Site of Action.

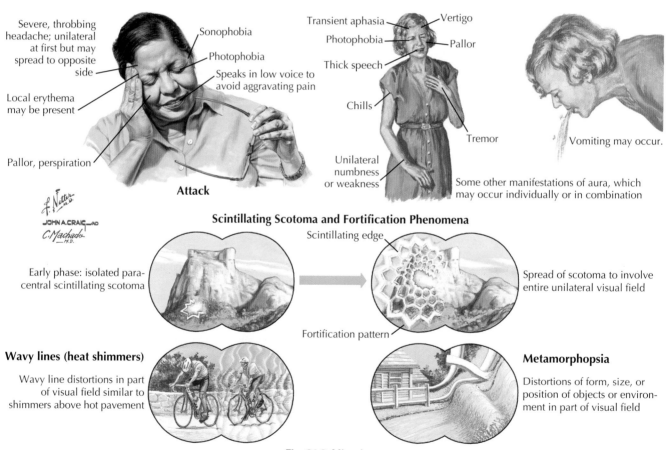

Fig. 21.3 Migraine.

depolarization wave (spreading depression) results clinically in negative phenomena like a transient scotoma, numbness, or even weakness.

Visual auras can occur in a homonymous or hemifield distribution and include scintillating flashes or stars (phosphenes) and geometric patterns known as fortification spectra (see Fig. 21.3), with an absolute or relative transient scotoma. Sensory symptoms typically consist of tingling/pins and needles anywhere in the body (often face or arm), and spread gradually, often leaving behind transient numbness. Less frequent, and often more dramatic, auras include language disturbances (any type of aphasia), brainstem auras (dysarthria, vertigo, tinnitus, hyperacusis, diplopia, ataxia, decreased level of consciousness) and hemiplegic migraine presenting with transient weakness or hemiplegia. Hemiplegic migraine is often familial (familial hemiplegic migraine) and is caused in many cases by various mutations of the voltage-gated calcium channel $Ca_V 2.1$. Oculomotor nerve palsies are the hallmark of ophthalmoplegic "migraine"; however this might represent a recurrent demyelinating neuropathy rather than a true migraine variant.

Careful neurologic evaluation is critical, and brain MRI is typically obtained for a first-time presentation of an aura. This is especially true if the aura is not followed by a headache (aura without headache), but presents as an isolated focal neurologic deficit.

Special Considerations

Ischemic strokes as well as other cardiovascular events (ischemic hemorrhage, coronary events) have been shown to have a higher prevalence in patients with migraines, especially in migraine with aura. Based on epidemiologic studies, the relative risk for ischemic stroke is double in female migraineurs with aura, and the risk increases with more frequent migraine attacks. However given the low prevalence in this typically young and healthy population, absolute numbers remain very low. In addition, several neuroimaging studies have shown an up to four-fold increased prevalence of white matter hyperintensities especially in the posterior circulation ("white spots") in people with migraine, as well as an increased risk for white matter lesions with increased attack frequency. Whether the association of migraine and cardiovascular events is causative remains uncertain; rather, there are several known diseases which present with both migraine type headaches as well as increased cardiovascular risk. For example, gene mutation of *NOTCH3* causes cerebral autosomal dominant arteriopathy with subcortical infarcts and leukoencephalopathy (CADASIL), a hereditary small-artery disease of the brain that is characterized by multiple ischemic strokes; however in 40% of patients, migraine headaches precede the first stroke by 10–20 years.

Patent foramen ovale (PFO) and migraines have sometimes been linked together; however, two population-based studies showed that the prevalence of a PFO was similar in patients with and without migraine. In addition, three randomized clinical trials did not show significant improvement of migraines other than in small subpopulations 1 year after PFO closure surgery.

Estrogen levels likely play a significant role as a migraine trigger in females. About two-thirds of female migraineurs primarily experience migraines just before or during menses, likely caused by the timing and rate of estrogen withdrawal. In many cases, first time migraine onset occurs around the time of menarche, and frequency often significantly decreases after menopause. In addition, migraines often worsen early in pregnancy but tend to improve during the second and third trimesters, particularly in women with migraine primarily related to their menstrual cycle.

Management and Therapy

Two types of treatment exist for migraine therapy: abortive treatment for acute headaches, and prophylactic treatment to decrease frequency and intensity of future migraine attacks.

Prophylaxis is indicated if migraine attacks are frequent and/or disabling despite use of abortive medications overuse/misuse of abortive medication occurs; auras are frequent and disabling, or for specific migraine conditions (e.g., hemiplegic migraine). Prophylactic treatment can be preemptive, short term, or continuous. If defined migraine triggers exist, preemptive treatment 30–60 minutes before the anticipated trigger is useful (e.g., indomethacin before exercise-induced headache). Time-limited exposure to a provoking factor can be treated with short-term daily prophylaxis, such as daily nonsteroidal antiinflammatory drug (NSAID) intake a few days prior and into menstruation for menstrual-related migraines. Continuous, daily prophylactic medication is necessary if trigger factors are unpredictable, unknown, or absent. Most commonly used daily prophylactic drug classes include tricyclic antidepressants, β-blockers, calcium channel blockers, antiepileptics, and gabapentinoids. Of these, certain β-blockers (especially propranolol and metoprolol), divalproex sodium, and topiramate have the best evidence. Other antiepileptics, including gabapentin, pregabalin, carbamazepine, oxcarbazepine, lamotrigine, levetiracetam, vigabatrin, and zonisamide, do not have high-quality evidence to support their use; however they might be worth trying in otherwise refractory patients. Given the similar efficacy of first-line preventatives in studies, the initial choice of medication is often based on comorbidities, side-effect profile, medication interaction, patient and prescriber preference, medication cost, and insurance coverage. For instance, difficulty with sleep may prompt prescribing of medications that are more sedating like amitriptyline. Topiramate may be preferable over valproic acid or tricyclics for those in whom weight gain is a concern. A concomitant mood disorder may prompt the use of antidepressants or medications with mood-stabilizing properties. β-blockers may help in controlling coexisting hypertension in some patients but should be avoided in those with reactive-airway disease or preexisting depression. To improve efficacy and to lower side effects, combination therapy of two different class agents is often advisable, such as the combination of β-blockers and a tricyclic, or the addition of topiramate. The empirical approach to find the right medication or medication combination can often be frustrating for patient and provider alike.

"Natural" treatments might sometimes be preferable due to their very favorable side-effect profile or patient preference, and substances with some evidence include riboflavin 400 mg daily, coenzyme Q10 300 mg daily, magnesium 400–600 mg daily, and a combination of simvastatin with vitamin D3. Nonpharmacologic prophylactic treatments are also advisable, and may include avoiding certain foods (typically caffeine overuse, chocolate, alcohol, cheese, processed meat containing nitrates) and environmental triggers, regular sleep, physical activity, regular meals, and appropriate hydration.

Interventional headache treatments should be considered if oral medications of different classes fail to control migraine attacks, or if use is limited due to side effects, comorbidities, or allergies. Occipital nerve blocks with or without steroids can be effective in reducing migraines for 1–3 months. The administration of 155 units of onabotulinumtoxin A every 12 weeks is FDA approved and has been shown in two large randomized controlled trials to be a safe and effective way to reduce migraine frequency and improve quality of life. The likely mechanism of action is inhibition of release of pronociceptive substances like substance P and CGRP from peripheral nociceptive trigeminal terminals, as well as (via retrograde axonal transport) decreasing central sensitization at the trigeminal spinal nucleus. Neurostimulation represents yet another modality, and daily supraorbital transcutaneous neurostimulation using the Cefaly device has been FDA approved for reduction of migraine frequency in episodic migraines. There might also be a modest effect from occipital nerve stimulation implant for chronic migraine prevention; however complication rate and surgical risk must be carefully weighed against potential benefit.

Regarding abortive therapy, mild to moderately intense migraines are best treated with oral NSAIDs, acetylsalicylic acid (aspirin), or acetaminophen. Opiates should be avoided as should butalbital-containing medications due to their association with medication overuse headache (MOH) and tendency to cause dependency. While many different NSAIDs are used for acute treatment, the soluble powder formulation of diclofenac potassium (Cambia in the United States, Voltfast in Europe) is the only FDA-approved NSAID for migraine. Caffeine may enhance the effect of these various medications or can be helpful by itself. Antiemetics such as prochlorperazine, metoclopramide, or ondansetron are often useful in conjunction with analgesics.

For more severe migraine attacks, serotonin 1B/1D receptor agonist ("triptan") preparations are the medications of choice. Their success is attributed to several sites of action on the migraine cascade, including peripheral mechanisms (vasoconstriction, nociceptor inhibition, inhibition of peripheral release of vasoactive peptides) as well as likely central mechanisms (decreasing neurotransmitter release at central nociceptive terminals, decreasing neuronal excitability) (see Fig. 21.2). Seven different triptans are available, which differ by their available route of administration (oral, quick-dissolve sublingual, injectable, or intranasal) as well as their bioavailability, plasma half-life, and lipophilicity, all of which does not translate into meaningful increased efficacy or decreased headache recurrence. The rapidly acting triptans include almotriptan, eletriptan, rizatriptan, sumatriptan, and zolmitriptan. The slower acting/longer acting triptans include naratriptan and frovatriptan. Sumatriptan is the only triptan available as subcutaneous injectable, which results in ultra-fast absorption and a quick onset of migraine relief. There are marked interindividual differences for both effect and side effects for different triptans, and changing triptans on a trial-and-error basis often results in better migraine control. Varying the administration route (e.g., from oral to subcutaneous in patients with severe nausea or the concomitant intake of an anti-nausea medication like metoclopramide) can increase the efficacy by improving triptan absorption. Despite the limited evidence for cardiovascular events caused by triptan use, it is still recommended that triptans be avoided in patients with hemiplegic migraine, basilar migraine, ischemic stroke, ischemic heart disease, Prinzmetal's angina, uncontrolled hypertension, and pregnancy.

Butalbital, isometheptene/dichloralphenazone, and oral opioids are rarely recommended abortive therapies, as they have a higher risk of sedation, overuse, and dependence.

The alpha-adrenergic blocker and serotonin 1B/1D receptor agonist dihydroergotamine (DHE) is available as intravenous, intramuscular, subcutaneous, and intranasal formulations, and is often used in the emergency room setting in combination with an antiemetic for acute migraine attacks and status migrainosus. Intravenous ketorolac or opioids are other options for emergency treatment in the most refractory cases.

Future Directions

Of the new therapeutic targets for migraine treatment, CGRP has been the most extensively investigated. The release of CGRP after activation of the trigeminal system plays a key role in inducing meningeal vasodilation, inflammation, and nociceptive transmission to the trigeminal spinal nucleus. Monoclonal antibodies to either the CGRP receptor or CGRP ligand itself have shown promising efficacy as preventative treatment in episodic and chronic migraine in several randomized controlled trials, with only minimal side effects. Single dose, subcutaneous administration monthly or quarterly, makes them an attractive alternative to daily preventative medications or botulinum toxin injection.

Trigeminal Autonomic Cephalalgias
Cluster Headache

> **CLINICAL VIGNETTE** *A 34-year-old man presents to his internist for evaluation of severe pain above and behind his right eye. The pain began a few days ago and is intermittent. It occurs several times a day, usually lasting for 30–60 minutes, and often awakens him at night. The pain is associated with ipsilateral tearing, conjunctival injection, and nasal congestion. Alcohol triggers or exacerbates the pain. His wife reports that he has been irritable and agitated. On exam, he has right-sided periorbital edema and mild ptosis. He reports having similar symptoms 2 years ago and is concerned because that episode lasted for several weeks.*

Epidemiology and pathophysiology. Cluster headaches are much less common than migraines, to which they are unrelated, affecting only 0.1% of adults. However, they are usually more severe and debilitating and have been referred to as the "suicide headache." About 10%–15% of patients have chronic cluster headache without remission periods. Although cluster headaches are very distinctive and stereotyped, they tend to be underdiagnosed or misdiagnosed as migraine or sinus headache. Cluster headaches usually respond well to the appropriate therapy and therefore a very careful history that aids in making the correct diagnosis is important. Age at onset is usually 20–40 years and men are more commonly affected with a male-to-female ratio of 4.3:1.

The underlying pathophysiology of cluster headache is not fully understood but is felt to be related to activation of the trigeminal vascular and parasympathetic systems. Theories include vascular dilation, trigeminal nerve stimulation, and disruption of circadian rhythms; additionally, there may be a genetic predisposition. Positron emission tomographic scan studies have revealed activation of the medial hypothalamic gray matter, an area involved in the control of circadian rhythms. It is felt that dysfunction of neurons in this area leads to activation of a trigeminal-autonomic loop in the brainstem. These pathophysiologic mechanisms help explain the cardinal symptoms of cluster headache including the episodic/circadian nature of attacks, the distribution and quality of pain, and associated autonomic symptoms.

Clinical presentation. The distinctive clinical features, as summarized in the clinical vignette, assist in diagnosing cluster headaches (Fig. 21.4). The first two divisions of the trigeminal nerve are more commonly involved as opposed to trigeminal neuralgia which primarily involves the second and third divisions.

According to the International Headache Society's revised classification of cluster headache, there must be recurrent attacks of at least severe unilateral pain lasting 15–180 minutes. The pain must be orbital, supraorbital, and/or temporal. The headaches must be accompanied by at least one of the following: restlessness or agitation, ipsilateral conjunctival injection and/or lacrimation, nasal congestion and/or rhinorrhea, eyelid edema, forehead and facial sweating, ipsilateral miosis, and/or ptosis. Attacks have a frequency of one every other day to eight a day. Finally, other causes must be ruled out.

Management and therapy. Like migraine, the treatment algorithm includes short-term and preventive therapy. The two most effective abortive therapies for cluster headache are sumatriptan 6 mg subcutaneous and high-flow oxygen inhalation at 7–10 L/min for 15–20 minutes. Other triptan preparations, oral indomethacin three times daily, ergotamines (particularly intravenous DHE), and intranasal lidocaine are often beneficial. Preventive therapy may also be indicated depending on frequency and severity of attacks. Verapamil is the drug of choice for prophylaxis of cluster headaches. Other beneficial drugs include lithium, gabapentin, topiramate, and short-term corticosteroids. About 10%–15% of cluster headache patients develop chronic or relentless symptoms, and combined-drug therapy may be needed. In medically refractory patients ipsilateral greater occipital nerve injections may be effective. Very rarely, and only in well-selected medically refractory patients, is deep brain stimulation (DBS) or occipital nerve stimulation indicated.

Other Trigeminal Autonomic Cephalalgias
Paroxysmal Hemicranias

These are unusual primary headaches—unilateral and short-lived (2–30 minutes), which occur in a chronic or episodic manner. They are localized to the orbital, supraorbital, and/or temporal region. Typically, the pain has a severe throbbing or boring quality and often recurs several times throughout the day. These headaches are associated with ipsilateral cranial autonomic dysfunction but, unlike cluster headaches, occur more

Cluster headache

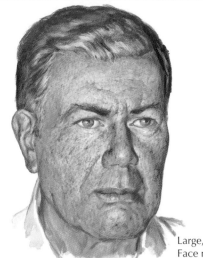

Temporal artery bulging and pulsating
Severe headache, pain behind eye
Unilateral ptosis, swelling, and redness of eyelid
Miosis, conjunctival injection
Tearing
Nasal congestion, rhinorrhea
Flushing of side of face, sweating

Attacks typically nocturnal; average frequency 1-3 in 24 hours, lasting 15 minutes-3 hours

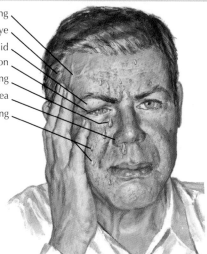

Large, strong, muscular man typical patient. Face may have peau d'orange skin, telangiectasis.

Chronic paroxysmal hemicrania (CHP)

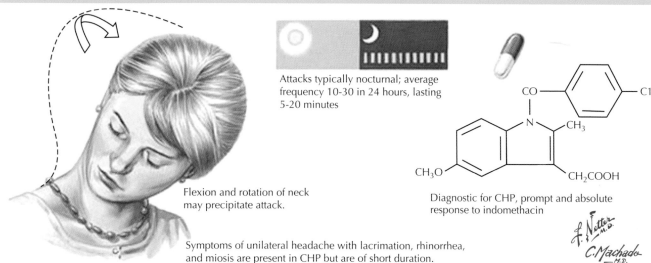

Attacks typically nocturnal; average frequency 10-30 in 24 hours, lasting 5-20 minutes

Flexion and rotation of neck may precipitate attack.

Diagnostic for CHP, prompt and absolute response to indomethacin

Symptoms of unilateral headache with lacrimation, rhinorrhea, and miosis are present in CHP but are of short duration.

Fig. 21.4 Cluster Headache and Chronic Paroxysmal Hemicrania.

often in women than in men. Furthermore, these headaches have daily recurrences and tend not to conglomerate over a few days such as in cluster headaches. They usually respond well to 25–50 mg indomethacin 2–3 times daily for at least 48 hours. Therefore these headaches by definition are "indomethacin responsive," and a trial is always warranted if there are no medical contraindications to its use (see Fig. 21.4). Agents proven effective for prophylactic treatment include lamotrigine, topiramate, and acetylsalicylic acid.

Short-Lasting Unilateral Neuralgiform Headache Attacks

Two subtypes of short-lasting unilateral neuralgiform headache attacks are recognized in the 3rd edition of the International Classification of Headache Disorders: short-lasting unilateral neuralgiform headache attacks with conjunctival injection and tearing (SUNCT) and short-lasting unilateral neuralgiform headache attacks with cranial autonomic symptoms (SUNA). They are syndromes of strictly unilateral headache attacks with the pain confined to the orbital/periorbital area. Most episodes are moderate to severe in intensity with a burning, stabbing, or electrical quality. The duration of the paroxysms usually ranges from

10–120 seconds distinguishing them from longer lasting headache syndromes. Prominent, ipsilateral conjunctival injection and lacrimation are present. Nasal congestion or rhinorrhea and ipsilateral forehead perspiration may also be present. In contrast to paroxysmal hemicranias, this headache syndrome predominates in middle-aged men and is not responsive to indomethacin. In fact, treatment efforts with numerous medications have been frustrating, with little or inconsistent responses. Antiepileptic drugs including lamotrigine, gabapentin, and topiramate may improve symptoms. At present, the drug of choice for SUNCT is lamotrigine whereas SUNA may respond better to gabapentin. Methylprednisolone therapy and intravenous lidocaine may be of benefit in severe cases. A few SUNCT patients who have undergone deep brain hypothalamic stimulation have had substantial and persistent relief.

Tension-Type Headache
Epidemiology and Pathophysiology

Tension headache is the most common headache type with lifetime prevalence in the general population ranging from 30%–78% in different studies. They affect ~1.4 billion people or 20.8% of the population. The female-to-male ratio is 3:2. The precise pathophysiology is unknown. It is likely a heterogeneous disorder with various etiologic factors that ultimately leads to pericranial and nuchal muscular tension or spasm (Fig. 21.5). Disrupted sleep, psychosocial stress, anxiety, depression, and analgesic drug overuse are common contributing factors.

Clinical Presentation

A diagnosis of tension headache requires the presence of at least two of the following pain characteristics: nonpulsatile steady pressure-like quality, nondisabling mild to moderate intensity, bilateral location, and no aggravation with routine physical activity. In addition, these patients do not experience nausea or vomiting and do not typically have photophobia or phonophobia. Their frequency varies from occasional to daily. If they occur more than 15 days per month, the diagnosis of chronic tension-type headache applies.

Careful evaluation is indicated in every patient suspected of having tension-type headache. Exclusion of structural, infectious, or metabolic disorders is essential. Although sometimes features of migraine are present, they are a minor part of the clinical picture. Specific triggers are less common than with migraine.

Management and Therapy

The treatment of tension headache usually requires only over-the-counter analgesics including NSAIDs, nonpharmacologic interventions that include relaxation and biofeedback techniques, massage, and heat application. Treatment of contributing factors including disrupted sleep and mood disorders should be addressed. Prophylactic medication is indicated for frequent recurrence or when abortive therapies are ineffective or contraindicated. The best available evidence supports the use of tricyclic antidepressants, specifically amitriptyline. There is also some evidence to support the use of other antidepressants including venlafaxine and mirtazapine and anticonvulsants including topiramate and gabapentin.

Chronic Daily Headaches

CLINICAL VIGNETTE *A 45-year-old man complains of daily headache for 10 years. His headache lasts all day but is worse on awakening. He notes a dull, sometimes pulsatile, moderate, bifrontal head pain with mild nausea that responds to an over-the-counter combination of aspirin, acetaminophen, and caffeine. He currently takes two of these pills every 6 hours around the clock*

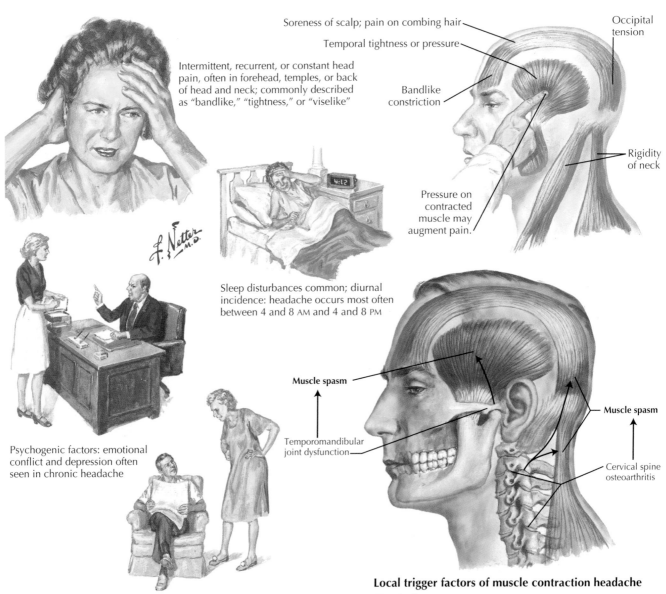

Soreness of scalp; pain on combing hair

Temporal tightness or pressure

Occipital tension

Bandlike constriction

Rigidity of neck

Pressure on contracted muscle may augment pain.

Intermittent, recurrent, or constant head pain, often in forehead, temples, or back of head and neck; commonly described as "bandlike," "tightness," or "viselike"

Sleep disturbances common; diurnal incidence: headache occurs most often between 4 and 8 AM and 4 and 8 PM

Psychogenic factors: emotional conflict and depression often seen in chronic headache

Muscle spasm

Temporomandibular joint dysfunction

Muscle spasm

Cervical spine osteoarthritis

Local trigger factors of muscle contraction headache

Fig. 21.5 Muscle Contraction Headache.

while awake. He has had numerous cranial scans and consultations for this problem. There is a longstanding history of intermittent headaches beginning in childhood. He is placed on a weaning schedule with eventual discontinuation of over-the-counter headache medications over 4 weeks and is advised to avoid all other forms of caffeine. His daily headache initially worsens, but then gradually improves. When seen in follow-up, he is improved and reports only intermittent, thrice-weekly tension-type headache. He is counseled on the hazards of medication and caffeine overuse and started on amitriptyline for prophylaxis.

The heterogeneous nature and numerous comorbidities associated with chronic daily headache represent a diagnostic and therapeutic challenge. The syndrome of chronic daily headache may evolve from a variety of primary and/or secondary headache types, with tension and migraine headaches being the most common. Frequent headaches of any type may lose their clinical distinctiveness and lead to an ill-defined vague head pain whose characteristics defy specific definition. The clinician must then uncover any previous history of intermittent or episodic headaches that may have transformed over time. Anxiety, mood, and sleep disorders are just a few of the common comorbid conditions. Medication overuse frequently contributes to chronic daily headache. Almost any short-acting analgesic may lead to "rebound" headaches, but vasoactive medications such as caffeine, triptans, and ergotamines are most likely to cause this phenomenon. Special care must be taken when patients overuse substances whose abrupt withdrawal may prove dangerous or life threatening, including butalbital, benzodiazepines, and opioids.

The treatment of chronic daily headache first requires that overused substances are weaned or discontinued. Many patients may resist this intervention out of fear that headaches will worsen. Careful education is necessary to explain the association between medication overuse and the chronic headaches. Support mechanisms to control anxiety and a clear management plan for headache recurrence are needed. Comorbid etiologic factors—depression, psychosocial stresses, and poor sleep—require attention. Nonpharmacologic interventions include emotional support, counseling, physical therapy, relaxation techniques, heat, and massage. Treatment with prednisone can assist in weaning patients off short-acting analgesics. The choice of prophylactic medication should be based on the underlying headache type and comorbidities. For example, the patient above suffers from transformed tension-type headache, and therefore amitriptyline is recommended. Recent trials have supported the use of botulinum toxin type A as a prophylactic agent for chronic daily headache.

Primary Headache Syndromes With Defined Triggers
Exertional Headache
Physical exercise is always the precipitating factor in primary exertional headaches. They may develop during acute straining, such as weight lifting, or after sustained exercise, such as running. These headaches are characterized by throbbing pain for minutes or hours after discontinuation of activity. They often respond to 25–50 mg of indomethacin three times daily taken either after the exercise or prophylactically once a typical pattern is established. β-Blockers may also be used for prophylaxis but may affect exercise tolerance. The possibility of a serious underlying disorder such as arterial dissection, intracranial aneurysm, and an intracranial mass lesion must be excluded. Computed tomography (CT), MRI, and magnetic resonance angiography (MRA) may therefore be indicated.

Headache Associated With Sexual Activity (Coital Headache)
Typically, these headaches develop as dull, generalized pain during sexual activity or as an acute, sometimes explosive, pain during orgasm. The headache lasts for minutes to hours after the cessation of sexual activity. Patients with coital headache often suffer from exertional headache as well. Clinicians may find patients suffering from this condition to be less than forthcoming about the circumstances surrounding the onset of headache. A careful history including questions about sexual symptoms is needed. Embarrassment and an unwillingness to address sexual concerns with a physician may lead patients with coital headache to go undiagnosed for years. As with other paroxysmal headaches, a search for underlying systemic or intracranial pathology, particularly a ruptured or unruptured aneurysm, is needed before diagnosing a benign process. NSAIDs, particularly indomethacin (25–50 mg), or propranolol, may be helpful when administered before sexual activity.

Others
Hypnic headaches tend to occur in women 50 years or older during rapid eye movement sleep and can recur several times at night. The pain is usually unilateral but can be bilateral and lasts 15 minutes to 4 hours after awakening. These headaches are not associated with cranial autonomic symptoms or restlessness. NSAIDs with caffeine or lithium have been used to control them. *Cough headaches* in contrast are sudden acute bilateral headaches usually occurring in older men and induced by straining or coughing. They last from 1 second to 2 hours and tend to be indomethacin responsive. Cough-induced headache is common in Arnold–Chiari type I malformations and this as well as cerebrovascular dissection and an intracranial aneurysm should be excluded before making a diagnosis of a primary cough-induced headache.

SECONDARY HEADACHE DISORDERS

Although most headaches occur in the absence of underlying intracranial or systemic pathology, some result from more serious illness. The neurologist is often the initial physician contacted, and a careful history is mandatory to achieve an accurate diagnosis and to institute proper management. The headache's temporal profile, pain characteristics, and precipitating factors as well as the patient's age, gender, family history, and associated systemic symptoms require analysis. The history should be followed by a careful neurologic and general examination. Often, immediate laboratory evaluation and neuroimaging are indicated. With the widespread availability of cranial CT and MRI, it is judicious to image patients who have experienced recent onset of a significant headache, including those with normal clinical examinations. Significant pathology, such as subarachnoid hemorrhage, subdural hematoma, and neoplasm, provides examples wherein cranial CT and MRI may diagnose serious neurologic conditions when even the most careful neurologic examination may, at times, be normal.

Giant Cell (Temporal) Arteritis

CLINICAL VIGNETTE *A 78-year-old man reports a constant, global headache for more than a month. He has felt generally unwell, with poor appetite, fatigue, and a 10-pound weight loss over the same time period. He experiences stiffness and pain in his shoulders and hips on awakening. A week prior to evaluation, he noticed a transient blurring of vision in his left eye for 20 minutes. His neurologic examination is normal, except for questionable temporal artery tenderness on the left. His C-reactive protein (CRP) is found to be elevated. He is placed on prednisone 60 mg daily with rapid improvement of his symptoms. A left temporal artery biopsy, performed several days later, demonstrates findings typical for giant cell arteritis (transmural inflammatory response with occasional multinucleated giant cells and areas of internal elastic lamina disruption). Eight months later, he remains on 5 mg of prednisone to control his stiffness and pain.*

Headache is the most common and prominent presenting symptom of giant cell or temporal arteritis, a serious disorder of the elderly with potentially devastating complications such as permanent blindness. As in the above vignette, early identification and prompt treatment prevents blindness from developing. The pain of temporal arteritis is usually bilateral and nonspecific, being throbbing or continuous, and with variable intensity, at times so mild that its potential significance is easily overlooked. Systemic complaints, including anorexia, general malaise, myalgias, and arthralgias, are common and serve as important diagnostic clues. Polymyalgia rheumatica, a condition characterized by proximal musculoskeletal pain and morning stiffness, frequently accompanies the headache. Jaw or tongue claudication and rarely facial tissue ischemia have been described and reflect external carotid artery involvement. Patients may have subtle and intermittent visual blurring or frank episodes of monocular visual loss mimicking transient ischemic attacks. Although often present, temporal artery tenderness may be relatively minor (Fig. 21.6). Early diagnosis is paramount as arteritis may precipitously cause unilateral or sequential bilateral anterior ischemic optic neuropathy with permanent visual loss. Although posterior ciliary arteries are most commonly involved, visual loss may less commonly result from ophthalmic artery involvement and rarely retinal artery involvement. Furthermore, the arteritis may be widespread with involvement beyond the temporal arteries to the aorta and its branches. Infrequently, ischemic stroke may occur as arteritis affects the extracranial carotid or vertebral arteries. The intracranial circulation is generally spared. Erythrocyte sedimentation rate (ESR) and c-reactive protein (CRP) provide the laboratory means to support the diagnosis. Typically, the ESR is increased to 60–110 mm/hour and CRP to 7–47 mg/L, although there are exceptions. Biopsy of a long temporal artery segment is indicated in every patient suspected of having temporal arteritis. Because the arteritis is patchy, a unilateral biopsy may fail to show the inflammatory changes of giant cell arteritis and bilateral biopsies may be required to make the diagnosis. A mixed infiltrate of neutrophils and T lymphocytes involves the media with concurrent intimal hyperplasia and gradual luminal narrowing. Granulomatous, inflammatory arteritis with giant cell formation, and marked disruption of the internal elastic lamina are classic for temporal arteritis (see Fig. 21.6).

Treatment

Because temporal arteritis is a chronic disorder, it requires relatively long-term oral corticosteroid treatment. Prompt diagnosis and treatment are required to prevent serious complications. Treatment must not be delayed because corticosteroids do not alter the pathologic findings if the biopsy is done within a few days of initiating therapy. Prednisone is begun at 40–60 mg/day, followed by a very gradual taper. When transient visual or neurologic symptoms occur, higher initial dosages of corticosteroid may be indicated. Steroids may be needed for 1–2 years at smaller doses to control associated symptoms. Treatment must be individualized, with frequent monitoring of ESR or CRP and symptoms. Long-term steroid side effects, such as truncal weight gain, glucose intolerance, electrolyte imbalance, hypertension, osteoporosis, potential immunosuppression, and cataract formation, to name just a few, need to be followed closely.

Future Directions

Giant cell arteritis is a chronic disease that requires prolonged immunosuppression. In selected patients with longstanding disease, the use of corticosteroid-sparing drugs like methotrexate, azathioprine, and tumor necrosis factor-α inhibitors may be necessary.

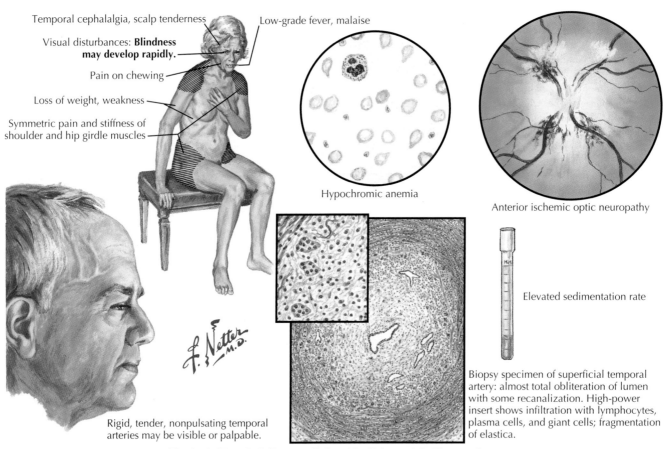

Temporal cephalalgia, scalp tenderness

Visual disturbances: **Blindness may develop rapidly.**

Pain on chewing

Loss of weight, weakness

Symmetric pain and stiffness of shoulder and hip girdle muscles

Low-grade fever, malaise

Hypochromic anemia

Anterior ischemic optic neuropathy

Elevated sedimentation rate

Biopsy specimen of superficial temporal artery: almost total obliteration of lumen with some recanalization. High-power insert shows infiltration with lymphocytes, plasma cells, and giant cells; fragmentation of elastica.

Rigid, tender, nonpulsating temporal arteries may be visible or palpable.

Fig. 21.6 Giant-Cell (Temporal) Arteritis, Polymyalgia Rheumatica.

Brain Hemorrhage, Infections, and Tumors

Subdural hematoma, intracerebral hemorrhage, subarachnoid hemorrhage, meningitis, and brain tumors are causes of secondary headaches. Each of these entities needs consideration in patients who experience the recent onset of headache without prior history or of a changing pattern of headache. Each of these important disorders is discussed elsewhere in this text; however, a few comments are warranted.

Every individual with a precipitous onset of "the worst headache of my life" warrants immediate careful medical and neurologic evaluation by their physician or in the emergency room. Funduscopic examination should evaluate for papilledema or subhyaloid hemorrhages. Regardless of the findings, emergency imaging is indicated. Cranial CT offers a rapid and readily available means to evaluate for hemorrhage and mass lesions. MRI and MRA may be indicated but are generally not required for the urgent evaluation of thunderclap headache. If no hemorrhage or mass lesion is found on imaging, cerebrospinal fluid (CSF) analysis may be indicated to evaluate for subarachnoid hemorrhage and infection in the appropriate clinical setting (Chapter 17 and Section XIII).

Idiopathic Intracranial Hypertension

> **CLINICAL VIGNETTE** *A 38-year-old overweight woman presents with recent onset of headaches and blurred vision. The headaches are increasingly severe and more bothersome to her when she bends forward. She notes intermittent double vision on lateral gaze.*
>
> *Neurologic examination demonstrates limitation of lateral eye movements compatible with CN-VI paresis and modest papilledema. Brain imaging demonstrates diminished size of the lateral ventricles. Spinal fluid pressure is elevated at 350 mm CSF; its hematologic, cytologic, and chemical components are normal.*

Idiopathic intracranial hypertension, also called pseudotumor cerebri, is a unique syndrome of severe, poorly defined, and often progressive headaches frequently associated with horizontal diplopia. In addition, transient visual obscurations and pulsatile tinnitus may be part of the clinical picture. It primarily presents in healthy, usually overweight, young women. Pseudotumor cerebri is associated with increased intracranial CSF pressure usually greater than 250 mm H_2O (Fig. 21.7).

Clinical Presentation and Diagnostic Studies

Neurologic examination usually demonstrates papilledema and visual field loss. Because of increased intracranial pressure (ICP), lateral rectus muscle weakness (sixth nerve palsy) may be seen but patients are otherwise awake, alert, and have no focal neurologic deficits.

Hypervitaminosis A or various antibiotics such as tetracycline, minocycline, nitrofurantoin, or ampicillin may induce this syndrome. Other possible offending medications include oral contraceptives, corticosteroids, estrogen and progestin therapies, NSAIDs, amiodarone, and the anesthetic agents ketamine and nitrous oxide.

Neuroimaging studies are mandatory to exclude other causes of increased intracranial pressure, such as cerebral masses or dural sinus thrombosis or stenosis. The CSF pressure is increased, usually greater than 250 mm H_2O in the decubitus position, but the cell count and chemical profile are normal.

Treatment

With idiopathic intracranial hypertension, treatment generally consists of weight loss, low-salt diet, diuretics, and symptomatic headache control. Discontinuation of the offending medication often reverses the clinical picture. Frequent visual monitoring with formal visual field testing is essential. Chronic increased intracranial pressure causes loss of vision secondary to optic nerve head swelling (i.e., papilledema) and eventual optic nerve fiber layer atrophy. The first sign of evolving optic nerve damage is inferonasal peripheral visual loss that gradually moves toward the center and forms a "nasal step." Very close follow-up with Goldmann perimetry is essential. Loss of central visual acuity is unusual early on and only occurs with long-term papilledema after significant peripheral visual loss has occurred. If there is evidence of visual loss, then repeated lumbar punctures to decrease ICP and more aggressive treatment are needed. A trial of corticosteroids may, paradoxically, be helpful but is likely not to be effective in the long run. Optic nerve sheath fenestration just behind the globe theoretically decompresses the optic nerve head and allows CSF to be shunted into the orbit and absorbed. This has been found successful in up to 80% of patients in arresting visual loss but has little effect in controlling the headache. In recalcitrant cases CSF shunting procedures may also be considered and they halt progressive visual loss in 30%–50% of cases and usually control the headache.

Low CSF Pressure Headache

> **CLINICAL VIGNETTE** *A 28-year-old woman with a history of tension headaches presents to her physician with change in quality of her headaches. Unlike her prior headaches, these do not occur upon awakening but rather after arising and when straining. They are aggravated by routine physical activity, such as bending over and during light exercise, and abate completely when lying down. These headaches are associated with nausea and vomiting, are more severe, and have lasted for 2 weeks, much longer than her usual headaches. She injured her neck in a car accident 3 weeks prior but has otherwise been feeling well.*
>
> *An MRI of her brain and spine with contrast reveals marked leptomeningeal enhancement. A subsequent myelogram reveals a dural tear at the cervicothoracic junction. CSF analysis demonstrates slightly elevated protein and a low opening pressure.*

Headache is often the presenting symptom in cases of intracranial hypotension. Precipitating factors include lumbar puncture, CSF shunt placement, spinal surgery, and skull base and spinal tumors. As in the above vignette, symptoms can also develop after spinal trauma. Sometimes a simple Valsalva maneuver or coughing can precipitate the condition. However, some cases occur spontaneously or after only minor trauma, and therefore often go undiagnosed or are misdiagnosed.

Intracranial hypotension is due to a continuous leakage of CSF. Typically, the headaches develop soon after a lumbar puncture. Spontaneous cases may be less precipitous, evolving over days, and are felt to be due to dural tears in the spine, most often in the cervical or thoracic regions along the nerve root dural sleeve. Generally, the headaches occur during the waking hours and are postural, worsening in the upright position, and improving or resolving with recumbence. Often, the headache is associated with nausea, vomiting, neck pain, and dizziness, which also clear on recumbence.

Leakage of CSF causes low pressure with sagging of the brain and traction on dural and vascular elements. This traction worsens in the upright position, explaining the postural nature of the headache.

Diagnosis

MRI with gadolinium demonstrates diffuse pachymeningeal enhancement in most low–CSF pressure headaches. This is often accompanied by dural thickening that can be striking and may be confused with leptomeningeal inflammatory or neoplastic processes (Fig. 21.8). In more severe cases, subdural fluid collections and descent of the brain

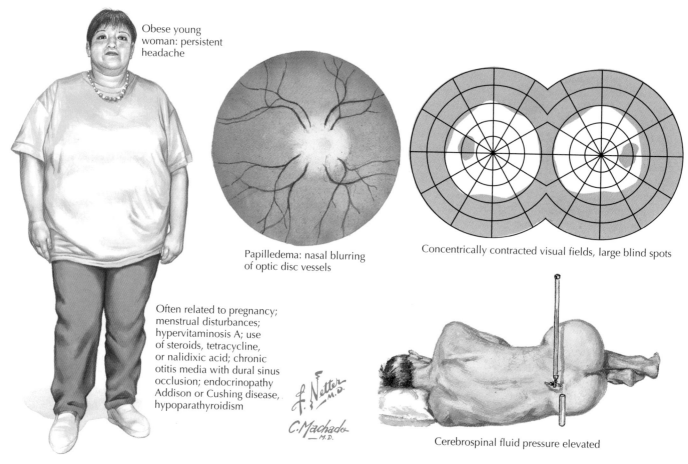

Obese young woman: persistent headache

Papilledema: nasal blurring of optic disc vessels

Concentrically contracted visual fields, large blind spots

Often related to pregnancy; menstrual disturbances; hypervitaminosis A; use of steroids, tetracycline, or nalidixic acid; chronic otitis media with dural sinus occlusion; endocrinopathy Addison or Cushing disease, hypoparathyroidism

Cerebrospinal fluid pressure elevated

Fig. 21.7 Pseudotumor Cerebri.

with downward displacement of the cerebellar tonsils can be seen. Lumbar puncture demonstrates decreased intracranial pressure, usually less than 50 mm H$_2$O. CSF analysis may be normal, but slight elevation of protein and a mild lymphocytic pleocytosis may be seen. Radioisotope cisternography or contrast myelography can be used to detect sites of CSF leakage.

Management and Therapy

Postlumbar puncture headache usually subsides with bed rest and hydration within a few days. An abdominal binder and caffeine may also be of benefit. If it persists, an epidural autologous blood patch injected at the lumbar puncture site, theoretically sealing the leak, almost universally improves postlumbar puncture headaches, providing credence to the theory that they are secondary to a CSF leak. Other options for treatment include prolonged bed rest and continuous intrathecal or epidural saline infusions. Surgical intervention is rarely necessary. In spontaneous cases, a blood patch in the lumbar region often provides relief despite no identifiable tear in that region. Occasionally, such headaches are resistant to therapy and become disabling.

In the above vignette, a diagnosis of traumatic leptomeningeal tear with CSF leak and subsequent low-pressure syndrome was made. A therapeutic trial of an autologous blood dural patch was successful, with relief of the headaches and associated symptoms within a week.

Cranial Neuralgias

This group of patients experiences brief but severe paroxysms of head pain in the distribution of a specific cranial nerve, particularly the trigeminal nerve.

Trigeminal Neuralgia

CLINICAL VIGNETTE *A 50-year-old woman develops pain in her left cheek. The pain begins as a dull ache, similar to a toothache. Soon she develops recurrent attacks of sudden sharp pain in the same distribution. The attacks are brief, lasting only a few seconds, but she describes them as the worst pain of her life. Brushing the teeth, a cold breeze, or any physical contact to the left side of her face frequently triggers the pain. She visits her dentist on several occasions, and eventually has two teeth extracted but without significant relief of symptoms. An MRI demonstrates tortuosity of the vertebrobasilar circulation with left trigeminal nerve neurovascular impingement. She is treated with varying dosages of carbamazepine and gabapentin, with only partial relief and side effects of lethargy and drowsiness. After 5 years, she undergoes microvascular decompression surgery and feels immediate relief. A year later the pain recurs, and she meets with her surgeon to discuss percutaneous radiofrequency ablation.*

Epidemiology and pathophysiology. The incidence of trigeminal neuralgia is 4–5 cases per 100,000 people. The female-to-male ratio is 3:1. In the majority of individuals, an idiopathic loss of myelin insulation within the posterior root of the trigeminal nerve causes the pain. When it occurs in a young adult, demyelination from multiple sclerosis is often the mechanism. Another cause is a tortuous or ectatic artery, often a branch of the superior cerebellar artery, compressing or pulsating against the trigeminal posterior rootlets. Trigeminal neuralgia can result from other conditions compressing the trigeminal nerve, such as acoustic neuroma (vestibular schwannoma), meningioma, arteriovenous

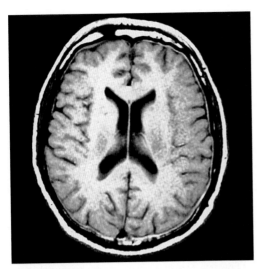

A. Axial FLAIR image with dural thickening.

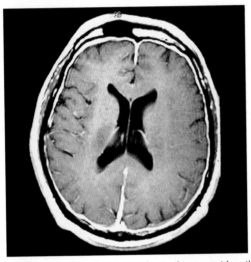

B. Axial T1-weighted, gadolinium-enhanced image with striking enhancement of the thickened dura.

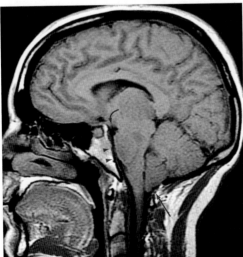

C. Intracranial hypotension. Sagittal T1-weighted MR: Cerebellar tonsillar descent (arrow), pons "flat tire sign" (arrowheads), and retroclival mammillary displacement (curved arrow).

Fig. 21.8 Low-Pressure Headache.

malformation, and rarely a carotid-posterior communicating or distal anterior inferior cerebellar artery aneurysm.

Clinical presentation. A careful history is the key to the diagnosis of this uncommon but eminently treatable facial neuralgia. Trigeminal neuralgia, also called tic douloureux, is a disabling, lancinating, or electrical facial pain that occurs in the trigeminal nerve distribution. It is one of the worst pains a human can experience. This condition is not defined by any test but requires the clinician to recognize it by its primary historical attributes. There are no associated neurologic deficits.

The patient, almost always an adult and usually a woman, experiences paroxysmal and frequently provocable intermittent unilateral facial pain. The stereotypical attacks that rarely occur during sleep are very brief, lasting anywhere from an indefinable instant to several minutes. In between sudden attacks, the patient may experience a more constant dull or aching pain, which may lead them to believe the problem is dental in origin. The frequency of attacks may fluctuate markedly, disabling a patient for weeks or months at a time before going into a remission.

Trigeminal neuralgia primarily involves the second or third division of the trigeminal nerve and occasionally the first division as opposed to cluster headache which primarily involves the first two divisions. Triggers include talking, chewing, shaving, drinking hot or cold liquids, or any form of sensory facial stimulation. The pain is usually unilateral; when it affects both sides of the face, it typically does not do so concomitantly.

Cranial scanning with MRI is indicated for all patients with trigeminal neuralgia. Bilateral symptoms, trigeminal sensory findings, and loss of corneal reflexes are strong indicators of secondary trigeminal neuralgia and should raise concern.

Management and therapy. Anticonvulsants are the mainstay of medical therapy for trigeminal neuralgia. Most patients respond to the use of carbamazepine, which stabilizes cell membranes and raises the threshold of neural stimulation. Carbamazepine and oxcarbazepine carry the best scientific evidence for efficacy. Phenytoin, gabapentin, lamotrigine, topiramate, and pregabalin may also be useful. Baclofen, an antispasmodic, may provide some relief as may certain antidepressants, including amitriptyline. Baclofen is advocated by some as an adjuvant treatment to carbamazepine if higher doses of carbamazepine alone are inadequate or cause side effects. The effectiveness of any agent may diminish over time. Some studies have shown that botulinum toxin type A injections may reduce pain when medications fail.

Several surgical approaches are available for patients who cannot tolerate or do not respond to medical therapy. Percutaneous approaches include trigeminal radiofrequency lesioning, glycerol injection, and balloon compression. Available open procedures such as posterior cranial fossa microvascular decompression and open trigeminal rhizotomy are much more invasive and may be less appropriate for elderly patients or those in poor health. However when appropriate, microvascular decompression often relieves the pain and causes less sensory loss than other procedures. Ipsilateral hearing loss is occasionally a complication of decompressive surgery, due to the delicate anatomic relationship between the auditory and trigeminal nerves. The operation carries a 1% risk of death or stroke. Focused-beam stereotactic radiosurgery by Gamma Knife is also available for this condition. Gamma Knife is successful in eliminating pain for the majority of people. In addition, if pain recurs, the procedure can be repeated. Facial numbness can be a side effect.

Trigeminal neuralgia can recur after any procedure at a lifetime rate of 15%–20%. Recurrences can be treated with subsequent radiofrequency ablation or stereotactic radiosurgery.

Accurate diagnosis is essential to successful surgical relief. Steady nonparoxysmal pain, posttraumatic pain, pain after dental procedures, and pain that is not in the trigeminal zone will not be effectively treated by radiofrequency ablation or other procedures mentioned above.

Knowledge of trigeminal nerve anatomy, its facial distribution, and an appreciation of the paroxysmal, provocable, and unilateral character of trigeminal neuralgia is essential for accurate diagnosis and management.

Glossopharyngeal Neuralgia

Glossopharyngeal neuralgia is less common than trigeminal neuralgia and generally located in the ear, tonsillar area, or deep within the throat in the CN-IX sensory distribution. The pain is paroxysmal, recurrent, and severe, usually with swallowing as the primary triggering mechanism. Occasionally, patients experience bradycardia during the pain paroxysms and, sometimes, loss of consciousness. Medical treatment is similar to that of trigeminal neuralgia. Rhizotomy or decompression of CN-IX may be necessary in severe, medically intractable cases.

Occipital Neuralgia

Although similar in pain characteristics to trigeminal neuralgia, occipital neuralgia is differentiated by location to the posterior scalp innervated by the greater and lesser occipital nerves from the C2 dermatome (Fig. 21.9). Occipital neuralgia is probably underdiagnosed. Pain is generally localized to the base of the skull but may extend to the vertex, behind the ear or into the neck and upper back. Pain may be initially incited by hyperextension of the neck or whiplash injury. Patients are commonly seen after motor vehicle accidents, sports trauma, or work-related injury. The neuralgia is usually unilateral and occurs in brief paroxysms of jabbing pain superimposed on a more chronic dull occipital ache, similar to trigeminal neuralgia.

Diagnosis is assisted by the identification of an occipital trigger point at the base of the skull between the mastoid process and the occipital protuberance. Although the pain and disability may be similar to trigeminal neuralgia, occipital neuralgia is more easily treated. Symptoms will often improve or resolve with heat, rest, physical therapy, and/or massage therapy. NSAIDs and muscle relaxants can be quite effective as well. Percutaneous nerve blocks may prove both diagnostic and therapeutic. When ineffective, carbamazepine, gabapentin, and other drugs commonly used in the treatment of neuropathic pain are often employed. For cases that are difficult to control, pulsed radiofrequency ablation and occipital nerve stimulation are procedures that may have some benefit. Microvascular decompression is an option in the most refractory cases.

Obstructive Sleep Apnea

Headache may be the presenting symptom in sleep apnea. Patients frequently complain of daily headaches that are worse upon awakening. Invariably, these patients are fatigued and experience excessive daytime sleepiness. A careful history, including discussion of snoring and the use of the Epworth Sleepiness Scale, may prove vital in making this diagnosis. The neurologic examination is generally normal, although certain clues on physical exam may include obesity and abnormalities or tissue redundancy of the palate, uvula, or tongue. When correctly identified, this headache syndrome may improve dramatically with nocturnal continuous positive airway pressure treatment. Sleep apnea is discussed in more detail in Chapter 24.

Infectious Mechanisms

Meningitis must be considered in anyone experiencing an acute-onset headache. Typically, these individuals have a concomitant fever and stiff neck (meningismus) as detailed in Section XIII.

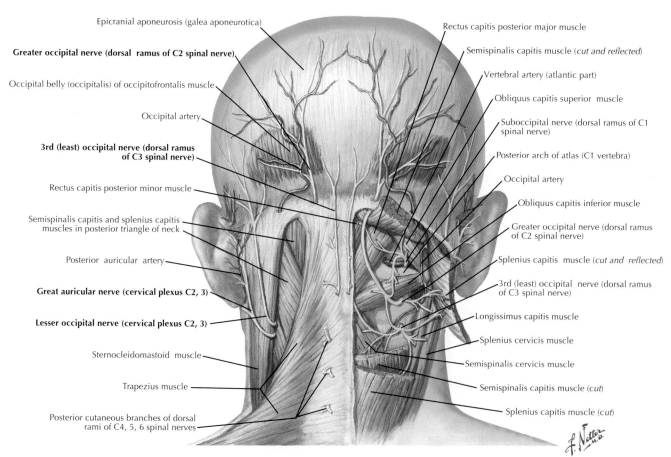

Epicranial aponeurosis (galea aponeurotica)

Greater occipital nerve (dorsal ramus of C2 spinal nerve)

Occipital belly (occipitalis) of occipitofrontalis muscle

Occipital artery

3rd (least) occipital nerve (dorsal ramus of C3 spinal nerve)

Rectus capitis posterior minor muscle

Semispinalis capitis and splenius capitis muscles in posterior triangle of neck

Posterior auricular artery

Great auricular nerve (cervical plexus C2, 3)

Lesser occipital nerve (cervical plexus C2, 3)

Sternocleidomastoid muscle

Trapezius muscle

Posterior cutaneous branches of dorsal rami of C4, 5, 6 spinal nerves

Rectus capitis posterior major muscle

Semispinalis capitis muscle (*cut and reflected*)

Vertebral artery (atlantic part)

Obliquus capitis superior muscle

Suboccipital nerve (dorsal ramus of C1 spinal nerve)

Posterior arch of atlas (C1 vertebra)

Occipital artery

Obliquus capitis inferior muscle

Greater occipital nerve (dorsal ramus of C2 spinal nerve)

Splenius capitis muscle (*cut and reflected*)

3rd (least) occipital nerve (dorsal ramus of C3 spinal nerve)

Longissimus capitis muscle

Splenius cervicis muscle

Semispinalis cervicis muscle

Semispinalis capitis muscle (*cut*)

Splenius capitis muscle (*cut*)

Fig. 21.9 Suboccipital Triangle.

Cranial herpes zoster (shingles) is a "reactivation" of the varicella-zoster virus within the gasserian ganglion or upper cervical dorsal root ganglion. Typically, these patients report severe, sometimes excruciating, boring head pain or neuralgia. The rash usually precedes the onset of the headache, but, in some instances, intense head pain can antedate skin lesions by a few days. The classic vesicles can vary from a few easily overlooked lesions to an extensive vesicular rash. After the dermatologic changes appear, treatment with antiviral medications, such as acyclovir, valacyclovir, and famciclovir, is indicated. When herpes zoster ophthalmicus occurs, an ophthalmology consultation should be obtained and along with antivirals, coadministration of corticosteroids may be considered, when no contraindication exists. There is an increased incidence of shingles in the elderly and the immunosuppressed. Postherpetic neuralgia may occur in the distribution of the trigeminal nerve or upper cervical roots and may require prolonged treatment. Treatment is discussed in Chapter 22.

Contiguous Structure Headaches

The last type of head pain involves secondary contiguous anatomic structures such as the nasal sinuses or teeth. Inherent brain, cerebrovascular, and leptomeningeal pathology is discussed in the sections on tumors, stroke, and infectious diseases, respectively.

Nasal Sinus Infection

This entity must be considered in all patients presenting with headache.

Often, a patient with tension headache presents with a self-diagnosis of "sinus headache" and a careful history and examination is needed. The typical patient with active nasal sinus infection experiences a deep boring discomfort in the maxillary or ethmoid facial region. With acute infections, there is often percussion tenderness, a purulent nasal discharge, and, if the infection is severe, fever. In contrast, sphenoid sinus infections are more easily masked, presenting with only deep-seated headaches, and pose the greatest risk for parameningeal seeding of the meninges and bacterial meningitis. Diagnosis depends on CT, MRI, or both. Appropriate antibiotic treatment, decongestants, and hydration are usually effective.

Dental Infection and Temporomandibular Joint Dysfunction

An abscessed tooth, primarily in the upper jaw, is a relatively common cause of facial pain or headache. Although the diagnosis is usually obvious to patients, on occasion they may present to a physician first. The neurologist must consider a primary dental source as an unusual cause for some instances of head and facial pain. A careful dental evaluation may be diagnostic when no other mechanism is identified. Temporomandibular joint dysfunction causes referred periorbital, temporal, zygomatic, and mandibular pain and is often mistaken for a primary or secondary headache syndrome. Joint clicking or crepitus, focal tenderness, limited jaw movement, and an altered bite are hints to its diagnosis.

ADDITIONAL RESOURCES

Pietrobon D, Moskowitz MA. Chaos and commotion in the wake of cortical spreading depression and spreading depolarizations. Nat Rev Neurosci 2014;15(6):379–93.
Review of migraine pathophysiology and cortical spreading depression.

Silberstein SD. Preventive migraine treatment. Continuum (Minneap Minn) 2015;21(4 Headache):973–89.
Review of preventive treatment for migraine.

Tariq N, Tepper SJ, Kriegler JS. Patent foramen ovale and migraine: closing the debate—a review. Headache 2016;56(3):462–78.
The connection between patent foramen ovale, migraines, and the utility of foramen closure.

Kurth T, Chabriat H, Bousser MG. Migraine and stroke: a complex association with clinical implications. Lancet Neurol 2012;11(1):92–100.
The connection between migraine and stroke.

Chole R, Patil R, Degwekar S, et al. Drug treatment of trigeminal neuralgia: a systemic review of the literature. J Oral Maxillofac Surg 2007;65:40–5.
Literature review of medical treatment of trigeminal neuralgia.

Headache Classification Committee of the International Headache Society. The international classification of headache disorders. 3rd ed. (Beta version). 2017.
Comprehensive classification of headache disorders based on pathophysiology and clinical presentation.

Lance JW, Goadsby PJ. Mechanism and management of headache. 7th ed. Philadelphia, PA: Elsevier; 2005.
Pathophysiology and management of different headache types.

Pareja A, Alvarez M, Montojo T. SUNCT and SUNA: recognition and treatment. Curr Treat Options Neurol 2013;15(1):28–39.
Definition, clinical presentation, and treatment of SUNCT and SUNA.

Pringsheim T. Cluster headache: evidence for a disorder of circadian rhythm and hypothalamic dysfunction. Can J Neurol Sci 2002;29(1):33–40.
Pathophysiology of cluster headache.

Silberstein S, Lipton R, Dodick D. Wolff's headache and other head pain. 8th ed. Oxford University Press; 2007.
Comprehensive overview of headache disorders.

Straube A, Empl M, Ceballos-Baumann A, et al. Pericranial injection of botulinum toxin type a (Dysport) for tension-type headache—a multicentre, double-blinded, randomized, placebo-controlled study. Eur J Neurol 2008;15(3):205–13.
Study on the use of botulinum toxin type A for tension headache.

US Headache Consortium. Multispecialty Consensus on Diagnosis and Treatment of Headache. Available from: www.aan.com.
Provides practice guidelines for the diagnosis and treatment of different headache types.

Weaver-Agostoni J. Cluster headache. Am Fam Physician 2013;88(2):122–8.

22

Pain Pathophysiology and Management

Daniel Vardeh

CLINICAL VIGNETTE *Tracy, a 65-year-old right-hand–dominant receptionist is referred to orthopedic surgery for right carpal tunnel release following progressively worsening pain and paresthesia in her right hand. Surgery is performed under conscious sedation without complications, and the patient is discharged home that afternoon to follow up with physical therapy for rehabilitation. However, the patient fails to keep her physical therapy appointment and returns to work 4 weeks later.*

Seven weeks postoperatively, the patient presents back to the orthopedic surgeon complaining of swelling, redness, and stiffness of her right hand. She also notes that her hand has become more sensitive to painful stimuli and that she experiences significant discomfort when her hand contacts virtually anything. On exam, the hand is warm, red, and swollen, with hyperhidrosis noted on the palmar surface. Despite admission to the hospital for empiric treatment of postoperative infection, the patient fails to improve and develops exquisite pain even to light touch and beyond the area of initial injury. The patient is eventually diagnosed with chronic regional pain syndrome (CRPS).

DEFINITION AND EPIDEMIOLOGY

According to the International Association for the Study of Pain (IASP), pain is defined as "an unpleasant sensory and emotional experience associated with actual or potential tissue damage." Chronic pain is defined as "persistent or recurrent pain lasting longer than 3 months." Per the current version of the *International Classification of Diseases (ICD)* of the World Health Organization (WHO), "Chronic Pain" is divided into 7 clinical pain syndromes: (1) chronic primary pain, (2) chronic cancer pain, (3) chronic posttraumatic and postsurgical pain, (4) chronic neuropathic pain, (5) chronic headache and orofacial pain, (6) chronic visceral pain, and (7) chronic musculoskeletal pain.

In the United States, chronic pain is estimated to affect about 20%–30% of the adult population, accounting for more patients than diabetes, heart disease, and cancer combined. Not surprisingly, pain is the most common reason Americans access the health care system, the most common cause of long-term disability, and a tremendous socioeconomic burden. The US healthcare cost associated with pain is estimated in the range of $300 billion, with another approximately $300 billion resulting from lost productivity at work. The most common pain conditions are chronic low back pain, neck pain, and headaches, followed by large joint pain (hip, knee, shoulder); at least 50% of all cancer patients name pain as one of the major symptoms of their disease. Except for headache, the prevalence of most chronic pain conditions increases with age often due to progression of osteoarthritis.

PAIN CLASSIFICATION

Nociceptive pain due to activation of nociceptors from actual or threatened damage of nonneuronal tissue can be distinguished from neuropathic pain, which is a result of direct damage to the peripheral or central nervous system. **Nociceptive pain** arises in either the somatosensory or viscerosensory afferents from mechanical damage or by tissue inflammation. **Neuropathic pain** in contrast is caused by intrinsic damage to the sensory components of the nervous system, either in the peripheral (nerve, nerve root, nerve plexus) or central nervous system (spinal cord and brain). Clinical examples for nociceptive/inflammatory pain include any kind of trauma, postsurgical pain, osteoarthritis, rheumatologic disease, visceral inflammatory disease, and infection-related pain. Examples of peripheral neuropathic pain include mechanical nerve/nerve root damage; toxic-metabolic nerve injury as seen in diabetic, alcoholic, nutrition-deficiency neuropathies; nerve entrapments; and demyelinating peripheral disease like chronic inflammatory demyelinating polyneuropathy (CIDP). Central neuropathic pain is caused by damage to the nerve root entry zone, the spinothalamic tract, or the sensory thalamus by any process. For development of central neuropathic pain, the underlying pathology of the central lesion is less important than the location in the nociceptive system. Common conditions include ischemic and hemorrhagic stroke, brain or spinal cord tumor, or trauma, spinal syringomyelia, and demyelination due to multiple sclerosis.

PAIN FUNCTION

The ability to sense pain evolved from the most primitive of nervous systems and has been preserved throughout evolution to avoid actual or impeding tissue damage and to increase survival. The congenital inability to sense pain due to gene mutations of a voltage-gated sodium channel ($Na_v1.7$) results in early mutilations, trauma, and sometimes early death. This type of pain, indicating an acute threat to tissue integrity, is termed **nociceptive** pain, and it requires a high-intensity stimulus to activate pain-sensing fibers. Once tissue damage has occurred, inflammatory mediators released by the damaged tissue and the immune system result in hypersensitivity of the injured area, discouraging further physical contact and promoting the healing process. This **inflammatory** pain, mediated by a lowered activation threshold of pain-sensing structures, is triggered by mild- to moderate-intensity stimuli and persists until inflammation has resolved. In contrast to nociceptive and inflammatory pain, **pathological pain** is a chronic pain condition which does not serve any protective purpose, but rather represents a maladaptive state of the nociceptive system and a disease in its own right. This can be due to detectable injury to the peripheral or central nervous system (neuropathic pain) or changes in pain processing and perception (centralized or dysfunction pain disorder).

PAIN PATHOPHYSIOLOGY

The mechanism of pain perception (**nociception**) is carried out by specialized sensory neurons called nociceptors, located in the dorsal root ganglion (DRG). Nociceptors carry specific membrane receptors (**transducers**) at their free nerve endings which translate a variety of stimuli—including temperature and mechanical and chemical irritants—into membrane depolarization (Fig. 22.2). Examples of well-researched transducer molecules expressed in nociceptive neurons include **TRPV1** (activated by heat and capsaicin), **TRPM8** (cold), acid-sensing ion channels (**ASICs**) sensing free protons, and **Piezo2** (mechanical stimuli). The initial depolarization signal results in activation of several voltage-gated sodium channels in the nociceptive neuron (e.g., $Na_{v1.7}$, $Na_{v1.8}$, and $Na_{v1.9}$), which ultimately translate stimulus intensity into action potential frequency.

Thinly myelinated **A-δ and unmyelinated C-fibers** represent the major contributors to physiological nociception. In pathological pain states, high threshold **A-β fiber neurons,** typically sensing touch and vibration, can lower activation thresholds and contribute to pain perception in the form of mechanical allodynia (painful perception of touch). Once activated, nociceptors transmit the pain signal to central neurons located in the superficial laminae (mostly LI and LII, some contribution to deeper LV) of the spinal dorsal column (Fig. 22.1B). At these central projection neurons, the pain signal can be modified by inhibitory (Gamma-Amino Butyric acid [GABA]ergic and glycinergic) descending pathways, which originate in the periaqueductal grey (PEG), the serotoninergic nucleus raphe, and the norepinephrinergic locus coeruleus (Fig. 22.1A). A complex network of inhibitory and excitatory spinal interneurons as well as competing incoming sensory information from A-β fibers (gate control theory) can further modulate the nociceptive signal at the spinal level.

This modified information travels via the **anterior and lateral spinothalamic tracts (STT)** to the **ventral posterior lateral (VPL)** subnucleus of the thalamus, carrying sensations of pain, temperature, and itch from the contralateral side of the body, which ultimately reaches the **primary sensory cortex** (see Fig. 22.1B). **Trigeminothalamic axons** from the spinal nucleus of the trigeminal nerve (located in the brainstem and the high cervical spinal cord C1-3) decussate in the ventral trigeminothalamic tract to the contralateral STT to convey equivalent sensations from the face to the **ventral posterior medial (VPM)** subnucleus (see Fig. 22.1C). Nociceptive information is also received in other thalamic nuclei and further projected to different areas of the brain to modulate autonomic responses (e.g., projection to the posterior insula where integration with visceral afferents occur), arousal/attention (spinoreticular tract to intralaminar thalamic nuclei projecting to widespread brain areas), and the emotional component of pain perception (e.g., projection to the anterior cingulate cortex).

The nociceptive pathway from peripheral nociceptor activation to its complex computation in the brain is not a hard-wired entity of the kind "same stimulus, same response," but rather a highly adaptive system to both external and internal conditions. Changes in the stimulus-response curve of the nociceptive system are exemplified by the clinical conditions of **allodynia** (pain due to a stimulus that does not usually provoke pain) and **hyperalgesia** (increased pain from a stimulus that usually provokes pain). These changes in nociceptive responsiveness can occur at the site of primary injury (**primary hyperalgesia**) as well as in intact tissue surrounding or far from the primary injury site (**secondary hyperalgesia**). Primary hyperalgesia is mainly driven by changes in the peripheral nociceptor (peripheral sensitization), whereas secondary hyperalgesia is primarily triggered by central changes in spinal cord and brain processing (central sensitization). **Peripheral sensitization** results in a decreased threshold and increased responsiveness of nociceptors, caused by posttranslational changes and altered trafficking of transducer receptors (e.g., TRPV1) and voltage-gated ion channels (e.g., Na_v channels). These changes are often triggered by an inflammatory immune response due to tissue damage or infection, where inflammatory cytokines like bradykinin, histamine, and prostaglandins cause phosphorylation of transducer molecules or voltage-gated sodium channels, therefore altering their activation threshold (Fig. 22.2). The profound effect of voltage-gated sodium channels in nociception is exemplified by the rare but dramatic human mutation of $Na_{v1.7}$, which results in loss of channel function and complete inability to sense pain. In contrast, autosomal dominant mutation of $Na_{v1.7}$ with gain of function causes erythromelalgia, a condition characterized by spontaneous episodes of burning pain in feet and hands, and erythema. **Central sensitization** in contrast is a change in central pain processing due to increased responsiveness of nociceptive neurons in the spinal cord and brain. Mechanisms include:

1. **Ongoing peripheral nociceptor activation,** which results in strengthening of the synapse between the nociceptor and the central spinal dorsal horn neuron (**homosynaptic potentiation**), as well as eventually between activated central spinal dorsal horn neurons and non-nociceptive afferents (e.g., A-β fibers) (**heterosynaptic potentiation**). The latter results in recruitment of typically high-threshold touch sensing A-β fibers into the nociceptive pathway, causing the clinical phenomenon of mechanical allodynia (painful sensation upon light touch).

2. **Reduced inhibition/spinal disinhibition** due to reduction of inhibitory tone from the descending spinal pain pathways as well as from loss of inhibitory (GABAergic and glycinergic) spinal interneurons, which occurs, for example, after peripheral nerve damage.

3. **Central nervous system (CNS) inflammation** as a response to peripheral or central neuronal injury. Microglia activation occurs in the spinal cord and brain, which triggers astrocyte activation, invasion of T cells, and as a net result enhancement of glutamatergic neurotransmission.

4. **Widespread, complex changes in pain sensing brain areas,** including gray matter trophic changes, neurotransmitter alterations, and changes in connectivity.

PAIN ASSESSMENT

As in any other medical field, identifying a specific underlying condition is most satisfying for both patient and provider, and will likely result in the most specific and effective treatment (and avoidance of unnecessary tests and treatments). In pain medicine, this is particularly challenging, since pain is an entirely subjective, multimodal experience, which cannot be objectively quantified or otherwise measured. It is further complicated by the low specificity of symptoms. For example, pain quality from the same condition can be completely different from one patient to another (burning, aching, stabbing, pressure, etc.), the pain quality can change for the same patient depending on external factors (weather changes, movement, etc.), and two different conditions can cause very similar pain symptoms (e.g., lumbar radiculopathy from disc herniation can present similar to piriformis syndrome). Physical exam findings (see below) can be helpful in neuropathic pain conditions, but are less reliable for finding a specific musculoskeletal pain source. Imaging, including x-ray, computed tomography (CT), and magnetic resonance imaging (MRI), can help to exclude serious underlying disease and facilitate surgical planning, but often has poor correlation with chronic pain conditions, such as low back pain or radiculopathies.

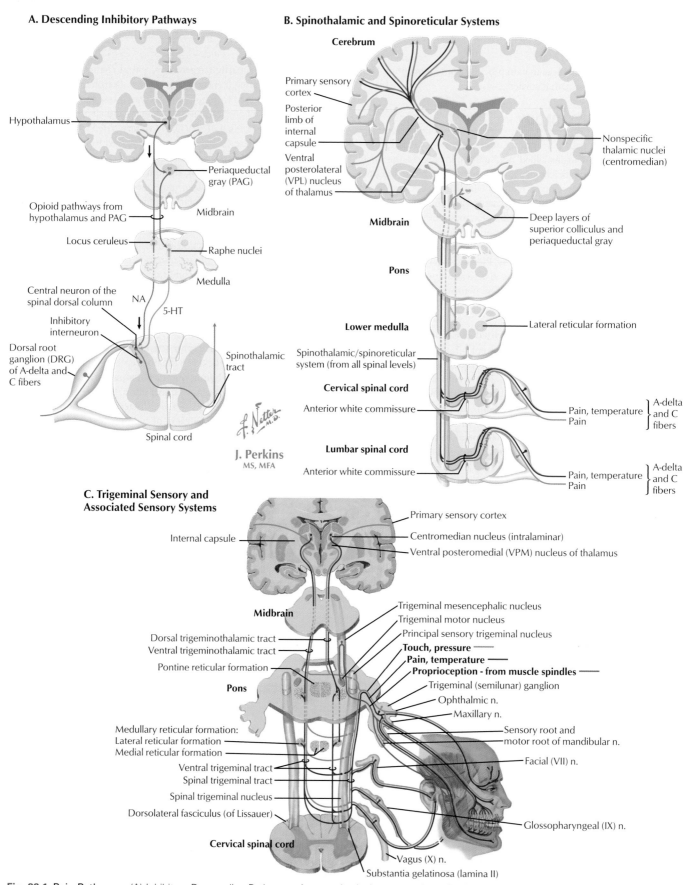

A. Descending Inhibitory Pathways

Hypothalamus

Periaqueductal gray (PAG)

Midbrain

Opioid pathways from hypothalamus and PAG

Locus ceruleus

Raphe nuclei

Medulla

Central neuron of the spinal dorsal column

NA

5-HT

Inhibitory interneuron

Dorsal root ganglion (DRG) of A-delta and C fibers

Spinothalamic tract

Spinal cord

J. Netter M.D.

J. Perkins
MS, MFA

B. Spinothalamic and Spinoreticular Systems

Cerebrum

Primary sensory cortex

Posterior limb of internal capsule

Ventral posterolateral (VPL) nucleus of thalamus

Nonspecific thalamic nuclei (centromedian)

Midbrain

Deep layers of superior colliculus and periaqueductal gray

Pons

Lower medulla

Lateral reticular formation

Spinothalamic/spinoreticular system (from all spinal levels)

Cervical spinal cord

Anterior white commissure

Pain, temperature } A-delta and C fibers
Pain

Lumbar spinal cord

Anterior white commissure

Pain, temperature } A-delta and C fibers
Pain

C. Trigeminal Sensory and Associated Sensory Systems

Internal capsule

Primary sensory cortex

Centromedian nucleus (intralaminar)

Ventral posteromedial (VPM) nucleus of thalamus

Midbrain

Trigeminal mesencephalic nucleus

Trigeminal motor nucleus

Dorsal trigeminothalamic tract

Principal sensory trigeminal nucleus

Ventral trigeminothalamic tract

Touch, pressure

Pain, temperature

Pontine reticular formation

Proprioception - from muscle spindles

Pons

Trigeminal (semilunar) ganglion

Ophthalmic n.

Maxillary n.

Medullary reticular formation:

Lateral reticular formation

Sensory root and motor root of mandibular n.

Medial reticular formation

Ventral trigeminal tract

Facial (VII) n.

Spinal trigeminal tract

Spinal trigeminal nucleus

Dorsolateral fasciculus (of Lissauer)

Glossopharyngeal (IX) n.

Cervical spinal cord

Vagus (X) n.

Substantia gelatinosa (lamina II)

Fig. 22.1 Pain Pathways. (A) Inhibitory Descending Pathways. At central spinal neurons, the pain signal can be modified by inhibitory (GABAergic and glycinergic) interneurons as well as by descending pathways, which originate in the periaqueductal grey (PEG), the serotoninergic nucleus raphe, and the norepinephrinergic locus coeruleus. (B) Spinothalamic and Spinoreticular Systems. Displayed is the major pathway of nociceptive fibers, which mostly decussate at the spinal level and run in the spinothalamic tract to the VPL nucleus of the thalamus. Ipsi- and contralateral nocicpetive information runs also in the spinoreticular tract to the reticular formation and to nonspecific thalamic nuclei, where it generates nonspecific pain responses such as arousal and autonomic responses. (C) Trigeminal and associated sensory systems. Nociceptors of the trigeminal nerve and other sensory nerves of the head/neck region project to central dorsal column neurons in the brainstem and high cervical spine (spinal trigeminal nucleus) and then decussate in the ventral trigeminothalamic tract to reach the VMP thalamic nucleus. These fibers join the spinothalamic tract and carry equivalent nociceptive information of the face. A smaller portion runs ipsilateral in the dorsal trigeminothalamic tract to the VPM.

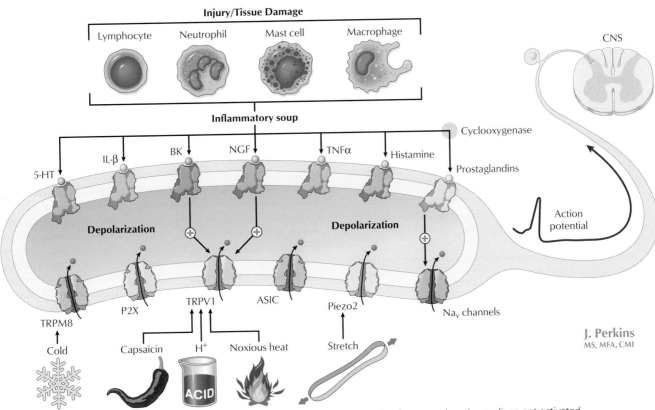

Fig. 22.2 Physiology of Nociceptor Activation. Transducer molecules on nociceptive endings get activated by intense mechanical, thermal, or chemical stimuli. This initial depolarization is amplified by voltage gated channels including Nav channels, coded in action potential frequency and conveyed to nociceptive neurons in the spinal cord. Changes in activation threshold or expression pattern of both transducer molecules and voltage gated channels, as often seen during inflammation or injury, result in altered responsiveness of the nociceptor and can lead to peripheral sensitization.

For all these reasons, the exact underlying pain mechanisms remain often unknown and treatment occurs on a "trial and error" basis. It is important to distinguish the biological process of nociception from the multimodal pain experience, which is influenced by cognitive and affective factors. Although the underlying structural disease might be irreversible, evaluating and reshaping the patient's perception of pain (e.g., by using cognitive behavioral therapy) can significantly change pain-related disability and quality of life.

NEUROPATHIC PAIN SYNDROMES

Neuropathic pain syndromes are a heterogeneous group of painful disorders, which by definition are caused by "disease of the somatosensory nervous system" (IASP). Common examples for *peripheral neuropathic pain* syndromes can be very focal as in mononeuropathies or radiculopathies, or more widespread, typically as a result of systemic diseases, toxicities, or deficiency states causing polyneuropathy or mononeuritis multiplex. Common conditions include postsurgical pain (e.g., after mastectomy or inguinal hernia repair), mechanical nerve compression (e.g., entrapment neuropathies, trigeminal neuralgia), nerve ischemia (e.g., due to vasculitis or diabetes), axonal degeneration (e.g., alcohol, diabetes), demyelinating (e.g., CIDP, Guillain-Barré syndrome [GBS]), infectious and postinfectious conditions (e.g., syphilis, HIV, postherpetic neuralgia). Intrinsic nerve damage as well as concomitant perineural inflammation (e.g., nerve root inflammation from disc extrusion, tissue inflammation after surgery) result in peripheral sensitization and

sometimes secondary central sensitization. At the site of traumatic nerve injury, a tangled mass of regenerating axons embedded within nerve connective tissue called **neuroma** can form, which shows abnormal electrical hyperexcitability and can generate spontaneous pain outbursts.

Central neuropathic pain syndromes occur due to a structural lesion disrupting nociceptive pathways anywhere in the CNS. Damage to the nerve root entry zone, the spinothalamic tract, the sensory thalamus, or somatosensory cortex by any process can result in central neuropathic pain. Common conditions include ischemic and hemorrhagic stroke, brain or spinal cord tumor, trauma and demyelinating disease such as MS.

Ultimately, the maladaptive response of the peripheral and central nervous system to disease or trauma results in structural and functional changes in the nociceptive system and manifests as the pathological state of chronic neuropathic pain.

EVALUATION OF NEUROPATHIC PAIN

Several symptomatic features as well as examination findings can help establish the presence of a neuropathic pain syndrome. In contrast to nociceptive/inflammatory pain, neuropathic pain often shows the presence of mechanical and temperature-evoked allodynia (painful sensation to low-threshold, nonpainful stimuli), numbness to several modalities (pinprick, touch, temperature), burning/tingling/electric shocklike paresthesias, and intermittent pain attacks rather than persistent pain. Validated pain questionnaires have been developed to capture these features and identify patients with neuropathic pain, such as the Douleur

Neuropathique 4 (DN4), Neuropathic Pain Questionnaire (NPQ), and painDETECT questionnaire.

Important physical examination findings include:

- Sensation
  - diminished or absent sensibility of small fibers (pinprick, temperature) and/or large fibers (vibration, position sense)
  - presence of hyperesthesia at the injury site (indicative of peripheral sensitization), hyperesthesia beyond the injury site (secondary hyperalgesia), or the presence of mechanical allodynia (indicative of central sensitization)
  - straight leg (high sensitivity) and crossed straight leg raise (high specificity) test, which can indicate a lumbar radiculopathy, plexopathy, or sciatic nerve disease
  - Spurling's test (laterally flexing, rotating, and compressing the patient's head toward the symptomatic side), which can be suggestive of cervical radiculopathy
- Weakness
  - important, more objective marker of (more severe) root, plexus, or peripheral nerve damage
- Location of sensory or strength deficit
  - symmetrical distal stockinglike distribution (e.g., axonal polyneuropathy)
  - peripheral nerve distribution (mononeuropathy)
  - dermatomal/myotomal distribution (nerve root, plexus)
  - symmetric proximal distribution (e.g., ganglionopathy)
  - sensory trunk level (spinal cord syndrome)
- Neuraxial symptoms
  - sensory trunk level, increased tone/spasticity, Babinski sign, bowel or bladder incontinence
- Autonomic findings
  - vasomotor (swelling, color, and temperature changes) and sudomotor (sweating) changes; particularly important for diagnosing autonomic/small fiber neuropathies and CRPS
- Ancillary testing
  - **Imaging:** Advanced imaging such as MRI and CT can be helpful to exclude/confirm more severe disease in patients with, for example, a history of cancer, neurological deficits, or help with surgical planning. In patients with no neurological deficit or other "red flags," imaging of common conditions such as low back pain, neck pain, or painful radiculopathies almost never advances diagnosis or changes treatment.
  - **Nerve conduction studies (NCS) and electromyography (EMG)** can help better define neurological dysfunction in terms of anatomic location (compression site of a peripheral nerve, root disease, muscle disease), etiology of nerve damage (axonal versus demyelinating), and chronicity of the disorder (acute, subacute, chronic). NCS will only measure large fiber function, so that isolated small fiber/autonomic neuropathies will result in a normal study.
  - **Autonomic testing and skin biopsy** for small fiber count can be helpful in the evaluation for autonomic/small fiber neuropathy. These patients often present with rather widespread neuropathic sensory symptoms as well as autonomic dysfunction, with otherwise normal imaging and NCS findings.

TREATMENT OF NEUROPATHIC PAIN

For most neuropathic pain conditions, the underlying etiology and nerve damage may be irreversible, so that treatment is geared toward symptomatic relief. As for any pain condition, expectations should be set to partial pain relief (e.g., 30%–50% pain decrease) and modest, defined functional improvement, rather than a pain-free state on a pain scale. To achieve this goal, it is important to treat psychiatric and other comorbidities, such as depression, anxiety, or poor sleep, which commonly results in increased disability as well as pain amplification. Psychological treatments which include biofeedback, relaxation techniques, and cognitive behavioral therapy can often reshape the experience of pain favorably and decrease disability.

The choice of a pharmacological agent is based on several factors, including efficacy for neuropathic pain conditions, side-effect profile, patient comorbidities, drug interactions, patient preference, and insurance coverage/expense, and most often remains an empirical endeavor.

First-line agents for neuropathic pain include tricyclic antidepressants, gabapentinoids, and SNRIs; **second-line agents** include topical lidocaine and capsaicin formulations (sometimes used as first line given excellent side-effect profile) and tramadol; and **third-line agents** include stronger opioids and botulinum toxin for peripheral neuropathic pain. Carbamazepine and the related drug oxcarbazepine are traditionally used as first-line therapy for trigeminal neuralgia, although strong evidence is lacking. All other antiepileptic drugs, including phenytoin, sodium valproate, lamotrigine, lacosamide, levetiracetam, and topiramate, lack convincing evidence of benefit in neuropathic pain treatment.

Antidepressants such as **tricyclic antidepressants (TCAs)** and **serotonin–norepinephrine reuptake inhibitors (SNRIs)** are among the most effective treatments for both peripheral and some central neuropathic pain conditions, and are the treatment of choice for patients with comorbid depression. Mechanism of action includes serotonergic and noradrenergic reuptake inhibition in descending inhibitory pain pathways, therefore increasing inhibitory tone on central spinal projection neurons. Amitriptyline is the best-studied TCA and has the highest efficacy for neuropathic conditions. Other commonly used TCAs are nortriptyline and desipramine, which have generally fewer side effects and are less sedating. Common side effects include anticholinergic effects (constipation and urinary retention, dry mouth), as well as postural hypotension, sedation, nausea, blurred vision, and weight gain. Commonly used SNRIs include duloxetine, milnacipran, and venlafaxine, which are preferred for comorbid anxiety as well as for centralized/dysfunction pain states (e.g., fibromyalgia). Common side effects include nausea, dizziness, diaphoresis, agitation, diarrhea, hypertension (not seen with duloxetine), and sexual dysfunction.

Gabapentinoids (gabapentin, pregabalin) have the best evidence of all antiepileptics for neuropathic pain conditions, especially for painful diabetic neuropathy, postherpetic neuralgia, and centralized pain states. Their mechanism of action is by binding to the α-2-δ-1 subunit of neuronal presynaptic voltage-gated calcium channels, which influences the release of excitatory neurotransmitters. They can often be helpful for patients with comorbid anxiety and restless legs syndrome. Common side effects include dizziness, somnolence, peripheral edema, and gait disturbance.

Topical **lidocaine** formulations including creams, ointments, and patches have excellent side-effect profiles and have shown good efficacy for diabetic neuropathy and postherpetic neuralgia. Topical **capsaicin** strongly activates TRPV1 ligand-gated cation channels expressed on nociceptors, which results in desensitization and substance P depletion of nociceptive neurons. Desensitization with capsaicin of any localized neuropathic pain area can be attempted, including conditions like postherpetic neuralgia, diabetic/HIV/cancer–related neuropathy, and postsurgical pain. An 8% capsaicin patch is sometimes used for postherpetic neuralgia and HIV polyneuropathy, but application can be very painful.

CHRONIC REGIONAL PAIN SYNDROME

Chronic regional pain syndrome (CRPS) has been known under many different names, including causalgia (Greek: kausis [fire] + algos [pain]),

Sudeck dystrophy, and reflex sympathetic dystrophy (RSD), and still remains a poorly understood condition. Diagnosis is purely clinical, and is defined by the Budapest criteria (Box 22.1).

The condition is more common in the middle-aged female, and rare to occur in children or the elderly. Based on the presence of a measurable nerve lesion, CRPS is divided into type I (no nerve damage) and type II (nerve damage present). Sympathetic dysregulation is likely responsible for vasomotor changes resulting in temperature changes and edema of the extremity, as well as sudomotor dysregulation causing changes in sweat. Typically, symptoms of sensory disturbance/pain, motor disturbance, and autonomic changes occur distally in one extremity and do not follow any particular peripheral nerve or radicular distribution. Involvement of the head/face region is exceedingly rare; however ipsilateral spread to the upper/lower extremity has been described. Temporal evolution of symptoms over months and years has been described as distinct clinical stages; however there is large interindividual variability among CRPS patients (Fig. 22.3):

- **Stage I** (acute, 0–3 months): pain/sensory abnormalities, edema
- **Stage II** (dystrophic, 3–9 months): more pain/sensory dysfunction, motor/trophic changes

- **Stage III** (atrophic, >9 months): less pain, increased motor/trophic changes

Although the diagnosis is purely clinical, **ancillary testing** can sometimes help to support the clinical picture or exclude alternative diagnoses. Sympathetic dysregulation can be measured as temperature differences of >1°C, measurement of edema, or dedicated sweat testing. X-ray of both hands can sometimes show patchy areas of deossification of the affected hand (see Fig. 22.3). Maybe most specific is a three-phase bone scan which can show increased delayed tracer uptake around the MCP joints of the affected hand in the first 5 months of CRPS onset.

The cornerstone of treatment remains early and aggressive physical and occupational therapy to counteract pain avoidance behavior and prevent progression to a chronic pain state. This includes **mirror therapy,** a technique in which a mirror image of the healthy limb is used to mimic pain-free movement of the affected side, and over time induces central neuronal reorganization which can help recovery. Medication therapies in the early stages of CRPS supported by evidence include oral steroid taper, oral and intravenous (IV) bisphosphonate medications (e.g., alendronate, clodronate), and possibly high-dose vitamin C and NSAIDs. Symptomatic oral treatment is generally similar to the guidelines for neuropathic pain management (see above). IV infusion of the NMDA-antagonist ketamine at subanesthetic doses has been used in an attempt to tackle central sensitization in CRPS. While there is some anecdotal evidence of long-term success with ketamine and the mechanism is intriguing, no high-quality evidence exists for its use; the difficulty with long term IV administration (poor oral availability, has to be given IV) as well as psychomimetic side effects limits its use for refractory cases only. Interventional therapies including stellate ganglion block for the upper extremity and lumbar sympathetic chain block for the lower extremity can be considered, but do not show consistent benefit in meta-analyses. Spinal cord stimulation therapy remains another option for refractory cases; however, treatment efficacy often declines after the first few years.

CENTRAL POSTSTROKE PAIN

Central poststroke pain (CPSP) is a central neuropathic pain condition which can occur after ischemic or hemorrhagic stroke. The prevalence in stroke patients is estimated around 8% and up to 18% in patients

---

BOX 22.1 Budapest Criteria 2010

a. Continuing pain, which is disproportionate to any inciting event
b. At least one symptom in three of the four following categories must be reported:
- Sensory: hyperesthesia and/or allodynia
- Vasomotor: temperature asymmetry and/or skin color changes and/or skin color asymmetry
- Sudomotor/Edema: edema and/or changes in sweating
- Motor/Trophic: decreased range of motion and/or motor dysfunction (weakness, tremor, dystonia) and/or trophic changes (hair, nail, skin)
c. At least one sign on exam in two or more of the above categories must be present at time of evaluation
d. There is no other diagnosis that better explains the signs and symptoms

Reused with permission from Harden RN, Bruehl S, Perez RS, et al. Validation of proposed diagnostic criteria (the "Budapest Criteria") for complex regional pain syndrome. *Pain.* 2010;150(2):268–274.

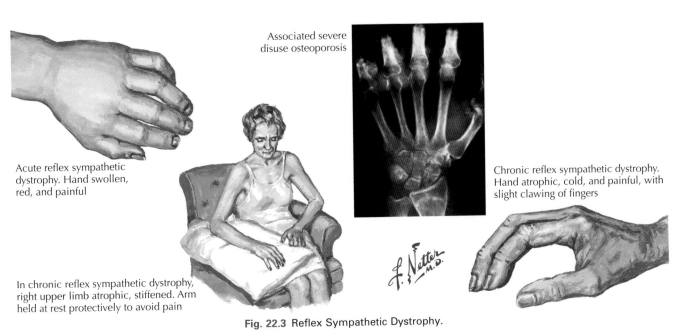

Associated severe disuse osteoporosis

Acute reflex sympathetic dystrophy. Hand swollen, red, and painful

Chronic reflex sympathetic dystrophy. Hand atrophic, cold, and painful, with slight clawing of fingers

In chronic reflex sympathetic dystrophy, right upper limb atrophic, stiffened. Arm held at rest protectively to avoid pain

Fig. 22.3 Reflex Sympathetic Dystrophy.

presenting initially with sensory deficits. Diagnosis is made when pain occurs at or after stroke onset in the body area which corresponds to the stroke lesion in the brain.

The phenomenon was first described in patients with a constellation of neurological symptoms and severe pain due to a vascular lesion in the thalamus, which was named after the authors "Dejerine-Roussy syndrome" or "thalamic pain syndrome." As later observations showed, the stroke location within the somatosensory system, rather than stroke type, is important for CPSP development, with lesions in the lower brainstem, the opercular-insular region, and thalamus bearing the greatest risk. Other risk factors include early onset of pain, initial sensory disturbances in the body area affected by the stroke, and severity of the stroke. Pain typically develops immediately after or gradually within 1–3 months after the stroke, can range anywhere from mild to severe, and can be spontaneous, triggered by external stimuli, or both. Sensory changes typically include a combination of negative (numbness) and positive sensory symptoms (dysesthesia, mechanical or cold allodynia), and pain qualities are typically described as burning, painful cold, electric shocks, aching, pressing, stinging, and pins and needles. In a poststroke patient, many confounding factors exist which expand the poststroke pain phenotype well beyond a purely central neuropathic pain condition, but also offer opportunity for symptomatic treatment. These conditions include musculoskeletal pain from decreased mobility and change in posture, spasticity, frozen shoulder syndrome/hemiplegic shoulder pain, and chronic headaches as well as coexisting painful conditions like diabetic neuropathy.

No specific treatment for CPSP exists; therefore treatment recommendations are along the general guidelines for treatment of neuropathic pain (see above), and first-line treatments based on small controlled trials include tricyclic antidepressants (e.g., amitriptyline), selective serotonin reuptake inhibitors (SSRIs) (e.g., fluvoxamine), gabapentinoids, and lamotrigine. In the poststroke population, side-effect profile, comorbidities, and drug interactions are particularly important factors in determining the initial treatment choice. A combination of different classes can be tried to avoid side effects from higher doses of monotherapy, as can second- and third-line agents (tramadol and stronger opioids, respectively). Nonpharmacological treatment options which have been successfully used in selected patients, but with inconclusive evidence for effectiveness, include repetitive transcranial magnetic stimulation (rTMS), deep brain stimulation (DBS), and motor cortex stimulation (MCS). Treating contributing pain conditions is typically helpful as well, and this includes botulinum toxin injections to reduce upper and lower extremity spasticity, physical therapy, as well as treatment of comorbid depression.

PHANTOM LIMB PAIN

Phantom limb pain (PLP) is defined as a painful sensation which is felt in the location of the missing limb and can occur after amputation or deafferentation of any limb. Related conditions include nonpainful phantom sensations and stump pain/sensations (restricted to the amputation stump). While stump sensations occur in almost all amputees, PLP occurs in 50%–80% of cases, with 10%–15% being severe. Symptoms start days to weeks after the initial injury and can range from a constant, intensely painful, vivid perception of the missing limb to an occasional, brief, shocklike sensation in the missing body part. Pain qualities are manifold, but typically include a burning, stabbing, cramping, or throbbing sensation, and are often more severe in the distal imaginary limb areas. Risk factors for developing PLP include age, with adults most often affected, children seldom, and congenital amputees virtually never. Optimization of perioperative pain control by using epidural opioid and local anesthetic infusions, as well as perineural

anesthesia, is likely beneficial. Whether the mechanism of injury, for example, traumatic versus medically indicated amputation, constitutes a risk factor is uncertain. The pathophysiology of PLP likely is a combination of peripheral and central mechanisms, as in many other neuropathic pain conditions. Peripheral mechanisms include the formation of a **neuroma** (a tangled mass of regenerating axons embedded within nerve connective tissue) at the site of nerve transection, as well as injury-induced changes of ion channel properties and expression patterns in the affected nerve and DRG. These changes result in decreased pain threshold in the affected area (**peripheral sensitization**) as well as spontaneous, ectopic discharges at the site of the neuroma or DRG, causing easily triggered or spontaneous pain attacks. Evidence in support of this theory includes the "Tinel sign" in the stump (provocation of PLP by direct pressure on the neuroma) and transient pain relief of PLP after local anesthetic block of the DRG/nerve root in some patients. Increased peripheral firing eventually results in secondary changes in the central somatosensory processing systems (**central sensitization**). Reorganization of the somatotopic representation occurs in the primary sensory cortex by invasion of adjacent areas into the representation zone of the deafferented limb, with the degree of remapping proportional to pain intensity. In addition, it is likely that reorganization occurs within a wider range of the pain processing matrix, including affective–motivational processing areas such as the insula, anterior cingulate, and frontal cortices.

Treatment remains challenging for these patients, and medications used for other neuropathic pain conditions are typically used first line, including tricyclic antidepressants, gabapentinoids, SNRIs, anticonvulsants, and opioids. Some evidence exists for long-term benefit from oral morphine and gabapentin, and weaker evidence for topiramate, amitriptyline, NMDA-antagonist memantine, and high-dose capsaicin patch. Nonpharmacological measures are mainly aimed to reverse central changes of cortical reorganization by mimicking the use of the missing body part, or by using direct stimuli to "activate" the missing body part. For example, the regular use of a myoelectric prosthesis reduces both phantom limb pain and the related cortical reorganization. Similar effects were observed using daily discrimination training of electric stimuli to the stump. Mirror treatment is yet another modality which has been successfully applied to CRPS patients and holds promise for PLP. During this treatment, a mirror is used to project the intact limb over the corresponding missing side, so that movements of the healthy side are perceived by the brain as movements of the missing limb, which can result in decrease in pathological somatotopic reorganization. As with other neuropathic pain syndromes, rTMS has been reported to be successful in some cases. In terms of interventional treatment, botulinum toxin stump injections have been proven ineffective. Spinal cord as well as peripheral nerve stimulation techniques can be considered for refractory cases, but good-quality evidence is missing.

ADDITIONAL RESOURCES

Costigan M, Scholz J, Woolf CJ. Neuropathic pain: a maladaptive response of the nervous system to damage. Annu Rev Neurosci 2009;32:1–32.
Overview of mechanisms of central and peripheral sensitization.
Finnerup NB, Attal N, Haroutounian S, et al. Pharmacotherapy for neuropathic pain in adults: a systematic review and meta-analysis. Lancet Neurol 2015;14(2):162–73.
Evidence-based review of neuropathic pain medications.
Birklein F, O'Neill D, Schlereth T. Complex regional pain syndrome: an optimistic perspective. Neurology 2015;84(1):89–96.
Diagnostic allorhythmia and criteria for CRPS, as well as useful ancillary testing for CRPS.

Harden RN, Oaklander AL, Burton AW, et al. Reflex sympathetic dystrophy syndrome association. Complex regional pain syndrome: practical diagnostic and treatment guidelines. Pain Med 2013;14(2):180–229.
Treatment guidelines for CRPS.
Klit H, Finnerup NB, Jensen TS. Central post-stroke pain: clinical characteristics, pathophysiology, and management. Lancet Neurol 2009;8(9):857–68.
Review and diagnostic criteria for central poststroke pain.
Treister AK, Hatch MN, Cramer SC, et al. Demystifying poststroke pain: from etiology to treatment. PM R 2017;9(1):63–75.
Treatment options for central poststroke pain.

Flor H, Nikolajsen L, Staehelin Jensen T. Phantom limb pain: a case of maladaptive CNS elasticity? Nat Rev Neurosci 2006;7(11):873–81.
Review of mechanisms underlying phantom limb pain.
McCormick Z, Chang-Chien G, Marshall B, et al. Phantom limb pain: a systematic neuroanatomical-based review of pharmacologic treatment. Pain Med 2014;15(2):292–305.
Treatment review for phantom limb pain.

Epilepsy and Sleep Disorders

Claudia J. Chaves

23

Epilepsy

Ritu Bagla, Joanna Suski

Epilepsy is generally defined as an illness of recurrent seizures. The prevalence of epilepsy is estimated at 1 in 200 persons. It affects all ages and is generally a chronic problem with significant personal, social, and economic impact, often affecting the ability to hold jobs and drive. Poor epilepsy control and the seizures themselves can lead to significant cognitive and personality changes as well as chronic depression. The incidence is about 200,000 new cases yearly in the United States. The clinical manifestations are initiated by abnormal electrical discharges within the brain. The underlying pathophysiology is complex and not completely defined, but ultimately involves repetitive cortical potentials leading to altered modulation of excitatory inputs and suppression of inhibitory feedback circuits (Fig. 23.1). Epilepsy remains a clinical diagnosis. It is made with a detailed history from the patient and any witnesses. The neurologic examination is often normal. An abnormal electroencephalogram (EEG) can confirm the diagnosis of epilepsy and help with classification and location of the seizure focus. Laboratory tests are generally done initially to correct an underlying metabolic abnormality. Magnetic resonance imaging (MRI) is the preferred imaging test in patients that need investigation for an underlying structural lesion (Fig. 23.2). Once the diagnosis of epilepsy is certain, most patients require treatment with antiepileptic medication. The goal of treatment is to stop seizures with one medication and minimal side effects. When seizures persist despite treatment with two antiepileptic medications, patients should be referred to an epilepsy specialist to confirm the diagnosis, classification, and consideration of epilepsy surgery.

DIFFERENTIAL DIAGNOSIS

All paroxysmal disorders of consciousness or perception may be included in the differential of seizures. Migraine with aura (classic migraine) is differentiated by generally distinct and recurrent positive visual or sensory phenomenon evolving gradually, then resolving over minutes and followed by a throbbing often unilateral headache. Transient ischemic attacks are characterized by negative (loss of function) neurologic symptoms often consistent with a single vascular territory that start maximally and resolve gradually over seconds to minutes. Syncope is usually preceded by prodromal symptoms of lightheadedness, limpness, pale complexion, and diaphoresis. Once the patient falls or lies down and cerebral circulation is restored, full consciousness is regained with little or no persistent confusion or disorientation, unlike the postictal period following seizures. Parasomnias with stereotyped nocturnal movements and psychiatric disorders can also be confused with seizures. One disorder that continues to be difficult to classify is transient global amnesia (TGA). It is considered by most to be a distinct benign entity that does not warrant any specific long-term treatment. A brief discussion follows.

TRANSIENT GLOBAL AMNESIA

TGA is a term that was first used by Fisher and Adams in the 1960s to denote a syndrome of abrupt onset of severe anterograde amnesia with other elements of neurologic function remaining intact. Retrograde amnesia may be present to a variable degree. Patients appear anxious or even agitated but are able to communicate and often ask the same exact questions repeatedly even when answered promptly. It is usually seen in patients 50–70 years of age. Patients recover fully within 24 hours without residual memory problems but have no recollection of the spell. Often there is no precipitating event, but sometimes the episode is preceded by stress, Valsalva maneuver, sexual intercourse, or pain. Associated altered level of consciousness, ataxia, dysarthria, visual changes, headache, abnormal movements, and vomiting strongly suggest an alternative diagnosis such as basilar ischemic etiology or seizure. Several etiologies have been proposed including seizure, migraine, ischemia, venous congestion, and psychogenic disturbances, but the exact etiology remains unknown.

Typically, a brain magnetic resonance imaging and routine electroencephalogram are considered the diagnostic tests in TGA mainly to exclude other diagnoses. TGA may show subtle neuroimaging changes with transient intense diffusion-weighted imaging (DWI) signal seen within the hippocampus. These changes are usually reversible and not in arterial distributions commonly seen with strokes arguing against it being due to ischemia. A comprehensive stroke workup (vascular imaging, echocardiogram, or heart monitor) is not necessary for typical cases of TGA as long as DWI changes are only seen in the hippocampus. An EEG can be helpful if transient epileptic amnesia (TEA) is considered. Typically TEA causes shorter episodes of amnesia, are recurrent events, and are accompanied by oral or motor automatisms. During TGA episodes, the EEG is normal. TGA is typically a benign condition and rarely will reoccur.

PARTIAL SEIZURES

Simple Partial Seizures

> **CLINICAL VIGNETTE** *A 40-year-old woman experiences episodic numbness that spreads from the left thumb to the hand, arm, and then to the face over a period of about 30 seconds. These occur sporadically and are stereotypical in nature. She maintains alertness throughout the events. Since starting antiepileptic medications, these events have abated.*

This history represents the typical simple partial seizure (SPS). During the episodes, patients are conscious, aware of their surroundings, and

Normal firing pattern of cortical neurons

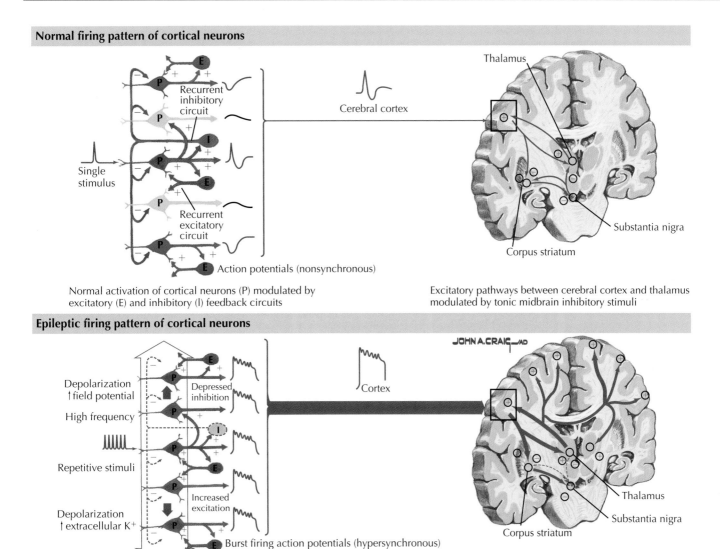

Normal activation of cortical neurons (P) modulated by excitatory (E) and inhibitory (I) feedback circuits

Excitatory pathways between cerebral cortex and thalamus modulated by tonic midbrain inhibitory stimuli

Epileptic firing pattern of cortical neurons

Repetitive cortical activation potentiates excitatory transmission and depresses inhibitory transmission, creating self-perpetuating excitatory circuit (burst) and facilitating excitation (recruitment) of neighboring neurons.

Cortical bursts to corpus striatum and thalamus block inhibitory projections and create self-perpetuating feedback circuit.

Fig. 23.1 Origin and Spread of Seizures.

able to respond appropriately. Partial seizures originate and develop within a discrete area of the cerebral cortex (Fig. 23.3). They may have a "Jacksonian march" wherein the cortical epileptic discharges spread along contiguous cortical regions. The brain area involved determines the clinical signature of the event. Symptoms may be somatosensory, as in the above vignette, when the origin is in the parietal lobe, motor when discharges arise from the frontal or motor cortex, and visual when they begin in the occipital lobe. However, the relation of focal cortical location to clinical expression is not absolute. Seizures may start in a "silent" cerebral cortical area with the manifest ictal symptoms representing the result of the discharge spreading to neighboring cortical areas. SPSs may occasionally have autonomic, psychic, or cognitive manifestations. Other seizure types may start off as SPS and then evolve into broader disruptions. By definition, these simple ictal events do not include any change in level of consciousness, and it is this preserved responsiveness to the external environment that characterizes SPSs. Auras, a warning that a patient experiences prior to altered or loss of consciousness, are, in effect, SPSs.

Clonic phases of partial motor seizures that continue uninterrupted for prolonged periods, with no progression into other body segments,

are known as epilepsia partialis continua, or Kojevnikov syndrome, and are discussed below.

The clinical evaluation of patients with partial epilepsy must include an EEG, a neuroimaging test, and laboratory testing. Although routine EEG recordings may often be normal in patients with unequivocal seizure disorders, it remains of paramount importance for the correct diagnosis and classification of the ictal events. Even when the neurologist suspects a seizure disorder from the clinical description, the EEG, if positive, may serve as an important confirmatory test when the episode is not well described. It should be remembered, however, that a routine EEG represents only a limited time sample and that sporadically firing interictal discharges can, therefore, be easily missed in patients with unequivocal seizure disorders. Long-term seizure telemetry units and ambulatory EEG monitoring are now available to increase recording time and enhance detection rates. The EEG hallmark of partial epilepsy is focal spikes or spike-and-wave discharges. Because delta-wave non-rapid eye movement sleep activates or disinhibits epileptiform discharges, the EEG is preferably recorded during both wakefulness and sleep to increase the probability of making the correct diagnosis and defining the focal origin (Fig. 23.4). A definitive result is often obtained only

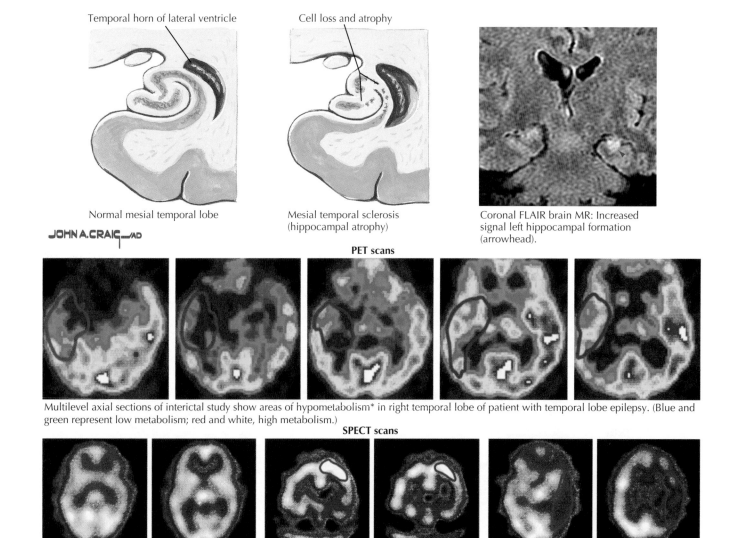

Normal mesial temporal lobe

Temporal horn of lateral ventricle

Mesial temporal sclerosis (hippocampal atrophy)

Cell loss and atrophy

Coronal FLAIR brain MR: Increased signal left hippocampal formation (arrowhead).

JOHN A.CRAIG—AD

PET scans

Multilevel axial sections of interictal study show areas of hypometabolism* in right temporal lobe of patient with temporal lobe epilepsy. (Blue and green represent low metabolism; red and white, high metabolism.)

SPECT scans

Interictal (baseline) study shows symmetric blood flow.

Ictal study shows increased left frontal blood flow* in patient with frontal lobe epilepsy.

Postictal study shows decreased left temporal blood flow* in patient with temporal lobe epilepsy.

*Areas of interest circled in red.

Fig. 23.2 Neuroimaging Studies.

during sleep recordings. Repeated recordings may be necessary if the nature of the episode is unclear or if psychogenic nonepileptic seizures are suspected. In contrast, the EEG in patients with epilepsia partialis continua contains spike-wave discharges in a variably continuous manner, often in the contralateral frontal lobe. A small number of individuals in the healthy population have abnormal EEG containing focal spikes but do not go on to have seizures later in life. This emphasizes that an abnormal EEG can only be interpreted in light of the presenting clinical symptoms and that it does not, on its own, define a seizure syndrome or dictate treatment. At best, the EEG may capture an ongoing seizure and greatly clarify its origin. It may also help to localize the epileptogenic pathology, guiding surgery if medical treatment fails.

Neuroimaging studies, especially MRI, are vital to the evaluation of new-onset or changing-pattern seizures. Brain computed tomography is a useful screening technique when MRI is not available. The onset of new partial seizures strongly suggests the development of a new pathologic process, including tumors (primary or metastatic) or abscess in the adult population, stroke from emboli or rarely vasculitis in older age groups, and focal encephalitis such as Rasmussen encephalitis in

children, herpes simplex encephalitis in children or adults, or head trauma (Fig. 23.5). However, sometimes a patient with a lesion, for example, mesial temporal sclerosis or an arteriovenous malformation (AVM), does not present with partial seizures until adulthood. Rarely, acute-onset partial seizures may be caused by metabolic abnormalities, such as nonketotic hyperglycemia or hypoglycemia.

Complex Partial Seizures

> **CLINICAL VIGNETTE** *A 37-year-old patient experiences episodic events that start with a rising feeling in the stomach followed by a blank stare with loss of awareness. Subsequently, he has nonpurposeful movements of the hands lasting several minutes followed by somnolence.*

This patient's history represents a typical example of complex partial seizures (CPSs). The clinical manifestations of this seizure type include changes in alertness or level of consciousness, partial amnesia, and

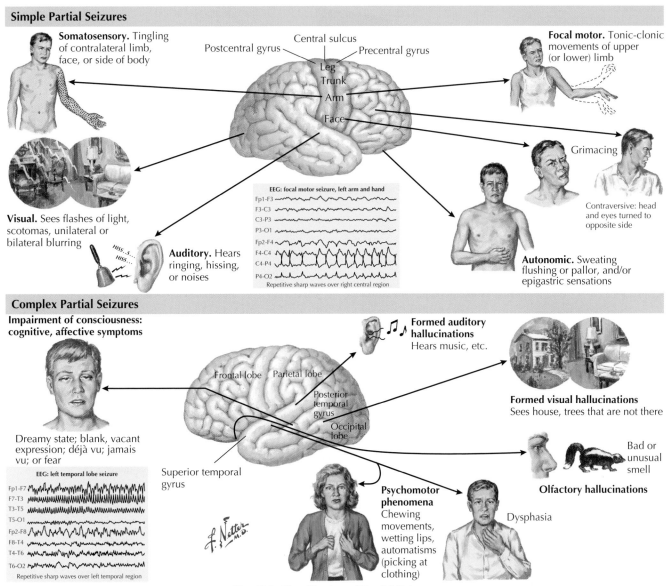

Simple Partial Seizures

Somatosensory. Tingling of contralateral limb, face, or side of body

Central sulcus
Postcentral gyrus
Precentral gyrus
Leg
Trunk
Arm
Face

Focal motor. Tonic-clonic movements of upper (or lower) limb

Grimacing

Contraversive: head and eyes turned to opposite side

Visual. Sees flashes of light, scotomas, unilateral or bilateral blurring

HISS..S..
HISS...

Auditory. Hears ringing, hissing, or noises

EEG: focal motor seizure, left arm and hand
Fp1-F3
F3-C3
C3-P3
P3-O1
Fp2-F4
F4-C4
C4-P4
P4-O2
Repetitive sharp waves over right central region

Autonomic. Sweating flushing or pallor, and/or epigastric sensations

Complex Partial Seizures

Impairment of consciousness: cognitive, affective symptoms

Formed auditory hallucinations
Hears music, etc.

Frontal lobe Parietal lobe
Posterior temporal gyrus
Occipital lobe

Formed visual hallucinations
Sees house, trees that are not there

Dreamy state; blank, vacant expression; déjà vu; jamais vu; or fear

Bad or unusual smell

Superior temporal gyrus

Olfactory hallucinations

EEG: left temporal lobe seizure
Fp1-F7
F7-T3
T3-T5
T5-O1
Fp2-F8
F8-T4
T4-T6
T6-O2
Repetitive sharp waves over left temporal region

Psychomotor phenomena
Chewing movements, wetting lips, automatisms (picking at clothing)

Dysphasia

Fig. 23.3 Classification of Partial Seizures.

automatisms (see Fig. 23.3). Patients often perform simple motor tasks and even may walk during the seizure. CPSs usually arise from mesial temporal structures but can also originate in other extralimbic temporal structures or the inferior frontal lobe and spread via the uncinate fasciculus and other pathways to the mesial temporal area.

Partial seizures of frontal lobe origin are frequently confused with a CPS of temporal origin but are distinguished by brief auras with rapid generalization or versive head and eye movements with tonic posturing of the arms. Rarely, a fall is the only clinical feature. Nocturnal frontal lobe seizures often produce odd complex behaviors suggestive of psychogenic nonepileptic seizures but should be kept in mind in those with fairly consistent patterns and no obvious secondary gain.

Because complex partial seizures are of focal origin, patient evaluation is similar to that undertaken for SPS. Typically, the interictal EEG (i.e., obtained between seizures) reveals spike discharges in one or both anterior temporal lobes. The ictal EEG is usually abnormal, with recurrent focal spikes or rhythmic activity. Brain MRI with special attention given to the temporal lobes shows that these patients often have mesial temporal lobe sclerosis with cell loss and atrophy (see Fig. 23.2).

Partial Seizures With Secondary Generalization

At times, an SPS or a CPS develops into a generalized tonic–clonic convulsion. Careful attention to the history is necessary to distinguish this secondarily generalized seizure from a primary generalized convulsion, especially when the event goes unwitnessed or the initial partial symptom may be brief or not recalled. Capturing a seizure with continuous EEG recordings may be the only way to differentiate a seizure with partial from a generalized onset.

GENERALIZED SEIZURES

Tonic–Clonic Seizures

CLINICAL VIGNETTE *A 40-year-old patient experiences events in which he suddenly stiffens, cries out, loses consciousness, and progresses to have rhythmic tonic–clonic movements of all four extremities lasting several minutes. The events are associated with incontinence, tongue bites, muscle soreness, and ultimately a state of somnolence. Several hours later, the patient was awake and back to normal but had no recollection of the event.*

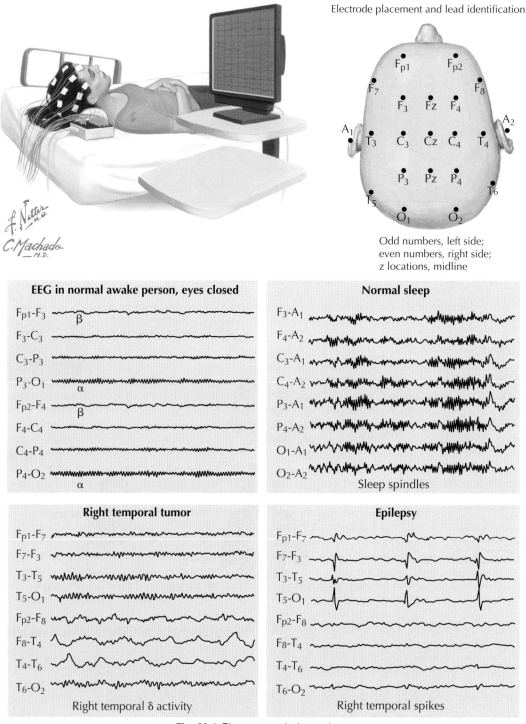

Electrode placement and lead identification

Odd numbers, left side;
even numbers, right side;
z locations, midline

EEG in normal awake person, eyes closed

Fp1-F3 β

F3-C3

C3-P3

P3-O1 α

Fp2-F4 β

F4-C4

C4-P4

P4-O2 α

Normal sleep

F3-A1

F4-A2

C3-A1

C4-A2

P3-A1

P4-A2

O1-A1

O2-A2

Sleep spindles

Right temporal tumor

Fp1-F7

F7-F3

T3-T5

T5-O1

Fp2-F8

F8-T4

T4-T6

T6-O2

Right temporal δ activity

Epilepsy

Fp1-F7

F7-F3

T3-T5

T5-O1

Fp2-F8

F8-T4

T4-T6

T6-O2

Right temporal spikes

Fig. 23.4 Electroencephalography.

This type of seizure represents the classic picture that the public and medical community generically perceives as epilepsy. Generalized seizure begins with simultaneous and almost equal involvement of both hemispheres from the onset and, unlike partial seizures with focal cortical abnormalities, involve the deeper thalamic, subcortical, and brainstem structures in a feedback loop to the cortices. Tonic–clonic seizures are often preceded by nonspecific, vaguely defined prodromes lasting at times up to hours or have no promontory symptoms at all. Seizures with specific auras, on the other hand, usually are of a focal origin with secondary generalization.

Generalized tonic–clonic seizures start with loss of consciousness, an ictal cry, generalized tonic muscle contraction, and a fall (Fig. 23.6). Autonomic signs are often present during the tonic phase, including tachycardia, hypertension, cyanosis, salivation, sweating, and incontinence. The tonic muscle contraction becomes interrupted relatively soon and is followed by the clonic phase of the seizure with brief relaxation periods progressively lengthening until the seizure eventually abates. Patients may remain stuporous for a moment and eventually awaken confused with postictal headaches, lethargy, disorientation, and myalgia that may persist for up to a few days.

Primary

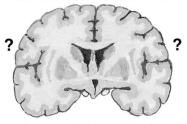

Unknown (genetic or biochemical predisposition)

Intracranial

Focal onset seizures with or without secondary generalization

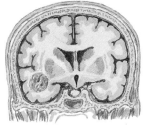

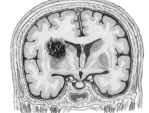

Tumor

Vascular (infarct or hemorrhage)

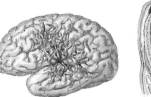

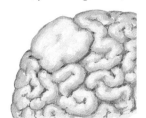

Arteriovenous malformation

Trauma (depressed fracture, penetrating wound)

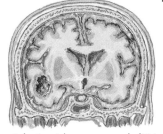

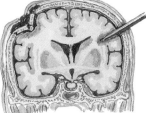

Infection (abscess, encephalitis)

Congenital and hereditary diseases (tuberous sclerosis)

Extracranial

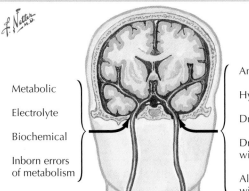

Metabolic

Electrolyte

Biochemical

Inborn errors of metabolism

Anoxia

Hypoglycemia

Drugs

Drug withdrawal

Alcohol withdrawal

Fig. 23.5 Causes of Seizures.

A single generalized tonic–clonic seizure does not warrant the diagnosis of epilepsy. In the vignette above, the patient later admitted that during the previous year, he was worried about his business and had been abusing alcohol and sedatives. He had recently discontinued these and had not had alcohol or sedatives for 48 hours. EEG and neuroimaging studies were normal. The seizure described above represents a reactive type of generalized tonic–clonic seizure secondary to drug withdrawal otherwise known as a provoked seizure. Similar seizures may occur from severe sleep deprivation, withdrawal from other drugs, trauma, central nervous system (CNS) infection, and various metabolic conditions.

Absence Seizures

> **CLINICAL VIGNETTE** *A 10-year-old boy is noted to have abrupt and brief (~10-second) episodes of impaired alertness. These can be brought out particularly when he hyperventilates. Eye fluttering is often noted during the episodes and occasional lip movements. The child returns to normal right after the episodes and the neurologic examination is normal.*

This is the typical history of a child with generalized absence (petit mal) seizures. Absence epilepsy is the classic example of benign primary generalized epilepsy, which occurs during 4–8 years of age and tends to remit in adulthood. Brief lapses in consciousness without an aura or any postictal symptoms are the main features (Fig. 23.7). Automatic movements, fluttering of the eyes, and transient loss of tone may be observed but are generally simple and brief. The neurologic examination is usually normal.

EEG provides the best diagnostic confirmation and typically demonstrates generalized bilaterally synchronous 3-Hz spike-and-wave discharges and a normal background. Hyperventilation may precipitate absence seizures and the classic EEG changes described above.

Atypical Absence Seizures

Atypical absence seizures differ from typical absence seizures because motor symptoms are more prominent and sometimes have a focal preponderance. Additionally, some patients have postictal confusion. Usually beginning during childhood, atypical absence seizures tend to occur over a longer lifetime period than typical absence seizures. Children with atypical absence seizures tend to have multifocal or generalized cerebral pathology, clinically associated with a lag in attaining normal developmental milestones.

The EEG demonstrates a slow (1.5–2.5 Hz) generalized bilaterally synchronous spike-and-wave pattern. This clinical constellation with its associated seizures and EEG pattern are characteristic of the Lennox–Gastaut syndrome. Generally, these patients also have other seizure types, and treatment of the seizures is difficult, usually requiring multiple anticonvulsants.

Myoclonic Seizures

> **CLINICAL VIGNETTE** *A 20-year-old college student reports a history of muscle jerks involving either arm for the past several years, which tended to occur in the morning. She also had two recent unexplained falls, without lapse of consciousness during the falls. Her neurologic examination results were normal. On two occasions, once after staying up late studying for exams, and another after drinking alcohol to excess and missing her medications, she had a generalized tonic–clonic seizure.*

The above-described patient has juvenile myoclonic epilepsy (JME), a primary generalized epilepsy syndrome that usually begins during the teenage years and is associated with morning myoclonic jerks soon

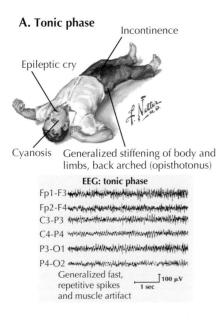

A. Tonic phase

Incontinence

Epileptic cry

Cyanosis

Cyanosis   Generalized stiffening of body and limbs, back arched (opisthotonus)

EEG: tonic phase

Fp1-F3
Fp2-F4
C3-P3
C4-P4
P3-O1
P4-O2

Generalized fast, repetitive spikes and muscle artifact

$100 \mu V$
$1 sec$

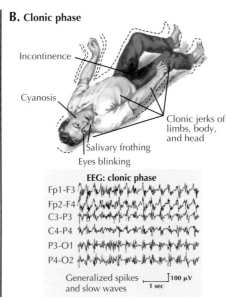

B. Clonic phase

Incontinence

Cyanosis

Clonic jerks of limbs, body, and head

Salivary frothing
Eyes blinking

EEG: clonic phase

Fp1-F3
Fp2-F4
C3-P3
C4-P4
P3-O1
P4-O2

Generalized spikes and slow waves

$100 \mu V$
$1 sec$

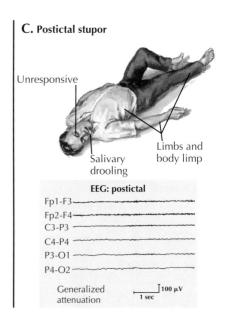

C. Postictal stupor

Unresponsive

Salivary drooling

Limbs and body limp

EEG: postictal

Fp1-F3
Fp2-F4
C3-P3
C4-P4
P3-O1
P4-O2

Generalized attenuation

$100 \mu V$
$1 sec$

Fig. 23.6 Generalized Tonic–Clonic Seizures.

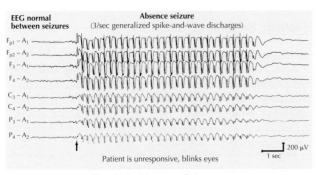

Between seizures patient normal

Seizure: vacant stare, eyes roll upward, eyelids flutter (3/sec), cessation of activity, lack of response

EEG normal between seizures   **Absence seizure** (3/sec generalized spike-and-wave discharges)

$F_{p1} - A_1$
$F_{p2} - A_2$
$F_3 - A_1$
$F_4 - A_2$
$C_3 - A_1$
$C_4 - A_2$
$P_3 - A_1$
$P_4 - A_2$

Patient is unresponsive, blinks eyes

$200 \mu V$
$1 sec$

Fig. 23.7 Absence Seizures.

after awakening. Many of these patients have occasional generalized seizures, especially under periods of physiologic stress. The EEG typically demonstrates generalized bilaterally synchronous 4–6-Hz polyspike and wave discharges. Paradoxically, the EEG discharges usually have no clinical myoclonic accompaniment. This condition responds generally well to antiepileptic medication and in a small percentage of patients remits spontaneously in later years.

Myoclonic seizures also may occur in children with a variety of epileptic syndromes such as the Lennox–Gastaut syndrome, infantile spasms (West syndrome), and early myoclonic encephalopathy. Myoclonus also may be a part of CNS storage diseases. In the past, myoclonus occurred as a significant manifestation of a rare late form of measles or subacute sclerosing panencephalitis. This illness presented with poor school performance, mental changes, and myoclonus in teenagers, with periodic EEG complexes occurring regularly every several seconds.

In contrast to myoclonic seizures, myoclonus is a nonspecific term that describes brief nonepileptic muscle jerks. They may involve a body segment or be generalized, may be single or repetitive, and may be spontaneous or provoked by sensory stimulation (reflex) or limb action. Myoclonus may be mediated by cortical, subcortical, brainstem, or spinal cord mechanisms.

Myoclonus may be due to the postanoxic syndrome (Lance–Adams syndrome) following prolonged cardiac arrest and resuscitation. Prognosis for full recovery in those who display myoclonus is generally poor. In the adult population, myoclonus is one of the classic findings in the prion-induced dementing illness or transmissible spongiform encephalopathy (Creutzfeldt–Jakob disease). This disease usually occurs in mid to later ages of life. The EEG in Creutzfeldt–Jakob disease has a classic appearance with generalized periodic sharp and slow wave complexes recurring usually at 1–2 Hz. The background EEG is abnormal.

EPILEPTIC SYNDROMES

Stereotypic seizures at a particular age associated with fairly distinct EEG abnormalities or a symptom complex constitute the epileptic syndromes. The seizures in these syndromes may be classified into reactive, the best known being benign febrile convulsions; primary or idiopathic, exemplified by childhood absence epilepsy; and secondary or symptomatic, for example, infantile spasms or West syndrome.

Simple Febrile Convulsions

Simple febrile convulsions occur in otherwise healthy children at the age of 6 months to 5 years. Up to 5% of healthy children in the United States experience at least one febrile convulsion, usually early during a benign febrile illness. The seizures are brief, lasting less than 15 minutes, and without any focal symptoms or signs. Interictal EEGs are always normal. If not, other seizure mechanisms should be considered. The long-term prognosis is usually excellent if seizures are generalized, not afebrile and last less than 15 minutes.

Benign Childhood Epilepsy With Centrotemporal (Rolandic) Spikes

Benign childhood epilepsy with centrotemporal (rolandic) spikes is an idiopathic focal epileptic syndrome that develops during the first decade of life. Typically, these children have partial seizures characterized by unilateral perioral sensory or minor motor activity associated with dysarthria or speech arrest, salivation, and preserved consciousness. Nocturnal generalized convulsions may occur. Children have normal intelligence and neurologic examination.

The EEG here demonstrates distinctive high-amplitude spikes or sharp waves with maximum electronegativity in the centrotemporal regions and positivity in the frontal regions. These epileptiform discharges, which increase during sleep, are commonly bilateral, shifting in preponderance from side to side, or occur independently. Although the etiology is unknown, autosomal dominant inheritance is suggested. The prognosis is excellent for this benign type of epilepsy.

West Syndrome

West syndrome is an example of a secondary (symptomatic) generalized epileptic syndrome occurring during the first year of life. West syndrome consists of a triad of infantile spasms, arrest of psychomotor development, and hypsarrhythmia. The spasms are characterized by brief jerks followed by a tonic phase and a subsequent period of generalized atonia lasting approximately 1 minute or associated with flexion–extension spasms.

The chaotic appearance of a typical EEG, called hypsarrhythmia, shows high-amplitude slow-wave activity with mixed high-amplitude sharp or spike discharges. The EEG correlate of the spasm is a sudden appearance of high-amplitude slow waves followed by an electrodecremental period with low-voltage fast activity. West syndrome is most often symptomatic but a small group is idiopathic. Usually the prognosis is poor. The primary treatment is corticotropin administration or oral steroids.

STATUS EPILEPTICUS

> **CLINICAL VIGNETTE** *A 60-year-old patient has a witnessed tonic–clonic seizure. 911 is called, and en route to the local hospital, he has repeated tonic–clonic seizures, without regaining consciousness between episodes. He becomes cyanotic with labored breathing and requires emergent intubation.*

Generalized convulsive status epilepticus (GCSE) is defined as recurrent seizures without recovery of consciousness lasting more than 30 minutes or when seizure activity becomes unremitting (Fig. 23.8). One of the most common and life-threatening neurologic emergencies, GCSE mandates immediate treatment because of the potential for irreversible CNS damage, that is, neuronal loss secondary to anoxia and systemic metabolic and autonomic dysfunction. Medical complications such as cardiac arrhythmias, pulmonary edema, and renal failure sometimes occur in association with GCSE. The GCSE mortality rate approaches 30%. Unfortunately, the

history in the above vignette in this chapter is common in patients with partial seizures with secondary generalization who do not comply with antiepileptic therapy and progress to status epilepticus.

Treatment of GCSE requires the maintenance of an adequate airway, ventilation, and circulatory support and the termination of seizures. Etiologic mechanisms include anticonvulsant or other medication withdrawal, illicit toxic drugs, hypoglycemia, hyponatremia, and hypocalcemia. GCSE may be the first manifestation of acute cerebral pathology.

The initial therapy, a benzodiazepine or phenytoin, often depends on whether the patient is actively seizing. Both first-line medications are frequently utilized within a short time. Intravenous lorazepam at 1–2 mg every 1–2 minutes up to 8 mg or diazepam 5 mg up to 20 mg is most often the initial therapy. A load of fosphenytoin (at 150 mg/min) up to 20 mg/kg must also be started promptly because of the short-term effect of benzodiazepines. Phenytoin is given with normal saline and not with glucose as it precipitates out of solution in this vehicle. ECG monitoring is required to monitor the effects of phenytoin on cardiac conduction, especially if infused too rapidly. Hypotension is also a serious side effect, especially in patients showing evidence of hemodynamic instability. The propylene glycol and alcohol content of the intravenous preparation is thought to be partially responsible for these effects and is dependent on the infusion rate. Fosphenytoin, a water-soluble phosphate ester rapidly converted to phenytoin, can be administered at a more rapid rate (150 mg/min of phenytoin equivalent) while minimizing the risk of cardiovascular instability in unstable patients. Fosphenytoin also has a lower incidence of pain and burning at the infusion site, but its routine use remains restricted because of its high cost. If seizures persist and serum phenytoin levels drawn 20 minutes after the initial infusion are less than 20 mg/dL, then additional phenytoin or fosphenytoin (5–10 mg/kg) to control seizure and maintain the level around 20–30 mg/dL may be given. Sodium valproate IV, at a loading dose of 20 mg/kg, has also been used successfully to control status epilepticus, especially in patients on regular regimens of oral valproic acid.

Barbiturates have been traditionally used as second-line agents in status epilepticus. Long-acting phenobarbital (at 50–100 mg/min, up to 20 mg/kg) or short-acting pentobarbital (3–5 mg/kg loading dose, followed by an infusion of 3–5 mg/kg per hour) may be added. Intubation for airway protection and continuous EEG monitoring are usually required at this stage. Over the years, however, many centers have shifted to using continuous infusions of other agents, such as the short-acting benzodiazepine midazolam or the hypnotic propofol (decreases excitatory effect of glutamate) for control of recurrent seizures. Many centers now use continuous infusion of benzodiazepines such as midazolam or propofol before barbiturate anesthesia is initiated.

Nonconvulsive status epilepticus or absence status epilepticus is another form of continued seizures without motor accompaniments. Typically, patients are poorly responsive with decreased alertness or obtundation. EEG reveals mostly continuous generalized spike-and-wave activity, the so-called spike–wave stupor. Intravenous benzodiazepine administration, the treatment of choice, is generally effective.

Complex partial seizures may occasionally evolve into complex partial status epilepticus, in which patients do not regain full consciousness between seizures. Prompt treatment as prescribed for GCSE is necessary. An SPS may evolve into epilepsia partialis continua, as described above. Long-term anticonvulsant therapy is usually needed in patients who have experienced status epilepticus.

ANTIEPILEPTIC THERAPY

The goal of antiepileptic treatment is the control of seizures. The most important step in seizure treatment is identification and treatment of the primary pathophysiologic mechanism. Examples include resection

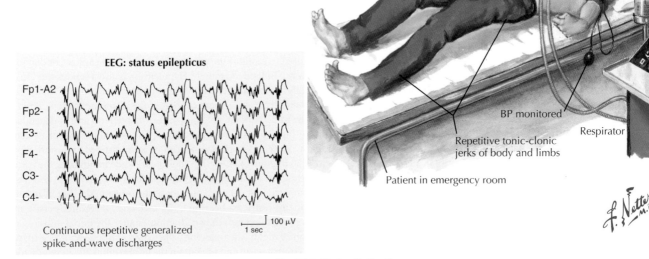

Stepwise Treatment Options in Status Epilepticus
1. Benzodiazepines (e.g., lorazepam, diazepam)
   Fosphenytoin

2. Barbiturates
   Consider:
       Valproic acid
       Newer AEDs (e.g., levetiracetam, topiramate)

3. Intubation, EEG monitoring, and continuous infusion of
   pentobarbital
   Midazolam
   More recently considered agent in adults: propofol

Fig. 23.8 Status Epilepticus.

of a tumor, correction of a metabolic imbalance, and treatment of a CNS infection. Appropriate therapy may stop seizure recurrence.

Unfortunately, most seizures occur with chronic neurologic processes and are not amenable to specific curative therapy and therefore require long-term treatment. The ideal seizure medication would have high efficacy across a broad range of seizure types, with no adverse effects and little interaction with other drugs. Unfortunately, no such anticonvulsant exists, and treatment must balance seizure control with quality of life. Choosing an anticonvulsant must be done on an individual basis, considering seizure or epilepsy type, side effects, comorbidities, and psychosocial factors such as age, sex, ease of use, and cost.

There is no single approach to medication selection, and good knowledge of the available drugs and their basic properties is essential. Seizure-free rates have been shown to be similar between the older and newer antiseizure medications. Newer agents are well tolerated, require less monitoring, and may be safer in the long term. With time and increasing regulatory approval, these anticonvulsants, initially approved for use as adjunctive agents, may soon replace the older ones as first-line agents in seizure management. Still, the newer medications are often more costly and may present various drug-specific side effects or issues. In addition, the therapeutic ranges are not as well established as compared to the older agents. With the exception of levetiracetam and lacosamide, the newer agents are not available in parenteral form. The variety of mechanisms of action of the newer medications has allowed these preparations to be possibly useful in other neurologic conditions such as for bipolar disease, headache, and neuropathic pain.

Phenobarbital and primidone are among the oldest antiseizure medications and are effective in all types of partial seizures and secondary generalized tonic–clonic seizures. Primidone is metabolized to phenobarbital and phenylethylmalonamide (PEMA) and has similar pharmacokinetics as phenobarbital. Both medications bind to the β-2 subunit of the γ-aminobutyric acid (GABAa) receptor, allowing GABA to bind to the β-1 subunit and increase chloride conductance. They are metabolized by the hepatic cytochrome p-450 system. The half-life is about 72 hours. Adverse effects are sedation and rash. To minimize sedation, phenobarbital can be given in once a day doses of 1.5–4 mg/kg per day. Primidone is usually given in doses of 750–1500 mg/day in 3–4 divided doses.

Phenytoin is another long-established anticonvulsant used for more than 50 years initially as a superior less-sedating alternative to barbiturates. It is effective for partial onset seizures of all types and secondary generalized tonic–clonic seizures. Phenytoin's presumed mechanism of action is through the blockade of membrane voltage-dependent sodium channels to increase transmembrane potential recovery time and limit high-frequency firing. At higher concentrations, phenytoin delays efflux of potassium and prolongs neuronal refractory periods. It is metabolized by the hepatic cytochrome p-450 system and its half-life is 12–36 hours, thus allowing twice-a-day dosing (5–7 mg/kg or about 300–500 mg/day). Optimum seizure control occurs with blood levels of 10–20 mg/mL. When plasma levels are higher there is a shift from first-order to zero-order kinetics with a longer half-life and with rapid increases in concentration levels and subsequent toxicity caused by small increases in the dose. Acute side effects mimic alcohol intoxication with dizziness, nystagmus, ataxia, slurred speech, and confusion. Prolonged use may produce coarsening facial features, gingival hyperplasia, acne, hirsutism, cerebellar impairment, megaloblastic anemia, and, at times, polyneuropathy. Acute idiosyncratic reactions occur in approximately 10% of patients and vary from a mild morbilliform rash to a rare severe exfoliative dermatitis. As with other anticonvulsants, teratogenic effects may occur. Phenytoin interacts with numerous drugs of many classes and close monitoring of the levels is advised whenever such medications are prescribed.

Carbamazepine is effective for partial seizures of all types and secondary generalized tonic–clonic seizures. It acts presumably by blocking Na channels in the brain and inhibiting depolarization of seizure foci in the brain without affecting the normal neuronal function. The usual dose is 400–1200 mg/day and the therapeutic blood serum level is between 4 and 12 mg/L. Adverse reactions relate to CNS depression and dizziness, nausea, as well as reversible and dose-dependent neutropenia and hyponatremia. Hypersensitive allergic reactions and Stevens–Johnson syndrome can occur early on within a few weeks of treatment.

Oxcarbazepine has a similar mechanism of action to carbamazepine via its rapid and complete metabolism to an active 10-monohydroxy derivative. Oxcarbazepine has linear pharmacokinetics, no autoinduction, minimal interaction with other seizure medications, and does not cause neutropenia. Hyponatremia sometimes occurs. Adverse reactions include psychomotor slowing and sedation but, on the whole, it may be better tolerated than carbamazepine. The typical starting dosage is 300 mg twice daily, increased gradually to 450 mg twice daily, and the therapeutic blood serum level is between 12 and 25 mg/L. Occasionally, higher dosages are used but should not exceed 2400 mg daily.

Divalproex sodium is an extremely effective drug for absence, myoclonic, and primary generalized tonic–clonic seizures. It can also be used for partial seizures. It inhibits calcium ion influx through T-type calcium channels and inhibits sodium ion influx through voltage-gated sodium channels. The therapeutic blood level ranges from 50 to 150 µg/mL, and it is given in doses of 1000–3000 mg/day. Divalproex sodium inhibits the hepatic cytochrome p-450 system and will therefore diminish the metabolism of other drugs. Adverse effects are gastrointestinal upset, somnolence, dizziness, tremor, weight gain, and hair loss. More serious effects include hepatotoxicity, pancreatitis, thrombocytopenia, polycystic ovarian disease, and teratogenic effects (neural tube defects and lowered IQ).

Ethosuximide is the first antiseizure drug used to treat absence (petit mal) seizures. It is thought to inhibit calcium ion influx through T-type calcium channels. Adverse effects are gastrointestinal and CNS related, but this drug is generally well tolerated. A common dose is 250–2000 mg/day according to age and response. The therapeutic blood level is 40–100 µg/mL.

Felbamate blocks voltage-dependent sodium channels and N-methyl-D-aspartate (NMDA) receptors and was found to be more effective than divalproex sodium in partial seizures and had a significant benefit for Lennox–Gastaut syndrome. It is better tolerated than other drugs, with relatively minor gastrointestinal and cognitive adverse effects. Unfortunately, its relatively high rates of (at times fatal) hepatotoxicity and aplastic anemia have severely restricted its use to those with severe epilepsy, such as Lennox–Gastaut syndrome.

Several other agents such as lamotrigine, gabapentin, topiramate, levetiracetam, tiagabine, pregabalin, and zonisamide as well as newer drugs such as lacosamide, perampanel, brivaracetam, eslicarbazepine, and rufinamide are recommended as adjunctive to the first-line medications of carbamazepine, phenytoin, phenobarbital, primidone, or valproate. Because they have different mechanisms of action, they may complement the traditional first-line drugs. However, many of these drugs such as lamotrigine, topiramate, levetiracetam, zonisamide, lacosamide, brivaracetam, eslicarbazepine, and perampanel have been used successfully as monotherapy in selected patients.

Lamotrigine is a newer antiepileptic drug recommended as an adjunct medication for partial seizures, primary generalized tonic–clonic seizures for patients of all ages, and Lennox–Gastaut syndrome. It is indicated for conversion to monotherapy in adults with partial seizures treated with the older anticonvulsants, carbamazepine, phenytoin, phenobarbital, primidone, or valproate. Lamotrigine blocks voltage-gated sodium and calcium channels and inhibits the presynaptic release of glutamate and aspartate. Metabolized by glucuronidation, it is not an enzyme inducer or inhibitor. When prescribed with an enzyme-inducing antiseizure medication, lamotrigine serum concentration may decrease by up to 40%. Frequent monitoring is therefore needed when switching to lamotrigine monotherapy. It has a half-life of about 12–60 hours, and typical adult doses are 300–500 mg/day divided twice a day with a therapeutic target range of 3–15 mg/L. It must be introduced at low doses with slow titration to the desired maintenance level over months to reduce the risk of Stevens–Johnson syndrome. Adverse effects are gastrointestinal and CNS related. There is a 10% risk of an idiosyncratic rash and a 3 in 1000 risk of Stevens–Johnson syndrome in adults, and the risk is more common in patients receiving valproic acid. There are no known long-term effects.

Levetiracetam is another antiepileptic medication whose mechanism of action is not completely understood but may involve modulating neurotransmitter release at the SV2A binding receptor complex. It is indicated for partial seizures and primary and secondary generalized seizures. The usual adult maintenance dose is between 1000 and 1500 mg divided twice a day. Doses higher than 3000 mg/day may not add benefit. An intravenous formulation is also available. It is not an enzyme inducer or inhibitor and has few drug interactions with other medications. Levetiracetam is eliminated renally with a half-life of 6–8 hours. Adverse effects include sedation, lethargy, or ataxia. Not to be overlooked are behavioral changes seen at higher doses around 3000 mg/day with aggression, depression, suicidal ideation, and, in extreme cases, frank psychosis.

Gabapentin is usually used as adjunctive therapy for partial seizures with or without secondary generalization. There is concern that it may worsen absence and myoclonic seizure and should generally be avoided in primary generalized epilepsy syndromes. It is an analogue of GABA; however, its exact mechanism of action is unknown. It is not an enzyme inducer or inhibitor and is eliminated through the renal system with a half-life of about 5–6 hours. It is given in doses of 900–3600 mg/day in divided doses. Adverse effects are somnolence, dizziness, ataxia, fatigue, weight gain, and behavioral changes, especially in children.

Topiramate blocks voltage-gated sodium channels, enhances GABA-mediated synaptic inhibition, and antagonizes the excitatory effect of glutamate on NMDA receptors. It has limited hepatic metabolism with a half-life of about 20 hours, and typical doses are 100–400 mg/day divided twice a day. Topiramate can increase phenytoin levels. It is indicated as an adjuvant treatment or monotherapy of partial, primary, and secondary generalized tonic–clonic seizures as well as in Lennox–Gastaut syndrome. Adverse effects are CNS related, including cognitive impairment or word-finding difficulty, weight loss, decreased sweating, glaucoma, and a 1%–1.5% risk of kidney stones.

Zonisamide blocks voltage-gated sodium channels and inhibits calcium ion influx through T-type calcium channels. It is not an enzyme inducer or inhibitor, has hepatic metabolism followed by glucuronidation, and has a half-life of about 63 hours. It is recommended for partial seizures and secondary tonic–clonic generalized seizures. It is usually given in doses of 200–400 mg once a day. Adverse effects are CNS related, rash, decreased sweating, weight loss, and a 0.6% risk of kidney stones.

Tiagabine is indicated for use as adjunctive therapy for refractory partial seizures. It is a GABA uptake inhibitor, is not an enzyme inducer or inhibitor, has hepatic metabolism, and a half-life of about 7–9 hours. Adverse effects are CNS related, rash, and nonconvulsive status.

Pregabalin is usually used as adjunctive therapy for partial seizures. Its exact mechanism of action is not known, is not an enzyme inducer or inhibitor, has renal metabolism, and has a half-life of about 6 hours. Adverse effects are CNS related, weight gain, and peripheral edema.

Lacosamide is an antiseizure medication approved as adjuvant therapy for partial-onset seizures but is also used in some cases as monotherapy. It is available in oral and IV formulations and is thought to work by the unique mechanism of selectively modulating the slow inactivation of voltage-gated sodium channels. It is renally excreted, has few drug interactions, and it is usually given in doses of 200–400 mg per day divided twice a day. CNS and behavioral adverse effects have been described but are thought to be less frequent than with levetiracetam.

Perampanel is a selective, noncompetitive AMPA receptor antagonist, used as monotherapy or adjunctive treatment for patients with partial seizures and as adjunctive treatment for patients with primary tonic–clonic generalized seizures. It has a long half-life between 53 and 136 hours. It is usually given in doses of 4–12 mg once daily at bedtime. Common side effects include CNS-related symptoms and there is a warning for psychiatric symptoms including aggression.

Ideally, a single antiepileptic drug is used. If adequate control of seizures is not achieved with one drug, another drug is substituted. Discontinuing antiseizure medications should be done gradually over 2–3 months to avoid withdrawal seizures from rebound.

Anticonvulsant Treatment Considerations

The decision to treat with antiepileptic drugs a first-time unprovoked seizure remains an individualized process that takes into account the structural integrity of the brain, the EEG findings, the circumstances surrounding the seizure, past history of provoked or unprovoked seizures, as well as the potential side effects of medications prescribed.

The incidence of recurrence after a single unprovoked seizure varies widely from 10% to 70%. Within the first 2 years the chances of a recurrent seizure is highest (21%–45%). Predictors of recurrent seizures are an abnormal EEG demonstrating epileptiform discharges (especially generalized patterns), focal spikes or sharp waves, nocturnal seizures, abnormal MRI scans, and an abnormal neurologic examination. Although only about 30% or fewer of EEGs done in adults will yield significant abnormalities, these have a strong predictive power of recurrent seizures in up to 50%–60% of patients within 2–3 years.

Any patient presenting with a first-time seizure will require, in addition to a detailed neurologic history and examination, imaging of the brain (preferably an MRI) and an EEG in the awake and sleep states. Other studies such as a toxic screen and lumbar puncture have a low general yield but may be helpful in specific clinical situations.

The decision to start an antiepileptic medication after a first-time unprovoked seizure is individualized and should be based on the risk of recurrent seizures. Patients with abnormal EEG, MRI, or a nocturnal seizure are at higher risks and should start treatment. Immediate short-term antiepileptic medication reduces the likelihood of recurrent seizures by half to two-thirds but does not affect the long-term prognosis of seizure remission over 3 years. If the risk of recurrent seizures is low, as seen in patients with normal exam, EEG, and MRI, then treatment may be deferred. Although immediate treatment may delay the loss of driving privileges, quality of life did not seem to improve over 2 years in patients treated early.

It is recommended that patients remain seizure free for about 2–5 years before considering discontinuation of antiepileptic drugs (AEDs). The recurrence rate and the predictive factors are similar to those mentioned above for first-time seizures. However, strong consideration should be given to the impact that a recurrent seizure, no matter how unlikely, may have on the life of active and productive patients under good seizure control and the impact on those who rely on them.

WOMEN WITH EPILEPSY

There are special considerations regarding management of women with epilepsy. Seizures and AEDs may impact menstruation, contraception, bone health, menopause, pregnancy, and breast feeding. The majority of women with epilepsy have routine pregnancies and deliver healthy babies. However, detailed discussions with patients about the potential teratogenic effects and the risks of seizures must begin prior to conception. About 25% of women experience an increase in seizures during pregnancy because of poor compliance, lowered anticonvulsant levels and protein binding, hormonal changes, or sleep deprivation. The incidence of preeclampsia (pregnancy-induced hypertension), preterm delivery, intrauterine bleeding, hyperemesis gravidarum, and abruptio placenta is increased twofold in women with epilepsy.

Generalized tonic–clonic seizures are harmful to a developing fetus and can cause seizure-related trauma, intrauterine death, and miscarriage. The risk of major fetal malformations for women with epilepsy is 4%–6% compared to 2%–3% in the healthy population. The major congenital anomalies include cleft lip or palate and urogenital, cardiac, and neural tube defects. Most antiseizure medications have potential teratogenic effects caused by varying degrees of folate deficiency. The risk is highest with valproic acid and increases with polypharmacy as well as higher concentration levels of antiseizure medication. The risk of major malformations, particularly neural tube defects, with valproic acid is 9.3%, phenobarbital 5.5%, topiramate 4.2%, carbamazepine 2.0%, phenytoin 2.9%, levetiracetam 2.4%, and lamotrigine 2.0%, with these data coming from the North American pregnancy registry.

Some women with medically refractory epilepsy consider epilepsy surgery to attain seizure freedom before planning pregnancy. In many circumstances, seizure-free women may be tapered off their antiseizure medication before conception. Women may choose not to take antiepileptic medications in the first trimester during organogenesis, especially if the seizure type is minor and infrequent. Not all patients can do this safely and there is evidence to suggest adverse effects of recurrent complex partial seizures on fetal growth and development. The goal throughout pregnancy is to remain seizure free while exposing the fetus to the least number of drugs and the lowest possible levels of antiseizure medication.

The neural tube closes between the 24th and the 27th day after conception. Folate reduces the risk of neural tube defects in the general population. Because neural tube closure defects occur early, before many women may realize they are pregnant, prophylaxis with folic acid is recommended in all epileptic women of childbearing age. The optimal dose of folic acid is not known but ranges from 0.4 to 5 mg/day. Tests to assess for neural tube and other anticonvulsant-induced congenital defects should be considered routine prenatal care.

Antiepileptic medications during pregnancy require close monitoring and often frequent adjustments to maintain the desired therapeutic levels. Serum levels decrease during pregnancy because of accelerated hepatic metabolism, changes in plasma volume, absorption, and protein binding. With the exception of lamotrigine, the newer antiseizure medications may be less prone to fluctuating levels during pregnancy. Pregnant women with epilepsy should be under the care of a high-risk obstetrician. Maternal serum alpha fetoprotein and a high-level ultrasound are recommended at 14–18 weeks and may be repeated at 22–24 weeks to screen for anomalies. About 3%–4% of epileptic women experience a seizure around delivery. The risk is highest in women with subtherapeutic drug levels, idiopathic generalized epilepsy, or a history of seizures during pregnancy.

Infants should be given 1 mg of vitamin K intramuscularly at birth to prevent fetal hemorrhage. Antiseizure medication levels need to be monitored postpartum because levels will gradually return to baseline 8–10 weeks after delivery. Lamotrigine levels decrease markedly during pregnancy because of increased clearance and need to be monitored closely after delivery to avoid postpartum toxicity. The concern of exposing nursing infants to antiseizure medication should be discussed with the mother. Most antiseizure medications have a milk-to-plasma ratio of less than 1, but the serum level below which there are no clinical effects on the neonate is unknown. Other than congenital malformations, children exposed in utero to phenobarbital and valproic acid may be at increased risk of cognitive deficits with lower verbal IQ and greater need for special education. The Neurodevelopmental Effects of Antiepileptic Drugs study is currently under way to assess children's neurobehavioral outcomes in mothers with epilepsy and those exposed to antiseizure medications.

Estrogen may have proconvulsant effects by reducing GABAa inhibition, whereas progesterone may have anticonvulsant effects by increasing GABAa inhibition. Women are prone to seizures during ovulation as a result of increased estrogen midcycle. Seizures may also increase a few days before or occur during the first days of menses, because of the rapid decline of progesterone that triggers menstruation. Women with anovulatory cycles fail to form a progesterone-secreting corpus luteum and can experience an increase in seizures during the second half of their cycle because of low progesterone levels. If a pattern can be documented, an increase in the daily dose of medication at the expected time of seizures may help control seizures. Use of acetazolamide, around the time of expected increase in seizures, has had some limited success.

Contraceptive pills are less effective in women taking hepatic enzyme–inducing antiseizure medications (carbamazepine, oxcarbazepine, phenobarbital, phenytoin, primidone) with a 6% failure rate. Topiramate in doses of >200 mg/day increases the clearance of estradiol and thus reduces its effectiveness. The American Academy of Neurology suggests that women on the above-mentioned antiseizure medication take higher doses of estradiol, but the lower progesterone dose may still lead to hormonal failure. Depo-Provera may be an alternative if given every 10 weeks instead of 12 weeks. Patients should be referred to their gynecologist to discuss and manage these issues long term. On the other hand, oral contraceptives in their turn may reduce lamotrigine and valproic acid levels. Levels should be monitored when oral contraceptives are initiated or discontinued. Intrauterine devices are effective in patients taking enzyme-inducing drugs and may be a safer alternative to oral contraceptives in preventing pregnancy.

Women with epilepsy may experience early menopause. There is some concern that estrogen replacement therapy might be associated with increased seizures. Although estrogen is not strictly contraindicated in women with epilepsy, selective estrogen receptor modulators may be a better alternative.

Patients with epilepsy are at increased risk for osteoporosis and fractures. Bone loss is caused by virtually all the anticonvulsants and is not restricted to the hepatic enzyme–inducing drugs. The mechanism remains obscure and no clear data exist as to which agent may be preferable. A dual-energy x-ray absorptiometry (DEXA) scan is generally recommended after 2 years of treatment with an anticonvulsant. Patients with osteopenia are advised calcium 1200 mg/day and vitamin D 800 IU/day, and lifestyle changes that include weight-bearing exercise, decreased alcohol consumption, and smoking cessation. Patients with osteoporosis should be referred to a specialist and followed closely.

All pregnant women with epilepsy, whether or not taking any antiseizure medication, should be encouraged to enroll in the North American Pregnancy Registry (www.aedpregnancyregistry.org), a prospective study to assess the risk of major fetal malformations.

SURGICAL TREATMENTS FOR EPILEPSY

Surgical treatment may be an option for individuals whose seizures are unresponsive to medical therapy or those who cannot take medications because of significant adverse effects or quality-of-life issues. Some of the first craniotomies on record were performed to treat refractory seizure disorders. Cerebral localization was grossly defined by the specific characteristics of a seizure, and cerebral tumors were localized and removed based on these techniques. Many aspects of cortical mapping and function were derived from work related to surgery for epileptic activity.

Surgical Candidates

> **CLINICAL VIGNETTE** *A 36-year-old woman had febrile seizures as an infant followed by a latent period of about 12 years. Complex partial seizures characterized by a rising epigastric sensation and staring with oral automatisms and unresponsiveness returned at menarche, and continued 2–4 times monthly despite several medication trials. The patient could not drive, experienced medication side effects, and worsening short-term memory. MRI identified right mesial temporal sclerosis without any other overt structural abnormality.*
>
> *Inpatient video EEG monitoring revealed interictal right temporal spikes and concordant complex partial seizures. Positron emission tomographic imaging revealed right temporal lobe hypometabolism.*

The above vignette identifies the typical clinical scenario of a patient with medically refractory mesial temporal lobe epilepsy with hippocampal sclerosis. Seizures are not fully controlled by medical therapy in about 30%–40% of patients with epilepsy. Once a patient fails to respond to two antiseizure drugs, the chance of achieving control on a third drug is small. The initial response to medication seen in the above vignette does not mean permanent seizure control. In a randomized controlled study of patients with refractory temporal lobe epilepsy, patients who underwent temporal lobectomy were more likely to be seizure free than the patients randomized to AED therapy (58% vs. 8%). Patients who underwent surgery had a significant improvement in their quality of life. Successful surgery not only can provide seizure control in patients, but also can arrest or reverse cognitive decline, lower the mortality, and relieve psychiatric disorders. Any patient in whom seizures persist after trials of two appropriate AEDs should be referred to a tertiary epilepsy center for surgical evaluation. Surgical evaluation consists of confirming a diagnosis of epilepsy and defining the location and extent of the epileptogenic zone. The above vignette represents a patient who is likely a candidate for an anterior temporal lobectomy that can often stop or completely cure the epilepsy.

Preoperative Assessments

Video EEG analysis is one of the mainstays of preoperative evaluations and is used to localize the ictal onset zone. The video is used to determine if the ictal semiology represents seizure origin or propagation. Often, seizures cannot be localized to one region of the brain but can be lateralized to one hemisphere, requiring invasive monitoring prior to surgical resection (Fig. 23.9). Invasive monitoring can also be utilized for functional mapping to define the boundaries of the epileptogenic zone in relation to eloquent cortex or key somatomotor regions that may be close to the potential resective zone. MRI is one of the most important structural neuroimaging tools in the presurgical evaluation of patients with medically refractory epilepsy. The presence of a structural abnormality may suggest site of seizure origin and surgical pathology. It can suggest a more favorable surgical outcome and help tailor the resection. The most common imaging finding in patients undergoing surgical evaluations is hippocampal atrophy best seen using T1-weighted coronal images and an increased mesial temporal signal intensity on T2-weighted or fluid-attenuated inversion recovery (FLAIR) coronal images. Magnetic resonance spectroscopy, positron emission tomography, single photon emission computed tomography, functional MRI, and magnetoencephalography are functional imaging tests that could better define the epileptogenic zone. In select cases, a Wada test can be

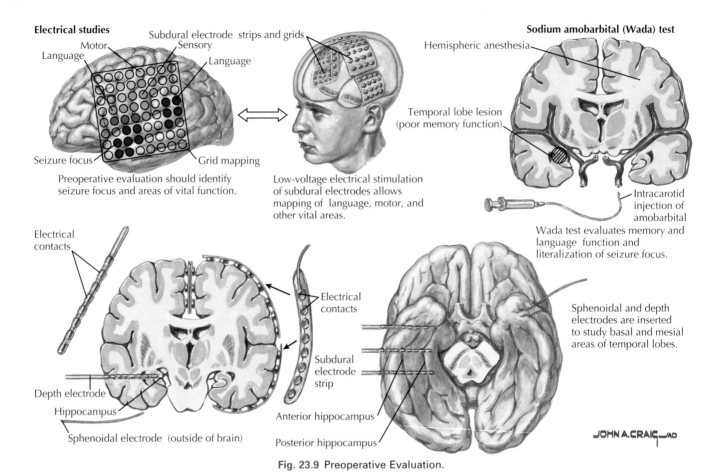

Fig. 23.9 Preoperative Evaluation.

performed for language and memory lateralization. Neuropsychological testing is performed to determine a patient's risk for postoperative memory decline. Ultimately, a decision regarding surgical treatment is based on a convergence of all these neurodiagnostic tests.

Types of Surgery
Temporal Lobectomy

Temporal lobectomy is the most common operation for epilepsy. When coupled with anatomic evidence of mesial temporal sclerosis, it has the best chance (~85%) for eliminating seizures. Typically, the resection includes a 3- to 6-cm section of neocortex from the superior, middle, inferior, and basal temporal gyri and the amygdalohippocampal complex (Fig. 23.10). Smaller-sized resections, usually less than 5 cm, should be considered on the dominant side, whereas a larger 6- or 7-cm segment may be removed from the nondominant temporal lobe. Larger resections risk damage to the optic radiation fibers (Meyer loop) and can result in contralateral superior quadrantanopia.

The precise location of the resected edge in the temporal cortex is often determined visually by appreciating the venous anatomy of the cortical surface, cortical arteries, and the sulcal pattern. A hippocampal resection, often performed separately, typically removes 3–4 cm of the hippocampus.

Focal Resection

If a relatively small area of extratemporal cortex can be defined as a specific seizure focus (typically with subdural grid electrodes, intraoperative cortical recordings of interictal spikes, or both), its removal can successfully eliminate focal seizures. Functionally relevant brain tissue, such as the visual or language cortex, known as the "eloquent" *cortex,* must be distinguished from less functional or "noneloquent"

areas. It is important that the focus to be resected is in a relatively "noneloquent" region of cortex, such as part of the anterior frontal lobe, and intraoperative mapping of motor or language areas may help avoid undue significant neurologic postoperative morbidity. Epileptogenic lesions such as cavernous malformations, or small tumors, may be removed using similar techniques.

> **CLINICAL VIGNETTE** *A 40-year-old patient with mental retardation has tonic and generalized tonic–clonic seizures, many of which result in falls with serious injuries. Video EEG reveals interictal slow generalized spike and wave and paroxysmal fast activity, and nonlocalized seizure onset. The seizures and falls continue despite medication trials.*

Corpus Callosotomy

Occasionally, surgical division of this important interhemispheric connector is helpful for controlling seizures that spread quickly from one side to the other. Drop attack seizures are good examples. The extent of surgery is debatable; generally an approximate 60%–80% resection is appropriate for the best outcome and the lowest degree of deficit. Left-handed patients with potential crossed dominance should undergo Wada's test before surgery because significant behavioral or language deficits may occur if language and handedness are entirely in opposite hemispheres.

Functional Hemispherectomy

Functional isolation of specific cerebral regions within each hemisphere is possible by dividing the fiber connections between frontal, temporal, and parietal lobes while avoiding large resection of cortex and sparing

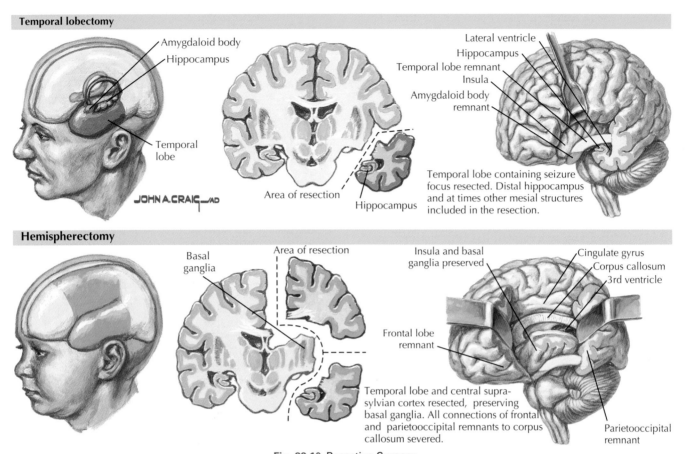

Temporal lobectomy

Amygdaloid body
Hippocampus
Temporal lobe

JOHN A.CRAIG—AD

Area of resection
Hippocampus

Lateral ventricle
Hippocampus
Temporal lobe remnant
Insula
Amygdaloid body remnant

Temporal lobe containing seizure focus resected. Distal hippocampus and at times other mesial structures included in the resection.

Hemispherectomy

Basal ganglia
Area of resection

Insula and basal ganglia preserved
Cingulate gyrus
Corpus callosum
3rd ventricle

Frontal lobe remnant

Temporal lobe and central suprasylvian cortex resected, preserving basal ganglia. All connections of frontal and parietooccipital remnants to corpus callosum severed.

Parietooccipital remnant

Fig. 23.10 Resective Surgery.

the deeper nuclei and structures such as the basal ganglia (see Fig. 23.10). Typically, these patients already have widespread contralateral neurologic deficits. Although this procedure is primarily used only in extremely severe generalized seizure disorders, such as Lennox–Gastaut syndrome, some children often regain significant neurologic function as new pathways develop in the years after surgery.

Multiple Subpial Transections

The multiple subpial transection procedure was developed to treat seizure foci localized to eloquent cortex. Surgical incisions with specially angled blades are made parallel to each other, 5 mm apart, across the cortex of interest, to section horizontally connected u-fibers while preserving many of the vertically oriented output fibers. Theoretically, it prevents spread of seizures through the cortex from this area. Although clinical outcomes vary, it may provide significant seizure control in settings where resection would be neurologically devastating. Often in the immediate postoperative period, a profound focal deficit occurs that resolves during a period of hours to weeks.

Vagus Nerve Stimulator

Stimulation of afferent fibers within the left vagus nerve can modify seizure activity. (The left contains approximately 80% afferent fibers, whereas stimulation of the right interferes with the cardiac cycle and may provoke asystole.) A set of three electrodes are coiled around the nerve after it has been dissected free within the carotid sheath in the neck. The electrodes are connected to a battery/pulse generator placed under the skin just below the clavicle. This appealing methodology does not require an intracranial procedure, although it is still prone to complications such as infection, bleeding, occasional hoarseness or coughing, and breathing dysregulation such as dyspnea and sleep apnea. Results vary, but some

patients have excellent seizure control or are seizure free. Cure rates of vagal nerve stimulation are approximately 5%–15% but may offer many patients the opportunity to reduce medications and enhance seizure control. This procedure warrants consideration in poorly controlled patients without a well-defined or accessible focus for resection.

Laser Ablation

MRI-guided laser interstitial thermal therapy stereotactically targets epileptogenic areas and heats cerebral structures to eliminate epileptogenic foci. Compared to a standard temporal lobectomy, laser ablation is less invasive, with lower risk of complications and a shorter hospitalization, but is less effective in stopping seizures.

Responsive Neurostimulation/NeuroPace

The responsive neurostimulation (RNS) contains two small implantable neurostimulators that are placed on the surface of the brain or deep in the brain. It records electrical activity and is able to detect seizures and deliver electrical pulses to terminate seizures. This is an option for patients that are not candidates for resective surgery such as in bitemporal epilepsy or epilepsy with onset in eloquent cortex. Treatment is palliative with a reduction in seizure frequency over a few years.

Deep Brain Stimulator

Other procedures being evaluated require placing electrodes in deep brain structures such as the anterior nucleus of the thalamus or hippocampus to control seizures. The requisite electrodes have been successfully used for treating tremors and Parkinson disease. For patients with uncontrolled epilepsy, the electrodes may be programmed or activated automatically when seizure activity is recorded. Less invasive procedures such as this may become more effective than focal resective procedures, with fewer risks of postoperative deficits in the future. This has not yet been approved in the United States for this indication.

Common Pathologies Found in Surgical Resections

Mesial temporal sclerosis, appreciated histologically as a gliosis and cell loss within the mesial temporal structures, indicates previous long-term damage. There is usually no inciting event predisposing to this pathologic finding. However, it is often seen in patients who have had temporal lobe seizures for years, birth trauma, evidence of anoxic damage, or previous head injuries. Hippocampal atrophy is often seen with mesial sclerosis.

Cortical dysplasia is a general term covering many cortical developmental architectural variants. Classified by the etiology of the dysplasia (proliferation, migration, or reorganization), up to 20%–30% of the normal population have such changes. Dysplastic abnormalities are often found microscopically in idiopathic cases in which no overt lesion is identified by MRI. Such alterations may comprise up to 40% of extramesial seizure foci.

Dysembryoplastic neuroectodermal tumor and low-grade glioma are two tumor types often associated with seizure generation. Typically slow growing, they can be barely perceptible on MRI or other imaging modalities. With complete resection, patients often become seizure free.

FUTURE DIRECTIONS

Future directions in the treatment of epilepsy include the development of more-sensitive MRI techniques and multimodal imaging that will combine anatomic detail with functional and metabolic mapping delineating dysfunctional regions of the brain likely responsible for the pathogenesis of seizures and potential surgical targets. Many genetic components are being investigated that could have the potential for therapies. Clinical trials are currently under way with implantable stimulators and sensing devices that may detect, modulate, and prevent seizure discharges.

ADDITIONAL RESOURCES

Akanuma N, Koutroumanidis M, Adachi N, et al. Presurgical assessment of memory-related brain structures: the wada test and functional neuroimaging. Seizure 2003;12:346–58.

American Academy of Neurology, American Epilepsy Society. Practice parameter: evaluating an apparent unprovoked first seizure in adults (an evidence-based review): report of the quality standards subcommittee of the American Academy of Neurology and the American Epilepsy Society. Neurology 2015;84(16):1705–13.

Evidence-based guideline: Management of an unprovoked first seizure in adults.

Arena J, Rabinstein A. Transient global amnesia. Mayo Clin Proc 2015;90: 264–72.

Asadi-Pooya AA, Sperling M. Antiepileptic drugs: a clinician's manual. Oxford University Press; 2009.

This handbook provides practical, up-to-date information on how to select, prescribe, and monitor AEDs.

Chen JW, Wasterlain CG. Status epilepticus: pathophysiology and management in adults. Lancet Neurol 2006;5(3):246–56.

Engel J Jr. Seizures and epilepsy. 2nd ed. New York: Oxford University Press; 2013.

Engel J Jr, Pedley TA. Epilepsy: a comprehensive textbook. 2nd ed. Philadelphia, PA: Lippincott-Raven; 2008.

Engel J Jr, Wiebe S, French J, et al. Practice parameter: temporal lobe and localized neocortical resections for epilepsy: report of the quality standards subcommittee of the American Academy of Neurology, in association with the American Epilepsy Society and the American Association of Neurological Surgeons. Neurology 2003;60:538–47.

Harden CL. The adolescent female with epilepsy: mood, menstruation, and birth control. Neurology 2006;66(S3).

An excellent supplement that addresses the challenges in treating women with epilepsy including the link between epilepsy and depression, risk of reproductive disorders, efficacy of hormonal contraceptives, and interactions between oral contraceptives and AEDs.

Kwan P, Brodie MJ. Early identification of refractory epilepsy. N Engl J Med 2000;342(5):314–19.

Meador KJ, Baker GA, Finnell RH, et al. In utero antiepileptic drug exposure: fetal death and malformations. Neurology 2006;67(3):407–12.

More adverse outcomes were observed with in utero exposure to valproate compared to other AEDs suggesting that valproate poses the greatest risk to the fetus.

Morrell MJ, et al. In: Levy RH, editor. Antiepileptic drugs. 5th ed. Lippincott Wilkins & Williams; 2002. pp. 132–48.

An excellent reference of the mechanisms of action, chemistry, biotransformation, pharmacokinetics, interactions, use, and adverse effects of AEDs.

Motamedi GK, Meador KJ. Antiepileptic drugs and neurodevelopment. Curr Neurol Neurosci Rep 2006;6(4):341–6.

Porter RJ, Meldrum BS. Antiseizure drugs. In: Katzung BG, editor. Basic & clinical pharmacology, Lange medical book. 10th ed. McGraw-Hill; 2006. pp. 374–94, [Chapter 24].

An up-to-date and complete pharmacology textbook.

Rosenow F, Luders H. Presurgical evaluation of epilepsy. Brain 2001;124:1683–700.

Siegel AM. Presurgical evaluation and surgical treatment of medically refractory epilepsy. Neurosurg Rev 2004;27:1–18.

Sperling MR, Barshow A. Reappraisal of mortality after epilepsy surgery. Neurology 2016;86(21):1938–44.

Wiebe S, Blume WT, Girvin JP, et al. A randomized controlled trial of surgery for temporal lobe epilepsy. N Engl J Med 2001;345(5):311–18.

Zahn CA, Morrell MJ, Collins SD, et al. Management issues for women with epilepsy. A review of the literature. Neurology 1998;51:949–56.

A review of the recommendations concerning contraception, folate supplementation, vitamin K use in pregnancy, breast feeding, bone loss, catamenial epilepsy, and reproductive endocrine disorders.

24

Sleep Disorders

Paul T. Gross, Joel M. Oster

Primary sleep disorders, such as sleep apnea syndrome, narcolepsy, periodic limb movements (PLMs), and rapid eye movement (REM) behavior disorder, are common and often underdiagnosed. These conditions result in excessive daytime sleepiness (EDS) and/or disrupted sleep, may have a profound effect on quality of life, and may predispose patients to cardiovascular diseases or other comorbidities. Many people are sleep deprived and EDS plays a significant role in automobile accidents and lost work productivity.

NEUROTRANSMITTERS AND SLEEP

Fig. 24.1 outlines the primary neurochemistry and physiology of the sleep-wake cycle. Several cell groups located in various areas of the brain, mostly in the brainstem and hypothalamus, regulate the sleep-wake cycle.

Wakefulness and consciousness are promoted by different pathways and neurotransmitters located in the basal forebrain (acetylcholine), posterior hypothalamus (histamine and orexin/hypocretin), and brainstem (norepinephrine, dopamine, glutamate, and serotonin). These different groups of cells have widespread projections throughout the brain, including forebrain, cerebral cortex, and brainstem contributing to brain arousal. On the other hand, non-REM sleep depends mostly on GABAergic circuitry located in the ventrolateral preoptic area, anterior hypothalamus, and basal forebrain. An arrangement of reciprocal inhibition between the arousal and non-REM sleep systems allows periods of sustained wakefulness and sleep that are best optimized when aligned with the individual circadian rhythm. A circadian-mediated decrease in body temperature at nighttime activates GABA neurons and promotes sleep, while the increased body temperature in early morning inhibits GABA neurons with consequent activation of the arousal pathways.

Regarding REM sleep, there are two major pathways involved. The most important one involves activation of the glutamatergic subcoeruleus nucleus in the pons, once the inhibition of GABAergic pontine neurons is released. The accessory pathway comprises cholinergic neurons located in the pontine reticular formation; those are activated when the monoaminergic neuron activity is decreased. In addition, during REM sleep, there is recruitment of glycine pathways, leading to suppression of spinal motor activity.

Other substances including melatonin and adenosine can also influence the awake-sleep cycle. Melatonin gets released from the pineal gland when light-detecting cells within the retina identify darkness and it influences the hypothalamic suprachiasmatic nucleus, modulating the biologic clock and the circadian system. Adenosine accumulates in the basal forebrain and preoptic hypothalamus during progressive sleep deprivation, while sleeping reverses this. Prostaglandins and other neuropeptides modulate the wake-sleep cycle as well.

Stimulant medications such as methylphenidate and amphetamines facilitate noradrenergic pathways to promote alertness, while benzodiazepines, barbiturates, and ethanol activate GABA circuits causing sedation. Over-the-counter melatonin is used to phase-shift the circadian system in patients with disrupted rhythms while caffeine blocks the effects of adenosine, providing a neurologic basis for why humans have cultivated coffee and used caffeine socially to promote wakefulness.

INSOMNIA

Insomnia, the most common sleep disorder, is defined as the inability to initiate or maintain sleep. Typically, adults require 7–9 hours of sleep daily. Disorders such as depression, musculoskeletal pain, and heart failure may significantly interfere with sleep and produce secondary insomnia. This section focuses on insomnia as a primary illness.

A small percentage of people with a complaint of insomnia have a **sleep state misperception** disorder. These individuals believe that they do not have an adequate amount of sleep but, when tested, they do not lack appropriate sleep. Another small subset of individuals sleeps reasonably well at night, but for a more limited period of time, perhaps 5–7 hours. Although they may feel restored and function reasonably well during the day, they are unlikely to be functioning at their best.

The most common long-term insomnias are **primary insomnia** and **psychophysiologic insomnia.** Patients with **primary insomnia** have a history of sleeping poorly since childhood. They are unable to sleep enough to meet their needs, and this is not secondary to depression, anxiety, or an underlying illness.

Psychophysiologic insomnia is the most common cause of the inability to initiate or maintain sleep. It is defined as the inability to relax sufficiently to fall asleep, which, through repetition, then becomes reinforced as a behavior. Multiple factors contribute to this condition, including anxiety, stress, and inability to relax, resulting in a learned behavior of poor sleep.

Good sleep hygiene: keeping regular sleep hours, using the bedroom only for sleep and sex, and avoidance of stimulants, excessive alcohol, and daytime naps, is often helpful. When additional treatment is needed, cognitive behavioral therapy for insomnia (CBT-I) is most useful.

If CBT-I fails, medication can be considered. Some patients sleep well when given a prescription for a hypnotic that, even if never filled or taken, removes the anxiety about sleep. For others, a program of taking a hypnotic on three predetermined nights each week, such as every Sunday, Tuesday, and Thursday, allows for sleep on some nights. This may eventually lead to reasonably good sleep without any need for medication.

Numerous neurotransmitters, nuclei, and fiber projections mediate
arousal and cortical activation, as well as the sleep-wake cycle.

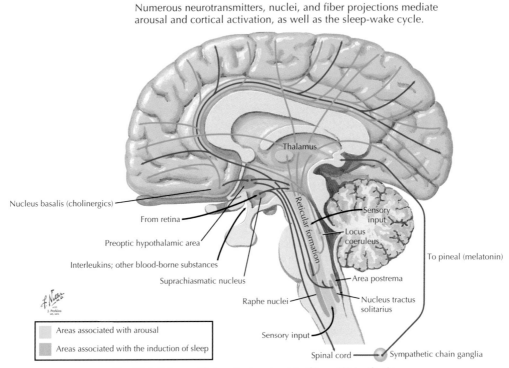

Fig. 24.1 Primary Networks Involved in Sleep-Wake Cycle.

SLEEP APNEA SYNDROME

CLINICAL VIGNETTE *A 37-year-old man was seen, at the request of his wife, for loud snoring. She noticed occasional snoring when they were first married 10 years earlier. Since then, however, he gained 15 pounds, and his shirt collar size had increased from 16 to 17. If he has two or more alcoholic beverages and sleeps on his back, the snoring can be heard in a room down the hall. The patient's wife was not certain whether he stops breathing in his sleep. He initially denied daytime sleepiness, but his wife reminded him that he tended to fall asleep with visitors present, and he confessed that he was having trouble staying awake during his 30-minute drive to work. He had hypertension and a family history of stroke in both parents. On examination, he appeared fatigued and modestly overweight. He was 5 feet 11 inches tall, and weighed 220 pounds (body mass index of 30.7). His blood pressure was 154/95. An all-night sleep test demonstrated 245 apneas, with an apnea/hypopnea index (number of apneas and hypopneas/hour) of 33. His oxygen saturation during the apneas decreased to 88% from a baseline of 92%, although occasionally it was as low as 81%. Subsequently, he had a second night in the sleep laboratory for continuous positive airway pressure (CPAP) titration. The repeat all-night sleep test demonstrated that a CPAP of 9 cm H_2O eliminated his apneas and hypopneas. After using CPAP, he and his wife noted a distinct change in his alertness. In retrospect, he had not realized how sleepy he was until he was treated.*

Disorders causing EDS include sleep disruption at night, such as sleep apnea syndrome or PLMs in sleep, or a disorder of the brain's sleep-wake system, such as narcolepsy, idiopathic hypersomnolence, or a circadian rhythm disorder. The patient in the preceding vignette had severe obstructive sleep apnea. Many similar patients with disrupted sleep may be impaired objective observers of their symptoms. Often they come at the bed partner's insistence, or the patient may present with nonspecific fatigue and weakness.

During obstructive sleep apneas, the soft palate and tongue relax excessively, producing upper airway obstruction, which results in snoring, apneas, and hypopneas (partial apneas). Predisposing factors include male gender; excessive weight; abnormal structure of the palate, uvula, tongue, and jaw; increasing age; use of alcohol; use of testosterone or reduction in female hormones; and positive family history.

Clinical Presentation

Loud snoring, caused by upper airway tissue vibration, is a warning sign of sleep apnea syndrome. When the obstruction becomes complete, an apneic event occurs and blood oxygen saturation decreases and a sleep arousal occurs. Although the patient is usually unaware of the event, often the partner is aroused and frightened by the individual's having ceased to breathe. Loud snoring, in combination with daytime sleepiness, raises the suspicion of clinically significant obstructive sleep apnea (Fig. 24.2A). Paradoxically, the majority of patients with obstructive sleep apnea do not report choking or gasping for breath, may be unaware of their apneas, and often believe that they have had an adequate night's sleep.

The cumulative effect of hundreds of such nighttime arousals is EDS. Patients with severe ($\geq$30 episodes per hour) or moderate (15–29 episodes per hour) sleep apnea are at increased risk for cardiovascular complications of hypertension, myocardial infarction, arrhythmias, and stroke.

Sleep fragmentation may lead to arousal with higher levels of catecholamines nocturnally which may lead to hypertension. Increased respiratory effort may increase negative intrathoracic pressure which increases secretion of aldosterone or catecholamines, promoting increased intravascular fluid volume and central venous pressure, and may also lead to abnormal transmural forces on the heart and conducting system leading to arrhythmias. Metabolic syndrome may develop with resultant insulin resistance and further weight gain, which may worsen the above cascade. Fortunately, CPAP supports the airway by pneumatic pressure, eliminating airway collapse; oxygen desaturation no longer occurs, and

Sleep Apnea

Narcolepsy

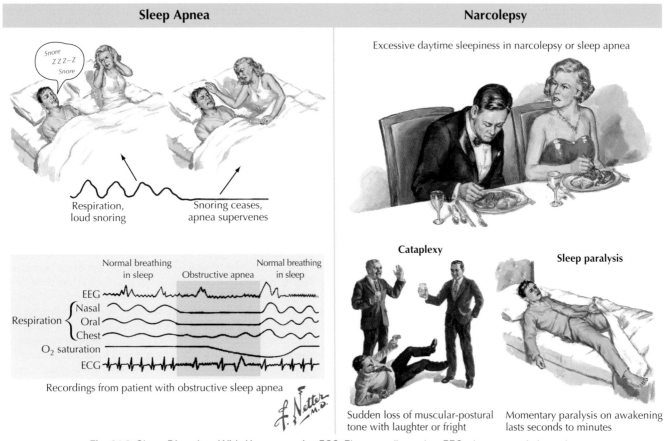

Excessive daytime sleepiness in narcolepsy or sleep apnea

Respiration, loud snoring

Snoring ceases, apnea supervenes

Normal breathing in sleep | Obstructive apnea | Normal breathing in sleep

EEG
Respiration { Nasal / Oral / Chest
O₂ saturation
ECG

Recordings from patient with obstructive sleep apnea

Cataplexy

Sleep paralysis

Sudden loss of muscular-postural tone with laughter or fright

Momentary paralysis on awakening lasts seconds to minutes

Fig. 24.2 Sleep Disorders With Hypersomnia. *ECG*, Electrocardiography; *EEG*, electroencephalography.

the above-defined pathophysiologic cascade is aborted with improvement in symptoms, hypertension, and cardiovascular risks.

Diagnosis and Treatment

Polysomnography is the best means to detect and quantitate apneic events. Treatment by reduction of risk factors, such as obesity and eliminating alcohol in the evening, may help. CPAP treatment, especially in patients with moderate, and especially severe, sleep apnea is the most reliable and effective treatment. Dental appliances may be helpful, particularly for mild to moderate sleep apnea.

Although surgical efforts to restructure the oropharynx are often helpful for relieving snoring, they are not as useful as CPAP for obstructive sleep apnea and are considered secondary treatment measures. Maxillo-mandibular advancement surgery, a major reconstruction of the maxilla and mandible, is usually successful, but is reserved for patients with severe apnea refractory to other treatments.

NARCOLEPSY

CLINICAL VIGNETTE *A 22-year-old man began having difficulty staying awake during college. Even with 8–9 hours of sleep at night, he fell asleep during class or when he was trying to study at home. Sometimes, he had a "second wind" and would be alert later in the evening. He found that a 5- to 10-minute nap was moderately refreshing, at least for an hour or two. The patient had noticed that he would lean against a wall or sit when he was laughing, as he otherwise might precipitously drop to the floor as his legs unexpectedly collapsed. On another occasion, he had a very frightening episode, when he woke from a nap but was unable to move. At that time, he had the sense of*

an evil stranger peering over him and tried to scream, but could not. After 45 seconds, he was able to move and talk. Results of an all-night sleep test were normal, aside from a borderline early rapid eye movement (REM) latency of 51 minutes. A multiple sleep latency test (MSLT), containing five daytime naps, showed a reduced average latency to sleep onset of 3.2 minutes and three of the naps contained REM sleep. He was treated with modafinil, with some improvement in his sleepiness. However, he continued to have episodes of cataplexy and sleep paralysis. The addition of fluoxetine, 10 mg daily, helped to ameliorate those symptoms.

Narcolepsy is a primary sleep disorder wherein the central nervous system (CNS) regulation of sleep, and particularly REM sleep, is impaired. Patients with narcolepsy tend to be much sleepier than the average person, and have episodes of an overwhelming urge to sleep, although even in narcolepsy it is unusual to fall asleep under extreme circumstances, such as when crossing a street or answering a question. Depending on the severity of the illness, the external circumstances, and the patient's willpower, he or she may or may not succumb to a severe urge to sleep. Narcolepsy is categorized as type 1 (with cataplexy) or type 2 (without cataplexy).

Clinical Presentation

The symptoms of the narcolepsy tetrad include EDS, which is present in almost all patients, and the ancillary symptoms of cataplexy, sleep paralysis, and hypnagogic hallucinations (see Fig. 24.2B). One or more of these ancillary symptoms are present in about 50%–60% of narcoleptics, and they are due to the inappropriate occurrence of episodes of partial REM sleep. During REM sleep, healthy individuals are often dreaming, and except for the extraocular and respiratory musculature, most muscles are paralyzed. This paralysis is subclinical in healthy individuals because it occurs while they are asleep.

In contrast, patients with narcolepsy may enter partial REM sleep at inappropriate times. Typically these events occur in specific settings: *cataplexy*, which is sudden paralysis occurring in response to strong emotions including laughter or anger, and *sleep paralysis*, which includes waking during the night with paralysis and often hallucinations. *Hypnagogic hallucinations* are realistic—often frightening—dreams that occur at sleep onset while the patient retains some degree of consciousness.

The etiology of narcolepsy is multifactorial. There is an association with reduced hypocretin or orexin levels in the hypothalamus, and genetic, autoimmune, and environmental factors may play a role. Most cases of narcolepsy are sporadic. HLA-DQB1*0602 is present in most narcoleptics, although it is also present in many unaffected individuals.

Diagnosis and Treatment

Narcolepsy is diagnosed clinically by the combination of a classic history of EDS relieved by brief naps, associated in about half of cases with other portions of the narcolepsy tetrad: cataplexy, sleep paralysis, and hypnagogic hallucinations. By measuring the average latency to sleep onset and the appearance of REM sleep on the multiple sleep latency test (MSLT) during the naps in a sleep lab, a diagnosis of narcolepsy can be supported. An all-night sleep test needs to be done on the night preceding an MSLT, because the MSLT cannot be properly interpreted unless the quality and quantity of the preceding night's sleep are assessed.

Treatment includes CNS stimulants, such as modafinil or amphetamines, for sleepiness. Ancillary symptoms are treated with selective serotonin reuptake inhibitors (SSRIs) such as fluoxetine, or serotonin norepinephrine reuptake inhibitors (SNRIs) including venlafaxine. Sodium oxybate is the only drug approved for treatment of both sleepiness and cataplexy.

Idiopathic hypersomnolence is a disorder seen in a small percentage of patients who have EDS but do not meet diagnostic criteria for narcolepsy or another nocturnal sleep disturbance. In contrast to narcolepsy, these individuals have prolonged periods of sleep at night as well as prolonged daytime naps. This is documented by a combination of an all-night sleep study showing adequate sleep and no significant sleep disruption, and an MSLT demonstrating EDS but no daytime REM sleep. Similar to narcolepsy, it is treated with stimulants.

PERIODIC LIMB MOVEMENTS

> **CLINICAL VIGNETTE**   *A 45-year-old woman saw her physician for excessive daytime sleepiness. She was tired much of the day but, if necessary, could stay awake. Her husband noted that she had trouble sitting still in the evening. She remarked that if she tried to sit and read or watch television, she needed to move her legs or get up and walk around. This provided momentary relief, but after she sat or lay down, the symptoms recurred. Her sister has similar evening symptoms. Physical examination and neurologic examination were unremarkable. Blood tests demonstrated a low ferritin level, but no anemia. Depression and hypothyroidism were ruled out by her primary care physician. An all-night sleep test showed frequent periodic limb movements (PLMs) of sleep associated with arousals. The PLM index was 59 episodes per hour, 46/hour of which were associated with arousals. A diagnosis of restless leg syndrome (RLS) and periodic limb movement syndrome (PLMS) was made. Treatment with iron resulted in 50% symptomatic improvement. Treatment with 0.25 mg pramipexole at 6:00 PM and again at 9:00 PM led to additional significant improvement.*

PLMs are another important consideration in the differential diagnosis of EDS. They consist of repeated brief episodes of limb movements, usually of the lower extremities. These movements range from simple dorsiflexion of the great toe to violent movements of the whole lower extremity. Many patients and their bed partners are unaware that they have PLMs during sleep. Individuals with PLMS may present with EDS because each episode disrupts their sleep.

Many of these patients also have RLS (an irresistible urge to move the legs while sitting or lying down). Patients who are anemic or have low ferritin may benefit from iron. Symptoms are also treated with dopamine agonists or with gabapentin. Antidepressants and stimulants may exacerbate RLS and PLMS.

PARASOMNIAS

> **CLINICAL VIGNETTE**   *A 72-year-old man was brought to the neurologist by his wife for violent activity in his sleep that concerned her for both of their safety. She recently noted him waving his fists, kicking, and occasionally banging his head against the headboard, all in his sleep. On one occasion, he fell out of bed, but, fortunately, did not hurt himself. Once, she had to wake him because he was punching her, completely contrary to his character and past behavior. When she woke him after this episode, he told her that he had dreamt that someone was trying to attack him. During the day, he was becoming more clumsy, took a long time to dress, and occasionally had a tremor of his right hand at rest. On exam, he had findings of subtle right hemiparkinsonism. An all-night sleep test demonstrated abundant tonic muscle activity during rapid eye movement (REM) sleep. The diagnosis of REM behavior disorder was made on the basis of the wife's history and the abnormal all-night sleep study. He was treated with clonazepam 0.5 mg nightly, and the spells resolved by approximately 90%. A diagnosis of possible Parkinson disease was also entertained, with a plan to follow him for any additional Parkinson symptoms.*

Parasomnias, characterized by abnormal symptoms or behaviors occurring during nighttime sleep, are another major category of sleep disorders.

Rapid Eye Movement Behavior Disorder

The vignette above has a typical history for REM sleep behavior disorder (RBD). The patient is unaware of the episodes during sleep. Some of these patients have RBD as a first manifestation of degenerative neurologic disease, particularly synucleinopathies, such as Parkinson disease, Lewy body disease, and multiple system atrophy, and in this case, the patient may have early Parkinson disease.

Usually, normal individuals are paralyzed and dreaming during REM sleep. The characteristic paralysis, sparing both eye movements and respiratory muscles, is from activation of reticulospinal pathways, which results in an inhibition of anterior horn cells within the spinal cord, preventing patients from acting out dreams. In sleep paralysis, mentioned earlier, this otherwise normal phenomenon occurs while the patient is awake. In RBD, this activation fails to occur, and patients act out their dreams. Elevated muscle or chin tone and movement artifacts may be manifest on the polysomnogram (Fig. 24.3) during these episodes.

Most of the patients respond positively to treatment with clonazepam or melatonin at bedtime.

Night Terrors

Night terrors are common in children and occasionally persist into adult life. The patient suddenly sits up in bed, has dilated pupils, a frightened expression, and a rapid pulse. Occasionally, affected individuals dash from the bed, sustaining injury. Children often return to sleep without memory of the event. If awakened, they describe a frightened feeling or image but not a complex dream, because these episodes

Patients with REM sleep behavior disorder lack reticulospinal inhibition that normally induces paralysis during REM sleep. Patients act out their dreams without any recollection in the morning. The episodes are usually witnessed by the spouse.

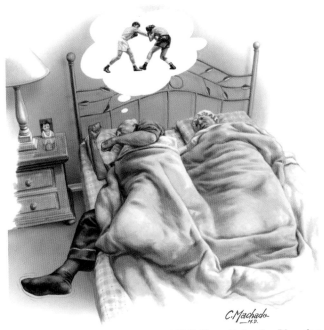

Fig. 24.3 Rapid Eye Movement (REM) Sleep Behavior Disorder.

arise during slow-wave sleep, in which dreams do not usually occur. Somnambulism tends to occur in the same patients, also during slow-wave sleep. Often an explanation of the problem is sufficient, but tricyclic antidepressants or benzodiazepines may be helpful.

Delayed Sleep Phase Syndrome

Delayed sleep phase syndrome is a **circadian rhythm disorder.** Individuals are not able to adjust their circadian clock to the time used by the rest of the world.

Most people can delay their sleep-wake cycle 1 hour or more daily and can advance it to an earlier time by approximately a half-hour daily. Therefore it is commonly easier to sleep and awaken later than to sleep and awaken earlier.

Some people have particular difficulty advancing to an earlier time. For example, a student with delayed sleep phase syndrome who spends 2 weeks staying up late studying for exams may find it impossible to learn to go to bed early and wake up early for a summer job. She will report insomnia because she cannot fall asleep at night, or daytime sleepiness because she cannot awaken before 11:00 AM. Treatments include medication, light therapy, or a program to delay sleep by 3 hours every day until sleep time returns to the new desired bedtime.

ADDITIONAL RESOURCES

Horner RL, Peever JH. Brain circuitry controlling sleep and wakefulness. Continuum (N Y) 2017;23:955–72.

Qaseem A, Holty J-E, Owens DK, et al. For the clinical guidelines committee of the American College of Physicians. Ann Intern Med 2013;159:471–83.

Winkelman JW. CLINICAL PRACTICE. Insomnia disorder. N Engl J Med 2015;373:1437–44.

Cognitive and Behavioral Disorders

Brian J. Scott

25

Neurocognitive Examination

Yuval Zabar, Dana Penney, Caitlin Macaulay

This chapter is an overview of the examination of higher cortical function as it relates to cortical anatomy and associated functions. Detailed anatomic drawings of the cerebral cortex are provided for one's review while reading this chapter. By the end of the chapter, the reader should gain a basic understanding of cognitive function, anatomical localization, and the neurocognitive examination.

her left hand when both hands were in front of her working in the kitchen. She again misidentified the right hand as someone else's hand. Her language abilities were relatively normal, thus she was able to describe her experience. Hypothetically, her dominant hemisphere was verbalizing severely distorted sensory information coming from the nondominant hemisphere.

CLINICAL VIGNETTE *A 78-year-old, right-handed woman presents with a fixed delusional syndrome with increasing paranoia developing over the previous year. There is no past history of psychiatric illness, trauma, surgery, or hospitalizations. There is no history of alcohol or substance abuse. Her behavior becomes increasingly volatile, at times extremely anxious, tearful, or aggressive. She believes there is a female stalker following her everywhere. She would be with her in the bathroom, closet, outside the house, etc. She is always behind her and sometimes would touch the back of her head or her left ear. She would interrupt her in the kitchen, reaching in to grab things without warning. Whenever the patient would look in the mirror, the stalker would hide. The patient is not certain if this intruder is human or not and sometimes thinks the intruder could be her, the patient. She is treated by several psychiatrists, including an inpatient psychiatric hospital stay, with no response to antipsychotic therapy.*

On examination she is awake, alert, oriented to person, place, but not to the year or the month. She is attentive to conversation and demonstrates normal comprehension. She speaks fluently, although speech is notable for occasional word finding difficulty. Short-term memory is mildly impaired, recalling only 1 out of 3 words in 5 minutes. The rest of the neurologic examination is notable for visual and tactile extinction to double simultaneous stimulation on the left side. She has finger agnosia on the right. She has partial agnosia of her right hand, sometimes identifying it as someone else and sometimes as her own hand. In fact, she cannot identify her left hand as her own when holding both hands in front of her. The rest of the neurologic examination demonstrates normal cranial nerve, motor, and primary sensory function bilaterally. There are no signs of parkinsonism. Her brain magnetic resonance imaging (MRI) is notable for bi-parietal and mesial temporal atrophy, worse on the right. Blood work is normal. Metabolic brain positron emission tomography (PET) scan shows marked hypometabolism in the right parietal lobe, as well as milder hypometabolism in the left parietal lobe. Comment: This case demonstrates an atypical presentation of dementia affecting posterior cortical function and presenting with pronounced behavior changes and less obvious cognitive decline. However, a detailed cognitive examination was crucial in delineating the basis for her delusion. A combination of sensory extinction on the left and limb misidentification on the right led to her delusional state. She did not recognize her right hand when rubbing her head or touching her ear and misidentified it as someone else's hand. Similarly, she visually extinguished

INTRODUCTION

Cognition is a complex neurologic function involving multiple neural networks distributed throughout the brain. The neurocognitive examination strives to determine deficits in specific cognitive domains and to localize deficits to corresponding neuroanatomic regions. As in all aspects of neurology, localization of deficits is imperative in making the correct diagnosis.

Behavior often reveals underlying cognitive impairment. The patient's mood, affect, level of cooperation, and distractibility during the interview should be noted. Patients with cognitive deficits commonly develop symptoms of anxiety, depression, even suspiciousness. The emotional consequences of cognitive dysfunction are often mistaken as the primary cause of cognitive symptoms when, in fact, the behavioral changes reflect cognitive impairment. Conversely, there may be limited subjective concern or awareness of underlying cognitive impairment. For example, the early stages of Alzheimer disease may go unnoticed in social situations and patients may not be fully aware of their memory impairment. Without some screening examination of mental status, these cases of early dementia or mild cognitive impairment go undetected until their dementia reaches more severe stages.

The human cerebral cortex, a network of billions of interconnections, is the most complex part of the nervous system. Anatomically, the cortex is grossly classified into four major functional areas: frontal, temporal, parietal, and occipital lobes (Fig. 25.1, Table 25.1). These anatomic regions serve different functions, are processed in parallel, and are interconnected in a complex network integrating sensory, motor, memory, and emotional information (Fig. 25.2, Table 25.2). Although these cortical areas are traditionally discussed as functionally and anatomically isolated, in reality they are components of a larger neural network processing input, output, and feedback from one another. The interconnectedness of cortical regions is critical for "higher cortical" function.

COGNITIVE TESTING

Assessment of cognitive function requires direct testing of various cognitive domains in a structured, hierarchical fashion. The major cognitive domains included in a routine mental status examination include level of

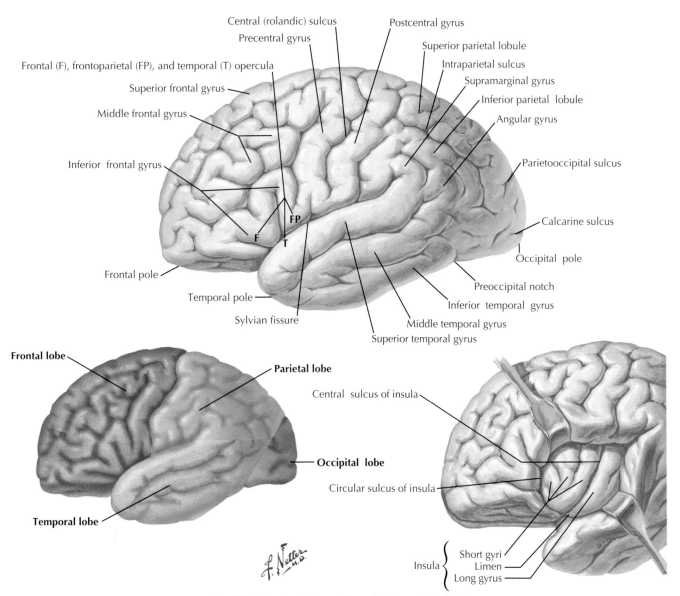

Fig. 25.1 Cerebral Cortex (Superior Lateral Surface).

From Rubin M, Safdieh J. *Netter's Concise Neuroanatomy.* Philadelphia: Saunders; 2007:32.

TABLE 25.1 **Lateral Surface of the Brain: Notable Lateral Sulci**	
Structure	**Anatomic Significance**
Lateral (Sylvian) fissure	Separates temporal lobe from frontal and parietal lobes
Central (Rolandic) sulcus	Separates frontal lobe from parietal lobe

consciousness, orientation, attention, language, memory, visuospatial processing, and executive function. These are operationally defined as follows.

Level of Consciousness

Level of consciousness underlies all aspects of mental status and must be considered immediately. A stuporous patient may be difficult to examine fully due to waxing and waning level of consciousness; obviously it is not possible to make a full cognitive assessment in a comatose patient. Generally, patients may be described as awake and alert, drowsy or lethargic, stuporous (needs stimulation to stay awake and responsive), obtunded (needs stimulation to awaken but not responsive), or comatose (not awake, not responsive).

Attention

Attention is a complex brain function allowing the individual to focus and register specific information from external and internal environments. Impaired attention may affect the patient's performance in other cognitive tasks, such as reading, writing, or memorizing lists. Digit span testing is a good means to test attention. The examiner may ask the patient to repeat a list of five digits following the same sequence. Next, a list of three digits is provided and the patient is instructed to repeat the sequence in reverse order. This test elicits the patient's ability to give immediate focus and avoid distraction. Fewer than five digits forward or three digits backward would indicate attention problems.

Orientation

Orientation allows an individual to identify when, where, and who they are at any given moment. This requires intact attention, memory,

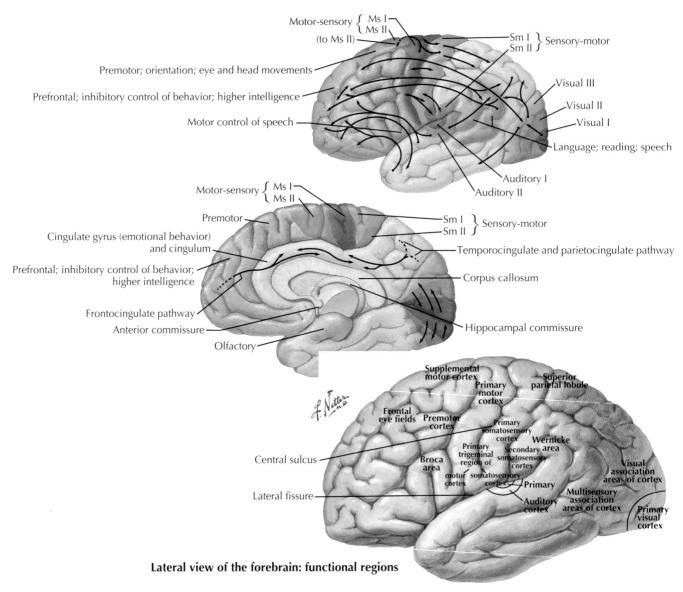

Lateral view of the forebrain: functional regions

Fig. 25.2 Cerebral Cortex: Localization of Function and Association Pathways.

TABLE 25.2	Lateral Surface of the Brain: Cortical Lobes, Lateral View		
Lobe	**Notable Gyri**	**Notable Sulci**	**Notable Functions**
Frontal	Superior frontal gyrus Middle frontal gyrus Inferior frontal gyrus Precentral gyrus	Superior frontal sulcus Inferior frontal sulcus Precentral sulcus	Motor control, expressive speech, personality, drive
Parietal	Postcentral gyrus Superior parietal lobule Inferior parietal lobule Supramarginal gyrus Angular gyrus	Postcentral sulcus Intraparietal sulcus	Sensory input and integration, receptive speech
Temporal	Superior temporal gyrus Middle temporal gyrus Inferior temporal gyrus	Superior temporal sulcus Inferior temporal sulcus	Auditory input and memory integration
Occipital		Transverse occipital sulcus Lunate sulcus	Visual input and processing

From Rubin M, Safdieh J. *Netter's Concise Neuroanatomy*. Philadelphia: Saunders; 2007:32.

language, and recognition involving widespread cortical regions as well as high-order cognitive processing. Testing this simple modality provides an efficient means to survey general cognitive function. *Disorientation* to time and/or place may occur in either widespread or focal cortical dysfunction. Of note, not knowing the current year suggests greater severity of disorientation than not knowing today's date. Similarly, not knowing the town or state at present is more concerning than not knowing the floor of the building. Several orientation questions are necessary to identify mild disorientation. Disorientation for person may be seen in severe stages of dementia, although by this point cognitive function may be severely impaired in general and testing specific domains becomes very difficult.

Language Function

Language function includes the patient's ability to monitor and to comprehend language-related sounds and visual symbols and to generate meaningful verbal or written responses. Most interaction with patients is language-based, and therefore it is crucial to ascertain whether language function is impaired early in the course of the examination. For example, a patient with an expressive aphasia may not be able to express three words during memory testing, express the date, or name of a place. Such a deficit would not necessarily indicate impaired short-term memory or inattention, but rather, a primary impairment of language. Impairment of language typically follows left hemispheric damage, although right hemispheric lesions may also impair language function, as discussed later in this chapter.

Language encompasses multiple cortical regions and is not classifiable within strict cortical anatomic borders. Impairment of language function is a common neurologic symptom presenting acutely, as in

stroke, or more insidiously, as in neurodegenerative disease. The classic nomenclature of the aphasia syndromes (Fig. 25.3) is largely based upon lesion analysis in cases of stroke or tumor. These syndromes postulate distinct, interconnected cortical regions responsible for the various phases of language processing from comprehension to expression. Broca syndrome is characterized by stuttering, agrammatical, effortful, and telegraphic language. This was thought to be an expressive language disorder typical of anterior frontal lesions (so-called motor aphasia). Wernicke aphasia, characterized by impairment of comprehension, is characterized by fluent expression of wrong or nonexistent words and syllables (neologisms and semantic paraphasic errors) that is sometimes referred to as a "word salad." Receptive language disorders were thought to be related to lesions of the more posterior temporal parietal cortex. Other aphasia syndromes, such as conduction aphasia, anomic aphasia, and the transcortical aphasias, emerged to describe syndromes that did not fit neatly into the broader forms of Broca and Wernicke aphasias. These syndromes were traditionally associated with various left middle cerebral artery (MCA) territory strokes or left hemispheric tumors and were thought to arise from disconnection between distinct cortical regions. However, exceptions to the traditional classification of aphasia occur commonly. For example, it is not unusual for a posterior MCA division stroke with no injury to the inferior frontal cortex to produce a nonfluent aphasia. Moreover, the progressive aphasia syndromes often produce characteristic language disorders that do not fit any of the traditional aphasia paradigms. Indeed, even in the acute stroke setting, the classification of aphasia as expressive or receptive, motor or sensory, or nonfluent or fluent is too simplistic and often inaccurate. Very few patients present with pure aphasia syndromes.

Clinical syndromes related to site of region

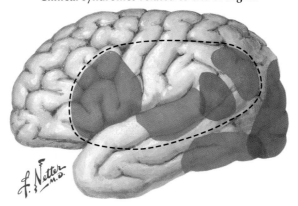

	Broca aphasia	Wernicke aphasia	Angular gyrus	Global aphasia
Pronunciation, speech rhythm	Dysarthria, stuttering, effortful	Normal, fluent, loquacious	Normal	Very abnormal
Speech content	Missed syllables, agrammatical, telegraphic	Use of wrong or nonexistent words	Often normal	Very abnormal
Repetition of speech	Abnormal but better than spontaneous	Abnormal	Normal	Very abnormal
Comprehension of spoken language	Normal	Very abnormal	Normal	Very abnormal
Comprehension of written language	Not as good as for spoken language	Abnormal but better than for spoken	Very abnormal	Very abnormal
Writing	Clumsy, agrammatical, misspelling	Penmanship OK but misspelling and inaccuracies	Very abnormal, spelling errors	Very abnormal
Naming	Better than spontaneous speech	Wrong names	Often abnormal	Very abnormal
Other	Hemiplegia, apraxia	Sometimes hemianopsia and apraxia	Slight hemiparesis, trouble calculating, finger agnosia, hemianopsia	Hemiplegia

Fig. 25.3 Dominant Hemisphere Language Dysfunction.

As mentioned earlier, patients commonly present complaining of gradual onset of word-finding difficulty; this is a general symptom that is not always the result of a primary language disorder. Rather, it may be a manifestation of either inattention or a memory impairment. Therefore the assessment of language must distinguish primary language disorders from other cognitive deficits or secondary language impairment. The patient presenting with progressive primary language disturbance often does not fit neatly into the traditional neuroanatomic aphasia classifications.

Newer descriptions of language impairment elucidated through study of patients with primary progressive aphasia have emerged. There are three main types of primary progressive aphasia, namely, primary nonfluent expressive aphasia, logopenic aphasia, and semantic aphasia. Primary nonfluent expressive aphasia is characterized by progressive impairment in verbal output, the mechanics of speech, or structure of words and sentences. The patient knows what to say but not how to say it. Logopenic aphasia is a progressive loss of verbal content. Vocabulary is reduced and speech becomes emptier. As with primary nonfluent expressive aphasia, the patient knows the meaning

to convey but has no words to convey the message. Semantic aphasia may be described as a loss of meaning. The patient's words do not correspond to the meaning of the message. Moreover, the patient does not comprehend the words or the messages of others, or their own message.

Language may be defined as the attempt to convey a message in verbal, spoken, or written form. This appears to occur in four interconnected stages, including speech initiation, speech content, speech structure, and motor programming of speech. These stages correlate with specific anatomical regions (Fig. 25.4).

Stage I: Initiation of Speech

Initiation of speech involves the ability to generate and plan a spoken message. Patients with speech initiation problems are quiet, as though they have nothing to say, so-called dynamic aphasia. Responses are terse and elaboration is absent. Patients speak only in response to conversation, not to initiate conversation. Although the amount of speech is reduced, the content and structure of spoken language are normal. This is often seen in patients with anterior frontal and subcortical abnormalities.

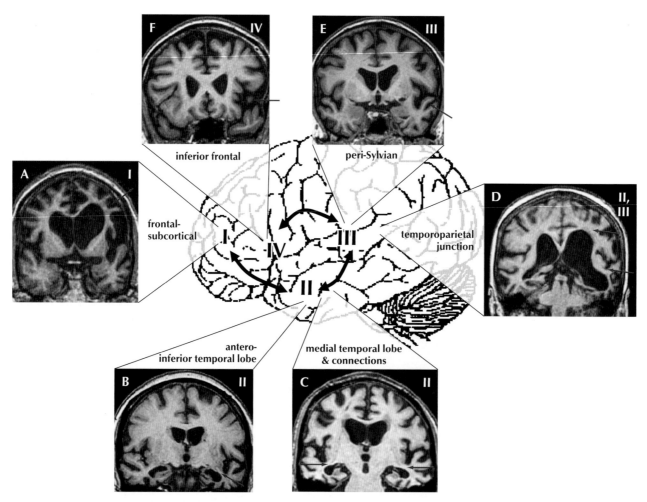

Roman numerals I through IV indicate proposed operational stages in the pathway for language output. Key anatomical areas are indicated along with superimposed MRI images as follows: (A) asymmetric (left greater than right) frontal lobe atrophy, dynamic aphasia; (B) focal left anterior/inferior temporal lobe atrophy, semantic dementia; (C) bilateral mesial temporal atrophy, Alzheimer's disease (anomia); (D) left posterior superior temporal/inferior parietal atrophy, progressive 'mixed', logopenic or jargon aphasia; (E) focal left superior temporal lobe/insular atrophy, progressive nonfluent aphasia; (F) focal left inferior frontal gyrus/frontal opercular atrophy, progressive apraxia of speech. Bidirectional arrows suggest reciprocal communications between key anatomical regions.

From Rohrer JD, Warren JD, Omar R, et al. Brain 2008. January; 131(Pt 1):8-38. By permission of Oxford University Press.

Fig. 25.4 Structural Anatomy of Word-Finding Difficulty in Degenerative Disorders.

These individuals often appear inert and slow to respond in general, sometimes referred to as appearing as a "bump on a log."

Stage II: Content

The content of the message comes next once the mental plan for speech is set. This includes vocabulary and concepts. Content is assessed at the level of single words or in the way words are combined. Loss of vocabulary is the major abnormality encountered in this setting. The patient substitutes approximate words or imprecise expressions for words they cannot conjure. Speech seems vague and deficient of meaning in more severe cases. Errors of meaning (semantic paraphasias) may occur. Stereotyped expressions, such as clichés, are overutilized. This is characteristic of semantic dementia, a variant of frontotemporal lobar degeneration. A variation of this occurs in Alzheimer disease, where the patient cannot retrieve words from storage, gradually and progressively developing logopenic aphasia. Here the content of the message is impaired because of a loss for words, rather than a loss of the meaning of words. At the level of word combinations, there is a lack of coherence due to incomplete sentences, tangentiality, fragmented phrases, etc. It is hard to follow the patient's train of thought in these cases. This also occurs acutely, most commonly in states of delirium such as alcohol withdrawal.

Stage III: Grammar and Phonology

Grammar and phonology are the basis for the structure of spoken language. Grammar is the ordering of words into normal sentence structure, that is, subject and predicate. It also includes the use of function words such as prepositions and conjunctions. Phonology refers to the selection of individual sounds and syllables to form spoken words. Agrammatism leads to telegraphic speech, composed of single words or phrases, often omitting connector words. Phonologic errors lead to errors in particular sounds within words, also known as phonemic paraphasic errors. For example, saying "aminal" for "animal," or "nucular" for "nuclear." These types of errors are common in progressive nonfluent aphasia.

Stage IV: Language Expression

Once the structure of the message is defined, the message is conveyed to the motor areas for speech where phonetics, articulation, and prosody are applied and the message is spoken. Impairment at this phase is often characterized by apraxia of speech, or the loss of learned motor programming for speech production. This often produces great frustration and effortful speech, with severe loss of fluency, phonetic errors, and impaired speech timing and rhythm.

The most important aspect of language assessment is carefully listening to conversational language during the patient interview, and performing a detailed characterization of speech sounds, grammatical structure, content, and comprehension. If the patient is not very talkative, the examiner may present him or her with a picture to describe, or questions about themselves, their life experiences, etc. Further tests of naming, repetition, writing, and reading all provide additional important information. In the case of progressive aphasia, the nature of language disturbance has a significant role in identifying the underlying neurodegenerative disease. Indeed, assessment of language in this way has proven reliable in localizing cortical regions attributed to various primary progressive aphasic syndromes (see Fig. 25.4). This approach complements the classic aphasia exam, providing a better description of language processing and improving localization during examination.

Memory

Memory is the ability to register, store, and retrieve information. The brain's innate capacity for memory is enormous. It continuously records what we hear and see, feel and think, in real time, from the moment we awaken to the moment we fall asleep, with very little conscious effort. Normally, we can retrieve recent experiences, conversations, and thoughts after some amount of time passes, without having to make a conscious effort to memorize. For example, most people may easily recall a conversation from earlier in the day. However, it will be harder to recall a week later. At the bedside, the brain's ability to record information may be tested using a short list of unrelated words. To successfully complete this task, the patient must be able to *register* the words (often by repeating the words immediately after the examiner), *store* them, and then *retrieve* them from storage. Registration requires intact attention, intact hearing or vision depending on the material being tested, and intact language comprehension. Storage of information may be facilitated with repetition/practice or cuing during the learning phase of the test. Similarly, retrieval may be facilitated with cuing. The patient with retrieval memory impairment will benefit from cuing more than the patient with storage problems. The latter patient will not benefit from cuing or practice. Storage memory deficits are typical of *medial temporal/hippocampal dysfunction,* such as in early Alzheimer disease. Impaired storage function is considered abnormal regardless of age. Retrieval memory deficits are often attributed to *frontal and subcortical dysfunction.* These limitations are characterized by increasing inefficiency and delay in retrieving information and occur more frequently with advancing age.

Executive Function

Executive function refers to the brain's ability to coordinate multimodal cortical processes for the purpose of solving problems, planning and executing tasks, keeping track of multiple tasks at once, and organizing one's thoughts. This is analogous to an orchestra conductor, directing the various sections of the orchestra to achieve a cohesive and meaningful whole. Executive function may be assessed by asking the patient to draw a clock with all the numbers and to indicate a specific time. The patient's approach to drawing the clock given those instructions may provide hints regarding impairment in planning and organizing the task. For example, the circle may be too small, the number placement may be haphazard or incomplete, or the hands may indicate concrete processing, such as pointing to the 10 and the 11 to indicate the time at 11:10. Clock drawing may also demonstrate impairment of spatial processing.

Praxis (Procedural Memory)

Praxis (procedural memory) is the brain's memory for skilled motor function. This encompasses a host of learned motor programs ranging from simple tasks, such as brushing one's teeth or using a spoon, to far more complex motor activities such as using a smartphone, operating an appliance, or playing the piano. Once learned, with practice, an individual performs these tasks implicitly without the need for explicit recall of the procedure. Praxis per se probably involves several cerebral cortical regions, but when abnormal (apraxia) it is most often associated with *dominant frontal lobe dysfunction.* Tests for apraxia include having the patient perform certain tasks. For example, "show how a soldier salutes," or "show how you blow out a candle," or "snap your fingers." These are common, well-known actions that an average person should be able to demonstrate. Another way to test for apraxia is to give a common object to the patient and ask him or her to demonstrate how to use it. For example, the object might be a pen, a hairbrush, a paperclip, etc.

Gnosis (Nonverbal Recognition)

Gnosis (nonverbal recognition) refers to the sensory identification and recognition of all aspects of our surroundings. We recognize objects, people, sounds, etc. in very complex sensory environments without needing verbal definition of those items. We can navigate through our world safely and effectively without using language, much like we do while driving home from work, or moving through the hallways of one's workplace. Agnosia is an acquired failure to recognize things normally. This may affect a single sensory modality (as in visual object agnosia), content specific (as in prosopagnosia/loss of facial recognition), or multimodal (as in semantic dementia). Gnosis likely involves bilateral posterior temporal, occipital, and parietal cortical regions, although cases of unilateral *right hemisphere lesions* have been described. A patient with visual object agnosia would know that an apple is a fruit that grows on trees, but would not recognize an apple visually.

A routine bedside mental status exam should include a description of level of consciousness, behavior, attention, language function, and memory. When following patient's cognitive status over time, for example, in cases of dementia, it is helpful to standardize the exam. This allows for direct comparison of findings from one visit to the next. There are several standardized assessments of cognition, including the Mini Mental State Exam (MMSE) and the Montreal Cognitive Assessment (MOCA). These tests are particularly useful for assessing memory problems in the elderly. The MOCA is available online at https://www.mocatest.org along with normative data translation into multiple languages and script for administration. It can detect very subtle impairment as in Mild Cognitive Impairment or the very earliest stages of dementia. The MMSE is less sensitive than the MOCA but may be a better tool for staging dementia severity over time, particularly in patients with Alzheimer disease.

FRONTAL LOBE DYSFUNCTION

The frontal lobe comprises the major portion of the adult brain occupying approximately 30% of brain mass. This includes the *motor area* (Brodmann area 4), the *premotor cortex* (Brodmann areas 6 and 8), and *significant prefrontal* areas (Fig. 25.5). A **Brodmann area** is a region of the cortex that is defined by the organization of its cells, or cytoarchitecture, as opposed to gross anatomic landmarks such as sulci or gyri. Reference to Brodmann areas provides more precise clinic-anatomic correlation localization.

The *prefrontal* areas are distinct from the adjacent motor and premotor areas, particularly in their connections with other cortical areas and the thalamus (see Fig. 25.2). Most of the prefrontal–thalamic connections are made with the *dorsal medial nucleus,* a prime relay center for limbic projections originating from the amygdala and the basal forebrain. The reciprocal inputs are the most prominent cortical connections, originating from second-order sensory association and paralimbic association areas, including the cingulate cortex, temporal pole, and parahippocampal area. The frontal lobe is an integrator and analyzer of highly complex multimodal cortical areas, including information processed by the limbic system.

Ablation of both frontal lobes in experimental animals leads to very unusual behaviors. Some of the most dramatic symptoms, including automatic nonpurposeful behaviors with a tendency to chew randomly on objects, led to the conclusion that the frontal lobe was important for the integration of goal-directed movement. Investigations in the 1950s began to define the importance of the frontal lobe for analyzing various stimuli. Frontal lobe lesions led to loss of normal social interchange, personal internal reinforcement, and judgment. Therefore patients sustaining frontal lobe lesions are unable to modify behavior despite the potentially harming or embarrassing effects of their actions. Additionally, these individuals tend to perseverate by repeating automatic behaviors that do not result in conclusive actions; these may be identified on perseveration testing.

Humans sustaining frontal lobe disorders may develop significant personality changes and "release of animal instincts." One of the earliest

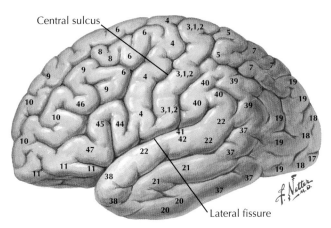

The numbers superimposed on the above brain images are what constitute the Brodmann map of cytoarchitectonics. Brodmann assigned numbers to various brain regions by analyzing each area's cellular structure starting from the central sulcus (the boundary between the frontal and parietal lobes).

Brodmann Functional Brain Cytoarchitecture Areas			
Function	Primary	Secondary	Tertiary
Motor	4	6	9, 10, 11, 45, 46, 47
Speech	44		
Eye Movement	8		
Sensory; Body	1, 2, 3	5, 7	7, 22, 37, 39, 40
Auditory	41	22, 42	
Vision	17	18, 19, 20	21, 37

Table provides a general view of brain function that refers to the Brodmann map shown above.

Fig. 25.5 Brodmann Areas: Lateral View of the Forebrain: Cytoarchitecture of the Brain Based on Neuronal Organization.

descriptions of frontal lobe damage described patients with apathy and disturbed emotions. Elucidation of the frontal lobe connections, particularly the medial-basal portion, demonstrates that the limbic system provides significant input to that area. Autonomic centers originating in the brainstem and hypothalamus also have significant connections with the basal frontal lobe. When these connections are disrupted, aggressive, impulsive, and uncontrolled behavior results.

From a neuropsychological perspective, the frontal lobes are responsible for executive functions. Frontal lobe syndromes are typically classified clinically, anatomically, and neuropsychologically into lateral, medial, and mesial groups. Prefrontal syndromes that affect these anterior areas have been described as dysexecutive, disinhibited, and apathetic–akinetic. From an anatomic perspective, the *dysexecutive syndrome* is due to damage of the dorsolateral prefrontal area. The *disinhibited syndrome* is due to disorders affecting the orbital frontal region of the brain, while the *apathetic–akinetic* syndrome is due to medial frontal lobe dysfunction.

Patients with damage to the *dorsolateral prefrontal* cortex typically exhibit *stereotyped* and *perseverative behaviors* with mental inflexibility (i.e., stuck in set). Additionally, one will note that these patients demonstrate poor self-monitoring, deficient working memory, difficulty generating hypotheses, and reduced fluency. These patients often demonstrate an associated inefficient/unorganized learning strategy, with impaired retrieval for learned information as well as a loss of set. Such individuals are typically apathetic, exhibiting reduced drive, depressed mentation, and motor programming deficits.

Damage to the *orbital–frontal* area is characterized by patients presenting with prominent *personality changes*. They are often disinhibited, impulsive, perseverative, and have potential to be socially inappropriate with poor self-monitoring. Inappropriate euphoria, affective lability with quick onset, poor judgment, and tendency to confabulate are other characteristic personality changes. Typically, these patients exhibit impaired sustained and divided attention, increased distractibility, and anosmia.

Patients with damage to the *anterior cingulate gyrus* typically experience difficulty reacting to stimuli. They have an impaired initiation of action as well as impaired persistence, reduced arousal, and akinesia, with loss of spontaneous speech and behavior. Such individuals may present with monosyllabic speech, appear apathetic, have a flat or diminished affect, and may be docile.

Although these various prefrontal lobe syndromes pertain to localized lesions, it is not uncommon for patients to display overlapping behaviors as it is relatively uncommon to have isolated areas of precise frontal lobe pathology. Also, some behaviors are not due to specific localized deficits. There are some nonspecific frontal signs that can be elucidated during neurologic examination of the patient with disorders of this nature. These include various frontal release signs, particularly involuntary grasping, and suck reflexes. However, one must take care when interpreting these findings, especially with elderly individuals, many of whom will have an increased incidence of such findings with normal aging or in the presence of generalized neurologic encephalopathy.

Language dysfunction is a common finding of some frontal lobe lesions. *Broca aphasia* is the classic form of frontal lobe language dysfunction with dominant hemisphere lesions. It is characterized by a nonfluent, effortful, slow, and halting speech. This language dysfunction is typically of reduced length, that is, few words with reduced phrase length, simplified grammar, and impaired naming. Repetition is characteristically intact. These individuals often have associated apraxia (buccofacial, speech, and of the nonparalyzed limb) and right-sided weakness of the face and hand. *Transcortical motor aphasia* is another characteristic of frontal lobe language dysfunction. These patients often have very limited spontaneous speech as well as delayed responsiveness. They also tend to be perseverative, akinetic, and may also have contralateral leg weakness and urinary incontinence because of a mesial lesion. This may result from a lesion either in the distribution of the anterior cerebral artery or in the watershed area between the middle and anterior cerebral artery territories. Proximal extremity weakness very rarely, if ever, occurs with a vascular watershed lesion. Auditory comprehension (barring complex syntax), repetition, and naming are intact in transcortical motor aphasia.

Various diseases or injuries that result in executive dysfunction do not necessarily have to directly affect the frontal lobes per se. This is due to the presence of widespread subcortical–frontal cortical as well as other cortical–frontal cortical connections wherein a distant nonfrontal lesion can impact primary frontal lobe function. When someone sustains an acceleration/deceleration brain injury wherein the brain strikes the bony prominences of the skull, there is an increased incidence of frontal lobe injury. This is particularly the situation with injuries either at the basal orbital frontal regions lying directly adjacent to the skull's cribriform plate or at the frontal poles adjacent to the frontal bone. Frontal lobe injury may also result indirectly because of shearing of white matter tracts.

Dementing illness, particularly those referred to as frontal-temporal lobar dementias and Lewy Body disease, present with executive dysfunction. This similarly occurs with various subcortical dementias. These occur with Parkinson disease, Huntington disease, acquired immune deficiency syndrome (AIDS)-related dementia, and demyelinating disorders that lead to involvement of subcortical white matter connections.

Additionally, there is a high incidence of executive dysfunction with vascular disease, whether due to large vessel stroke, small vessel ischemic disease, or ruptured aneurysm (typically of the anterior communicating artery). The anterior cerebral artery and MCA supply the anterior and medial portions and the lateral dorsal frontal cortex, respectively. Primary brain tumors, for example, gliomas, oligodendrogliomas, meningiomas, and pituitary adenomas, may typically affect executive functioning. Various causes of hydrocephalus, particularly normal-pressure hydrocephalus, may present in a similar fashion, although a gait disorder may often presage the dementia-associated normal-pressure hydrocephalus.

TEMPORAL LOBE DYSFUNCTION

Because of the complexity of the temporal lobe regions and the high interconnectivity with other brain regions, damage or injury can result in a wide variety of deficits involving many cognitive functions. It is impossible to assess all of them during an office visit or bedside consult. However, it is important to recognize some of the major symptom complexes that may occur with lesions in this elegant portion of our brains. One needs to be able to quickly evaluate the patient for lesions at this critical level through specific interview questions with the patient and family or in either the office or bedside setting. The primary manifestations that are addressed here are personality and affect alterations, language and naming deficits, visuoperceptual difficulties, and lastly memory learning problems.

An understanding of temporal lobe anatomy helps one appreciate the various clinical deficits that can arise from lesions at this level. The temporal lobe is defined as encompassing all brain regions below the Sylvian fissure and anterior to the occipital cortex (see Fig. 25.1). These also include subcortical structures such as the hippocampal formation, the amygdala, and limbic cortex (Fig. 25.6). The temporal lobe is divided into three distinct regions: the *lateral area* consisting of the superior, middle, and inferior temporal gyri; the *inferior temporal cortex* containing the auditory and visual areas; and the *medial area* including the fusiform gyrus and parahippocampal gyrus.

The temporal lobe is characterized by a high prevalence of multisite brain connections through efferent projections extending to the limbic system, basal ganglia, frontal and parietal association regions, as well as afferent projections from the sensory areas. The right and left temporal lobes are connected by the corpus callosum and anterior commissure. This interconnectedness contributes to the diverse cognitive and behavioral changes that can result from injury to the temporal lobes. Each of the temporal lobe regions is important for specific cognitive functions and modifies cognition specific to other regions through the many inherent temporal lobe interconnections.

Personality

Disorders affecting the limbic structures (amygdalae) within the temporal lobes can result in alterations of personality and affect. Head injury, neurodegenerative dementias, central nervous system infections, particularly herpes simplex encephalitis, and temporal lobe epilepsy are some of the common insults that may be associated with acute to episodic chronic emotional lability or dysregulation. Personality and emotional changes are best assessed by patient as well as family interview. Very often the family first notices the emergence of angry or aggressive outbursts, irritability, or depression that is disproportionate to the patient's life situation. Frequently, relatives report that the patient has become "different" or "difficult." Often, there are changes in sexual comportment. The development of hyperreligiosity, hypergraphia, and clingy behavior (temporal lobe personality) is witnessed among patients with temporal lobe epilepsy.

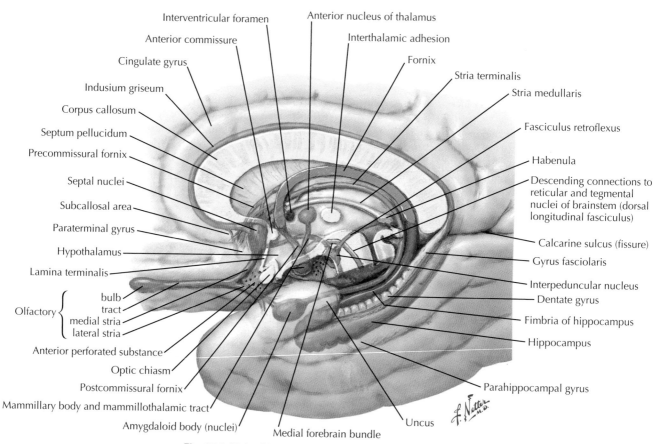

Interventricular foramen

Anterior commissure

Cingulate gyrus

Indusium griseum

Corpus callosum

Septum pellucidum

Precommissural fornix

Septal nuclei

Subcallosal area

Paraterminal gyrus

Hypothalamus

Lamina terminalis

Olfactory { bulb / tract / medial stria / lateral stria

Anterior perforated substance

Optic chiasm

Postcommissural fornix

Mammillary body and mammillothalamic tract

Amygdaloid body (nuclei)

Medial forebrain bundle

Anterior nucleus of thalamus

Interthalamic adhesion

Fornix

Stria terminalis

Stria medullaris

Fasciculus retroflexus

Habenula

Descending connections to reticular and tegmental nuclei of brainstem (dorsal longitudinal fasciculus)

Calcarine sulcus (fissure)

Gyrus fasciolaris

Interpeduncular nucleus

Dentate gyrus

Fimbria of hippocampus

Hippocampus

Parahippocampal gyrus

Uncus

Fig. 25.6 Major Limbic Forebrain Cingulate Cortex Areas.

The patient who becomes excessively irritable or angry during mental status testing may have limbic involvement. It is common for some individuals to complain a bit about bedside testing (too tired, not able to draw well, bad at math, feel "stupid"). Furthermore, it is understandable that worried or sick patients might be depressed or cranky. However, excessive, abrupt, or unanticipated emotional outbursts, rage, or erratic behavior are not typical; these need to be both noted and equated with the clinical question at hand. A sudden refusal to cooperate, throwing the pen, crumpling response paper, change in voice such as ranting, or yelling, or even abrupt tearfulness are each suggestive of limbic involvement. The key elements are poor modulation and a change from the patient's baseline personality.

Language

Functions of the right and left hemispheric regions have individual variations that are contingent upon hemispheric language dominance. Population studies estimate that 90%–95% of adults are right-handed. Estimates of left-hemisphere dominance for language have been determined by various studies of stroke patients, functional magnetic resonance imaging (fMRI), and intracarotid sodium amobarbital (a.k.a. Wada) investigations. Left-brain dominance occurs in more than 95% of right-handers and in almost 20% of left-handers. Right hemisphere or bilateral language distribution is found in approximately 20% of left-handers. The likelihood of right hemisphere language dominance increases with the strength of a patient's left-handedness and increased frequency of familial left-handedness. Thus a transient ischemic attack with left-hand weakness could cause temporary speech disruption or naming problems, particularly in a left-handed patient or a right-hander with left-handed relatives. Knowing which hemisphere is most likely dominant for language is critical to the diagnosis of various cognitive problems.

Left dominant temporal lobe injury leads to major language deficits. *Wernicke aphasia* is the most classic example occurring with lesions of the left superior temporal gyrus (see Fig. 25.2). Typically, these patients demonstrate spontaneous speech that is *fluent* with *phonemic* (mixed syllables) and *verbal* (incorrect words) *paraphasic* errors at times referred to as a *word salad*. In addition, these patients have problems with naming, comprehension, repetition, reading, and writing. There may be total lack or incomplete awareness of these various impairments. Such language changes can be accompanied by emotional symptoms that are associated with the limbic region.

Circumscribed deficits in language functions sometimes emerge if the temporal lobe is disconnected from other brain regions. One of these disconnection syndromes, *Pure Word Deafness,* can occur when an intact Wernicke area is disconnected from both auditory cortices. The deafness is only for words, and the patient can hear and interpret normally meaningful nonverbal sounds like a baby crying or phone ringing. Bilateral destructive temporal lobe lesions including the transverse oriented Heschl gyrus impair word comprehension and also the identification of meaningful sounds and result in the syndrome of *cortical deafness*. These syndromes can result from a number of medical conditions, including bilateral strokes, herpes simplex encephalitis, and other infectious disorders. Patients may also have subtle problems discriminating speech sounds, suggestive of left temporal damage. These patients may complain that people are talking "too fast" or that they "can't hear." The problem is not actually the rate of speech; it is difficulty discriminating sounds that are presented quickly. To test this, simply speak more slowly with distinct pauses between each word without changing voice volume or simplifying the words that you are using.

Patients frequently complain of "short-term memory" problems that they describe as a failure to "remember" words (typically nouns) although they can recognize the word that they are searching for if it is provided by someone else. "Forgetting words" is not a memory problem; it is a disorder of language typically associated with impairment of the temporal lobe that may occur with or without a true memory impairment. Object naming is disrupted in all of the aphasic syndromes, and is also a common early symptom in dementias affecting the temporal lobes. It was an early symptom in the patient with *frontal temporal dementia* described at the beginning of this chapter and is a common early complaint for patients with degenerative disorders such as *mild cognitive impairment* (amnestic or nonamnestic), *Alzheimer disease,* and *vascular dementia.* Lesions in the nonlanguage temporal lobe can result in *amusia.* This is a collection of disorders wherein patients are unable to recognize musical melodies or specific aspects of music (including even dramatic changes in pitch).

Naming deficits are easily tested using the MMSE naming items as well as objects available in the patient's room or your office. If a patient cannot name the specified object that you point to, then provide the first sound of the object name (phonemic cue), such as *com* for the word computer or *laa* for the word laptop. If the patient is then able to say the name of the object, then they do know the word but have a problem with retrieval. Word fluency tests are also useful in measuring naming problems associated with temporal lobe dysfunction. A word generation task that asks the patient to generate in 1 minute as many words as he or she can beginning with a particular letter serves as a test of frontal lobe function. A variation of that task requires the patient to generate words pertaining to a specific category (i.e., proper names, musical instruments, animals). This task requires the patient to retrieve nouns rapidly. Problems generating *restricted category words* are suggestive of *temporal lobe* damage, while problems with generating *restricted letter words* suggest *frontal lobe* damage.

Damage to the *inferior temporal cortex* can result in disorders of visual perception; frequently this occurs without the physician being able to demonstrate precise visual field deficits. The temporal lobes help in processing the visual information. Damage to the right temporal lobe can result in a wide variety of deficits, including inattention to the contralateral left side of visual space (more frequent in right temporal lesions), problems with visual object recognition, and the ability to recognize anomalous aspects of pictures and discriminate faces. There may be problems with perceiving and understanding social cues, such as understanding that their appointment is over when you glance at your watch or when you stand up at the end of an appointment.

Perceptual deficits arising from the temporal lobe are difficult to test because other functions, including attention, organization, spatial orientation, and memory, overlap with tasks of perception, making the perceptual component of a deficit difficult to isolate. Damage to either or both temporal lobes may result in perceptual impairment. When using visual material to test perception, the language hemisphere may be helping to process pictures, and the nondominant hemisphere may be contributing to understanding the shapes of words. Patients with acquired alexia are sometimes taught to use visuospatial techniques to help them relearn to read. The nonlanguage hemisphere role in reading is demonstrated below. One of the groups of lines below represents the word "horses" and the other represents the word "elephant." Can you determine which grouping represents the word "elephant" (Fig. 25.7)?

Notice that there are no letters, but because of the right hemisphere contribution you can still identify the word on the left as "elephant" from the contour created by the lines. Similarly, the nonlanguage temporal lobe can also help decode words that are seemingly nonsense if you attend strictly to the letters and rules of phonics. In fact, it *deosn't mttaer in waht oredr the ltteers in a wrod are, the olny iprmoetnt tihng is taht the frist and lsat ltteer be at the rghit pclae.*

Assessing a handwriting sample is helpful. Damage to the left temporal region may result in wider right-side margins, spaces, or wide separations between letters or syllables and disrupt the continuity of the writing line. Patients with damage to the left temporal region may also be noted to have a decline in ability to write in script, as opposed to a better-preserved ability to print.

The clock-drawing test used to identify frontal lobe deficits is also useful in identifying temporal lobe deficits. In order to draw a clock, there must be a mental visual representation of which features are essential. Visuospatial abilities are essential for determining the layout and proportions and for making sure that features are accurate on both sides of space. Visuospatial perception is also a component of evaluating the output and making corrections.

In the clock drawing below (Fig. 25.8), the entire left side is neglected, and the right side is drawn twice because the patient did not attend to his first attempt. This patient had a right temporal lesion causing perceptual problems on the left side of space within the context of intact visual fields.

The clock drawing below demonstrates several types of errors associated with the temporal lobes (Fig. 25.9). The patient has added additional structure (lines that look like spokes in a wheel) in an attempt to compensate for perceptual problems in spacing the numbers. There is a numbering error in the upper left quadrant and the hands are missing. These errors are suggestive of right temporal involvement. In addition, the patient wrote a cue to help remember the time, suggesting compensation for a memory problem. Note, too, that the time cue is incorrect: Rather than 10 past 11, the patient wrote 10 to 11, suggesting a language-processing problem. Memory loss, language problem, and time concept error are all suggestive of temporal lobe deficit.

The temporal lobes are essential in the learning of new information. Damage here will affect memory. The ability to retain information starts with *acquisition* (attention, sustaining focus, organization), *encoding* (information processing), *storage* (retention of information through consolidation), and *retrieval* (accessing the information that is in storage) of the information that is stored. *Explicit or episodic memory* is information

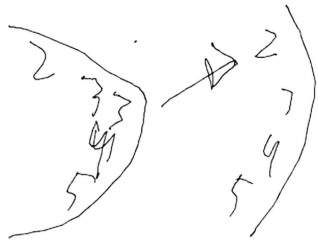

Fig. 25.8 Clock Drawing in a Patient With Right Temporal Lobe Dysfunction.

Fig. 25.7 Groups of Lines Representing the Words "Horses" and "Elephant."

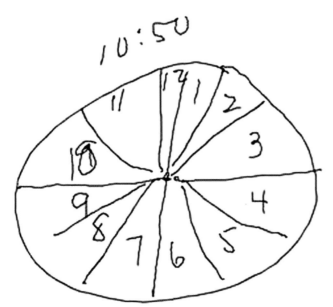

Fig. 25.9 A Different Example of Clock Drawing in a Patient With Right Temporal Lobe Dysfunction.

that can be specifically stated (contextual knowledge, autobiographical information, events, the knowledge in this book). Information that is recalled or influences behavior per se, without conscious intention, that is, procedures such as how to drive a car or ride a bicycle, is called *implicit memory*. Memory deficits may result if any of these complex stages fail. Damage to different regions of the temporal lobe can result in various breakdowns in the memory encoding and storage process. Damage to the mesial temporal regions, the hippocampal complex, can result in profound memory deficits as is well demonstrated by the famous case of Patient HM.

CLINICAL VIGNETTE *On December 2, 2008, Henry Gustav Molaison, age 82, died of respiratory failure. If the name is unfamiliar, that's because for the past 55 years, he was known to the world only as HM. In 1953 Mr. Molaison underwent temporal lobe surgery for severe epilepsy with uncontrolled seizures. Although the surgery was largely successful in reducing seizure frequency, it left him with a profound memory loss and essentially no ability to learn new things. For 55 years after the surgery, he could recall almost nothing that happened subsequently: births and deaths of family members, the events of 9–11, or what he did that morning. Each time he met a friend, each time he ate at a restaurant, each time he walked into his own home, it was for him, the first time.*

Damage to the *inferior temporal regions* interferes with the intentional retrieval of information. Lesions of the *left hemisphere* tend to preferentially compromise retrieval of *verbal* information (e.g., conversations, word lists), whereas *right hemisphere* damage tends to impair the retrieval of *visual information* (e.g., misplacing items). Assessment of memory is an important aspect of the mental status exam. Patients with memory deficits frequently have difficulty accurately reporting the type and extent of their memory problems. Interviews with the family are the best way to quickly determine the type of memory impairment and the implication of the memory deficit for that patient. The terminology for memory functions may be confusing and may be used differently by different physicians. Effective communication of results and accurate retesting at a later date require both the use of descriptive terms

for documenting memory complaints stated by the family, including examples, and a detailed description of the procedure's amount and type of information presented, interval delay, and instructions that you use to test memory. One must specify the number of learning trials or types of problems observed during the learning trials, that is, acquisition. It is important to attend to any strategies, for example, rehearsal, that a patient may use to learn the information, referred to as encoding. Note how much information is freely recalled after at least a 10- to 15-minute delay retention, and the improvement in the amount of information recalled with cues when compared to the amount freely recalled, or retrieval.

Information and orientation questions are useful in assessing episodic memory. Knowing where you are, the date and the time of day, without looking at a clock, have clinical utility. If the patient is not oriented to time, within 30 minutes, then there are likely to be medication compliance problems. The key to assessing information storage is to ensure that registration and encoding have taken place and to allow sufficient time for memory to decay, that is, forgetting, prior to testing retention. The memory problems in disorders like early Alzheimer disease may not be apparent when tested following a few minutes' delay, but they may be evident when tested 15 minutes later. The MMSE registration and recall of three objects is often used to assess memory function. Although a reasonable brief bedside task for the very impaired patient, it is insensitive to impairment in the young or mildly impaired and can result in the underestimation of memory deficits because of the abbreviated list to be learned and short interval delay between registration and recall. The addition of a second recall condition, 10–15 minutes later, at the completion of your examination affords additional time for storage as well as memory decay. This may be very important for detecting modest memory impairment.

PARIETAL LOBE DYSFUNCTION

The parietal lobe is situated between the frontal and occipital lobes. The central sulcus separates frontal from parietal cortex, while the parieto-occipital sulcus separates parietal from occipital cortex (see Fig. 25.1). The Sylvian fissure forms the lateral boundary separating parietal from temporal cortex. The most anterior portion of the parietal lobe, sitting immediately behind the central sulcus, is the primary somatosensory cortex, Brodmann area 3. More posteriorly, the parietal lobe may be divided into the superior parietal lobule (Brodmann areas 5 and 7) and the inferior parietal lobule (Brodmann areas 39 and 40) (see Fig. 25.5). These areas are separated by the intraparietal sulcus.

The primary role of the parietal lobe is to process unimodal tactile somatosensory information and to integrate multimodal sensory information, creating a sensory map of one's self, the surroundings, and the relationship of the self within the surrounding perceived environment. Recent research in primates elucidated the functional anatomy of the parietal lobe. The *posterior parietal lobe* is thought to primarily integrate visual and somatosensory data allowing proper hand–eye coordination; spatial localization of objects; proper targeting of eye movements; and accurate gauging of the shape, size, and orientation of objects. Further functional subdivision identifies that the *posterior (dorsal)* portion provides integration of spatial vision via occipital-parietal connections, the *"where" stream*, whereas the *inferior (ventral)* regions involve *visual recognition* of objects and actions via occipital and temporal connections, the *"what" stream*. There is a further specialization of function within the parietal lobes determined by lateralization. *Number processing and calculation* are primarily represented within the *left* hemisphere, whereas *sensory integration* is predominantly defined within the *right* hemisphere.

Somatosensory integration begins in the primary somatosensory cortex, where basic tactile localization is appreciated. This is evaluated by testing both joint position and two-point discrimination sensory modalities. Once sensory information is received in the primary somatosensory cortex, this then streams posteriorly toward the somatosensory association cortex (see Fig. 25.2). Here, tactile information is integrated to provide discriminatory sensation over larger areas of the body surface for sensory definition of object weight, size and shape, texture, etc. This allows for specialized tactile sensation, such as graphesthesia and stereognosis. Most importantly, this allows the integrative *mapping* of the spatial, tactile, and visual aspects of one's body. The sensory *mapping* of the external world takes place posteriorly in the parietal lobe. There are two "functional maps," one of the self and the other of the world. These are also integrated, presumably in the heteromodal association area in the right parieto-temporal-occipital junction.

Right Parietal Lobe

Patients with lesions at this level develop unilateral neglect of sensory events occurring on their left side when sensory input from those areas seemingly appears to vanish. The patient is unaware of those events, as though they were not happening at all. The patient may be completely unaware of the examiner standing on his left side. Sometimes, this occurs

in a milder form, whereby events on the left side of the patient extinguish when competing with sensory events on the right side. Double simultaneous stimulation tests this at the bedside. When the examiner touches the patient on either side individually, the patient detects each stimulus correctly. However, when the stimuli are presented simultaneously, the patient with neglect will "extinguish" the stimulus on the left side. This may also occur with simultaneous visual stimuli of both visual fields.

A related condition, called *asomatognosia*, affects the patient's ability to recognize his or her own body part. When viewing his or her own hand, the patient does not recognize it as his or her own. Moreover, the patient may identify it as someone else's limb. *Anosognosia* refers to the patient's absent recognition of illness or disability, which is not mediated by psychological denial and is not associated with a disturbance of mood (Fig. 25.10). A milder version of neglect may occur while writing or drawing. The patient may draw a clock and place all the numbers and even the hands within the right hemispace of the clock face. *Visuospatial impairment* is relatively common following right parietal lesions. This may be seen on construction tests, where the patient is asked to copy shapes, such as a clock, a cube, or overlapping geometric figures (Fig. 25.11, also see Fig. 25.10).

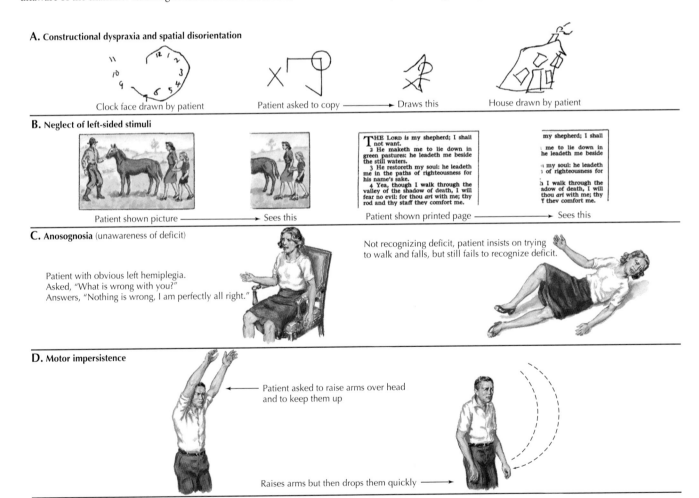

A. Constructional dyspraxia and spatial disorientation

Clock face drawn by patient   Patient asked to copy ⟶ Draws this   House drawn by patient

B. Neglect of left-sided stimuli

Patient shown picture ⟶ Sees this   Patient shown printed page ⟶ Sees this

C. Anosognosia (unawareness of deficit)

Patient with obvious left hemiplegia.
Asked, "What is wrong with you?"
Answers, "Nothing is wrong, I am perfectly all right."

Not recognizing deficit, patient insists on trying to walk and falls, but still fails to recognize deficit.

D. Motor impersistence

Patient asked to raise arms over head and to keep them up

Raises arms but then drops them quickly ⟶

E. Abnormal recognition of nonlanguage cues (facial expression, voice tone, mood)

Patient shown picture.
Asked, "Which is the happy face?"

Patient answers, "I don't know, they are all the same."

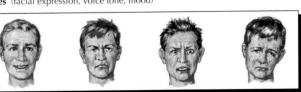

Fig. 25.10 Nondominant Hemisphere Higher Cortical Function.

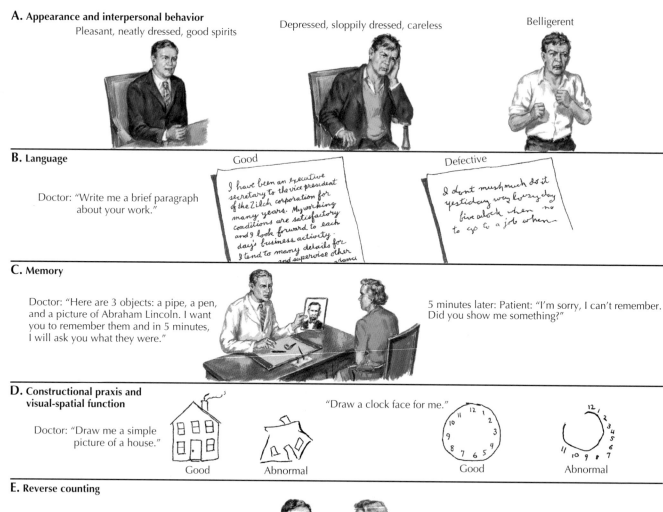

A. **Appearance and interpersonal behavior**

Pleasant, neatly dressed, good spirits

Depressed, sloppily dressed, careless

Belligerent

B. **Language**

Doctor: "Write me a brief paragraph about your work."

Good

I have been an executive secretary to the vice president of the Zilch corporation for many years. My working conditions are satisfactory and I look forward to each day's business activity. I tend to many details for and supervise other...

Defective

I dont mush much do it yestiday way busy day five oclock when ...no to go to a job when...

C. **Memory**

Doctor: "Here are 3 objects: a pipe, a pen, and a picture of Abraham Lincoln. I want you to remember them and in 5 minutes, I will ask you what they were."

5 minutes later: Patient: "I'm sorry, I can't remember. Did you show me something?"

D. **Constructional praxis and visual-spatial function**

Doctor: "Draw me a simple picture of a house."

Good   Abnormal

"Draw a clock face for me."

Good   Abnormal

E. **Reverse counting**

Doctor: "Count backward from 5 to 1 for me."
Patient: "5...3...4..., sorry, I can't do it."

Doctor: "Spell the word *worlds* backward for me."
Patient: "W..L..R..D..S."

Fig. 25.11 Testing for Defects of Higher Cortical Function.

Dressing apraxia is the inability to dress, in the absence of weakness or primary sensory loss. There is impairment of spatial processing and body mapping. Typically, these individuals are unable to distinguish where to place their arm or leg within an article of clothing. This may be demonstrated by asking the patient to put on a shirt—for example, rolling it up, turning a sleeve inside out, and asking the patient to put it on appropriately. The patient cannot rearrange the shirt and insert his or her arms correctly into the sleeves. This is not a true apraxia because the motor program for dressing is presumably intact, although difficult to prove. Praxis for other common tasks may be intact. Sometimes, the dressing difficulty occurs only on the left side due to a right parietal lesion. In this circumstance, this finding could be part of the neglect syndrome.

Left Parietal Lobe

Gerstmann syndrome is the classic representation of left parietal cerebral dysfunction. This includes four different sets of symptoms that emerge in comparison to those occurring with right-sided parietal lesions. These patients may exhibit an (1) inability to perform arithmetic, *acalculia;*

(2) *left–right confusion,* an inability to distinguish left from right side; (3) inability to identify specific fingers such as index, middle, or ring, termed *finger agnosia;* and (4) inability to write, *agraphia.* When all four of these symptoms occur together, the condition is known as Gerstmann syndrome. It is debatable whether it ever presents in a pure form given the high proportion of patients with left parietal dysfunction who also have some degree of aphasia. It is intriguing whether the agraphia related to left parietal dysfunction is qualitatively different from agraphia with more anterior lesions, although this is very difficult to determine in aphasic patients.

Balint syndrome is representative of disorders related to posterior parietal dysfunction and includes three specific forms of visual disorientation. (1) *Simultanagnosia* is evident when the patients are unable to perceive their surroundings as a whole. They literally perceive their environment just one object at a time. Often, they have trouble detecting movement. (2) *Optic ataxia* occurs when the patient is unable to shift gaze toward a target accurately. There is a tendency to overshoot or undershoot the target. (3) *Ocular apraxia* is the inability to shift gaze at will toward a new target; this is commonly seen together with simultanagnosia. Cases of Balint syndrome typically follow bilateral posterior parietal lesions, but there are several reports of unilateral right posterior parietal lesions with Balint syndrome as well.

Classically, these syndromes were described in cases of stroke or tumor. However, a gradual presentation of such symptoms also occurs in cases of *posterior dementia*, a primary neurodegenerative disease affecting posterior parietal lobes initially before spreading to involve other cortical regions. An interesting cognitive syndrome in these patients is *topographical amnesia*, a condition defined by loss of memory of familiar places and routes. In such cases, patients may get lost in their own home but memory for stories, conversations, and lists of things to do may be normal.

OCCIPITAL LOBE DYSFUNCTION

The primary function of the occipital cortex is to process and organize visual information. The *calcarine area*, Brodmann area 17 (see Figs. 25.1 and 25.5), is the primary visual cortex. It is located within the medial side of the occipital cortex along the calcarine sulcus (Fig. 25.12). This region is also called the *striate cortex* because of prominent myelin striation, called the *stria of Gennari*. The portion of the occipital cortex that lies beyond the primary visual area is termed *extra-striate* cortex; it is the site of higher order visual processing, including color discrimination, motion perception, shape detection, etc. Each visual area contains a full map of the mentally perceived visual world.

The primary visual cortex provides a low-level description of visual object shape, spatial distribution, and color properties. Projections from the extra-striate cortex branch ventrally toward temporal lobes and dorsally toward parietal lobes. The visual information from the ventral stream integrates with temporal lobe association areas to allow recognition of objects, people, and places. Visual information traveling through the dorsal stream merges with parietal association areas to allow proper visual orientation of objects in the environment and of the self within the environment (Fig. 25.13). There are few cognitive syndromes attributable to disorders placing the occipital lobe in isolation.

Cortical blindness follows bilateral occipital lobe injury. Patients are completely blind but, paradoxically, may deny their symptom. Frequently these individuals describe scenes with extraordinary detail, often with bizarre contextual information. These patients function as though delusional, insisting their vision is intact despite clear evidence to the contrary, lying down, or being unable to manipulate any object they see. This condition, also known as *Anton syndrome*, most commonly occurs after bilateral posterior cerebral artery strokes, progressive multifocal leukoencephalopathy, or posterior reversible leukoencephalopathy.

Pure alexia without agraphia is a classic *disconnection syndrome* that occurs when a lesion within the left occipital lobe extends to involve fibers traversing across the splenium of the corpus callosum from the right occipital lobe. This disconnection causes loss of the ability to read while sparing all other language function. All cases include a right homonymous hemianopia (hemi-field cut). Visual information recorded by either or both occipital lobes is relayed to the posterior left temporal lobe in order for the individual to detect and process the visual symbols of language. Therefore a lesion affecting the left occipital lobe and splenium together effectively blocks visual language data—both from the left and the right visual cortex lobe—from being sent to the dominant temporal lobe. Even though patients see objects in their left hemi-field, utilizing their still intact right occipital lobe, they cannot read. Although the left hemi-field remains intact, its potential language information cannot be "seen" by the dominant left temporal lobe. This condition could also be called *pure word blindness*.

Cerebellum

There is a longstanding debate regarding the cerebellum and the role it plays in cognition and behavior. During the 17th century, debates occurred as to whether the cerebellum was critical for vegetative functions and survival. During the 18th century, some considered whether the cerebellum was the center for sexual function or pure motor functioning, a more limited approach. In the 19th century, the sole proposed focus was directed at its role in coordinated movement. More recently, in the latter half of the 20th century, neuroscientists have come to recognize that the cerebellum may be responsible for more than just a balance and coordination function; however, for some this is still a debatable topic. Most think of motor symptoms when considering cerebellar disorders, and these would consist of ataxia, dysmetria, disordered eye movement, scanning dysarthria, dysphagia, and tremor. Bedside testing of cerebellar motor dysfunction requires observation of gait and balance, the presence of dysmetria with use of the extremities, tendency to overshoot or overcorrect, and eye movement abnormalities.

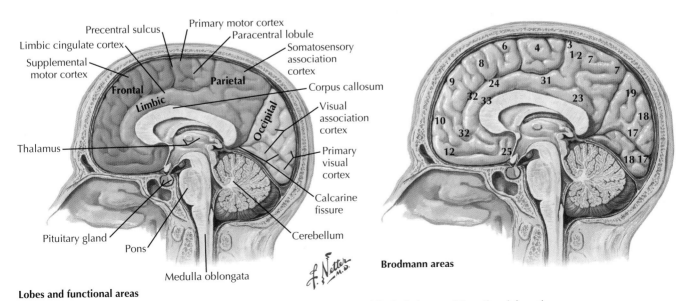

Lobes and functional areas

Brodmann areas

Fig. 25.12 Cerebral Cortex (Medial Surface of Brain Lobes and Functional Areas).

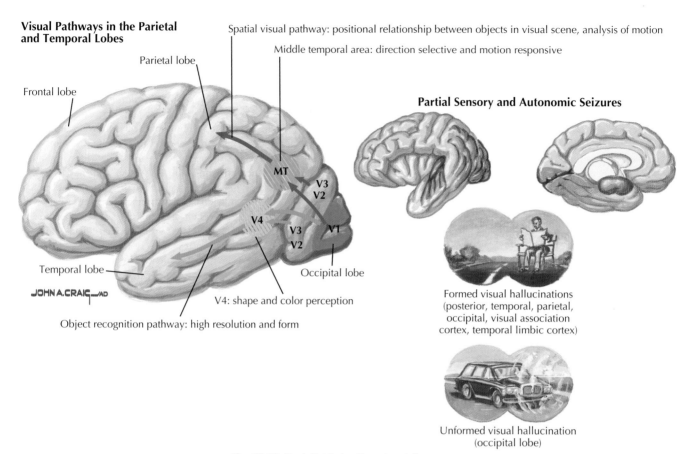

Visual Pathways in the Parietal and Temporal Lobes

Spatial visual pathway: positional relationship between objects in visual scene, analysis of motion

Middle temporal area: direction selective and motion responsive

Frontal lobe

Parietal lobe

MT

V3
V2

V4

V3
V2

V1

Temporal lobe

JOHN A.CRAIG_AD

V4: shape and color perception

Occipital lobe

Object recognition pathway: high resolution and form

Partial Sensory and Autonomic Seizures

Formed visual hallucinations (posterior, temporal, parietal, occipital, visual association cortex, temporal limbic cortex)

Unformed visual hallucination (occipital lobe)

Fig. 25.13 Occipital Lobe Functional Anatomy.

However, the cerebellum is connected to the contralateral cerebral hemispheres, the dorsolateral prefrontal cortex, posterior parietal and superior temporal areas, and occipital lobes, as well as limbic structures. Thus it is not surprising that there is an increased focus on the cerebellum having an important role in cognitive functioning. Kalashnikova et al. studied 25 patients with isolated cerebellar infarcts and found that 88% exhibited cognitive impairment. Based on the pattern of deficits, they divided them into two groups: dysfunction of the prefrontal and premotor areas and dysfunction of the posterior parietal/temporal/occipital area.

Schmahmann and Sherman have postulated that there is a *cerebellar cognitive affective syndrome* (CAS). They attribute this to cerebellar lesions that are connected with the associative zones. CAS is associated with executive dysfunction (e.g., planning, set-shifting, abstract reasoning, divided attention, working memory, perseveration, verbal fluency, and memory deficits due to executive dysfunction), speech disorder (agrammatism, dysprosody, mild anomia), visual spatial dysfunction (difficulty copying and conceptualizing drawings), and personality changes (flat affect, disinhibition, impulsivity, pathologic laughing/crying).

The degree of impairment tends to depend on the location of cerebellar damage. Specifically, those with slowly progressive cerebellar degenerations, or small strokes within the cerebellum, primarily supplied by the superior cerebellar artery, tended to exhibit very subtle deficits. In contrast, those with bilateral or large unilateral strokes in the territory of the posterior inferior cerebellar arteries, or those with subacute onset of pancerebellar disorders, exhibited more striking deficits. There is a wide range of possible etiologies for cerebellar disorders, including developmental, genetic, toxic, vascular, metabolic, infectious, tumor, trauma, degenerative, and autoimmune. Thus these patients not only

have cerebellar involvement but frequently also have dysfunction of other areas of the cerebrum that may contribute to cognitive symptoms.

Understanding the neurophysiologic role of the cerebellum in cognition is still in relative infancy. It is likely that some study findings will be replicated and it will become more widely accepted that the cerebellum does have a significant role in cognitive functioning.

ADDITIONAL RESOURCES

Benson DF. Aphasia, alexia, and agraphia. New York: Churchill Livingstone Inc.; 1979.

Carey BHM. An unforgettable amnesiac, dies at 82. New York Times Obituaries. December 4, 2008.

Feinberg TE, Farrah MJ. Behavioral neurology and neuropsychology. New York, NY: McGraw-Hill; 1997.

Freedman M, Leech L, Kaplan E, et al. Clock drawing: a neuropsychological analysis. New York: Oxford University Press, Inc.; 1994.

Goodglass H, Kaplan E. The assessment of aphasia and related disorders. 2nd ed. Philadelphia: Lea & Febiger; 1983.

Heilman KM, Valenstein E. Clinical neuropsychology. 4th ed. New York, NY: Oxford University Press, Inc.; 2003.

Jeffrey P, Nussbaum PD. Clinical neuropsychology: a pocket handbook for assessment. Washington, DC: American Psychological Association; 1998.

Kalashnikova LA, Zueva YV, Pugacheva OV, et al. Cognitive impairments in cerebellar infarcts. Neurosci Behav Physiol 2005;35(8):773–9.

Kaplan E. Right hemisphere contributions to reading: horse and elephant example. Personal communication. 2000.

Kolb B, Whishaw IQ. Fundamentals of human neuropsychology. 6th ed. New York, NY: Worth Publishers; 2008.

Lezak MD, Howieson DB, Loring DW. Neuropsychological assessment. 4th ed. New York, NY: Oxford University Press, Inc.; 2004.

Mesulam MM. Principles of behavioral neurology. Philadelphia: FA Davis; 1985.

Rawlinson G. The significance of letter position in word recognition. PhD Thesis, Nottingham University; 1976. Available from: www.mrc-cbu.cam.ac.uk/~mattd/Cmabridge/rawlinson.html.

Rizzo M, Eslinger PE. Principles and practice of behavioral neurology and neuropsychology. Philadelphia: Saunders; 2004.

Rohrer JD, Knight WD, Warren JE, et al. Word-finding difficulty: a clinical analysis of the progressive aphasias. Brain 2008;131(Pt 1): 8–38.

Schmahmann JD. Disorders of the cerebellum: ataxia, dysmetria of thought, and the cerebellar cognitive affective syndrome. J Neuropsychiatry Clin Neurosci 2004;16(3):367–78.

Schmahmann JD, Sherman JC. The cerebellar cognitive affective syndrome. Brain 1998;121:561–79.

Schmahmann JD, Weilburg JB, Sherman JC. The neuropsychiatry of the cerebellum—insights from the clinic. Cerebellum 2007;6:254–67.

Strauss E, Sherman EMS, Spreen O. A compendium of neuropsychological tests. 3rd ed. New York: Oxford University Press, Inc.; 2006.

Strub RL, Black FW. The mental status examination in neurology. Philadelphia: FA Davis; 2000.

26

Delirium and Acute Encephalopathies

Matthew E. Tilem

CLINICAL VIGNETTE *A 19-year-old woman is brought to the emergency room after she experiences her first ever generalized seizure. An unenhanced brain computed tomography (CT) and basic blood work are normal. She is initially drowsy and disoriented but gradually awakens, becoming increasingly irritable and impulsive. Both the patient and her parents deny that she used alcohol or recreational drugs. She begins pacing the halls and accosting the nurses, who find it difficult to redirect her or to keep her out of other patients' rooms. Her mental state remains disoriented and inattentive; she is incapable of making her own medical decisions. Over the next 12 hours she becomes aggressive and combative, eventually requiring restraints to protect the safety of hospital staff and other patients. With no explanation for her rapid deterioration and with the consent of her parents acting as her proxies, she is sedated for neurologic testing. After a normal contrast-enhanced magnetic resonance imaging (MRI) scan and lumbar puncture, her parents return home to inspect her room, where they find a stash of stolen clonazepam. She is treated for benzodiazepine withdrawal and makes a full recovery over the next 48 hours.*

Delirium is among the most common neuropsychiatric disorders in clinical practice. Virtually every practitioner who treats hospitalized patients will encounter patients suffering from this condition. Various terms are used interchangeably and arbitrarily to describe this diagnosis. Neurologists frequently use the term "toxic metabolic encephalopathy," whereas psychiatrists prefer "delirium." Some practitioners reserve the term "delirium" for patients who demonstrate irritability or hypersympathetic activity. "Acute confusional state" and "change in mental status" (abbreviated "Δ MS") are also frequently used terminologies. The lack of agreement on nomenclature adds a degree of imprecision to the description of these patients. Here, the terms *encephalopathy* and *delirium* are used interchangeably.

As encephalopathy often presents within the context of a complex medical or surgical illness, it is often not appreciated as a clinically independent entity. Nevertheless delirium is associated with considerable morbidity and mortality, delaying or interfering with proper care as well as promoting great distress for nursing staff, physicians, and families.

DEFINITION

There are no universally accepted criteria for a diagnosis of encephalopathy. The most often cited criteria are found in the fifth edition of the *Diagnostic and Statistical Manual of Mental Disorders* (DSM-5). The onset is acute to subacute, within hours or days. It involves a change from baseline that disproportionately affects attention, level of consciousness, and awareness. The state is brought on by a medical condition, intoxication, or withdrawal and follows a fluctuating course. Other elements of cognition may also be affected, including memory, language, visuospatial ability, and/or perception. Patients may experience psychotic features such as delusions or hallucinations.

CAUSES

The list of conditions that may provoke encephalopathy is seemingly endless. Frequently multiple provocations are present in the same patient and the inciting event becomes impossible to distinguish. Common causes of encephalopathy include central nervous system or systemic infection, single-organ or multiorgan failure, electrolyte disturbances, dysglycemia, nutritional deficiencies, drug intoxication or withdrawal, ischemic or hemorrhagic stroke, and brain trauma.

It is a common misconception that encephalopathy is not caused by structural brain disease. For this reason, patients suffering from stroke, a brain tumor, or intracranial hemorrhage may be treated for a presumed infection or metabolic disturbance until an alternative diagnosis is considered and confirmed with brain imaging. Patients with brain lesions in the nondominant hemisphere are particularly prone to encephalopathy, especially when localized to the parietal lobe or thalamus. Ischemic stroke is a commonly overlooked cause for encephalopathy because it is presumed to be focal. However, embolic stroke may be multifocal or diffuse, as with a "shower of emboli." Such presentations are more likely to present with encephalopathy. Embolism to the artery of Percheron, causing bilateral thalamic and hypothalamic infarction, may result in a drowsy, inattentive state that is clinically indistinguishable from other, more common encephalopathies. Similarly, spontaneous or traumatic subdural hematoma or "butterfly" glioma (crossing the corpus callosum) may affect both hemispheres, leading to a "nonfocal" syndrome that is most consistent with encephalopathy.

EPIDEMIOLOGY

Nearly 30% of all patients 65 years of age or older will experience some degree of delirium during hospitalization. The risk varies from 10% to more than 50% depending on comorbidities, severity of illness, and hospital setting. For example, as many as 70% of intensive care patients experience delirium. Delirium prolongs hospitalization, delays rehabilitation, and promotes functional decline and increased risk of institutionalization, all with associated increased costs. According to pooled data from several studies, mortality associated with delirium is high.

The incidence of delirium within the hospitalized patient population ranges from 10% to 20% overall and increases in direct relation to age. This age-related increased prevalence of delirium is more common in the setting of an underlying brain disease. In some instances this may not have been previously identified, as in the individual with occult

Alzheimer disease. Sensory impairment (including poor hearing and vision) heightens the potential for delirium to develop in the elderly.

Despite such a high prevalence, some studies suggest that delirium is neither detected nor documented in up to 66% of these patients. Precipitants of delirium include polypharmacy, infection, metabolic disturbance, malnutrition, and dehydration. Other inciting clinical settings include hospitalization in the intensive care unit, immobility (particularly when restraints are used), frequent room changes, absence of environmental cues such as a clock or watch, and lack of reading glasses.

Another group at very high risk are those in palliative care settings, where delirium is found in close to half the patients. Delirium is also common as a postoperative complication, occurring in up to 52%, and again preferentially in elderly individuals. Certain procedures are associated with a greater risk of delirium, such as coronary bypass and emergency hip surgery. The specific type of anesthesia does not influence risk. Severe postoperative pain increases the propensity for delirium. This may pose a clinical quandary, as the clinician must reconcile the benefits of pain management in preventing encephalopathy with the inherent risk that opioids present in promoting the very same problem. It is essential to aim for the best possible balance between adequate pain control and medication side effects.

DIAGNOSIS AND CLINICAL FEATURES

The core elements of encephalopathy can be evaluated at the bedside with a few easily mastered skills. Special consideration must be given to the assessment of attention and awareness and the detection of clinical fluctuations.

Encephalopathy patients are prototypically inattentive and distractible. They demonstrate difficulty in maintaining focus and directing their attention to particular stimuli in the environment. Consequently the affected patient cannot coherently follow a conversation or train of thought. Responses seem random, tangential, or provided in an inconsequential manner. A commonly used bedside test of attention involves recitation of the months of the year or days of the week in reverse. Patients with impaired attention find it difficult to complete the task and frequently become distracted. Often, they revert to the more familiar forward recitation. Digit span testing is another sensitive way to assess impaired attention. The examiner lists a series of digits in random order and asks the patient to repeat them in the same sequence. Then the examiner lists three digits and asks the patient to repeat them in reverse sequence. A normal forward digit span in an adult is at least seven.

Alteration of awareness, commonly manifesting clinically as disorientation, is universally present. Patients are most frequently disoriented to time but may also be disoriented to location, self, or situation. It is also not uncommon for patients to misidentify close relatives or loved ones. This sort of misidentification can provoke distress and anxiety among family, which far exceeds its clinical significance relative any other disorientation.

Patients often have impaired recall and an inability to learn new information. Consequently they may be very repetitive or may confabulate. Encephalopathic patients are usually amnestic. The memory deficit can be both antegrade and retrograde, although the process of memory creation is most prominently affected and patients rarely remember the details or events that have occurred during the delirium. This can be of great comfort to family, who will usually suffer the lone burden of recalling the sometimes dramatic confusion and abnormal behavior of their loved one. Short-term memory may be tested at the bedside with three-word registration and delayed (≥5 minutes) recall.

Fluctuation in the level of consciousness is the norm in patients suffering from encephalopathy. It may be helpful to conceptualize a normal level of consciousness as the median point of a linear scale. Below the median are patients suffering from drowsiness, stupor, or more severe depression of the level of consciousness. Irritability, aggressiveness, and hypervigilance lie above the median and represent an elevated level of consciousness. Patients withdrawing from alcohol or sedatives usually fall into the hypervigilant category, whereas those suffering from sedative intoxication or hepatic encephalopathy present with a depressed level of consciousness. In practice, patients often fluctuate through a variable level of consciousness. These fluctuations may run counter to the circadian rhythm. The term "sundowning" is applied to patients who are drowsy during the day and awake but irritable at night. It is not uncommon for patients "sundowning" at night to receive a visit from a neurologist or psychiatrist the following morning, who then finds the patient to have shifted to a drowsy or stuporous state (Fig. 26.1). It is important to observe the patient at various times during the day to understand the degree and nature of fluctuating consciousness.

Typically language function is relatively spared in the context of an episode of encephalopathy. In some cases the mechanics of articulation are disrupted, causing slurred speech, as occurs in many cases of intoxication. It is uncommon but not impossible for encephalopathy to mimic aphasia.

The classic tremor associated with encephalopathy is asterixis (Fig. 26.2). Because of its particular association with hepatic encephalopathy, it is often referred to as a "liver flap." The tremor involves a transient loss of extensor tone, which is easily tested at the bedside by having the patient hold up both hands with wrists extended "as if stopping traffic." In patients with limited mobility, the tremor may be elicited in the index fingers by holding them in extension. Some patients may be too inattentive to perform these maneuvers, making it difficult to identify the tremor. If the tremor is exclusively unilateral, a structural brain process should be suspected.

Multifocal myoclonus carries similar clinical significance and may occur in the same patients who experience asterixis. Multifocal, rapid twitches and jerks are observed in the limbs, trunk, or head. These are generally more prominent with arousal and with volitional activation of the affected muscles. The myoclonus may be misconstrued as an epileptic seizure, which frequently leads to urgent neurologic consultation and/or monitoring with electroencephalography (EEG) to distinguish seizure activity from myoclonus. Periodic generalized myoclonic jerks are frequently seen following hypoxic brain injury. Focal or generalized myoclonus is more likely epileptic than multifocal myoclonus.

Delusions and hallucinations occur commonly in the setting of encephalopathy. Visual hallucinations predominate, although tactile, olfactory, and auditory hallucinations do occur. Delusional misidentification may also occur. There are many variations of delusional misidentification, and these are often associated with paranoia, anxiety, and agitation. When patients present with psychosis as the initial manifestation of encephalopathy, they may be misdiagnosed as having a primary psychiatric illness. In these circumstances, the presence of disorientation can be a useful early marker for encephalopathy.

EVALUATION

Evaluation of the encephalopathic patient begins with a search for the underlying medical, surgical, or neuroanatomic abnormality responsible for provoking the altered state (Table 26.1).

Brain imaging should be performed on all patients with newly diagnosed encephalopathy. Unenhanced brain CT is readily available and remains the best way to quickly assess for structural brain abnormalities. Although speed and availability are its strengths, CT is insensitive in the detection of many abnormalities, the most notable of which in this context is acute ischemic stroke. For this reason, additional imaging

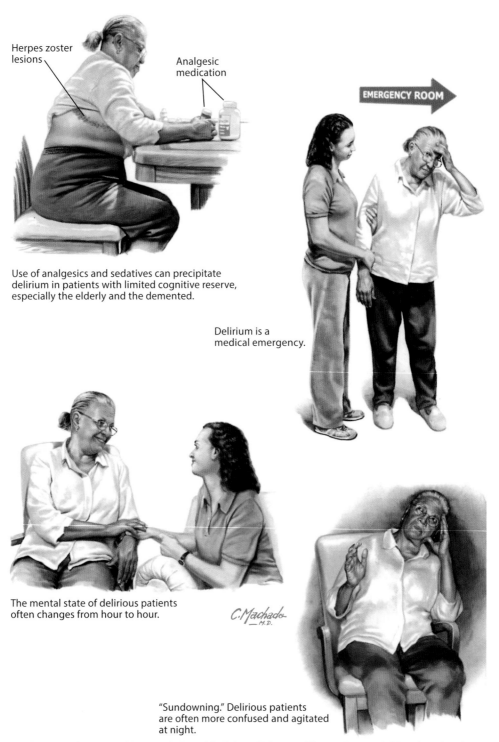

Herpes zoster lesions

Analgesic medication

Use of analgesics and sedatives can precipitate delirium in patients with limited cognitive reserve, especially the elderly and the demented.

EMERGENCY ROOM

Delirium is a medical emergency.

The mental state of delirious patients often changes from hour to hour.

C. Machado
M.D.

"Sundowning." Delirious patients are often more confused and agitated at night.

Fig. 26.1 Common Characteristics of Delirium: Triggers, Fluctuation, and "Sundowning."

with either a brain MRI or repeat head CT 24 hours or more after the initial study is appropriate and may detect abnormalities not seen on initial imaging.

Encephalopathic patients should be evaluated for common infectious and metabolic disturbances as potential inciting factors for their altered mental status. This should include blood work to check electrolytes, glucose, renal function, and hepatic function as well as a complete blood count. Common causes of infection should be explored, especially in patients with fever or leukocytosis. Chest x-ray should be performed.

Urinalysis, although commonly obtained, is of uncertain utility in patients who lack symptoms of urinary tract infection. It is not clear that isolated cystitis can cause encephalopathy, and the high prevalence of asymptomatic bacteriuria, especially among the elderly, can lead to misdiagnosis of urinary tract infection.

The patient's medication history must be thoroughly scrutinized to uncover potential intoxicants or causes of withdrawal. Newer illicit or synthetic intoxicants may not be included in the routine blood or urine toxicology screen. Sometimes friends and family must be questioned

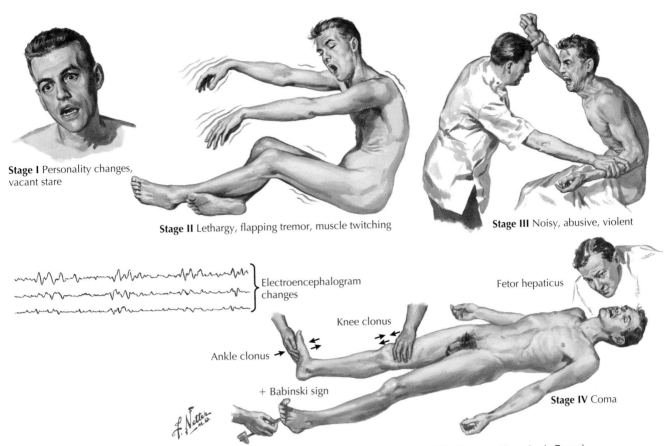

Stage I Personality changes, vacant stare

Stage II Lethargy, flapping tremor, muscle twitching

Stage III Noisy, abusive, violent

Electroencephalogram changes

Fetor hepaticus

Knee clonus

Ankle clonus

+ Babinski sign

Stage IV Coma

Fig. 26.2 Stages of Delirium in Hepatic Encephalopathy and Associated Findings on Neurologic Examination and Electroencephalography.

TABLE 26.1 Clinical Differences Between Delirium and Dementia		
	Delirium	**Dementia**
Onset	Acute to subacute	Subacute to chronic
Level of consciousness	Impaired, fluctuates	Unaffected until late stages
Cognition	Poor attention, disorientation	Poor memory; attention and orientation affected later
Motor behavior	Variably increased or reduced	Usually normal
Psychotic features	Common and prominent	Less common and usually less prominent

to uncover an intoxicant that the patient will not admit to taking. The patient's pharmacy can be a useful resource to identify medication overuse or interactions. More recently, state-run databases have come online and can provide the clinician with a snapshot of controlled substance usage in the recent past.

EEG can be a useful test in the diagnosis of encephalopathy. Patients presenting with a seemingly unprovoked encephalopathy may be experiencing nonconvulsive seizures with a postictal state or with ongoing status epilepticus. There are patterns of EEG, such as generalized slowing or triphasic waves, that correspond with metabolic encephalopathy and may serve to support the diagnostic impression. EEG may be useful in excluding encephalopathy in patients who present with a psychiatric disturbance. A patient suffering from a primary psychiatric illness such as schizophrenia or a mood disorder should have a largely normal EEG.

Lumbar puncture is undertaken early in the workup of encephalopathy when there is suspicion for central nervous system infection or subarachnoid hemorrhage. Lumbar puncture is also indicated when no underlying cause for encephalopathy can be identified. Care must be taken to exclude an intracranial mass lesion with brain imaging before performing lumbar puncture on an encephalopathic patient.

MANAGEMENT

The most important steps in the management of encephalopathy are the identification and treatment of the underlying triggers. When the trigger is adequately addressed, the superimposed encephalopathy can be expected to gradually improve. There is frequently an imperfect correlation between resolution of the encephalopathy and the underlying trigger. The encephalopathy may persist for days or even weeks beyond the apparent correction or resolution of the initial medical or surgical provocation. In these circumstances it is important to review the patient's medication list in order to remove any drugs that are likely to prolong encephalopathy.

Encephalopathic patients frequently experience behavioral disturbances that require management. As a general rule, nonpharmacologic interventions are preferred and should be exhausted before medications are initiated. This is because medications frequently exacerbate and prolong the encephalopathic state. Nonpharmacologic interventions begin with the prevention of disorientation. The patient's eyeglasses and hearing aids must be readily available. The hospital room must include a prominent clock, an easily readable calendar, and proper lighting, ideally including exposure to natural sunlight. Consistency in care providers with limited changes in personnel, frequent reorientation, one-to-one monitoring, and a structured environment to avoid triggers of agitation may reduce the need for chemical and physical restraint in many cases. Every attempt should be made to preserve the integrity of the circadian rhythm. Lighting should reflect the time of day and unnecessary nocturnal arousals should be avoided. The presence of familiar individuals can have a calming effect and help to reduce the need for sedating medication. Providers should work with the patient's support network to bring calming and familiar media into the hospital room.

The pharmacologic management of encephalopathy centers on the maintenance of patient safety and the relief of disturbing symptomatology. The patient's sensitivity to medication should be assessed based on advanced age, a history of dementia, or a previous adverse reaction to sedatives or neuroleptics. Frequently medications are initiated to control agitation, especially as pertaining to patient safety. In particular, patients who remove their intravenous lines or feeding tubes and those who risk falling by getting out of bed may require medical management of agitation. Treatment must be tailored to the individual patient. For example, patients with diffuse Lewy body dementia or Parkinson disease can be expected to react poorly to typical neuroleptics. Patients withdrawing from alcohol would be expected to respond well to benzodiazepines.

Commonly used treatment options for agitation include benzodiazepines and neuroleptics. Atypical neuroleptics are preferred as a scheduled intervention for encephalopathic patients who are not withdrawing from alcohol or sedatives. Parenteral haloperidol or lorazepam are administered when agitation must be addressed urgently owing to safety concerns and/or the patient's inability to swallow oral medications.

When medications fail to preserve patient safety or patients are intolerant of these drugs, physical restraints may become necessary. However, restraints should always be an intervention of last resort and the need for restraints should be reevaluated frequently.

SUMMARY

Encephalopathy is a common diagnosis among hospitalized patients and one that is associated with poor clinical outcome. It is characterized by an acute alteration in mental status that disproportionately affects awareness and attention. The condition occurs among patients who suffer from an underlying toxic or medical condition. Prompt diagnosis and resolution of the inciting event is critical to the management of encephalopathy. Nonpharmacologic management of agitation is preferred in encephalopathic patients, but neuroleptics and benzodiazepines are sometimes needed, especially to maintain patient safety.

ADDITIONAL RESOURCES

Andrew MK, Freter SH, Rockwood K. Prevalence and outcomes of delirium in community and non-acute care settings in people without dementia: a report from the Canadian Study of Health and Aging. BMC Med 2006;4:15.

Brown TM, Boyle MF. ABC of psychological medicine: delirium. BMJ 2002;325:644–7.

Francis J, Young GB. Diagnosis of delirium and confusional states; 2009. Available from: www.uptodate.com.

Johnson MH. Assessing confused patients. J Neurol Neurosurg Psychiatry 2001;71(Suppl. 1):i7–12.

Meagher DJ. Delirium: optimising management. BMJ 2001;322:144–9.

27

Dementia: Mild Cognitive Impairment, Alzheimer Disease, Lewy Body Dementia, Frontotemporal Lobar Dementia, Vascular Dementia

Yuval Zabar

The diagnosis and management of dementia in older adults presents major challenges to the clinician and to society at large. The age-related increase in prevalence of dementia combined with increasing life expectancy is expected to result in a worldwide epidemic within the next few decades. Many of the diseases underlying dementia are definitively diagnosed only at autopsy, including the most common cause of dementia, namely Alzheimer disease (AD). In addition, many neurodegenerative dementias develop without producing symptoms for many years, so-called preclinical disease. Consequently, many patients move through an early phase of illness that does not meet standard diagnostic criteria for dementia. This intermediate clinical phase is called mild cognitive impairment (MCI), reflecting the presence of significant cognitive decline minus the expected loss of function typical of dementia. As our clinical acumen improves and as public awareness of dementia increases, the number of MCI cases is also likely to increase. With this in mind, this chapter reviews the definition of dementia and MCI and discusses the commonest causes of dementia.

Standardized diagnostic criteria for dementia in epidemiologic studies reveal three groups of patients, namely, those who meet the diagnostic criteria of dementia, those who are normal, and those who cannot be classified as normal or demented. The third group of patients represents individuals with isolated cognitive deficits (usually memory) or individuals without disability related to their cognitive deficits. This group of patients includes individuals with MCI.

MILD COGNITIVE IMPAIRMENT

Longitudinal follow-up of these patients reveals a substantially increased risk of cognitive decline and eventual "conversion" to dementia. This risk is estimated to be between 12% and 15% per year. The sensitivity and specificity of screening tools for dementia and MCI vary greatly. The more sensitive diagnostic instruments usually require more time to administer. Consequently, they are not helpful for routine screening. Current brief cognitive screening instruments, including the Mini Mental State Exam (MMSE) or the 7-Minute Screen, are more useful for detecting dementia than MCI when used in populations with elevated prevalence rates of dementia, particularly in the elderly. Other brief, more focused cognitive screening tools such as the Clock Drawing Test or the Time and Change Test may offer additional sensitivity in screening for dementia.

The utility of these tests in detecting MCI is less reliable. Indeed, most patients with MCI score within the normal range on the MMSE.

Interview-based dementia assessments, such as the Clinical Dementia Rating scale (CDR), provide a more sensitive means for reliable detection of MCI but may require considerably more time to administer. Another brief screening tool, the Montreal Cognitive Assessment Test (www.mocatest.org), may provide greater sensitivity in detecting MCI. The definitive diagnosis of MCI requires formal neuropsychological assessment. However, neuropsychological test batteries take several hours to administer and interpret. Therefore they are not practical as screening tools. In the hands of an experienced neuropsychologist, formal neuropsychological tests provide the most sensitive means of detecting cognitive impairment. They may also provide greater specificity in identifying the underlying cause, although there may be significant variability among neuropsychologists' interpretations.

Neuropsychological batteries can differentiate MCI subtypes depending upon the predominant cognitive domain(s) involved. *Amnestic MCI* involves deficits in short-term memory localizable to mesial temporal structures. Neuropathologically, this subtype of MCI is most often associated with AD. *Nonamnestic MCI* includes patients with isolated nonmemory-related cognitive deficits, such as aphasia, apraxia, executive dysfunction, or agnosia. The neuropathology associated with nonamnestic MCI is more variable but also includes AD. Although detection of MCI is relatively easy, treatment of MCI remains controversial. In the largest randomized clinical trial to date, donepezil was shown to delay "conversion" of amnestic MCI to AD better than placebo or vitamin E over 18 months' duration. Very disappointingly after 3 years of follow-up there was no difference in the rate of "conversion" nor in the severity of cognitive impairment.

DEMENTIA

The most common feature of dementia is impairment in short- and long-term memory, with additional impairment in at least one of the following: abstract thinking, impaired judgment, other disturbances of higher cognitive function, or personality change. The disturbance causes disability in usual social, occupational, or personal function. Of course, any two cognitive domains may be involved, and memory loss is not essential for every type of dementia. The diagnosis of dementia is not made if these symptoms occur in delirium (DSM IIIR).

Although this standard definition is adequate for diagnosis of dementia, it is limited in scope. Defined in this way, the diagnosis of dementia requires disability secondary to cognitive losses. However, an 80-year-old retired businessman with progressive deficits in multiple cognitive domains, but functioning independently, may not be considered "disabled," and therefore his condition does not technically meet the diagnostic criteria for dementia. Further refinements of diagnostic criteria, aimed at identifying the underlying neuropathologic disease process, require the presence of more specific cognitive deficits for diagnosis. For example, the National Institute of Neurological and Communicative Disorders and Stroke–Alzheimer Disease and Related Disorders Association (NINCDS-ADRDA) Work Group criteria for a diagnosis of probable AD require deficits in short-term memory plus at least one additional cognitive domain. In this context, a 55-year-old businessman who can no longer work because of isolated short-term memory impairment also would not technically meet diagnostic criteria for dementia, despite having a disabling cognitive problem. Such cases should be monitored for future decline. Formal neuropsychological assessment must be considered in such cases to assess for more subtle deficits that standard bedside examination often misses. Additional diagnostic criteria may be applied to diagnose the underlying disease process once dementia is identified. In the future, there may be additional studies to improve the accuracy of diagnosis, such as cerebrospinal fluid (CSF) protein analysis for amyloid and tau proteins, and brain positron emission tomography (PET) imaging.

Various comorbidities should be assessed to address potentially treatable factors contributing to cognitive impairment. Depression is particularly important because it commonly coexists with dementia in the elderly. Often, depression may be a harbinger of impending dementia in many cases of late life onset of depression. Validated depression assessment instruments, such as Geriatric Depression Scale–Short Form or the Hamilton Depression Scale, may facilitate office screening for depression.

Certain nutritional, endocrinologic, or infectious processes must also be considered in the evaluation of the demented patient. Vitamin B_{12} (cobalamin) deficiency is common in the elderly, although a specific causative relationship with dementia is not known. On rare occasions, vitamin B_{12} deficiency is associated with cognitive impairment that may reverse with vitamin supplementation. Hypothyroidism is also common in the elderly, and it is associated with impaired performance on cognitive tests. Although there is no well-established association with dementia, coincident hypothyroidism may impact dementia severity. The incidence and prevalence of tertiary syphilis in the United States is now virtually zero. Therefore, routine screening for syphilis as a cause of dementia in the elderly is no longer recommended in most US population groups.

The increasing recognition of possible biomarkers for various dementing diseases may also improve diagnostic accuracy. These include various CSF protein assays, such as protein 14-3-3 in prion disease, and amyloid and tau proteins in AD. Imaging modalities such as fluorodeoxyglucose (FDG)-PET scans or ligand-based PET scans (detecting β-amyloid deposition in AD) may reveal the molecular changes in the brains of living dementia patients. However, the newer assays and brain imaging techniques still do not provide a definitive diagnosis of dementia and are not used routinely. The definitive diagnosis of most dementing illnesses requires pathologic confirmation. Therefore diagnosis of dementia currently remains largely clinical.

Dementia Management

The treatment of dementia requires pharmacologic and nonpharmacologic approaches. We will review general treatment strategies here. The target of treatment typically falls into one or more of three interdependent factors, namely (1) cognition, (2) behavior, and (3) functional capacity. Treatment of one factor may negatively impact the other factors. The literature on dementia treatments is too expansive for full review here. More detailed discussion of specific dementia treatment strategies follows in subsequent sections.

It is imperative to recognize and treat dementia as early as possible, with a goal to maximize and preserve quality of life for both patient and caregiver. Treatment of cognitive impairment involves intervention either to reverse, slow, or delay progression of cognitive decline. For the most part, currently available pharmacologic agents prove valuable only in delaying decline, perhaps preventing more severe disability and behavior problems. Behavior problems range from disturbances of mood to psychotic symptoms, apathy to agitation, anxiety, and stereotypic, purposeless, rituals. Treatment of behavioral disturbance must address the behavior that proves disabling for the patient or the caregiver. In many cases, nonpharmacologic approaches may suffice. This may include diverting the patient's attention, changing the subject of conversation, comforting the patient affectionately, or occupying the patient with a task. Environmental manipulation, caregiver support, and day programs all provide structure and routine for the patient with behavior problems and for his or her caregiver. In cases where such interventions prove less effective for behavior management, or safety is compromised by aberrant behavior, pharmacologic treatments should be used. The chosen medication should address the primary aspect of behavior aberration, such as antidepressants for low mood and vegetative symptoms, mood stabilizers for emotional lability, or antipsychotics for psychotic symptoms and combativeness. Prevention of functional decline requires comprehensive management of both cognitive and behavioral disturbances, as well as provision of support and education to the caregiver. Routine follow-up of patients with their primary caregiver is essential to maximize quality of life for all involved.

Dementia and Driving

One of the most difficult aspects of counseling dementia patients and families relates to safety of operating a motor vehicle. Driving safety in AD is well studied, and there is clear evidence that relative risk of crashes for drivers with AD, from mild to severe stages of dementia, is greater than accepted societal standards. Drivers with MCI seem to have risk for crashes similar to teenage drivers. Several studies link driving risk with dementia severity using the CDR scale. The CDR is an informant-based scale that includes direct assessment of the patient and information given by a knowledgeable informant. The CDR scores increase from 0 (normal) to 0.5 (possible dementia) to 1.0–3.0 (mild, moderate, severe dementia). Most clinicians do not routinely use this scale in their everyday practice, and therefore translating the scale scores into everyday terms may be difficult. For practical purposes, the CDR score of 0.5 loosely translates into MCI, whereas a CDR score of 1.0 or greater translates to dementia. There may be exceptions to these findings, and further research is required to find more specific patterns of cognitive impairment that lead to driving risk. Risk of driving in non-Alzheimer dementia is relatively unstudied. However, it is safe to assume that driving risk is increased also in this population.

ALZHEIMER DISEASE

CLINICAL VIGNETTE *A 75-year-old man became lost driving to his daughter's house; he was subsequently referred for cognitive evaluation. He is a retired accountant, college graduate, and competitive bridge player. The patient has no specific complaints, stating he came to the doctor's appointment because of family members' concerns about increasing short-term memory loss. He expresses frustration with family members' "overblown concerns," but he acknowledges occasionally forgetting people's names and trouble finding words during conversation. He excuses his recent driving error, stating "it could happen to anyone."*

His wife paints a direful picture. She reports the patient's mentation is declining progressively. Two to three years earlier he began forgetting friends' and neighbors' names. Subsequently, he became increasingly repetitive and easily frustrated when she would try reminding him of recent conversation. Approximately 1 year earlier, he made mistakes with the bills and bounced several checks, prompting her to take over the checkbook. He gave up playing bridge and reading. He spends increasing amounts of time sitting in front of his computer but does not seem to be accomplishing anything. When she tries to get him to go out to visit friends or family, he refuses and, occasionally, becomes angry with her. The patient recalls becoming angry but cannot recall the details of the events. She is concerned he may be mismanaging his medications because of recent changes in blood sugar levels. When he misplaces things, such as his wallet, he accuses her of taking it. He is reluctant to let her supervise his medications. Within the past 6 months, while driving he has had trouble finding his way around town.

On examination, he appears well. His mood is good and his affect is appropriate. He is fully awake and alert. He scores 18/30 on the MMSE, losing points on orientation items, all three memory items, and on serial seven subtractions. In addition, he could not copy the intersecting pentagon figure. There was no evidence of apraxia or agnosia. His remaining neurologic examination was completely normal.

Brain magnetic resonance imaging (MRI) showed mild, diffuse atrophy, bilateral periventricular/subcortical white matter "microvascular" changes, and two chronic lacunar strokes in the right striatum and cerebellar hemisphere. Thyroid, vitamin B$_{12}$, folate, and rapid plasma reagin (RPR) studies were normal. Hemoglobin A1C was elevated.

Initially donepezil was prescribed and memantine added 6 months later. His MMSE scores remained relatively stable over the next 3 years. He never resumed bridge playing, but he is more engaged and outgoing during this time. His wife enrolls him in a day program 4 days per week. There is a gradual decline in daily activities and, 4 years later, his MMSE score is 12/30. He now requires assistance with personal hygiene and with dressing. He continues to decline slowly until entering a nursing home approximately 10 years after disease onset.

Epidemiology

AD is the most common cause of dementia in adults, accounting for approximately 5 million cases of dementia in the United States. Age-specific disease incidence increases exponentially with advancing age; the risk of development of AD doubles every 5 years, beginning at 65 years of age. AD affects approximately 50% of the population aged 85 years and older. Given the growing elderly population in developed countries, projections of future AD prevalence show a fourfold increase through 2050. Because dementia is a major factor in healthcare costs, morbidity, and mortality, the high prevalence of AD places enormous burdens on the healthcare system. In many cases, diagnosis is delayed until an advanced stage, at which point caregiver stress is already high and treatment options are limited. Of the 5 million prevalent cases, only 3 million are diagnosed and only one-third of diagnosed cases receive treatment. Of those who receive treatment, the percentage receiving adequate doses and follow-up is unknown. It is very important for clinicians to understand the natural history of AD, recognize early warning signs, implement appropriate screening and diagnostic tools, prescribe appropriate treatment, and follow patients regularly.

Pathogenesis

There is pronounced gross cerebral atrophy clearly evident on both imaging studies and postmortem. Typically, the dementia of AD preferentially affects the frontal, temporal, and parietal cortex. This is particularly evident in the temporoparietal and frontal association areas and the olfactory cortex. In contrast, other primary sensory cortical areas are unaffected. In addition, the limbic system, subcortical nuclei, and the nucleus basalis of Meynert are preferentially affected. Microscopically, there is clear loss of both neurons and neuropil. The classic findings include senile plaques and neurofibrillary tangles (Figs. 27.1 and 27.2). The white matter sometimes demonstrates a secondary demyelination.

β-Amyloid

AD is a neurodegenerative disorder thought to result from deposition of the protein β-amyloid in the brain. β-Amyloid is formed by processing of the amyloid precursor protein (APP), a protein that may help to regulate synaptic integrity and function, possibly by regulating excitotoxic activity of glutamate. APP is encoded on chromosome 21. It is processed at the cell membrane by secretase enzymes, called α-, β-, and γ-secretases. Two known membrane-bound proteins, called presenilins, comprise the active domains of the membrane-bound γ-secretase protein: presenilin 1 and presenilin 2 are encoded on chromosomes 14 and 1, respectively. Numerous genetic mutations of the presenilin and APP genes are known to cause familial, early-onset cases of AD. The familial forms of AD account for fewer than 5% of all AD cases. The known mutations account for approximately 50% of familial AD. In all cases the genetic mutation leads to an overproduction of β-amyloid that may be the first step in the subsequent cascade of neurodegeneration.

β-Amyloid is a short fragment of the APP, typically 40–42 amino acids in length, which accumulates outside the cell during APP processing (Figs. 27.3 and 27.4). The tertiary structure of the 42–amino acid fragment is a β-pleated sheet that renders it insoluble. Consequently, it accumulates slowly, over many years, in the extracellular space and within synapses. In vitro studies confirm that β-amyloid is toxic to surrounding synapses and neurons, causing synaptic membrane destruction and eventual cell death. Transgenic mouse models show a clear association between accumulation of β-amyloid fragments, formation of amyloid plaques, and development of cognitive impairment.

In vivo, β-amyloid fragments coalesce to form *"diffuse"* or immature *plaques,* best seen with silver-staining techniques. However, diffuse plaques are not sufficient to produce dementia; many nondemented elderly patients have substantial depositions of diffuse plaques throughout the cortex, a condition termed pathologic aging. It is when these plaques mature into *"senile"* or neuritic plaques that dementia becomes more likely (Fig. 27.5, top). Senile plaques consist of other substances in addition to β-amyloid, including synaptic proteins, inflammatory proteins, neuritic threads, activated glial cells, and other components. Unlike diffuse plaques, senile plaques are composed of a central core of β-amyloid surrounded by a myriad of proteins and cellular debris. Senile plaques are distributed diffusely in the cortex, typically starting in the hippocampus and the basal forebrain. Senile plaque formation correlates with increasing loss of synapses, which correlates with the earliest clinical sign, namely, short-term memory loss. The anatomic pattern of progression gradually spreads to neocortical and subcortical gray matter of the temporal, parietal, frontal, and, eventually, occipital cortex. Subcortical nuclei become involved relatively late in the process.

Neurofibrillary Tangles

The second pathologic hallmark of AD is the neurofibrillary tangle (see Fig. 27.5, bottom). These lesions develop and conform to an anatomic pattern that correlates with the clinical syndrome; the number and distribution of tangles are directly related to the severity and clinical features of the dementia. Neurofibrillary tangles form intracellularly, consisting of a *microtubule-associated protein, tau,* which has a vital role in the maintenance of neuronal cytoskeleton structure and function. Tau is hyperphosphorylated in AD, causing it to dissociate from the cytoskeleton and accumulate, forming a paired helical filament protein structure. The cytoskeleton is compromised structurally and functionally, disrupting normal cell function. The most commonly used

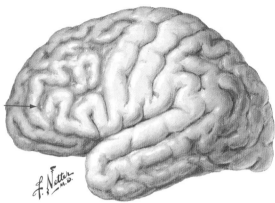

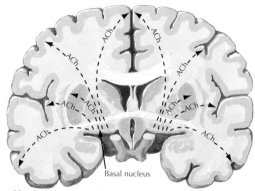

Regional atrophy of brain with narrowed gyri and widened sulci (arrow), but precentral and postcentral, inferior frontal, angular, supramarginal, and some occipital gyri fairly well preserved. Association cortex mostly involved.

Section of brain schematically demonstrating postulated normal transport of acetylcholine (ACh) from basal nucleus of Meynert (substantia innominata) to cortical gray matter

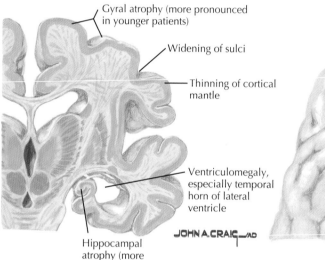

Gyral atrophy (more pronounced in younger patients)

Widening of sulci

Thinning of cortical mantle

Ventriculomegaly, especially temporal horn of lateral ventricle

Hippocampal atrophy (more pronounced in older patients)

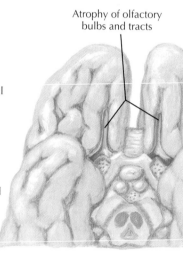

Atrophy of olfactory bulbs and tracts

JOHN A. CRAIG _AD

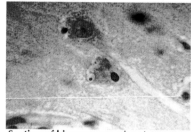

Senile plaque (center) made up of argyrophil fibers around core of pink-staining amyloid (Bodian preparation). Neurons decreased in number, with characteristic tangles in cytoplasm.

Section of hippocampus showing granulovacuolar inclusions and loss of pyramidal cells

Fig. 27.1 Alzheimer Disease: Pathology.

pathologic criteria for definitive AD diagnosis at autopsy require the presence of senile plaques and neurofibrillary tangles. Other lesions, such as Hirano bodies, are also seen in AD but have little diagnostic specificity.

Neurotransmitters

In addition to neuronal and synaptic loss, there is a gradual loss of various neurotransmitters. *Acetylcholine* synthesis is the earliest and most prominently affected. Most acetylcholinergic neurons arise within the *nucleus basalis of Meynert* in the basal forebrain (see Fig. 27.2). This nucleus is affected relatively early in the process; acetylcholine levels within the brain and spinal fluid of patients with AD quickly decline with disease progression. This observation supported the cholinergic hypothesis—that acetylcholine depletion results in the cognitive decline observed in patients with AD—eventually leading to the first symptomatic treatment of AD.

Risk Factors

Epidemiologic studies identify several potential risk factors for AD. The most consistent risk factors include advanced age, family history

(especially in first-degree relatives), and apolipoprotein E (ApoE) genotype. Other risk factors include hypertension, stroke, and fasting homocysteine levels (Fig. 27.6). Because vascular risk factors are modifiable, they may affect risk reduction and treatment for patients with AD and those at risk for development of AD.

1. *Advanced age* is the single consistently identified risk factor for AD across numerous all-international studies. AD incidence and prevalence increase with advancing age, leading to the hypothesis that AD would develop in all individuals if they lived long enough. The true incidence in persons older than age 85 years is difficult to ascertain because of sharp decline in life expectancy. However, there are many instances of nondemented elders where no pathologic evidence of AD is found at autopsy, including in centenarians. Therefore dementia is not considered a "normal" part of aging.

2. *Family history* of dementia is another consistent risk factor in many studies; however, the most common form of AD occurs sporadically. Establishing accurate family history of dementia is difficult because many of these patients' relatives may not have survived into older ages where dementia risk is greatest. Rare, early-onset, presenile (before age 65 years) forms of AD occur with an autosomal-dominant pattern

In neocortex, primary involvement of association areas (especially temporoparietal and frontal) with relative sparing of primary sensory cortices (except olfactory) and motor cortices

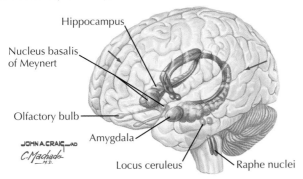

Pathologic involvement of limbic system and subcortical nuclei projecting to cortex

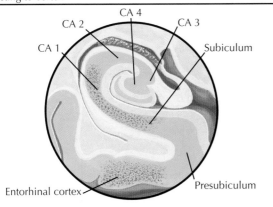

In hippocampus, neurofibrillary tangles, neuronal loss, and senile plaques primarily located in layer CA1, subiculum, and entorhinal cortex

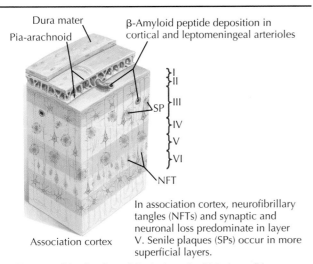

In association cortex, neurofibrillary tangles (NFTs) and synaptic and neuronal loss predominate in layer V. Senile plaques (SPs) occur in more superficial layers.

Fig. 27.2 Distribution of Pathology in Alzheimer Disease.

of inheritance. The genetic basis for many hereditary AD forms is identified. Most mutations affect the genes that encode APP and the presenilins. Each mutation leads to increased deposition of amyloid in affected individuals, predisposing to earlier onset. Individuals with trisomy 21 (Down syndrome) also have a high deposition of β-amyloid. AD develops in all patients with Down syndrome by age 35 years.

3. *ApoE genotype* is another genetic risk factor (Fig. 27.7). The three common allelic forms of this gene, epsilon 2 through 4, are encoded on chromosome 19. The presence of an e4 allele is associated with increased risk of AD and younger age at onset. This risk is greatly increased in e4 homozygotes. Conversely, the e2 allele appears to impart a protective, risk-lowering effect, as replicated in numerous international, population-based studies. The association between the ApoE e4 allele and AD seems to be disease specific. There is no clear association between e4 and other neurodegenerative or amyloid-based diseases.

The mechanism underlying this increased risk associated with the Apo e4 allele is not well understood but may relate to the role of ApoE in cell membrane repair. Phenotypically, the e4 cases have greater amyloid deposition than do the non-e4 cases. Although ApoE genotyping is available, it is not a diagnostic test for AD, nor is it recommended for routine testing. Most patients with AD are non-e4 carriers. ApoE genotyping is largely used in research, primarily as a biologic marker to differentiate cases. Some studies suggest differential response to medications in cases stratified by ApoE genotypes.

4. In recent years, cerebrovascular disease and vascular disease risk factors have emerged as significant risk factors for AD. The presence of stroke increases the likelihood of dementia in old age. Diabetes, hypertension, and hyperlipidemia consistently elevate relative risk of dementia across international epidemiologic surveys of AD and dementia. Moreover, multiple observational studies show reduced risk among individuals receiving treatment for these conditions. This connection between AD and cerebrovascular disease may provide an important focus for premorbid dementia prevention. It is unknown whether secondary stroke prevention reduces the likelihood of dementia or its rate of progression. Nevertheless, assessment of stroke risk factors may become increasingly important for the management of dementia patients.

Clinical Presentation

The early signs of AD may be subtle (Fig. 27.8). In the initial stages of AD, memory losses can be clinically distinguished from normal aging, although formal memory testing is often required to confirm suspicion of early dementia. The early signs of AD begin insidiously, progress slowly, and are often covered up by patients. Detection may be challenging even for close family members. The physician may observe changes in the patient's pattern of behavior, such as missing appointments or poor compliance with medications. It is important to discuss such issues openly with family members given the patient often cannot recall examples of memory problems. Indeed, it is common for patients to have limited insight into their deficit and for family members to initiate an evaluation for memory loss. In these early stages, patients maintain their social graces. It is not uncommon during mental status testing to discover the significant cognitive problems concealed by a patient's friendly and sociable affect. "Very pleasant" patients sometimes fool even seasoned geriatricians. The Alzheimer's Association lists 10 key warning signs of AD.

Commonly, AD begins with short-term memory loss, although atypical presentations sometimes develop. Often, patients have increasing forgetfulness of words and names, relying more on lists, calendars, and family members for reminders. Disorganization of appointments, bills, and medications becomes commonplace. Family members often notice increasing repetitiveness, patients asking the same question or repeating the same conversation minutes after it was completed. Patients may forget to convey telephone messages or turn off the stove, or lose track of where they place things. Moreover, their ability to recall these incidents is impaired. They "forget that they forget." Affected individuals may become suspicious of others (e.g., thinking that misplaced items were stolen).

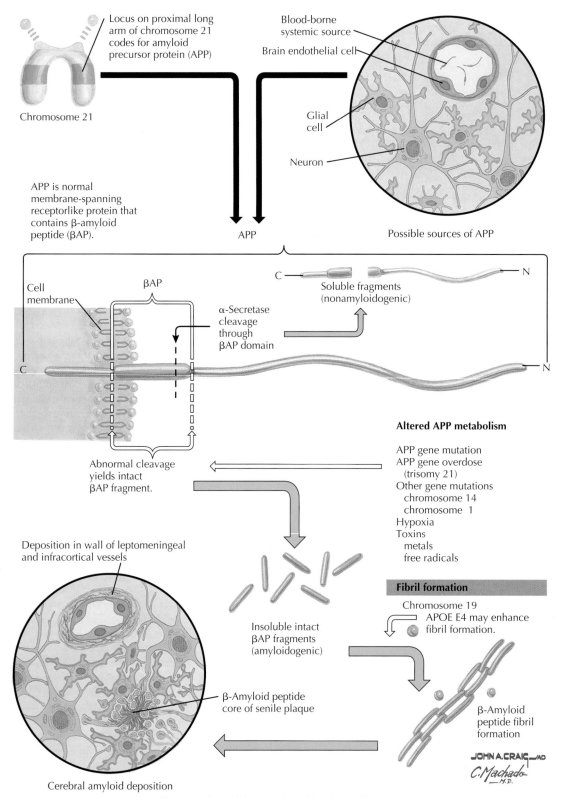

Locus on proximal long arm of chromosome 21 codes for amyloid precursor protein (APP)

Chromosome 21

Blood-borne systemic source

Brain endothelial cell

Glial cell

Neuron

APP is normal membrane-spanning receptorlike protein that contains β-amyloid peptide (βAP).

APP

Possible sources of APP

Cell membrane

βAP

Soluble fragments (nonamyloidogenic)

α-Secretase cleavage through βAP domain

C

N

C

N

Abnormal cleavage yields intact βAP fragment.

Altered APP metabolism

APP gene mutation
APP gene overdose (trisomy 21)
Other gene mutations
   chromosome 14
   chromosome 1
Hypoxia
Toxins
   metals
   free radicals

Fibril formation

Chromosome 19
APOE E4 may enhance fibril formation.

Deposition in wall of leptomeningeal and infracortical vessels

Insoluble intact βAP fragments (amyloidogenic)

β-Amyloid peptide fibril formation

β-Amyloid peptide core of senile plaque

JOHN A. CRAIG—AD
C. Machado
—M.D.

Cerebral amyloid deposition

Fig. 27.3 Amyloidogenesis in Alzheimer Disease.

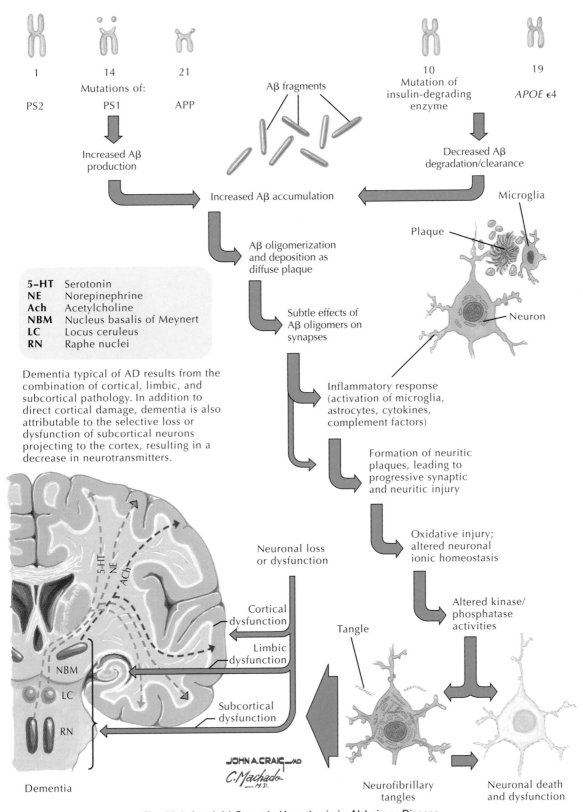

Fig. 27.4 Amyloid Cascade Hypothesis in Alzheimer Disease.

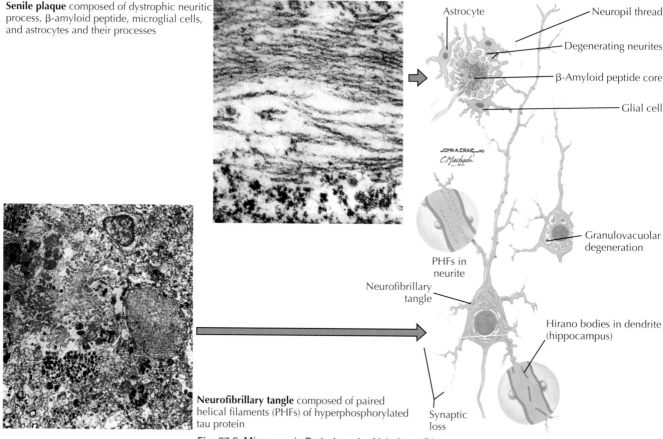

Senile plaque composed of dystrophic neuritic process, β-amyloid peptide, microglial cells, and astrocytes and their processes

Astrocyte
Neuropil thread
Degenerating neurites
β-Amyloid peptide core
Glial cell

PHFs in neurite

Neurofibrillary tangle

Granulovacuolar degeneration

Hirano bodies in dendrite (hippocampus)

Neurofibrillary tangle composed of paired helical filaments (PHFs) of hyperphosphorylated tau protein

Synaptic loss

Fig. 27.5 Microscopic Pathology in Alzheimer Disease.

Language function gradually declines. Word-finding and name-finding difficulties are common even in very early stages. Naming impairment and gradual loss of comprehension, expression, or both are universal. The perception of the temporal sequence of events is affected and disorientation eventually becomes pervasive. Geographic orientation declines, first affecting patients' ability to navigate in unfamiliar environments and later within their homes. Visuospatial skills decline and construction deficits may occur early.

Behavior and personality in patients with AD are often affected; combativeness, irritability, frustration, and anxiety become extremely common. Many patients seek medical attention only when family members are alarmed by behavioral changes, rather than because of their earlier progressive memory loss. Psychotic features may become prominent. Some patients also develop delusional thoughts and hallucinations, most commonly visual or auditory in nature. These may be benign, understated, hidden, or frightening and may lead to severe agitation. Family members may not speak freely in the patient's presence about these symptoms.

As cognitive and behavioral changes appear, the patients' ability to maintain personal independence declines. Altered activities that may occur early include medication mismanagement, financial disorganization, burnt pots on the stove, and driving errors. Eventually patients require assistance with activities of daily living: personal hygiene/bathing, eating, dressing, and toileting. Often, by this stage, patients exhibit signs of parkinsonism characterized by midline rigidity, symmetric bradykinesia and hypokinesia, stooped posture, and shuffling stride. The risk of falling increases. Seizures occur in up to 20% of cases. Myoclonic jerks are increasingly noted in advanced stages.

Later stages of AD are characterized by loss of bladder and then bowel control, failure to recognize family members, and eventually severe akinesia, requiring total nursing care. The most common cause of death is aspiration pneumonia. On average, AD has a duration of approximately 8 years. However, this varies substantially. Some patients live 20 years or more. Nursing care marks an important endpoint for many patients and their caregivers. The most common causes for nursing home placement include behavioral problems, immobility, and incontinence.

The Alzheimer's Association provides a staging system to allow doctors and caregivers a frame of reference when discussing the patient's level of impairment and possible future progression. It is important to emphasize that not every patient will follow through these stages in the same way or at the same rate.

Differential Diagnosis

The *absence of motor deficits* early in AD differentiates it from most other dementias. Other dementias lacking motor signs include amnestic syndrome (Korsakoff encephalopathy), Pick disease, vascular dementia, and human immunodeficiency virus (HIV) dementia complex. Depression can also produce dementia-like symptoms without motor deficits. Poor concentration and short-term memory impairment result from lack of effort, disinterest, or distractibility. "Pseudodementia" due to depression is usually not progressive, and functional loss is often disproportionately severe relative to cognitive impairment (Fig. 27.9).

Reversible causes of dementia without motor signs include toxic and metabolic causes of chronic delirium. Chronic use of medication with anticholinergic side effects (e.g., antihistamines and tricyclic antidepressants) is a possible cause of chronic delirium that may mimic AD. β-Blockers, digoxin, H_2 blockers, and various antibiotics may also contribute to chronic delirium. Chronic mass effect, caused

Increased Risk

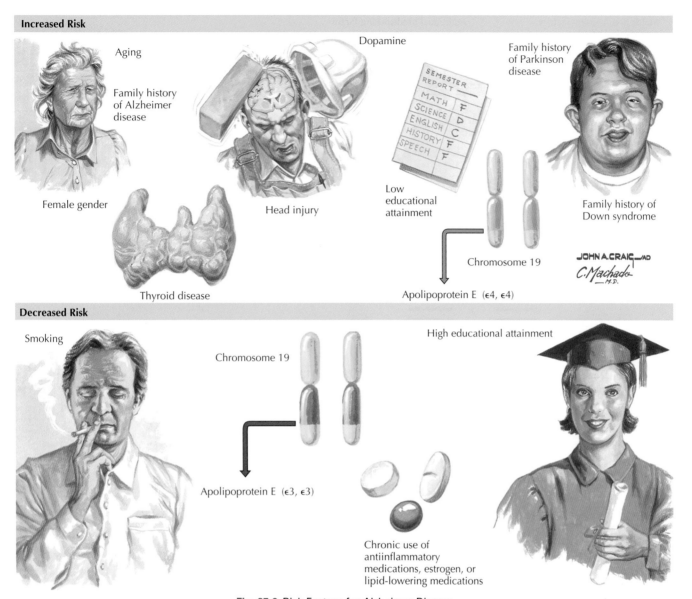

Aging

Family history of Alzheimer disease

Female gender

Dopamine

Head injury

Thyroid disease

Low educational attainment

Chromosome 19

Family history of Parkinson disease

Family history of Down syndrome

JOHN A. CRAIG—AD
C. Machado
—M.D.

Apolipoprotein E (∈4, ∈4)

Decreased Risk

Smoking

Chromosome 19

High educational attainment

Apolipoprotein E (∈3, ∈3)

Chronic use of antiinflammatory medications, estrogen, or lipid-lowering medications

Fig. 27.6 Risk Factors for Alzheimer Disease.

by a slow-growing tumor (see Fig. 27.9), may also produce reversible cognitive impairment.

Dementia *with motor deficits* includes a longer list of possibilities. Thyroid disease, vitamin B_{12} deficiency, and tertiary neurosyphilis are often considered; however, these conditions rarely cause dementia and usually present with characteristic metabolic or sensorimotor symptoms.

Normal pressure hydrocephalus is a relatively uncommon condition that late in its course may be characterized by a significant dementia (see Fig. 32.2). Typically, these individuals present with a broad-based magnetic gait as if their feet were partially glued to the ground. Eventually these patients may become unwittingly incontinent, unaware of their loss of sphincter control as the dementing process evolves. Although these patients most often have no identifiable cause, on occasion, they have previously sustained a subarachnoid hemorrhage or meningitis leading to poor CSF reabsorption. This leads to the characteristic hydrocephalus without an associated loss of cortical mantel. A CSF shunt may lead to a remarkable improvement.

The presence of spastic hemiparesis or dysarthria raises suspicion of cerebrovascular disease. Parkinsonism is associated with Parkinson

disease (PD) and dementia with Lewy bodies (DLBs). Progressive ataxia occurs with multisystem atrophy. Chorea characterizes Huntington disease. As AD progresses to late stages, parkinsonism often becomes evident, making clinical differentiation from other parkinsonian diseases more difficult. AD may also coexist with cerebrovascular or Lewy body (LB) pathology to produce dementia with motor signs.

Dementia may be further characterized by cortical and subcortical cognitive features, which also helps to differentiate between different dementing diseases. Subcortical features include slower mental processing, slow retrieval of information, and often significant extrapyramidal motor signs, including bradykinesia or adventitious movements.

Diagnosis

The subjective complaint of memory impairment is not useful for dementia screening because it is a common complaint in older adults. Prospective evaluation of individuals aged 65 years who have complaints of memory loss show that dementia develops in fewer than 9% within a 5-year follow-up. However, dementia develops during a 5-year prospective follow-up in 50% of patients aged 85 years who had no

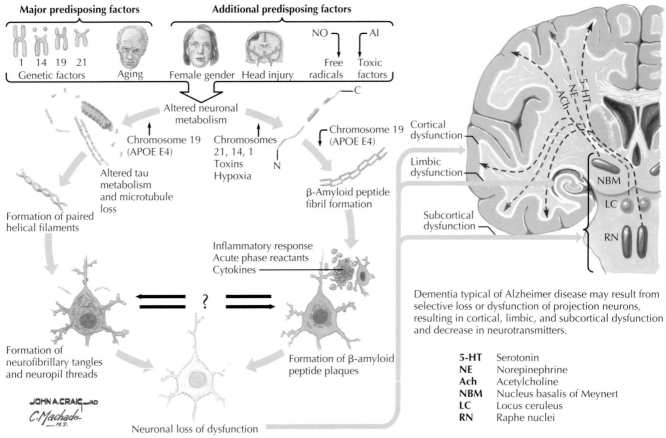

Fig. 27.7 Possible Factors in Development and Progression of Alzheimer Disease.

Dementia typical of Alzheimer disease may result from selective loss or dysfunction of projection neurons, resulting in cortical, limbic, and subcortical dysfunction and decrease in neurotransmitters.

5-HT	Serotonin
NE	Norepinephrine
Ach	Acetylcholine
NBM	Nucleus basalis of Meynert
LC	Locus ceruleus
RN	Raphe nuclei

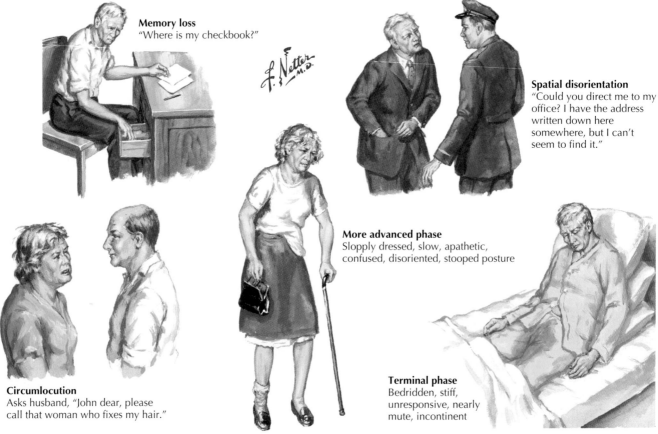

Memory loss
"Where is my checkbook?"

Spatial disorientation
"Could you direct me to my office? I have the address written down here somewhere, but I can't seem to find it."

More advanced phase
Slopply dressed, slow, apathetic, confused, disoriented, stooped posture

Circumlocution
Asks husband, "John dear, please call that woman who fixes my hair."

Terminal phase
Bedridden, stiff, unresponsive, nearly mute, incontinent

Fig. 27.8 Alzheimer Disease: Clinical Manifestations, Progressive Phases.

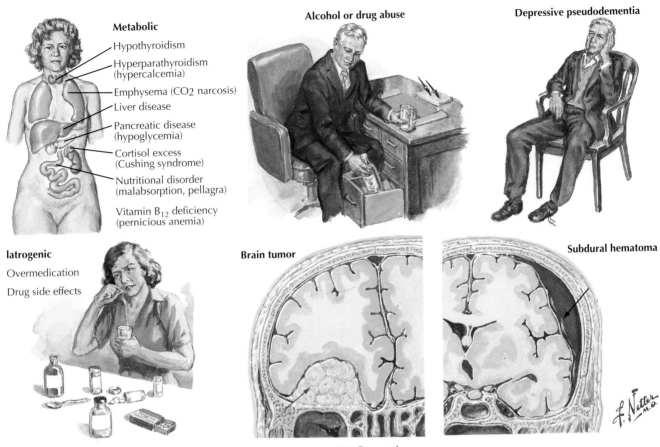

Fig. 27.9 Treatable Dementias.

complaints of memory loss at baseline. Consequently, clinicians must be proactive, particularly with patients aged 85 years or older, and screen for cognitive impairment.

Proper clinical assessment requires a detailed history, preferably provided by a trustworthy, knowledgeable informant particularly a spouse or child. The history should describe the cognitive decline, in temporal sequence, from earliest suggestion of cognitive impairment to most recent events. Examination in early stages may reveal no neurologic deficits other than cognitive impairment. In later stages, or in patients with coexisting neuropathology, such as stroke, there may be motor deficits or other focal central nervous system (CNS) findings on physical examination.

Mental Status Exam

The mental status examination (see Chapter 2) should assess all major cognitive domains, including *M*emory, *A*ttention, *L*anguage, *C*onstruction, *O*rientation, *P*raxis, and *E*xecutive function (MALCOPE). Standardized global measures of cognitive function such as the MMSE are of limited diagnostic value. The widely used MMSE is relatively insensitive to the milder stages of AD. Other tests, such as the Montreal Cognitive Assessment Test, include test items more suited to detecting earlier stages of cognitive impairment, allowing improved sensitivity for detecting MCI. Another measure, the Alzheimer Disease 8 (AD8) is an informant-based tool that may shorten screening considerably. It must be emphasized that such instruments are not diagnostic tests, and interpretation of results must take into consideration level of education, native language, and physical or sensory impairment that might affect performance.

Impaired recording of information characterizes the memory loss of early AD. The inability to record information occurs when patients cannot recall information even with practice and when given hints or cues. Additional early cognitive deficits in AD include *dysnomia, reduced verbal fluency (especially in word categories), orientation to time,* and *construction impairment.* Having the patient list as many category words as possible within 1 minute provides a test of *verbal fluency.* For example, patients try to list animals or words beginning with the letter *s.*

Clock drawing is useful when testing *construction and executive function* (Fig. 27.10). Patients draw a clock, for example, indicating 1:45 on a blank sheet of paper. Their performance is observed from beginning to end, including the shape and size, number order and placement, hand size and placement, etc. The strategy (or lack thereof) used to draw the clock manifests itself readily, indicating impaired executive function in following a set of rules or organizing and executing a multistep task. When patients finish, they should try copying a clock that the examiner draws in front of them. The numbers 12, 6, 3, and 9 are placed first, and the hands drawn accurately. If *construction problems* exist, patients have difficulty with the copy task, as well as with the command task. If the copy is good, construction problems may not be a factor in cognitive impairment. There are many standardized, brief mental status tests like these available to clinicians. Routine use of such tests allows for longitudinal assessment and staging of dementia severity.

Additional Testing

Brain imaging. All patients with evidence of cognitive impairment should undergo structural brain imaging with MRI or when not available, computed tomography (CT). This may show findings of non–AD-related changes such as stroke, subdural hematoma, tumor, or hydrocephalus (see Fig. 27.9, bottom).

Quantitative or volumetric imaging may provide more accurate assessment of regional atrophy and provide better imaging resolution of AD-related changes. These modalities are not yet ready for routine

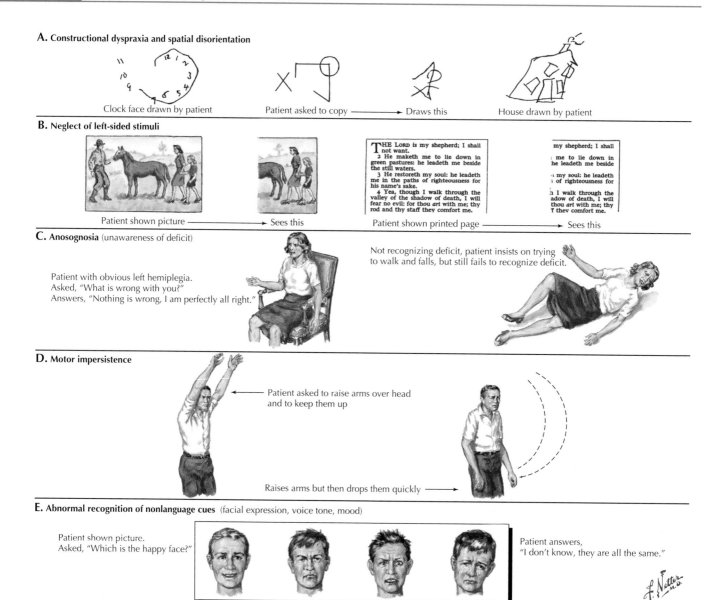

A. Constructional dyspraxia and spatial disorientation

Clock face drawn by patient   Patient asked to copy ———→ Draws this   House drawn by patient

B. Neglect of left-sided stimuli

Patient shown picture ———→ Sees this   Patient shown printed page ———→ Sees this

C. Anosognosia (unawareness of deficit)

Patient with obvious left hemiplegia.
Asked, "What is wrong with you?"
Answers, "Nothing is wrong, I am perfectly all right."

Not recognizing deficit, patient insists on trying to walk and falls, but still fails to recognize deficit.

D. Motor impersistence

Patient asked to raise arms over head and to keep them up

Raises arms but then drops them quickly ———→

E. Abnormal recognition of nonlanguage cues (facial expression, voice tone, mood)

Patient shown picture.
Asked, "Which is the happy face?"

Patient answers,
"I don't know, they are all the same."

Fig. 27.10 Nondominant Hemisphere Cortical Dysfunction.

clinical use. Functional imaging, such as FDG-PET and single-photon emission computed tomography (SPECT) scans, may also be considered. FDG-PET scanning may be useful in differentiating AD from frontotemporal dementia (FTD) and could be considered in select cases as a diagnostic tool (Fig. 27.11). The role of PET in MCI remains controversial, although PET imaging detects the changes of AD very early in the course. Eventually, PET scanning may provide a way to predict decline in MCI. Most recently, PET scanning using biomarkers for β-amyloid have allowed researchers to image the presence and distribution of amyloid plaque in AD patients. SPECT scans do not provide a significant improvement in detecting AD beyond routine assessment and are not recommended.

Cerebrospinal fluid biomarkers. Decreased β amyloid and increase tau/phosphotau concentrations in spinal fluid may be detected very early in the disease. However, the sensitivity and specificity of these assays are not a proven improvement over routine noninvasive, diagnostic approaches. More research into these tests is needed before they can be recommended for routine assessment of AD in most patients.

Blood tests. There is no standard test panel to diagnose AD. Traditionally, levels of vitamin B₁₂, folate, thyroid-stimulating hormone (TSH), and often serum RPR are measured. These tests may reveal a reversible cause of cognitive impairment that may contribute to overall dementia severity. The routine screening for syphilis is no longer recommended given the virtual absence of tertiary cases in the United States. Fasting homocysteine levels have been linked to increased risk of AD. The effect of decreasing homocysteine on the disease course of patients diagnosed with AD is unknown. However, premorbid reduction of homocysteine levels may decrease the risk of development of AD.

Genetic tests. ApoE genotyping is not diagnostic of AD. Moreover, ApoE genotyping should not be used routinely in family members because there is no specific genetic counseling to offer. The presence of an ApoE e4 genotype may only heighten anxiety unnecessarily.

TREATMENT

Treatment of Mild Cognitive Impairment

There are currently no Food and Drug Administration–approved therapies for MCI. Several studies of currently available AD medications in MCI have shown mixed results. Prescriptions for patients with MCI may not be covered by insurance. The largest of these studies suggested

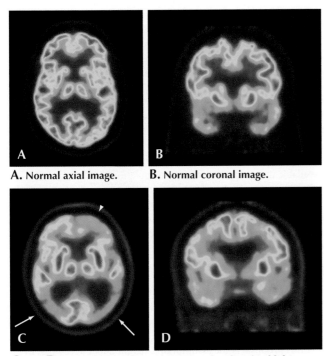

A. Normal axial image. **B.** Normal coronal image.

C. and D. Reduced activity within temporal and parietal lobes (arrows) and early decreased activity in left frontal lobe consistent with advancing disease (arrowhead).

Fig. 27.11 Fluorodeoxyglucose–Positron Emission Tomography Typical Pattern for Alzheimer Disease.

limited benefit for donepezil in MCI for all study participants. It is noteworthy that the effect of donepezil was more pronounced and long-lived in patients with the ApoE e4 allele. The risks and benefits should be discussed carefully with MCI patients before initiating treatment.

Treatment of Alzheimer Disease
General Approach

Much of the management of the patient with AD revolves around family interactions. Caregivers should provide patients with a comforting and respectful living environment. As their cognitive abilities slip away, it is important to provide a setting that preserves patient dignity. AD patients particularly benefit from a structured simple approach to daily life, maintaining a routine of social and physical activities (Fig. 27.12).

MCI patients and those with very *early AD* and their caregivers should be counseled regarding driving risk as compared with cognitively healthy elder drivers. It is recommended that a driving performance evaluation be carried out. Even if felt to be safe, these patients should be reassessed on a regular basis, because progression of the disease will unequivocally require them to stop driving at a later stage of their illness.

Once an Alzheimer diagnosis is confirmed, it is imperative to protect the patient and the public from potential motor vehicle accidents. It is emphasized that the family and the treating physician assume responsibility for restricting the patient with AD from driving.

The assignment of simple daily chores where the individual can feel productive such as setting the table, folding clothes from the dryer, or sweeping the sidewalk is recommended. Use of scheduled bathroom breaks or providing diapers keeps the incontinent patient from the

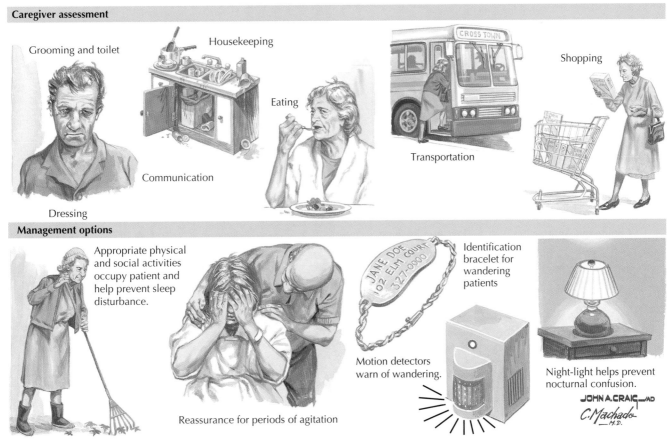

Caregiver assessment

Grooming and toilet

Housekeeping

Communication

Dressing

Eating

Transportation

Shopping

Management options

Appropriate physical and social activities occupy patient and help prevent sleep disturbance.

Reassurance for periods of agitation

Identification bracelet for wandering patients

Motion detectors warn of wandering.

Night-light helps prevent nocturnal confusion.

JOHN A. CRAIG_MD
C. Machado_M.D.

Fig. 27.12 Daily Living Assessment.

embarrassment of having soiled clothes that are socially obvious. Helping these individuals with simple activities of daily living such as dressing or feeding is eventually required. It is very important for the patient to have an easily seen identification bracelet. These patients have a tendency to "sun down," becoming easily confused in the dark; a simple bedlight can be very helpful for preventing this problem. Have the patient flip through an old photo album to comfort them with familiar, pleasant memories of their younger years, their childhood home, and their parents.

As they become increasingly confused, it is typical for Alzheimer patients to be more easily agitated; reassurance by relatives is often the best treatment. At times, simple anxiolytic medications, such as the SSRIs, may be useful. Eventually, a number of Alzheimer patients require long-term care to protect their family from the increasingly demanding nursing support that will eventually totally consume them emotionally and physically. The family should be reassured that the patient's cognitive decline prevents them from harboring any resentment for such a placement, otherwise their feelings of guilt may be overwhelming. This is a most challenging and sad experience for any family; their physicians and caregivers need to be very proactive and supportive.

Cholinesterase Inhibitors

The various agents available include donepezil, rivastigmine, and galantamine. Several studies show these medications reduce the decline on standardized tests better than placebo when used for 6–12 months but do not slow the degenerative process. These drugs may provide some benefit if taken consistently over time. When initiating therapy, patients need to increase the dose gradually. In addition, the eventual maximum required doses of these medications are not predictable. **Cholinesterase**

inhibitors are generally used in patients with mild to moderate AD (Fig. 27.13).

If these medications are stopped, patients may experience decline to the severity level that they would have reached without the medication. In such cases, restarting the medication may not regain lost ground. These medications are primarily effective at maximal doses. Rivastigmine is most effective at 4.5 or 6 mg twice daily. Recently, rivastigmine became available in transdermal patch form, significantly reducing the rate of side effects. Donepezil is only mildly effective at 5 mg/day, but greater benefit occurs with 10 mg/day doses. Similarly, galantamine should always be titrated to 12 mg twice daily to maximize benefit. Galantamine is available in an extended-release formulation to allow for once-daily dosing. If patients do not tolerate these drugs at lower doses, it is prudent to try a different agent. It is unusual for patients to be unable to tolerate at least one of these three drugs. Typical adverse effects that may cause discontinuation include cholinergic effects, especially vomiting and persistent loose stools.

Memantine

Memantine is an *N*-methyl-D-aspartate (NMDA) receptor antagonist that is approved for patients with moderate to severe AD. The involvement of glutamate-mediated neurotoxicity in the pathogenesis of AD is a hypothesis that is gaining increased acceptance. The keystone underlying this proposal is the assumption that glutamate receptors, in particular of the NMDA type, are overactivated in a tonic rather than a phasic manner in AD. Such continuous, mild, chronic activation may lead to neuronal damage/death. Memantine may improve memory by restoring homeostasis in the glutamatergic system—too little activation is bad, too much is even worse. Furthermore, memantine shows promise

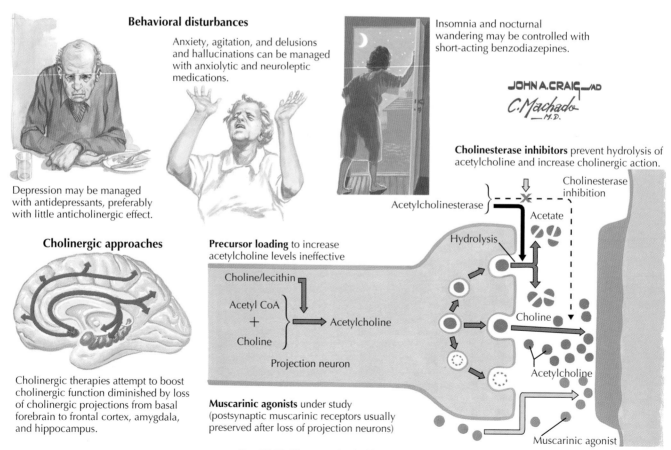

Behavioral disturbances

Anxiety, agitation, and delusions and hallucinations can be managed with anxiolytic and neuroleptic medications.

Insomnia and nocturnal wandering may be controlled with short-acting benzodiazepines.

JOHN A. CRAIG_AD
C. Machado _M.D.

Cholinesterase inhibitors prevent hydrolysis of acetylcholine and increase cholinergic action.

Cholinesterase inhibition

Acetylcholinesterase

Acetate

Hydrolysis

Depression may be managed with antidepressants, preferably with little anticholinergic effect.

Cholinergic approaches

Cholinergic therapies attempt to boost cholinergic function diminished by loss of cholinergic projections from basal forebrain to frontal cortex, amygdala, and hippocampus.

Precursor loading to increase acetylcholine levels ineffective

Choline/lecithin

Acetyl CoA + Choline → Acetylcholine

Projection neuron

Choline

Acetylcholine

Muscarinic agonists under study (postsynaptic muscarinic receptors usually preserved after loss of projection neurons)

Muscarinic agonist

Fig. 27.13 Pharmacologic Management.

when used in combination with cholinesterase inhibitors. Memantine is primarily used as a supplemental medication in moderate to severe stages of AD. Clinical trials demonstrated that in combination with donepezil, there is improved stability of cognitive performance for 6–12 months compared with donepezil or memantine alone.

The current pharmacologic treatment of AD is purely symptomatic. Long-term benefits of these medications may include a delay in need for nursing home placement. For example, using donepezil for 9–12 months may delay nursing home placement by approximately 20 months. However, functional decline continues and reasonable expectations for the effects of these medications must be emphasized to patients and their families. These treatments are associated with reduced behavioral problems and may reduce the need for sedatives in some patients. Determination of medication efficacy is challenging. When the maximum dosage is reached, annual follow-up examination is beneficial.

Repeated standardized mental status examinations are helpful. For example, the average rate of decline on the MMSE in AD is approximately three points per year. When a patient shows less than three points of decline, the medication may be helping. This method approximates the same measurements used in clinical trials of AD to assess medication efficacy. Such tests, in combination with the caregivers' subjective impressions, can help to determine whether to continue or change medications.

Other potential therapies do not have unequivocal evidence to support their use. **Ginkgo biloba** may be useful with various unspecified (mixed) dementia, but efficacy data are lacking. Ginkgo showed no benefit versus placebo for treatment of AD in a large National Institutes of Health (NIH)-sponsored clinical trial. There is no reproduced clinical study to support use of antiinflammatories (shown to lower the risk of AD in epidemiologic studies) or antioxidants. Estrogen treatment is not effective in the treatment of AD, and postmenopausal estrogen replacement in midlife may increase the risk of dementia.

AD treatments in the future will likely focus on preventive strategies, including cerebrovascular risk factors in premorbid individuals at risk. For patients already demonstrating overt AD, there is increasing interest in disease-modifying therapies. Most noteworthy are a group of drugs that reduce accumulation of β-amyloid in the brain. These include a range of agents from γ-secretase inhibitors to monoclonal antibodies against amyloid.

DEMENTIA WITH LEWY BODIES

> **CLINICAL VIGNETTE** *A 78-year-old man is referred for evaluation of intermittent confusion. During the past 3 years, he had developed depression with prominent psychotic features requiring two psychiatric hospitalizations. The patient was initially very depressed and withdrawn. A trial of fluoxetine led to some disorientation and anxiety. When his hallucinations became persistently threatening, and his family could no longer distract his attention, he was switched to quetiapine. Initially, he had a poor response to low doses; gradual increases in dosage led to severe drowsiness and stiff gait. His first inpatient stay was related to increasing agitation at home because of vivid hallucinations characterized by a sensation of intruders coming into his home. During this hospitalization, he was treated with risperidone. Although his psychotic symptoms seemed to improve, he developed severe stiffness and a shuffling gait, prone to falling. Despite such, he remained on this drug for nearly a year.*
>
> *Once the medication was discontinued, the patient became more alert and his gait improved. However, he never returned to baseline, remaining slower than his baseline. Moreover, he appeared more forgetful, needing frequent reminders and prompts to complete tasks. Some days he seemed intoxicated,*

confused, disoriented, lethargic, and withdrawn. On other days, he appeared brighter, more alert, and competent. Subsequently, his psychotic symptoms returned; this led to his second psychiatric hospitalization. Formal mental status testing demonstrated significant impairment of both memory and visuospatial processing. A second trial of low-dose risperidone subdued the patient once again, but his mobility deteriorated to the point of needing a wheelchair.

During neurologic assessment, his wife revealed he had experienced severe nightmares over the past 10 years, causing him to yell, punch, and kick in his sleep. This forced his wife to sleep in another room. He fell out of bed a number of times. The patient never recalled these events. His exam was notable for an MMSE score of 22/30 and moderate symmetric extrapyramidal motor signs, including retropulsion, bradykinesia, and rigidity. There was no significant tremor. He did not initiate conversation, and his affect was generally flat. Brain MRI showed diffuse atrophy and minimal microvascular changes. There were no metabolic signs of toxic/metabolic encephalopathy. Electroencephalography (EEG) revealed bitemporal slowing without epileptiform discharges or rhythmic abnormality.

Treatment with rivastigmine, a cholinesterase inhibitor, led to significant reduction in confusion and hallucinations. He was then taken off risperidone and remained psychiatrically stable for over a year. Although his parkinsonism persisted, he no longer needed an assistive device to get around. Attempts at treatment with levodopa failed due to confusion and recurrent hallucinations. This patient's neurologic status slowly declined, with occasional bouts of agitated confusion. After a 5-year period, nursing home placement was necessitated.

Pathogenesis

LBs, originally described at the turn of the 20th century in the substantia nigra of patients with PD, also occur in widespread areas of the cortex and other subcortical nuclei in many cases of parkinsonism with dementia. Neurodegenerative changes with LB formation were first linked with dementia in the 1960s. Early case descriptions noted LBs distributed diffusely within the cerebral cortex and brainstem and were termed *diffuse Lewy body disease*. Subsequent neuropathologic studies found a surprisingly high frequency of LB pathology in the brains of patients with AD. These cases commonly show coexisting AD lesions and LBs and were classified as LB variant of AD.

In general, "variant" cases demonstrated relatively less AD pathology (especially NFTs) than pure AD cases matched for clinical dementia severity. Reports of Lewy neurites located in the CA2 region of the hippocampus suggest that DLB is a unique neurodegenerative cause of dementia, independent of AD pathology. Interestingly, LBs are also found in the brains of patients with hereditary AD, suggesting a possible pathophysiologic link between these disorders. In addition, LBs are occasionally found in the brains of nondemented elders. Few familial cases of DLB are described, and there are no known mutations associated with hereditary DLB.

A definitive pathologic diagnosis of DLB requires only the presence of cortical LB pathology, regardless of coexisting AD pathology. Many of these cases also fulfill pathologic criteria for a definitive diagnosis of AD and clinical criteria for a diagnosis of probable or possible AD. Consequently, controversy surrounds this diagnosis, and no agreement exists on a single-disease classification of cases with concomitant LB and AD pathology. Dementia autopsy series suggest that DLB is the second most common cause of elderly dementia after AD. Clinical epidemiologic studies are lacking.

LBs are intracytoplasmic inclusion bodies. They are the hallmark histopathologic lesions of primary PD where these occur within neurons of the substantia nigra and other brainstem nuclei. A spherical shape and eosinophilic staining properties characterize LBs morphologically (Fig. 27.14). The center stains densely, and a pale halo surrounds it. In

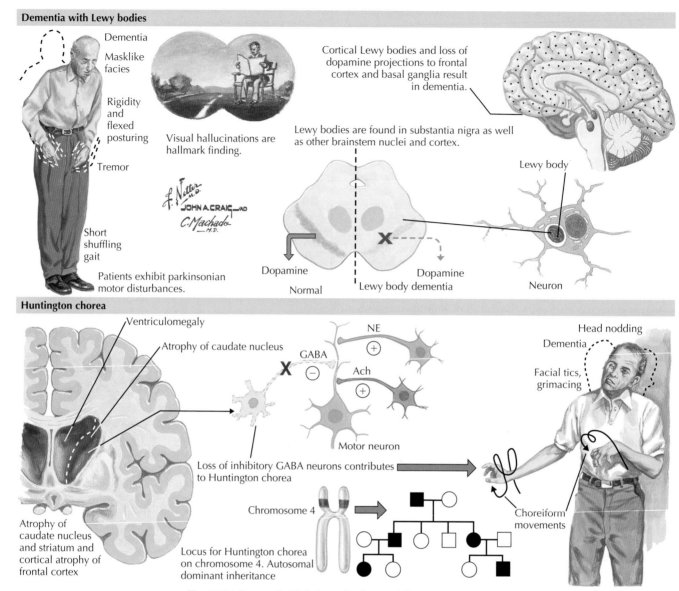

Fig. 27.14 Dementia With Lewy Bodies and Huntington Chorea.

cases of PD with dementia, LBs occur in cortical neurons and other gray matter regions. Cortical LBs are characterized by irregular shapes and do not have the characteristic pale halo seen with PD. Hence cortical LBs can easily be missed with routine neuropathologic staining techniques. Moreover, LBs do not stain with silver-based stains often used to identify neuropathologic lesions in AD. A synaptic protein called *alpha-synuclein* is the major LB component. Specific immunohistochemical stains for alpha-synuclein greatly improve LB detection throughout the brain. *Ubiquitin* staining also detects these lesions well. The function of alpha-synuclein is not completely understood. It may have a role in regulating presynaptic, nerve-terminal vesicular function. Mutations in the alpha-synuclein gene produce a mixed phenotype within members of affected kindred. Symptoms are predominantly PD-like, with cases of dementia occurring less frequently. Alpha-synuclein appears to be the main pathologic substrate in multiple system atrophy (MSA) as well.

Clinical Presentation and Differential Diagnosis

DLB patients characteristically have cognitive decline, behavioral change, and motor dysfunction. The most crucial component for this clinical diagnosis is dementia, although the initial manifestations of DLB may be characteristically motor or behavioral impairment. A critical clinical feature of DLB is fluctuating mental status, which may be dramatic, ranging from relatively lucid to severe confusion. Episode duration and frequency vary greatly, lasting minutes, days, or weeks. Awareness and arousal levels may vary and include periodic somnolence and unresponsiveness. Transient neurologic symptoms (i.e., dysarthria, dizziness, or unexplained falls) may occur. Such episodes may suggest complex partial seizures, delirium, or transient ischemic attacks. Although patients with AD have "good and bad days," the fluctuations of patients with DLB are more pronounced. Clinical assessments may vary significantly from visit to visit. Caregivers often become stressed by the unpredictability of symptoms.

The cognitive impairment in DLB may be similar to that in AD, although there are some important differences. The memory loss in DLB tends to be less severe than in AD; however, retrieval deficits are more pronounced than encoding deficits. Therefore patients with DLB have a greater problem retrieving previously learned information and show a greater benefit with cueing than do patients with AD. In AD, encoding difficulty predominates, and consequently, patients do not benefit as much from practice or from cueing. In DLB, visuospatial and construction skills may be impaired earlier than in AD. Patients with DLB may present with geographic disorientation in familiar neighborhoods or even in their own homes while their memory is mildly impaired. Executive function is also impaired significantly earlier in DLB than in AD, manifested as impaired problem solving, inability to complete tasks, and marked disorganization of daily activities. Formal neuropsychological tests help to differentiate AD from DLB, particularly in early disease stages.

Prominent psychotic features, including hallucinations and delusions, also develop in patients with DLB, although such symptoms are not typically seen early in the disease course. In DLB, psychosis can be an early and severely disabling feature, sometimes heralding the onset of dementia. Recurrent vivid and detailed visual hallucinations are particularly prevalent in DLB. The emotional response to these hallucinations ranges from relative indifference to severe agitation and combativeness. Agitation typically occurs when the patient has little insight or the hallucinations are perceived as threatening. Hallucinations having other sensory (i.e., nonvisual) also occur but are less specific for DLB. Delusions are frequently bizarre, complex, and unrelated to cognitive impairment. In contrast, delusions in patients with AD often occur from misinterpretation secondary to forgetfulness. For example, patients with AD may become suspicious of others when they cannot find things they misplaced. Other behavioral problems such as depression and anxiety also occur frequently but are not unique to DLB (Table 27.1).

Motor signs of DLB include all the typical features of PD; however, here the bradykinesia and rigidity are more characteristic, whereas tremor is relatively uncommon. Signs tend to be distributed more symmetrically and axially than they are in PD. Unexplained falls occur early and often in patients with DLB, unlike postural instability in PD, which tends to mark more advanced disease. Response to dopaminergic medications is limited or absent with DLB, although they may exacerbate hallucinations. Parkinsonism is also seen in advanced AD and in FTD. When parkinsonism occurs within 1–2 years of dementia, either before or after the onset of cognitive decline, DLB is a prime consideration in the differential diagnosis.

Diagnosis

The clinical evaluation for DLB is similar to that for AD. Formal neuropsychological tests can be useful early in the course to differentiate DLB from AD or other dementing illnesses. There are no specific findings on blood or spinal fluid analysis. Brain MRI and CT do not reveal any specific abnormalities. Volumetric MRI studies suggest there is relative sparing of hippocampal volumes in DLB cases. EEG shows nonspecific abnormalities, including focal or diffuse brain wave slowing. PET imaging may be helpful in the future, particularly in highlighting affected dopaminergic systems.

Treatment

Cholinergic CNS deficits occur in DLB as they do in AD. Some studies suggest that DLB is associated with greater cholinergic deficit than is AD. In theory, cholinesterase inhibitors—donepezil, rivastigmine, and galantamine—should be effective, and small, controlled clinical trials show that these medications have a favorable effect on cognitive outcome measures in DLB. The duration of drug benefit is not established but may be similar to that in AD. Cholinesterase inhibitors offer only symptomatic benefits, having no known effect on the degenerative process. Therefore patients can delay cognitive progression for a limited amount of time only. It is not clear when these drugs truly lose their efficacy. As in AD, drug discontinuation, especially after several years of treatment, may result in rapid cognitive and functional decline. These drugs may reduce the extent and severity of cognitive fluctuations and behavioral problems throughout the disease course.

When psychotic features are disabling, use of atypical neuroleptic agents is common, similar to their efficacy in cases of PD with psychotic features. The efficacy of these drugs for DLB has not been studied in controlled clinical trials. Because atypical neuroleptics produce fewer extrapyramidal adverse effects than "typical" neuroleptics, this must be an important consideration when treating DLB patients. However, these atypical neuroleptics are associated with increased morbidity and mortality in nursing home patients. Therefore their use in the elderly population with dementia requires careful assessment of risk and benefit and close monitoring if used at all.

In addition, patients with DLB often exhibit sensitivity to various centrally acting drugs, most prominently to neuroleptic medications, and may become completely incapacitated by severe akinesia, dystonia, or delirium. The incidence of neuroleptic malignant syndrome in DLB is unknown. Good clinical judgment and conservative dosing strategies should be used in every case. The treatment of psychotic features in DLB is one of the most challenging management issues. If at all possible, neuroleptic medication should be avoided.

Often, psychotic symptoms distress caregivers more than patients, but this should not prompt immediate initiation of such medications. Recently, use of cholinesterase inhibitors, such as rivastigmine, was shown to reduce hallucinations in patients with DLB. Therefore cholinesterase inhibitors remain the first line of treatment in DLB, including cases with prominent psychotic features. Treatment of motor symptoms is based largely on anecdotal reports. Dopaminergic drugs may be tried

TABLE 27.1 Comparison of Dementia With Lewy Bodies and Alzheimer Disease Manifestations

Manifestation	DLBs	AD
Memory loss	Less pronounced, poor retrieval	Characteristic, poor encoding
Visuospatial and construction skills	Severely impaired early	Mildly impaired early
Executive function	Impaired earlier	Impaired later
Fluctuating mental status	Pronounced	Less pronounced
Psychotic features	Can be prominent early	Not typical early
Delusions	Bizarre, unrelated to impaired cognitive function	Often related to memory loss
Depression and anxiety	Common	Common
Parkinsonism	Within 1–2 years of dementia	Later in disease course

AD, Alzheimer disease; *DLBs,* dementia with Lewy bodies.

with caution in selected cases; however, psychosis may be exacerbated, and efficacy is often minimal.

As in AD, caregiver counseling about the disease course and realistic treatment expectations is paramount for successful monitoring, intervention, and improved quality of life. The most common causes for nursing home placement in the demented population include psychosis with behavioral problems and parkinsonism. Patients with DLB are therefore at high risk for early nursing home placement. As in AD, use of cholinesterase inhibitors may help to delay nursing home placement.

FRONTOTEMPORAL LOBAR DEMENTIA

CLINICAL VIGNETTE *During the preceding 2-year period, a 55-year-old man previously regarded by his family as "thoughtful, accomplished, and intelligent," began neglecting both his home and occupational responsibilities. He became increasingly inflexible and uncaring. At work he missed several deadlines, and clients complained that he "forgot" about them. Consequently, he stopped working. He became more impulsive, driving late at night without reason. He obsessively checked his furnace numerous times each day and night.*

Concomitantly his wife became increasingly tearful and anxious; however, he seemed unconcerned about her turmoil and unaware of his own personality changes. His personal hygiene declined; he stopped shaving and dressed sloppily. At social functions, he interrupted conversations, touched people inappropriately, and spoke in a tasteless and loud fashion, often embarrassing his wife. Despite these changes, he continued to garden and perform other favored activities, albeit with less attention to detail.

On examination, he was disheveled, malodorous, and unshaven, wearing unwashed clothes. He spoke out of turn and repeatedly said, "I have to go." At times he attempted to leave the examination room but returned with gentle coaxing. His affect was otherwise flat. He gave concrete, terse responses to questions, mostly affirmative, negative, or stating, "I don't know." Naming was impaired. He followed some simple commands, but more complex sequences were incomplete or disorganized. His memory was relatively intact, although retrieval of relatives' names was impaired. He listed only five animals in 1 minute, a significant impairment given his postgraduate education level. Other than motor impersistence and a mild rooting reflex, bilaterally, the results of his primary neurologic examination were relatively unremarkable. During the next 2 years, he became increasingly withdrawn, spoke less, and required prompting for virtually every activity.

A brain MRI demonstrated lateral frontal lobe atrophy, albeit slightly asymmetric, because it affected the left side slightly more than the right. Blood work, CSF studies, and EEG results were unremarkable.

Pathogenesis

This case exemplifies evolving dementia related to a degenerative process primarily confined to the frontal and temporal lobes. A previously accomplished individual initially demonstrated signs of intellectual decline, diminished sense of responsibility, and loss of social graces punctuated by a disinhibited personality. More than a century ago, Arnold Pick was the first to describe behavioral and personality changes associated with frontotemporal atrophy. He subsequently also was the first to recognize progressive aphasia and progressive apraxia syndromes on the basis of focal lobar atrophy. Concomitantly, Alois Alzheimer described the histopathology of what came to be known as Pick disease or FTD.

FTD features were subsequently described in other, pathologically different processes, including corticobasal degeneration (CBD), motor neuron disease (MND)-type dementia, primary progressive aphasia

(PPA), and dementia lacking distinctive histology. In addition, the presence of diseased subcortical regions leads to extrapyramidal features, including akinesia and rigidity. In other cases, similar pathologic features appear in cortical regions other than the frontal or temporal lobes. For example, in PPA, parietal cortical involvement may predominate. The term *frontotemporal dementia* does not fully account for the spectrum linking pathology and clinical phenomenology. As the disease progresses, lobar degeneration occurs, often asymmetrically and bilaterally. The term Pick complex has been suggested, instead of FTD, to provide a more inclusive diagnostic entity to encompass the pathologic and clinical features of these dementias inclusively. Perhaps, more specifically, the term frontotemporal lobar degeneration (FTLD) encompasses the myriad pathologic substrates of this primary neurodegenerative dementia, whereas the terms FTD, PPA, CBD, etc. describe the corresponding clinical syndromes.

The basic histopathology of FTLD is rather nonspecific, characterized by gliosis, neuronal loss, and spongiform degeneration in superficial cortical layers, with predilection for frontal and temporal lobes. However, the molecular pathology involves several proteins (tau and TDP-43) distributed in different cortical and subcortical distributions and corresponds to specific clinical manifestations of various FTD syndromes. The formation of Pick bodies and Pick cells occurs in less than 25% of cases. Pick bodies are round, argyrophilic intracytoplasmic inclusions, easily detected by most silver-staining techniques and mildly eosinophilic on standard hematoxylin and eosin staining. Cortical Pick bodies form in small neurons; they are pathognomonic for Pick disease when they occur in the dentate gyrus. Pick cells are large, ballooned neurons that affect superficial cortical cells. In many cases, evidence exists of complement and microglial activation, suggesting that inflammatory mechanisms may play a role in pathogenesis. In Pick disease, degeneration is restricted to frontal and temporal lobes, producing a characteristic "knife-edge" atrophy of sulci.

A *positive labeling for pathologic tau protein within Pick bodies, astrocytes, and oligodendrocytes* is a common thread in the pathogenesis of these disorders, termed *tauopathies*. Associated dementias of the tauopathy group (FTLD-tau), besides Pick disease, include progressive supranuclear palsy (PSP), CBD, and amyotrophic lateral sclerosis–parkinsonism complex of Guam (ALS-PDC). Tau is involved in the pathogenesis of AD. However, the mechanism by which tau is affected in AD and Pick disease differs. A range of mechanisms may transform tau, determining the final pathologic and clinical picture.

Other FTD cases demonstrate no significant tau labeling. Many of these conditions are associated with *intracytoplasmic and intranuclear aggregates of the ubiquinated protein called TDP-43*. These forms of FTLD (FTLD-U) occur in the behavioral subtype of FTD (bvFTD), FTD in MND (FTD-MND), semantic dementia (SD), and progressive nonfluent aphasia (PNFA).

There are other *nontauopathy- and non-TDPopathy–related* molecular pathologies producing FTD syndromes. Familial forms of FTLD are quite common (up to 40% of cases). Four genes for FTLD are identified: the microtubule-associated protein tau (MAPT) gene associated with tau aggregates, the progranulin (PGRN) gene associated with TDP-43 aggregates, the charged multivesicular body protein 2B (CHMP2B) gene, and the valosin-containing protein (VCP) gene.

Clinical Presentation

FTD/Pick disease accounts for approximately 15%–20% of all degenerative dementias. The typical age of onset is broad, ranging from 21 to 75 years, usually affecting persons aged 45–60 years. Men and women are equally affected. The median illness duration is 8 years, although this ranges from 2 to 20 years. Family history is present in more than 50% of cases.

Behavior Subtype of Frontotemporal Dementia

The distinguishing clinical features of bvFTD and Pick disease are striking behavioral and personality changes. Most patients are unaware of their problem. There is often a major breakdown in social behavior, personal hygiene, and affect. Mental processes become concrete and perseverative (Fig. 27.15). *Three major behavioral subtypes* include disinhibition, apathy, and stereotypic behavior.

1. *Disinhibited patients* exhibit overactivity, restlessness, inattention and distractibility, impulsivity, lack of application, and impersistence. There is mental disorganization and frequent set shifting, moving unproductively from one activity or conversation topic to the next. Demeanor is often inappropriately jocular and socially inappropriate. Some exhibit signs of the Klüver-Bucy syndrome, namely, hyperorality, hypersexuality, and utilization behavior. These patients frequently gain weight rapidly as a result of overeating. They may impulsively touch or pick up objects within sight or within reach. In extreme cases, incontinence of stool and urine may be associated with coprophagia, sometimes in an otherwise alert and oriented patient.

2. *Apathetic patients* lack motivation and appear pseudodepressed. Left alone, they spend the day sitting or lying in bed. They stop bathing and grooming and dress sloppily. Behavior is "economical," with minimal expenditure of energy or mental effort. These patients often have prolonged response latency to questions, although the eventual answer is often accurate. There is economy of speech, with many responses characterized by single words or short phrases with no attempt at elaboration. Speech prosody may be lost. Perseveration of verbal and motor activity is common. There may be a loss of concern for self and others because patients become emotionally shallow. Apathetic states are commonly mistaken for depression, and treatment with antidepressants is typically not effective.

3. *Stereotypic behavior* includes repetitive, ritualistic, and idiosyncratic behaviors. These individuals require a rigid daily routine, becoming agitated when their routine is interrupted. They may repeat, perseverate, the same story verbatim and with the same prosodic inflection numerous times during a single clinic visit. This is akin to "listening to a broken record." They evidence mental inflexibility and difficulty shifting mindset. Ritualistic behaviors, picking lint from the floor, rearranging the silverware drawer, rewriting a letter, etc., have a compulsive quality absent the anxiety associated with obsessive-compulsive disorder. The clinical features often overlap during the course of illness.

Patients may present with predominant apathetic features only to later develop increasingly disinhibited or stereotypic behavior or both. As symptoms progress, most patients experience akinesia, progressive rigidity, mutism, and incontinence, requiring total nursing care. Features of disinhibition are associated with degeneration within the orbital frontal and adjacent temporal lobes. Apathetic features correlate with degenerative changes within the dorsolateral frontal lobes. Stereotypic behavior type seems to correlate with more widespread involvement of frontal and temporal lobes, although greater emphasis may exist in the region of the cingulate gyrus.

Cognitive function may be relatively spared initially, so that mental status examination may be notable only for distractibility, inattentiveness, or perseveration rather than clear impairment of memory or

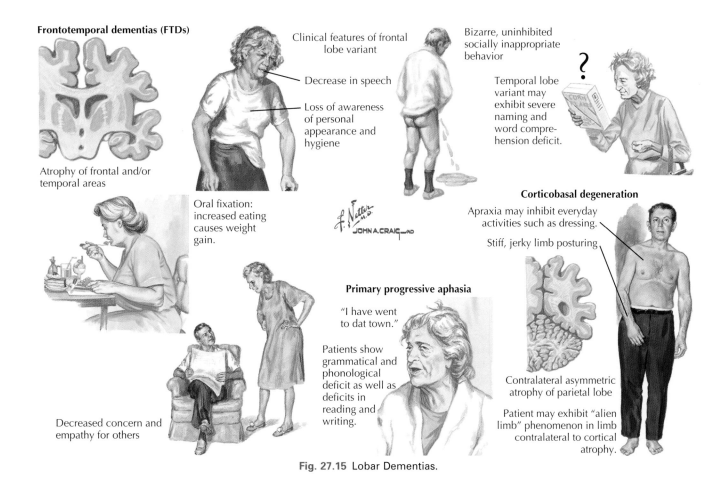

Fig. 27.15 Lobar Dementias.

constructional apraxia. One of the more striking cognitive features of bvFTD is executive dysfunction seen on sorting and sequencing tasks, loss of verbal fluency, and impairment in general problem-solving skills.

Frontotemporal Lobar Degeneration With Motor Neuron Disease

FTLD with MND presents most often in men younger than age 65 years. Characteristic FTD typically precedes onset of motor neuron symptoms, and disinhibited-type behaviors predominate. The motor neuron component leads to a more rapid decline and death in these cases. Consequently, akinesia and mutism are not often seen. The duration of illness is typically 2–3 years. A family history of disease is only occasionally found.

Primary Progressive Aphasia

PPA presents in fluent and nonfluent subtypes. In both conditions, progressive aphasia is the predominant clinical feature, often remaining the only feature throughout the illness. Typically women, patients with fluent PPA usually present between the ages of 50 and 65 years. Illness duration ranges from 3 to 15 years. There is gradual loss of comprehension and naming, with relatively less impairment in reading and writing. Behavioral features include mental rigidity, stereotypic behaviors, self-centeredness, and disregard for personal safety. Many patients are easily agitated. Memory, calculations, and constructional skills are relatively spared, whereas visual agnosia and prosopagnosia may occur relatively early.

SD may present as a fluent progressive aphasia and visual agnosia. Nonfluent PPA patients typically present at the same ages. Men and women are affected equally. Illness duration is between 4 and 12 years. There is overall good comprehension, with impaired verbal expression. Patients have effortful, agrammatic, stuttering speech, with impaired repetition and word retrieval. Reading and writing are also affected but less so than speech. These individuals are aware of their impairment and become frustrated and depressed easily. Behavioral problems develop later in the disease and may include any FTD symptoms. Nevertheless, the focal characteristic of PPA clinically differentiates it from classic FTD.

Diagnosis

Brain MRI, important for excluding other mechanisms for frontal lobe syndromes such as tumor or infection, may demonstrate atrophy predominating within frontal and temporal lobes in neurodegenerative disease. Brain imaging may show focal lobar or asymmetric atrophy in PPA cases. EMG in cases of FTD/MND may be diagnostic. Brain SPECT may show deficits in a similar distribution, although it does not have a sensitivity that provides a definitive diagnosis. Brain FDG-PET scans are useful in distinguishing FTLD from AD. EEG is normal, especially early in the disease course. Blood work and CSF studies are not helpful. Formal neuropsychological tests are helpful in localizing deficits in cortical function.

Treatment

Treatment of FTD is supportive. There is no proven benefit to using the cholinesterase inhibitors, commonly used in AD. Caregiver education and reduction of caregiver stress are essential in successful management of agitation and other behavioral problems. When patients become aggressive and combative, caregivers tend to oppose their behavior. Distraction and redirection are more effective than verbal instruction in these instances.

Limited use of sedatives is recommended to avoid overmedication. Paradoxically, benzodiazepines may exacerbate agitation in some patients. SSRIs may reduce anxiety and restlessness. Other drugs, including mood stabilizers, and atypical anxiolytics (e.g., trazodone, buspirone), sometimes help with problematic behavior when used as monotherapy or in combination. There are few randomized clinical trials of classic and atypical neuroleptics in FTD, but they may be necessary in cases of aggressive or violent behavior.

VASCULAR COGNITIVE IMPAIRMENT

> **CLINICAL VIGNETTE** *A 67-year-old man with a history of hypertension and coronary artery disease, who had lived alone since his wife's death 3 years previously, came to the clinic at his daughter's insistence because he had become increasingly complacent and inactive. The daughter noted that he had stopped fixing his own meals and might not eat unless she brought something to him. He tended to eat junk food and sweets. She was unsure whether he was taking his antihypertensive medications regularly. He had neglected housework and the yard, stopped balancing his checkbook, and decreased participation in social activities.*
>
> *The patient reported dizziness and gradually worsening unsteady gait. Although he had not fallen, he felt off balance especially when turning. He also reported urinary frequency and occasional incontinence. He denied depression but was not particularly happy. He gave up previous interests because they were "too much to keep track of."*
>
> *Five years previously, the patient had experienced a stroke causing transient weakness on the right side but no residual deficit. Approximately 1 year previously, he had stayed in the hospital for a transient ischemic attack characterized by transient right-sided weakness and dysarthria. Brain MRI showed extensive subcortical and periventricular white matter changes and numerous microvascular infarcts in the basal ganglia.*
>
> *On exam, his affect was flat; he was slow to respond. Mental status examination results showed impaired motor sequencing, executive dysfunction, and memory impairment. He could not spell "world" backward. He was able to register four words but recalled only one of four spontaneously. With cueing, he recalled all four items. He could not draw a clock to command but copied a clock, drawn by the examiner, well. He had evidence of a wide-based, spastic gait, with bilateral Babinski signs. Stride and arm-swing amplitudes were reduced. Muscle stretch reflexes were brisk throughout. His blood pressure was 160/86 mm Hg. Repeated MRI demonstrated progressive subcortical and periventricular microvascular changes. Blood test results revealed normal cell counts, a normal B_{12} level, and a normal TSH level. Serum RPR was nonreactive. The fasting serum homocysteine level was slightly increased, at 17 mol/L.*

Pathogenesis

The association between cerebrovascular disease and dementia has been recognized for many years. Some authors propose using the term *vascular cognitive impairment* (VCI) to describe the contribution of cerebrovascular disease to various dementia syndromes. This applies whether the dementia is primarily related to cerebrovascular disease or mixed with another dementing disorder. Indeed, in the early and mid-20th century, cerebrovascular disease was postulated to be the specific etiology for senile dementia. It was not until the 1960s that AD was recognized to be the most common pathophysiologic mechanism for the majority of individuals who have dementia. In subsequent decades, the concept of VCI underwent several revisions. Given the wide array of clinical syndromes possible with stroke, VCI presentation varies considerably. The heterogeneity of stroke complicates one's ability to specifically define VCI as a single clinical entity with specific diagnostic criteria. Autopsy series show cerebrovascular disease coexisting with AD, and influencing clinical dementia, in approximately 20% of dementia cases.

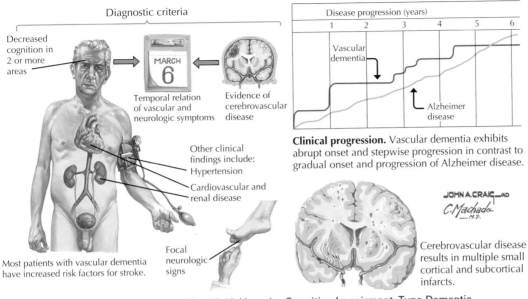

Diagnostic criteria

Decreased cognition in 2 or more areas

MARCH 6

Temporal relation of vascular and neurologic symptoms

Evidence of cerebrovascular disease

Other clinical findings include: Hypertension

Cardiovascular and renal disease

Focal neurologic signs

Most patients with vascular dementia have increased risk factors for stroke.

Disease progression (years)

Vascular dementia

Alzheimer disease

Clinical progression. Vascular dementia exhibits abrupt onset and stepwise progression in contrast to gradual onset and progression of Alzheimer disease.

JOHN A. CRAIG—AD
C. Machado M.D.

Cerebrovascular disease results in multiple small cortical and subcortical infarcts.

Axial FLAIR image demonstrates moderately severe confluent white matter, T2 hyperintensities, some regions with black holes consistent with cystic change.

Fig. 27.16 Vascular Cognitive Impairment–Type Dementia.

VCI occurs when multiple cerebral infarcts or hemorrhages cause enough neuronal or axonal loss to impair cognitive function. The core pathologic VCI syndromes include (1) *lacunar disease* (penetrator-vessel disease), (2) *multiinfarct* dementia (MID; medium- and large-vessel disease), (3) *strategic single-infarct* dementia (e.g., thalamus, angular gyrus), and (4) *Binswanger* dementia. These conditions are not mutually exclusive; there are many instances wherein the patient has a mixture of small-vessel and medium-vessel infarcts. Furthermore, age-related microvascular disease, frequently defined by brain MRI scans of elderly patients, may also contribute to the onset, progression, and symptoms of old-age dementia.

Epidemiology

The risk of VCI increases with age just as the risk of stroke increases with age. Most epidemiologic studies of dementia do not differentiate among AD, cerebrovascular, and mixed dementia. The prevalence of a pure vascular cause of dementia in autopsy studies is probably less than 10% of old-age dementia cases. However, the prevalence of VCI may be much greater. There is often a prevalence of patients with mixed dementia, including the effects of both vascular and neurodegenerative disorders; this in fact may be much higher than current estimates. In general, diagnostic criteria for VCI lack sufficient sensitivity and specificity to recognize cases of VCI reliably. Many patients may also have other dementia types, such as AD, DLB, or normal pressure hydrocephalus. Interestingly, cerebrovascular disease is extremely common and shares several risk factors for AD. These include hypertension, diabetes, and hyperlipidemia. Recent investigations also suggest a link between AD and metabolic syndrome. Stroke is identified more commonly in AD patients than in age-matched controls. Therefore it is reasonable to suspect that cerebrovascular disease contributes significantly to old-age dementia.

Clinical Presentation and Differential Diagnosis

The potential for prevention of VCI highlights the importance of recognizing and treating the various vascular causes that may predispose to or contribute to dementia. Standard criteria for diagnosing vascular dementia are difficult to define given the variable nature of cognitive deficits following stroke, mainly depending upon the anatomic location of the stroke. The most common dementia is AD, typically characterized by short-term memory loss in the early stages. Although vascular dementia may present in this way, it is not necessarily the "cardinal" feature of VCI. The cognitive consequence of stroke may include executive dysfunction, neglect, or aphasia. In addition, the degree of cerebrovascular disease progression varies greatly. Residual symptoms following acute stroke may seem to initially but incompletely improve and then later on contribute to eventual cognitive dysfunction in the setting of mixed dementia. Moreover, there is now considerable evidence that stroke increases the risk of AD. "Silent" lacunar infarcts are particularly associated with increased risk of AD.

Almost all standard diagnostic criteria for VCI require imaging studies demonstrating evidence of stroke (Fig. 27.16). However, there is no specific characteristic appearance on imaging studies that provides a diagnosis of VCI per se. The absence of specific cerebrovascular lesions of course mitigates this diagnosis. MRI is more sensitive than CT in showing subcortical and periventricular white matter changes consistent with small-vessel disease and smaller infarcts. Therefore a VCI diagnosis requires recognition of various syndromic features to correlate with findings on imaging studies.

Clinical presentation is arbitrarily divided into large-vessel and small-vessel disease, which are not mutually exclusive clinically. Large-vessel disease tends to affect large vascular territories, producing well-known clinical syndromes. For example, frontal lobe involvement may produce aphasia, apraxia, disinhibition, or apathy. Mesial temporal involvement produces amnesia, angular gyrus lesions lead to constructional apraxia, and parietal lesions produce alexia or apraxia.

The clinical syndrome of MID typically proceeds in a stepwise fashion with clear-cut stroke events leading to successive, cumulative impairment of various cognitive domains. Small-vessel disease typically eventuates in subcortical infarcts. These are sometimes localized within strategic locations, such as the thalamus or basal ganglia, and involve white matter tracts such as frontosubcortical and thalamocortical tracts.

Moreover, small-vessel pathology is often seen in the context of "normal" aging, where the smallest branches become increasingly tortuous, producing twists and loops along paths deep in the brain. Morphologic changes are amplified by hypertension and diabetes. This results in diffuse myelin loss within deep vascular territories such as periventricular and subcortical white matter regions. The clinical correlates of small-vessel disease may include executive dysfunction, apathy, inattentiveness, and personality changes typical of frontal lobe syndromes as occur with hydrocephalus and FTD (see Fig. 27.15). Involvement of specific circuits correlates with recognized clinical manifestations.

Dorsolateral prefrontal circuit dysfunction correlates with executive dysfunction, decreased verbal fluency, poor performance on sequencing tasks, impersistence, set shifting, and perseveration. *Subcortical orbito-frontal* circuits are associated with disinhibition, manic behavior, and compulsive behavior. *Medial frontal* circuits produce apathy, psychomotor retardation, and mood lability.

Binswanger Disease

This is the clinical representation of VCI dementia resulting from small-vessel disease. Characteristically, patients are aged between 50 and 70 years; more than 80% have a history of hypertension, diabetes, or both. Initial symptoms vary but often include behavioral changes such as depression, emotional lability, or abulia. Gait disturbances are characterized by lower extremity parkinsonism, ataxia, or spasticity. Dysarthria and other focal motor signs may be present. Urinary incontinence is common. Patients often have histories of dizziness or syncope. Progressive executive dysfunction, slow mental processing, and memory impairment affecting information retrieval rather than encoding characterize cognitive impairment.

Binswanger disease follows a clinical course having intermittent progression, often without clear strokelike events. Typically, this follows a 3- to 10-year course. Pathologically, one finds numerous subcortical and periventricular infarcts that spare cortical U-fibers. When patients present with the clinical picture typical for Binswanger disease but do not have hypertension or diabetes, a diagnosis of cerebral autosomal-dominant arteriopathy with subcortical infarcts and leukoariosis (CADASIL) should be considered. It is one of the few hereditary causes of VCI.

In the elderly, the possibility of mixed dementia exists when patients exhibit clinical features of AD and VCI. Imaging studies reveal evidence of infarct, widespread microvascular disease, or both. Silent brain infarction, especially in the basal ganglia and thalamic regions, and significant ischemic white matter changes enhance the clinical presentation and progression of AD. In addition, various vascular risk factors, such as hypertension, hypercholesterolemia, and hyperhomocysteinemia (levels 14 mmol/L), also increase the risk of AD. Brains with mixed pathologies, matched for dementia severity, reveal fewer AD lesions compared with pure AD cases. Clearly the specific clinical presentation is influenced by cerebrovascular disease in these cases. Finally, the risk of developing poststroke dementia increases with advancing age, recurrent stroke, and larger periventricular white matter lesions on MRI. Hypoxic and ischemic stroke complications, such as pneumonia or seizure, also increase the risk of poststroke dementia.

Prevention and Treatment

Primary prevention must be pursued aggressively. When at-risk patients are identified, treatment of arterial hypertension, cardiac disease, lipid abnormality, and diabetes is important in reducing dementia risk. Secondary prevention (i.e., treatment when cerebrovascular disease is initially recognized) begins with appropriate acute management of stroke and its complications. Prevention of stroke recurrence by appropriate antiplatelet or anticoagulant therapy and addressing primary risk factors are also very important. Use of calcium channel blockers in the treatment of hypertension may be more effective in dementia prevention than other antihypertensive medications. Dietary supplementation with folic acid and vitamins B_6 and B_{12} may help to reduce the levels of homocysteine, a possible contributory precursor to VCI. The role of "neuroprotective agents" in prevention of poststroke dementia is unknown.

To date, evidence-based controlled trials have not yet identified any pharmacologic agents for treatment of ischemic vascular (multiinfarct)

dementia. However, when dementia develops, cholinesterase inhibitors may be helpful. As in AD, titration of these medications to maximum doses is recommended; their long-term efficacy in VCI is unknown. The efficacy of cholinesterase inhibitor treatment may be greater in cases of mixed dementia. However, acetylcholine deficits may be significant in VCI as well as in AD. Subcortical vascular disease often interrupts major cholinergic pathways from the basal forebrain to widespread regions of the cerebral cortex. Deficits of CSF acetylcholine levels are found in VCI cases when compared with healthy controls. As in all dementia cases, caregiver education and support are essential to long-term success and quality of patient life.

ADDITIONAL RESOURCES

Alzheimer Disease

Alzheimer's Association. www.alz.org.

Cummings JL. Alzheimer's disease. N Engl J Med 2004;351(1):56–67, *Review*.

Dubinsky RM, Stein AC, Lyons K. Practice parameter: risk of driving and Alzheimer's disease (an evidence-based review): report of the quality standards subcommittee of the American Academy of Neurology. Neurology 2000;54:2205–11.

Klafki HW, Staufenbiel M, Kornhuber J, et al. Therapeutic approaches to Alzheimer's disease. Brain 2006;129(Pt.11):2840–55, *Review*. [Epub 2006 Oct 3].

Knopman DS, Dekosky ST, Cummings JL, et al. The American Academy of Neurology. Practice parameter: diagnosis of dementia (an evidence-based review—report of the quality standards subcommittee of the American Academy of Neurology). Neurology 2001;56:1143–53.

Lesser JM, Hughes S. Psychosis-related disturbances. Psychosis, agitation, and disinhibition in Alzheimer's disease: definitions and treatment options. Geriatrics 2006;61(12):14–20, *Review*.

Raina P, Santaguida P, Ismaila A, et al. Effectiveness of cholinesterase inhibitors and memantine for treating dementia: evidence review for a clinical practice guideline. Ann Intern Med 2008;148(5):379–97, *Review*.

Small BJ, Gagnon E, Robinson B. Early identification of cognitive deficits: preclinical Alzheimer's disease and mild cognitive impairment. Geriatrics 2007;62(4):19–23, *Review*.

Dementia With Lewy Bodies

Fantini ML, Ferini-Strambi L, Montplaisir J. Idiopathic REM sleep behavior disorder: toward a better nosologic definition. Neurology 2005;64(5):780–6, *Review*.

Huey ED, Putnam KT, Grafman J. A systematic review of neurotransmitter deficits and treatments in frontotemporal dementia. Neurology 2006;66(1):17–22, *Review*.

McKeith IG, Dickson DW, Lowe J. Consortium on DLB. Diagnosis and management of dementia with Lewy bodies: third report of the DLB consortium. Neurology 2005;65(12):1863–72, *Review*. Erratum in: Neurology. 2005.

Murphy J, Henry R, Lomen-Hoerth C. Establishing subtypes of the continuum of frontal lobe impairment in amyotrophic lateral sclerosis. Arch Neurol 2007;64:330–4, *Review*.

Sleegers K, Kumar-Singh S, Cruts M, et al. Molecular pathogenesis of frontotemporal lobar degeneration: basic science seminar in neurology. Arch Neurol 2008;65(6):700–4, *Review*.

van der Zee J, Sleegers K, Van Broeckhoven C. Invited article: the Alzheimer disease–frontotemporal lobar degeneration spectrum. Neurology 2008;71:1191–7, *Review*.

Frontotemporal Dementia

Josephs KA. Frontotemporal dementia and related disorders: deciphering the enigma. Ann Neurol 2008;64:4–14.

Vascular Dementia

Bronge L, Wahlund LO. White matter changes in dementia: does radiology matter? Br J Radiol 2007;80(Spec2):S115–20, *Review*.

Farlow MR. Use of antidementia agents in vascular dementia: beyond Alzheimer disease. Mayo Clin Proc 2006;81(10):1350–8, *Review*.

Knopman DS. Cerebrovascular disease and dementia. Br J Radiol 2007;80(Spec2):S121–7, *Review*.

Papademetriou V. Hypertension and cognitive function. Blood pressure regulation and cognitive function: a review of the literature. Geriatrics 2005;60(1):20–2, 24. *Review*.

Viswanathan A, Rocca WA, Tzourio C. Vascular risk factors and dementia: how to move forward? Neurology 2009;72(4):368–74, *Review*.

Movement Disorders and Gait

Claudia J. Chaves

28

Parkinson Disease

Diana Apetauerova

> **CLINICAL VIGNETTE** *This 64-year-old auto mechanic noticed intermittent tremor in his right hand while working. His wife reported he was not swinging his right arm when walking, and she was also observing tremor in his right hand when they were sitting quietly watching movies. The patient himself noted slowness and clumsiness of the right hand when shaving, writing, and typing on the computer or smartphone. Soon he lost normal range of motion of that limb; eventually this arm became stiff, and he had increasingly limited motion at the shoulder. He also loved to cook and realized that he slowly lost his sense of smell. He became much more anxious, and his tremor worsened during any stressful situation. He also described constipation. One year after onset, he began to drag his right foot.*
>
> *Neurologic examination demonstrated moderate masking of his face, a positive Myerson sign, a mild 6-Hz resting tremor of his right hand, cogwheel rigidity of the right wrist and elbow, and diminished right arm swing, and his stride length had been reduced. Extraocular muscle function was full, with no limitation of vertical gaze. The diagnosis of Parkinson disease (PD) was made, and he was treated with carbidopa-levodopa.*
>
> *Head magnetic resonance image (MRI) scan was normal. No other investigations were indicated because the diagnosis of PD is primarily a clinical one. Within 3 weeks, he demonstrated marked improvement. He was able to move faster, and his fine motor activities and tremor were improved. This excellent response made idiopathic PD the most likely diagnosis.*

In 1817 James Parkinson made the seminal observations on this disorder, defining a specific neurodegenerative illness characterized by bradykinesia, resting tremor, cogwheel rigidity, and postural reflex impairment. Parkinson disease (PD) has a relatively stereotyped clinical presentation that now bears the name of this early 19th-century neurologist.

PD is the second most common neurodegenerative disease after Alzheimer disease, affecting approximately 10 million people worldwide. PD prevalence increases steadily with age. PD prevalence rises from 107/100,000 in people 50–59 years of age to 1087/100,000 in those 70–79 years of age. Incidence is greater in men than in women.

Usually the patient's clinical status progresses from a relatively modest limitation at diagnosis to an ever-increasing disability over 10–20 years in many but not all patients. The primary neuropathologic features are loss of pigmented dopaminergic neurons mainly in the substantia nigra (SN) and the presence of Lewy bodies—eosinophilic, cytoplasmic inclusions found within the pigmented neurons, the primary structural component of which is alpha-synuclein (Fig. 28.1).

These dopaminergic neurons' primary projection is to the striatum (putamen and caudate). From there the neurotransmission is sequentially directed to other structures of the basal ganglia, thalamus, and primary motor cortex, via the direct and indirect pathways (Figs. 28.2 and 28.3).

ETIOLOGY

The etiology of PD is multifactorial and still poorly understood. Numerous studies point to environmental poisons, such as synthetic toxins, pesticides, and heavy metals, as potential risk factors. The environmental hypothesis of PD was born in the early to mid-1980s, when Langston and colleagues discovered that the toxin, 1-methyl 4-phenyl 1,2,3,6-tetrahydropyridine (MPTP) could cause parkinsonism. 1-methyl-4-phenylpyridinium (MPP+) accumulates in mitochondria and interferes with the function of complex I of the respiratory chain. A chemical resemblance between MPTP and some herbicides and pesticides suggested that an MPTP-like environmental toxin might be a cause of PD, but no specific agent has been identified. Nonetheless, mitochondrial complex I activity is reduced in PD, suggesting a common pathway with MPTP-induced parkinsonism. The oxidation hypothesis suggests that free radical damage, resulting from dopamine's oxidative metabolism, plays a role in the development or progression of PD. The oxidative metabolism of dopamine by monoamine oxidase (MAO) leads to the formation of hydrogen peroxide, which may lead to the formation of highly reactive hydroxyl radicals that can react with cell membrane lipids to cause lipid peroxidation and cell damage.

Humans are exposed to numerous pesticides and toxins in nature, yet not everyone develops PD, suggesting that the factors required for disease development are more complex. Many studies, using animal models or patients, point to interactions between an individual's genetic background and exposure to environmental toxins, which has led to the multiple hit hypothesis of PD (i.e., more than one risk factor contributes to disease development and progression). In addition, oxidative stress, protein mishandling, and inflammation are recognized as important features that may contribute to the neurodegenerative process.

GENES FOR PARKINSON DISEASE

A genetic predisposition has been recognized in PD in the past 20 years. Since the discovery of the first disease-causing mutation in the *SNCA* gene, investigations into the role of genetics in PD have grown exponentially. Presently known mendelian forms of PD with autosomal dominant and recessive inheritance account for less than 10% of PD cases (Table 28.1). A 2014 meta-analysis of genome-wide association studies, with data from more than 13,700 PD cases and 95,000 controls, identified and replicated 28 independent risk variants for PD across 24 loci.

- *Autosomal dominant and autosomal recessive: SNCA* and *LRRK2* are the two dominantly inherited genes that have been studied most in depth. A base pair change in the *SNCA* gene was the first mutation identified as causing PD in 1997. Subsequently multiplication mutations in the *SNCA* gene were described, with the number of copies

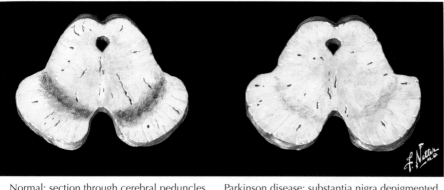

Normal: section through cerebral peduncles and substantia nigra

Parkinson disease: substantia nigra depigmented

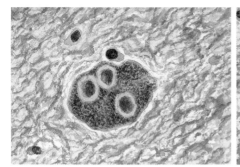

Lewy inclusion bodies in cell of substantia nigra in Parkinson disease; may also appear in locus ceruleus and tegmentum, cranial motor nerve nuclei, and peripheral autonomic ganglia

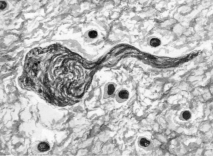

Neurofibrillary tangle in nerve cell of substantia nigra as seen in postencephalitic parkinsonism, progressive supranuclear palsy, and parkinsonism-dementia complex

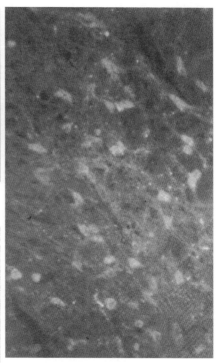

Section of substantia nigra of normal animal: treatment of section with formaldehyde vapor causes formation of polymers with monoamines (dopa and norepinephrine) that fluoresce to bright green under ultraviolet light

Fig. 28.1 Neuropathology of Parkinson Disease.

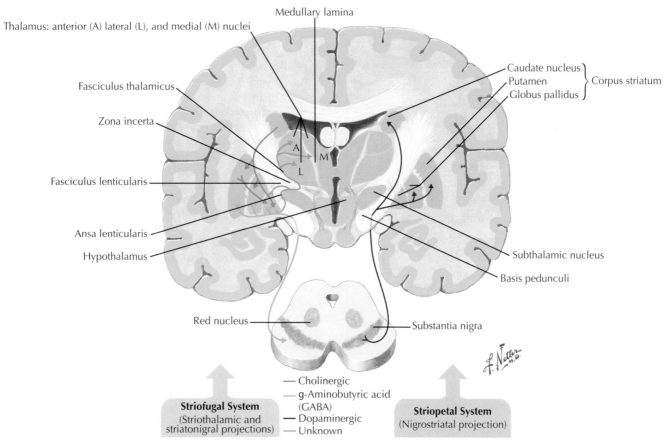

Medullary lamina

Thalamus: anterior (A) lateral (L), and medial (M) nuclei

Fasciculus thalamicus

Zona incerta

Fasciculus lenticularis

Ansa lenticularis

Hypothalamus

Caudate nucleus
Putamen   } Corpus striatum
Globus pallidus

Subthalamic nucleus

Basis pedunculi

Red nucleus

Substantia nigra

Cholinergic
g-Aminobutyric acid (GABA)
Dopaminergic
Unknown

Striofugal System
(Striothalamic and striatonigral projections)

Striopetal System
(Nigrostriatal projection)

Fig. 28.2 Parkinson Disease (PD)—Anatomy With Biochemical Pathways.

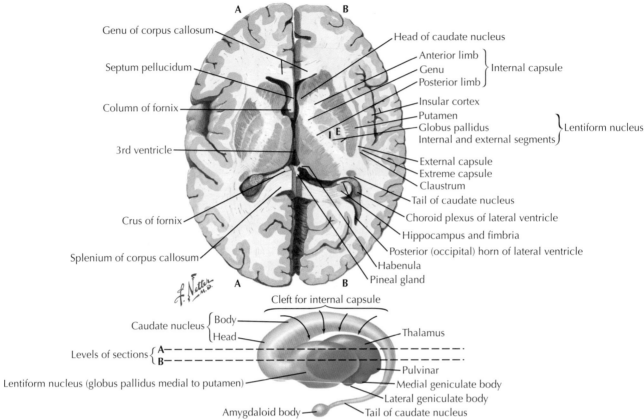

Schematic illustration showing interrelationship of thalamus, lentiform nucleus, caudate nucleus, and amygdaloid body (viewed from side).

Fig. 28.3 Horizontal Brain Sections of Basal Ganglia.

TABLE 28.1	Genetic Forms of Parkinson Disease		
Locus	**Chromosome**	**Gene**	**Inheritance**
PARK1/4	**4q21**	**SNCA**	**AD**
PARK2	**6q25.2–q27**	**PARK2**	**AR**
PARK3	2p13	?	AD
PARK5	4p14	UCHL1	?
PARK6	**1p36**	**PINK1**	**AR**
PARK7	**1p36**	**DJ-1**	**AR**
PARK8	**12q12**	**LRRK2**	**AD**
PARK9	**1p36**	**ATP13A2**	**AR**
PARK10	1p32	?	?
PARK11	2q37	GIGYF2	?
PARK12	Xq21–q25	?	X-linked
PARK13	2p12	HTRA2	?
PARK14	22q13.1	PLA2G6	?
PARK15	22q12–q13	FBX07	AR
PARK16	1q32	?	?

AD, Autosomal dominant; *AR,* autosomal recessive.

of the *SNCA* gene appearing to correlate with disease severity. The significance of the *SNCA* gene is related to the subsequent discovery of the encoded protein alpha-synuclein (α-Syn), which is the major component of Lewy bodies. Mutations in **LRRK2** are the most frequent cause of dominantly inherited PD. It accounts for 2% of all PD and 5% of familial cases. The clinical presentation of the parkinsonian phenotype caused by *LRRK2* is often indistinguishable from sporadic PD. Mutations in **Parkin, PINK1, and DJ-1** have been identified to cause autosomal recessive forms of PD, characterized by pure parkinsonism, early onset, slow progression, and good response to levodopa. Other genes (*PARK9, PARK14, PARK15*) with autosomal recessive inheritance have been associated with more complex phenotypes and additional neurologic findings such as hyperreflexia, spasticity, dystonia, and dementia.

- *Glucocerebrosidase (GBA) mutations:* Clinical observations of frequent occurrence of PD in relatives of patients with Gaucher disease, an autosomal recessive lysosomal storage disorder, led to the discovery that heterozygous mutations in *GBA* gene increase PD risk by fivefold.
- *Mitochondrial mutations:* Mitochondrial dysfunction has been recognized as a part of PD pathogenesis. Frequent mitochondrial DNA mutations and reduced mitochondrial function in complex I of the respiratory chain have been detected in the SN pars compacta (SNc) of PD brains.

PATHOLOGY/PATHOPHYSIOLOGY

The pathologic hallmark of PD is degeneration of the SNc. Neurons within the SN synthesize the neurotransmitter dopamine (Figs. 28.2 and 28.4). These cells contain a dark pigment called neuromelanin. Parkinson symptoms develop when approximately 60% of these cells die. Concomitantly, direct inspection of the SN in PD demonstrates an abnormal pallor when compared with that characteristically seen with the normal hyperpigmented melanin-containing cells.

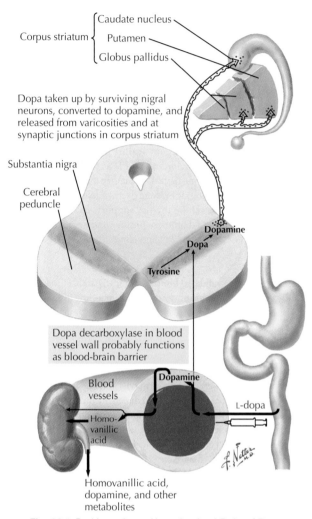

Corpus striatum {
Caudate nucleus
Putamen
Globus pallidus
}

Dopa taken up by surviving nigral neurons, converted to dopamine, and released from varicosities and at synaptic junctions in corpus striatum

Substantia nigra

Cerebral peduncle

Dopamine

Dopa

Tyrosine

Dopa decarboxylase in blood vessel wall probably functions as blood-brain barrier

Dopamine

Blood vessels

L-dopa

Homo-vanillic acid

Homovanillic acid, dopamine, and other metabolites

Fig. 28.4 Parkinsonism—Hypothesized Role of Dopa.

Microscopically, the SNc and other regions of the central and peripheral nervous system (PNS) in PD patients contain intraneuronal protein accumulation in the form of Lewy bodies and Lewy neurites. α-Syn is the principal component of Lewy pathology and thought to play an important role in PD pathogenesis. The significance of α-Syn in PD originates from discovery of rare mendelian forms of PD caused by mutations in *SNCA*. Genetic variations in *SNCA* are linked to an increased risk for sporadic PD. With advances in immunostaining, the extent of Lewy pathology in PD is now known to be more widespread than originally thought. Neurodegeneration with Lewy pathology is also found in the nucleus basalis of Meynert, locus coeruleus (LC), median raphe, and nerve cells in the olfactory system, upper and lower brainstem, cerebral cortex, spinal cord, and peripheral autonomic system. Perhaps one of the greatest pathologic advancements in PD was when *Braak* and colleagues examined α-Syn distribution in brains of PD patients and controls (Fig. 28.5). They proposed a sequential pattern of Lewy pathology distribution, beginning in the olfactory system and dorsal motor nucleus of the vagus, progressing to involve the peripheral autonomic nervous system, extending to involve SNc in the mid-stage of the disease, later involving the upper brainstem, and finally affecting the cerebral hemispheres. The findings of Lewy bodies in the olfactory cells and autonomic nerves of the heart and gastrointestinal tract prior to neurodegeneration in SNc and the development of classic motor symptoms of PD support the concept of a *prodromal (premotor) phase* of PD.

The pathologic spreading scheme in the brains of PD raised the possibility of prionlike mechanism of α-Syn in disease progression called the ***Prion Hypothesis.*** Autopsy studies in PD patients with fetal brain tissue grafts found Lewy pathology similar to that of PD in the grafted neurons more than 10 years after the transplant procedure, suggesting a possible transmissible nature of α-Syn. Under certain circumstances, α-Syn undergoes conformational change from α-helical structure to β-sheet–rich fibrils, similar to prion proteins. Recent studies using animal models have demonstrated a "seeding" phenomenon of α-Syn fibrils inducing endogenous α-Syn protein to misfold, aggregate,

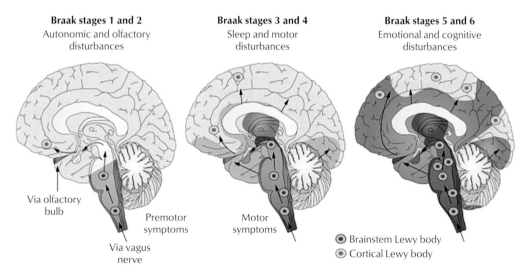

Braak stages 1 and 2
Autonomic and olfactory disturbances

Braak stages 3 and 4
Sleep and motor disturbances

Braak stages 5 and 6
Emotional and cognitive disturbances

Via olfactory bulb

Premotor symptoms

Via vagus nerve

Motor symptoms

◉ Brainstem Lewy body
◉ Cortical Lewy body

Fig. 28.5 Stylized representation of the Braak staging of Lewy pathology showing initiation sites in the medulla oblongata and olfactory bulb, progressing to midbrain, and finally to cortical regions. (Reused with permission from Halliday G, Lees A, Stern M. Milestones in Parkinson disease: clinical and pathologic features. *Mov Disord* 2011;26:1015–1021.)

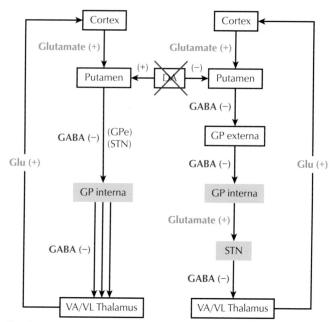

Fig. 28.6 Direct and Indirect Pathway. *GABA,* Gamma-aminobutyric acid; *GP,* globus pallidus; *STN,* subthalamic nucleus; *VA,* ventral anterior nucleus; *VL,* ventral lateral nucleus.

form Lewy body–like inclusions, and cause neuronal death. The prion hypothesis has challenged the traditional way that we view PD.

Human Gut Microbiota (GM) has now been accepted as a potential modulator of cognition, learning, and behavior and can directly or indirectly modify brain neurochemistry. GM can influence dopamine turnover, dopaminergic cell expression, striatal gene expression, etc. The GM's composition is altered in PD, and this dysbiosis has been related to motor fluctuations. More studies are needed to establish a cause and effect relationship between GM and PD.

Anatomy

The pathologic sites responsible for the parkinsonian disorders reside in a group of brain gray matter structures known as the extrapyramidal system or basal ganglia. The prevailing model of basal ganglia function states that two circuits, the direct and indirect pathways, originate from distinct populations of striatal medium spiny neurons (MSNs) and project to different output structures. These circuits are believed to have opposite effects on movement. Specifically, the activity of direct pathway MSNs is postulated to promote movement, whereas the activation of indirect pathway MSNs is hypothesized to inhibit it. An important pathway that modulates the direct and indirect circuits is the dopaminergic nigrostriatal projection from the SNc to the striatum. D1 dopamine receptors are present in the striatal neurons of the direct pathway and are depolarized by dopamine, whereas D2 dopamine receptors predominate in the striatal neurons from the indirect pathway and are inhibited by the presence of dopamine. Therefore, in the presence of dopamine, the cortex is stimulated by both direct and indirect circuits. The loss of dopamine neurons in PD causes impairment of movements due to the development of an imbalance between direct and indirect pathways, in favor of the latter, with consequent inhibition of motor cortex regions (Fig. 28.6).

DIAGNOSIS AND BIOMARKERS

It has been increasingly recognized that PD has a long prodromal phase during which early symptoms can occur years before the appearance of motor symptoms. Our current method of diagnosing PD during life

remains clinical, whereas definitive diagnosis is obtained through pathologic confirmation of α-Syn deposition and neurodegeneration in the SNc. Clinical diagnostic accuracy ranges from 75% to 95% depending on disease duration and stage and clinician expertise. In 2015 the International Parkinson and Movement Disorder Society (MDS) created new Clinical Diagnostic Criteria for PD (Box 28.1). The MDS-PD criteria incorporated nonmotor symptoms (NMSs) while retaining the central features of parkinsonism as bradykinesia in combination with either rest tremor, rigidity, or both. MDS-PD criteria proposed a list of absolute exclusions and red flags that argues against the diagnosis of PD, and supportive criteria that argue in favor of PD as the etiology of parkinsonism. Two ancillary diagnostic tests, olfactory loss and metaiodobenzylguanidine (MIBG) scintigraphy, were deemed reliable, with specificity greater than 80%; these can be used as supportive criteria. Two levels of diagnostic certainty based on these positive and negative factors were proposed: *clinically established PD* and *clinically probable PD.*

Biomarkers

There is no definitive validated biomarker for PD at this time. A number of candidates are undergoing evaluation, including fluid and tissue analysis, genetic susceptibility, clinical evaluations such as olfactory testing, and neuroimaging. Positron emission tomography (PET) and single-photon emission computed tomography (SPECT) using radiolabeled tracers have allowed functional assessment of the nigrostriatal pathway. Neurodegeneration in the SN leads to decreased striatal density of presynaptic dopaminergic nerve terminals and dopamine transporters (DATs), which can be reflected by reduced ligand binding on DAT SPECT imaging. SPECT with DAT radiotracers can help to distinguish neurodegenerative parkinsonism from nonneurodegenerative parkinsonism (Fig. 28.7). PET imaging measuring cerebral glucose metabolism and cerebral blood flow may have some potential application for the differential diagnosis of parkinsonian syndromes. Transcranial sonography (TCS), a noninvasive and low-cost ultrasound imaging method, has shown potential usefulness in the clinical diagnosis of PD by assessing the echogenicity of the SNc. Novel MRI techniques have been developed to evaluate the SNc in PD.

CLINICAL PRESENTATION

The clinical course or temporal profile of PD is quite variable. It usually progresses slowly and inexorably (Fig. 28.8). Typically, the illness begins unilaterally with focal tremor or difficulty using one limb. Eventually, the symptoms become more generalized and occur on the contralateral side, interfering with activities of daily living (ADLs). Clinical features can be divided into motor and NMSs.

Motor Symptoms

The four *primary signs* of PD are bradykinesia, tremor, rigidity, and gait disturbance (see Fig. 28.8).

Bradykinesia is a decreased ability to initiate movement (akinesia is the extreme manifestation). This may affect multiple functions, particularly fine motor tasks such as buttoning a shirt or handwriting, the latter becoming micrographic. Other individuals may present with a masked facies, expressionless, which later becomes associated with decreased blink frequency, muted speech, and slowed swallowing. Typically, the gait is shuffling with decreased arm swing, stooped posture, and en bloc turning, The *Myerson sign,* or glabellar tap sign, is elicited by having the patient look straight ahead while the examiner gently taps with her or his index finger tip between the medial ends of the eyebrows. Normally the patient blinks for the first few taps and then such movement is inhibited. In contrast, the PD patient persistently blinks as long as the tapping is maintained and thus a positive test.

BOX 28.1 Movement Disorder Society Diagnostic Criteria for Parkinson Disease

Diagnosis of Clinically Established Parkinson Disease Requires

1. Absence of absolute exclusion criteria
2. At least two supportive criteria, and
3. No red flags

Diagnosis of Clinically Probable Parkinson Disease Requires

1. Absence of absolute exclusion criteria
2. Presence of red flags counterbalanced by supportive criteria
   If 1 red flag is present, there must also be at least 1 supportive criterion
   If 2 red flags, at least 2 supportive criteria are needed
   No more than 2 red flags are allowed for this category

Supportive Criteria

1. Clear and dramatic beneficial response to dopaminergic therapy. During initial treatment, patient returned to normal or near-normal level of function. In the absence of clear documentation of initial response, a dramatic response can be classified as:
   a. Marked improvement with dose increases or marked worsening with dose decreases. Mild changes do not qualify. Document this either objectively (>30% in UPDRS III with change in treatment), or subjectively (clearly documented history of marked changes from a reliable patient or caregiver).
   b. Unequivocal and marked on/off fluctuations, which must have at some point included predictable end-of-dose wearing off.
2. Presence of levodopa-induced dyskinesia
3. Rest tremor of a limb, documented on clinical examination (in past, or on current examination)
4. The presence of either olfactory loss or cardiac sympathetic denervation on MIBG scintigraphy

Absolute Exclusion Criteria: The Presence of Any of These Features Rules Out Parkinson Disease

1. Unequivocal cerebellar abnormalities, such as cerebellar gait, limb ataxia, or cerebellar oculomotor abnormalities (e.g., sustained gaze evoked nystagmus, macro square wave jerks, hypermetric saccades)
2. Downward vertical supranuclear gaze palsy or selective slowing of downward vertical saccades
3. Diagnosis of probable behavioral variant frontotemporal dementia or primary progressive aphasia, defined according to consensus criteria within the first 5 years of disease
4. Parkinsonian features restricted to the lower limbs for more than 3 years
5. Treatment with a dopamine receptor blocker or a dopamine-depleting agent in a dose and time-course consistent with drug-induced parkinsonism
6. Absence of observable response to high-dose levodopa despite at least moderate severity of disease
7. Unequivocal cortical sensory loss (i.e., graphesthesia, stereognosis with intact primary sensory modalities), clear limb ideomotor apraxia, or progressive aphasia
8. Normal functional neuroimaging of the presynaptic dopaminergic system
9. Documentation of an alternative condition known to produce parkinsonism and plausibly connected to the patient's symptoms, or the expert evaluating physician, based on the full diagnostic assessment, believes that an alternative syndrome is more likely than PD

Red Flags

1. Rapid progression of gait impairment requiring regular use of wheelchair within 5 years of onset
2. A complete absence of progression of motor symptoms or signs over 5 or more years unless stability is related to treatment
3. Early bulbar dysfunction: severe dysphonia or dysarthria (speech unintelligible most of the time) or severe dysphagia (requiring soft food, NG tube, or gastrostomy feeding) within first 5 years
4. Inspiratory respiratory dysfunction: either diurnal or nocturnal inspiratory stridor or frequent inspiratory sighs
5. Severe autonomic failure in the first 5 years of disease. This can include:
   a. Orthostatic hypotension—orthostatic decrease of blood pressure within 3 min of standing by at least 30 mm Hg systolic or 15 mm Hg diastolic, in the absence of dehydration, medication, or other diseases that could plausibly explain autonomic dysfunction, or
   b. Severe urinary retention or urinary incontinence in the first 5 years of disease (excluding long-standing or small amount stress incontinence in women) that is not simply functional incontinence. In men, urinary retention must not be attributable to prostate disease and must be associated with erectile dysfunction
6. Recurrent (>1/year) falls because of impaired balance within 3 years of onset
7. Disproportionate anterocollis (dystonic) or contractures of hand or feet within the first 10 years
8. Absence of any of the common nonmotor features of disease despite 5-year disease duration. These include sleep dysfunction (sleep-maintenance insomnia, excessive daytime somnolence, symptoms of REM sleep behavior disorder), autonomic dysfunction (constipation, daytime urinary urgency, symptomatic orthostasis), hyposmia, or psychiatric dysfunction (depression, anxiety, or hallucinations)
9. Otherwise-unexplained pyramidal tract signs, defined as pyramidal weakness or clear pathologic hyperreflexia (excluding mild reflex asymmetry and isolated extensor plantar response)
10. Bilateral symmetric parkinsonism. The patient or caregiver reports bilateral symptom onset with no side predominance, and no side predominance is observed on objective examination

Criteria Application

1. Does the patient have parkinsonism, as defined by the MDS criteria?
If no, neither probable PD nor clinically established PD can be diagnosed. If yes:
2. Are any absolute exclusion criteria present?
If "yes," neither probable PD nor clinically established PD can be diagnosed. If no:
3. Number of red flags present _____
4. Number of supportive criteria present _____
5. Are there at least two supportive criteria and no red flags?
If yes, patient meets criteria for clinically established PD. If no:
6. Are there more than 2 red flags?
If "yes," probable PD cannot be diagnosed. If no:
7. Is the number of red flags equal to, or less than, the number of supportive criteria?
If yes, patient meets criteria for probable PD

MDS, Movement Disorder Society; *MIBG,* metaiodobenzylguanidine; *PD,* Parkinson disease; *UPDRS,* Unified Parkinson Disease Rating Scale. Reused with permission Postuma RB, Berg D, Stern M, et al. MDS clinical diagnostic criteria for Parkinson's disease. *Mov Disord* 2015;30(12):1591–1599, Table, p. 1596. John Wiley and Sons.

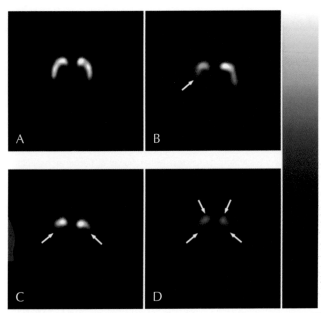

Fig. 28.7 DaTscan (Dopamine Transporter scan) performed in four different patients with worsening degrees of clinical Parkinson disease. The color scale is shown—black representing lowest activity and white highest activity. (A) Normal symmetric uptake in the head of caudate and putamen. (B–D) Sequential progressive reduction in uptake in the putamen and head of caudate as the disease worsens *(arrows)*. (Reused with permission from McArthur C, Jampana R, Patterson J, Hadley D. Applications of cerebral SPECT. *Clin Radiol* 2011;66(7):651–661. Copyright © 2011 The Royal College of Radiologists [Fig. 9]).

Rigidity is a resistance to passive movement throughout the entire range of motion occurring in flexor and extensor muscles. This contrasts with spasticity, wherein there is an initial marked resistance to passive movement and then a sudden release (e.g., *clasp-knife* phenomena). The classic cogwheel quality (stop-and-go effect) is from a tremor superimposed on the altered muscle tone. Very early on, patients are often concerned about stiffness, "weakness," or fatigue. Initially, the patient will just note a limitation in his or her daily activities or exercise capacity—unable to hike as long a distance, inability to get to the ball when playing tennis, or simply walking from the car to the store. When more pronounced, these bradykinetic symptoms may represent the combination of bradykinesia with rigidity.

Tremor occurs in 75% of patients. Typically, it is prominent at rest, having a frequency of 3–7 Hz. Although this tremor usually does not significantly interfere with ADLs, such as eating or writing, the patient finds it very embarrassing. Tremor is often seen while the patient is walking; not only is the arm swing lost but a minor pill rolling tremor may become amplified as the hand comes away from the body. Occasionally a PD tremor has a significant postural or action component complicating distinction from the more benign essential tremor (ET).

Gait disturbance, postural instability, or both usually present at later stages of PD characterized by a change in the center of gravity typified by falling forward (propulsion) or backward (retropulsion) and a festinating (shuffling, slowly propulsive) petit pas (small steps) gait.

Typically PD progresses in stages (see Fig. 28.8). There are two commonly used rating scales to measure the degree of disability that these patients manifest: (1) Unified Parkinson Disease Rating Scale (UPDRS) and (2) Hoehn and Yahr (H&Y) scale (Box 28.2).

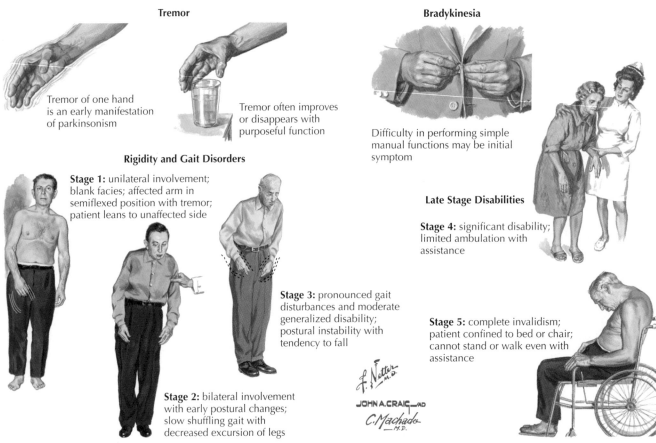

Tremor

Tremor of one hand is an early manifestation of parkinsonism

Tremor often improves or disappears with purposeful function

Bradykinesia

Difficulty in performing simple manual functions may be initial symptom

Rigidity and Gait Disorders

Stage 1: unilateral involvement; blank facies; affected arm in semiflexed position with tremor; patient leans to unaffected side

Stage 2: bilateral involvement with early postural changes; slow shuffling gait with decreased excursion of legs

Stage 3: pronounced gait disturbances and moderate generalized disability; postural instability with tendency to fall

Late Stage Disabilities

Stage 4: significant disability; limited ambulation with assistance

Stage 5: complete invalidism; patient confined to bed or chair; cannot stand or walk even with assistance

Fig. 28.8 Clinical Signs of Parkinson Disease.

Nonmotor Symptoms (Box 28.3)

NMSs occur throughout the course of the disease. Some may appear at the earliest stage or precede the motor symptoms by years and then are called premotor symptoms (olfactory dysfunction, rapid eye movement [REM] sleep behavior disorder [RBD], constipation, depression, and pain) (Fig. 28.9A).

BOX 28.2 Parkinson Disease Rating Scales

Hoehn and Yahr
- Stage I: unilateral disease
- Stage II: bilateral disease with preservation of postural reflexes
- Stage III: bilateral disease with impaired postural reflexes but preserved ability to ambulate independently
- Stage IV: severe disease requiring considerable assistance
- Stage V: end-stage disease, bed or chair confined

United Parkinson Disease Rating Scale (UPDRS)
Four major subsets:
- Cognitive
- Activities of daily living
- Motor examination
- Complications of treatment

Mood Disturbance and Apathy

Depression and anxiety. Depression occurs at any stage of the disease. Predominant features are somatic (lack of energy, psychomotor slowing), with irritability, often associated with sleep disorders, lack of refreshing sleep, decrease of libido, and feeling of poor physical appearance. Anxiety appears to be frequent in PD and is two times more frequent compared with the general population. During the course of the disease, 30%–50% of PD patients experience anxiety, which can be partly explained by the burden of the disease.

Apathy. Apathy consists in a loss of motivation, which appears in emotional, intellectual domains and in the behavior. Prevalence is estimated to be 30%–40%. Apathy is one of the major determinants of a reduced quality of life in PD.

Dopamine Dysregulation Syndrome and Impulse Control Disorders

Dopamine dysregulation syndrome (DDS) has been defined as compulsive use of dopaminergic drugs, associated with severe behavioral symptoms, and impaired social functioning. DDS consists of a craving or intense desire to obtain medication, even in absence of motor parkinsonian symptoms.

Impulse control disorders (ICDs) are behavioral disorders characterized by failure to resist an impulse, inability to cut down, and unsuccessful

---

BOX 28.3 Major Nonmotor Symptoms in Parkinson Disease

Neuropsychiatric Symptoms
- Depression
- Anxiety
- Apathy
- Hallucinations, delusions, illusions
- Delirium (may be drug induced)
- Cognitive impairment (dementia, mild cognitive impairment [MCI])
- Dopaminergic dysregulation syndrome (usually related to levodopa)
- Impulse control disorders (related to dopaminergic drugs)

Sleep Disorders
- REM sleep behavior disorder (possible premotor symptoms)
- Excessive daytime somnolence, narcolepsy type "sleep attack"
- Restless legs syndrome, periodic leg movements
- Insomnia
- Sleep disordered breathing
- Non-rapid eye movement (REM) parasomnias (confusional wandering)

Fatigue
- Central fatigue (may be related to dysautonomia)
- Peripheral fatigue

Sensory Symptoms
- Pain
- Olfactory disturbance
- Hyposmia
- Functional anosmia
- Visual disturbance (blurred vision, diplopia; impaired contrast sensitivity)

Autonomic Dysfunction
- Bladder dysfunction (urgency, frequency, nocturia)
- Sexual dysfunction (may be drug induced)
- Sweating abnormalities (hyperhidrosis)
- Orthostatic hypotension

Gastrointestinal Symptoms
- Dribbling of saliva
- Dysphagia
- Ageusia
- Constipation
- Nausea
- Vomiting

Dopaminergic Drug-Induced Behavior Nonmotor Symptoms
- Hallucinations, psychosis, delusions
- Dopamine dysregulation syndrome
- Impulse control disorders

Dopaminergic Drug-Induced Other Nonmotor Symptoms
- Ankle swelling
- Dyspnea
- Skin reactions
- Subcutaneous nodules
- Erythematous

Nonmotor Fluctuations
- Dysautonomia
- Cognitive/psychiatric
- Sensory/pain
- Visual blurring

Other Symptoms
- Weight loss

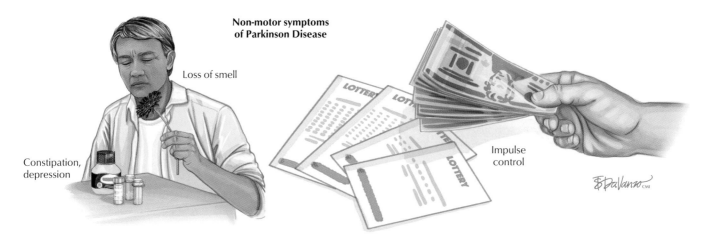

Fig. 28.9 Nonmotor Symptoms of Parkinson Disease.

attempts to control a specific behavior. ICDs include pathologic gambling, hypersexuality, compulsive shopping, and binge or compulsive eating (see Fig. 28.9B). Another repetitive and compulsive behavior, the punding, has been described.

ICDs occur in 15%–20% of PD patients, and their prevalence has been found increased among patients treated with a dopamine agonist (DA), or if combined with l-dopa. The identified risk factors consist of a younger age, male gender, family history of addictive problems, depression, anxiety, and specific traits such as impulsivity and novelty seeking.

Cognitive Decline

In PD, very subtle cognitive disorders can develop insidiously within the first years of the disease. They consist first of an intellectual slowing and difficulties organizing and managing the intellectual capacities, with preservation of global cognitive efficiency. Eventually, these disturbances can progressively increase. Dementia can be present in advanced stages of PD, with an estimated prevalence between 20% and 30%.

Hallucinations, Delusions, and Psychosis

Psychosis is defined as hallucinations, delusions, or both, in patients with clear sensorium.

Hallucinations occur usually in a normal state of consciousness, without delirium, and have a chronic course. Benign hallucinations are limited to presence sensation, passing lights or visions at periphery of the visual field, with great tolerance by the patient. Conversely, elaborated hallucinations are usually disabling because of their disturbing nature (wild animals, fantastic human creatures). Illusions consist of transformation of a real image and occur more often in the dark. Auditory, olfactory, or tactile hallucinations are less frequent. Hallucinations are mostly induced by dopaminergic therapies.

Pain

Pain may precede the onset of motor parkinsonian symptoms. The prevalence of all types of pain is high but variably assessed. Pain is estimated to be twice as frequent in PD patients than in patients without PD. A common type of pain is musculoskeletal pain, dystonic pain, and neuropathic pain. Factors such as rigidity, skeletal deformity, and mechanical factors play a role.

Sleep Disorders

Sleep disorders are present in approximately 66%–90% of PD patients and are more frequent in advanced disease. RBD is a substantial risk

factor for development of PD and occurs in one-third of patients with PD. Nocturnal disturbances can be related to motor symptoms (nocturnal akinesia, dystonia), nocturnal behavioral disturbances (agitation, confusion), and others, such as fragmentation of sleep, RBD, restless leg syndrome (RLS), periodic leg movements in sleep (PLMS), and excessive daytime sleepiness.

Dysautonomia

Autonomic symptoms in PD include orthostatic hypotension, constipation, bladder and sexual dysfunction, and sweating abnormalities. Autonomic failure may be an early feature of PD, although it is more typically associated with advanced stage of the disease.

Genitourinary Dysfunction

Lower urinary tract symptoms, such as urinary frequency, nocturia, and urinary incontinence are caused by detrusor hyperactivity. Aspects of sexual function can be altered, including decreased libido and difficulties with erection, ejaculation, and orgasm.

Orthostatic Hypotension

Orthostatic hypotension is defined as a fall of at least 20 mm Hg in systolic pressure and/or 10 mm Hg in diastolic pressure within 3 minutes of standing. There is an orthostatic hypotension in 20%–58% of PD patients. PD is a cause of primary autonomic failure with presence of peripheral postganglionic sympathetic dysfunction, which can be demonstrated by MIBG cardiac scintigraphy. Symptoms of autonomic dysfunction correlate with disease duration and severity.

Constipation

Constipation is seen early in the course of the disease and commonly precedes diagnosis by several years. Disabling constipation predominates on the later stage of the disease, with difficulty in defecation and reduced number of bowel movements, in comparison with early stages

DIFFERENTIAL DIAGNOSES (Box 28.4)

Symptoms and signs of parkinsonism can be prominent in neurodegenerative disorders other than idiopathic PD, including atypical parkinsonian syndrome (Table 28.2) Furthermore, parkinsonism is seen in a wide variety of other conditions (secondary parkinsonism). Distinguishing PD from these parkinsonian syndromes can be difficult, particularly in the early stages of disease. ET may also be confused with PD.

BOX 28.4 Differential Diagnoses of Parkinson Disease

1. Essential tremor
2. Secondary parkinsonism
   a. Dopamine-blocking agents
   b. Vascular parkinsonism
   c. Normal-pressure hydrocephalus
   d. Infectious or postinfectious
   e. Toxic
   f. Metabolic
3. Atypical ("Parkinson plus"):
   a. PSP (Progressive supranuclear palsy)
   b. CBD (Corticobasal degeneration)
   c. MSA (Multisystem atrophy)
   d. DLBD (Dementia Lewy body disease)
4. Familial
5. Normal-pressure hydrocephalus
6. Other degenerative causes of parkinsonism

TABLE 28.2 Degenerative Causes of Parkinsonism

Alpha-Synuclein Deposition	Tau Deposition	Polyglutamine Tract Deposition
Parkinson disease	Progressive supranuclear palsy	Juvenile Huntington disease
Multiple-system atrophy	Corticobasal ganglionic degeneration	Autosomal dominant cerebellar ataxia (SCA-3)
	Parkinsonism dementia complex of Guam	Dentato-rubro-pallido-luyusian atrophy
	Postencephalitic Parkinson syndrome	Sporadic neuronal intranuclear inclusion disease
	Frontotemporal dementia with parkinsonism linked to chromosome 17	
	Posttraumatic parkinsonism	

SCA, Spinocerebellar atrophy.

Essential Tremor

ET is the most common neurologic cause of action tremor. ET usually affects both hands and arms and can also involve the head, voice, chin, trunk, and legs. Isolated tremor of the chin or lips is more likely to be a manifestation of PD. ET typically becomes immediately apparent in the arms when they are held outstretched or when they are engaged in activities such as writing or eating. ET is most often symmetric. A small drink of an alcoholic beverage may clarify the diagnostic issue because ETs are commonly greatly inhibited by some ethanol derivative.

Dementia With Lewy Bodies

Dementia with Lewy bodies (DLB) is characterized clinically by visual hallucinations, fluctuating cognition, and parkinsonism. Other associated symptoms include repeated falls, syncope, autonomic dysfunction, neuroleptic sensitivity, delusions, and hallucinations in nonvisual modalities, sleep disorders, and depression. Dementia in DLB usually occurs concomitantly with or before the development of parkinsonian signs or no more than a year after onset of motor symptoms.

Multiple System Atrophy

Multiple system atrophy (MSA) commonly presents with parkinsonism, but patients also have varying degrees of dysautonomia, cerebellar involvement, and pyramidal signs. The prominence of these manifestations along with symmetry of onset and poor response to levodopa suggest this diagnosis rather than PD. Cognitive function in MSA tends to be relatively well preserved.

Corticobasal Degeneration

This is a rare, progressive asymmetric movement disorder with symptoms initially affecting one limb, including various combinations of akinesia and extreme rigidity, dystonia, focal myoclonus, ideomotor apraxia, and alien limb phenomenon. Cognitive impairment is a common manifestation of corticobasal degeneration (CBD) and may be a presenting feature and includes executive dysfunction, aphasia, apraxia, behavioral change, and visuospatial dysfunction. The distinctive clinical phenotype and the lack of clear response to an adequate trial of levodopa are typical for CBD and help to distinguish it from PD.

Progressive Supranuclear Palsy

Progressive supranuclear palsy (PSP) is an uncommon but not rare parkinsonian syndrome that can mimic PD in its early phase. The most common "classic" phenotype of PSP, known as Richardson syndrome, presents with a disturbance of gait resulting in falls. Supranuclear vertical ophthalmoparesis or ophthalmoplegia is the hallmark of PSP. Dysarthria, dysphagia, rigidity, frontal cognitive abnormalities, and sleep disturbances are additional common clinical features. The phenotype known as PSP-parkinsonism can be confused with idiopathic PD and is characterized by asymmetric onset of limb symptoms, tremor, and a moderate initial therapeutic response to levodopa.

Idiopathic and Familial Basal Ganglia Calcification

Idiopathic and familial basal ganglia calcification (IBGC) is also known as bilateral striatopallidodentate calcinosis, Fahr syndrome, or Fahr disease and is a rare neurodegenerative condition characterized by the accumulation of calcium deposits in the basal ganglia and other brain regions, most easily visualized on CT scan, and a variable phenotype that can include one or more features of parkinsonism, chorea, dystonia, cognitive impairment, or ataxia. Onset of symptoms usually occurs between ages 20 and 60.

Other Neurodegenerative Disorders

Parkinsonism may develop in late stages of Alzheimer disease. The relative timing of the appearance of dementia and parkinsonism is usually obvious, such that the late onset of parkinsonism in itself does not lead to confusion about the diagnosis of Alzheimer disease.

Parkinsonism may also occur in several other disorders: Huntington disease (rigid form), frontotemporal dementia with parkinsonism linked to chromosome 17, spinocerebellar ataxias, and dentatorubral pallido-luysian atrophy.

Secondary parkinsonism—a wide variety of conditions can cause secondary parkinsonism. Most common is drug-induced parkinsonism caused by classic or atypical antipsychotic agents, metoclopramide, prochloperazine, and reserpine (Table 28.3). Other causes include toxins (e.g., carbon disulfide, carbon monoxide, cyanide, MPTP, manganese, organic solvents), head trauma—isolated or repeated (e.g., boxing), structural brain lesions that affect striatonigral circuits (e.g., hydrocephalus, chronic subdural hematoma, tumor), and metabolic and miscellaneous disorders (e.g., Wilson disease, hypoparathyroidism and

TABLE 28.3 Medications Causing Secondary Parkinsonism

Generic	Trade Name
Acetophenazine	Tindal
Amoxapine	Asendin
Chlorpromazine	Thorazine
Fluphenazine	Permitil, Prolixin
Haloperidol	Haldol
Loxapine	Loxitane, Daxolin
Mesoridazine	Serentil
Metoclopramide	Reglan
Molindone	Lidone, Moban
Perphenazine	Trilafon or Triavil
Piperacetazine	Quide
Prochlorperazine	Compazine, Combid
Promazine	Sparine
Promethazine	Phenergan
Thiethylperazine	Torecan
Thioridazine	Mellaril
Thiothixene	Navane
Trifluoperazine	Stelazine
Triflupromazine	Vesprin
Trimeprazine	Temaril

BOX 28.5 Pharmacologic Therapy for Parkinson Disease

1. Dopaminergic
   a. Levodopa
   b. Dopamine agonist
2. Anticholinergics
3. MAO inhibitors
4. COMT inhibitors
5. Amantadine

COMT, Catechol-*O*-methyltransferase; *MAO,* monoamine oxidase.

pseudohypoparathyroidism, chronic liver failure, extrapontine myelinolysis). Certain infections can also cause parkinsonism (e.g., encephalitis lethargica or Economo encephalitis, HIV/AIDS, neurosyphilis, prion disease, progressive multifocal leukoencephalopathy, toxoplasmosis). Vascular parkinsonism is another cause of parkinsonism induced by small vessel disease, particularly multiple lacunar infarcts in the basal ganglia, and/or Binswanger disease.

TREATMENT

Treatment of PD patients can be divided into nonpharmacologic, pharmacologic, and surgical. In this chapter, only pharmacologic therapy will be discussed. Pharmacologic treatment options in PD may involve manipulating dopamine, or using nondopamine, symptom-related strategies. To improve motor symptoms, dopamine can either be "replaced," dopamine receptors can be stimulated, or the metabolism of dopamine can be prevented. Alternatively, medications that may specifically address tremor, dyskinesia, dystonia, or rigidity may be used. Patients with PD typically experience a smooth and even response to the early stages of levodopa treatment. However, as the disease advances, the effect of levodopa begins to wear off several hours after some or even all doses, leaving patients aware that the duration of action of a dose of levodopa is not being sustained. Many patients who are treated with levodopa for several years will experience motor complications. Motor complications include motor fluctuations and dyskinesias, in which the duration of benefit from a dose of medication is offset by involuntary hyperkinetic movements (dyskinesia). Motor fluctuations are alterations between periods of being "on," during which the patient has a positive response to medications, and being "off," during which the patient experiences reemergence of PD symptoms. Combinations of multiple medications are often required to optimize symptom control. The unpredictability of response to medications can be quite disabling

and is attributed to the pulsatile stimulation of dopamine receptors. By contrast, the strategy of continuous dopaminergic stimulation emphasizes the maintenance of regular concentrations of dopamine in the striatum and has gained acceptance as a potential mechanism by which to avoid or delay the development of motor complications.

PD treatment remains symptomatic; there is no neuroprotective therapy available.

Patient management requires careful consideration of the patient's symptoms and signs, stage of disease, degree of functional disability, and levels of activity and daily productivity. Most patients with idiopathic PD have a significant therapeutic response to levodopa. The complete absence of a clinical response to a dose of 25/100 mg of carbidopa/levodopa 6–10 times a day strongly suggests that the original diagnosis was incorrect and should prompt a search for other causes of parkinsonism.

Pharmacologic therapy for PD consists of five types of medication (Box 28.5). First-line initial symptomatic therapies (class A evidence) include levodopa (most effective), DAs, and monoamine oxide B (MAO-B) inhibitors. Second-line initial symptomatic therapies (class B evidence) include amantadine and anticholinergic medications, but these drugs are weaker and often poorly tolerated. Initiating therapy with a DA rather than levodopa may delay the onset of motor complications but is less effective and increases the risk of neuropsychiatric complications such as ICDs and psychosis. Long-term outcomes appear to be the same with early levodopa versus levodopa-sparing strategies, suggesting that disease progression (rather than initial medication choice) may be the primary risk factor for motor complications.

An important principle for early treatment of PD is that the introduction and use of medication must be tailored to the patient's individual needs. As a general rule, for younger patients and having no cognitive dysfunction, the choice of initial drug may lie between MAO-B inhibitor and a DA. Carbidopa/levodopa is started in older Parkinson patients who have a significant motor disability. Older patients with PD may also be considered for MAO-B inhibitor or DA if they are cognitively intact and lack any significant comorbidity. As PD progresses, the provision of effective symptom control becomes more challenging, and additional drugs may need to be added. *For wearing off,* evidence-based treatments include catechol-O-methyltransferase (COMT) inhibitors (entacapone is most commonly used; tolcapone is used infrequently due to the risk of hepatotoxicity and need for blood monitoring) or MAO-B inhibitors (rasagiline; selegiline is also used but lacks evidence-based data). Reducing the interval between levodopa doses is another common approach. Traditional carbidopa/levodopa controlled-release (CR) tablets have not been shown to reduce wearing off. *For dyskinesias,* evidence-based treatments include adjustment of dopaminergic medications; amantadine (not always tolerated due to side effects); and clozapine (rarely used due to the potential for severe neutropenia and need for blood monitoring). Advanced therapies such as deep brain stimulation

(DBS) and carbidopa/levodopa intestinal gel are also effective treatments for motor complications.

Management of Motor Symptoms
Dopaminergic

Levodopa. Levodopa with carbidopa is the most commonly used, most potent antiparkinsonian medication and is equally beneficial for all symptoms. L-dopa is the precursor to dopamine, norepinephrine, and epinephrine, which are collectively known as catecholamines (Fig. 28.10). Carbidopa-levodopa is available in immediate-release form as oral tablets (Sinemet) or sublingual pills (Parcopa) and CR formulations (Sinemet CR). Combined preparation of carbidopa-levodopa and entacapone (Stalevo) and combined immediate-release and CR levodopa capsules (Rytary) are also available and they reduce "off" time as compared with immediate-release levodopa.

For carbidopa/levodopa intestinal gel (Duopa), levodopa is delivered via percutaneous endoscopic gastrostomy (PEG)/jejunostomy tube (J-tube) using an infusion pump that runs for 16 hours/day. This represents an alternative to DBS for patients with advanced PD, particularly those with contraindications to DBS such as mild to moderate cognitive impairment. Benefits include the reduction of motor complications and potential simplification of the oral medication regimen.

Dopaminergic Agonists

DAs directly stimulate dopaminergic receptors. They are particularly indicated for monotherapy in younger patients, who are more prone to the early development of levodopa-related clinical fluctuations and who require long-term treatment. At least two general classes of DAs exist: D_1, which activates the enzyme adenylate cyclase, and D_2, which inhibits it. Most effective antiparkinsonian DAs stimulate predominantly D_2 receptors.

DAs often provide satisfactory relief of mild symptoms. Commonly used preparations include pramipexole, ropinirole, and rotigotine (Box 28.6). ICDs or dysfunctional behaviors are problems that have been increasingly recognized with dopaminergic agonists but that occur much less commonly with levodopa. These disorders include hypersexuality, compulsive gambling, meaningless and repetitive activities (punding), hypomanic states, and addictive overuse of levodopa.

Anticholinergic

Anticholinergic agents are the oldest drug class used for PD. They act as muscarinic receptor blockers by penetrating the CNS to antagonize acetylcholine transmission by striatal interneurons. Anticholinergics are most effective for tremor, but because of their innate side effects these medications must be used with significant caution in the elderly. Usually used as monotherapy or an adjunct to dopaminergic therapy, the most commonly used anticholinergic agents include benztropine and trihexyphenidyl.

Side effects, resulting from both peripheral and central cholinergic blockade, include dry mouth, narrow-angle glaucoma, constipation, urinary retention, memory impairment, and confusion with hallucinations.

Catechol-O-Methyltransferase Inhibitors

Inhibition of the enzyme COMT blocks dopamine metabolism. COMT inhibitors prolong levodopa's benefits by extending the life span of the

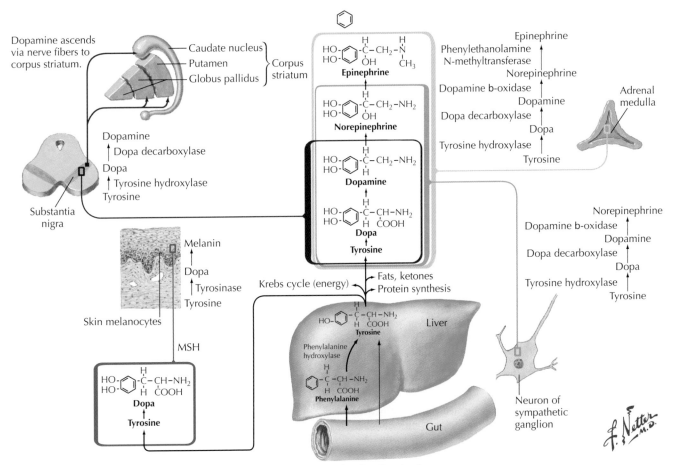

Fig. 28.10 Catecholamine Synthesis.

BOX 28.6 Advantages and Disadvantages of Dopamine Agonists

Advantages
- Some antiparkinson effect
- Reduced incidence of levodopa-related adverse events (dyskinesia and motor fluctuations)
- Selective stimulation of dopamine receptor subtypes and longer duration of action
- Levodopa-sparing effect

Disadvantages
- Limited antiparkinson efficacy, always require levodopa adjunctive therapy
- Specific side effects (nausea, vomiting, postural hypotension, drowsiness, constipation, psychiatric reactions—hallucinations, confusion)
- Do not completely prevent development of levodopa-related adverse events. Once patients have developed dyskinesias, dopamine agonists exacerbate them further
- Do not treat all features of Parkinson disease, such as freezing, postural instability, autonomic dysfunction, dementia
- Unable to prevent disease progression

Scale 0–4 (0 = *normal*, 4 = *most severe*)

dopamine to which it is converted. There are two major COMT inhibitors. Entacapone is generally used adjunctively to levodopa. Tolcapone can cause severe hepatotoxicity, requires regular laboratory monitoring, and thus is used less frequently.

Monoamine Oxidase B Inhibitors

Selegiline is a selective inhibitor of MAO-B. Its primary mechanism of action is blockade of central dopamine metabolism. It is available as a swallowed pill (Eldepryl) and as an orally disintegrating tablet (Zelapar ODT). It may improve response to levodopa, especially in patients with mild dose-related fluctuations.

Rasagiline is a newer MAO-B inhibitor also available as Azilect commonly used as initial monotherapy and as adjunct therapy to levodopa. As monotherapy, it may reduce parkinsonian disability. As adjunctive therapy, it may reduce off time and increase dyskinesia-free on time. Side effects include insomnia, hallucinations, and orthostatic hypotension.

Amantadine

Amantadine is an antiviral agent that was serendipitously found to have an antiparkinsonian effect. Its mechanism of action, thought to include blocking an *N*-methyl-D-aspartate receptor, is controversial. Amantadine has a mild beneficial effect on tremor, bradykinesia, and rigidity. It is the only antiparkinsonian medication that can decrease the severity of levodopa-induced dyskinesias. Common side effects include livedo reticularis and lower extremity edema.

Management of Nonmotor Symptoms

PD is not just an illness of dopamine depletion, but a complex illness with impacts throughout and beyond the central nervous system. Detecting and treating NMSs can reduce the burden of the disease and improve quality of life of PD patients.

Depression

Amitriptyline may be considered in nondemented patients (American Academy of Neurology [AAN], level C). Pramipexole is efficacious and likely also nortriptyline and desipramine. Insufficient evidence for selective serotonin reuptake inhibitors (SSRIs), nefazodone, atomoxetine, pergolide, Ω-3 fatty acids, or repetitive transcranial magnetic stimulation (TMS).

Cognitive Impairment/Dementia

Donepezil or rivastigmine should be considered (AAN, level B). Rivastigmine is efficacious; insufficient evidence exists for donepezil, galantamine, or memantine. Note that cholinesterase inhibitors have limited benefit and may worsen motor function in PD.

Hallucinations and Psychosis

Clozapine should be considered (AAN, level B). Quetiapine may be considered (AAN, level C), but olanzapine should not (AAN, level B). Clozapine requires frequent blood monitoring due to the risk of severe neutropenia and is not commonly used. Recommended doses of quetiapine do not worsen motor symptoms, but efficacy data are limited, and both short- and long-term side effects are common. Pimavanserin (Nuplazid) is a new option to treat psychosis in PD patients. Pimavanserin is a selective serotonin (5-HT2A) receptor inverse agonist and a first-in-class drug for PD psychosis. In clinical trials, it was well tolerated and did not cause sedation or worsen PD motor symptoms. Like other antipsychotics, it has a black box warning about increased mortality when used in elderly patients with dementia-related psychosis.

Sialorrhea

Botulinum toxin A and B (AAN—should be considered, level B). Glycopyrrolate (anticholinergic that does not cross the blood-brain barrier) is possibly useful.

Constipation

Polyethylene Glycol (Macrogol)—(AAN—may be considered).

Orthostatic Hypotension

Droxidopa (Northera)—Approved for the short-term management of symptomatic neurogenic orthostatic hypotension in PD.

Nonmotor Complications of Dopaminergic Therapy

For DA-related ICDs, there is insufficient evidence for the use of amantadine in pathologic gambling and no evidence-based treatments for other ICDs such as compulsive eating, compulsive buying/shopping, or hypersexuality. There are no evidence-based treatments for DA withdrawal syndrome, DDS, or punding.

FUTURE DIRECTIONS

The main goal in the early diagnosis is finding the biomarker. Our recent advances on PD genetics and pathophysiology have researchers looking at new targets to delay disease progression, such as immunotherapies for synucleinopathies, and the modulation of glucacon-like peptide and GBA/glycoceramide activity. There continues to be development of many new forms of levodopa, as well as newer medications for motor and NMSs (inhaled levodopa, extended-release amantadine, novel reversible MAO-B inhibitor, COMT inhibitor, apomorphine infusion), among others. In the surgical field, a potential alternative to DBS is MRI-guided high-intensity focused ultrasound (MRgFUS) thalamotomy or pallidotomy for PD, as well as TMS.

ADDITIONAL RESOURCES

Connolly BS, Lang AE. Pharmacological treatment of Parkinson disease: a review. JAMA 2014;311(16):1670–83.
This review provides an evidence-based review of the initial pharmacologic management of the classic motor symptoms of Parkinson disease; describes management of medication-related motor complications and other medication adverse effects. It also discusses the management of selected nonmotor symptoms of Parkinson disease.

Ferreira JJ, Katzenschlager R, Bloem BR, et al. Summary of the recommendations of the EFNS/MDS-ES review on therapeutic management of Parkinson's disease. Eur J Neurol 2013;20(1):5–15.

This review summarizes the 2010 EFNS/MDS-ES evidence-based treatment recommendations for the management of early and late PD.

Fox SH, Katzenschlager R, Lim SY, et al. The Movement Disorder Society evidence-based medicine review update: treatments for the motor symptoms of Parkinson's disease. Mov Disord 2011;26(S3):S2–SS41. And 2015 online update: http://www.movementdisorders.org/MDS/Resources/Publications-Reviews/EBM-Reviews1.htm.

Seppi K, Weintraub D, Coelho M, et al. The Movement Disorder Society evidence-based medicine review update: treatments for the non-motor symptoms of Parkinson's disease. Mov Disord 2011;26(Suppl. 3):S42–80. And 2012 online update. See http://display.mds.prod.titanclient.com/MDS-Files1/PDFs/EBM-Papers/EBM_NMS_Updated_15Jan2014.pdf.

The objective of this work was to update previous EBM reviews on treatments for PD with a focus on nonmotor symptoms.

Marras C, Lang A, van de Warrenburg BP, et al. Nomenclature of genetic movement disorders: recommendations of the International Parkinson and Movement Disorder Society task force. Mov Disord 2016;31:436–57.

This system provides a resource for clinicians and researchers that, unlike the previous system, can be considered an accurate and criterion-based list of confirmed genetically determined movement disorders at the time it was last updated.

McCann H, Cartwright H, Halliday GM. Neuropathology of alpha-synuclein propagation and Braak hypothesis. Mov Disord 2016;31:152–60.

This article reviews neuropathology of PD.

Fernandez HH. Part I: 2017 update on our current understanding of Parkinson's disease. AAN; 2017.

Postuma RB, Berg D, Stern M, et al. MDS clinical diagnostic criteria for Parkinson's disease. Mov Disord 2015;30:1591–9.

29

Atypical Parkinsonian Syndromes

Diana Apetauerova

Atypical parkinsonian syndromes, previously called *Parkinson-plus syndromes,* are chronic, progressive neurodegenerative disorders characterized by rapidly evolving parkinsonism in association with other signs of neurologic dysfunction beyond the spectrum of idiopathic Parkinson disease (PD). These include early dementia, postural instability, supranuclear gaze palsy, early autonomic failure, and pyramidal, cerebellar, or cortical signs. The most common disorders (Table 29.1) are progressive supranuclear palsy (PSP), corticobasal degeneration (CBD), multiple-system atrophy (MSA), and dementia with Lewy bodies. Unlike idiopathic PD, these uncommon syndromes have poor or transient responses to dopaminergic therapy and consequently a worse prognosis. These disorders are classified as *tauopathies* and *synucleinopathies* based on the accumulation of the abnormal proteins tau or alpha-synuclein within neurons and glial cells having various anatomic distributions within the brain.

Tau is found in a hyperphosphorylated form in both PSP and CBD. In normal human brains, tau functions as a microtubule-binding protein as well as a stabilizer of the neuronal cytoskeleton. In the diseased brain, tau is found in glial cells and neurons, where it produces a special cluster of fibrils called neurofibrillary tangles (NFTs). Generally there are six isoforms of tau made by alternative splicing from the tau gene. Tau also accumulates in the less common tauopathy, frontotemporal dementia with parkinsonism (FTPD). This is linked to chromosome 17 (FTPD-17).

Alpha-synuclein is a highly soluble synaptic protein found in the normal human brain. In MSA it typically accumulates as insoluble aggregates within white matter oligodendrocytes as glial cytoplasmic inclusions (GCIs) and in the form of Lewy bodies in DLB. There are no effective therapies for these syndromes.

PROGRESSIVE SUPRANUCLEAR PALSY

> **CLINICAL VIGNETTE** *A 65-year-old writer presented with poor balance starting 2 years earlier. He tripped easily and fell backward multiple times. He also described changes in his speech and in the swallowing of liquids, which was accompanied by coughing. His wife described change in his facial expression and stated that he looked as though he were staring and always had to turn his whole body in turning to the side.*
>
> *He had described blurred vision while typing on the computer. He was squinting and occasionally had difficulties opening his eyes.*
>
> *Neurologic examination demonstrated hypertonic facial muscles, which produced facial folds and a worried, astonished expression, dysarthric speech, a vertical more than horizontal supranuclear gaze palsy with preserved oculocephalic reflexes. Blepharospasm, prominent axial rigidity, and mild bradykinesia in all four extremities with minimal cogwheel rigidity and brisk muscle stretch reflexes were also identified. He stood up quickly, nearly falling backward if not assisted. He walked with erect posture and a stiff, wide-base gait. He had no postural reflexes and, during a pull test, fell backward easily.*

PSP is a sporadic tauopathy that has a progressive clinical course characterized by parkinsonism with supranuclear gaze palsy (Fig. 29.1), early postural instability, falls, bradykinesia, and dysarthria, all of which are illustrated in this vignette. PSP typically does not respond to dopaminergic therapy. Its prognosis is poor, with a median survival of 5 to 8 years. PSP's etiology, like that of CBD, is unknown. A genetic susceptibility combined with environmental risk factors is suspected. To date, only the H1 MAPT haplotype has been consistently associated with a risk of developing PSP. A recent genome-wide association study identified three additional putative genes associated with PSP: *STX6, EIF2AK3,* and *MOBP.*

Pathophysiology

PSP is primarily a subcortical neurodegenerative tauopathy, in contrast to both CBD and FTPD-17, having involvement of the cerebral cortex. Macroscopically, depigmentation is observable within the substantia nigra (SN) and locus coeruleus (LC), as is atrophy of the pons, midbrain, and globus pallidus. Microscopically the most affected regions are brainstem nuclei III, IV, IX, and X; the red nucleus; LC; SN; globus pallidus; and cerebellar dentate nucleus. Tau protein accumulates within neurons as NFT and in glia as spherical neuropil threads (Fig. 29.2).

Clinical Presentation

PSP typically occurs between the sixth and seventh decades of life. Onset before age 40 years is rare. Prevalence is estimated to be about 5 per 100,000. PSP is sporadic in most individuals, but rarely an autosomal dominant inheritance is suggested.

The most common form of PSP is known as the *Richardson variant.* Patients with this form present with gait instability and a tendency to fall backward unexpectedly; in contrast, neither of these symptoms occurs early on in PD. The parkinsonism of PSP is typically axial and symmetric, unlike the asymmetric often single-limb presentation of PD. Most patients with PSP carry an erect posture, in contrast to the flexed PD stance (see Fig. 29.1). Often they lack the typical PD tremor. Dystonia is a common finding, affecting the neck (in the form of retrocollis), limbs, and eyelids (blepharospasm). However, at least five phenotypic variants have recently been described: PSP-parkinsonism, PSP-pure akinesia with gait freezing, PSP-corticobasal syndrome (PSP-CBS) (or primary nonfluent aphasia), PSP-behavioral variant of frontotemporal dementia (FTD), and two other possible PSP variants with features that overlap with either primary lateral sclerosis (PLS) or cerebellar ataxia.

The hallmark of PSP is the classic and characteristic finding of limited vertical eye movements; eventually horizontal supranuclear gaze palsy may also become evident. In this clinical setting, the patient usually does not recognize the loss of eye movement per se but rather perceives these limitations as blurry vision, particularly manifested by difficulties with routine activities such as reading or walking down stairs. Dysarthria

TABLE 29.1 Atypical Parkinsonian Syndromes

Syndrome	Abnormal	Clinical Features	Age at Onset (Years)	Genetic	Pathology	Therapy
PSP	Tau	Gait disorder, falls Abnormal eye movements Akinetic-rigid asymmetric parkinsonism Cortical signs Dystonia Action/postural tremor Myoclonus	55–70	Sporadic? Familial	Atrophy of BG and brainstem regions Normal cerebral cortex Globose, NFT	Poor response to dopaminergic medication Botulinum toxin for blepharospasm Supportive therapy
CBD	Tau	Alien limb phenomenon Symmetric axially predominant parkinsonism Dysarthria and dysphagia Frontal lobe abnormalities Cognitive impairment	60	Sporadic	Atrophy in FP cortex Tau-positive neurons in cortex Swollen and achromatic neurons (ballooned neurons)	Poor response to dopaminergic medication Botulinum toxin for blepharospasm Supportive therapy
FTDP-17	Tau	Highly variable: behavioral disturbance Cognitive impairment Motor disturbance (later in the disease) Positive family history	50	Autosomal dominant	Atrophy in FT cortex, BG, SN, LC Neuronal loss Argentophilic neuronal inclusions	Poor response to dopaminergic therapy
MSA	Alpha-synuclein	Parkinsonism Cerebellar signs Autonomic features Pyramidal features	60	Sporadic	Glial and neuronal cytoplasmic inclusions Absence of Lewy bodies	Poor or marginal response to dopaminergic therapy Fludrocortisone or midodrine for orthostatic hypotension

BG, Basal ganglia; *CBD*, corticobasal degeneration; *FP*, frontoparietal; *FT*, frontotemporal; *FTDP-17*, frontotemporal dementia with parkinsonism linked to chromosome 17; *LC*, locus ceruleus; *MSA*, multiple system atrophy; *NFT*, neurofibrillary tangle; *PSP*, progressive supranuclear palsy; *SN*, substantia nigra.

and dysphagia are also commonly experienced early in the disease course. Cognitive dysfunction is a later development for most PSP patients.

Diagnosis

PSP and other atypical parkinsonian syndromes—including CBD, MSA, and dementia with Lewy bodies—are often misdiagnosed as PD in the early stages. The most important diagnostic clues are (1) the results of a careful clinical evaluation and (2) a poor response to dopaminergic therapy. There are proposed diagnostic criteria for each disorder, which are used in neurology and movement disorders practice. To date there is no available biomarker for PSP, and brain magnetic resonance imaging (MRI) remains most helpful, showing atrophy of the midbrain and superior cerebellar peduncles. As a result, the brainstem is often beaked and takes on the appearance of a hummingbird or penguin body (Fig. 29.3). Metabolic positron emission tomography (PET) has demonstrated global reduction in cerebral metabolism; ^{18}F-fluorodopa PET uptake studies have revealed reduced caudate and putamen uptake. Single photon emission computed tomography (SPECT) revealed bifrontal hypometabolism. Other newer methods including diffusion-tensor imaging (DTI) and recent tau PET ligands show promise for detecting tau in PSP.

Treatment

There are no effective specific therapies available for the PSP patient. Although some of these individuals with slowness, stiffness, and balance problems initially may respond to antiparkinsonian therapies such as levodopa or levodopa combined with anticholinergic agents, this

effect is usually limited and at best a temporary one. Visual limitations, dysarthria, and dysphagia are usually unresponsive to pharmacologic intervention.

Antidepressant drugs have had modest success in PSP; fluoxetine, amitriptyline, and imipramine are the most commonly used, although their benefit seems to be unrelated to their ability to relieve depression. Botulinum toxin injections are used when blepharospasm is an issue. Physical and occupational therapy are the most important aspects of patient management.

Multiple research studies with potential disease-modifying therapies for PSP have not been successful. PSP has an inexorably progressive course. The average PSP patient has a survival from symptom onset to death of 5–6 years. Head injury and fractures from falls are common. Because of dysphagia, PSP patients are predisposed to other serious complications such as choking and pneumonia, the most common cause of death.

CORTICOBASAL DEGENERATION

CLINICAL VIGNETTE *Two years earlier, a 68-year-old retired orthopedic surgeon began having difficulties with fine motor coordination of the right hand. His hand felt stiff and uncoordinated and was occasionally doing things on its own. His family described it as, "His hand elevates and wanders around without a purpose." When an object was placed in his right hand, he had*

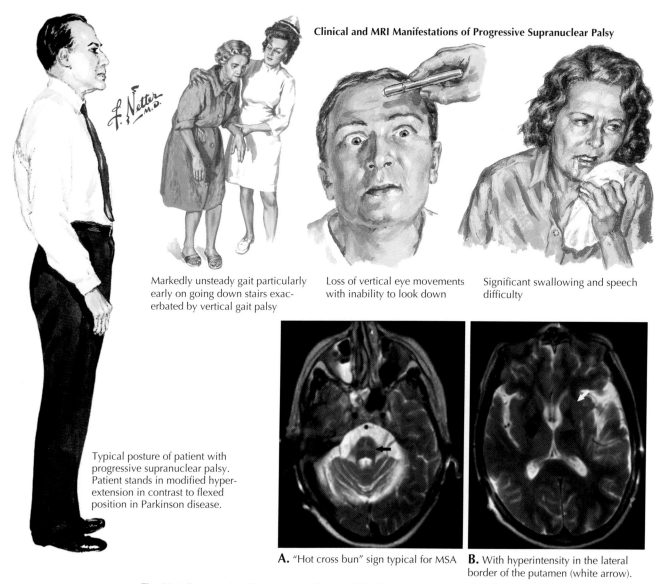

Clinical and MRI Manifestations of Progressive Supranuclear Palsy

Markedly unsteady gait particularly early on going down stairs exacerbated by vertical gait palsy

Loss of vertical eye movements with inability to look down

Significant swallowing and speech difficulty

Typical posture of patient with progressive supranuclear palsy. Patient stands in modified hyperextension in contrast to flexed position in Parkinson disease.

A. "Hot cross bun" sign typical for MSA

B. With hyperintensity in the lateral border of the putamen (white arrow).

Fig. 29.1 **Progressive Supranuclear Palsy.** *MRI*, Magnetic resonance imaging.

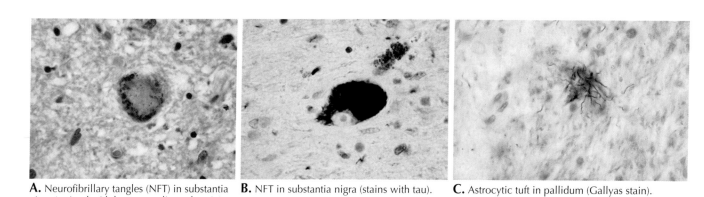

A. Neurofibrillary tangles (NFT) in substantia nigra (stained with haematoxylin and eosin).

B. NFT in substantia nigra (stains with tau).

C. Astrocytic tuft in pallidum (Gallyas stain).

Fig. 29.2 Pathology of Progressive Supranuclear Palsy.

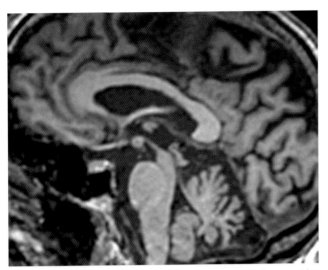

Sagittal T1-weighted MR image shows atrophy of the midbrain, with preservation of the volume of the pons. This appearance has been called the "penguin sign." There is also atrophy of the tectum, particularly the superior colluculi. These findings suggest the diagnosis of progressive supranuclear palsy.

Fig. 29.3 Magnetic Resonance (MR) Imaging in Progressive Supranuclear Palsy.

difficulty releasing it. Later, his right hand tended to close involuntarily and appeared swollen. Eventually he was unable to perform any fine motor tasks with this hand. Treatment with high doses of carbidopa/levodopa (Sinemet) 25/100, total of 15 tablets a day, was ineffective. One year later, he also noted poor balance and started to fall down. His gait was slow and shuffling, and his right arm was held close to his body in a flexed position. A jerky intention-type tremor developed in the right hand; it was particularly noticeable when he attempted to reach for an object. Concomitantly, his family began to observe that he was experiencing word-finding difficulties, memory problems, slurred speech, and swallowing difficulties.

His neurologic examination demonstrated very dysarthric bulbar speech, word-finding difficulties with anomia for uncommonly utilized objects, and an apraxia wherein he could not appropriately use a body part as illustrated or demonstrate how to perform certain common functions such as combing his hair. On cranial nerve examination, he had mild difficulty generating vertical more than horizontal saccadic eye movements. He had a reduced blink frequency. Right arm levitation, dystonic posture of the right arm with irregular jerky tremor, striking rigidity and bradykinesia on the right side, brisker right muscle stretch reflexes, and a right Babinski sign were also seen. He also had positive snout and grasp reflexes. His gait was very stiff and so limited that he was unable to walk without the assistance of two people.

CBD is a rare sporadic neurodegenerative tauopathy. It occurs mainly after age 60 years and shows no population clusters; its incidence, prevalence, and etiology are unknown. The typical presentation is that of an asymmetric progressive akinetic rigid syndrome, dystonia, and alien-hand phenomenon as well as signs of cerebral cortical dysfunction. All of these various CBD manifestations are poorly responsive to levodopa therapy.

Pathophysiology

In contrast to PSP, CBD primarily affects the cerebral cortex. The patient's clinical presentation correlates well with the later finding of an asymmetric cortical atrophy contralateral to the involved limb (Fig. 29.4). The frontoparietal cortex is the most involved, with most prominent changes of cortical atrophy demonstrated within the perirolandic area. A reduction in the amount of cerebral white matter is also apparent in the cerebral peduncles and corpus callosum. Additionally, neuronal loss is present within the SN and LC.

Typical microscopic features include neuronal loss (cortex, subcortical regions, SN), astrocytic gliosis, ballooned (achromatic) neurons, NFT, and tau-positive glial inclusions. The microscopic hallmarks of CBD are the ballooned, swollen, or achromatic neurons lacking Nissl substance.

Clinical Presentation

An asymmetric akinetic-rigid parkinsonism, primarily affecting the arm and hand, is often the major feature. Patients usually present with limb clumsiness; awkward, slow voluntary movements of one arm; with dystonic posturing and tremor. Cortical signs include apraxia, cortical sensory disturbance, and finger myoclonus. The alien-limb phenomenon, a failure to recognize ownership of a limb without visual cues, is also a common clinically appreciable sign (see Fig. 29.4). Gradually a gait disorder develops, characterized by limb rigidity and impaired position sense. Dementia usually develops late in the course of CBD; however, relatively early on, declining cognitive function is sometimes a predominant feature. Less commonly, there is an overlap with some similar atypical parkinsonian syndromes. This is particularly related to the typical vertical eye movement abnormalities of the type characteristically associated with PSP. Slowed speech production, dysarthria, swallowing difficulties, and cognitive deficits occur later in this disease. Less common CBD presentations include dementia and altered behavior.

Diagnosis

CBD is relatively easy to diagnose because of its stereotypic clinical presentation, particularly the alien-limb phenomenon. Some conditions clinically mimic CBD, including PSP, Pick disease, Alzheimer disease, some vascular lesions, and rarely adult-onset leukodystrophies. Neuropathologic evaluation is necessary to confirm the diagnosis.

Imaging studies are not diagnostic. MRI and CT can show asymmetric cortical atrophy in the frontoparietal region, maximal on the side contralateral to the involved limb. The asymmetrically reduced pattern in frontoparietal cerebral cortical metabolism, CBF, or both, coupled with bilateral reduction of fluorodopa uptake in the caudate and putamen on PET scanning, provide strong evidence for CBD.

Treatment

There is no definitive treatment; dopaminergic therapy is of limited benefit, clonazepam can be used for finger myoclonus, and botulinum toxin improves dystonia. Occupational, physical, and speech therapy may also help. There is a significant average survival of usually 5–6 years from symptom onset to death.

FRONTOTEMPORAL DEMENTIA PARKINSONISM–CHROMOSOME 17

Frontotemporal dementia parkinsonism–chromosome 17 (FTDP-17) type dementia is an autosomal dominant tauopathy caused by a tau gene mutation located on chromosome 17q21. Many different mutations located in the microtubule-binding region of the tau gene are now identified. FTDP-17 has both a significant clinical phenotypic expression as well as neuropathologic variability. Behavioral changes and parkinsonism are the most common features.

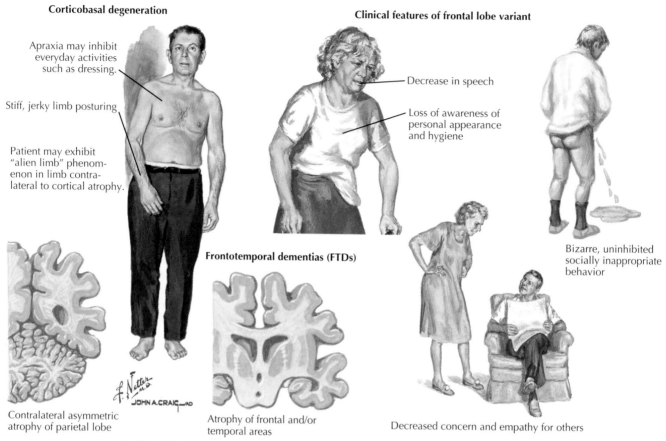

Corticobasal degeneration

Apraxia may inhibit everyday activities such as dressing.

Stiff, jerky limb posturing

Patient may exhibit "alien limb" phenomenon in limb contralateral to cortical atrophy.

Clinical features of frontal lobe variant

Decrease in speech

Loss of awareness of personal appearance and hygiene

Bizarre, uninhibited socially inappropriate behavior

Frontotemporal dementias (FTDs)

Contralateral asymmetric atrophy of parietal lobe

Atrophy of frontal and/or temporal areas

Decreased concern and empathy for others

Fig. 29.4 Other Tauopathies, Corticobasal Degeneration, and Frontotemporal Dementia.

Pathophysiology and Clinical Presentation

Pathologically the neocortex is degenerated, with marked frontal and temporal lobe atrophy. The subcortical basal ganglia and brainstem nuclei are also concomitantly affected.

FTDP-17 is a highly variable neurodegenerative disease. The first symptoms typically occur in the fifth decade of life but this can range from the third to the sixth decades. The clinical onset is an insidious one. Often there is significant history of similar problems among multiple family members. Behavioral disturbances are often the initial and typical features; they include disinhibition, inappropriate behavior, and poor impulse control (see Fig. 29.4). Other individuals present with apathetic, socially withdrawn behavior and often neglect personal hygiene. In some individuals a prominent psychosis—similar to schizophrenia with auditory hallucination, delusion, and paranoia—may be apparent.

Cognitive impairment affecting executive function, judgment, planning, and reasoning may be the initial sign of FTDP-17. Surprisingly, patients with this variant do have preservation of memory, orientation, and visuospatial functions. The typical patient develops disinhibited behavior in the fifth decade without impairment of memory or orientation. However, there is progressive worsening over several years, eventually associated with severe dementia, bradykinesia, rigidity, and evidence of frontal or temporal atrophy or both.

Motor disturbance usually does not occur early on in this disorder. Later, patients have parkinsonism-type findings, including bradykinesia, axial and limb rigidity, and postural instability. Resting tremor is uncommon.

Diagnosis and Treatment

Other conditions that present with parkinsonism and dementia include Pick disease, CBD, PSP, and Alzheimer disease. The prominent family history of FTDP-17 is usually lacking in these other disorders. Careful attention to the family history and the clinical presentation per se provide the diagnostic keys. DNA genetic testing demonstrates the chromosome 17 gene mutation. PET scanning, used infrequently, shows a reduction of caudate and putamen fluorodopa uptake.

There is no therapy for FTDP-17. As with other tauopathies, the response to dopaminergic therapy is poor. The disease duration averages 10 to 12 years.

MULTIPLE SYSTEM ATROPHY

CLINICAL VIGNETTE *The patient, a 60-year-old man, first noted poor balance and right-hand clumsiness during his job as a painter 2 years earlier. He observed poor fine motor control of the right hand as well as several unexpected falls while climbing a ladder. His wife noted his poor balance with a tendency to walk "as a drunk person." He also described a feeling of lightheadedness when he stood up quickly, urinary urgency, and sexual dysfunction. He had to retire from his job. An initial trial of low doses of levodopa produced no benefit. When the dose of levodopa was increased to Sinemet 25/100, nine tablets a day, he noted some benefit in fine motor control, but within several months prominent orofacial and lower extremity dyskinesia developed. Despite a continued response of his right upper extremity akinesia to levodopa, his gait and balance deteriorated and he started to have slowness* *on the opposite left side of his body. Because his balance deteriorated rather quickly, leading to multiple falls, he became wheelchair-bound within the next year. He also experienced several fainting spells later in the course of the disease.*

His examination was notable for hypophonic speech, stridor, square wave jerks seen during an eye movement exam, orofacial dyskinesia, and antecollis. He had asymmetric akinetic rigid syndrome with more involvement of the right-sided extremities with brisker muscle stretch reflexes and the presence of a right Babinski sign. Bilateral right greater than left finger-to-nose-to-finger and heel-to-shin ataxia was identified, right more prominent than left. He was unable to ambulate independently and required two people to support him. His gait was characterized by a wide base with significant slowness, bilateral loss of arm swing, and poor postural stability. MRI demonstrated lateral putamen and pontine cruciate patterns of T2 hyperintensity (Fig. 29.5). He had abnormal autonomic testing.

MSA is a sporadic, degenerative CNS disease classified as a *synucleinopathy*. It presents with a combination of extrapyramidal, pyramidal, cerebellar, and autonomic symptoms and signs. Its clinical manifestations may change as it evolves.

MSA comprises three clinical conditions previously classified as (1) striatonigral degeneration (SND) with predominant parkinsonism and a *poor response to levodopa*; (2) Shy-Drager syndrome (SDS), parkinsonism or cerebellar syndrome, or both with predominant *autonomic* dysfunction; and (3) sporadic *olivopontocerebellar atrophy* (OPCA) with predominant cerebellar dysfunction. MSA is a specific condition with a specific pathology regardless of previous SND, SDS, or OPCA labels. It is characterized by oligodendro GCIs that stain for alpha-synuclein. The etiology of MSA is unknown.

Pathophysiology

Macroscopically, *neuronal loss and gliosis* are primarily seen in many subcortical areas such as the SN, LC, putamen, globus pallidus, inferior olive nucleus, pons, cerebellar cortex, autonomic nuclei of the brainstem, and intermediolateral columns of the spinal cord. *GCIs are major microscopic findings that are characteristic of but not specific for MSA*. These GCIs represent the accumulation of the protein alpha-synuclein within previously normal oligodendrocytes. These inclusions are distributed selectively within the basal ganglia, motor cortex, reticular formation, middle cerebellar peduncle, and the cerebellar white matter.

Clinical Presentation

MSA affects a slightly younger age group than PD, with peak onset in the sixth decade. The clinical syndromes are characterized by parkinsonism, cerebellar dysfunction, and autonomic failure. The motor presentations of MSA are classified into two separate but overlapping clinical subtypes—MSA with predominant parkinsonism (MSA-P) and MSA with predominant cerebellar ataxia (MSA-C). Any one of these subcategories may be clinically predominant but would still fall within the clinical spectrum of MSA.

The parkinsonism of MSA-P tends to be more symmetric, rest tremor is less common, and postural instability develops earlier than in classic PD. Early stages, however, can be identical to the presentation of idiopathic PD. Similarly, an initial positive response to levodopa as well as negative fluctuations and dyskinesias may occur. Clinical "red flags" that should alert the clinician to a diagnosis of possible MSA include orthostatic hypotension, urinary retention or incontinence, ataxia, unexpected falls, stimulus-sensitive myoclonus, antecollis, slurred speech, stridor, and corticospinal tract signs. In contrast to MSA-P, the motor features of MSA-C involve predominant cerebellar dysfunction that manifests as gait ataxia, limb ataxia, ataxic dysarthria, and cerebellar disturbances of eye movements. Ocular abnormalities may include gaze-evoked nystagmus, impaired smooth pursuits with saccadic intrusion, and/or ocular dysmetria.

MSA is a chronically progressive disorder characterized by the gradual onset of symptoms. Patients who present initially with extrapyramidal features commonly progress to develop autonomic disturbances, cerebellar disorders, or both. Conversely, patients whose first symptoms are cerebellar dysfunction often later develop extrapyramidal or autonomic disorders or both.

Diagnosis

Distinguishing MSA from idiopathic PD and PSP is often challenging early in the illness. Some features—such as autonomic dysfunction, poor or marginal response to levodopa with early clinical fluctuations, and dyskinesia—can help to differentiate MSA from early PD. Autonomic failure is common in MSA and rare in early PD, whereas dementia and psychiatric features are more common in PD.

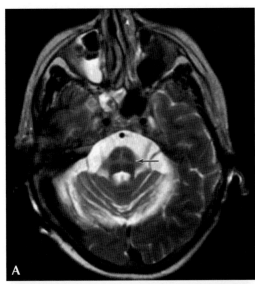

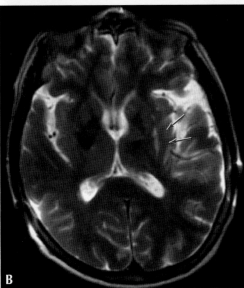

Typical brain MRI in MSA patient showing "hot cross bun" sign in the pons (arrow in A) and putaminal hyperintensity (arrows in B) .

Fig. 29.5 Diagnosis of Multiple-System Atrophy. *MRI,* Magnetic resonance imaging; *MSA,* multiple-system atrophy.

Neuroimaging can be helpful in excluding other conditions. MRI abnormalities include hypointensity on T1 or hyperintensities on T2 in the lateral border of the putamen or putaminal atrophy. Cerebellar and pontine atrophy with the "hot cross bun" sign (see Fig. 29.5) in the pons is seen; however, MRI is not specific and is often normal. Cerebellar atrophy can be demonstrated even with brain CT scans. Presynaptic dopaminergic denervation in the striatum on functional imaging with SPECT or PET can also be helpful.

Other tests used in the diagnosis of MSA include autonomic testing, external anal or urethral sphincter electromyography (EMG), and dopamine transporter scan.

Treatment

Only symptomatic therapy is available. Parkinsonism is treated with levodopa, despite its inconsistent efficacy. Orthostatic hypotension may respond to conservative measures such as raising the head of the bed, binding stockings, and liberal salt intake. Medications such as fludrocortisone or midodrine and the newer droxidopa are commonly required. Urinary dysfunction can be treated with antispasmodics such as oxybutynin and self-catheterization. Typical disease duration is 3–10 years. Breathing problems such as aspiration and cardiopulmonary arrest are common causes of death.

ADDITIONAL RESOURCES

Boxer AL, Yu JT, Golbe LI, et al. Advances in progressive supranuclear palsy: new diagnostic criteria, biomarkers, and therapeutic approaches. Lancet Neurol 2017;16:552.

Buee L, Delacourte A. Comparative biochemistry of tau in progressive supranuclear palsy, corticobasal degeneration, FTDP-17 and Pick's disease. Brain Pathol 1999;9:681–93.

Dickson DW, Rademakers R, Hutton ML. Progressive supranuclear palsy: pathology and genetics. Brain Pathol 2007;17(1):74–82.

Frank S, Clavaquera F, Tolnay M. Tauopathy models and human neuropathology: similarities and differences. Acta Neuropathol 2008;115(1):39053.

Gibb RG, Luthert PJ, Marsden CD. Corticobasal degeneration. Brain 1989;112:1171–92.

Gilman S. Multiple system atrophy. In: Jankovic J, Tolosa E, editors. Parkinson's disease and movement disorders. Lippincott Williams & Wilkins; 1998. pp. 245–95.

Gilman S, et al. Second consensus statement on the diagnosis of multiple system atrophy. Neurology 2008;71(9):670–6.

Houghton DJ, Litvan I. Unraveling progressive supranuclear palsy: from the bedside back to the bench. Parkinsonism Relat Disord 2007; 13(Suppl. 3):S34106.

Lamb R, Rohrer JD, Lees AJ, et al. Progressive supranuclear palsy and corticobasal degeneration: pathophysiology and treatment options. Curr Treat Options Neurol 2016;18:42.

Litvan I, Cummings JL, Mega M. Neuropsychiatric features of corticobasal degeneration. J Neurol Neurosurg Psychiatry 1998;65:717–21.

McFarland NR. Diagnostic approach to atypical parkinsonian syndromes. Continuum (Minneap Minn) 2016;22:1117.

Melquist S, Craig DW, Huentelman MJ, et al. Identification of a novel risk locus for progressive supranuclear palsy by a pooled genome wide scan of 500,288 single-nucleotide polymorphisms. Am J Hum Genet 2007;80(4):769–78.

Rebeiz JJ, Edwin MD, Kolodny H, et al. Corticodentatonigral degeneration with neuronal achromasia. Arch Neurol 1986;18:20–34.

Respondek G, Stamelou M, Kurz C, et al. The phenotypic spectrum of progressive supranuclear palsy: a retrospective multicenter study of 100 definite cases. Mov Disord 2014;29:1758.

Sailer A, Scholz SW, Nalls MA, et al. A genome-wide association study in multiple system atrophy. Neurology 2016;87:1591.

Savoiardo M, Grisoli M, Girotti F. Magnetic resonance imaging in CBD, related atypical parkinsonian disorders, and dementias. In: Litvan I, Goetz CH, Lang A, editors. Advances in neurology, 82. Corticobasal degeneration and related disorders. Lippincott Williams & Wilkins; 2000. pp. 197–208.

Seppi K, Schocke MF, Wenning GK, et al. How to diagnose MSA early: the role of magnetic resonance imaging. J Neural Transm 2005;112(12):1625–34.

Stefanova N, Bücke P, Duerr S, et al. Multiple system atrophy: an update. Lancet Neurol 2009;8:1172.

Wadia PM, Lang AE. The many faces of corticobasal degeneration. Parkinsonism Relat Disord 2007;13(Suppl. 3):S336–40. Review.

Wenning GK, Stefanova N, Jellinger KA, et al. Multiple system atrophy: a primary oligodendrogliopathy. Ann Neurol 2008;64(3):239–43. Review.

30

Tremors

Julie Leegwater-Kim

CLINICAL VIGNETTE *A 31-year-old woman had the spontaneous onset of a relatively mild horizontal ("no-no") head tremor. She had no family history of neurologic disorders. This tremor was initially inconsequential but it gradually increased in severity. Turning her head to the right seemed to increase the tremor, whereas turning her head to the left decreased the tremor. Mild finger pressure on her left chin dampened the tremor and the involuntary movements of her head. Beta blockers, primidone, and alcohol had little effect. Eighteen months later, driving had become difficult because her head tended to turn to the left involuntarily. Attempts to hold her head in the neutral position as well as stress markedly increased the tremor, leading to neck discomfort. Over time, the involuntary movements were continuously present. Neurologic examination demonstrated right sternocleidomastoid muscle hypertrophy. A trial of anticholinergic medication increased the tremor and precipitated a psychotic reaction. Eventually, the patient was treated with botulinum toxin in the right sternocleidomastoid muscle and some of the left paracervical muscles. This treatment controlled the involuntary movements and dampened the involuntary tremor.*

Tremor is defined as a rhythmic, oscillatory movement of a body part that is produced by alternating contractions of reciprocally innervated antagonist muscles. Tremor is the most common involuntary movement encountered in the neurology clinic and is usually distinguishable from other movement disorders because of its rhythmic quality.

The pathophysiology of tremor is not completely understood but is thought to result from complex interactions between central nervous system oscillators and peripheral mechanical–reflex mechanisms. Central oscillators are groups of neurons which can fire rhythmically and are present in the thalamus, basal ganglia, and inferior olive. Different tremor types have different pathophysiologies. The tremor of Parkinson disease (PD) may have its origin in the basal ganglia while essential tremor (ET) is associated with dysfunction in the cerebellothalamocortical network and possibly the inferior olive-cerebellar network.

Tremor can be classified using multiple criteria: phenomenology, frequency, anatomical distribution, and etiology. Tremors are phenomenologically divided into two broad categories based on the context in which they occur: rest tremor and action tremor (Table 30.1). Rest tremor is present when the involved body part is in repose and supported against gravity (i.e., arm tremor when arms are resting in the lap). Action tremor occurs during voluntary contraction of muscles and encompasses four subcategories: postural, kinetic, task-specific, and isometric. Postural tremor is produced with maintenance of an antigravity posture (i.e., when arms are held in sustention in an outstretched position). Kinetic tremor is triggered by voluntary movement of the affected body part. It can be observed during the course of

movement and when approaching a target (in which it is referred to as an intention tremor). Task-specific tremor, as its name implies, occurs with performance of a specific action (i.e., writing) but not with other actions. Isometric tremor appears during voluntary contraction of muscles not accompanied by a change in position of the involved body part, such as, prolonged fist clenching or standing (orthostatic tremor).

Tremor frequency can vary considerably, depending on etiology (Table 30.2). Most tremors encountered in the clinic are in the 4–12 Hz range. Slow tremors of 1–3 Hz are usually seen in cerebellar or brainstem disorders (i.e., Holmes tremor) and are sometimes referred to as myorhythmia. Parkinsonian tremor is typically 4–6 Hz and the tremor of ET has a wide range of 4–12 Hz, though it is usually faster than the tremor of Parkinson disease. Examples of fast tremors (11–20 Hz) are enhanced physiologic tremor (EPT) and orthostatic tremor. Tremors can be classified according to anatomic distribution (e.g., head, tongue, limb, voice). The tremor of early Parkinson disease is usually a unilateral arm tremor. Patients with ET can have involvement of the arms, head, or voice. Palatal tremor, as the name implies, involves the soft palate though other cranial muscles may be involved.

Tremor has myriad causes including metabolic, neurodegenerative, genetic, and iatrogenic disorders. The following is a review of the more common tremor syndromes (Table 30.3).

ENHANCED PHYSIOLOGIC TREMOR

It is important to recognize that not all tremor is pathologic. A physiologic tremor is a normal phenomenon that occurs in all subjects. It is a fast (8–12 Hz), low-amplitude, postural, and kinetic tremor that is frequently not appreciated with the naked eye. Physiologic tremor may be detected when the arms are held in sustention and a piece of paper is placed over them. When physiologic tremor is intensified to the degree that it is easily visible, it is referred to as EPT. Physiologic tremor can be exacerbated by stress, fatigue, stimulants such as caffeine, exposure to certain drugs (i.e., lithium, valproic acid), metabolic disturbances (hyperthyroidism), and alcohol withdrawal. EPT is usually reversible provided a cause is discovered and corrected. In cases in which EPT is functionally impairing or socially embarrassing, low-dose propranolol can be used as needed.

PARKINSONIAN TREMOR

The tremor of PD is classically a 4–6 Hz rest tremor. It usually presents unilaterally in a limb, most commonly the arm, but over time can spread to the contralateral side. Though rest tremor is considered a cardinal sign of PD it can be absent in up to 30% of patients with this disorder. The arm tremor is often characterized by flexion-extension of the elbow, pronation-supination of the forearm, and movements of

TABLE 30.1   Classification of Tremors

Type of Tremor	Clinical Characteristics	Examples of Underlying Disorder
Rest	Occurs when body part is in repose, supported against gravity	Parkinson disease Holmes tremor
Action	Occurs with voluntary contraction of muscles	
1. Postural	Produced by maintenance of antigravity posture	Enhanced physiologic tremor Essential tremor
2. Kinetic a. Intention	Triggered by movements Increases with approach of target	Essential tremor Cerebellar tremor Holmes tremor
3. Task-specific	Occurs with performance of specific action	Primary writing tremor Embouchure tremor/dystonia
4. Isometric	Appears during voluntary contraction of muscles without accompanying change in body part position	Orthostatic tremor

TABLE 30.2   Approximate Frequencies of Tremor Types

Tremor Types	Frequency Range (Hz)
Palatal	1.5–3
Cerebellar	<4
Holmes	<4.5
Tardive	2.5–6
Parkinsonian	4–6
Essential	4–12
Enhanced physiologic	8–12
Orthostatic	13–18

TABLE 30.3   Treatment of Tremor

Tremor Types	Treatment
Parkinsonian	• Dopaminergic drugs: levodopa, dopamine agonists, MAO-B inhibitors, amantadine • Anticholinergics • Deep brain stimulation surgery
Essential	• Propranolol, primidone • Topiramate, benzodiazepines, gabapentin • Botulinum toxin • Deep brain stimulation surgery • Focused ultrasound thalamotomy
Dystonic	• Botulinum toxin • Anticholinergics • Clonazepam • Deep brain stimulation surgery
Orthostatic	• Clonazepam • Gabapentin, primidone, levodopa, pramipexole.
Cerebellar	• Clonazepam • Deep brain stimulation
Holmes	• Levodopa • Deep brain stimulation • Stereotactic thalamotomy
Palatal	• Clonazepam, valproic acid • Botulinum toxin
Tardive	• Tetrabenazine
Neuropathic	• Propranolol, primidone, pregabalin • Deep brain stimulation
Psychogenic	• Psychotherapy • Physical Therapy • Antidepressants, anxiolytics

the thumb across the fingers producing the "pill-rolling" phenomenon (Fig. 30.1). The tremor disappears with action but can reemerge when the arm is held in sustention ("re-emergent postural tremor"). Anticholinergic drugs and dopaminergic medications are the treatments of choice in the management of PD tremor though they are frequently not as effective in treating tremor as other manifestations of parkinsonism such as bradykinesia and rigidity. For severe, drug-resistant parkinsonian tremor, deep brain stimulation (DBS) can be considered. Rest tremor can also occur in atypical parkinsonism (i.e., progressive supranuclear palsy, multiple-system atrophy) and secondary parkinsonism (i.e., vascular parkinsonism, drug-induced parkinsonism). Treatment of tremor in atypical parkinsonism is similar to that in PD. In drug-induced parkinsonism, withdrawal of the offending agent and/or addition of anticholinergic medication is recommended.

ESSENTIAL TREMOR

ET is the most common pathologic tremor type. ET is typically a 4–12 Hz, upper limb, action (postural and/or kinetic) tremor though it can also involve the head, voice, and, less commonly, the face, jaw, and legs (see Fig. 30.1). The tremor is largely symmetric, though in one study, 50% of 487 ET patients had asymmetric disease with more prominent tremor on the dominant side. Age at onset shows a bimodal distribution with two peaks—adolescence and late adulthood (50–70 years of age). Approximately 50% of ET cases are familial with autosomal dominant inheritance and nearly complete penetrance by age 65. In 50%–70% of ET patients, symptoms improve with alcohol ingestion. The severity of tremor gradually progresses over time though there is no correlation

between age at onset and severity or disability. Although tremor is usually the sole neurologic sign in ET, a subset of ET patients can exhibit impaired tandem gait or postural instability. Recent data suggest nonmotor symptoms such as cognitive impairment may be associated with ET, though this remains controversial.

A number of treatments are available for ET and the decision to begin therapy is dependent on the patient's subjective assessment of functional impairment and severity of tremor. Nonpharmacologic

Rest tremor

Usually called parkinsonian tremor, occurs in a limb that is not voluntarily activated. It is suppressed with voluntary movement. It may appear as "pill rolling."

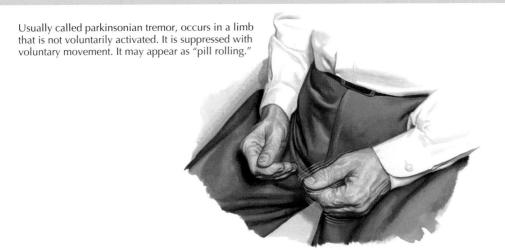

Action tremor (example: essential tremor)

Typically bilateral, this movement disorder is the most common. It may be accentuated with goal-directed movement of the limbs. Essential tremor commonly affects the hands, head, and voice. Although considered benign, it can become incapacitating.

In the severe forms the patient may not be able to perform essential daily activities, such as drinking from a cup or dressing

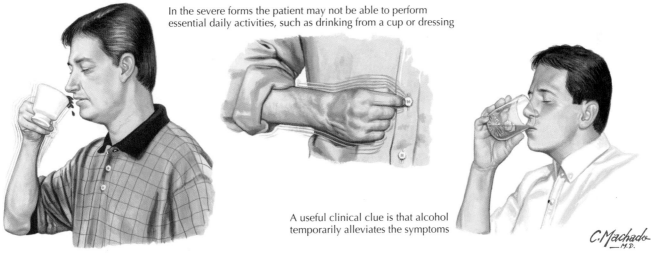

A useful clinical clue is that alcohol temporarily alleviates the symptoms

C. Machado — M.D.

Fig. 30.1 Tremor.

treatments such as wrist weights or the use of weighted utensils can be explored in mild cases. If tremor causes significant disability or social embarrassment, medications can be prescribed. First-line agents include propranolol and primidone. Propranolol can be initiated at 10 mg once or twice per day and titrated to effect. Therapeutic doses range from 40 mg/day to 320 mg/day. Primidone is generally started at 25 mg/day and titrated slowly to avoid side effects such as sedation and dizziness. Effective doses range from 50 mg/day to 750 mg/day. If there is inadequate response to either propranolol or primidone, then combination therapy can be tried. If primidone or propranolol is not effective or contraindicated, topiramate is often recommended as the next option. Typical starting dose is 25 mg/day with titration upward to effect. Topiramate is contraindicated in patients who have a history of nephrolithiasis. Other agents that have been shown probably to be effective in ET include alprazolam, gabapentin, and sotalol. In ET patients, especially those with head tremor, who do not respond to oral therapies, botulinum toxin injections can be considered.

For severe, medication-refractory ET, surgical treatment with DBS of the ventral intermediate nucleus (VIM) of the thalamus can be very effective. Recently, focused ultrasound thalamotomy was approved as a therapy for ET.

CLINICAL VIGNETTE *A 13-year-old boy was evaluated for a long-standing hand tremor that was accentuated by stress and physical activity, particularly having an essential quality. He had a grandmother with a head tremor and a grandfather with PD. Neurologic examination demonstrated intermittent bilateral action tremor of his hands most pronounced by finger-to-nose testing. His muscle stretch reflexes were hypoactive and he evidenced bilateral pes cavus. He refused an EMG. A trial of propranolol was considered. He returned 2 years later while attending vocational high school where he was studying welding. His tremor had increased and now involved his lower extremities and his head. He now had minimal distal weakness and sensory loss.*

DNA testing was negative for Charcot-Marie-Tooth (CMT) polyneuropathy. Nerve conduction studies demonstrated multifocal demyelinating motor and sensory conduction slowing typical for an acquired chronic inflammatory demyelinating polyneuropathy (CIDP). Cerebrospinal fluid protein was 107 mg/dL.

Treatment with intravenous immunoglobulin led to clinical improvement. Serendipitously, his mom had an EMG that had some findings similar to his. Further DNA testing was carried out and demonstrated X-linked CMT polyneuropathy associated with 13-basepair deletion in the coding region of connexin-32.

Comment: Although this is a very uncommon clinical scenario, this patient's clinical presentation emphasizes the need to take a broad perspective when evaluating a patient with an ET as it can be mimicked by either acquired or hereditary demyelinating polyneuropathies.

NEUROPATHIC TREMOR

Tremor can be a manifestation of peripheral neuropathy. Tremor has been associated most frequently with acute and chronic demyelinating neuropathies, paraproteinemic neuropathies (i.e., IgM neuropathy), and hereditary sensory and motor neuropathy. Neuropathic tremor is usually an action tremor similar to the tremor of ET. In addition to the tremor, signs of peripheral neuropathy are present on exam. Propranolol, primidone, and pregabalin may be helpful. Some patients have reported improvement of their tremor following treatment of the neuropathy (intravenous immunoglobulin [IVIg], rituximab). DBS of VIM in the thalamus has been shown to be beneficial in hereditary neuropathy.

DYSTONIC TREMOR

Dystonic tremor is a postural/kinetic tremor that occurs in a body part affected by dystonia. Dystonic tremor tends to be more irregular and variable than ET. Sometimes tremor can be the presenting manifestation of dystonia with dystonic signs developing later. In cases of dystonia in which tremor predominates, it may be challenging to distinguish it from ET (i.e., differentiating mild cervical dystonia with prominent tremor from head tremor in ET). Unlike other tremor types, dystonic tremor can be suppressed by employment of sensory tricks (gestes antagonistes). Dystonic tremor tends to occur when the affected body part is placed in a position opposing the direction of dystonic pull (i.e., a patient with left torticollis turning his head to the right). Some cases of task-specific tremor (i.e., primary writing tremor and embouchure tremor) may be forms of dystonia. Botulinum toxin injections are the treatment of choice for dystonia and dystonic tremor. Anticholinergics and clonazepam may be beneficial.

CEREBELLAR TREMOR

The most common form of cerebellar tremor is intention tremor which is characterized by an increase in tremor amplitude during visually guided movement toward a target. Postural tremor, but not rest tremor, can be present. Tremor tends to be slow—less than 4 Hz. The tremor is produced by lesions in the dentate nucleus and its efferent pathway through the superior cerebellar peduncle. Common causes include multiple sclerosis and the spinocerebellar ataxias. Another cerebellar tremor syndrome is titubation—slow-frequency rhythmic oscillation of the head and/or trunk caused by hypotonia of axial muscles. Cerebellar tremors are notoriously difficulty to treat but may respond to low-dose benzodiazepines, particularly clonazepam. DBS surgery targeting portions of the thalamus has shown some promise.

HOLMES TREMOR (MIDBRAIN OR RUBRAL TREMOR)

Holmes tremor is a unique tremor that consists of both rest and intention tremor produced by CNS lesions in proximity to the red nucleus

which affect the cerebellothalamic and nigrostriatal pathways. Postural tremor can also be present. The tremor has a slow frequency of less than 4.5 Hz and is often irregular with a jerky appearance. The affected limb can also display dysmetria and dysdiadochokinesia. Stroke, trauma, and demyelinating lesions are the most common causes of this tremor type. There is often a latency period (2 weeks–2 years) between the initial insult and the development of tremor. Because of the involvement of the dopaminergic pathways, levodopa may be of some benefit. DBS surgery of VIM or stereotactic thalamotomy have been shown to be effective treatments.

PALATAL TREMOR (PALATAL MYOCLONUS)

Palatal tremor, also termed palatal myoclonus, is characterized by rhythmic 1.5–3 Hz movements of the soft palate. Palatal tremor can be associated with synchronous movements of the face, tongue, and larynx. Movements are typically bilateral and symmetric. There are two main subtypes of palatal tremor/myoclonus: essential and symptomatic. In symptomatic palatal tremor/myoclonus, a focal brainstem lesion is identified which interrupts the Guillain-Mollaret triangle. Hypertrophy of the inferior olive can be seen on brain MRI. It is caused by contractions of the levator veli palatini and usually persists in sleep. By contrast, in essential palatal tremor/myoclonus a cause is not evident and the contractions result from involvement of the tensor veli palatini. Because this muscle opens the Eustachian tube, the palatal movements are associated with an ear click. Essential palatal tremor/myoclonus disappears in sleep. Clonazepam, valproic acid, and botulinum toxin injections may provide benefit.

TARDIVE TREMOR

Tardive tremor is a rare subtype of drug-induced tremor. It is associated with long-term use of dopamine-receptor blocking agents such as neuroleptics and metoclopramide. It is a 2.5–6 Hz predominantly action tremor which can emerge 2–20 years after drug exposure and often during drug withdrawal. Unlike the tremor of drug-induced parkinsonism, tardive tremor persists after removal of the offending drug. Tardive tremor can coexist with other tardive movement disorders including dystonia, chorea, and akathisia. Treatment with a dopamine depleting drug such as tetrabenazine can improve tremor.

CLINICAL VIGNETTE *A 72-year-old man had experienced difficulty playing golf during the past 6 months. When he would step to the tee standing still to get ready to hit the ball, his legs became increasingly tremulous. Although he could walk all 18 holes without difficulty, he was eventually unable to maintain his balance when he tried to stand still to make his shots. To compensate, he assumed an ever-widening posture, but this gradually became less helpful. Similarly, he had routinely begun to sit down when he urinated. Neurologic examination demonstrated an alert, pleasant man with normal facial expression. He arose from his chair without difficulty, walking with a normal gait, including a good arm swing. However, when he stopped and tried to stand still, he stood with an abnormally wide base and would soon develop an 18- to 20-Hz tremor involving both legs. It became necessary for him to hold on to someone to keep from falling. While seated, he had no rest tremor. He had no cogwheeling or rigidity, and his neurologic examination was otherwise normal.*

Various medications were tried, including primidone, but no effective remedies were found.

ORTHOSTATIC TREMOR

Orthostatic tremor (OT) is a rare entity characterized by a pronounced feeling of unsteadiness with standing that is relieved by sitting or walking. OT is a high-frequency tremor—13–18 Hz which is not always visible but may be palpated as a rippling of leg muscles (quadriceps) or auscultated by placing a stethoscope to the gastrocnemius or quadriceps muscles. The sound has been described as that of a helicopter. Diagnosis of OT can be confirmed with EMG recordings of leg muscles when the patient is standing. High-frequency rhythmic discharges of 13–18 Hz can be demonstrated. A number of pharmacotherapies have been used to treat OT. Clonazepam has been shown to be effective in ~1/3 of patients and is started at 0.5 mg/day and can be titrated up to 2 mg tid. A number of agents have demonstrated variable efficacy in OT including gabapentin, primidone, valproic acid, levodopa, and pramipexole.

PSYCHOGENIC TREMOR

Tremor, like other movement disorders, can be psychogenic in origin. Differentiating psychogenic from neurogenic tremor can be difficult but a number of "red flag" symptoms and signs can point to a psychogenic cause. Abrupt onset of tremor, spontaneous remission, selective disability, and remission with psychotherapy may be present in the history. On exam, reduction of tremor with distractibility, variability in amplitude, frequency and direction of tremor, responsiveness to placebo, coactivation of antagonist muscles either during passive flexion or extension, and entrainment (adaptation of tremor frequency to the frequency of repetitive movements in the contralateral limb) can suggest a psychogenic tremor. Psychiatric comorbidities are frequently seen in this tremor type, but it should be emphasized that the presence of a psychiatric disorder does not prove the tremor is psychogenic. Appropriate workup should be done to rule out organic causes of tremor. Ultimately, accurate diagnosis of psychogenic tremor is based on both the exclusion of neurogenic disorders and the presence of positive clinical signs. A multidisciplinary treatment approach including psychotherapy, physical therapy, and pharmacotherapy (antidepressants, anxiolytics) can be beneficial.

ADDITIONAL RESOURCES

Fahn SA, Jankovic J, Hallett M. Principles and practice of movement disorders. 2nd ed. 2011.

Puschmann A, Wazolek ZK. Diagnosis and treatment of common forms of tremors. Semin Neurol 2011;31:65–77.

Schneider SA, Deuschl G. The treatment of tremor. Neurotherapeutics 2014;11:128–38.

31

Dystonia

Julie Leegwater-Kim

CLINICAL VIGNETTE *A 22-year-old previously healthy woman developed slurred speech, difficulty walking, and hand tremors over the course of 1 month after a severe psychologic trauma. She had mild neck pain and took cyclobenzaprine without benefit. She denied any history of fever, head trauma, or exposure to dopamine receptor blocking agents. There was no family history of neurologic disease. Exam revealed lower facial dystonia, including risus sardonicus and tongue dystonia, dysarthria, bradykinesia, mild cogwheel rigidity, mild rest and kinetic tremor, dystonic gait, and loss of postural reflexes. After several weeks her symptoms plateaued. A trial of carbidopa/levodopa was ineffective. She reported slight benefit on high doses of trihexyphenidyl.*

Workup included blood glucose, creatinine, electrolytes, complete blood count, liver function tests, thyroid-stimulating hormone, erythrocyte sedimentation rate, antinuclear antibodies test, vitamin B_{12}, ceruloplasmin, and 24-hour urine copper, all of which were within normal limits. Slit-lamp exam was negative for Kayser-Fleischer rings. Genetic testing for spinocerebellar ataxia was negative. Magnetic resonance imaging of the brain was unremarkable, as were electroencephalography and electromyography. ATP1A3 genetic sequencing revealed a mutation, confirming the diagnosis of rapid-onset dystonia-parkinsonism (RPD).

Dystonia is a hyperkinetic movement disorder characterized by involuntary sustained muscle contractions that frequently cause twisting and repetitive movements or abnormal postures. Dystonic movements are patterned, meaning that they repeatedly involve the same group of muscles. There is simultaneous contraction of agonist and antagonist muscles. In general the duration of dystonic muscle contractions is longer than other hyperkinesias (i.e., chorea), though sometimes the movements can be rapid enough to resemble repetitive myoclonic jerking. One of the characteristic features of dystonia is that it is often temporarily diminished by tactile sensory tricks *(gestes antagonistes)*. For example, a patient with cervical dystonia may be able to reduce dystonic movements by placing a hand on his or her chin or side of the face. Patients with orobuccolingual dystonia often experience improvement by touching their lips or placing an object, such as a toothpick, into their mouths. In some patients, simply thinking about performing the sensory trick diminishes the dystonia. The efficacy of sensory tricks can be exploited in the development of therapies. For example, some patients with lower cranial dystonia may benefit from wearing a mouth guard.

The initial presentation of dystonia is usually focal (affecting one body part) and task-specific—the dystonia occurs with a particular action. For example, a subject with foot dystonia may initially note dystonia when walking forward but not walking backward or running. In the majority of patients, the dystonia remains focal without spreading to other parts of the body. If dystonia spreads, it tends to involve contiguous body parts and becomes a segmental dystonia. In more severe cases, the dystonia can become generalized. As a rule, the younger the age at onset, the more likely it is that the dystonia will spread. Recent data have also suggested that in the primary dystonias there is a caudal-to-rostral anatomic gradient in the site of onset as a function of age.

As dystonia progresses, it emerges with other actions of the affected body part, therefore becoming less task-specific. For example, the patient with foot dystonia may experience it when walking forward and backward, running, or tapping the foot. Further progression can lead to "overflow dystonia," in which movement of a distant body part elicits the dystonia. As dystonia worsens, it can occur at rest. In the most severe cases of dystonia, contractures may develop.

Dystonia is frequently worsened by fatigue and stress and diminished with relaxation and sleep. Pain is generally uncommon in dystonia except for cervical dystonia, in which approximately 75% of patients report pain.

CLASSIFICATION OF DYSTONIA

There are several recognized classification schemes for dystonia: (1) age at onset, (2) anatomic distribution, and (3) etiology.

Age at Onset

Early-onset dystonia is defined as dystonia developing at or before the age of 26 years; late onset is defined as dystonia developing after the age of 26 years. Age at onset is an important factor determining prognosis in patients with dystonia, with earlier age at onset correlating with an increased likelihood that the dystonia will spread to other body parts. In general, young-onset dystonia tends to begin in a limb and become generalized, whereas adult-onset dystonia tends to be craniocervical and to remain focal or become segmental.

Anatomic Distribution

The topographic characteristics of dystonia are useful in defining its severity and guiding treatment. Focal dystonia affects a single body part. Virtually any part of the body can be involved in dystonia, and many types of focal dystonia have specific names: *blepharospasm* (dystonic eye closure), *spasmodic torticollis* (rotational cervical dystonia), and *writer's cramp* (focal hand dystonia). When dystonia involves two or more contiguous body parts/regions, it is referred to as *segmental dystonia*. *Multifocal dystonia* refers to the involvement of two or more noncontiguous body parts. *Generalized dystonia* represents a combination of crural dystonia (one or both legs plus trunk) and any other area of the body. *Hemidystonia*, as its name implies, affects one-half of the body. Hemidystonia suggests a symptomatic (secondary) rather than primary dystonia.

Etiology

The growth in our understanding of the genetics of dystonia has contributed significantly to the etiologic classification of this disorder. There are essentially two broad categories of dystonia: primary and secondary.

PRIMARY DYSTONIA

Primary dystonias are characterized by isolated dystonia (with the exception that tremor can be present) and may be sporadic or familial. Most primary dystonias are sporadic, with onset in adulthood and a focal or segmental presentation. The most common focal dystonia presenting to movement disorder clinics is cervical dystonia (Fig. 31.1). After cervical dystonia, the most common focal dystonias are blepharospasm, spasmodic dysphonia, oromandibular dystonia, and hand dystonia.

A minority of primary dystonias have an identified genetic etiology (Box 31.1). Perhaps the best studied of the primary dystonias is DYT1 dystonia, or Oppenheim dystonia, a generalized torsion dystonia that usually begins in childhood and affects the limbs first. DYT1 dystonia is caused by a deletion in the *DYT1* gene, which encodes for the *torsin A* protein. The disease is inherited in an autosomal dominant fashion and has 30% to 40% penetrance. Phenotype can vary widely within an affected family. The *DYT1* mutation is estimated to account for 90% of the cases of limb-onset dystonia in the Ashkenazi Jewish population and 50% to 70% of cases in the non-Jewish population. A number of other primary dystonias have had their genetic loci mapped (Table 31.1).

BOX 31.1   Classification Schemes for Dystonia

Age at Onset
- Young-onset: up to 26 years
- Late-onset: later than 26 years

Anatomic Distribution
- Focal—single body part
- Segmental—two or more contiguous body parts
- Multifocal—two or more noncontiguous body parts
- Generalized—segmental crural dystonia plus one other body part
- Hemidystonia—dystonia affecting one-half of the body

Etiologic
- Primary (idiopathic)
  - Familial
  - Sporadic
- Secondary
  - Heredodegenerative
  - Degenerative-sporadic
  - Dystonia-plus syndromes (inherited nondegenerative)
  - Drug-induced
  - Injury/trauma
  - Structural lesions
  - Psychogenic

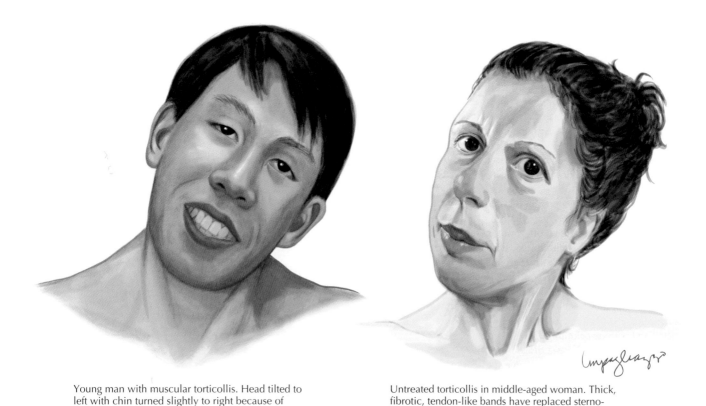

Young man with muscular torticollis. Head tilted to left with chin turned slightly to right because of contracture of left sternocleidomastoid muscle.

Untreated torticollis in middle-aged woman. Thick, fibrotic, tendon-like bands have replaced sterno-cleidomastoid muscle, making head appear tethered to clavicle. Two heads of left sternocleidomastoid muscle are prominent.

Fig. 31.1 Cervical Dystonia.

TABLE 31.1 Selected Dystonias With an Established Genetic Cause

Dystonia Designation	Etiologic Type	Inheritance	Clinical Features	Gene	Protein
DYT1	Primary	Autosomal dominant	Early onset (age < 40 years) Generalized dystonia Limbs affected first	TOR1A	TorsinA: ATPase
DYT3	Secondary	X-linked recessive	Dystonia/parkinsonism (Lubag)	TAF1	Transcription initiation factor TFIID subunit 1
DYT5	Secondary (dystonia-plus)	Autosomal dominant	Dopa-responsive dystonia (DRD)	GCH1	GTP cyclohydrolase
DYT6	Primary	Autosomal dominant	Adolescent-onset mixed type dystonia	THAP1	Transcription factor
DYT11	Secondary (dystonia-plus)	Autosomal dominant	Myoclonus-dystonia (MD)	SGCE	Episolon sarcoglycan
DYT12	Secondary (dystonia-plus)	Autosomal dominant	Rapid-onset dystonia-parkinsonism (RPD)	ATP1A3	ATPase subunit
DYT24	Primary	Autosomal dominant	Late-onset craniocervical dystonia	ANO3	Calcium activated chloride channel
DYT25	Primary	Autosomal dominant	Adult-onset segmental dystonia	GNAL	Guanine nucleotide-binding protein

SECONDARY DYSTONIA

Secondary dystonia encompasses a broad clinical category that includes inherited degenerative disorders, degenerative disorders of unknown etiology, acquired dystonias (i.e., drug-induced, structural lesions, trauma), and psychogenic dystonia. Patients with secondary dystonia frequently display associated clinical abnormalities including other movement disorders besides tremor (i.e., parkinsonism) as well as dementia, spasticity, ataxia, weakness, reflex changes, eye movement abnormalities, or seizures. Other historical and clinical features that suggest secondary dystonia include history of trauma, perinatal anoxia, toxin or drug exposure, onset of dystonia at rest, and hemidystonia.

A number of heredodegenerative disorders may present with dystonia. Autosomal dominant disorders (Huntington disease, spinocerebellar ataxia type 3, neuroferritinopathy), autosomal recessive disorders (Wilson disease, pantothenate kinase–associated neurodegeneration), X-linked recessive disorders (DYT3 or Lubag), and mitochondrial disorders (Leigh disease) have been described and are listed in Box 31.2.

Dystonia can also be seen in various neurodegenerative parkinsonian syndromes, including Parkinson disease (PD), as well as the atypical parkinsonian syndromes such as progressive supranuclear palsy and corticobasal ganglionic degeneration (CBD). Adult-onset focal foot or leg dystonia can be the initial presentation of PD. Patients with PD may also develop dystonia as an off-symptom or as part of levodopa-induced dyskinesias. A dystonic apraxic limb is a hallmark of CBD.

Dystonia-plus syndromes are a rare group of inherited nondegenerative diseases that include dopa-responsive dystonia (DRD), myoclonus–dystonia (MD), and RDP. These diseases are considered neurochemical disorders because they are due to biochemical defects not associated with neuronal loss. Dystonia is associated with parkinsonism in DRD and RDP and with myoclonus in MD.

1. **DRD,** also called Segawa disease or DYT5, is characterized by the onset of progressive dystonia and parkinsonism in mid-childhood. Patients exhibit a diurnal variation in symptoms and the feet and legs are predominantly involved. The disease is inherited in an autosomal dominant pattern and is caused by genetic mutations in the GTP-cyclohydrolase I *(GCHI)* gene. GCHI is the rate-limiting enzyme in the synthesis of tetrahydrobiopterin, an essential cofactor for tyrosine hydroxylase. Patients respond dramatically to small doses of levodopa.

BOX 31.2 Heredodegenerative Disorders Causing Dystonia

Autosomal Dominant
- Huntington disease
- Spinocerebellar ataxias (SCA3)
- Dentatorubro-pallidoluysian atrophy (DRPLA)

Autosomal Recessive
- Wilson disease
- Neuroacanthocytosis
- Niemann–Pick type C
- Glutaric aciduria
- GM1 gangliosidosis
- GM2 gangliosidosis
- Metachromatic leukodystrophy
- Homocystinuria
- Friedreich ataxia
- Pantothenate-kinase–associated neurodegeneration (PKAN)
- Neuronal intranuclear hyaline inclusion disease (NIHID)

X-Linked Dominant
- Rett syndrome

X-Linked Recessive
- DYT3 (Lubag)
- Deafness–dystonia syndrome

Mitochondrial
- Leigh disease
- Leber disease

2. **RDP** is an autosomal dominant disorder characterized by young-onset dystonia and parkinsonism. The symptoms appear dramatically over days to weeks and can often emerge in the setting of a stressor. Bulbar symptoms are very common. Symptoms tend to plateau after weeks. Patients exhibit little if any response to levodopa. The gene for RDP has been identified as *ATP1A3,* which encodes an Na+/K+ATPase. **Myoclonus-dystonia (MD)** is

an autosomal dominant disorder characterized by alcohol-responsive myoclonus and dystonia. Symptoms can emerge in childhood or in adulthood. Psychiatric disorders such as obsessive-compulsive disorder and alcohol abuse are frequently seen. This disorder has been associated with mutations in the epsilon sarcoglycan gene.

3. *Iatrogenic dystonia* can occur with exposure to dopamine receptor blocking agents, levodopa, and selective serotonin reuptake inhibitors. Tardive dystonia may be focal, segmental, or generalized and is often characterized as retrocollis and opisthotonic posturing. Acute dystonic reactions may also develop in association with exposure to dopamine receptor blocking agents.

A variety of lesions causing damage to the basal ganglia are associated with dystonia. These include perinatal hypoxia, stroke, head trauma, brain tumor, infection, and autoimmune disorders.

Psychogenic dystonia is perhaps the most diagnostically challenging type of secondary dystonia, as illustrated by the record that many patients now recognized as having organic dystonia were initially thought to have a primary psychiatric disorder. It is also important to recognize that a minority of patients with organic movement disorder may have a superimposed psychogenic movement disorder including dystonia. Features on history and examination that can suggest a psychogenic dystonia include abrupt onset, spontaneous remission, distractible or entrainable movements, variability and inconsistency of movements (i.e., nonpatterned dystonic movements), false weakness or sensory complaints, multiple somatizations, the presence of secondary gain, and concomitant psychiatric disease.

PATHOPHYSIOLOGY

Although the genetics of a number of primary dystonias have been elucidated, the pathophysiology of dystonia remains unclear. Lesions in the basal ganglia, particularly the thalamus and putamen, point to these structures as having key roles in the development of dystonia. Models of basal ganglia circuitry suggest that there is an imbalance between direct and indirect pathways leading to reduced pallidal inhibition of the thalamus with subsequent overactivity of the premotor cortex. However, this hypothesis does not square with the finding that pallidotomy and deep brain stimulation (DBS) of the globus pallidus internus can improve dystonia. A more complex pathophysiologic model

of dystonia is emerging that incorporates not only rate but also the pattern, synchronization, and somatosensory responsiveness of neuronal activity.

TREATMENT

Treatment of dystonia is determined by etiology and the anatomic region or regions involved. All children and young adults presenting with dystonia should be given a trial of levodopa to rule out DRD.

The most effective treatment for focal dystonias such as cervical dystonia, blepharospasm, limb dystonia, and spasmodic dysphonia is botulinum toxin. Both serotypes A and B are available in the United States. Botulinum toxin and baclofen can be beneficial for oromandibular dystonia. In addition to medications, physical therapy is an important adjunct in the treatment of dystonia.

For patients with generalized dystonia, trihexyphenidyl at high doses (~90 mg/day) can provide some benefit. Baclofen may also be tried for generalized dystonia and can be given at high doses orally or delivered intrathecally. The benzodiazepines may provide adjunctive benefit. Variable results have been found for diphenhydramine, carbamazepine, dopamine agonists, and dopamine antagonists. Tetrabenazine can be helpful, especially in tardive dystonia.

For medication-refractory dystonia, surgery can be considered. DBS of the globus pallidus internus has been shown to significantly improve primary generalized dystonia by 50% on average. DBS also appears to be effective in reducing the severity of cervical dystonia. DBS has been less beneficial in treating secondary dystonias with the exception of tardive dystonia, where the degree of improvement is similar to that seen in primary dystonias.

ADDITIONAL RESOURCES

Crowell JL, Shah BB. Surgery for dystonia and tremor. Curr Neurol Neurosci Rep 2016;16:22.

Fahn S, Bressman SB, Marsden CD. Classification of dystonia. Adv Neurol 1998;78:1–10.

Fahn S, Jankovic J, Hallett M. Principles and practice of movement disorders. 2nd ed. Saunders; 2011.

Lohmann K, Klein C. Update on the genetics of dystonia. Curr Neurol Neurosci Rep 2017;17:26.

Tarsy D, Simon DK. Dystonia. N Engl J Med 2006;355:818–29.

32

Chorea

Diana Apetauerova

CLINICAL VIGNETTE *Sylvia is a 59-year-old, right-handed teacher who developed jerky movements in her body within the past 3–4 years and was now "fidgety" all the time. Her family observed intellectual changes; she seemed withdrawn and forgetful, was occasionally inappropriate in her behavior, had to retire early due to inability to "concentrate," and appearing "nervous" all the time. She had no other past medical history. Her mother died at the age of 55 and reportedly had a "mental breakdown" and was forgetful and always fidgety. Her father died at the age of 70 from a heart attack. Her grandmother had a "mental disorder." Sylvia did not have any siblings and was a single mother of a 27-year-old son. When seen in movement disorders clinic, she was unable to sit still. She had constant grimacing in her face, motor impersistence of her tongue, and piano-like playing movements in her hands. Brief, jerky choreiform movements were present in her trunk and extremities. When ambulated, she appeared very disorganized and unsteady. She also had mild bradykinesia predominantly with testing of her hands. Her demeanor was jovial, and she had no signs of depression. The movements were not under any voluntary control, and she had no urge to do them. Because of the combination of cognitive decline and generalized chorea, Huntington disease (HD) was suspected. Her genetic testing revealed 45 CAG repeats in the HD gene. She was treated with low doses of tetrabenazine, with substantial improvement in her chorea. However, her intellectual and behavioral decline continued. Her son was single and was not interested in being tested for HD.*

Chorea (from Latin *choreus*, dance) is an abnormal involuntary movement usually distal in location, brief, nonrhythmic, abrupt, and irregular, that seems to flow from one body part to another. The movements are random, unpredictable in timing, direction, and distribution. Chorea can be partially suppressed; some patients can incorporate these into semipurposeful movements called *parakinesia*. Motor impersistence, the inability to maintain a sustained contraction, is a typical feature of chorea.

Athetosis and **ballism** are sometimes confused with chorea. *Athetosis* is a slow, writhing, continuous set of involuntary movements, usually affecting limbs distally, but it can involve the axial musculature (neck, face, and tongue). If athetosis becomes faster, it sometimes blends with chorea (i.e., *choreoathetosis*). *Ballism* is large-amplitude, involuntary movements affecting the proximal limbs, causing flinging and flailing limb movements.

Patients with chorea are often initially unaware of these involuntary movements. The chorea is often first interpreted by observers as fidgetiness. The patients are usually frustrated by their own incoordination or clumsiness.

ETIOLOGY

Chorea results from disruption of the basal ganglia's modulation of thalamocortical motor pathways. Multiple pathophysiologic mechanisms may be implicated. These include neuronal degeneration in selective regions, neurotransmitter receptor blockade, other metabolic factors within the basal ganglia, and exceedingly rarely a structural lesion. Chorea is classified into inherited, primarily Huntington disease (HD), immunologic Sydenham chorea, drug-related, structural, and various miscellaneous etiologies (Table 32.1).

PATHOPHYSIOLOGY

The putamen, globus pallidus, and subthalamic nuclei are the key pathologic sites related to the development of chorea. Normal movement patterns depend on the presence of a critical physiologic balance between the direct and indirect motor pathways, with the direct pathway promoting and the indirect pathway inhibiting movements. The direct pathway consists of inhibitory projections (gamma-aminobutyric acid [GABA] mediated) from the striatum to the internal portion of the globus pallidus and substantia nigra pars reticulata (GPi/SNr) and from the GPi/SNr to the thalamus, and excitatory projections (glutamate-mediate) from the thalamus to the cortex. In the indirect pathway, there are inhibitory GABA pathways from the striatum to the external portion of the globus pallidus (GPe) and from the GPe to the subthalamic nucleus (STN). This double inhibition causes stimulation of the STN that, in turn, through its excitatory glutaminergic projections, stimulates the GPi/SNr. These two structures once stimulated, produce inhibition (GABA mediated) of the thalamus and consequently inhibition of the excitatory thalamocortical pathway.

In HD, the major neurodegenerative pathology occurs within the caudate nuclei and the putamen (striatum). These changes primarily affect *medium-sized "spiny" neurons* that secrete the inhibitory neurotransmitter GABA. It has been proposed that in the earlier stages of HD the indirect pathway is mainly affected, resulting in loss of inhibition from the striatum to the external portion of the globus pallidus and consequent increase inhibition of the STN and decreased excitation of GPi/SNr, with overall decreased inhibition to the thalamus. This disinhibition of the thalamus allows for enhanced excitatory outflow to the cortex, resulting in the disorganized, excessive (hyperkinetic) movement patterns of chorea. As HD progresses into the later stages, the direct pathway also becomes affected causing a hypokinetic or akinetic stage.

Concomitantly, HD patients also have a prominent associated temporal and frontal lobe cerebral cortex neuronal degeneration.

TABLE 32.1 Causes of Chorea

Type of Chorea	
Inherited	Huntington disease
	Neuroacanthocytosis
	Wilson disease
	Benign hereditary chorea
	Olivopontocerebellar atrophy
	Ataxia telangiectasia
	Idiopathic torsion dystonia
	Tic disorder
	Myoclonic epilepsy
	Dentatorubropallidoluysian degeneration
	Gerstmann-Sträussler-Scheinker syndrome
Metabolic	Amino acid disorders (glutaric academia)
	Leigh disease
	Lesch-Nyhan disease
	Lipid disorders (gangliosidoses)
	Mitochondrial myopathy
	Nonketotic hyperglycemia
	Disorders of calcium, magnesium, or glucose
Immunologic	Sydenham chorea
	Systemic lupus erythematosus
	Antiphospholipid antibody syndrome
	Chorea gravidarum
	Reaction to immunization
Drug related	Tardive dyskinesia (neuroleptics, serotonin reuptake inhibitors, others)
	Withdrawal emergent syndrome
	Sympathomimetics
	Cocaine
	Anticonvulsants
	Contraceptives
	Lithium
	Tricyclic antidepressants
	Levodopa
	Amantadine
	Dopamine agonist
	Theophylline and beta-adrenergic agents
	Ethanol
	Carbon monoxide
	Gasoline inhalation
Structural	Cerebrovascular disease
	Multiple sclerosis
	Traumatic brain injury
	Anoxic encephalopathy
	Pseudochoreoathetosis (spinal cord injury, peripheral nerve injury)
	Delayed onset following perinatal injury
Miscellaneous	Encephalitis (herpes simplex, HIV, Lyme disease)
	Endocrine dysfunction (e.g., hyperthyroidism)
	Metabolic disturbance (e.g., hypocalcemia, hyperglycemia, hypoglycemia)
	Kernicterus
	Nutritional (e.g., B_{12} deficiency)
	Postpump chorea (cardiac bypass)
	Normal maturation

With Sydenham chorea, various streptococcal proteins or antigens (streptococcal M proteins) induce the body's production of antineuronal immunoglobulin G (IgG) antibodies. These antibodies cross-react against the body's own cells that provide the neuronal antigens within the basal ganglia, such as the caudate nuclei and STN.

CLINICAL PRESENTATION

The spectrum of clinical findings in chorea varies, presenting in isolation or with other involuntary movements. At the simplest level, chorea appears as semipurposeful movements resembling fidgetiness. This is exemplified by the flitting movements of the fingers, wrists, toes, and ankles so characteristic of HD. The movements can be focal, as in tardive dyskinesia (TD), where they are more repetitive and stereotypical. They may present as lip pouting or pursing, cheek puffing, lateral or forward jaw movements, or tongue rolling or protruding.

Asymmetric chorea, such as hemichorea, primarily affects the limbs on one side of the body. Sometimes, chorea affects only specific functional muscle groups, such as respiratory chorea. When there is a more diffuse basal ganglia dysfunction, chorea is often accompanied by parkinsonism, tics, and dystonia. Later, chorea can interfere with activities of daily living; for example, limb chorea can cause falls and interfere with dressing and eating. Chorea of the face, jaw, larynx, and respiratory muscles may eventually limit verbal communication.

On neurologic examination, there is altered finger-to-nose testing. Rapid alternating movements are executed with a jerky and interrupted performance. When patients with significant chorea grasp an examiner's fingers, a squeezing motion called *milkmaid's grip* is sometimes noted. This is a sign of motor impersistence. As with other adventitious movements, seen with the various movement disorders, chorea is frequently aggravated while walking. Various oculomotor abnormalities may be observed. These include slow and hypometric saccades and saccadic pursuit, convergence paresis, and gaze impersistence. Parkinsonian features, particularly bradykinesia and dystonia, are sometimes evidenced with more advanced disease.

Huntington Disease

This hereditary, progressive neurodegenerative disorder is the most common cause of chorea. The classic signs of HD include the development of chorea, neurobehavioral changes, and gradual dementia (Fig. 32.1). Symptoms typically become evident during the fourth or fifth decade of life, although onset varies from early childhood to late adulthood. HD symptoms vary among patients in range and severity, as well as by age at onset, and in rate of clinical progression. An early onset is associated with increased severity and more rapid progression. For example, adult-onset HD typically lasts approximately 15–20 years, whereas the course of juvenile HD tends to last approximately 8–10 years.

The initial clinical presentation may be either neurologic or psychiatric. Characteristic early presentations include the gradual onset of subtle personality changes, forgetfulness, clumsiness, and development of choreiform, fidgeting movement of the fingers or toes. Neurobehavioral changes include both emotional and behavioral disturbance. Patients present with increased irritability, suspiciousness, impulsiveness, lack of self-control, and anhedonia. Sometimes anxiety, depression, mania, obsessive-compulsive behaviors, and agitation are seen early in the disease. Later, a severe distortion in thinking and occasionally hallucinations, such as the perception of sounds, sights, or other sensations without external stimuli, may develop. The juvenile form of HD more often presents with dystonia, rigidity, or cerebella ataxia than chorea per se.

Cognitive decline is characterized by progressive dementia or gradual impairment of the mental processes involved in comprehension, reasoning, judgment, and memory. Typical early signs include forgetfulness, inattention, increased difficulty in concentrating, and various forms of disinhibition manifested by emotional outbursts, financial irresponsibility, or sexual promiscuity. Communication difficulties develop, including problems expressing thoughts in words, initiating conversations, or comprehending others' words and responding appropriately.

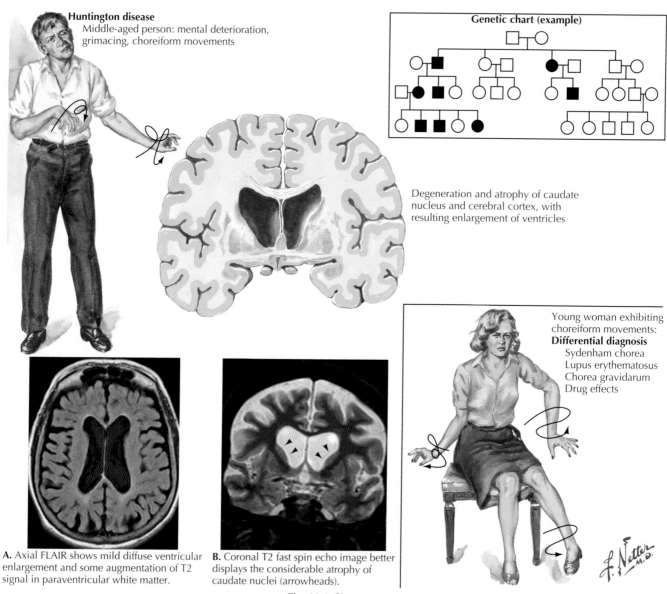

Huntington disease
Middle-aged person: mental deterioration, grimacing, choreiform movements

Genetic chart (example)

Degeneration and atrophy of caudate nucleus and cerebral cortex, with resulting enlargement of ventricles

Young woman exhibiting choreiform movements:
Differential diagnosis
Sydenham chorea
Lupus erythematosus
Chorea gravidarum
Drug effects

A. Axial FLAIR shows mild diffuse ventricular enlargement and some augmentation of T2 signal in paraventricular white matter.

B. Coronal T2 fast spin echo image better displays the considerable atrophy of caudate nuclei (arrowheads).

Fig. 32.1 Chorea.

Motor disturbances are characterized by the gradual onset of clumsiness, balance difficulties, and fidgeting movements. Early chorea may be limited to the fingers and toes, later extending to the arms, legs, face, and trunk. Eventually, chorea tends to become widespread or generalized. Parkinsonism and dystonia are sometimes seen later in the disease. Many patients with HD develop a distinctive manner of walking that may be unsteady, disjointed, lurching, and dancelike. Eventually, postural instability, dysphagia, and dysarthria appear.

Later disease stages are characterized by severe dementia and progressive motor dysfunction; patients usually become unable to walk, have poor dietary intake, become unable to care for themselves, and eventually cease to talk, leading to a persistent vegetative state. Life-threatening complications may result from serious falls, sometimes even leading to subdural hematomas, poor nutrition, infection, choking, aspiration pneumonia, or heart failure.

Sydenham Chorea

This is the other well-recognized form of chorea. It is related to an autoimmune response to infection with group A beta-hemolytic streptococci leading to acute rheumatic fever (ARF). This is currently very

uncommon in economically developed countries with the widespread availability of antibiotics for *Streptococcus* A infection. The initial illness is usually characterized by pharyngitis, followed within approximately 1–5 weeks by the sudden onset of ARF. Chorea primarily occurs in patients between the ages of 5 and 15 years. It usually does not present until 1–6 months after the initial sore throat. Sydenham chorea may occur as an isolated condition or subsequent to other characteristic features of ARF. Initially, these children often are described as unusually restless, aggressive, or "excessively emotional." The distribution of chorea is usually generalized, and these movements consist of relatively fast or rapid, irregular, uncontrollable, jerky motions that disappear with sleep and may increase with stress, fatigue, and excitement (Fig. 32.2). Occasionally, the choreiform movements are so severe that they have a ballistic character. Some children also evidence emotional and behavioral disturbances.

Typically, in a significant majority of children, Sydenham chorea is a self-limited condition, resolving spontaneously within an average duration of 9 months to 2 years. However, sometimes residual signs of chorea and behavioral abnormalities fluctuate over a year or more. In approximately 20% of patients, Sydenham chorea may recur, usually

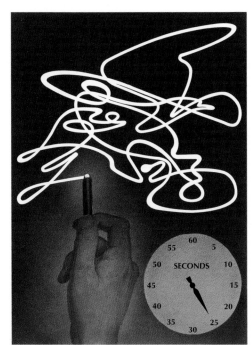

Sydenham chorea: spontaneous uncoordinated movements demonstrated by electric penlight held in patient's hand

Fig. 32.2 Choreiform Movements.

BOX 32.1   **Initial Laboratory and Imaging Investigation of Chorea**

Thyroid hormone assay
Electrolyte panel
Complete blood count (look for acanthocytes)
Antinuclear antibody test (SLE)
Antistreptolysin-O antibody test
Urine toxicological screen for illicit drugs
Brain MRI/PET

MRI, Magnetic resonance imaging; *PET,* positron emission tomography; *SLE,* systemic lupus erythematosus.

or hemorrhage or an associated polycythemia rubra vera, leads to an acute focal chorea, or hemiballismus.

If the onset of chorea occurs during childhood, other inheritable disorders, including the leukodystrophies and gangliosidosis, require differentiation. *Neuroacanthocytosis* is another hereditary movement disorder also manifested by mild chorea, tics, parkinsonism, and dystonia. Laboratory findings include increased serum creatine phosphokinase and red cell acanthocytes. In all age groups, possible reactions to drugs or toxins must always be investigated.

DIAGNOSTIC EVALUATION

Huntington Disease

The evaluation of patients with chorea includes detailed family history and tests to exclude other possible pathophysiology (Box 32.1). Genetic testing is the most accurate test for HD. The mutation that is responsible for the disease consists of an unstable enlargement of the CAG repeat sequence. The gene is located at 4p16.3 and encodes for a protein called huntingtin.

Genetic testing is available for presymptomatic individuals at risk for HD; it requires careful pretest and posttest counseling to guard against suicidal risk in individuals who request the study and find out they have the illness. Other investigations are less important, but magnetic resonance imaging (MRI) or computed tomography (CT) is commonly performed. Head MRI is preferable to CT for better delineation of the affected subcortical tissue. Atrophy of the caudate nucleus may be demonstrated. Positron emission tomography (PET) typically demonstrates glucose hypometabolism within the striatum.

Sydenham Chorea

Diagnosis primarily relies on the recognition of acute chorea in a child or adolescent who recently had a streptococcal pharyngitis. The combination fulfills the criteria for a diagnosis of ARF. Other manifestations of ARF are not mandatory for the diagnosis. Tests for acute-phase reactions are less helpful because of the latency between the early infection and the onset of the movement disorder. These include erythrocyte sedimentation rate, C-reactive protein, and leukocytosis. Supporting evidence of preceding streptococcal infections include positive throat culture for group A *Streptococcus,* increased antistreptolysin-O titer, or other antistreptococcal antibodies. Brain CT usually fails to display abnormalities. Head MRI is often normal but occasionally shows reversible hyperintensity in the basal ganglia. PET and single photo emission computed tomography (SPECT) demonstrate reversible striatal hypermetabolism.

Chorea Gravidarum

A chorea of any etiology beginning during a pregnancy is referred to as chorea gravidarum (CG). This is most common in younger woman,

within approximately 2 years of the initial occurrence. Recurrences are also reported during pregnancy and in association with certain medications in women who had ARF during childhood.

DIFFERENTIAL DIAGNOSES

Diagnostic considerations in a patient presenting with chorea is a broad one (see Table 32.1). HD, the most common cause of chorea, is usually easily diagnosed when an adult has the typical triad of chorea, dementia, and family history. Several neurodegenerative disorders, some also having expanded trinucleotide repeats, are phenocopies of HD. These include spinocerebellar atrophy (SCA2, SCA3) and dentatorubral-pallidoluysian atrophy (DRPLA). In addition, there are some other HD-like diseases (HDL1, HDL2, HDL3) that may present with an HD-like phenotype. Sydenham chorea has an earlier onset, lacks the characteristic mental disturbances, and is usually self-limiting. Chorea with mental dysfunction may also occur as a manifestation of systemic lupus erythematosus (SLE). These patients usually have a more acute onset, with more localized chorea, and the characteristic SLE clinical and serologic abnormalities. There is a prior history of recurrent vascular thrombosis or spontaneous abortions and disappearance after therapy with prednisone.

Involuntary movements occurring in psychiatric patients receiving long-term treatment with neuroleptic agents occasionally pose a diagnostic problem when they present with TD. Usually repetitive, these TD movements contrast with the nonrepetitive and flowing nature of chorea. Patients with TD usually have a predominant oral-lingual-buccal dyskinesia. Unlike in those with HD, these patients' gait is usually normal. Similar mental dysfunction occurs with some of the dementing disorders, particularly Alzheimer or Pick disease where language is more involved. Myoclonus is more typical than chorea with dementia, especially with spongiform encephalopathies (e.g., Creutzfeldt-Jakob disease). Very rarely, a structural basal ganglia lesion, particularly an infarction having an average age of 22 years. CG is frequently associated with eclampsia. At least 35% of CG individuals have a prior history of ARF with associated Sydenham chorea. CG is now quite uncommon, probably attributable to a decline in the incidence of RF with the more widespread use of antibiotics. It is postulated that estrogen and progesterone may sensitize dopaminergic receptors, inducing chorea in an individual with preexisting basal ganglia pathology.

TREATMENT

Readily reversible causes of chorea need to be excluded before considering pharmacologic intervention. Therapy depends on the severity of symptoms; mild chorea does not usually require any treatment. Chorea is treated with either dopamine-blocking or dopamine-depleting medications. Benzodiazepine drugs and amantadine are another possible therapeutic modality, offering a nonspecific means to suppress chorea.

The overall treatment of HD patients requires an integrated, multidisciplinary approach, including symptomatic and supportive medical management; psychosocial support; physical, occupational, or speech therapy; and genetic counseling. Often more specific additional supportive services are helpful for individual patients and their families. There is no specific treatment available that slows, alters, or reverses the progression of HD. Tetrabenazine is a dopaminergic-depleting medication that effectively lessens chorea. Newer deutetrabenazine is a deuterated form of tetrabenazine. The potential advantages of deutetrabenazine include attenuated metabolism and a prolonged plasma half-life, permitting less frequent and lower dosing and a more favorable risk-benefit profile compared with tetrabenazine. In patients who do not respond to tetrabenazine or deutetrabenazine, the choice among neuroleptics is largely empiric and based on clinical experience. In cases of severe chorea, treatment with the more potent typical neuroleptic agents such as haloperidol or chlorpromazine may be helpful. In patients with moderate chorea, the use of typical neuroleptics has been largely replaced by the use of newer atypical neuroleptics, such as risperidone and olanzapine, which may have fewer side effects.

Sydenham chorea is usually not a disabling disorder; however, the more severely affected patients with more severe chorea, requiring short-time treatment, may respond to dopamine antagonists or valproic acid. Severely affected patients may improve with immunosuppressants, plasmapheresis, or intravenous immunoglobulin. Drug treatment should be withdrawn after a short period because remission invariably occurs. Penicillin prophylaxis for ARF is advisable.

Prognosis depends on the cause of chorea. Drug-induced chorea is usually transient. Patients with a past history of rheumatic chorea are more susceptible to developing chorea during pregnancy or drug-induced chorea (e.g., from phenytoin or oral contraceptives).

FUTURE DIRECTIONS

Current research is directed at better definition of the genetics, pathophysiology, symptoms, and progression of HD. Neuroprotection is the preservation of neuronal structure, function, and viability, and neuroprotective therapy is thus targeted at the underlying pathology of HD, rather than at its specific symptoms. Thus ultimately the development of disease-modifying neuroprotective therapies that can delay or even prevent the clinical presentation of HD is ideal for those individuals who are at genetic risk. Preclinical discovery research in HD is identifying numerous distinct targets, along with options for modulating them. Some of these are now proceeding into large-scale efficacy studies in early symptomatic HD subjects. Cell models also offer a very important means to study early, direct effects of mutant huntingtin mRNA changes to identify groups of genes that could play a role in the early pathology of HD. In the meantime, alternative therapeutic agents that can slow progression for those who are already clinically affected with HD will be very welcome.

ADDITIONAL RESOURCES

Cardoso F, Seppi K, Mair KJ, et al. Seminar on choreas. Lancet Neurol 2006;5:589.

Gövert F, Schneider SA. Huntington's disease and Huntington's disease-like syndromes: an overview. Curr Opin Neurol 2013;26:420.

Harper PS. The epidemiology of Huntington's disease. Hum Genet 1992;89:365.

O'Toole O, Lennon VA, Ahlskog JE, et al. Autoimmune chorea in adults. Neurology 2013;80:1133.

Schneider SA, Walker RH, Bhatia KP. The Huntington's disease-like syndromes: what to consider in patients with a negative Huntington's disease gene test. Nat Clin Pract Neurol 2007;3:517.

Shannon KM. Treatment of chorea. Continuum (N Y) 2007;13:72.

33

Myoclonus

Diana Apetauerova

CLINICAL VIGNETTE *A 73-year-old, right-handed man with history of coronary artery disease, myocardial infarction, peripheral vascular disease, and hypertension presented with cardiac arrest followed by resuscitation with subsequent development of anoxic brain injury. He was seen by a neurologist in the intensive care unit (ICU) setting 1 week after his cardiac arrest. His family was very concerned about constant "jerkiness" of his body. Those movements seemed to worsen when people were touching the patient, which affected all four extremities as well as his trunk. He appeared very uncomfortable because of these jerks. Neurologic examination demonstrated an elderly man who was intubated without any sedation. He was restless, inconsistently able to open his eyes to verbal commands, and followed very simple yes-and-no questions. His examination was notable for multiple, irregular, large-amplitude, brief shocklike jerks of the trunk, arms, and legs. These movements occurred randomly, and many of them were stimulus sensitive. His magnetic resonance image (MRI) was unremarkable, and electroencephalography (EEG) showed multifocal spike discharges. A diagnosis of postanoxic generalized myoclonus (Lance-Adams syndrome) was made, and the patient was started on sodium valproate, which significantly diminished those movements.*

Myoclonus is characterized by sudden, abrupt, brief, involuntary, jerk-like contractions of a single muscle or muscle group. They are related to involuntary muscle contractions (positive myoclonus) or sudden inhibition of voluntary muscular contraction, with lapses of sustained posture (negative myoclonus or asterixis). Myoclonus may affect any bodily region, multiple bodily regions, or the entire body, interfering with normal movements and posture.

There are various classifications of myoclonus; these include (1) etiology (Table 33.1), (2) affected body region (focal, segmental, multifocal, or generalized forms), (3) the presence or absence of specific provocative factors, and (4) specific site of nervous system origin of the abnormal neuronal discharges (Table 33.2). Spontaneous myoclonus has no clinically identifiable mechanism. Reflex myoclonus occurs in response to specific external sensory stimuli. Voluntary movement or attempts to perform specific movements induce action or intention myoclonus.

A neurophysiologic classification links the myoclonus to the anatomic origin for the abnormal neuronal discharge within the central nervous system (CNS). Cortical myoclonus arises from the cerebral cortex and is considered epileptic, often being associated with other seizure types. Subcortical myoclonus usually arises from the brainstem. Spinal myoclonus originates within the spinal cord. Clinically, differentiation is often impossible, but electromyography may help.

Another classification, based on etiology, categorizes myoclonus into physiologic or pathologic forms. Common examples of "normal," nonpathologic, physiologic myoclonus include hiccups or "sleep starts" occurring as one drifts into sleep. In pathologic myoclonus, the brief muscle jerks may occur infrequently or repeatedly. Examples include essential myoclonus, myoclonic epilepsy, and secondary myoclonus. Postanoxic encephalopathy and spongiform encephalopathy (i.e., Creutzfeldt-Jakob disease) are the best-known examples of pathologic myoclonus. Additional rare forms include (1) palatal myoclonus, (2) periodic limb movements of sleep, and (3) psychogenic myoclonus. Although pathologic myoclonus is always a sign of CNS dysfunction, its pathophysiologic mechanism often remains enigmatic. Myoclonus may be an important clinical indicator in determining the proper diagnosis. It is also sometimes a nonspecific feature within more widespread neurologic abnormalities.

PATHOPHYSIOLOGY

The pathophysiologic mechanism leading to myoclonus is not well understood, thus complicating anatomic correlation. Cortical myoclonus is possibly a disorder of decreased cortical inhibition, although the reason for the reduced inhibition is unknown. Its frequent association with seizure disorders suggests a common pathophysiologic mechanism for myoclonus and some forms of epilepsy. Mechanisms for subcortical and spinal myoclonus are even less well appreciated.

CLINICAL PRESENTATION

Physiologic Nonpathologic Myoclonus

Shocklike contractions of the arms or legs during sleep or as individuals drift off to sleep are a common form of physiologic myoclonus, sometimes described as *physiologic sleep myoclonus*.

Pathologic Myoclonus

It is essential to distinguish the various forms of presumed pathologic myoclonus (see Table 33.1).

Essential myoclonus is an isolated neurologic finding that has no association with seizures, dementia, or ataxia. It is nonprogressive, usually multifocal in distribution, typically induced by voluntary movements (action myoclonus), and usually responds to alcohol (Fig. 33.1).

Although often familial, essential myoclonus can occur sporadically. Familial essential myoclonus appears to be an autosomal dominant trait with reduced penetrance and variable expressivity. Symptoms typically begin before the age of 20 years. Essential myoclonus often occurs in association with other movement disorders, particularly tremor and dystonia.

Various forms of epilepsy may be accompanied by myoclonus. For example, in forms of idiopathic epilepsy, such as juvenile myoclonic epilepsy and benign myoclonus of infancy, myoclonus may be a primary finding.

TABLE 33.1   Etiologies of Pathologic Myoclonus

Type of Myoclonus	Etiologies
Essential	Autosomal dominant trait with reduced penetrance and variable expressivity
Myoclonic epilepsy	Juvenile myoclonic epilepsy, benign myoclonus of infancy
Secondary	Brain trauma, infection, inflammation, tumors (neoplasms), or cerebral hypoxia due to temporary lack of oxygen (i.e., postanoxic myoclonus or Lance-Adams syndrome)
Spinal	Spinal cord trauma, infection, inflammation, or lesions may produce segmental myoclonus
Inborn biochemical errors	Inborn errors of metabolism (lysosomal storage diseases: Tay-Sachs disease, Sandhoff disease, sialidosis)
Infectious	Creutzfeldt-Jakob disease, subacute sclerosing panencephalitis (SSPE), Whipple disease (facial myoclonus—oculofacial masticatory monorhythmia)
Neuroimmunologic	Stiffman variant: encephalomyelitis with rigidity
Neurodegenerative	Parkinsonism, Huntington disease, Alzheimer disease, Lafora disease, corticobasal degeneration, progressive supranuclear palsy, or olivopontocerebellar atrophy
Metabolic	Metabolic conditions, such as kidney, liver, or respiratory failure, hypokalemia, hyperglycemia, etc.
Mitochondrial	Mitochondrial encephalomyopathy, particularly myoclonic epilepsy with ragged red fibers (MERFF) syndrome (myoclonus epilepsy with ragged-red fibers), or other progressive myoclonic encephalopathies, including those characterized by epilepsy and dementia (e.g., Lafora disease) or epilepsy and ataxia (e.g., Unverricht-Lundborg disease)
Medications: drug-induced myoclonus	Serotonin receptor inhibitors: serotonin syndrome; toxic levels of anticonvulsants, levodopa, and certain antipsychotic agents (tardive myoclonus)
Toxins	Exposure to toxic agents, such as bismuth or other metals

TABLE 33.2   Classification of Myoclonus

Classification Bases	Classifications
Affected body part	Focal
	Segmental
	Multifocal
	Generalized
Provoking symptom	Spontaneous
	Reflex
	Action
Neurophysiology	Cortical
	Subcortical
	Spinal
Etiology	Physiologic
	Essential
	Myoclonic epilepsy
	Secondary
Additional forms	Palatal myoclonus
	Periodic limb movements of sleep
	Psychogenic myoclonus

In psychogenic myoclonus, symptoms have a mental or emotional basis rather than an organic origin. In most patients, the condition worsens with stress or anxiety. The myoclonus can be segmental or generalized.

DIFFERENTIAL DIAGNOSIS

Myoclonus must be differentiated from other movement disorders, including tics, tremors, ataxia, and chorea. When the jerks are single or repetitive but arrhythmic, a tic diagnosis should be considered. A history of an urge associated with tics is helpful in the diagnosis. In contrast, organic myoclonus is usually briefer and less coordinated or patterned than tics.

Rhythmic forms of myoclonus may be confused with tremors. The pattern of myoclonus is more repetitive, abrupt-onset, square-wave movements, unlike the smoother sinusoidal activity of tremor. Rhythmic myoclonus usually ranges from 1 to 4 Hz, differing from faster tremor frequencies.

Myoclonus, particularly action (intention) myoclonus, is often confused with cerebellar ataxia. Myoclonic jerking occurs during voluntary motor activity, especially when patients attempt to perform a fine motor task, such as reaching for a target.

DIAGNOSTIC EVALUATION

A diagnosis of myoclonus is based on a thorough clinical assessment, evaluation of the nature of the myoclonus (e.g., electrophysiologic characteristics), bodily distribution, provocative factors, and a careful family history. Examination and observation of patients with myoclonus are important diagnostic steps. However, patients with myoclonus can have entirely normal examination results, particularly with physiologic and essential myoclonus. When myoclonus is present during examination, characterization of its rhythm, repetitiveness, onset, and frequency is important. Because myoclonus may occur with other movement disorders, it is important to look for evidence of dystonia, tremor, ataxia, or spasticity.

The clinical distribution of the myoclonus is also helpful. Focal myoclonus is more commonly associated with CNS lesions. Segmental

Any underlying disease process or cause of CNS dysfunction may lead to secondary myoclonus (see Fig. 33.1).

Additional Forms of Myoclonus

Palatal myoclonus has rapid, rhythmic jerking of muscle of one or both sides of the soft palate. It is more appropriately classified as a form of tremor despite continued use of the term *palatal myoclonus.*

Periodic limb movements of sleep differ from physiologic sleep myoclonus in that they typically consist of repeated, stereotypic, upward extension of the great toe and foot, possibly followed by flexion of the hip, knee, or ankle. These usually involve both legs, tend to occur in repeated episodes lasting a few minutes to several hours, and occur during non-REM sleep. An association with restless legs syndrome is common.

Essential Myoclonus

Usually multifocal in distribution, often familial, typically induced by voluntary movements causing a single jerk of the extremity (action myoclonus). Symptoms begin before age 20 and frequently occur associated with tremor, dystonia, and other movement disorders.

Commonly, essential myoclonus responds to ingestion of alcohol.

Lance-Adams Syndrome

Prolonged hypoxia may result in posthypoxic myoclonus, which is usually stimulus sensitive.

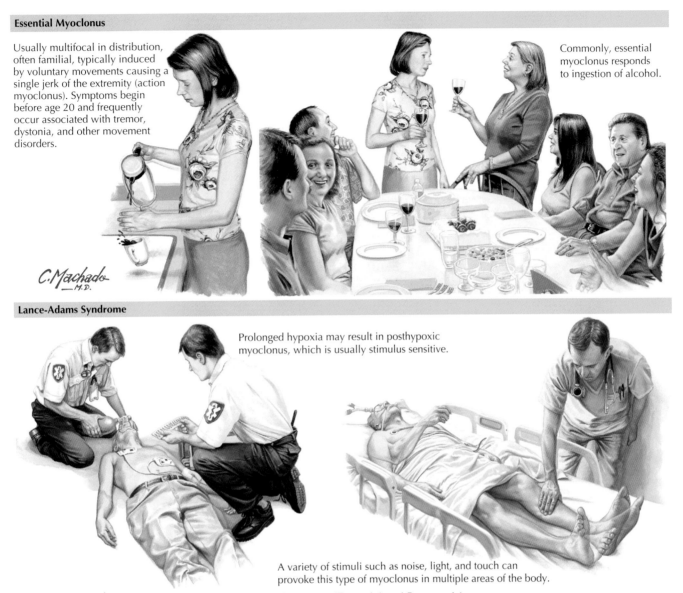

A variety of stimuli such as noise, light, and touch can provoke this type of myoclonus in multiple areas of the body.

Fig. 33.1 Myoclonus (Essential and Postanoxic).

involvement may suggest brainstem or spinal cord lesions. Multifocal or generalized myoclonus suggests a more diffuse disorder, as seen in diffuse postanoxic insults. This particularly involves the reticular substance of the brainstem. Precipitating factors are important for stimulus-sensitive myoclonus. Therefore somesthetic sensory input testing is needed. It is important to determine whether the myoclonus occurs spontaneously and whether symptoms improve or worsen with voluntary activity.

During testing for negative myoclonus (asterixis), patients are asked to extend their arms with the wrists back or to perform another movement that requires holding the limb against gravity. In this way, a sudden loss of muscle contraction causes the hand or the arm to fall downward.

Specialized testing can be used to determine the site of the abnormal neuronal discharge within the CNS (e.g., cerebral cortex, brainstem, or spinal cord) and establish the underlying cause. These studies typically primarily include EEG, and less commonly electromyography, or somatosensory evoked potential testing. Neuroimaging studies such as MRI or computed tomography can on rare occasions demonstrate structural lesions. Other specialized diagnostic tests may help to exclude particular conditions such as hereditary, metabolic, mitochondrial, infectious, vascular, neoplastic, toxic, or neurodegenerative processes.

TREATMENT AND PROGNOSIS

The treatment of myoclonus varies depending on the type. If a specific cause is found, myoclonus usually resolves with effective treatment of the underlying disease. A good example is juvenile myoclonic epilepsy. This usually responds to valproate and may require lifelong treatment. Less specific symptomatic therapy typically includes medications to reduce the severity of the myoclonus, such as benzodiazepines. Cortical myoclonus may respond to valproate, piracetam, levetiracetam, or lamotrigine. Myoclonus from an anoxic event may respond to 5-hydroxytryptophan, and this may help in other causes. Carbamazepine may worsen myoclonus and should be avoided.

Prognosis depends on the form of myoclonus. In general, although myoclonus is not a life-threatening condition, it may be secondary to serious, debilitating fatal diseases such as individuals with

Creutzfeldt-Jakob disease. Postanoxic myoclonus is another disorder that is associated with an extremely poor prognosis in the postcardiac arrest individual.

Researchers are attempting to clarify the genetic and molecular aspects of myoclonus. Newer physiologic techniques, such as magnetoencephalography, are being used to study cortical activity in cortical reflex myoclonus.

ADDITIONAL RESOURCES

Carr J. Classifying myoclonus a riddle, wrapped in a mystery, inside an enigma. Parkinsonism Relat Disord 2012;18(Suppl. 1):S174–6.

Caviness JN. Myoclonus. Parkinsonism Relat D 2007;13(Suppl. 3):S375–84.

Caviness JN. Treatment of myoclonus. Neurother 2014;11(1):188–200.

Caviness JN, Truong DD. Myoclonus. Handb Clin Neurol 2011;100:399.

Freund B, Kaplan PW. Post-hypoxic myoclonus: differentiating benign and malignant etiologies and prognosis. Clin Neurophysiol Pract 2017;2:98–102.

Hallet M. Neurophysiology of brainstem myoclonus. Adv Neurol 2002;89:99–102.

Levy A, Chen R. Myoclonus: pathophysiology and treatment options. Curr Treat Options Neurol 2016;18(5):21.

Rubboli G, Tassinari CA. Negative myoclonus. An overview of its clinical features, pathophysiological mechanism, and management. Neurophysiol Clin 2006;36(5–6):337–43.

Shafiq M, Lang AE. Myoclonus in parkinsonian disorders. Adv Neurol 2002;89:77–83.

34

Tic Disorders

Julie Leegwater-Kim

CLINICAL VIGNETTE *A 9-year-old boy presented to the neurology clinic with 1 year of excessive eye blinking. He was accompanied by his parents. His past medical history was unremarkable; he was born at term and reached all developmental milestones appropriately. Schoolwork has been average; he frequently loses pencils and articles of clothing. He has difficulty finishing his homework. During the past year, his parents have noticed a significant increase in his eye blinking and mention that he grimaces often. The patient is aware of the blinking and has been told by his classmates that he "squints" and "makes funny faces." He is embarrassed by the movements. His neurologic exam was notable for eye blinking, sniffing, nose wrinkling, and contraction of the platysma. He was able to suppress the movements volitionally. He was prescribed guanfacine. After 8 weeks, he returned to the office with his parents. He reported lessening of his tics. His parents felt he was performing better in school.*

PHENOMENOLOGY AND CLASSIFICATION

Tics are sudden, relatively quick, stereotyped movements (motor tics) or sounds (phonic tics) that are repeated at irregular intervals. Tics are often preceded by a premonitory urge or inner sensory stimulus and can be suppressed at will. Therefore they are referred to as semivoluntary, or unvoluntary, movements.

Tics are categorized as simple or complex (Box 34.1). Simple motor tics involve only one group of muscles and are characterized by quick, jerklike movements. Usually they are abrupt in onset and brief *(clonic tics)*, but they can also be slower and sustained *(dystonic tics)*. Examples of *simple motor tics* include eye blinking, nose twitching, and shoulder shrugging. Simple phonic tics include sniffing, throat clearing, and grunting. *Complex motor tics* are sequenced and coordinated movements that can resemble gestures or fragments of normal behavior (e.g., kicking, jumping) and, rarely, inappropriate behavior (e.g., showing the middle finger). Complex phonic tics have a semantic basis, including words, parts of words, and obscene words (coprolalia).

It is important to distinguish tics from other hyperkinetic movement disorders. For example, simple motor tics can resemble myoclonus. However, clonic tics are stereotyped, rather than random, are suppressible, and are typically accompanied by a premonitory sensation.

The most common tic disorder is *Tourette syndrome* (**TS**), which is characterized by motor and phonic tics. The Tourette Syndrome Classification Study Group has formulated diagnostic criteria for TS that include the presence of both motor and phonic tics, although not necessarily concurrently; the presence of tics for at least 1 year; fluctuation in tic type, frequency, and severity; and onset before age 21 years. Tics of duration less than a year are classified as *transient tic disorder.* When only one category of chronic tics can be identified, the term *chronic motor tic disorder* or *chronic vocal tic disorder* is used.

CAUSES OF TIC DISORDERS

Tic disorders can be primary or secondary (Box 34.2). Primary tic disorders are discussed in the previous section and include transient tic disorder, chronic motor tic disorder, chronic vocal tic disorder, and TS. Less commonly, tics can be secondary to other causes, including neurodegenerative illnesses (i.e., Huntington disease, neuroacanthocytosis), infection (i.e., viral encephalitis), global developmental syndromes (i.e., static encephalopathy, autism spectrum disorders), and drugs (i.e., amphetamines, lamotrigine). Secondary causes should always be considered in adult-onset tic disorders.

The pathogenesis of tic disorders is unknown, but biochemical, neuroimaging, and genetic data suggest an abnormality in the cortico-striato-thalamocortical circuits and their neurotransmitter systems. One hypothesis suggests that there is disinhibition of excitatory neurons in the thalamus resulting in hyperexcitability of the cortical motor areas. Dysfunction of dopamine neurotransmission has been implicated, with recent evidence suggesting excessive dopaminergic activity via abnormal presynaptic terminal function, dopamine hyperinnervation, and/or dopamine receptor supersensitivity.

CLINICAL COURSE AND NATURAL HISTORY OF TOURETTE SYNDROME

In TS, symptoms typically begin in childhood, usually by age 7 years. Early in the course, tics frequently involve the face, head, and neck (Fig. 34.1). Vocal tics tend to start later (ages 8–15 years). The frequency and severity of tics fluctuate over time, with peak severity occurring at approximately 10 years of age. The anatomic locations and complexity of tics also tend to change over time. The vast majority of TS patients (85%) experience reduction in tics during and after adolescence. Tics can be exacerbated by stress, fatigue, central nervous system (CNS) stimulants, and caffeine. Alleviation of tics can occur with focused mental and physical exercise, relaxation, and exposure to nicotine and cannabinoids.

Tic disorders are frequently associated with a wide range of neuropsychiatric disorders. Approximately 50% of patients with TS have obsessive-compulsive disorder (OCD), and 50% exhibit attention-deficit/hyperactivity disorder (ADHD). In addition, affective disorders, impulse control disorders, anxiety, and rage attacks can be seen in patients with TS.

THERAPIES

There are both nonpharmacologic and pharmacologic treatments for tics. It is important to recognize that the mere presence of tics does not necessarily imply a need to initiate pharmacologic treatment. One initially needs to determine the degree to which tics are interfering with functioning at school, at work, or at home and any disability associated

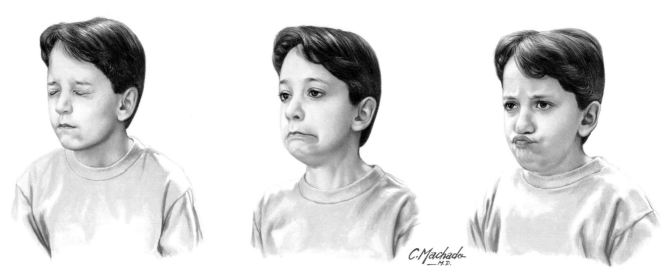

Tics involving the eyes, i.e., eye-blinking, are the most common tics in childhood-onset tic disorders. Patients with tic disorders frequently develop other motor tics of the head and neck, including grimacing and frowning.

Fig. 34.1 Common Motor Tics.

BOX 34.1 Tic Types—Examples

Simple Motor
Eye blinking
Nose twitching
Head jerking
Shoulder shrugging
Tensing of abdominal muscles

Simple Vocal
Sniffing
Grunting
Throat clearing
Screaming

Complex Motor
Touching
Throwing
Hitting
Jumping
Obscene gestures (copropraxia)

Complex Vocal
Repetition of words
Repetition of obscenities (coprolalia)
Repetition of parts of words (palilalia)
Repetition of another person's words (echolalia)

BOX 34.2 Tic Disorders—Causes

Primary
Transient tic disorder
Chronic motor or vocal tic disorder
Tourette syndrome

Secondary
Infectious
  • Encephalitis
Neurodegenerative
  • Pantothenate kinase–associated neurodegeneration
  • Huntington disease
  • Wilson disease
  • Neuroacanthocytosis
Autoimmune
  • Sydenham chorea
  • Antiphospholipid antibody syndrome
Drug Induced
  • Side effect: lamotrigine, carbamazepine, methylphenidate, cocaine
  • Tardive syndrome: typical and atypical neuroleptics
Toxins
  • Carbon monoxide
Developmental
  • Mental retardation
  • Autism spectrum disorders

---

with tics. In addition, comorbidities such as ADHD, OCD, and mood disorders need to be assessed. If tics are mild, educational and psychosocial interventions can be implemented for treatment of tics. Habit reversal training, a behavioral approach, has been shown to reduce tic severity. If tics are more severe and disabling, medication treatment should be considered (Box 34.3).

The *alpha-agonists* clonidine and guanfacine have moderate efficacy in treating tic disorders and are often considered as *first-line treatments* because of their relatively low side effect burden. In addition, they can be helpful in treating concomitant ADHD.

Dopamine receptor–blocking agents are effective in the treatment of tics. These drugs include both typical (haloperidol, fluphenazine,

---

BOX 34.3 Pharmacologic Treatment for Tics

Alpha agonists: clonidine, guanfacine
Neuroleptics
  Atypical neuroleptics: risperidone, olanzapine, aripiprazole
  Typical neuroleptics: pimozide, haloperidol, fluphenazine
Dopamine depletor: tetrabenazine
Benzodiazepine: clonazepam
Dopamine agonists: pergolide, ropinirole
Botulinum toxin injections

BOX 34.4   Tourette Syndrome (TS) DBS Guidelines

Inclusion Criteria

- DSM-V diagnosis of TS by expert clinician
- No specific age requirement but ethics committee should be involved in TS cases younger than 18 years of age
- Severe tic disorder with functional impairment with Yale Global Tic Severity Scale (YGTSS) score >35/50
- Tics are primary cause of disability
- Comorbid neuropsychiatric and medical conditions stably treated × 6 months
- Tics refractory to conservative therapies: failed trials of medications from three pharmacologic classes; Cognitive Behavioral Intervention Therapy (CBIT) offered
- Optimization of treatment of comorbid medical conditions for >6 months prior to DBS
- Psychosocial environment is stable
- Demonstrated ability to adhere to recommended treatments
- Neuropsychological profile indicates candidate can tolerate demands of surgery, postoperative follow-up, and possibility of poor outcome

Exclusion Criteria

- Active suicidal or homicidal ideation within 6 months
- Active or recent substance abuse
- Structural lesions on brain magnetic resonance imaging (MRI)
- Medical, neurologic, or psychiatric disorders that increase the risk of a failed procedure or interference with postoperative management
- Malingering, factitious disorder, or psychogenic tics

DBS, Deep brain stimulation; *DSM-V,* Diagnostic and Statistical Manual of Mental Disorders, Fifth Edition.

pimozide) and atypical (risperidone, olanzapine) neuroleptics. Although these drugs are often highly effective, they can cause numerous side effects, including sedation, weight gain, metabolic syndrome, and tardive dyskinesia. The atypical neuroleptics, quetiapine and clozapine, are associated with lower risk of tardive syndrome, but they tend to be less effective in treating tics.

Tetrabenazine, a *dopamine-depleting* agent, has also shown efficacy in treatment of tics and is often preferred over neuroleptics because of the negligible risk of tardive dyskinesia. Common dose-related side effects include depression, akathisia, parkinsonism, and sedation.

Other agents that have tic-suppressing effects include clonazepam, dopamine agonists (low-dose ropinirole and pergolide), and levetiracetam.

Botulinum toxin injections into the affected muscles can be considered for simple motor tics, especially dystonic tics. Reduction in premonitory urge, as well as reduction in tic frequency, has been reported with botulinum toxin therapy.

In patients with severe tic disorders that are disabling and refractory to medication and behavioral therapies, deep brain stimulation (DBS) surgery has been used. Although the most effective anatomic target for DBS in tic disorders has not been established, clinical improvement has been reported in cases targeting the centromedian-parafascicular complex of the thalamus, the globus pallidus internus, the nucleus accumbens, and the anterior limb of the internal capsule. Guidelines for the selection of TS candidates for DBS have been proposed based on data from the Tourette Syndrome International DBS Database/Registry (Box 34.4). Further controlled trials of DBS in TS are needed to confirm the efficacy of DBS in TS and the optimal surgical target.

ADDITIONAL RESOURCES

Gunduz A, Okun MS. A review and update on Tourette's syndrome: where is the field headed? Curr Neurol Neurosci Rep 2016;16:37.

Schrock LE, Mink JW, et al. Tourette syndrome deep brain stimulation: a review and updated recommendations. Mov Disord 2015;30:447–71.

Shprecher D, Kurlan R. The management of tics. Mov Disord 2009;24:15–24.

35

Medication-Induced Movement Disorders

Diana Apetauerova

CLINICAL VIGNETTE *A 52-year-old Caucasian woman presented to a psychiatrist with her first manic episode. Patient had never been treated with any antipsychotic medication in her life. During the current episode, she was treated with aripiprazole 30 mg/day. During a follow-up visit 3 months later, the patient was found to have developed involuntary orofacial movements. She was not taking any other antipsychotic or antidopaminergic medications. The patient's psychiatrist immediately discontinued aripiprazole, but unfortunately involuntary movements persisted. Physical exam showed involuntary chewing movements of jaw, lip smacking, infrequent tongue protrusion, and twisting and side-to-side movement of the tongue. Her routine laboratory examinations (complete blood count, liver function test, and urine analysis), serum copper, ceruloplasmin, and thyroid-stimulating hormone levels were within normal limits. Computed tomography (CT) scan of head (without contrast) was negative for any acute changes. She was diagnosed with tardive dyskinesia (TD) and was then treated with various psychotropics including quetiapine, lamotrigine, and sodium valproate to control her mood symptoms. Unfortunately, TD symptoms persisted prompting initiation of tetrabenazine with subsequent improvement of tongue and lip movements.*

There are a large number of pharmaceutical agents with the potential to cause a movement disorder (Table 35.1). These medications primarily interfere with dopaminergic transmission within the basal ganglia (levodopa, dopamine agonists, dopamine receptor–blocking agents [DRBs]). Other classes of these movement disorder–inducing agents do not have as precisely defined biochemical mechanisms. These medications include central nervous system (CNS) stimulants, anticonvulsants, tricyclic antidepressants, and estrogens. From a clinical perspective, the medications most commonly responsible for iatrogenic movement disorders are the various neuroleptics and pharmacologic agents that block or stimulate dopamine receptors.

The clinical temporal profile of drug-induced movement disorders can be acute, subacute, or chronic. Acute syndromes include dystonia, choreoathetosis, akathisia, and tics. Subacute syndromes include drug-induced parkinsonism and tremor. Chronic syndromes include levodopa-induced dyskinesias in Parkinson disease and tardive dyskinesia (TD). There is no direct evidence of precise CNS pathology predisposing to the development of drug-induced movement disorders. Because no precise pathoanatomic correlation or model is known, a primary biochemical mechanism is therefore the likely responsible pathophysiologic mechanism here.

CLINICAL SYNDROMES

Neuroleptic Malignant Syndrome

Neuroleptic malignant syndrome (NMS) is a very unusual complication and is one of the most severe reactions to neuroleptic therapy. It has a relatively high incidence (0.5%–1%) considering the very large numbers of patients taking neuroleptic medication. Symptoms typically occur shortly after institution of neuroleptic therapy or at the time of initiating increased dosage. Young men are at higher risk than the general population. Pathogenesis is thought to involve both central and peripheral effects of dopamine receptor blockade.

Typically, NMS patients present with an acute onset of a severe movement disorder characterized by rigidity, tremor, and dystonia. There are often manifestations of very significant dysautonomic disturbances, including fever, diaphoresis, and cardiovascular/pulmonary dysfunction. Often the patients are stuporous, and a very intense concomitant myonecrosis usually accompanies the NMS; this leads to significant elevation of serum creatine kinase (usually >1000 IU/L) with its own innate risk of significant renal compromise. There is an associated leukocytosis. The fatality rate in NMS may reach as much as 20% because of the various associated complications, including dehydration, cardiac arrhythmias, pulmonary embolism, and renal failure. As soon as this clinical setting of NMS is recognized, it is very important to begin treatment. Medications that are frequently useful include levodopa, dopamine agonists, and the antispastic agent dantrolene.

Acute Dystonic Reactions

These very dramatic movement disorder syndromes usually develop within 5 days after initiation of various neuroleptic medications. This clinical picture typically presents very rapidly after initiation of the responsible therapeutic agent. The craniocervical region is the most commonly affected site. These patients are sometimes thought to have tetanus because the facial spasms may mimic the classic trismus with risus sardonicus (Fig. 35.1).

Pathophysiologically, these disorders are related to a sudden imbalance between the striatal dopamine and cholinergic systems. Typically these disorders are diagnosed by their relatively acute resolution either spontaneously subsequent to drug withdrawal or more immediately by parenteral administration of an antihistamine, such as diphenhydramine, or sometimes anticholinergics.

Medication-Induced Parkinsonism

Various medications have the potential to interfere with the synthesis, storage, and release of dopamine, as well as the varied dopamine-blocking agents, and may precipitate an akinetic-rigid syndrome that is nearly indistinguishable from idiopathic Parkinson disease (Fig. 35.2). Substituted benzamides, particularly metoclopramide, used to treat gastrointestinal disorders, and calcium channel blockers particularly have the potential to produce a medication-induced parkinsonism. The basic pathophysiologic mechanism here is related to a predominant presynaptic effect on dopamine and serotonin neurons.

TABLE 35.1 Types of Drug-Induced Movement Disorders and Responsible Medications

Syndrome	Responsible Medication	Syndrome	Responsible Medication
Postural tremor	Sympathomimetics	Chorea, including tardive and orofacial dyskinesia	Antipsychotics
	Levodopa		Metoclopramide
	Amphetamines		Levodopa
	Bronchodilators		Direct dopamine agonists
	Tricyclic antidepressants		Indirect dopamine agonists and other catecholaminergic drugs
	Lithium carbonate		Anticholinergics
	Caffeine		Antihistaminics
	Thyroid hormone		Oral contraceptives
	Sodium valproate		Phenytoin
	Antipsychotics		Carbamazepine
	Hypoglycemic agents		Ethosuximide
	Adrenocorticosteroids		Phenobarbital
	Alcohol withdrawal		Lithium carbonate
	Amiodarone		Methadone
	Cyclosporin A		Benzodiazepines
	Others		Monoamine oxidase inhibitors
Acute dystonic reactions	Antipsychotics		Tricyclic antidepressants
	Metoclopramide		Methyldopa
	Antimalarial agents		Digoxin
	Tetrabenazine		Alcohol withdrawal
	Diphenhydramine		Toluene sniffing
	Mefenamic acid		Flunarizine and cinnarizine
	Oxatomide	Dystonia, including tardive dystonia (excluding acute dystonic reactions)	Antipsychotics
	Flunarizine and cinnarizine		Metoclopramide
Akathisia	Antipsychotics		Levodopa
	Metoclopramide		Direct dopamine agonists
	Reserpine		Phenytoin
	Tetrabenazine		Carbamazepine
	Levodopa and dopamine agonists		Flunarizine and cinnarizine
	Flunarizine and cinnarizine	Neuroleptic malignant syndrome	Antipsychotics
	Ethosuximide		Tetrabenazine with α-methyl-*para*-tyrosine
	Methysergide		Antiparkinsonian drugs withdrawal
Parkinsonism	Antipsychotics	Tics	Levodopa
	Metoclopramide		Direct dopamine agonists
	Reserpine		Antipsychotics
	Tetrabenazine		Carbamazepine
	Methyldopa	Myoclonus	Levodopa
	Flunarizine and cinnarizine		Anticonvulsants
	Lithium		Tricyclic antidepressants
	Phenytoin		Antipsychotics
	Captopril	Asterixis	Anticonvulsants
	Alcohol withdrawal		Levodopa
	MPTP (1-methyl-4-phenyl-1,2,3,6-tetrahydropyridine)		Hepatotoxins
	Other toxins (manganese, carbon disulfide, cyanide)		Respiratory depressants
	Cytosine arabinoside		

In contrast to Parkinson disease, where the presentation often has a focal distribution, therapeutic medication–induced parkinsonism is often characterized by a symmetric bilateral presentation. Bradykinesia predominates over typical rigidity and resting tremor. When a tremor is present, it is usually postural instead of resting. Although drug-induced parkinsonism may persist long after withdrawal of the offending drug, eventually most patients improve without further therapeutic interventions if use of the offending drug can be stopped.

Akathisia

This unusual disorder is typified by an inability to keep still; subjectively, it is often accompanied by feelings of restlessness, primarily resulting from the initiation of neuroleptic therapy. Akathisia is the most poorly understood, acute drug-induced syndrome; no neuroanatomic correlates explain it. Dose reduction or withdrawal of the offending drug is the most effective treatment. At times, introduction of other medications, such as propranolol and clonidine, can provide reasonable treatment. The

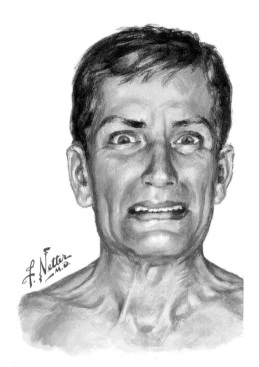

Spasm of jaw, facial, and neck muscles (trismus [lockjaw], risus sardonicus), and dysphagia are often early symptoms after variable incubation period.

Fig. 35.1 Acute Dystonic Reaction.

pathophysiologic mechanisms are not well defined. It is known that these neuroleptics have little or no direct effect on beta-adrenergic receptors.

Tardive Dyskinesia Syndromes

The prevalence of TD varies between 0.5% and 65%, making it the most feared complication of long-term neuroleptic therapy. These syndromes present after a latency period following initiation of these various inciting medications. They usually do not present until at least 3 months after—or, more commonly, 1–2 years after—the patient begins taking the responsible medication. The timing of presentation for these disorders can be varied during treatment per se, after dose reduction, or subsequent to medication withdrawal. Unfortunately, some of these syndromes are irreversible. Neuroleptics are the most common offending drugs, particularly because of dopamine receptor blocking.

Most commonly, TD clinically affects the orofacial region, in particular, various chewing movements, tongue protrusion, vermicular tongue motion, lip smacking, puckering, and pursing (Fig. 35.3A). TD

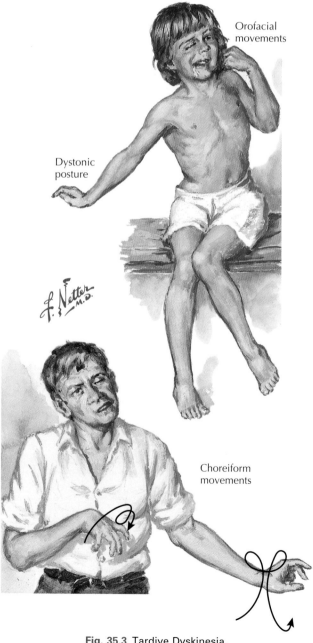

Orofacial movements

Dystonic posture

Choreiform movements

Fig. 35.3 Tardive Dyskinesia.

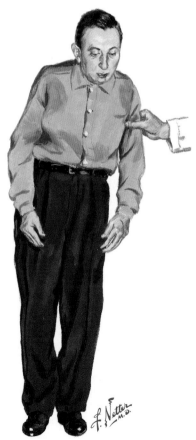

Fig. 35.2 Medication-Induced Parkinsonism.

patients also have hyperkinesias, including chorea (see Fig. 35.3B), athetosis, dystonia, and tics affecting the limb and truncal regions, or paroxysms of rapid eye blinking. Various risk factors are thought to be operative, including female sex, older age, and duration and dosage of therapy. It may take months for TD to resolve if it is going to do so, and sadly this is not predictable.

The primary pathophysiology of TD is only partly appreciated. Currently it is thought that striatal dopamine receptors are chronically blocked by DRBs. Subsequently, these receptors develop supersensitivity to small amounts of dopamine that would be too small to induce dyskinesia in an otherwise healthy individual. An updated version of the dopamine hypothesis suggests that an imbalance between D1 and D2 receptor-mediated effects in the basal ganglia may also be responsible for TD. According to this theory, traditional antipsychotic drugs preferentially block D2 receptors, resulting in excessive activity of D1-mediated striatopallidal output, altered firing patterns in medial globus pallidus, and eventual evolution of the clinical features of TD. The persistence of TD after drug withdrawal also suggests that there is underactivity of gamma-aminobutyric acid (GABA)-mediated inhibition of the thalamocortical pathway and an excitotoxic DRB mechanism.

DIAGNOSIS

Careful clinical observation and review of the patient's medication history are the primary keys to the diagnosis of drug-induced movement disorders. When there is no well-defined pharmacologic predisposition defined, the possibility of other etiologic mechanisms must be considered to exclude hereditary or systemic illness. Extraordinarily rare structural basal ganglia lesions require consideration, and a magnetic resonance image (MRI) needs to be performed.

The differential diagnosis of TD is sometimes a difficult one, including idiopathic movement disorders such as psychotic patients having stereotypic behavior, Tourette syndrome, simple or complex motor tics, and possible dental problems. Other drug-induced dyskinesias deserve consideration, particularly with the acute dystonic reaction secondary to antiemetics such as chlorpromazine. Here intravenous diphenylhydramine can be both therapeutic and diagnostic. Inheritable disorders including Huntington disease, Wilson disease, and pantothenate kinase–associated neurodegeneration with brain iron accumulation type 1 disease also require consideration in the differential diagnosis. Some systemic illnesses are also associated with various dyskinesias: hyperthyroidism, hypoparathyroidism, hyperglycemia, chorea of pregnancy, and Sydenham chorea. Inflammatory or space-occupying brain lesions may rarely cause a pseudo-TD.

TREATMENT

No single therapeutic strategy is significantly effective for TD. Thus prevention, early detection, and management of potentially reversible causes are the cornerstones of modern treatment. Reduction or withdrawal of medication, when possible, is advisable. Drugs most commonly used in its treatment include vesicular monoamine transporter 2 (VMAT2) inhibitors such as tetrabenazine, velbenazine, and deutetrabenazine; benzodiazepines, anticholinergics (trihexyphenidyl, benztropine), and Botulinum toxin injections. It is unclear whether second-generation (atypical) antipsychotic drugs like clozapine and quetiapine have ameliorating effects on TD severity; they may have antipsychotic drug "sparing" effect, in which gradual improvement of TD occurs during treatment with weaker (second generation) rather than more potent (first generation) dopamine blocking agents.

PROGNOSIS

Medication-induced movement disorders have primarily been studied in individual case reports. Solid epidemiologic data are lacking. Although once considered a permanent condition, TD is often reversible, especially when identified early in younger populations. The associated remission rate is 50%–90% of the patients. Remission of TD usually occurs within several months after antipsychotic drug withdrawal but may occur as late as 1–3 years. The prognosis of TD in patients who require continued antipsychotic drug treatment is unknown.

ADDITIONAL RESOURCES

Esper CD, Factor SA. Failure of recognition of drug-induced parkinsonism in the elderly. Mov Disord 2008;23(3):401–4.

Fernandez HH, Friedman JH. Classification and treatment of tardive syndromes. Neurologist 2003;9:16.

Gershanik OS. Drug-induced dyskinesia. In: Anodic J, Tolosa E, editors. Parkinson's disease and movement disorders. Baltimore, Md: Williams & Wilkins; 1998. pp. 579–600.

Kiriakakis V, Bhatia K, Quinn NP, et al. The natural history of tardive dystonia: a long-term follow-up study of 107 cases. Brain 1998;121:2053–66.

Mena MA, de Yebenes JG. Drug-induced parkinsonism. Expert Opin Drug Saf 2006;5(6):759–71.

Pierre JM. Extrapyramidal symptoms with atypical antipsychotics; incidence, prevention and management. Drug Saf 2005;28(3):191–208.

Tarsy D, Indorf G. Tardive tremor due to metoclopramide. Mov Disord 2002;17:620.

36

Psychogenic Movement Disorders

Diana Apetauerova

CLINICAL VIGNETTE *A 25-year-old swimming champion presented with sudden onset of gait disturbance and tremor. She presented to the clinic with her boyfriend and mother. On examination, she walked slowly and gingerly with her arms held out and fell repeatedly in the arms of her boyfriend who shadowed her for fear that she would fall and injure herself. She also exhibited tremor which appeared when arms were raised and was distractible. When she was speaking about difficulties with her coach she developed a course tremor of her trunk which caused a chair she was sitting on to creak. However, she was able to dial numbers of her smartphone without any difficulties. Her symptoms continued to worsen over a period of 18 months. After 18 months, she was cured by a faith healer. She then walked quite normally for several years until she gave birth to her first child. At this time of great emotional stress and physical exhaustion, her tremor and gait disturbance returned. She was treated as an inpatient with rehabilitation and made a rapid recovery.*

Psychogenic, psychosomatic, hysterical, or functional movement disorders are conditions related to an underlying psychiatric illness with no evidence of any organic etiology. One has to be very cautious. There is a major inherent difficulty whenever one entertains a diagnosis of a psychogenic movement disorder, because studies demonstrate that this is a too common and poorly documented diagnosis, in that up to 30% of patients diagnosed with *psychogenic disorders* eventually are found to have an organic neurologic illness. Because, with just a few exceptions, most movement disorders have no specific diagnostic laboratory or imaging study available, beyond clinical observation, there is a temptation by the uninitiated to label a patient hysterical when the clinician cannot arrive at a definitive organic diagnosis. An important diagnostic caveat is for the evaluating physician to not rush to judgment when the patient's findings do not initially fit a specific diagnostic set, such as pill-rolling rest tremor, cogwheel rigidity, masked facies, and en bloc walking as is typical of Parkinson disease. Astute clinicians often use a "tincture of time" to prospectively and carefully follow patients by repeated clinical evaluations. Here one monitors the individual patient for the gradual development of recognized classic signs of an evolving and well-recognized neurologic process. Barring the later clinical evolution of symptoms and findings into a more classic organic movement disorder, the clinician will gradually acquire information from the patient or family to become more comfortable with the importance of underlying psychogenic factors.

A variety of underlying psychiatric diagnoses are found in patients with psychogenic neurologic movement disorders; these include various somatoform and factitious disorders, malingering, depression, anxiety, and histrionic personality disorders. Although a specific psychiatric diagnosis cannot always be confirmed for these various abnormal and consistently inconsistent motor symptoms, despite the clinician's high suspicion of psychogenicity, an emotionally based diagnosis is not totally precluded. Often it is only time and a cautious diagnostic approach that will allow one to sort out the majority of these challenging patients' specific diagnosis. In young women, one has to be particularly careful to not overlook sexual abuse, particularly incest.

Psychogenic tremor, dystonia, myoclonus, chorea, and parkinsonism are the typical means for a functional movement disorder to present and are particularly common in women (Fig. 36.1). These patients usually have multiplicity and variability of symptoms superimposed on a significant psychiatric background. The neurologic findings do not fit a specific diagnostic set typical of the classic organic movement disorders. These factitious patients present with movements that are consistently inconsistent and are particularly liable to change or decrease during distraction. Frequently, patients with psychogenic movement disorders display uneconomic postures demonstrating a most exaggerated effort during examination that may also produce fatigue. They may demonstrate marked slowness when asked to perform certain tasks such as rapid alternating movements.

Therapeutically, psychogenic movement disorders often respond to placebo or suggestion.

ETIOLOGY

Because the etiologies of psychogenic movement disorders are unknown, no anatomic correlation can be made. It is totally conjectural as to whether any neurochemical interplay exists or will later be recognized, between the effect of the presumed underlying psychiatric condition and the patient's clinical presentation.

CLINICAL PRESENTATIONS

Psychogenic Dystonia

Dystonia is an involuntary, sustained muscle contraction causing repetitive twisting and abnormal postures. Most patients with dystonia have no identified mechanism, although some have a genetic basis. Because no specific test for organic dystonia exists, the diagnosis of psychogenic dystonia is very difficult to initially confirm. There is a broad clinical presentation for the organic dystonias. And the neurologist must always take such into consideration, keeping an open mind before making a psychogenic diagnosis.

Patients with psychogenic dystonia may present with foot or leg involvement, a distribution that is relatively unlikely but not exclusive of an organic adult-onset idiopathic dystonia. An important clue to a diagnosis of a psychogenic dystonia is the presence of symptoms at

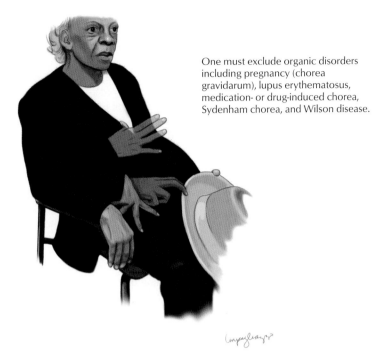

One must exclude organic disorders including pregnancy (chorea gravidarum), lupus erythematosus, medication- or drug-induced chorea, Sydenham chorea, and Wilson disease.

Fig. 36.1 Psychogenic Movement Disorder, Pseudochoreoathetosis.

rest; this often helps to differentiate such individuals from those with an action-specific organic dystonia.

Psychogenic Tremor

Tremors are rhythmic, bidirectional, oscillating movements resulting from contraction of agonist and antagonistic muscles. Tremors can be resting, postural, or action.

Psychogenic tremor usually varies in frequency and amplitude, is complex, and occurs at rest, during various postures, and with various actions. Psychogenic tremor often has amplitudes unlike that of even midbrain tremor. It typically lessens with distraction.

Psychogenic Myoclonus

Myoclonus is defined as brief, shocklike movements caused by muscle contraction or lapses in posture. The frequency, amplitude, body distribution, symmetry, and course differ with various etiologies. Psychogenic myoclonus decreases in amplitude during distraction and often occurs at rest, in contrast to organic myoclonus, which decreases at rest.

Psychogenic Parkinsonism

Parkinsonism is a symptom complex consisting of resting tremor, rigidity, bradykinesia, and impaired postural reflexes. Psychogenic tremor varies in frequency and rhythmicity, remitting with distraction. Rigidity related to psychiatric problems consists of voluntary resistance without any evidence of cogwheeling. As with other psychogenic movement disorders, the symptoms of psychogenic parkinsonism lessen with distraction. Gait is atypical, with extreme or bizarre postural instability.

DIFFERENTIAL DIAGNOSES

Psychogenic movement disorders have certain common characteristics, such as acute onset, static course, spontaneous remissions, consistently inconsistent character of their movements in amplitude, frequency, and distribution, and a selective disability. Furthermore, these psychiatrically affected individuals are unresponsiveness to appropriate medications, may sometimes respond to placebo, have their movements increase with attention while these same adventitious movements decrease with distraction. A remission may occur with psychotherapy, once a specific psychopathology is diagnosed. The clinician strives to make a distinction between these psychogenic clinical presentations and those of organic movement disorders. It is often a diagnostic challenge, and sometimes may take several years to sort out.

Certain factors support the possibility of a psychogenic movement disorder. This is particularly relevant when there is a patient history of multiple poorly defined, somatic complaints. Other supportive evidence for an emotional basis includes specific findings on neurologic examination. These include a nonanatomic sensory loss such as when one places a tuning fork on the forehead and the patient states he or she does not feel it when it is tilted to the left but does so when tilted to the right, while the examiner maintains the instrument's base in the precisely same anatomic spot for each testing. Similarly, a consistently inconsistent weakness and a seemingly deliberate slowness of movement are also typical of psychogenic movement disorders.

Questioning the individual or family to potentially uncover possible secondary gain is also important. This is especially true when one determines that there is a pending litigation or workman's compensation action. On some occasions, psychiatrically ill patients use a family member or friend with an organic movement disorder to serve as a subconscious model for their own adventitious movement or gait disorder. Thus one may sometimes find a positive family history by meeting with and observing family members important in the individual's daily life. These encounters may provide a good means for establishing the true identity of the patient's problem. Such a meeting may be overwhelming when one identifies the precise model for the specific movement.

DIAGNOSTIC EVALUATION

The diagnosis of psychogenic movement disorder usually requires a neurologist and a psychiatrist, as well as a direct meeting with family members. The initial step is a detailed clinical history and examination, review of current and previous medications, and subsequent exclusion of a true organic movement disorder. Diagnostic tests follow clinical assessment and may include brain magnetic resonance imaging (MRI), serum ceruloplasmin and urine copper excretion, thyroid functions, and other tests based on clinical suspicion. The diagnostic evaluation may also include an appropriate trial of specific medications typically used for various organic movement disorders and tailored to the patient's clinical picture. After these steps are taken, and certain clinical suggestions of psychogenicity are defined, a diagnostic psychiatric evaluation is needed. However, the definition of a psychiatric illness still does not absolutely prove that the movement disorder has a psychogenic basis, because patients with psychiatric disorders of course also develop organic neurologic diseases.

Thus careful neurologic as well as psychiatric follow-up is often mandated. Wilson disease is a good example of patients presenting with seemingly bizarre movements that have led to psychiatric diagnosis early on. Careful attention to search for a Kayser-Fleischer ring when looking at the patient's iris and obtaining copper screening studies may occasionally uncover this important but very rare movement disorder. There is no more grateful patient.

TREATMENT AND PROGNOSIS

These patients present a therapeutic challenge equal to the diagnostic challenge that led to a proper diagnosis. Treatment of these individuals is often very difficult. No specific treatment protocols exist. Periodic neurologic follow-up with the same neurologist, in conjunction with psychotherapy, is often necessary to alleviate residual concerns that an organic illness is present. These visits will also provide reassurance to the patient and subsequently lead to a reduction or remission of the adventitious motor symptoms. Careful neurologic follow-up can be exceedingly reassuring for not only the patient but often the physician. It is not appropriate to make a psychogenic diagnosis without providing for careful follow-up. Ongoing psychotherapy and physical therapy are important, as is treatment of the underlying psychiatric conditions

(antidepressants, anxiolytics, etc.). Finally, the use of placebo is debatable. Some physicians and patients interpret this as confrontational. Unfortunately, some patients resist accepting both the diagnosis and psychiatric treatment.

Prognosis depends on the psychodynamic specifics underlying the movement disorder. Generally good prognostic signs include acute onset, short duration of symptoms, healthy premorbid functioning, absence of coexisting organic and psychogenic disease, and presence of an identifiable stressor.

FUTURE DIRECTIONS

When specific laboratory tests, possibly neurochemical or autoimmune in type, become available for the diagnosis of organic movement disorders, psychogenic movement disorders will be easier to confirm. More research in the field of neurotransmitters, more specific brain studies, such as functional MRI, and genetic testing will eventually aid the understanding of this complex and difficult therapeutic problem. It is not out of the question that eventually some new previously misunderstood organic movement disorders will be identified in some of these individuals.

ADDITIONAL RESOURCES

Fahn S, Williams D. Psychogenic dystonia. Adv Neurol 1988;50: 431–55.

Hallett M, Fahn S, Jankovic J, et al. Psychogenic movement disorders. Neurology and neuropsychiatry. Baltimore, MD: Lippincott Williams & Wilkins; 2006.

Koller WC, Marjama J, Troster A. Psychogenic movement disorders. In: Jankovic J, Tolosa E, editors. Parkinson's disease and movement disorders. Baltimore, MD: Williams & Wilkins; 1998. pp. 859–68.

Ricciardi L, Edwards MJ. Treatment of functional (psychogenic) movement disorders. Neurotherapeutics 2014;11(1):201–7.

Thenganatt MA, Jankovic J. Psychogenic movement disorders. Neurol Clin 2015;33(1):205–24.

37

Surgical Treatment of Movement Disorders

Peter K. Dempsey

Medical treatment of movement disorders continues to be effective but has substantial limitations. For decades, the surgical treatment of movement disorders centered around the creation of lesions within the brain. Developments in technology made neuromodulation, in the form of deep brain stimulation (DBS), a more attractive option for many patients. Advantages of DBS include the ability to modulate the degree of stimulation over time, allowing for changes arising from the disease progression, and reversibility, with removal of the device if necessary. Patients with Parkinson disease (PD), essential tremor (ET), and dystonia have recognized the benefits of DBS and experience significantly improved quality of life after DBS surgery. This chapter will focus on the DBS procedure, including the risks of surgery and expected outcomes.

Surgical treatment of movement disorders was transformed in 1952 with the inadvertent ligation of the anterior choroidal artery by Dr. Irving Cooper. Following surgery, Dr. Cooper noted marked improvement in tremor and rigidity without substantial weakness in a patient with PD. This led to the development of lesioning deep cerebral nuclei as a method of treating the symptoms of PD. For many years, pallidotomy and thalamotomy were the most effective means of treating tremor and other symptoms of PD. These were invasive procedures, relying on generic anatomic atlases for localization, in which areas in the brain were heated and thermocoagulation was used to create a lesion. To confirm proper targeting, intraoperative testing was done with the patient's participation. The lesion size could be modulated by varying the time of the thermocoagulation. This technique was permanent and not able to be modified; however, the results for controlling tremor were quite good, with many patients achieving long-lasting results.

With the development of dopamine-replacement medications (levodopa), lesioning fell out of favor because the risks outweighed the benefits. Medical treatment with dopamine-agonist replacement became the mainstay for the treatment of PD symptoms, but limitations were soon recognized. Patients experience fluctuations in their symptoms between "on" states, in which the medication is effective, and "off" states, in which the symptoms return. Adverse responses to medication often result in undesired side effects such as dyskinesia. The advent of cross-sectional imaging such as computed tomography (CT) and magnetic resonance imaging (MRI) saw a resurgence in image-guided procedures in the brain. In the mid-1980s, surgeons began implanting electrodes into the globus pallidus interna (GPi) and the subthalamic nucleus (STN), which demonstrated dramatic improvements in parkinsonian symptoms with minimal risks. Today, DBS surgery is seen as an excellent alternative for patients with PD or ET, in whom the medical treatment has become ineffective or intolerable. Other treatments such as pallidotomy and thalamotomy, while still performed in some centers, have largely been abandoned. Patients with primary dystonia can also benefit from DBS. In addition, drug-induced (tardive) dystonia and cervical dystonia (torticollis) seem to respond well to DBS.

DEEP BRAIN STIMULATION PROCEDURE

Proper patient selection for DBS surgery is a critical first step, and it requires a team composed of movement disorder neurologists, neuropsychologists, and psychiatrists. Severe fluctuations in motor symptoms and the presence of medication-induced dyskinesias are the primary indications for DBS in patients with PD. Disabling tremor, refractory to medical treatment, is the primary indication for DBS for ET. Screening involves measuring symptoms when patients are on and off medication to assess the degree of improvement. MRI of the brain is also required to assess for any anatomic impediments to the DBS lead placement. Neuropsychological testing is performed to evaluate the patient's cognitive status and ability to understand the expected outcomes of the procedure. A multidisciplinary approach is essential to selecting the proper patients and selecting the proper target. PD patients typically have leads placed into the STN or, less commonly, the GPi, whereas the ventral intermediate (VIM) nucleus of the thalamus is typically the target in patients with ET. There is no clear evidence demonstrating superiority with implanting electrodes in the STN over the GPi for PD; however, results have shown that patients with electrodes in the STN often are able to reduce their medications after DBS surgery, whereas those with electrodes in the GPi may have greater improvement in control of dyskinesia. Bilateral placement of DBS leads is commonly done, although in patients older than 65 years of age, the procedures are done as separate operations because these patients seem to have more postoperative side effects after bilateral lead placement in a single surgical procedure.

The DBS procedure is often staged, with the intracranial lead(s) placed during the first stage and the implantable pulse generator (IPG) or battery placed at a later date. Critical to the procedure is proper placement of the electrode into the appropriate intracranial location. This requires precise imaging localization with a guiding device to ensure that the proper trajectory is followed. In many centers, physiologic monitoring is used to ensure proper lead placement.

The lead placement procedure begins with the application of a guiding device, or stereotactic frame, to the patient's head (Fig. 37.1A). Four pins are placed in the outer table of the skull, holding the frame securely in place. CT showing elements of the frame called *fiducial markers* is obtained and then fused via software to previously acquired MRI. This process provides the spatial accuracy of the CT with the anatomic resolution of the MRI. Using these fused data, the computer creates a three-dimensional reconstruction of the brain. Based on well-recognized intracranial structures (anterior and posterior commissures), the location of the STN, the GPi, and the VIM can be localized using standard anatomic atlases (see Fig. 37.1B). The target site for the DBS lead is selected on MRI, and the computer calculates coordinates in the x, y, and z planes. The trajectory of the lead placement is demonstrated on

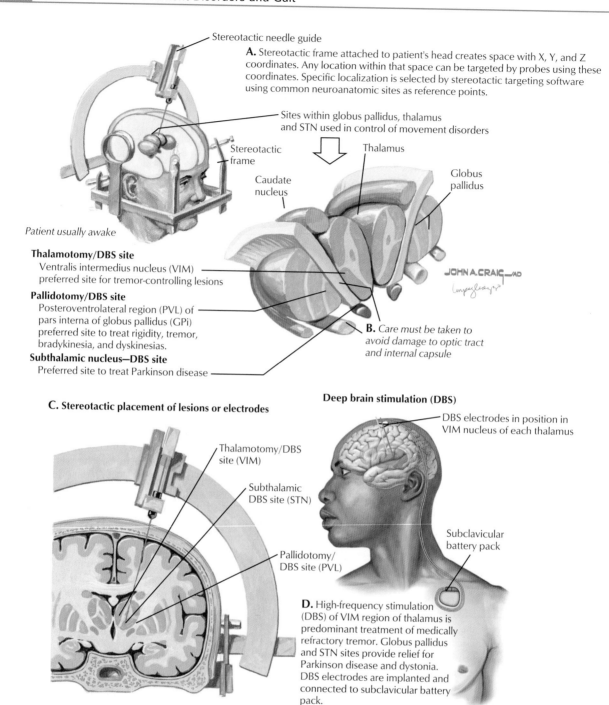

A. Stereotactic frame attached to patient's head creates space with X, Y, and Z coordinates. Any location within that space can be targeted by probes using these coordinates. Specific localization is selected by stereotactic targeting software using common neuroanatomic sites as reference points.

Stereotactic needle guide

Stereotactic frame

Patient usually awake

Sites within globus pallidus, thalamus and STN used in control of movement disorders

Thalamus

Globus pallidus

Caudate nucleus

Thalamotomy/DBS site
Ventralis intermedius nucleus (VIM) preferred site for tremor-controlling lesions

Pallidotomy/DBS site
Posteroventrolateral region (PVL) of pars interna of globus pallidus (GPi) preferred site to treat rigidity, tremor, bradykinesia, and dyskinesias.

Subthalamic nucleus—DBS site
Preferred site to treat Parkinson disease

B. Care must be taken to avoid damage to optic tract and internal capsule

JOHN A. CRAIG—AD

C. Stereotactic placement of lesions or electrodes

Thalamotomy/DBS site (VIM)

Subthalamic DBS site (STN)

Pallidotomy/ DBS site (PVL)

Deep brain stimulation (DBS)

DBS electrodes in position in VIM nucleus of each thalamus

Subclavicular battery pack

D. High-frequency stimulation (DBS) of VIM region of thalamus is predominant treatment of medically refractory tremor. Globus pallidus and STN sites provide relief for Parkinson disease and dystonia. DBS electrodes are implanted and connected to subclavicular battery pack.

Fig. 37.1 Surgical Management of Movement Disorders. *DBS,* Deep brain stimulation; *STN,* subthalamic nucleus

MRI, clearly depicting the anatomic structures and blood vessels to avoid. Selection of the proper trajectory not only includes the target point but also the angle of the lead within the target nucleus, allowing for maximum contact of the leads with the target.

In the operating room, the patient is placed in the supine position, and the localizing frame is attached to the operating room table. The patient is mildly sedated for the incision and creation of the burr hole. The computer-generated target coordinates and angles are set on the guiding device, and the entry point is selected on the scalp. After creation of a 1-cm burr hole, a microelectrode used for recording is then precisely and slowly passed to the target point (see Fig. 37.1C). Neuronal activity is mapped, confirming the proper target using physiologic parameters.

More than one pass is required to properly localize the target 60% of the time. Macrostimulation is then performed through the electrode, looking for adverse reactions, such as paresthesias, motor tract stimulation, speech impairment, and eye movements. The patient is awake and cooperates during this part of the procedure, providing real-time feedback for any subjective symptoms. The efficacy of the DBS electrode also can be assessed during the procedure, with immediate resolution of tremor and rigidity seen in many patients. Once the optimal location has been determined, the permanent lead is placed in the same location, and the distal part of the lead is tucked under the scalp in the retroauricular region (Fig. 37.2). The incision is closed, the guiding frame is removed, and the patient is admitted overnight to the hospital.

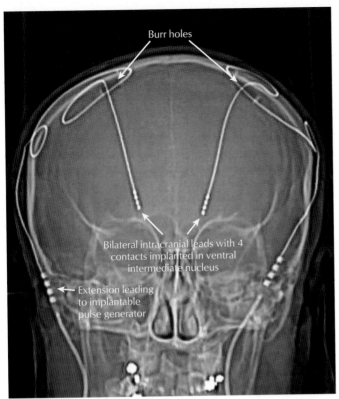

Fig. 37.2 Anteroposterior skull radiograph showing the intracranial deep brain stimulation electrodes implanted into the ventral intermediate nucleus.

Seven to ten days later, the patient returns for placement of an extension lead that connects the intracranial electrode that had been placed under the scalp to the IPG, which is placed in a pocket on the ipsilateral anterior chest wall (see Fig. 37.1D). This part of the procedure is performed with general anesthesia. The patient is discharged home on the same day, returning for programming within the next week.

DBS programming is an iterative process that often is completed in several outpatient sessions. The IPG is capable of creating current between the contacts at the end of the electrode implanted in the brain. The current can vary in pulse width, frequency, and amplitude, and the programmer tests many combinations of these parameters, looking for maximum benefit with minimal adverse effects.

RESULTS OF DEEP BRAIN STIMULATION

Many studies have shown the benefit of DBS in patients with movement disorders. Positive results are seen primarily in motor function and overall quality of life, with patients experiencing more "on" time and fewer fluctuations and dyskinesias. DBS surgery is safe and effective;

however, there are risks. The most problematic risk is infection, occurring in 5%–10% of patients. Despite perioperative antibiotics and meticulous surgical technique, the presence of the electrode wires, connectors, and IPG can create skin breakdown, leading to infection and possible removal of equipment. Other complications of DBS include brain injury from bleeding or passage of the electrode (1%–2%), not achieving the desired benefit of the DBS system, cognitive or psychiatric issues, and malfunctioning of the hardware, including IPG depletion. Depending on the settings, a typical IPG will last from 3 to 5 years and then require replacement.

Technological advancements will improve the outcome of DBS procedures. Improvements in programming capability and lead manufacturing will increase the beneficial effects and reduce side effects. Leads with eight or more contacts, which allow for directional programming, have been developed. With these new leads, electrical current can be steered away from areas in which adverse effects are noticed, allowing increased current in the beneficial regions. Closed-loop systems, in which the electrical activity of the brain is constantly recorded and used to modulate the output of the DBS system, are also in development.

SUMMARY

DBS is a safe and effective procedure that successfully reduces many symptoms of PD, ET, and dystonia, resulting in marked improvement in quality of life. Recent studies suggest that earlier intervention with DBS when medications first begin to lose their effect may be the best long-term option for patients with movement disorders.

ADDITIONAL RESOURCES

Das K, Benzil DL, Rovit RL, et al. Irving S. Cooper (1922-1985): a pioneer in functional neurosurgery. J Neurosurg 1998;89(5):865–73.
A paper about the surgeon and the surgical misadventure that led to the development of creating lesions in the deep nuclei for treating the symptoms of Parkinson disease.
Benabid AL, Pollak P, Gervason C, et al. Long-term suppression of tremor by chronic stimulation of the ventral intermediate thalamic nucleus. Lancet 1991;337:403–6.
This paper by the first surgeon to employ DBS for tremor describes the results of DBS compared to thalamotomy.
Volkmann J. Deep brain stimulation for the treatment of Parkinson's disease. J Clin Neurophysiol 2004;21:6–17.
Comprehensive comparison among various DBS targets.
Schuepbach WMM, Rau J, Knudsen K, et al. Neurostimulation for Parkinson's disease with early motor complications. N Engl J Med 2013;368:610–22.
The benefits of early use of DBS in PD patients are described. DBS patients had improved quality of life and overall lower cost of care compared with medically treated patients.
Martinez-Ramirez D, Hu W, Bona AR, et al. Update on deep brain stimulation in Parkinson's disease. Transl Neurodegener 2015;4:12.
Well-referenced recent paper that describes the mechanism of action and outcomes of DBS.

38

Gait Disorders

Julie Leegwater-Kim

CLINICAL VIGNETTE *A 70-year-old woman presented with a 2-year history of gait slowness and unsteadiness. She sustained several falls, usually backward. She began using a cane 1 year ago. She has noticed difficulty standing up or getting out of her car. Her husband described her walking as if "her feet are glued to the floor." In addition to her gait difficulties, she has developed urinary frequency and had one episode of urinary incontinence. She also described being more forgetful.*

Neurologic exam was notable for a slow, shuffled, broad-based gait with shortened stride length and en bloc turning. Arm swing was intact. When the patient was quickly pulled backward, she demonstrated marked postural instability with retropulsion. She could not arise from a chair without using her arms to push herself up. Cognitive testing was notable for limited object recall and executive dysfunction.

The patient underwent brain magnetic resonance imaging (MRI), which revealed an enlarged ventricular system out of proportion to the degree of brain atrophy. A large-volume lumbar puncture was performed, and the patient demonstrated marked improvement in her gait and balance afterward. A ventriculoperitoneal shunt was placed with subsequent sustained improvement in the patient's gait. She also experienced mild improvement in her urinary function. Her cognitive functioning was relatively unchanged.

Gait disorders are a common presentation of neurologic disease, and their prevalence increases with age. In a cross-sectional study of 488 community-residing subjects aged 60–97 years of age, 32.2% presented with an impaired gait. Twenty-four percent of participants exhibited neurologic gait disorders, 17.4% experienced nonneurological gait disorders, and 9.2% had combinations of both. Those with neurologic gait disorders were three times more likely to experience recurrent falls. Neurologic gait disorders were also significantly associated with cognitive dysfunction, depressed mood, and diminished quality of life.

ANATOMY AND PATHOPHYSIOLOGY

Normal gait requires the integration and coordination of the central and peripheral nervous systems and the musculoskeletal system. Gait consists of two key components: (1) locomotion, the generation and maintenance of rhythmic stepping, and (2) equilibrium, the ability to keep the body upright and maintain balance. In quadrupedal animals, locomotion is mainly dependent on spinal pattern generators, which produce rhythmic stepping movements. In contrast, locomotion in primates can be elicited by electrical stimulation of brainstem areas, including the posterior subthalamus, dorsal and ventral portions of the caudal pons, and the mesencephalic tegmentum. The latter includes the pedunculopontine nucleus (PPN), a group of cholinergic neurons that receives input from the basal ganglia and motor cortex and projects

to the spinal cord and reticular nuclei. Although the exact function of the PPN is not clear, it is uniquely situated to modulate the influence of the basal ganglia on locomotion and balance. Higher cortical centers are also important in the maintenance of gait and balance. The frontal cortex is implicated in the control, coordination, and planning of automatic and voluntary movements. In addition, the posterior parietal cortex is involved in the perception of body position and posture.

ETIOLOGY AND CLASSIFICATION

Because gait is dependent on the proper functioning and integration of different aspects of the nervous system, a variety of lesions in the central and/or peripheral nervous systems can produce walking difficulties. In a recent series of 120 patients presenting to an outpatient neurology clinic with gait disorder in which patients with hemiparesis, known Parkinson disease (PD), neuroleptic exposure, and orthopedic deformity were excluded, the distribution of etiologies was as follows: myelopathy (17%), sensory deficits (17%), multiple infarcts (15%), parkinsonism (12%), hydrocephalus (7%), cerebellar dysfunction (7%), psychogenic (3%) and toxic/metabolic causes (3%).

Gait disorders can be classified in a number of ways: etiologically (Box 38.1), anatomically (Box 38.2), and clinically (Table 38.1 and Fig. 38.1). Perhaps the most useful approach to understanding gait disorders is a clinicoanatomic one. According to this method, gait disorders can be divided into roughly three anatomic categories: cortical, subcortical, and peripheral. A variety of well-defined clinical gait syndromes can be described under each anatomic rubric.

CORTICAL GAIT DISORDERS

Frontal Gait

Bilateral frontal lobe dysfunction and/or disconnection between cortical and subcortical motor areas (i.e., basal ganglia, brainstem, cerebellum) leads to a distinctive gait, variously known as magnetic gait, "marche a petits pas," lower-body parkinsonism, and frontal apraxia of gait. It is characterized by a combination of gait initiation failure, impaired walking, and disequilibrium. The patient exhibits a wider than normal gait base, reduced stride length and heel strike, and shuffling steps (Fig. 38.2). There is often a pronounced hesitation to the initiation of the gait. Such patients frequently exhibit retropulsion, something that often leads to backward falls. Paradoxically, there is usually preservation of other types of leg movements—that is, pedaling or bicycling in the recumbent position (hence the term *apraxia of gait*).

Frontal gait, on initial clinical assessment, can resemble parkinsonian gait, although there is generally only involvement of the lower body (hence the term *lower-body parkinsonism*). Features that can help differentiate frontal gait from typical parkinsonian gait are more erect

BOX 38.1 Gait Disorders—Etiologic Classification

Myelopathy
- Cervical spondylosis
- Vitamin B_{12} deficiency
- Demyelinating diseases (e.g., multiple sclerosis)
- Infectious diseases (e.g., human T-lymphotropic virus type 1 infection)

Parkinsonism
- Parkinson disease
- Atypical parkinsonism
- Progressive supranuclear palsy
- Corticobasal ganglionic degeneration
- Dementia with Lewy body disease
- Secondary parkinsonism
- Neuroleptic-induced parkinsonism

Multiple Infarcts/Small Vessel Disease
- Stroke
- Vasculitis
- Mitochondrial disease

Hydrocephalus
- Communicating
  - Normal pressure hydrocephalus
- Noncommunicating

Cerebellar Disease
- Toxic-metabolic
  - Alcohol-induced cerebellar degeneration
  - Medications (e.g., phenytoin)
  - Thiamine deficiency
- Heredodegenerative disorders
  - Spinocerebellar ataxias
  - Fragile X-tremor-ataxia syndrome
- Infectious/postinfectious diseases
- Paraneoplastic disorders
- Celiac sprue

Sensory Deficits
- Peripheral neuropathy (e.g., diabetic neuropathy)
- Dorsal root ganglionopathy (e.g., Sjögren syndrome)
- Posterior column lesions (e.g., tabes dorsalis)
- Vestibular disorders
- Visual disorders

posture, wide base, lack of tremor, and preserved arm swing. Patients can sometimes also develop freezing of gait (FOG; see hypokinetic-rigid gait). Associated signs of frontal gait disorder include frontal release signs, behavioral changes, and executive dysfunction.

The most common cause of frontal gait is cerebrovascular disease (small vessel ischemic changes or infarcts), affecting the basal ganglia and/or periventricular white matter. Normal-pressure hydrocephalus (NPH) is another and very important etiology, particularly because it is potentially remediable. NPH is characterized by the clinical triad of frontal gait disorder, urinary incontinence, and dementia. Imaging of the brain demonstrates hydrocephalus (see Fig. 38.2). Diagnostic workup includes large-volume lumbar puncture, which reveals improvement of gait hours to days after removal of cerebrospinal fluid (CSF). Treatment involves placement of a ventriculoperitoneal shunt.

Cautious Gait

This is a very common disorder, especially among senior citizens who are beginning to show signs of being elderly. It is also seen among individuals made more cautious than usual after having experienced an unexpected or seemingly unprovoked fall. These patients assume a stance and gait pattern that *mimics walking on ice*. The base is widened and steps are slow, with reduced stride length. Turning is *en bloc*, and the arms are abducted. This relatively common gait significantly improves with minimal support (i.e., the assistance of a companion, a cane, or a walker). There is usually associated anxiety and fear of falling. Cautious gait can improve with physical therapy and an assistive device. However, on occasion a patient presenting with a cautious gait may be offering a precursor of a more specific and serious gait disorder that may soon show itself.

BOX 38.2 Gait Disorders—Anatomic Classification

Frontal/cortical
Subcortical-hypokinetic
Subcortical-hyperkinetic
Pyramidal
Cerebellar
Vestibular
Neuropathic
Myopathic
Orthopedic

TABLE 38.1 Clinical Gait Syndromes: Specific Examples

Gait Type	Clinical Features	Associated Findings
Frontal gait	Wide based Shortened stride length Reduced heel strike Start and turn hesitation Retropulsion	Frontal-release signs Cognitive impairment Behavioral changes Urinary disturbance
Cautious gait	Mildly wide based Shortened stride Improvement with assistive device	Anxiety Fear of falling Fear of open spaces
Psychogenic gait	Bizarre, inconsistent movements Lurching and knee-bucking but rare falls Distractibility/entrainment of movements	Abrupt onset/resolution Positive psychiatric features Secondary gain Wide fluctuations over short time periods

A. Cerebellar Gait Disorders

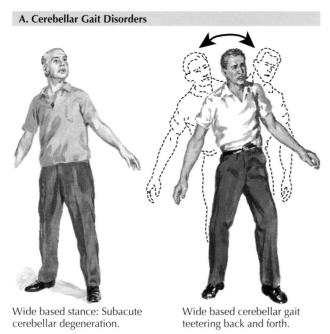

Wide based stance: Subacute cerebellar degeneration.

Wide based cerebellar gait teetering back and forth.

B. Spastic Gait

C. Peripheral Neuropathic Gait

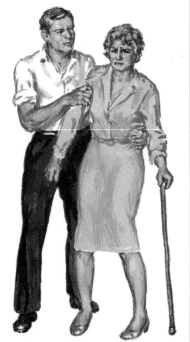

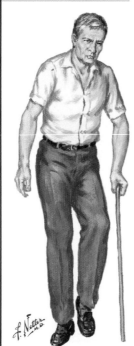

Cerebral, subcortical, or myelopathic lesions. Stroke, MS, or tumor at multiple sites: frontal lobe, internal capsule, pontine, or brainstem and cervical spinal cord, particularly spinal stenosis.

Painful burning feet with numbness and tingling. Foot drop.

Fig. 38.1 Clinical Classification of Gait Disorders. *MS,* Multiple sclerosis.

Psychogenic Gait

This is also termed *hysterical gait disorder* or *astasia-abasia*. It is a most unusual gait to witness, as it is not congruent with the features of any known organic gait disorder. The gait is marked by bizarre, consistently inconsistent, and distractible movements. Some movements may be dramatic and lurching, but subjects rarely fall. There are often significant clinical fluctuations over time. The diagnosis of psychogenic gait disorder relies on the exclusion of organic etiologies but also on the presence of positive signs such as abrupt onset or resolution of symptoms/signs, false or giveaway weakness, distractibility of movements, somatization, la belle indifference affect, and psychiatric history and symptoms. Treatment is challenging, but a combination of intensive physical therapy and various psychiatric treatments, including cognitive therapy, may be beneficial.

One needs to be extremely cautious in arriving at such a diagnosis, as is attested to by the following case history.

> **CLINICAL VIGNETTE** *A 28-year-old woman with depression had recently been evaluated by a psychiatrist; she began treatment using amitriptyline. Within a few weeks she appeared somewhat unsteady to others, who noted that she occasionally was bumping into furniture. Her internist stopped the antidepressant medication and scheduled a neurology consult. She reported to the neurologist that she was feeling significantly improved since the medication had been stopped. She still had a slightly abnormal poorly defined gait, which prompted the neurologist to pursue brain-imaging studies, but she failed to keep the appointment. Unbeknownst to the neurologist, she instead returned to see her psychiatrist; her depression worsened and noting her prior sensitivity to the amitriptyline, the psychiatrist elected to hospitalize her for electroconvulsive therapy (ECT).*
>
> *After a few ECT treatments, she began to complain about problems with coordination of her left arm and leg. Her psychiatrist did not consult the neurologist but made an assumption that her new difficulties were psychogenic. He continued the daily ECT explaining her deteriorating neurologic status as a post-ECT effect. The patient's family demanded a recheck by the neurologist.*
>
> *Unfortunately, the neurologist found that she had vertical nystagmus, left-hand finger to nose ataxia, and a spastic hemiparetic gait with brisk muscle stretch reflexes and a Babinski sign on the left. Imaging studies demonstrated a fourth-ventricle tumor. At surgery, this proved to be a malignant ependymoma with severe brainstem compression.*
>
> *Comment: One always needs to be very circumspect in evaluating any neurologic problem. Gait disorders can be prone to misinterpretation. Modern imaging studies generally prevent the unfortunate outcome experienced by this patient.*

SUBCORTICAL GAIT DISORDERS

Spastic Gait

This represents a pyramidal gait disorder, originating in the motor cortex or corticospinal tracts. Unilateral disease leads to a spastic hemiparetic gait characterized by stiff-legged extension and circumduction of the affected leg (see Fig. 38.1B) and flexion of the ipsilateral upper limb. In the case of bilateral involvement, the patient exhibits adduction and scissoring of the legs. Associated findings include leg weakness, hyperreflexia, and extensor plantar responses. Causes of hemiparetic gait include stroke, demyelinating lesion, mass, or trauma. Paraparetic gait can be caused by cerebral palsy, primary lateral sclerosis, and spinal cord lesions. Botulinum toxin and oral medications such as baclofen and tizanidine can be beneficial.

Ataxic Gait

The gait has a lurching or veering quality, imitating a "drunken gait" that is marked by a widened base of support and irregular stepping. These patients also exhibit increased truncal instability that is exacerbated with standing with one's feet together or tandem walking. Ataxic gait disorders signal cerebellar dysfunction (see Fig. 38.1A). On

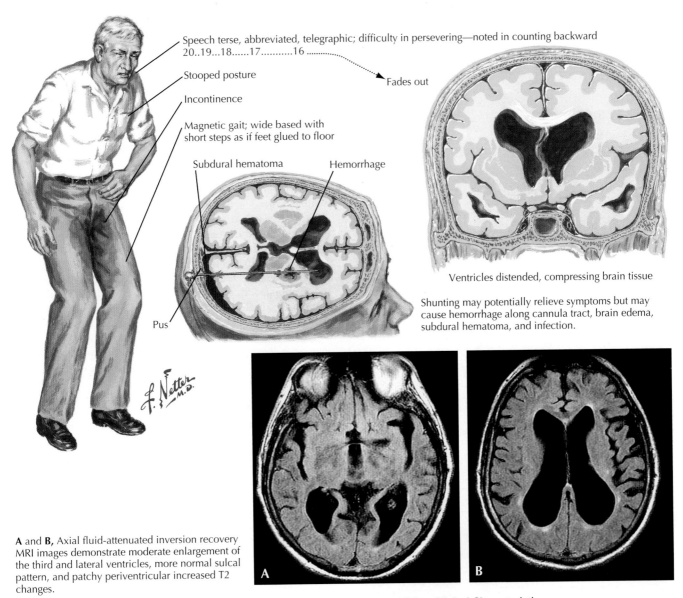

Speech terse, abbreviated, telegraphic; difficulty in persevering—noted in counting backward
20..19...18......17...........16 ....

Fades out

Stooped posture

Incontinence

Magnetic gait; wide based with short steps as if feet glued to floor

Subdural hematoma

Hemorrhage

Pus

Ventricles distended, compressing brain tissue

Shunting may potentially relieve symptoms but may cause hemorrhage along cannula tract, brain edema, subdural hematoma, and infection.

A and **B,** Axial fluid-attenuated inversion recovery MRI images demonstrate moderate enlargement of the third and lateral ventricles, more normal sulcal pattern, and patchy periventricular increased T2 changes.

Fig. 38.2 Normal-Pressure Hydrocephalus: Gait and Other Clinical Characteristics.

examination, other signs of cerebellar disease can be elicited: dysmetria, dysdiadochokinesia, nystagmus, hypermetric saccades, and scanning dysarthria.

Causes are myriad (see Box 38.1): toxic/metabolic disorders (i.e., acute or chronic alcoholism), neurodegenerative diseases such as the spinocerebellar ataxias, paraneoplastic disease, and ischemic (Fig. 38.3) or demyelinating disorders affecting the cerebellum or its connections. Pharmacologic treatments to date have been unsuccessful. Physical therapy is the main treatment available.

Hypokinetic-Rigid Gait

This is also known as akinetic-rigid gait or parkinsonian gait and is seen in any of the various parkinsonian syndromes. The gait is characterized by flexed posture, reduced arm swing and stride length, shuffled steps, turning en bloc, and postural instability. Patients frequently exhibit festination, an acceleration of gait in which the steps get shorter and faster as the patient attempts to keep pace with his or her displaced center of gravity. Associated parkinsonian features may include brady-kinesia, tremor, cogwheel rigidity, and FOG. FOG refers to motor blocks in which the subject is unable to initiate and maintain locomotion.

Common etiologies of hypokinetic-rigid gait include neurodegen-erative disorders such as idiopathic PD and atypical parkinsonian syn-dromes such as progressive supranuclear palsy (PSP) and corticobasal ganglionic degeneration (Fig. 38.4). One distinguishing feature between PD and other forms of parkinsonism is that the former is characterized by a normal or narrow base while the latter generally exhibits a broad-based gait. In addition, PD tends to start unilaterally versus the bilaterality seen with the atypical syndromes. Furthermore, the presence of a tremor is usually typical of idiopathic PD.

Patients with hypokinetic-rigid gaits should be given a trial of carbidopa/levodopa. A robust response to this medication supports a diagnosis of idiopathic PD. Patients with atypical parkinsonism may also benefit from carbidopa/levodopa; however, the effect, if any, is often temporary.

Hyperkinetic Gait

Hyperkinesias are excessive movements. Because many hyperkinesias represent abnormal movements, they are often termed dyskinesias. Hyperkinesias include chorea (random, brief movements that flow from one body part to another), dystonia (abnormal sustained involuntary

Acute gait ataxia, sometimes truncal ataxia, vomiting, headache, dysarthria, with occasional hiccups and tinnitus

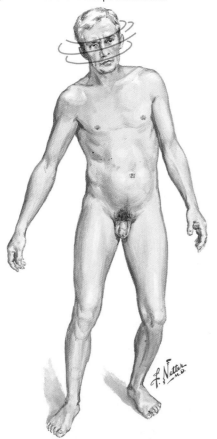

Acute gait disorder secondary to intracerebellar hemorrhage

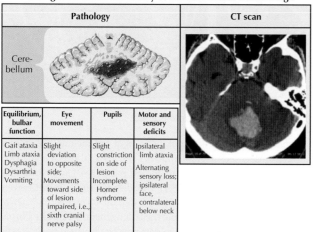

Pathology				CT scan
Cerebellum				

Equilibrium, bulbar function	Eye movement	Pupils	Motor and sensory deficits
Gait ataxia Limb ataxia Dysphagia Dysarthria Vomiting	Slight deviation to opposite side; Movements toward side of lesion impaired, i.e., sixth cranial nerve palsy	Slight constriction on side of lesion Incomplete Horner syndrome	Ipsilateral limb ataxia Alternating sensory loss; ipsilateral face, contralateral below neck

Fig. 38.3 Vertebrobasilar Stroke: Gait and Other Clinical Findings.

movements), and myoclonus (rapid, involuntary, jerklike movements). Patients with hyperkinesias often display distinctive gait patterns.

Choreic Gait

Choreic gait has a stuttering or dancelike quality that reflects superimposed choreic and choreoathetotic movements. Stride length and cadence are irregular and random. The base is variable. Steps often deviate from the direction of travel, giving the gait a somewhat ataxic quality. Choreic

gait can be seen in patients with Huntington disease and in patients with PD who experience medication-induced dyskinesias.

Dystonic Gait

These patients demonstrate lower extremity and/or trunk dystonia. When the dystonia involves the foot, the gait is usually characterized by foot inversion. In the early stages of dystonia, the gait pattern is task-specific. For example, a patient with foot dystonia may exhibit dystonic gait when walking forward but may walk backward or run normally. In our clinic we evaluated a middle-aged patient who could only move forward, emulating a cross-country skiing gliding movement, yet moved backward with impunity. In addition, dystonias can be temporarily improved with sensory tricks (i.e., placing hands in pockets, putting the hand on the back or hip). Isolated foot/leg dystonia can be due to early idiopathic PD, corticobasal ganglionic degeneration, or idiopathic torsion dystonia. Dystonia affecting the trunk can lead to retrocollis, anterocollis, Pisa syndrome (lateral flexion of the trunk), camptocormia, and opisthotonus. Causes of truncal dystonia include neurodegenerative disorders such as PSP (retrocollis) and multiple-system atrophy (Pisa syndrome, anterocollis), tardive syndromes (opisthotonus, retrocollis), and genetic disorders such as DYT-1 dystonia (generalized dystonia). Because dystonic gaits can appear unusual, be task-specific, and temporarily improve with sensory tricks, they are sometimes mistaken for psychogenic gaits. Treatments for dystonia include baclofen, trihexyphenidyl, and botulinum toxin. In severe cases, deep brain stimulation can be beneficial.

Myoclonic Gait

This is characterized by a bouncing gait and stance. This is due to the effects of positive myoclonus (quick jerklike movements) and negative myoclonus (sudden give in muscle tone). Negative myoclonus while walking can lead to drop attacks. The classic example of myoclonic gait is posthypoxic (Lance-Adams) myoclonus. Other causes include neurodegenerative disorders, myoclonic epilepsies, myoclonic ataxia syndromes, and myoclonus-dystonia. A variety of pharmacologic agents may improve myoclonus and include clonazepam, piracetam, levetiracetam, and valproic acid. Posthypoxic myoclonus is exquisitely sensitive to alcohol. Sodium oxybate has recently been studied as a treatment for alcohol-responsive myoclonus.

PERIPHERAL GAIT DISORDERS

Sensory Gait

These patients have a loss of proprioceptive input from the legs; they tend to walk with a wide base and reduced stride length. Arms are usually held in abduction. Gait unsteadiness is markedly worsened when visual input is reduced—that is, in the dark or closing the eyes. Lesions of the large-fiber sensory afferent nerves, including peripheral neuropathies, dorsal root lesions, sensory ganglionopathies, and posterior column damage, account for the typical sensory gait disorders (see Fig. 38.1C).

Steppage Gait

This gait disorder results from distal anterolateral leg muscle group weakness. Weakness of foot dorsiflexors causes foot drop, and patients compensate by adopting a high-stepping gait with excessive flexion of the hips and knees. When the foot touches down, the toe or anterolateral portion of the foot touches first. These patients cannot walk on their heels because of the weakness in the dorsiflexors of the feet and toes. Associated signs include distal muscle atrophy, reduced or absent ankle reflexes, and often sensory loss. The most common cause of steppage gait is peripheral neuropathy (see Fig. 38.1C).

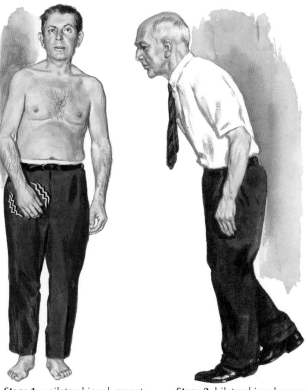
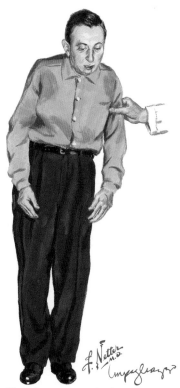

Stage 1: unilateral involvement; early masking of facial expression; affected arm in semiflexed position with tremor.

Stage 2: bilateral involvement with early postural changes; slow, shuffling gait with decreased excursion of legs

Stage 3: pronounced gait disturbances and moderate generalized disability; postural instability with tendency to fall

Fig. 38.4 Parkinson Disease: Gait Findings: Evolution of Disease Process.

Waddling Gait

As its name implies, this is characterized by the swinging of the hip and trunk from side to side. The base is widened, and lumbar hyperlordosis can develop. This type of gait arises from weakness affecting the proximal muscles of the leg and pelvic girdle muscles. Patients also have difficulty arising from a seated position and ascending stairs. Etiologies of waddling gait include myopathies, muscular dystrophies, neuromuscular transmission defects, particularly the Lambert-Eaton myasthenic syndrome, and on occasion a proximal peripheral nerve disorder such as chronic inflammatory demyelinating polyneuropathy.

Antalgic Gait

This classic gait is associated with orthopedic disorders such as arthritis. The gait is slow, limping, and painful (antalgic). Patients avoid weight bearing on the affected leg, and there is limited range of movement of the leg and hip.

ADDITIONAL RESOURCES

Jankovic J. Gait disorders. Neurol Clin 2015;33:248–68.

Jankovic J, Nutt JG, Sudarsky L. Classification, diagnosis, and etiology of gait disorders. Adv Neurol 2001;87:119–33.

Mahlknecht P, Kiechl S, et al. Prevalence and burden of gait disorders in elderly men and women aged 60–97 years: a population-based study. PLoS ONE 2013;8:e69627.

Snijders AH, van de Waarenburg BP, Giladi N, et al. Neurological gait disorders in elderly people: clinical approach and classification. Lancet Neurol 2007;6:63–74.

Multiple Sclerosis and Other Demyelinating Disorders

Claudia J. Chaves

39

Multiple Sclerosis

Claudia J. Chaves

INCIDENCE

Multiple sclerosis (MS) is the most common chronic disabling immunologic disease of the central nervous system among young people, typically presenting in the third to fifth decades of life, affecting women more than men. It is estimated that approximately 2.5 million individuals around the world have MS, more than 400,000 of them in the United States. Multiple sclerosis is more prevalent in northern latitudes, and that has been attributed not only to genetic factors but also to vitamin D deficiency, more common in populations living farther from the Equator.

PATHOPHYSIOLOGY

While its etiology is still unknown, it is believed that MS is the result of an abnormal autoimmune response against the central nervous system, likely the result of an exposure to certain environmental factors in genetically predisposed patients. Several environmental factors have been considered as potential culprits, such as early seroconversion to Epstein-Barr, smoking, low vitamin D, Western diet, and the intestinal microbiota.

While MS is not a hereditary disorder, the risk of developing MS is higher in individuals with a positive family history. For example, the risk for developing MS for a child with one parent with this condition is approximately 2% as compared to 0.1% risk in the general population. Studies have identified that the primary MS susceptibility locus is located within the major histocompatibility complex (MHC). The primary risk allele is HLA-DRB1*15, although other alleles of this gene and other genes within the MHC also contribute to the MS susceptibility. It is estimated that potentially there are as many as 200 genes involved in the susceptibility to development of MS, with the majority of the identified genes having known immunologic functions.

The abnormal autoimmune response in MS involves predominantly proinflammatory T lymphocytes (Th1 and Th17 cells) and B lymphocytes, with consequent development of acute inflammatory plaques in the white matter greater than that in the gray matter, leading to motor and cognitive disabilities over time. In addition to inflammation, degeneration is also present during the course of the disease, predominantly in its progressive stages. Important elements that likely drive neurodegeneration include activation of the microglia, oxidative injury, accumulation of iron in the brain, and mitochondrial damage in axons.

CLASSIFICATION

The first MS classification dated back in 1996 and included four different subtypes: relapsing-remitting, secondary progressive, primary progressive, and progressive relapsing forms.

In 2014, this classification was revised by the International Advisory Committee on Clinical trials of MS to better reflect the clinical aspects of the disease and separate active inflammation (based on clinical relapse rate and imaging findings) from gradual clinical progression. The new classification comprises relapsing-remitting, primary progressive, and secondary progressive MS, and includes disease activity and evidence of disease progression as modifiers. The progressive-relapsing MS category has been eliminated.

This classification also recognizes the two more recently described disease courses:

1. Clinically isolated syndrome (CIS)—defined as the initial inflammatory event involving the brain, spinal cord, or optic nerves in a patient who otherwise does not fulfill the diagnostic criteria for MS. CIS is now considered part of the MS disease spectrum, because studies have shown that patients with CIS and two or more typical MS lesions on imaging have a high risk of fulfilling the MS criteria over time (88% in 10 years).

> **CLINICAL VIGNETTE** *A 21-year-old woman developed pain in her right eye, which worsened with eye movement associated with blurry vision. The patient consulted her ophthalmologist and was diagnosed as having a right optic neuritis. She was recommended to have an MRI of her brain and orbits that showed enhancement of her right optic nerve, confirming the clinical impression of optic neuritis and also showed periventricular and infratentorial T2 hyperintense white matter abnormalities suggestive of MS (Fig. 39.1). The patient was treated with a 5-day course of intravenous (IV) steroids and referred to a neurologist. At the time of her visit to the neurologist, vision was much improved and examination was remarkable only for a pale disc, afferent defect, and red color desaturation on the right. The patient denied any prior neurologic symptoms. She was diagnosed as having CIS and placed on a disease modifying agent (DMA).*
>
> *Comment: This is a typical presentation for CIS in a young woman with brain MRI showing the presence of typical "silent" central nervous system demyelinating plaques. Because of her high risk of conversion to MS, she was promptly started on treatment.*

2. Radiologically isolated syndrome (RIS)—defined by clinically asymptomatic patients with incidental MRI findings consistent with MS. Because there is no clinical evidence of demyelination in these patients, RIS is not considered an MS subtype. However, one should be aware that the presence of gadolinium enhancement or spinal cord lesions increases the chances of an eventual MS diagnosis; therefore, in these patients, clinical and imaging monitoring is warranted.

CLINICAL VIGNETTE *A 44-year-old man with no significant past medical history presented to the office after having a brain MRI to investigate ongoing headaches. He was told that the MRI showed "some spots in his brain," with concerns about the possibility of MS (Fig. 39.2A). He denies ever having symptoms suggestive of MS in the past, but states that he has a maternal cousin who has this disease. Neurologic examination was normal. MRI of his spine showed a small nonenhancing cervical cord lesion, for which the patient was asymptomatic. Spinal fluid showed no oligoclonal bands. MS mimickers were checked and negative. The patient was diagnosed as having RIS and recommended to be followed up clinically every 6 months and by imaging yearly. One year later, he developed isolated numbness in his right leg with a sensory level at T4. MRI of his thoracic spine showed a new T4 enhancing lesion (Fig. 39.2B), and at that point, he was placed on a DMA.*

Comment: The widespread use of MRI to investigate other neurologic conditions, such as in this patient, has led to the identification of incidental typical MS lesions, and given rise to a newly defined syndrome termed RIS. The presence of spinal cord involvement in this case increases the risk for a first clinical event, reinforcing the importance of clinical and imaging monitoring of these patients over time.

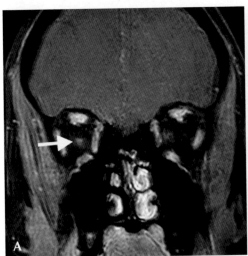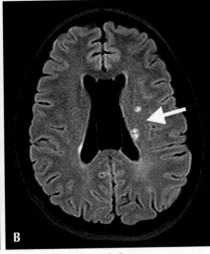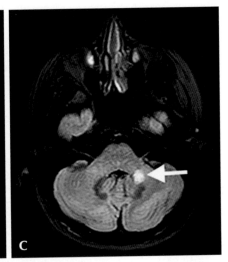

Fig. 39.1 CIS Case.

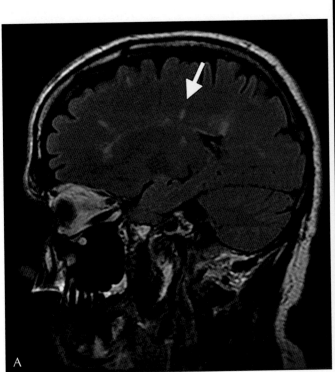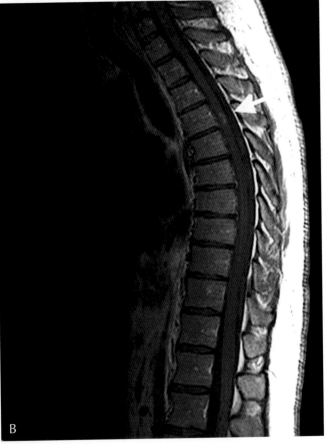

Fig. 39.2 RIS Case.

CLINICAL PRESENTATION

The clinical picture of MS varies according to the subtype of the disease.

1. Relapsing MS: This is the most common disease course, occurring in 85% of patients with MS and characterized by the development of relapses, also called exacerbations or "flare-ups." During the relapses, patients develop new or increasing neurologic symptoms that are followed by periods of remission in which symptoms can improve partially or completely. The clinical presentation will depend on the location of the active lesion(s) and can vary from sensory loss (usually an early complaint), weakness in one or more limbs (monoparesis, hemiparesis, or paraparesis), difficulties in controlling bowel and bladder, gait imbalance, blurry or double vision, facial pain (trigeminal neuralgia), and cognitive difficulties, particularly with attention and concentration problems as well as memory and judgment impairments. Aphasia and seizures can occur, but are not common. Onset of the disease is usually between the ages of 20 and 40, with a female preponderance.

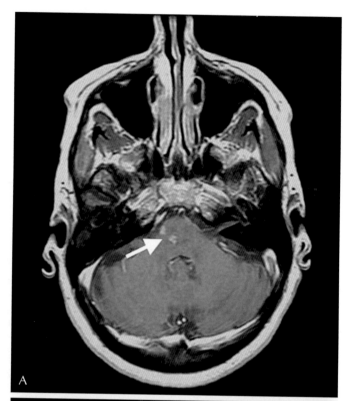

> **CLINICAL VIGNETTE** *A 40-year-old woman presents to the clinic; 6 years prior to the consultation, she was diagnosed as having a left optic neuritis by her ophthalmologist and treated with IV steroids. Brain MRI done at that time showed "nonspecific white matter abnormalities." Vision improved and she did well until 2 years later, when she developed double vision and gait unsteadiness. MRIs of her brain showed two enhancing lesions in the pons (Fig. 39.3A). She was diagnosed as having RRMS, treated with a 5-day course steroids, and started on a DMA. During treatment, she had another exacerbation presenting with leg weakness and urinary urgency, and MRIs done at that point showed two new enhancing lesions in her cervical cord (Fig. 39.3B). The patient was treated with IV steroids and switched to another DMA. Unfortunately, she continued to have exacerbations, prompting a referral for a second opinion to an MS clinic. During that evaluation, she was tested for JCV antibodies, and the finding was negative. At that point, she was placed on an intravenous monoclonal antibody and has been stable since then.*
>
> *Comment: This patient presented with a typical case of optic neuritis successfully treated with IV steroids with reported "nonspecific T2 hyperintensities" on initial brain MRI. No further diagnostic testing or treatment were recommended at that time, but 2 years later, she develops further neurologic symptoms with new enhancing lesions in her brainstem, fulfilling the diagnosis of RRMS. The first two DMAs were not able to control her disease, prompting escalation to a more aggressive treatment with the use of IV monoclonal antibody with subsequent stabilization of her condition.*

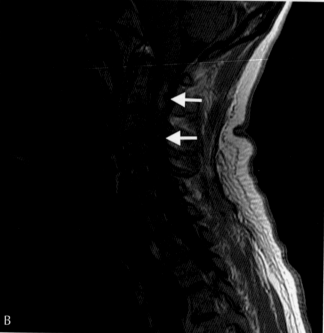

Fig. 39.3 RRMS Case.

2. Progressive MS—As the name suggests, this type of MS is characterized by progressive worsening of neurologic function with accumulation of disability over time, with much less inflammatory component. Progressive MS is subdivided in primary (PPMS) and secondary progressive MS (SPMS).

   a. PPMS—In PPMS, patients experience a progressive course from onset with no preceding relapses or remissions. The spinal cord is more commonly involved than the brain with consequent gait impairment early on in the course of the disease. Overall, there are less lesions and inflammation in PPMS than in relapsing MS. In addition, different from the other MS subtypes, men and women are affected equally. The average age of initial diagnosis is in the fifth to sixth decades of life.

> **CLINICAL VIGNETTE** *A 49-year-old man presents with gradual onset of gait difficulties for the past 4 years, initially attributed to "arthritis" in his knees. More recently, he started to trip while walking and having urinary urgency and frequency. He complained that his legs felt "tight," and because of two recent falls, he started using a cane to walk. Neuro examination was remarkable for a spastic gait, with weakness of bilateral iliopsoas and left tibialis anterior, brisk reflexes throughout with bilateral Babinski. Vibratory sensation was also lost in his toes and ankles. MRI of his brain showed*

approximately 9 T2 hyperintensities distributed in the periventricular and juxtacortical areas, none enhancing with contrast. MRI of his spinal cord showed two nonenhancing spinal cord lesions, one at C5 and another one at T8. Extensive blood work was done, including vitamin B12, copper, Lyme, HIV, HTLV-1, ESR, ANA with reflex, and long-chain fatty acids, all of which were normal or negative. Spinal fluid showed the presence of three oligoclonal bands, none present in the serum.

Comment: In approximately 15% of patients with MS, the clinical course is more chronically progressive from the beginning without any "flare-ups," as typically seen in patients with RRMS. Most of these patients have clinical evidence of significant spinal cord disease with high disability scores and very little intracranial findings. An initial misdiagnosis of an underlying orthopedic problem is common in these patients.

b. SPMS: The diagnosis of SPMS requires an initial relapsing-remitting course followed by progressive neurologic disability for at least 6 months that is independent of the relapses. In the preimmunomodulator area, patients would more often evolve to SPMS after having RRMS for an average of 15–20 years. Typically, patients present with gradual gait and cognitive decline associated with worsening of spasticity and of bladder control.

CLINICAL VIGNETTE *A 50-year-old woman presents with a 30-year history of MS. She recalls having numbness on her left side at age 25, but did not seek medical advice at that time as symptoms improved on their own after a couple of weeks. One year later, she developed diplopia and gait difficulties, prompting her first visit to a neurologist. She had a spinal tap that showed the presence of oligoclonal bands. She was diagnosed as having RRMS and treated with IV steroids with improvement. She reports having "flare-ups" every couple of years, with some of them treated with steroids. She was never treated with an immunomodulator as she "was doing so well" and was afraid of potential side effects. However, in the past 10 years, she has noted progressive gait difficulties, requiring her to use a cane initially and more recently a walker. She also noted urinary urgency and frequency, and has been more forgetful. MRIs of her brain and spine during this period of time showed extensive T2 hyperintensities in her brain with the presence of "black holes" and cerebral atrophy (Fig. 39.4) as well as extensive involvement of her spinal cord, but no new MS lesions.*

Comment: Typical case of an SPMS patient with a long preceding history of MS exacerbations for several years, treated only with intermittent pulse of IV steroids, with subsequent slow progression of difficulties with her gait, cognition and bladder control with MRIs showing extensive disease burden reflecting all the prior exacerbations, but no new lesions to account for the progression of symptoms. This is due to the fact that the progression is because of neurodegeneration and not because of new inflammatory lesions.

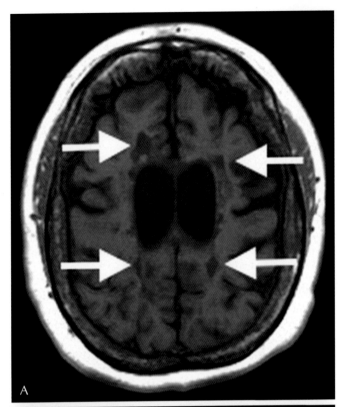

A

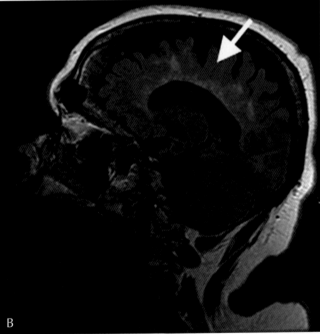

B

Fig. 39.4 SPMS Case.

Fatigue, pain, depression, and heat intolerance are also common symptoms in all types of MS.

The terms *benign* and *malignant/aggressive* MS should be used with caution, as they do not describe an MS phenotype, but simply provide an indication of disease severity. In addition, MS is an unpredictable disease, and its disease activity can significantly change over time. Therefore the term *benign* should only be used retrospectively, with the understanding that having a benign course up to the present time does not guarantee that it will continue to be the case in the years to come.

As MS is a condition that affects predominantly young women, it is not uncommon that patients will get pregnant during the course of

their disease. Patients should be informed that MS is not a contraindication for pregnancy, and that actually for the most part, patients do quite well during this period of time. However, the postpartum period has been associated with an increase in the number of relapses, particularly in patients who have had active disease within the year before getting pregnant. Therefore, ideally, patients with MS should plan their pregnancy during a period of time in which their disease is not active. In addition, all patients on DMA will need to discontinue their treatment prior to conceiving, with most DMAs being class C for pregnancy, while glatiramer acetate is class B and teriflunomide is class X. Current evidence suggests that breastfeeding is safe and potentially can be beneficial in patients with MS, with a meta-analysis study showing a 47% decrease in postpartum annualized relapse rate for women who breastfed their children as compared with the ones who did not. Patients who are breastfeeding should be off their DMA until weaning, with the exception of patients who are on glatiramer acetate and interferon. These two types of DMA are likely safe for use during lactation, as they are not likely to be transmitted into breast milk in large quantities due to their large molecular size. For patients who have decided not to breastfeed, a DMA should be started as soon as possible after delivery.

DIAGNOSIS

The diagnosis of MS is based on the clinical picture, as reported above and complemented by diagnostic testing such as neuroimaging, spinal fluid analysis, and evoked potentials.

Magnetic Resonance Imaging

In recent years, magnetic resonance imaging (MRI) of the brain and spinal cord has become the most important tool to support the diagnosis of MS as well as to monitor longitudinally treatment outcomes.

Typical MS lesions in the brain are ovoid hyperintensities involving the periventricular and juxtacortical regions, best seen on fluid-attenuated inversion recovery, also known as FLAIR (Figs. 39.1 and 39.2). The periventricular distribution is secondary to the distribution of the inflammatory process around the venules, as seen in histopathology and more recently with ultra-high-field-strength MRI. The corpus callosum as well as other infratentorial regions such as brainstem, cerebellar peduncles (see Fig. 39.1), and cerebellum are also commonly involved and better seen on sagittal FLAIR and T2-weighted images, respectively. T1-weighted images with contrast (gadolinium) can show contrast enhancement in acute demyelinating lesions due to the increased blood-brain permeability caused by the inflammation (Figs. 39.2 and 39.3). Enhancement can be punctate, nodular, or ringlike and tends to persist for 4–6 weeks, being more common in the relapsing-remitting than in the progressive phases of MS. Prominent T1 hypointensities, also called "black holes," can also be seen in patients with MS and are correlated with a greater axonal pathology on histopathology. In addition, atrophy of both gray and white matter can be detected, predominantly in the progressive phase of this disease (Fig. 39.4).

Abnormalities in the spinal cord can be noted in more than 80% of patients with MS with predominance of the cervical cord (see Fig. 39.3). Lesions are usually dorsal or lateral, tend to involve less than half of the axial cord, and span one vertebral body or less. The spinal cord MRI protocol often includes a sagittal T1-weighted and proton density, STIR or phase sensitive inversion recovery, axial T2-weighted or T2*-weighted images through suspicious lesions, and postcontrast gadolinium enhanced T1–weighted imaging.

Spinal Fluid

Spinal fluid analysis has become superfluous in patients with typical history and examination findings and supportive imaging studies. However, in cases in which the MRI is not typical, a spinal tap should be considered (Fig. 39.5). In most cases, the white blood count is normal; however, occasionally one may see MS patients with up to 50 lymphocytes per cubic millimeter. The CSF glucose level is usually normal, and protein can be normal or slightly elevated. The presence of a high IGG index and CSF-specific oligoclonal bands can be seen in approximately 70% and 90% of the patients with MS, respectively, reflecting the abnormal intrathecal immunoglobulin production. However, neither is specific for MS and may be present in other conditions that affect the CNS, such as sarcoidosis, SLE, Sjögren disease, and antiphospholipid antibody syndrome. Increased myelin basic protein is quite common in this population, which is a result of breakdown of the myelin, but is nonspecific.

Evoked Potentials

Advances in imaging technology in the past couple of decades have reduced the use of evoked potentials in clinical practice. However, visual evoked potentials are still used in some cases, when MRIs are not conclusive, to detect subclinical optic neuritis, thereby helping to fulfill the criteria for dissemination in space (Fig. 39.6).

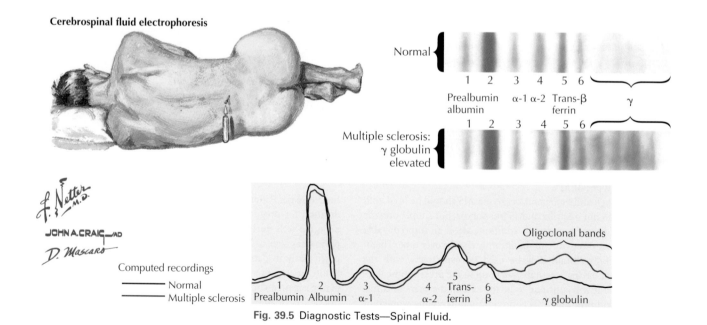

Cerebrospinal fluid electrophoresis

Normal
1 2 3 4 5 6
Prealbumin α-1 α-2 Trans-β   γ
albumin   ferrin

Multiple sclerosis:
γ globulin
elevated
1 2 3 4 5 6

Oligoclonal bands

Computed recordings
—— Normal
—— Multiple sclerosis

1 2 3 4 5 6
Prealbumin Albumin   α-1   α-2 Trans-   β   γ globulin
ferrin

Fig. 39.5 Diagnostic Tests—Spinal Fluid.

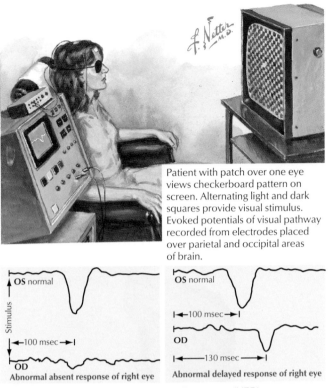

Patient with patch over one eye views checkerboard pattern on screen. Alternating light and dark squares provide visual stimulus. Evoked potentials of visual pathway recorded from electrodes placed over parietal and occipital areas of brain.

OS normal

OD

Stimulus

←100 msec→

Abnormal absent response of right eye

OS normal

←100 msec→

OD

←130 msec→

Abnormal delayed response of right eye

Fig. 39.6 Visual Evoked Response (VER).

DIAGNOSIS CRITERIA FOR MULTIPLE SCLEROSIS

Since its first description by Charcot, MS has had many versions of proposed diagnostic criteria, with the most recent one being the McDonald Criteria 2010, which will be discussed here.

RRMS

The current criteria to diagnose RRMS require dissemination in space and time. Dissemination in space can be satisfied only on clinical grounds, if there is evidence of involvement of two different CNS locations. In cases in which there is clinical evidence of only one lesion, MRI can be used to confirm the dissemination in space, by showing at least one T2 lesion in two of the following sites: periventricular, juxtacortical, infratentorial, or spinal cord. Dissemination in time can also be satisfied on clinical grounds only if a patient has a history of at least two exacerbations. In a patient who had only one clinical attack, dissemination in time can also be established by follow-up MRIs showing subsequent development of new T2 and/or gadolinium-enhancing lesions. Of note, the presence of simultaneous asymptomatic enhancing lesions and nonenhancing lesions on initial MRI after the first clinical attack will fulfill dissemination in time. In this case, a second clinical attack or new lesions on subsequent MRIs are not needed to confirm the diagnosis.

PPMS

The criteria for the diagnosis of PPMS include the following:
- One year of disease progression
- Two of the following:
  - Evidence of dissemination in space in the brain with at least one lesion in one of the characteristic MS locations: periventricular, juxtacortical, or infratentorial.
  - Evidence of dissemination in space in the spinal cord, with two or more typical MS lesions.

- Presence of oligoclonal bands or high IGG index in the spinal fluid.

SPMS

Secondary progressive MS is usually diagnosed when a patient demonstrates disease progression for at least 6 months independent of a clinical relapse or new inflammatory activity on imaging.

DIFFERENTIAL DIAGNOSIS

Depending on the clinical presentation, certain etiologies should be considered in the differential diagnosis of MS.

Optic Neuritis

The typical optic neuritis (ON) presentation is characterized by a subacute, painful, unilateral visual loss that can vary from mild to severe intensity and tends to improve over time (Fig. 39.7). Red flags such as an acute or chronic/progressive presentation, bilateral involvement, and severe visual loss with poor recovery should prompt consideration of an alternative etiologies, including vascular (anterior ischemic optic neuritis, giant cell arteritis), compressive (primary and metastatic tumors), infectious (Lyme, syphilis), inflammatory (sarcoidosis, SLE, Behçet syndrome, neuromyelitis optica), inherited (Leber), toxic (methanol intoxication, ethambutol toxicity), and nutritional (B12 deficiency) etiologies.

Brainstem and Cerebellar Syndromes

Internuclear ophthalmoplegia often bilateral, sixth nerve palsy, ataxia, nystagmus, facial sensory symptoms, and dizziness presenting subacutely, with at least partial recovery, are common MS presentations reflecting its infratentorial involvement (Fig. 39.8). Acute onset of symptoms should raise suspicion for a vascular cause, while a more progressive course, particularly if associated with persistent enhancement on MRI, should prompt further investigation to rule out inflammatory (sarcoidosis, Behçet syndrome) and infectious (Whipple, tuberculosis) etiologies as well as malignancies. Chronic lymphocytic inflammation with pontine perivascular enhancement responsive to steroids (CLIPPERS) should also be included in the differential of patients presenting with brainstem symptoms. This is a rare condition in which patients present with diplopia, facial paresthesias, and occasionally myelopathy, with typical MRI findings and good response to high-dose corticosteroids. In addition, in patients with progressive cerebellar presentation, paraneoplastic and hereditary spinocerebellar ataxias should be ruled out.

Spinal Cord Involvement

Typically patients present with an incomplete transverse myelitis, with predominance of sensory symptoms often associated with bladder difficulties and Lhermitte sign (Fig. 39.9). Symptoms usually progress for the first few days and last for a couple of weeks, and that is followed by at least some partial recovery. Acute presentations should prompt consideration for a vascular etiology, while in a more progressive course, other etiologies such as HTLV-1, cervical spondylosis, B12, and copper deficiency should be ruled out. Neuromyelitis optica must be considered in the differential diagnosis when there is an extensive cord involvement (three or more vertebral segments).

TREATMENT

Treatment of MS has significantly changed over the course of the past two decades. Not only has the drug armamentarium expanded greatly, with more than a dozen therapeutic options, but also the goals of treatment emphasize the "no evidence of disease activity" (NEDA) concept.

Optic neuritis

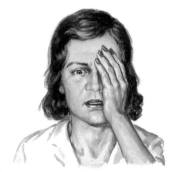

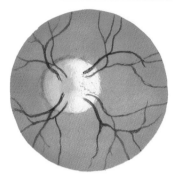

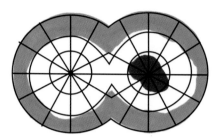

Sudden unilateral blindness, self-limited (usually 2 to 3 weeks). Patient covering one eye, suddenly realizes other eye is partially or totally blind.

Temporal pallor in optic disc, caused by delayed recovery of temporal side of optic (II) nerve

Visual fields reveal central scotoma due to acute retrobulbar neuritis

Internuclear ophthalmoplegia

(OD = right, OS = left)

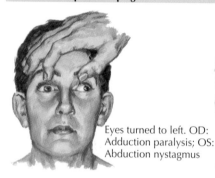

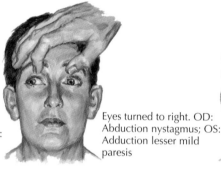

Eyes turned to left. OD: Adduction paralysis; OS: Abduction nystagmus

Eyes turned to right. OD: Abduction nystagmus; OS: Adduction lesser mild paresis

Convergence. Fully preserved adduction; both eyes have full medial movement

Fig. 39.7 Multiple Sclerosis: Visual Manifestations.

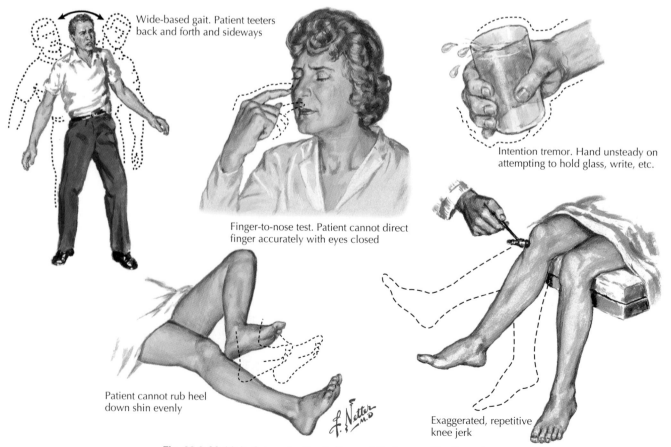

Wide-based gait. Patient teeters back and forth and sideways

Intention tremor. Hand unsteady on attempting to hold glass, write, etc.

Finger-to-nose test. Patient cannot direct finger accurately with eyes closed

Patient cannot rub heel down shin evenly

Exaggerated, repetitive knee jerk

Fig. 39.8 Multiple Sclerosis: Cerebellar and Brainstem Manifestations.

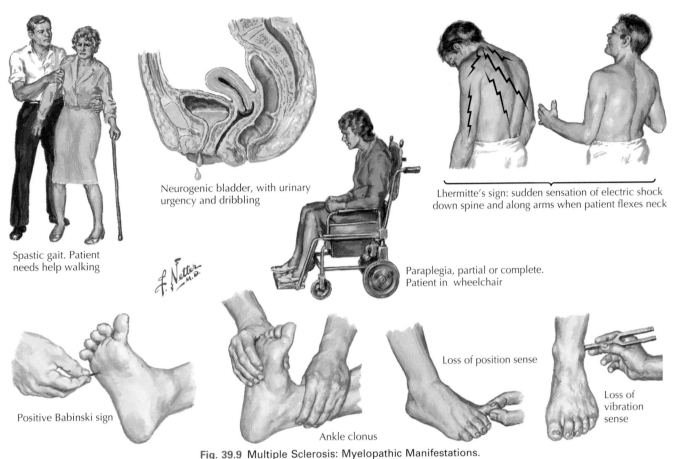

Spastic gait. Patient needs help walking

Neurogenic bladder, with urinary urgency and dribbling

Lhermitte's sign: sudden sensation of electric shock down spine and along arms when patient flexes neck

Paraplegia, partial or complete. Patient in wheelchair

Loss of position sense

Loss of vibration sense

Positive Babinski sign

Ankle clonus

Fig. 39.9 Multiple Sclerosis: Myelopathic Manifestations.

The original NEDA definition included lack of relapses and disability worsening, in addition to lack of new or active lesions on MRI scans (NEDA-3), and was weighted more toward the absence of inflammatory activity. More recently, this concept has been expanded to include the lack of brain volume loss, a surrogate of neurodegeneration, as its fourth parameter (NEDA-4). For the vast majority of relapsing MS, a stepwise approach model is appropriate, starting with safer treatments in the early stages of the disease (interferon beta, glatiramer acetate [GA], oral immunomodulators) and escalating to drugs with higher efficacy but also with greater side effects, such as monoclonal antibodies, if suboptimal response is detected. However, in patients who already present with very active disease initially, a more aggressive approach early on should be considered.

RELAPSING REMITTING MULTIPLE SCLEROSIS

The treatment for RRMS can be divided into treatment of acute relapses and preventive treatment.

Acute Phase Treatment

During acute MS exacerbations, intravenous corticosteroids such as methylprednisolone are frequently used due to their ability to decrease inflammation of the central nervous system. Even though the dose and duration of treatment tend to vary among different centers, a common dose is 1 g of intravenous methylprednisolone for 3–5 days, followed or not by a steroid taper. Adrenocorticotropic hormone (ACTH) has been approved for the treatment of MS exacerbations by the US Food and Drug Administration (FDA) in 1978 and is usually recommended

for patients who cannot tolerate or did not have a good response to corticosteroids in the past or have poor intravenous access. The dose varies from 80 to 120 units a day and is given intramuscular or subcutaneously for 2–3 weeks.

For patients with severe attacks that do not respond to corticosteroids, plasma exchange can be used. The treatment usually consists of plasma exchanges every other day for a total of five treatments. The severity of symptoms must warrant the potential side effects associated with plasma exchange.

Preventive Treatment

There are currently 14 FDA-approved preventive treatments for RRMS of six different classes, as listed below. They all have shown to decrease the number of relapses and new lesions on MRI, and some of them have also shown some impact in delaying disability progression. Unfortunately, none of the approved therapies have been shown to repair MS plaques or to improve preexisting symptoms or signs.

Interferon Beta

Betaseron, an interferon beta 1b (250 mcg SC every other day), was the first FDA immunomodulator approved for the treatment of MS in 1993. Since then, multiple interferons beta, both 1a and 1b, have been approved for the treatment of RRMS, including low-dose interferon 1a (Avonex: 30 mcg IM every week), high-dose interferon 1a (Rebif 44 mcg SC three times a week), and more recently, a pegylated form of interferon beta 1a (Plegridy 125 mcg SC twice a month). In addition, a generic form of Betaseron, named Extavia, was also added to the treatment armamentarium. Interferon beta reduces the annual relapse rate (ARR) by approximately a third as compared with placebo, and most of them are also approved for the treatment of CIS in high-risk patients for conversion to clinically definitive MS. The mechanism of action of interferons is still somewhat unclear, but it is believed that they promote a shift from inflammatory (Th1) to antiinflammatory (Th2) environment, in addition to stabilizing the blood-brain barrier. The most common side effects are flulike symptoms, more prominent within the first 3 months of treatment, and local site reactions, followed by cytopenias, abnormalities in the liver function, worsening depression, and thyroid abnormalities.

Glatiramer Acetate

GA was first approved for the treatment of RRMS in 1996 and later was also approved for CIS. The initial preparation (Copaxone) consisted of 20 mg of GA given daily. In 2013, another preparation with 40 mg of GA given three times a week was approved with the hope of increasing compliance with a less frequent dosing, and that was followed by the approval of the generic form of GA (Glatopa) in 2015. Like the interferons, the mechanism of action of GA is not well known, but likely also involved a shift from Th1 to Th2 antiinflammatory cells and upregulation of T-regulatory cells, with an annual relapse rate reduction of 29% as compared with placebo. Often considered the immunomodulator with less number of side effects, GA has been known to cause injection site reactions and postinjection systemic reactions. These are characterized by at least two of the following symptoms: chest pain, palpitations, shortness of breath, and flushing. Symptoms are transient, usually lasting 15 minutes, and have no known long-term effects.

Fingolimod (Gylenia)

The first oral immunomodulator for the treatment of RRMS, fingolimod (0.5 mg PO daily), was FDA approved in 2010, with an ARR of approximately 50% over 2 years as compared with placebo. It is a sphingosine-1-phosphate antagonist preventing the egress of both lymphocytes B and T from the lymph nodes, including autoreactive ones. Potential side effects include cardiac bradyarrhythmias and atrioventricular blocks, arterial hypertension, macular edema, abnormal liver function tests, dyspnea, and increased risk of herpetic infections. In addition, cases of PML have been reported, some of them after transition from natalizumab therapy. Because of the risk of cardiac arrhythmias and blocks, all patients starting fingolimod should be monitored with hourly pulse and blood pressure for at least 6 hours of initial dose, and have an ECG prior to and at the end of the observation period. This also includes patients who are reinitiating treatment after a hiatus of more than 14 days.

Teriflunomide (Aubagio)

Teriflunomide was the second oral immunomodulator approved by FDA for the treatment of RRMS in 2012 (14 mg oral daily) and subsequently for CIS. Teriflunomide is a dihydroorotate inhibitor preventing pyrimidine synthesis in rapidly dividing cells. It has been shown to decrease the ARR by 31%–36% over 1 year in placebo-controlled trials. Potential side effects include transaminase elevation, hair thinning, diarrhea, arterial hypertension, and infections. It is also a category X for pregnancy for both female and male patients; therefore effective contraception should be used if prescribed for child-bearing age patients.

Dimethyl Fumarate (Tecfidera)

In 2013, dimethyl fumarate (240 mg oral twice a day) became the third immunomodulator approved by FDA for the treatment of RRMS with an ARR reduction of 44%–53% over 2 years as compared with placebo. Its mechanism of action is unclear, but it is believed to have both neuroprotective and antiinflammatory properties. Common side effects

are flushing, gastrointestinal upset, leucopenia, and lymphopenia. Since its approval, a few cases of progressive multifocal leukoencephalopathy in patients with severe and prolonged lymphopenia have been described, leading to a label change in 2016, with the recommendation of frequent CBC with differential monitoring (q6 months) and considering interruption of dimethyl fumarate if a lymphocyte count less than $0.5 \times 10/L$ persists for more than 6 months

Monoclonal Antibodies

In MS, monoclonal antibodies work by selectively interfering with the immune response by blocking cell adhesion or by depleting specific immune cells. There are four approved mAbs for MS treatment; however, one of them, daclizumab, has been permanently removed from the market in 2018, due to the development of serious side effects (discussed later).

Natalizumab (Tysabri®)

Natalizumab is a humanized mAb that inhibits alpha-4-integrin with consequent reduction of the migration of VLA-4-positive lymphocytes to the central nervous system. This treatment consists of monthly IV infusions of 300 mg each and reduces the ARR by 68% and 55%, as compared with placebo and interferon beta 1a (Avonex), respectively. Its main concerning side effect is the potential risk for progressive multifocal leukoencephalopathy, a condition that can lead to severe disability and death, occurring in approximately 4 per 1000 patients. This risk can be further stratified, depending on the presence of positive JC virus antibodies, prior exposure to immunosuppressive drugs, and treatment duration.

Alemtuzumab (Lemtrada)

Humanized mAb against CD52, a surface antigen present in both B and T lymphocytes, leads to sustained depletion of those cells for up to 1 year with an ARR reduction of 49%–55% over 2 years, as compared with interferon beta 1a (Rebif). Even though this drug has been approved to treat RRMS patients with either naïve or breakthrough disease, the risks of developing other autoimmune disorders such as thyroid disease, idiopathic thrombocytopenic purpura, and Goodpasture syndrome after one or more treatments have limited its use for more aggressive forms of this disease.

Daclizumab (Zynbryta)

Daclizumab is a humanized mAb that binds to CD25, the alpha subunit of the IL-2 receptor of T cells with consequent reduction of T cell responses. In addition, daclizumab promotes the expansion of natural killer cells, which kill the activated autologous T cells, thus helping regulate the immune system. This drug (150 mg SC every month) was approved for RRMS treatment in May 2016 with a reduction of the ARR by 45% after nearly 3 years as compared with interferon beta 1a (Avonex). Main side effects include increased risk of infections, skin rashes, and liver complications. Because of its safety profile, this medication is generally recommended for patients who have failed two or more other DMAs. In March 2018, daclizumab was voluntarily withdrawn from the market due to new safety concerns related to reports of inflammatory encephalitis and meningoencephalitis.

Ocrelizumab (Ocrevus)

The most recent approved humanized mAb (March 2017), ocrelizumab targets CD20 on B lymphocytes and has shown a reduction of ARR by up to 47% as compared with interferon beta 1a (Rebif) over 2 years. This medication is administered intravenously, 600 mg every 6 months. However, the first dose is divided into two doses of 300 mg each and given 2 weeks apart. Most common side effects are infusion-related reactions and infections such as respiratory tract and herpes-related infections. In addition, an increased risk of malignancy, particularly of breast cancer, may exist.

In some selected patients with very aggressive forms of RRMS not responsive to any of the above treatment options, the use of chemotherapy agents can be considered. The most common chemotherapy agents used in those situations are as follows.

Cyclophosphamide

Cyclophosphamide is an alkylating agent with cytotoxic effects on both T and B lymphocytes. Its benefit in aggressive MS has been demonstrated in small studies over the years. Its significant toxicity, including possibility of development of hemorrhagic cystitis as well as bladder cancer associated with potential infertility, has limited its use. Induction, pulse, and high-dose protocols have been reported with this drug, with a lifetime maximal dose of 80–100 g.

Mitoxantrone

Mitoxantrone (12 mg/m^2 IV q3 months for 24 months, max dose of 140 mg/m^2) is an anthracycline that also inhibits both T and B cells, and similar to cyclophosphamide, its more widespread use has been disfavored due to its potential side effects, including cardiotoxicity, leukemia risk, liver toxicity, and infertility. However, it remains a potential option if other treatments fail.

Cladribine

The use of intravenous *cladribine* (0.875 mg/kg/d IV for 4 days q6 months for 2 years), an antimetabolite that selectively reduces lymphocytes, in particular CD4 and CD8, can be considered in selected cases, when other therapies have failed or are not available. However, as with any of the other chemotherapy agents listed above, the possibility of severe side effects such as infections and long-term risk of malignancies should be carefully considered during the decision-making process.

Stem Cell Transplant

The hope of potentially rebooting the immune system by eliminating pathogenic immune cells and replacing them with normal functioning ones has prompted the treatment of patients with aggressive forms of MS with autologous hematopoietic stem cell transplant. Various conditioning regimen intensities have been used, and as expected, less ablative treatments were associated with less toxicity but also with less efficacy. Mortality has been reported to be as high as 5% in earlier studies, but it has decreased to less than 1% more recently. Hematopoietic stem cell transplant is not currently FDA approved for the treatment of MS and, like the chemotherapy agents, should only be considered in selected relapsing MS patients with significant inflammatory disease not responsive to standard treatment and performed in centers with established experience in bone marrow transplantation.

Progressive Multiple Sclerosis

Contrary to the current wide variety of treatments available for patients with relapsing forms of MS, trials with different DMAs for patients with progressive MS have been quite disappointing.

In patients with SPMS, the only FDA-approved treatment is mitoxantrone, but it is rarely used in clinical practice due to its side effects.

Regarding patients with PPMS, ocrelizumab was recently FDA approved to treat those patients after showing a 24% reduction in the risk of progression of clinical disability as compared with placebo. Other benefits included decreased volume of brain lesions and reduced rate of brain atrophy.

Symptomatic Treatment

Beyond the use of DMAs, symptomatic treatment should be considered in all MS patients, with relapsing or progressive forms of this disease. Treatment should include not only pharmacotherapy but also behavior and lifestyle changes as well as rehabilitative strategies. The most common symptoms reported by MS patients are fatigue, paresthesias/pain, cognitive difficulties, mood disorder, spasticity, and lack of bladder control. Some options for the treatment of these symptoms are presented in Table 39.1.

In addition, smoking cessation, a healthy diet, good sleep quality, regular exercises, and vitamin D supplementation (when deficient) should be encouraged in all patients. The use of medical marijuana to treat spasticity, central pain, and overactive bladder is still controversial,

TABLE 39.1 Treatment of Commonly Reported MS Symptoms

Common Reported Symptoms	Pharmacologic Treatment	Lifestyle Changes/Rehab
Fatigue	Amantadine, modafinil, or armodafinil Stimulants (amphetamines, methylphenidate)	Treatment-associated depression and sleep problems, if present Regular exercises Cognitive behavior therapy, such as mindfulness
Paresthesias/pain	TN: carbamazepine, oxcarbazepine, gabapentin CNP: tricyclics, SNRIs, anticonvulsants	Meditation, mindfulness, biofeedback techniques
Cognitive impairment	Cholinesterase inhibitors (donepezil, rivastigmine, galantamine) NMDA receptor antagonist (memantine)	Cognitive rehabilitation
Mood disorder	SSRIs SNRIs	Psychotherapy
Spasticity	GABA-A receptor agonist (benzodiazepines) GABA-B receptor agonist (baclofen PO, baclofen pump) Central adrenergic agonist (tizanidine)	Physical therapy Botox treatment
Neurogenic bladder	Hyperactive bladder: anticholinergics, B$_3$ adrenergic receptor agonist (mirabegron) Bladder dyssynergia: α$_1$ adrenergic receptor antagonist	Bladder dyssynergia—Intradetrusor injections of Botox Hypotonic bladder—Intermittent or indwelling bladder catheterization

CNP, Chronic neuropathic pain; *SNRIs,* serotonin-norepinephrine reuptake inhibitors; *SSRIs,* selective serotonin reuptake inhibitors; *TN,* trigeminal neuralgia.

despite evidence of some benefit, mostly due to lack of data about potential risks, in particular with cognition.

FUTURE DIRECTIONS

Currently, we have a variety of medications that impact the inflammatory changes that occur in MS patients, with consequent decrease in the number of relapses, new lesions on MRIs, and delay in disease progression. However, there is a lack of therapeutic options to help improve patients' established disabilities and ongoing progression of symptoms, most noticeable in progressive forms of MS. Ongoing and upcoming trials to promote remyelination and axonal repair will hopefully be successful in addressing these challenges in the near future.

ADDITIONAL RESOURCES

Confavreux C, Hutchinson M, Hours MM, et al. Rate of pregnancy-related relapse in multiple sclerosis. Pregnancy in multiple sclerosis group. N Engl J Med 1998;339(5):285–91.

Multicenter study involving 254 women who were followed during their pregnancy up to 1 year after delivery to determine the relapse rate of MS per trimester as well as the effects of epidural analgesia and breast feeding on the frequency of relapse during the first 3 months postpartum.

Kappos L, De Stefano N, Freedman MS, et al. Inclusion of brain volume loss in a revised measure of "no evidence of disease activity" (NEDA-4) in relapsing-remitting multiple sclerosis. Mult Scler 2016;22(10):1297–305.

Revision of the concept of "no evidence of disease activity" (NEDA) with the inclusion of a fourth component, brain volume loss, to the other three measures: absence of MRI activity, absence of relapses, and disability progression.

Lublin FD, Reingold SC, Cohen JA, et al. Defining the clinical course of multiple sclerosis. The 2013 revisions. Neurology 2014;83:278–86.

New revised MS classification including disease activity based on clinical relapse rate and imaging findings as well as disease progression.

Okuda DT, Mowry EM, Beheshtian A, et al. Incidental MRI anomalies suggestive of multiple sclerosis: the radiologically isolated syndrome. Neurology 2009;72:800–5.

Initial study describing the characteristics of a new entity: the radiologically isolated syndrome.

Pakpoor J, Disanto G, Lacey MV, et al. Breastfeeding and multiple sclerosis relapses: a meta-analysis. J Neurol 2012;259(10):2246–8.

Meta-analysis of 12 studies assessing the annualized relapse rate of MS patients who breastfed versus those who did not.

Polman CH, Reingold SC, Banwell B, et al. Diagnostic criteria for multiple sclerosis: 2010 revisions to the McDonald criteria. Ann Neurol 2011;69(2):292–302.

Most recent revision of the McDonald criteria for the diagnosis of MS.

Yadav SK, Mindur JE, Ito K, et al. Advances in the immunopathogenesis of multiple sclerosis. Curr Opin Neurol 2015;28(3):206–19.

Review of the immunopathophysiology of multiple sclerosis.

40

Other Central Nervous System Demyelinating Disorders

Claudia J. Chaves

NEUROMYELITIS OPTICA (DEVIC DISEASE) AND NEUROMYELITIS OPTIC SPECTRUM DISORDER

> **CLINICAL VIGNETTE** *A 58-year-old woman was admitted to the hospital with a 5-day history of numbness and weakness in both lower extremities, a tight bandlike sensation across her chest associated with gait difficulties, and urinary urgency. The patient had similar but less severe symptoms 1 year prior that resolved within a few weeks. She did not seek medical attention at that time. In addition, she reported having an episode of left optic neuritis 3 years prior and since then has had extremely poor vision in that eye.*
>
> *Her neuro exam was remarkable for an afferent defect on the left, a pale left disk, visual acuity of 20/200 on the left, and lower extremity weakness with a T4 sensory level in all modalities. The patient had magnetic resonance images (MRIs) of her brain and spine that showed central predominant intramedullary T2 hyperintense signal abnormality from C7 through T5-T6, with peripheral enhancement from T2 through T4 (Fig. 40.1). Spinal fluid showed 8 white blood cells, 90% lymphocytes, protein of 55, and glucose of 71, with normal IGG index and no oligoclonal bands. She had positive aquaporin-4 in the blood and in the spinal fluid. Lyme, ACE, ANA screen, and HIV were negative. The patient was diagnosed as having neuromyelitis optic spectrum disorder with positive aquaporin-4 antibodies. She was treated with a 5-day course of 1000 mg of IV methylprednisolone with some improvement of her symptoms and subsequently placed on intravenous rituximab every 6 months without any recurrence of the neurologic symptoms.*
>
> *Comment: This is a typical clinical presentation and imaging studies in this 58-year-old woman presenting with a thoracic transverse myelitis with an extensive spinal cord lesion extending for more than three vertebral bodies. Of note, this patient had a prior episode of a severe optic neuritis that left her legally blind on the left as well as a prior demyelinating event involving her spinal cord the year before. A positive serum aquaporin-4 confirmed the diagnosis.*

Neuromyelitis optica (NMO) is an inflammatory disorder causing severe damage to the myelin and axons of the central nervous system, affecting mostly the optic nerves and spinal cord. First described by E. Devic in 1894, NMO was initially thought to be a variant of multiple sclerosis. However, recent advances have shown that NMO has its own distinct clinical and immunologic characteristics. The discovery over a decade ago of pathogenic IGG antibodies in patients with NMO that specifically target aquaporin-4 (AQPR-4), a water channel protein located in the astrocytic foot processes, has allowed an easier distinction between the two clinical entities, supporting a humoral rather than a cell-mediated mechanism. Furthermore, the increase in specificity of the AQPR-4 antibody due to improved assays have expanded the clinical and

radiologic spectrum of NMO, prompting the introduction in 2007 of the term neuromyelitis optic spectrum disorders (NMOSD) to include AQPR-4 antibody positive patients with limited or atypical forms of NMO.

Pathologically this syndrome is characterized by astrocytic damage, demyelination, neuronal loss, and frequently the presence of severe necrosis.

Revised criteria as of 2015 have simplified the terminology of these conditions, and currently the unifying term NMOSD stratified by presence, absence, or unknown status of AQPR-4 antibodies is recommended and will be used in this chapter. As expected, the criteria for patients with absent or unknown AQPR-4 antibodies are more stringent as compared with positive patients (Box 40.1).

Clinical Picture

Since AQPR-4, the main target of the NMOSD IGG antibodies, is highly concentrated in the optic nerves, spinal cord gray matter, periaqueductal, and periventricular regions, the following clinical manifestations can occur in those patients: optic neuritis, acute myelitis, acute brainstem, and diencephalic syndromes and symptomatic cerebral syndrome. In general, NMOSD has a relapsing course with more than half of the patients presenting with a relapse within the first year of the initial attack and 90% within the first 3 years. In contrast to multiple sclerosis, secondary progression phase is rare in this entity.

Optic Neuritis

Episodes of optic neuritis in patients with NMOSD are characterized by visual loss often associated with eye pain, similar to the attacks secondary to multiple sclerosis; however, simultaneous or sequential involvement of both optic nerves, accompanied by severe visual loss, is characteristic of NMOSD. Altitudinal defects as well as involvement of the optic chiasm are also very suggestive of NMOSD.

Acute Myelitis

Differently from multiple sclerosis (MS), patients with NMOSD often present with a complete transverse myelitis characterized by motor and sensory loss below the level of the lesion associated with bowel and bladder dysfunction, as well as severe pain and paroxysmal tonic spasms of the trunk or extremities. In addition, in contrast to MS, the lesions in NMOSD are usually extensive, involving more than three vertebral segments on MRI.

Brainstem Syndrome

The most common brainstem syndrome is due to the involvement of the area postrema and characterized by nausea, vomiting, and intractable hiccups. Oculomotor involvement and less commonly involvement of other cranial nerves have been reported.

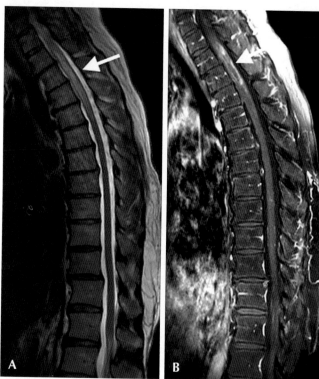

Fig. 40.1 (A) Sagittal T2 MRI of the thoracic spinal cord showing extensive abnormal T2 hyperintense signal in the lower cervical and upper thoracic cord with more than three segments involved, characteristic of NMO. (B) Sagittal T1 Fat Sat postcontrast image demonstrating peripheral intramedullary enhancement from T2 through T4.

Acute Diencephalic Syndrome

Hypothalamic involvement may lead to hypersomnia or symptomatic narcolepsy as well as temperature and appetite dysregulations.

Symptomatic Cerebral Syndrome

Large tumefactive or spindlelike lesions causing encephalopathy and/ or neurologic deficits have been reported in NMOSD.

Diagnosis

The workup of patients with clinical suspect NMOSD include AQPR-4 antibody status, MRI of brain and spine, and occasionally spinal fluid analysis.

Serum AQPR-4 Antibody

Due to its higher sensitivity (76%) and specificity (99%), a cell-based essay is recommended when evaluating suspected NMOSD patients and ideally should be tested during an exacerbation and before starting immunosuppressive treatment. In some patients who are negative for aquaporin-4, antibodies against myelin oligodendrocyte glycoprotein (MOG) have been detected. Those patients are usually male, present with optic neuritis more than with myelitis, and have a better prognosis than the patients with positive anti-AQPR-4. In addition, unlike anti-AQP4 antibodies, the pathogenic nature of anti-NMO is still under investigation.

MRIs of Orbits, Brain, and Spine

Extensive lesions involving the spinal cord (three or more vertebral segments) and the optic nerves are common in patients with NMOSD (Figs. 40.1 and 40.2). The spinal cord involvement tends to include the

BOX 40.1   Neuromyelitis Optic Spectrum Disorders Diagnostic Criteria for Adult Patients

Diagnostic criteria for NMOSD with AQP4 antibodies
1. At least one core clinical characteristic
2. Positive test for AQP4 antibodies using best available method (cell-based assay strongly recommended)
3. Exclusion of alternative diagnosis

Diagnosis criteria for NMOSD without or unknown AQP4 antibodies
1. At least two core clinical characteristics occurring as a result of one or more clinical attacks and meeting all the following requirements:
   a. At least one core clinical characteristic must be optic neuritis, acute myelitis with LETM, or area postrema syndrome
   b. Dissemination in space (two or more different core clinical characteristics)
   c. Fulfillment of additional MRI requirements, as applicable
2. Negative tests for AQP4 antibodies using best available detection method, or testing unavailable
3. Exclusion of alternative diagnosis

Core clinical characteristics
1. Optic neuritis
2. Acute myelitis
3. Area postrema syndrome episode of otherwise unexplained hiccups or nausea and vomiting
4. Acute brainstem syndrome
5. Symptomatic narcolepsy or acute diencephalic clinical syndrome with NMOSD-typical diencephalic MRI lesions
6. Symptomatic cerebral syndrome with NMOSD-typical brain lesions

Additional MRI requirements for NMOSD without or with unknown AQP4 antibodies
1. Acute optic neuritis: requires brain MRI showing:
   a. Normal findings or only nonspecific white matter lesions OR
   b. Optic nerve MRI with T2-hyperintense lesion or T1-W gado enhancing lesion extending over $\geq \frac{1}{2}$ optic nerve length or involving optic chiasma
2. Acute myelitis requires
   a. Associated intramedullary MRI lesion extending over ≥ 3 contiguous segments (LETM) OR
   b. ≥ 3 contiguous segments of focal spinal cord atrophy in patients with history compatible with acute myelitis
3. Area postrema syndrome: requires associated dorsal medulla/area postrema lesions
4. Acute brainstem syndrome: requires associated periependymal brainstem lesions

AQP4, Aquaporin-4; *LETM,* longitudinal extensive transverse myelitis; *MRI,* magnetic resonance imaging; *NMOSD,* neuromyelitis optic spectrum disorders.

entire cross-sectional segment of the cord and characteristically includes the central cord gray matter. Enhancement and edema of the cord are often present, with occasional enlargement of the cord, which may mimic a spinal cord tumor. MRI of the brain can be normal, particularly at presentation; however, over time, lesions in the periependymal regions adjacent to the ventricles, including the dorsal brainstem and diencephalon, can be seen. Nonspecific subcortical white matter T2 hyperintensities, usually asymptomatic, can also be detected in these patients.

Spinal Fluid

Can be helpful in cases where the diagnosis is unclear. Increases in protein and white blood cells with counts up to a couple of hundred cells/mm³, sometimes with neutrophilic predominance, are common during exacerbations, but can be normal during remissions. Abnormalities are more prominent in patients with transverse myelitis as compared with the ones with optic neuritis. Oligoclonal bands are often absent (up to three-fourths of the patients) in contrast to patients with MS. Antibodies against aquaporin-4 may be positive in the spinal fluid.

The criteria to fulfill the NMOSD diagnosis vary depending on the aquaporin status and are listed in Box 40.1.

Differential Diagnosis

The most common condition to be considered in the differential diagnosis of patients with NMOSD is multiple sclerosis, and the main differences are listed in Table 40.1. Acute disseminated encephalomyelitis (ADEM) and other autoimmune disorders, such as lupus, Sjögren's, Behçet's, and sarcoidosis, can sometimes have similar presentations and should be considered in the differential diagnosis. Other conditions that can potentially mimic NMOSD include lymphoma, CRMP-5 associated optic neuropathy, and myelopathy and chronic infections such as HIV and syphilis.

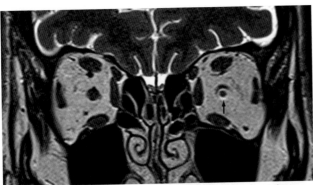

Coronal T2 fast spin echo with fat saturation demonstrates striking atrophy of left optic nerve resulting from previous optic neuritis (arrow).

Fig. 40.2 Optic Nerve Atrophy.

Treatment

The treatment of NMOSD includes acute phase and preventive therapies. During an exacerbation, intravenous corticosteroids such as methylprednisolone 1000 mg/day for 5 days and/or plasma exchange are commonly used. Intravenous immunoglobulin (0.4 g/kg for 5 days) can also be considered in patients who have a suboptimal response to steroids and have contraindications to plasma exchange.

Despite the lack of FDA-approved treatments to prevent further relapses in patients with NMOSD, immunosuppressive agents such as azathioprine, mycophenolate, and rituximab are commonly used and maintained for at least 5 years in patients who are aquaporin positive to prevent further attacks.

Of note, the common disease-modifying agents used to treat multiple sclerosis, such as the interferon beta, fingolimod, and natalizumab, have not shown any benefits in patients with NMOSD and may be harmful, making it imperative to correctly distinguish between these two conditions.

Prognosis

As compared with multiple sclerosis, the prognosis for NMOSD is worse, primarily due to accumulation of severe disabilities from the recurrent attacks. Mortality rates are high, mostly due to respiratory failure associated with lesions extending or involving the brainstem. Advances in diagnosis and treatment will hopefully improve morbidity and mortality in these patients.

Future Directions

Advances in drug development, such as anti-IL-6 therapy (tocilizumab), inhibitors of complement (eculizumab), and of neutrophil elastase (sivelestat), as well as monoclonal antibodies against the antibodies to aquaporin-4 (aquaporumab), will hopefully expand the therapeutic armamentarium for NMOSD.

TABLE 40.1 Differences Between Neuromyelitis Optic Spectrum Disorders and Multiple Sclerosis		
	NMOSD	**MS**
Age (mean)	40	30
Female : male ratio	9:1	2:1
Race	More common in Asians and blacks	More common in whites
Clinical features		
1. Optic neuritis	Often bilateral and severe with poor recovery. Optic chiasm and tracts commonly involved.	Usually unilateral with good recovery
2. Acute myelitis	Complete spinal cord syndrome	Partial spinal cord syndrome
3. Area postrema and diencephalon involvement	Common	Rare
Antibodies to aquaporin-4	Present in 75% of patients	Absent
Imaging	Extensive optic nerves and spinal cord (three or more segments) involvement. Central cord is commonly affected. Brain lesion can occur, but usually nonspecific T2 hyperintensities.	T2 hyperintensities perpendicular to ventricles and juxtacortical are common. Spinal cord lesions are smaller and tend to involve the dorsolateral cord.
Spinal fluid	Cell count often greater than 50 cells/mm³, with presence of neutrophils and eosinophils, oligoclonal bands often absent.	Cell count often less than 50 cells/mm³, with presence of lymphocytes, oligoclonal bands often present.

MS, Multiple sclerosis; *NMOSD,* neuromyelitis optic spectrum disorders.

ACUTE DISSEMINATED ENCEPHALOMYELITIS

CLINICAL VIGNETTE *A 37-year-old woman was admitted to the hospital after presenting with progressive language difficulties and right-sided weakness, 2 weeks after having Mycoplasma pneumonia. MRI of her brain showed extensive confluent T2 hyperintensity involving the left frontal and parietal lobes with extension to the internal capsule, midbrain, and pons. T1 postcontrast images demonstrated subtle peripheral enhancement (Fig. 40.3ABCD). Spinal fluid showed 17 white blood cells, 87% lymphocytes, protein of 52, normal glucose and IGG index, and no oligoclonal bands. Viral serologies, Lyme, and ACE were negative. Mycoplasma IGM was positive. The patient was diagnosed as having ADEM and treated with 1000 mg of methylprednisolone for 5 days followed by a course of intravenous immunoglobulin (IVIG) and an oral steroid taper. Symptoms improved overtime, and 1 year later her neuro exam was remarkable only for a right pronator drift and her follow-up brain MRI showed significant improvement of the T2 hyperintense signal abnormality with some residual abnormalities in the left peri-rolandic area and underlying white matter with no associated mass effect, edema, or enhancement. No new T2 hyperintensities were seen (Fig. 40.3EF).*

Comment: This case illustrates a severe case of ADEM after a bout of mycoplasma pneumonia successfully treated with steroids and IVIG. The patient continues to be monitored clinically and by imaging yearly to rule out the possibility that this could have been the first episode of multiple sclerosis, but so far no evidence for findings consistent with MS have been found.

ADEM is a rare autoimmune demyelinating disease, usually monophasic, that involves the central nervous system, more common in children than adults. It can occur after viral and bacterial infections, as well as after vaccinations, but also without any recognized prior cause.

Clinical Presentation

The typical presentation of ADEM includes the acute onset of severe focal or multifocal encephalopathy associated with pyramidal, cerebellar, and brainstem signs, starting a few days to a couple of months after a preceding illness or vaccination. Seizures are present in up to 25% of the patients. Optic neuritis, sometimes bilateral, and transverse myelitis can also occur.

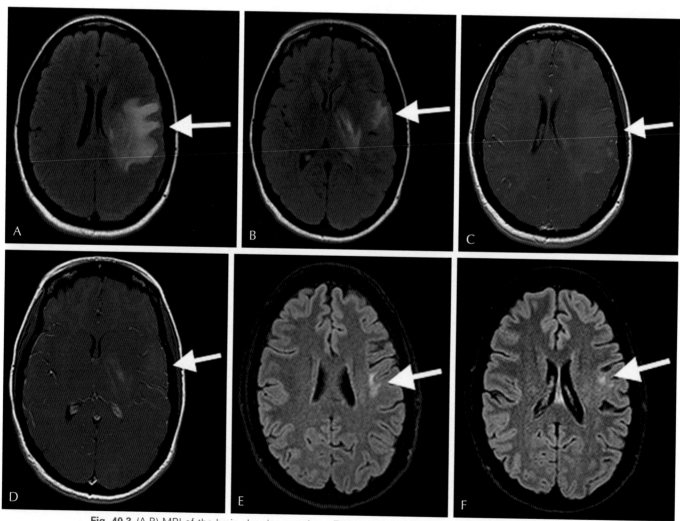

Fig. 40.3 (A,B) MRI of the brain showing prominent T2 hyperintensity involving the left frontal and parietal lobes with extension to the internal capsule, midbrain and pons. (C,D) Postgadolinium enhanced T1 showing peripheral enhancement. (E,F) MRI of the brain performed 1 year after the initial presentation showing significant improvement of the T2 hyperintensities with residual abnormalities in the left peri-rolandic area and underlying white matter.

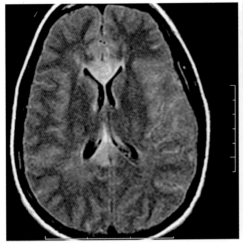
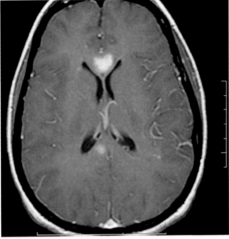

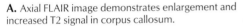
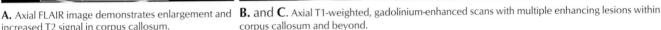

A. Axial FLAIR image demonstrates enlargement and increased T2 signal in corpus callosum.

B. and **C.** Axial T1-weighted, gadolinium-enhanced scans with multiple enhancing lesions within corpus callosum and beyond.

Fig. 40.4 Acute Disseminated Encephalomyelitis.

A hyperacute variant of ADEM with a more fulminant course, called acute hemorrhagic encephalomyelitis (AHEM), has also been reported and characterized by hemorrhagic lesions in the white matter.

Diagnostic Approach

MRI is usually the modality of choice to diagnose ADEM and AHEM. In ADEM, one often sees large ill-defined multifocal asymmetric gadolinium-enhancing lesions throughout the brain and spinal cord (Figs. 40.3 and 40.4), affecting subcortical and periventricular white matter as well as the gray matter, including cortex, basal ganglia, and thalamus. Brainstem, cerebellum, and spinal cord are also commonly involved. In AHEM, the lesions on MRI are usually larger, have a hemorrhagic component, and are more edematous than in ADEM.

The CSF findings in this condition are variable, with abnormalities reported in 50%–80% of cases. Typically a modest lymphocytic pleocytosis (<100 cells/mL) associated with increased protein and normal glucose is seen with positive oligoclonal bands identified in 20%–65% of the patients. In addition, an increase in RBC is often present in the hemorrhagic variant.

Electroencephalography often shows diffuse slowing compatible with an encephalopathic process and occasionally epileptiform abnormalities.

In some cases, cerebral biopsy is necessary to confirm the diagnosis of ADEM and typically shows perivenous sleeves of mononuclear cell infiltration associated with demyelination.

Differential Diagnosis

This includes the first attack of MS, various acute aseptic meningoencephalitides (herpes simplex virus, West Nile virus, mumps, Epstein-Barr), neurosarcoidosis, vasculitis, and very rarely metabolic leukoencephalopathies, such as Schilder disease or Leigh syndrome.

Therapy

The treatment of ADEM and its variant is based on empirical studies, since no randomized clinical trial has been conducted. The most common form of treatment is high doses of methylprednisolone (1 g a day for 5 days) followed by an oral steroid taper over 4–6 weeks. Intravenous immunoglobulins (0.4 g/kg/day for 5 days) or plasma exchange are often used in patients with poor response to IV steroids and in some cases IV cyclophosphamide.

Prognosis

ADEM is usually associated with a good prognosis, since demyelination and axonal injury is usually less severe than in other inflammatory disorders. Most patients sustain mild residual deficits or even achieve complete recovery. However, in fulminant cases, death can occur.

Approximately one-third of adults with ADEM can progress into multiple sclerosis overtime, supporting longitudinal clinical monitoring of these patients.

ADDITIONAL RESOURCES

Neuromyelitis Optica (Devic Disease) and Neuromyelitis Optic Spectrum Disorder

Lennon VA, Wingerchuk DM, Kryzer TJ, et al. A serum autoantibody marker of neuromyelitis optica: distinction from multiple sclerosis. Lancet 2004;364:2106–12.

Original report defining the presence of this specific antibody.

Roemer SF, Parisi JE, Lennon VA, et al. Pattern-specific loss of aquaporin-4 immunoreactivity distinguishes neuromyelitis optica from multiple sclerosis. Brain 2007;130:1194–205.

Study comparing the patterns of aquaporin-4 in the CNS tissues of patients with NMO, MS, infarcts, and controls.

Sato DK, Callegaro D, Lana-Peixoto MA, et al. Distinction between MOG antibody-positive and AQP4 antibody-positive NMO spectrum disorders. Neurology 2014;82:474–81.

This study reports the distinct clinical features of NMOSD with positive MOG antibodies.

Wingerchuk DM, Banwell B, Bennett JL, et al. International consensus diagnostic criteria for neuromyelitis optica spectrum disorders. Neurology 2015;85:177–89.

This article presents the most recent revised diagnostic criteria for NMOSD with and without aquaporin-4 antibodies.

Wingerchuk DM, Weinshenker BG. Neuromyelitis optica (Devic's syndrome). Handb Clin Neurol 2014;122:581–99.

Detailed review of neuromyelitis optica.

Trebst C, Jarius S, Berthele A, et al. Update on the diagnosis and treatment of neuromyelitis optica: recommendations of the neuromyelitis optica study group (NEMOS). J Neurol 2014;261:1–16.

In this review, the NEMOS group reports recent updates in the diagnosis and treatment of neuromyelitis optica.

Acute Disseminated Encephalomyelitis

Koelman DL, Chahin S, Mar SS, et al. Acute disseminated encephalomyelitis in 228 patients: a retrospective, multicenter US study. Neurology 2016;86(22):2085–93.

Recent retrospective study that analyzes the clinical, laboratorial, and imaging findings as well as long-term outcomes of 228 patients with ADEM.

Marin SE, Cllen DJ. The magnetic resonance imaging appearance of monophasic acute disseminated encephalomyelitis: an update post application of the 2007 consensus criteria. Neuroimaging Clin N Am 2013;23(2):245–66.

This article provides an updated overview of ADEM in children, with a main focus on its neuroimaging.

Tenenbaum SN. Acute disseminated encephalomyelitis. Handb Clin Neurol 2013;112:1253–62.

This article summarizes the available literature on ADEM in children, including its monophasic and relapsing forms.

Psychiatric Disorders

Jayashri Srinivasan

41

Mood and Psychotic Disorders

Patrick R. Aquino, Kenneth Lakritz

Mood and psychotic disorders account for a substantial burden of mental disease. These disorders are often first evaluated in primary care offices or emergency departments. This chapter will focus on a selection of these commonly encountered disorders: major depressive disorder, persistent depressive disorder, bipolar disorder, and schizophrenia.

MAJOR DEPRESSIVE DISORDER

> **CLINICAL VIGNETTE** *A 69-year-old man was brought to the emergency room by his family for evaluation of weight loss, inability to sleep, loss of interest in hobbies, and crying. He described himself as a useless individual whose productive life was over; he had become a burden to his family. In addition, he was experiencing intense anxiety, poorly localized back pain, difficulty concentrating, and insomnia. Ten years earlier he had been hospitalized for a depressive episode following a suicide attempt by overdose.*

Major depressive disorder is a very significant and common psychiatric disorder that usually begins in early adulthood. Physicians of all specialties encounter it frequently in many different guises. Major depressive disorder accounts for 5% of total disability worldwide in adults; comparatively, cardiovascular disease represents 6.6% and cancer 5.6%. Women have a higher prevalence. There is no gender difference in symptoms, course, or consequences of illness. When depression affects men, the long-term risk of suicide is more common. Familial clustering is apparent, especially for earlier onset and recurrent episodes; heritability is approximately 40%. Chronic medical conditions are associated with an increased risk of major depressive disorder. In addition, the risk of some chronic medical conditions (i.e., obesity, diabetes, cardiovascular disease) is increased in the setting of major depressive disorder; these interactions are bidirectional.

Certain medical conditions may provoke or mimic major depressive disorder. These can include adrenal insufficiency, neurodegenerative disorders, hypothyroidism, vitamin deficiencies, stroke, multiple sclerosis, cancers, obstructive sleep apnea, systemic lupus erythematosus, certain toxins, or brain injury. There are no reliable laboratory screening tests to diagnose major depressive disorder. Rather, laboratory examination should be guided by the medical history and physical examination (e.g., head imaging with focal neurologic deficits on exam).

Major depressive disorder presents clinically as a 2-week period of sad mood or anhedonia (loss of pleasure from normally enjoyable experiences), with at least five or more associated symptoms of impaired energy or concentration, insomnia, loss of appetite, feelings of worthlessness or guilt, or recurrent thoughts of death or suicide. The presence of predominant diurnal mood fluctuation—feeling worse in the morning—is almost pathognomonic of major depressive disorder. It is not uncommon to find disturbed sleep architecture with shortened rapid eye movement latency.

Suicidal ideation or suicide attempts are a major concern in the care of patients with major depressive disorder (Fig. 41.1). Although overt suicide attempts are notoriously difficult to predict, physicians must maintain a heightened sense of alertness to assessing suicide risk. Screening tools and assessment instruments are available that can support the clinical examination (e.g., Columbia-Suicide Severity Rating Scale). One must always stand by to offer help and intervene when necessary, especially with the patient having significant suicidal risk factors—previous suicide attempts, substance use, being male, intense anxiety or agitation, social isolation, advanced age, or psychosis.

Major depressive disorder has graded levels of severity from mild, moderate, to severe. The severe form is characterized by increasing numbers of symptoms or the presence of psychosis. The psychotic phenomena are typically characterized by delusions that are "affect consonant"—for example, delusions of poverty, moral depravity, or life-threatening illness. The recognition of psychotic thinking in the depressed patient has very definite therapeutic consequences. This subgroup of patients typically fails to respond to standard antidepressant medications and can instead benefit more robustly from electroconvulsive therapy or a combination of antidepressant and antipsychotic medication (Fig. 41.2).

Treatment of major depressive disorder combines specific pharmacologic medications with psychotherapy. Studies have repeatedly demonstrated the superiority of combined pharmacologic and psychotherapeutic intervention to either intervention alone. Goals of treatment of a major depressive episode are symptom remission and improving function. Treatment outcomes can be commonly monitored with patient reported or provider administered questionnaires and scales that are increasingly incorporated into general practice (e.g., Patient Health Questionnaire-9, Montgomery-Asberg Depression Rating Scale, and Beck Depression Inventory).

There are various psychological frameworks describing depression in individuals. Aaron Beck introduced the cognitive triad of depression, linking an individual's negative view of the world, pessimism of the future, and negative view of himself or herself. These elements provide a basis for the direct psychological interventions of cognitive-behavioral therapy (CBT), a validated and effective psychological treatment for major depressive disorder.

Serotonin reuptake inhibitors (SRIs) are the preferred pharmacologic agents for initial treatment. Other pharmacologic agents have demonstrated equal efficacy to SRIs, although with varying mechanisms of action that modulate combinations of monoamines: serotonin and norepinephrine reuptake inhibitors (SNRIs), norepinephrine and dopamine reuptake inhibitors (NDI), and serotonergic agonists or alpha-2 inhibitors. Newer agents with more specific receptor profiles continue to be developed. Large, multicentered pharmacologic trials have demonstrated the relative efficacy of these agents in the treatment of major depressive disorder.

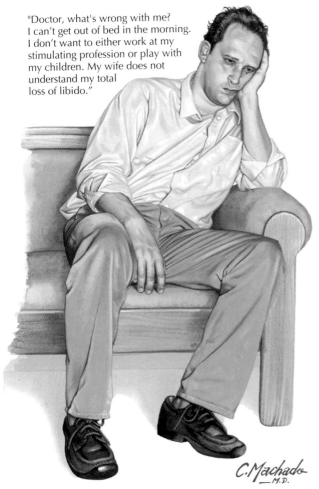

"Doctor, what's wrong with me? I can't get out of bed in the morning. I don't want to either work at my stimulating profession or play with my children. My wife does not understand my total loss of libido."

Fig. 41.1 Major Depressive Disorder.

Older agents, including tricyclic antidepressants and monoamine oxidase inhibitors (MAOIs), remain efficacious; unfortunately these agents have an increasing burden of side effects, including lethal toxidromes, cardiac conduction abnormalities, and a narrow therapeutic index. However, these agents may be useful in specific situations of major depression with comorbid illness (e.g., tricyclic use for a migrainous patient or selegiline for a patient with Parkinson disease).

Patients who have only a partial response to pharmacologic treatment may sometimes respond to various other therapeutic maneuvers. These include a switch to a different class of antidepressant, addition of a second antidepressant of a different class, or augmentation with lithium, triiodothyronine (T3), or atypical antipsychotic agent. However, likelihood of symptom remission is reduced with each subsequent failed therapeutic trial.

Bipolar disorder may be present in at least 10% of individuals presenting with what appears at first to be unipolar, major depressive disorder; this creates a unique diagnostic challenge. A heightened level of suspicion for the presence of underlying bipolar disorder is necessary for anyone with a family history of bipolar disorder, childhood onset of depressive illness, or poor therapeutic response to past antidepressant treatments. Similarly, if the patient experiences a sudden or immediate response to initiation of antidepressant medication—that is, "switching"—rather than following the usual delayed therapeutic response, a bipolar disorder requires further consideration. Efforts should be made to limit the exposure of patients with known or suspected bipolar disorder to the usual antidepressant medications.

Additional somatic therapies for major depressive disorder include electroconvulsive therapy (ECT), repetitive transcranial magnetic stimulation (rTMS), bright light therapy, and vagus nerve stimulation (VNS). ECT is indicated for severely depressed individuals or those who fail medication trials. It has more than a 90% response rate in well-selected populations. ECT is also the first-line treatment for severe major depressive disorder with psychotic features, intense suicidal ideation, and otherwise medically ill patients. Unilateral electrode placement can diminish the occurrence of post-ECT confusion. Although rTMS can be used in major depressive disorder and may have a less severe side-effect profile than ECT, it has not been adopted as a first-line treatment due to modest benefits from this treatment. Patients who get depressed in the winter (i.e., major depressive disorder with seasonal component) can respond to bright light therapy, typically at 10,000 lux daily for 20–30 minutes/day. Surgical VNS placement can be used for treatment-resistant major depressive disorder. However, controversy as to its effectiveness continues.

It is important to recognize that depression is a chronic illness with a propensity for recurrence. Therefore a maintenance and prophylactic treatment protocol should be considered at the time of diagnosis for each patient. Active treatment for first episodes should last at least 6 months, preferably 1 year. After three episodes, indefinite lifelong prophylaxis with full-dose antidepressant medication is indicated.

PERSISTENT DEPRESSIVE DISORDER (DYSTHYMIA)

> **CLINICAL VIGNETTE** A 47-year-old woman was referred to psychiatry by her internist who was caring for her chronic fatigue and diffuse, nonspecific achiness. Uncertain of the diagnosis, her internist wondered if the patient was depressed. Although resentful of the referral, the patient reluctantly agreed to a single consultation. She experienced inadequate and poor-quality sleep, impaired concentration, migratory chest pain, and migraine headaches. Over the years, the patient had sought treatment for chronic Lyme disease, fibromyalgia, chronic fatigue syndrome, and other syndromes; however, her symptoms continued unabated.
>
> Although she had been clearly depressed on two occasions, at age 19 years after her father's death and at age 26 years after the birth of her first child, she denied current feelings of sadness, guilt, or hopelessness. She described herself as overworked, justifiably pessimistic, socially isolated, and burdened with an unappreciative and unsympathetic husband. An extensive medical workup had revealed an iron deficiency anemia and hypothyroidism; however, their treatment was not helpful in resolving her many symptoms. As this woman was generally sedentary, her physician recommended aerobic exercise, but she felt too tired to try it.
>
> She reluctantly acknowledged that her pessimism and low mood might be contributing to her problems. She agreed to a trial of cognitive-behavioral therapy, which she found helpful.

Persistent depressive disorder (dysthymia) represents a consolidation of prior named disorders of chronic major depressive disorder, dysthymic disorder, minor depression, and subsyndromal depression. To establish the diagnosis, the *Diagnostic and Statistical Manual of Mental Disorders—Fifth Edition* (DSM-5) requires depressed mood for most of the day, for more days than not, for at least 2 years. The chronic low mood may be such a fixture of the patient's life as to be unrecognized by the patient. Two other symptoms must also be present from a list, including sleep disturbance, appetite disturbance, fatigue, hopelessness, low self-esteem, and impaired concentration. Dysthymic patients have fewer and less-intense depressive symptoms than patients with major depressive disorder

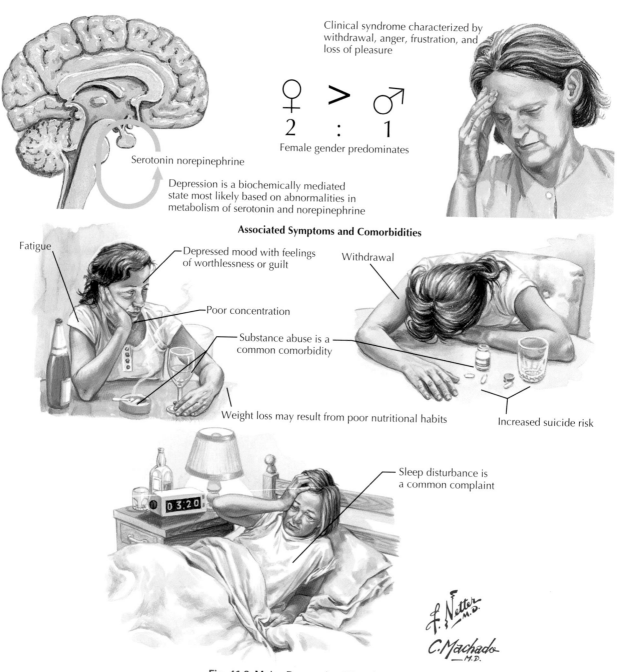

Clinical syndrome characterized by withdrawal, anger, frustration, and loss of pleasure

♀ > ♂
2 : 1
Female gender predominates

Serotonin norepinephrine

Depression is a biochemically mediated state most likely based on abnormalities in metabolism of serotonin and norepinephrine

Associated Symptoms and Comorbidities

Fatigue

Depressed mood with feelings of worthlessness or guilt

Withdrawal

Poor concentration

Substance abuse is a common comorbidity

Weight loss may result from poor nutritional habits

Increased suicide risk

Sleep disturbance is a common complaint

Fig. 41.2 Major Depressive Disorder.

(Fig. 41.3). Persistent depressive disorder usually has an early and insidious onset and a chronic course. Family history of mood disorder is common.

Individuals with persistent depressive disorder have a high risk of psychiatric comorbidity, especially anxiety and substance use disorders. DSM-5 does not recognize the existence of a depressive personality disorder. However, patients who are characterologically prone to depression may have an underlying conception (misconception) of themselves as defective or inadequate and are prone to feelings of guilt and shame. They symptomatically overlap partially with patients suffering from dysthymia.

Although dysthymic patients do not meet the criteria for a diagnosis of major depressive disorder, persistent depressive disorder is not a benign illness. As a chronic disease, it causes immense suffering and loss of potential. Patients do less well than they should at school, work,

and in personal relations. They overuse medical resources and substances, both legal and illegal. They are at high risk for the development of more severe affective disorders; one of the most common is double depression, a pattern of repeated major depressive episodes with partial recovery to a state of dysthymia.

Most physician practices include a number of patients with poorly characterized pain or other vague but persistent physical complaints. Even after excluding appropriate and specific medical diagnoses, illness anxiety disorder (hypochondriasis), malingering, and delusional disorder, certain puzzling cases remain unclassified or specifically diagnosed. These are best understood as disguised presentations of persistent depressive disorder. Neurologists, rheumatologists, and gastroenterologists are frequently sought out by these relatively common dysthymic patients. Both the patients and the clinicians can be frustrated during the diagnostic and treatment process.

Some of the common complaints of dysthymic patients may include:

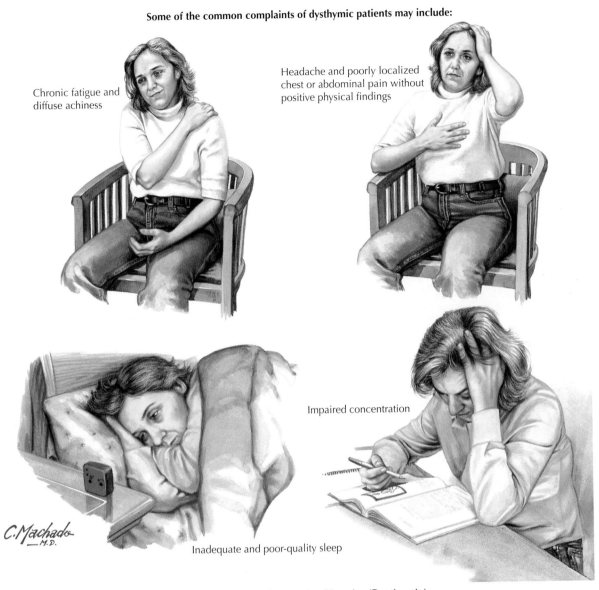

Chronic fatigue and diffuse achiness

Headache and poorly localized chest or abdominal pain without positive physical findings

Impaired concentration

Inadequate and poor-quality sleep

Fig. 41.3 Persistent Depressive Disorder (Dysthymia).

Patients with persistent depressive disorder deserve careful evaluation and intensive treatment. They often respond well to specific psychological interventions, such as CBT or interpersonal therapy. Often a combination of psychotherapy and antidepressant medication produces the best outcome.

BIPOLAR DISORDER

CLINICAL VIGNETTE *A 20-year-old woman was admitted to an inpatient psychiatric unit after a deliberate overdose with acetaminophen. She complained of sadness and anxiety, "for as long as I can remember," but in the preceding 3 months she had suffered from feelings of hopelessness, anhedonia, fatigue, and hypersomnia. Her family history was positive for major depression in three of five first-degree relatives and manic-depressive psychosis in her maternal grandmother.*

Treatment with an antidepressant was initiated for presumed major depressive disorder and the patient participated in individual and group psychotherapy. After 1 week, she announced that her energy had returned and that her need for sleep had decreased dramatically. She told staff that she was "cured," and developed a plan to move to leave school and start her own internet business. When she was prevented from leaving, she became agitated and threw chairs at the nursing staff, accusing them of a plot to keep her from succeeding. Despite this, she promised to buy everyone she knew a new car as soon as she left the hospital.

Less common than major depressive disorder, bipolar disorder can often have a dramatic presentation. Bipolar disorder has a typical onset in adolescence or early adulthood; mean age of first episode of mania, hypomania, or major depression is 18 years. Like other mood disorders, first onset in late life should prompt consideration of an underlying medical condition or substance toxidrome. Most individuals will have recurrent episodes of mania, with approximately 60% of manic episodes occurring immediately before a major depressive episode. Family history of bipolar disorder is the most consistent risk factor for development of bipolar disorder. There appear to be shared genetic vulnerabilities between schizophrenia and bipolar disorder. A first-degree relative with

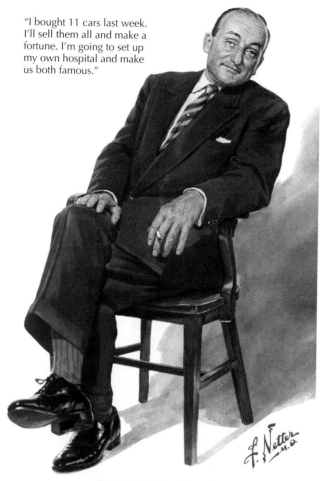

"I bought 11 cars last week. I'll sell them all and make a fortune. I'm going to set up my own hospital and make us both famous."

Fig. 41.4 Bipolar Disorder.

bipolar disorder has at least a 10% chance of developing bipolar disorder. When individuals with this background present with a complaint of depression, suspicion of bipolar disorder must be high.

Bipolar disorders encompass several separate entities, which vary in symptom severity and frequency: bipolar I disorder, bipolar II disorder, and cyclothymic disorder. The diagnosis of bipolar I disorder is defined by the lifetime presence of a single manic episode, itself defined by a period of abnormally expansive or irritable mood and persistently increased activity or energy lasting at least 1 week. During this discrete period, three additional associated symptoms must also be present, including grandiosity, decreased need for sleep, talkativeness, racing thoughts, distractibility, psychomotor agitation, or excessive risk-taking (Fig. 41.4). Bipolar II disorder is characterized by a prior hypomanic episode and a prior major depressive episode without lifetime evidence of a manic episode. Hypomania is characterized by the same symptom cluster that defines mania; however, symptoms last 4 days or less and are not severe enough to cause marked impairment in functioning. Cyclothymic disorder is characterized by recurrent periods over 2 years of hypomanic and depressive symptoms, without ever meeting full criteria for a hypomanic or depressive episode.

Although classic mania is hard to miss, it is an uncommon initial presentation. Early on, bipolar disorder is often misdiagnosed. In most studies, the time from initial presentation to correct diagnosis is over 5 years. There are several reasons for this high rate of misdiagnosis:

1. Patients most often seek treatment when they are depressed. They may not yet have suffered a manic episode or, if they have, may not have recognized it as a problem.

2. Previous "high episodes" may have been either relatively mild or not easily recognized as beyond the realm of normal behavior.

3. Patients often present with simultaneous features of mania and depression (i.e., mixed features) easily confounding the diagnosis.

Mood-stabilizing medications (i.e., lithium, anticonvulsants, and antipsychotics) provide the primary treatment modality. Severely ill patients with acute mania often require combination pharmacotherapy—lithium or valproate plus an antipsychotic. Because of its natural history, once the diagnosis is established, bipolar patients must be treated indefinitely.

Lithium is effective for both the manic and depressed phases, as well as for long-term prophylaxis. Lithium continues to be the only medication clearly shown to reduce suicide rates in bipolar disorder. Because lithium has a narrow therapeutic index and many side effects, frequent blood-level monitoring is required. One also needs to monitor renal and thyroid function.

Anticonvulsants are more effective than lithium in mixed or atypical cases, especially for patients with "rapid cycling"—more than four episodes of illness per year. Valproic acid, carbamazepine, and lamotrigine are all efficacious. Atypical antipsychotics also have mood-stabilizing properties. When these usual medications are ineffective, clozapine is sometimes helpful, although often it is the last medication that is tried given its high side-effect burden and need for hematologic monitoring.

The treatment of bipolar depression is especially challenging. Most patients with bipolar disorder experience depressive rather than manic symptoms a greater proportion of their lifetime. Unfortunately, antidepressants typically promote mood instability. There is little or no evidence that long-term use of antidepressant medication improves the outcome of bipolar depression. Currently lurasidone, quetiapine, and the combination of fluoxetine with olanzapine have US Food and Drug Administration (FDA) approval as treatments for bipolar depression. However, all mood stabilizers are routinely used in this phase of illness. Lamotrigine may be more effective than other anticonvulsants for bipolar depression. ECT is highly effective in both phases of bipolar disorder.

Dietary augmentation with omega-3 fatty acids from fish oils may have modest to moderate benefits for bipolar depression. Because these dietary supplements have few serious side effects and are known to benefit cardiovascular health, they can be widely recommended.

Maintenance pharmacotherapy typically continues the same medication regimen that produced remission of acute symptoms. Use of lithium, valproate, quetiapine, and lamotrigine as maintenance prophylaxis is consistent with treatment guidelines. Therapeutic noncompliance almost universally occurs, as most successfully treated bipolar patients eventually miss their high moods. Each patient must learn to recognize and report early signs of relapse, with sleep loss often an early harbinger of relapse.

SCHIZOPHRENIA

CLINICAL VIGNETTE *A 22-year-old man was brought to the emergency department by his parents for increasingly bizarre behavior. Over months his parents have endured long tales of his continued connection to "another dimension." He described frequent communication from other beings through radio transmissions, television programs, and bus advertisements with specific details meant solely for him. He frequently heard these other beings talking among themselves, commenting on him, his environment, or making plans for him in the future. He would often feel as if his body was not under his own control, or others could read his mind or hear his thoughts. He would frequently ask family and friends about the comments he heard and became increasingly frustrated with them when they dismissed his concerns. He grew increasingly isolated, withdrew from work, and stopped caring for his hygiene.*

Up until this time, he had been in perfect health with no outward signs of a thought disorder. He had never required any psychiatric treatment. He had done well in school and obtained steady employment.

Psychiatric examination demonstrated him to be exceedingly tense and fearful. Physical examination, brain MRI, and routine laboratory testing, including drug screen, were unremarkable.

He was involuntarily hospitalized. An atypical antipsychotic drug helped to significantly improve his anxiety and hallucinations. Although this medication did not significantly impact the presence and frequency of his delusional thinking, these thoughts seemed to be less bothersome to him and at times he could verbalize they may not be true.

More than 120 years ago, Emil Kraepelin delineated schizophrenia as a global impairment of psychic functioning (dementia praecox). It is distinguished from the affective psychoses (major depressive and bipolar disorders) by its unremitting course. Schizophrenia typically first occurs in late adolescence or early adulthood; this distinguishes it from the dementias. Sufferers, often initially odd or unsociable, eventually become progressively more isolated and eccentric, commonly failing to care for themselves. It is quite uncommon for schizophrenia to first appear in midlife. However, when it does occur at this time in life, it overwhelmingly affects women, usually presenting with prominent paranoid symptoms. Familial clustering is obvious, but even identical twins have only ~50% disease concordance. Other prenatal, perinatal, and birth seasonality effects have been linked to the incidence of schizophrenia, though not definitively.

Schizophrenia and the other psychotic disorders are all characterized by abnormalities in delusions, hallucinations, disorganized thought, grossly disorganized or abnormal motor behavior, and negative symptoms. Specifically, schizophrenia is defined by the presence of two or more of these symptoms over a 1-month period with a continuous disturbance in function of at least 6 months.

During their initial evaluation, these patients overtly express the positive symptoms of schizophrenia—hallucinations, disordered thinking, or delusional beliefs (Fig. 41.5). The delusions and hallucinations are positive symptoms, which are often more bizarre and illogical than those seen in individuals having an affective psychosis. Many experts consider certain "first-rank" symptoms—delusions of passivity or outside control, thoughts being withdrawn from the patient's brain, thoughts being broadcast by the patient to others—as pathognomonic for schizophrenia. Others maintain that only the long-term course of the illness reveals the diagnosis. Negative symptoms, though not as obvious, account for a majority of morbidity associated with schizophrenia. These typically include diminished speech (alogia), emotional flatness or lack of interest in activities (anhedonia), social withdrawal (asociality), and lack of initiative and self-care (avolition). When untreated, patients with schizophrenia exhibit declining cognitive function, especially during their first decade of the illness. Remissions and long-term improvement are eventually possible. Nevertheless, only a minority of patients with schizophrenia achieve functional recovery; many individuals are chronically disabled. Sadly, one of the major consequences of schizophrenia is a very high suicide rate, approaching 10%.

Patients with schizophrenia have more than the expected number of neurologic "soft signs." Specific findings include abnormalities of smooth eye movement pursuit, auditory evoked potentials, and olfactory deficits. At least 50% of these patients have gross central nervous system pathology visible on magnetic resonance imaging (MRI), including ventricular enlargement and decreased temporal and frontal lobe volume. Cerebellar abnormalities are also common. Ventricular enlargement appears to correlate with negative symptoms and treatment

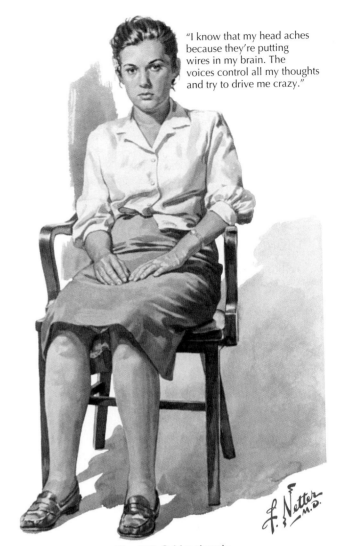

"I know that my head aches because they're putting wires in my brain. The voices control all my thoughts and try to drive me crazy."

Fig. 41.5 Schizophrenia.

resistance. The underlying mechanisms explaining brain volume changes in schizophrenia are not yet understood. Five-year follow-ups on patients with first-episode schizophrenia demonstrated an association between longer duration of psychosis, larger gray matter volume decrease, and larger ventricular volume increase. These findings strongly suggest that psychosis contributes to brain volume reductions found in schizophrenia. Despite these associations, there are no radiologic, laboratory, or psychometric tests diagnostic for the disorder.

Treating schizophrenia is challenging. Part of the difficulty is that patients are often strikingly unaware that they are ill. Because of this, they frequently stop their medications or drop out of treatment. Until neuroleptic medications were introduced in 1953, no effective biologic treatments existed. The classic neuroleptic agents (typical antipsychotics) that work by blocking dopamine D_2 receptors appear most effective against positive symptoms, but do not help and may exacerbate negative symptoms.

The first of the atypical antipsychotics, clozapine, was studied as early as the 1960s but was not introduced in the United States for more than 25 years because of its bone marrow toxicity—1% of patients develop potentially fatal agranulocytosis, and clozapine can only be prescribed when there is a mandatory monitoring of hematopoietic functions with regularly scheduled blood counts. Clozapine also lowers seizure threshold, induces metabolic syndrome, and causes weight gain.

Despite these problems, clozapine is superior in efficacy to all other currently available antipsychotic drugs. Subsequent atypical antipsychotics were developed to mimic clozapine's mechanism of action—thought to depend on weak D_2 antagonism combined with antagonism to the serotonin 5-HT2 receptor—without its inherent toxicity. The newer drugs are all, in varying degrees, less toxic, but none are quite as effective.

Our current treatments are largely based on the idea that schizophrenia is a disorder of excess dopamine. This idea has some clinical support; prodopaminergic drugs can cause or exacerbate psychosis, and antidopaminergic drugs treat psychosis. However, there is little direct evidence for this theory, and no one believes that it comprises the entire story. More recent research has implicated a more complex biology with dysregulation of other pathways, such as glutamatergic, opioid, GABAergic, serotonergic, cholinergic, and inflammatory systems.

ADDITIONAL RESOURCES

American Psychiatric Association. Diagnostic and statistical manual of mental disorders: DSM-5. Washington, DC: American Psychiatric Association; 2013.
Authoritative volume that defines and classifies mental disorders in order to improve diagnoses, treatment, and research.

Beck AT, Rush AJ, Shaw BF, et al. Cognitive therapy of depression. New York, NY: Guilford Press; 1987.
Classic book offers a definitive presentation of the theory and practice of cognitive therapy for depression.

Bowden CL, Perlis RH, Thase ME, et al. Aims and results of the NIMH systematic treatment enhancement program for bipolar disorder (STEP-BD). CNS Neurosci Ther 2012;18:243–9.
The Systematic Treatment Enhancement Program for Bipolar Disorder (STEP-BD) was funded as part of a National Institute of Mental Health initiative to develop effectiveness information about treatments, illness course, and assessment strategies for severe mental disorders.

Diane W, Rush AJ, Trivedi MH, et al. The STAR*D project results: a comprehensive review of findings. Curr Psychiatry Reports 2007;9(6):449–59.
*The Sequenced Treatment Alternatives to Relieve Depression (STAR*D) trial enrolled outpatients with nonpsychotic major depressive disorder treated prospectively in a series of randomized controlled trials. These results highlight the prevalence of treatment-resistant depression and suggest potential benefit for using more vigorous treatments in the earlier steps.*

Jamison KR. An unquiet mind: a memoir of moods and madness. New York, NY: Vintage; 1997.
Psychiatrist memoir and first-hand account as individual suffering from bipolar disorder.

Solomon A. The noonday demon: an atlas of depression. New York, NY: Scribner; 2015.
Book examines depression in personal, cultural, and scientific terms.

Stroup TS, Lieberman JA. Antipsychotic trials in schizophrenia: the CATIE study. New York: Cambridge University Press; 2010.
National Institute of Mental Health (NIMH) Clinical Antipsychotic Trials of Intervention Effectiveness (CATIE) study enrolled 1500 patients to compare effectiveness of various antipsychotics. This book archives the study's results and implications.

42

Other Psychiatric Disorders

Patrick R. Aquino, Kenneth Lakritz

The recognition and treatment of mental disorders are not confined to the specialty of psychiatry. Neuropsychiatric symptoms can mimic those of nonpsychiatric disorders that bring the patient to the attention of the nonpsychiatrist. This chapter reviews a number of important conditions that should be recognized in the nonpsychiatric setting because they are common, serious, and often overlooked: somatic symptom disorder, attention-deficit/hyperactivity disorder, panic disorder, posttraumatic stress disorder, obsessive-compulsive disorder, borderline personality disorder, and eating disorders.

SOMATIC SYMPTOM AND RELATED DISORDERS

> **CLINICAL VIGNETTE** At the age of 35 years, Barbara W. had already been a medical patient for 15 years. When she consulted a new rheumatologist for unexplained fatigue, arthralgias, and muscle tenderness, a thorough examination revealed only an overweight, deconditioned, angry woman demanding relief from her suffering. She was dependent on an oral opiate and a benzodiazepine, which she insisted were both ineffective and necessary for her continued functioning. She also consumed large quantities of nonsteroidal antiinflammatory drugs and over-the-counter hypnotics.
>
> A careful review revealed that she had seen at least 15 physicians in the previous 5 years, had been hospitalized at four different institutions, and had undergone an appendectomy, two subsequent exploratory laparotomies for unexplained abdominal pain, and numerous steroid injections of her knees, shoulders, and lower back. She was an avid consumer of medical literature and believed herself to be suffering from fibromyalgia, chronic fatigue syndrome, multiple chemical sensitivities, sick building syndrome, chronic Lyme disease, and mercury poisoning. When gently confronted about the absence of clinical findings and her lengthy history of unresponsiveness to medical intervention, she angrily accused the rheumatologist of labeling her "a mental patient" and left.

Somatic symptom disorder, formerly referred to as somatization disorder or Briquet syndrome, is a dramatic and severely disabling illness. It is widely encountered in medical and surgical practices rather than in psychiatric treatment settings. Previous diagnostic criteria focused on the necessity of multiple unexplained symptoms across multiple body sites. Newer diagnostic criteria from the *Diagnostic and Statistical Manual of Mental Disorders*—Fifth Edition (DSM-5) focus on the presence of one or more somatic symptoms that are distressing, resulting in significant disruption of an individual's life, and that are associated with excessive feelings or behaviors related to the symptoms, high levels of anxiety about the symptoms, or excessive time devoted to the symptoms. Somatic symptom disorder is related to other similar disorders, including illness anxiety disorder (excessive preoccupation and worry about illness) and functional neurologic symptom disorder (conversion disorder, with one or more symptoms affecting voluntary motor or sensory

function). When all forms of unexplained medical symptoms are lumped together, somatic symptom disorder is surprisingly common; one study found them in more than 30% of patients presenting to neurology clinics. However, the shift of focus away from the symptoms and toward the thoughts, feelings, and behaviors engendered by the symptoms provides an alternative means of addressing distress without "solving" the etiology of the symptoms.

Somatic symptom and related disorders are hard to diagnose. By definition, they are disorders of exclusion, and a full medical workup must precede the diagnosis. This is complicated by the common presence of concurrent physical illnesses in these patients. Additionally, somatic symptom disorders must be distinguished from deliberately feigned illness for secondary gain (malingering) and the intentional production of physical symptoms to obtain the role of patient (factitious disorder). This distinction is notoriously tricky.

Somatic symptom and related disorders, although rarely cured, can often be adequately managed. Such individuals need a primary doctor and should have regularly scheduled visits; if they get to see their doctor only when they are symptomatic, they become more symptomatic. These individuals must be protected from medical and surgical overtreatment. More importantly, these patients require close medical care, as significant disease states can arise over time that may easily be overlooked. Despite their preoccupation with illness, these patients often neglect their health.

Patients with somatic symptom and related disorders benefit from psychiatric treatment. They are often concrete in their thinking and alexithymic—deficient in verbalizing their emotional state—and are suitable targets for psychotherapy. The biggest barrier to treatment (apart from failing to diagnose the disorder) is finding a way to tell the patient that he or she has a psychiatric disorder. One way is to tell the patient that he or she has a chronic illness of unknown etiology whose symptoms are exacerbated by stress.

ATTENTION-DEFICIT/HYPERACTIVITY DISORDER

> **CLINICAL VIGNETTE** A 26-year-old engineer was referred to a psychiatrist for help with concentration. He had begun a job 3 months earlier but had been placed on probation for inattention to detail. This was his third job in 3 years.
>
> The patient acknowledged falling behind at work. He had difficulty maintaining focus when he found his work to be "boring." He had a tendency to procrastinate; despite having adequate funds, he was behind on his tax and mortgage payments. His wife reported that he occasionally abused alcohol and cocaine.
>
> He had been diagnosed with hyperactive-type attention deficit disorder at the age of 8 and treatment with methylphenidate had been successful. He maintained adequate academic progress until the age of 18, when the methylphenidate was discontinued.

Attention-deficit/hyperactivity disorder (ADHD) is a common, well-characterized, and treatable neuropsychiatric disorder that begins in childhood and manifests in multiple settings throughout an individual's life. It occurs in about 5% of children and about 2.5% of adults. Affected children are at increased risk for failing at school and developing antisocial personality disorders as well as substance abuse disorders. In most individuals, symptoms of motor hyperactivity lessen with advancing age, whereas problems with inattention, organization, and impulsivity persist. In adults, attentional disorders can present as apparent laziness, lack of focus, and procrastination (Fig. 42.1).

The core symptom domains necessary for the diagnosis of ADHD are (1) inattention and/or (2) hyperactivity and impulsivity. Clinical diagnosis of ADHD requires at least five symptoms from each domain over 6 months. ADHD by definition requires the presence of symptoms prior to age 12 years. Adults with ADHD must be distinguished from adults with new complaints of boredom or impaired attention and no past history of childhood ADHD. For the latter patients with new onset of cognitive complaints, a broader differential is generated to include neurodegenerative disease, vitamin deficiencies, affective disorders, endocrine disorders, or normal aging. Adult recollection of childhood symptoms is generally inaccurate; therefore clinical diagnosis should include neuropsychologic testing and review of records. Several screening tools are available for routine clinical use and monitoring.

ADHD must also be distinguished from mania or hypomania. Both groups of patients can be hyperactive with cognitive dysfunction; however, patients with mania or hypomania are also irritable, euphoric, and overtalkative. This distinction can be difficult, in part because of the coexistence of these disorders. Treatment of the affective disorder is generally prioritized.

Imaging studies may demonstrate anatomic abnormalities, such as atrophy or asymmetry in the prefrontal cortex, striatum, or cerebellum. Functional imaging may show decreased frontal and striatal perfusion, especially during tests of sustained attention.

Stimulant medications are the mainstay of treatment. They are highly effective and have few side effects when used correctly. Although there are legitimate concerns that these medications may promote illicit drug use, clinical studies demonstrate that appropriate treatment actually decreases future use of illicit drugs. Atomoxetine and other noradrenergic antidepressants are reasonable alternatives for patients who misuse or cannot tolerate stimulants.

Significant objections are raised to the current approaches for the diagnosis and treatment of ADHD. These stem from the fear that children are being overdiagnosed and then inappropriately medicated. In reality, some children are inappropriately treated, but many others are not diagnosed appropriately with ADHD. The failure to diagnose and treat ADHD in children is as undesirable as misdiagnosis and overtreatment.

PANIC DISORDER

CLINICAL VIGNETTE *A 33-year-old woman was referred to a psychiatric clinic after presenting to a hospital emergency department (ED) on four consecutive nights complaining of chest pain, dyspnea, and faintness. Each time, careful cardiac and pulmonary examinations were unremarkable and the patient was sent home with a benzodiazepine prescription and reassurance from the ED staff that she was not ill.*

She reported infrequent similar attacks in childhood. She felt a desperate need to have help available in case an attack occurred and rarely left home unaccompanied.

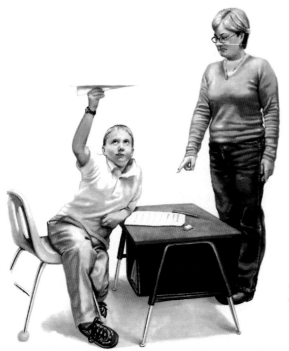

Attention-deficit disorder is a highly treatable neuropsychiatric disorder, common in school-age children, especially boys. Affected children are at increased risk for academic failure.

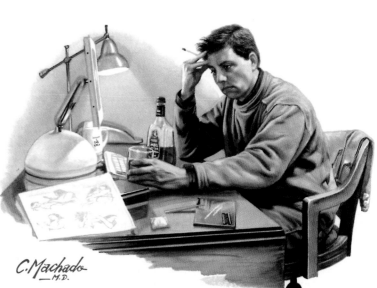

Hyperactivity improves or resolves spontaneously in adulthood, but 50% of patients maintain their cognitive disabilities. Substance abuse is commonly associated with ADHD.

Fig. 42.1 Attention-Deficit/Hyperactivity Disorder.

She had recently given up driving and air travel. She worked at an undemanding job near home. The lack of a substantial social life significantly troubled her, but despite this she felt helpless and was not able to socialize more. Caffeine made her feel "wired," and she presented to the psychiatrist a long list of medications to which she was "allergic." She acknowledged occasional excessive consumption of alcohol in order to lessen her anxiety.

ED staff members frequently encounter patients with panic disorder. These individuals experience unpredictable and sudden bouts of intense anxiety and frightening physical symptoms, leading them to fear they are having a heart attack, stroke, or other medical emergency. Patients with panic disorder are focused on the minute details of their symptoms and tend to make catastrophic self-diagnoses based on minor aches, palpitations, and shortness of breath (Fig. 42.2). They may present repeatedly to the ED with symptoms such as dyspnea, chest pain, tachycardia, and faintness. Typically these patients are not reassured by a negative examination and may present again a few days later with the same complaints. Between episodes they may feel entirely well, but more commonly they remain anxious and vigilant for signs of the next attack.

Many individuals with panic attacks develop agoraphobia. Agoraphobia is not solely—as the word would suggest—a fear of open spaces but also a fear of being isolated from help and support. Patients with agoraphobia avoid public transportation, open spaces, crowds, or being alone outside the home. Eventually such patients may become so fearful that they cannot leave home without being accompanied. The presence of panic or intense anxiety in patients with mood disorders is a well-established risk factor for suicide. It is unclear whether panic disorder in isolation, without a major depressive disorder, heightens this risk.

Intravenous lactic acid infusion, which mimics respiratory acidosis, reproduces the symptoms of panic attacks in many patients. This has led to postulation of the "suffocation alarm" theory of panic disorder—that affected individuals are overly sensitive to minor changes in blood pH and PCO_2. Hence asthma, the exacerbation of chronic obstructive pulmonary disorder, and pulmonary embolus are some of the respiratory disorders that must be excluded in these patients. Other conditions that must be excluded are cardiac arrhythmias, myocardial infarction, ingestion of sympathomimetics (particularly cocaine), excess caffeine, alcohol and sedative-hypnotic withdrawal, hypoglycemia, partial complex seizures, and, rarely, pheochromocytoma or carcinoid tumors.

Psychotherapeutic approaches to panic disorder include patient education about the syndrome's benign natural history and remediation of patients' catastrophic thinking. For some this is sufficient, although most phobic patients also need a course of graded exposure to feared situations.

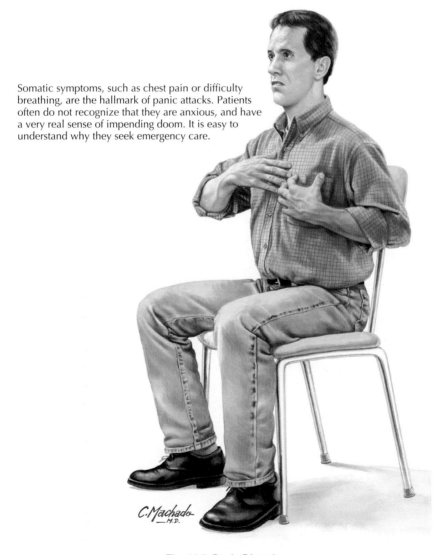

Somatic symptoms, such as chest pain or difficulty breathing, are the hallmark of panic attacks. Patients often do not recognize that they are anxious, and have a very real sense of impending doom. It is easy to understand why they seek emergency care.

Fig. 42.2 Panic Disorder.

Many patients also require pharmacologic management. Benzodiazepines abort panic attacks quickly and can be used as needed if attacks are infrequent. Serotonergic antidepressant medications are the first choice for extended treatment. Anxious patients are sensitive to the initial activating or anxiogenic effects of antidepressants; therefore treatment should begin with lower-than-usual doses. Monoamine oxidase (MAO) inhibitors may work when other antidepressants are ineffective. However, caution is needed with MAO inhibitors because of their potential for serious side effects.

POSTTRAUMATIC STRESS DISORDER

> **CLINICAL VIGNETTE** *Friends say that John W. was never the same after he returned from the war in Iraq. He had been wounded but seemed to recover uneventfully, was sent back for a second tour of duty, and was finally granted an honorable discharge.*
>
> *His troubles began after returning home. His previous civilian job had been permanently filled with no opportunity for him to return to that particular company, and he was uncharacteristically passive about finding a new position. His family found him to be distant, preoccupied, and jittery; they joked that he would dive under the kitchen table if a car backfired. They were unaware that John's sleep was chronically disrupted by vivid nightmares, replaying the worst of his combat experiences.*
>
> *After being home for a year, John developed a chronic dependence on alcohol. Eventually, after his second arrest for drunk driving, he was hospitalized for detoxification. Although Alcoholics Anonymous helped him to stop drinking, his anxiety and social withdrawal proved unresponsive to treatment and he was eventually granted a disability pension.*

Posttraumatic stress disorder (PTSD) is a syndrome of chronic maladaptation following unusual stress or trauma. Historically PTSD was associated with experiences in combat. In earlier versions of the DSM, PTSD was diagnosed only in individuals who had suffered trauma "outside the range of usual human experience" (Fig. 42.3). However, PTSD can develop as a consequence of other trauma or stress, including medical events (e.g., myocardial infarction, stroke, intensive care unit stay). Direct traumatic exposure, witnessing trauma, or learning about trauma can all lead to PTSD in susceptible individuals, making PTSD relatively common, with a lifetime prevalence in the United States of 8%.

Physical injury with high levels of pain has been associated with the development of PTSD. Low baseline cortisol levels may also be a risk factor for developing PTSD. For many of these patients, PTSD contributes to a lower quality of life and poorer health outcomes.

Patients with PTSD typically have four types of symptoms: (1) flashbacks, which are often very fearful, frightening thoughts, often occurring as night terrors or dreams; (2) avoidance, especially of any setting that reminds the patient of an inciting experience; (3) hyperarousal, characterized by the inability to sleep well, perpetually being edgy or tense, being easily startled and prone to angry, inappropriate outbursts; (4) withdrawal, a tendency to be emotionally numb, guilty, and anhedonic; these patients may appear to have depression.

Although such symptoms can be seen in any healthy individual after an acute stressful traumatic life experience, in PTSD it is the chronicity of these symptoms that leads to a state of virtual emotional paralysis. Interestingly, there may be a period of normal behavior immediately following the severe trauma, with the individual initially seeming to cope very well with the preceding disturbing experiences. There may

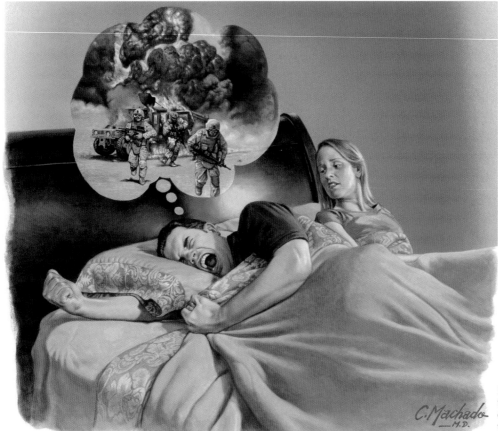

Individuals with PTSD may relive traumatic events in their thoughts during the day and in nightmares when they sleep

Fig. 42.3 Posttraumatic Stress Disorder.

be a latency of several months before PTSD begins to take its toll on the individual's activities of daily living.

Most patients with PTSD require intensive, sustained, multimodal therapy. Cognitive therapy is effective, as is exposure or reimagining.

Serotonin reuptake inhibitors (SRI) are the cornerstone of PTSD pharmacotherapy, but they rarely if ever produce full remission. Commonly used adjunctive treatments include atypical antipsychotics and mood stabilizers. The antiadrenergic agent prazosin appears to be especially effective in treating the nightmares and disordered sleep architecture characteristic of the disorder.

Once established, PTSD is stubborn and difficult to treat; thus effective prevention is essential. However, the previously intuitive idea of requiring trauma victims to "talk out" their experience by providing "critical incident debriefing" after trauma exposure has not proven to be useful and may even increase the risk of developing PTSD. Earlier evidence suggested that prophylactic administration of beta-adrenergic receptor blockers may prevent the development of PTSD. However, subsequent studies have not consistently demonstrated this effect and further research is required to support this intervention. Benzodiazepines, though commonly used in PTSD, have not been systematically studied. However, given the high comorbidity with substance use disorders, cautious use of benzodiazepines is advised. Once a patient has been stabilized, treatments should be continued for 6 to 12 months to prevent relapse.

OBSESSIVE-COMPULSIVE DISORDER

> **CLINICAL VIGNETTE** *A 36-year-old high school teacher consulted a psychiatrist because of difficulty driving to work. He had a long-standing fear that he would lose control of his car and accidentally run over a pedestrian. Recently this fear had intensified to the extent that he had to stop and examine his car's bumpers for signs of blood whenever he hit a bump on the road. It was taking him more than 2 hours each morning to complete a 20-minute commute. He also had to check the appliances and faucets at his home four times before leaving to make sure that they had been turned off, and he had a 1-hour ritual of washing and shaving that he needed to perform in strict order every morning.*
>
> *Despite his time-wasting habits and rituals, the patient had a successful career. He was well liked by friends and family, who worked around his "eccentricities." His symptoms gradually diminished with combined treatment with a serotonergic antidepressant and a behavioral program of exposure and response prevention.*

Patients with obsessive-compulsive disorder (OCD) complain of unwelcome, intrusive, and repetitive thoughts (obsessions) and/or urges to act in ways they find meaningless or inappropriate (compulsions). The thoughts and urges are "ego dystonic"—they are perceived as unreasonable and seemingly imposed upon the patient. People with OCD are tormented by their thoughts and behaviors, usually struggling with them for years before seeking help. OCD is closely related to body dysmorphic disorder, hoarding disorder, excoriation, trichotillomania, and other anxiety disorders, although each disorder varies in its diagnostic features, course, and treatment. These disorders frequently overlap, and screening for comorbid disorders is encouraged.

Patients with OCD usually fit into one of several categories. Some worry about germs or contamination and clean obsessively (Fig. 42.4). Some are obsessed with symmetry or arranging their possessions in exactly the right order and repeatedly check for the same. Often, patients with OCD are troubled by thoughts of violence; they may fear that they will injure someone or themselves (e.g., run someone over while driving) and repeatedly check to negate the fear and reassure themselves. Inexperienced clinicians sometimes err by seeing these obsessions as real threats, thereby exacerbating patients' fears. In fact, OCD patients are terrified of these thoughts and do not act on them.

Most diagnostic classifications employ a category of obsessive-compulsive personality disorder, to describe individuals who are highly controlled, formal, emotionally distant, parsimonious, perfectionistic, resistant to change, and intolerant of ambiguity. Despite the similarity in names, this personality constellation and OCD are unrelated.

Patients with OCD typically have no structural brain abnormalities; rarely subtle loss of frontal tissue has been described. In contrast, functional brain imaging reliably shows excess metabolic activity in the caudate and frontal regions. Patients typically exhibit minor difficulties on tests of executive function and less frequently have short-term memory dysfunction.

Patients with OCD share a unique pattern of response to medications. They improve when given serotonergic antidepressants. Typically higher doses of medication are required to treat OCD, the response is slower, and full remission with medication alone is uncommon. In contrast, antidepressants that block the reuptake of norepinephrine are ineffective for OCD. For patients with only a partial response, the addition of a low-dose neuroleptic medication can be helpful. Patients who are refractory to all other treatments and severely impaired by their illness are candidates for deep brain stimulation or other neurosurgical interventions.

Some form of behavioral therapy is almost always also required. The most effective of these is exposure and response prevention. If a patient has a compulsion to wash his or her hands, the quickest way to cure this is to get dirt on the hands and prevent the patient from washing it off. Naturally patients need support and encouragement to try this method. When patients improve, their functional imaging abnormalities resolve.

Some cases of childhood-onset OCD, especially those with abrupt onset or those associated with movement disorders, may be caused by streptococcal infections. A combination of antibiotic treatment and plasmapheresis, to remove antistreptococcal antibodies, may be helpful in these children.

BORDERLINE PERSONALITY DISORDER

> **CLINICAL VIGNETTE** *A 23-year-old woman was hospitalized after her parents brought her to the ED for an overdose of acetaminophen. Because of her history of illicit drug use, her parents had refused to underwrite a spring-break vacation and the patient took the overdose to "punish" her parents. The ingestion was minor and the patient was initially calm and friendly, but when ED staff expressed uncertainty about sending her home, the patient flew into a rage, accused staff of conspiring with her parents, and tried to bite a nurse.*
>
> *This was her fifth psychiatric hospitalization in 3 years; all but one had been preceded by a suicide gesture or attempt. She lived with her parents and sporadically took adult education courses with a vague ambition to direct films. Despite her high intelligence, she had failed three tries at college; in one instance, she had been dismissed for selling drugs. Although she had seen four respected therapists, she derided them as "only being in it for the money." Her arms showed multiple burn marks, and she admitted to burning herself with cigarettes "to relieve tension."*
>
> *Once admitted, she quickly established an alliance with a psychotic male patient and announced plans to move in with him when she was discharged. She was angry and sarcastic with some staff members but pleasant with others, leading to disagreements over her treatment and disposition.*

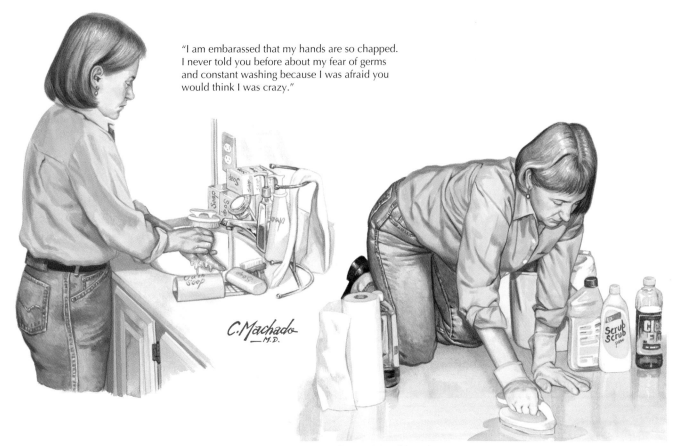

"I am embarassed that my hands are so chapped. I never told you before about my fear of germs and constant washing because I was afraid you would think I was crazy."

Fig. 42.4 Obsessive-Compulsive Disorder.

Psychoanalysts of the early 20th century described patients who appeared superficially healthy but could not be psychoanalyzed because of their inability to establish a stable therapeutic relationship. These patients tended to have tumultuous life histories, poor social and vocational adjustment, and occasional brief regressions to psychosis. They were called "ambulatory schizophrenics," "pseudoneurotic schizophrenics," or "borderline schizophrenics"; borderline personality disorder is now the accepted terminology.

Patients with borderline personality disorder are frequently described as "stably unstable." They have rapid and overwhelming mood fluctuations, can be strikingly angry, and react disastrously to minor slights and disappointments (Fig. 42.5). Their interpersonal relations are intense and stormy. They fail to establish consistent vocational identities, frequently misuse substances, injure themselves, and are liable to have brief psychotic episodes when stressed. High rates of childhood neglect and sexual abuse are found in hospitalized borderline patients.

Personality disorders develop in adolescence and early adulthood. Impairment from borderline personality disorder is greatest in early adulthood and gradually wanes with advancing age. Studies have demonstrated that after about 10 years, as many as half of individuals with borderline personality disorder still meet full criteria for the disorder.

These patients rely on two primitive psychologic defense mechanisms: splitting and projective identification. Splitting is the tendency to see oneself and others as either all good or all bad, often with rapid fluctuation between the two. Within a confined environment—as found in schools and hospitals—splitting often occurs among staff and authority figures; some are idealized, whereas others are hated and feared. This often leads to conflict between the two treatment groups, causing the patient's providers to enact the patient's conflict among themselves. Projective identification is the unconscious process of assuming that another person has an undesirable trait or attitude and then acting in such a way as to evoke those traits. Providers of borderline patients may find themselves overwhelmed with rage or contempt for their patients and will be tempted to act on these feelings.

Borderline patients are exhausting to treat because of their frequent crises, their simultaneous neediness and hostility, and their difficulty in establishing stable relationships. Dialectical behavioral therapy has demonstrated great efficacy. This is a comprehensive system of treatment with extensive institutional support for patients. Here therapists provide a persistent emphasis on diminishing unacceptable behavior as well as suicidal thinking.

No clear medication guidelines are available and none are likely to emerge, given the probable biologic heterogeneity of this disorder. On the whole, though, second-generation antipsychotic medications have the most research support. Low-dose lithium and other mood stabilizers sometimes help. In contrast, benzodiazepines may not only disinhibit patients but are also apt to be misused. Whatever treatment is proposed, it is important to first rule out active substance use and bipolar disorders, two conditions with specific treatments that may mimic borderline personality disorder.

EATING DISORDERS

CLINICAL VIGNETTE *Ellen W. gained 15 pounds during her freshman year at college and felt out of control. She began a strict diet, limiting her intake to 1000 calories daily. She also began to run every day. By summer's end she had returned to her baseline weight but decided to continue her diet and exercise regime. She was continually hungry and sometimes binged, but she soon discovered how to induce vomiting and settled into a regular pattern of*

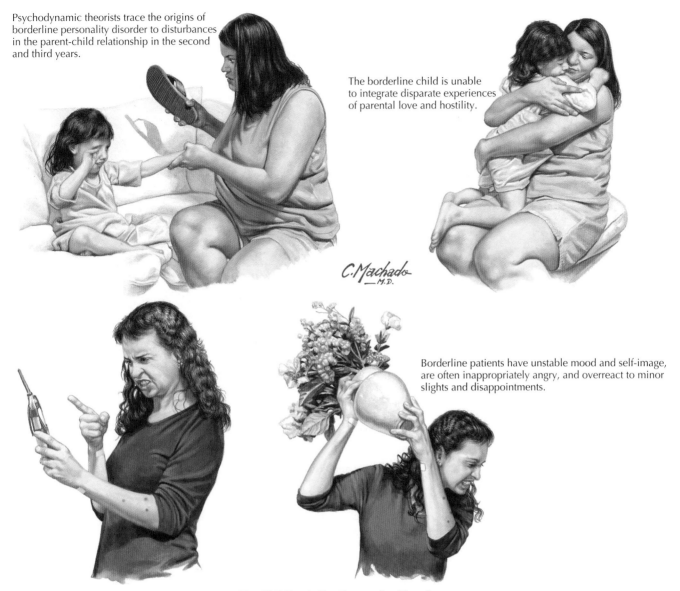

Psychodynamic theorists trace the origins of borderline personality disorder to disturbances in the parent-child relationship in the second and third years.

The borderline child is unable to integrate disparate experiences of parental love and hostility.

Borderline patients have unstable mood and self-image, are often inappropriately angry, and overreact to minor slights and disappointments.

Fig. 42.5 Borderline Personality Disorder.

bingeing and purging. After another year, she came to medical attention when she was brought, against her objections, to an ED after collapsing while running.

On examination she was cachectic, hypotensive, and bradycardic. Her teeth were eroded and she had parotid enlargement. Laboratory studies revealed microcytic anemia, metabolic alkalosis, and hypokalemia. She was admitted and required forced feeding to correct her life-threatening nutritional deficiencies. Throughout her hospitalization, she insisted that she was well but slightly overweight and needed to lose 10 more pounds. Five years later, she participated in regular individual and family psychotherapy. She had stopped bingeing and had negotiated a slightly less rigorous diet with her therapists, but she continued to monitor her caloric intake and weight every day.

The DSM-5 describes several feeding and eating disorders, including anorexia nervosa, bulimia nervosa, and binge-eating disorder. Eating disorders are primarily disorders of young women, though recognition in men is increasing. Anorexia nervosa is one of the deadliest of psychiatric disorders—a recent estimate is that 6% of such patients die from their illness.

Anorexia Nervosa

Anorexia nervosa is characterized by distorted body image, an unwillingness to maintain minimally normal body weight, and severely disordered eating habits. The etiology of anorexia nervosa is unknown, but patients typically display high levels of anxiety and perfectionism, and twin studies suggest comorbidity with major depression and a substantial inherited risk (Fig. 42.6). However, the prevalence of anorexia nervosa, unlike many other psychiatric illnesses, varies among different cultures; pressure to conform to cultural standards of thinness may play an important role in initiating this disorder.

The physical consequences of anorexia nervosa are directly related to weight loss and malnutrition. Therefore the basis of treatment is nutritional supplementation and restoration of healthy weight. Patients usually receive intensive individual and sometimes family psychotherapy. No medication is clearly effective.

Bulimia Nervosa

Bulimia is characterized by recurrent episodes of excessive food intake (binges) and loss of control, preoccupation with weight and body image,

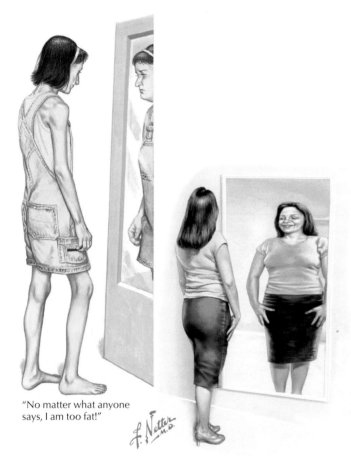

"No matter what anyone says, I am too fat!"

Two Forms	Restrictive anorexia nervosa. Bulimia nervosa; binge eating
Common Findings	Body image distortion @ ages 14-18; women > men Amenorrhea at least 3 months, and often precedes Weight loss >15% of ideal body weight Preserved secondary sex characteristics
Psychiatric Associated Disorders	Affective Anxiety OCD Personality Substance abuse
Differential Diagnosis	Adrenal insufficiency Inflammatory bowel and other GI disease Diabetes mellitus recent onset CNS posterior fossa lesions Primary depression
Endocrine Findings	Serum cortisol and growth hormone increased Serum LH & FSH low Insulin-like growth factor IGF-I low

Fig. 42.6 Eating Disorder.

and inappropriate compensatory behaviors to control weight, such as fasting, excessive exercise, induced vomiting, and ingestion of laxatives and diuretics. Unlike anorexia nervosa, patients with bulimia are usually obese or of normal weight.

Bulimia is less deadly than anorexia but much more common. There is a high rate of comorbidity with other mental disorders with an increased frequency of depressive disorders.

Like anorexia nervosa, the foundation of treatment for bulimia is nutritional rehabilitation and psychotherapy. Typical psychotherapies utilize a cognitive approach that addresses the all-or-none thinking that leads to binges.

Unlike the case in anorexia nervosa, most antidepressant medications are at least partially effective in treating bulimia (the exception is bupropion, which is contraindicated in eating disorder patients because of a heightened risk of seizures). Serotonergic antidepressants are considered first-line treatment. The anticonvulsant topiramate also appears to have a clinically useful antibingeing effect and can cause weight loss.

Binge-Eating Disorder

Binge-eating disorder (BED) is characterized by recurrent binges and loss of control. Unlike bulimia, patients with BED do not purge and do not typically use dietary restriction to lower body weight. BED is more prevalent than either bulimia or anorexia nervosa; moreover, remission rates and treatment outcomes appear better in BED.

Psychotherapy is generally more beneficial than pharmacotherapy, although medications can be efficacious. Serotonergic antidepressants are considered first-line treatment. Topiramate or lisdexamfetamine may be considered as alternative treatments.

ADDITIONAL RESOURCES

American Psychiatric Association. Diagnostic and statistical manual of mental disorders: DSM-5. Washington, DC: American Psychiatric Association; 2013.

This authoritative volume defines and classifies mental disorders in order to improve diagnosis, treatment, and research.

Asmundson GJG, Taylor S. It's not all in your head: how worrying about your health could be making you sick—and what you can do about it. New York, NY: Guilford; 2005.

This work focuses on understanding health anxiety and the role of stress, with examples of how to change thought and behavior patterns that contribute to aches, pains, and anxiety.

Barkley RA. Attention-deficit hyperactivity disorder. 4th ed. A handbook for diagnosis and treatment. New York, NY: Guilford; 2014.

This is the standard clinical reference on ADHD, addressing assessment, diagnosis, and treatment.

Clark DA. Cognitive behavioral therapy for OCD. New York, NY: Guilford; 2004.

This volume reviews cognitive-behavioral models of obsessive compulsive disorder and delineates an approach to assessment and treatment.

Forbes D, Creamer M, Bisson JI, et al. A guide to guidelines for the treatment of PTSD and related conditions. J Traum Stress 2010;23:537–52.

An examination of the various guidelines, comparing and contrasting methodologies and offering recommendations to aid clinicians.

Gunderson JG, Links P. Handbook of good psychiatric management of borderline personality disorder. Washington, DC: American Psychiatric Publishing, Inc.; 2014.

A review of evidence-based treatment and good psychiatric management (GPM) utilizing practical cognitive, behavioral, and psychodynamic interventions for borderline personality disorder.

Linehan M. Cognitive-behavioral treatment of borderline personality disorder. New York, NY: Guilford; 1993.

A reference book describing dialectical behavior therapy, a comprehensive, integrated approach to treating individuals with borderline personality disorder.

Wonderlich SA, Gordon KH, Mitchell JE, et al. The validity and clinical utility of binge-eating disorder. Int J Eat Disord 2009;42:687–705.

A review of the validity and clinical utility of the Diagnostic and Statistical Manual's binge-eating disorder diagnosis across a wide range of validating strategies.

Yager J, Devlin MJ, Halmi KA, et al. Guideline watch. 3rd ed. Practice guideline for the treatment of patients with eating disorders. Washington, DC: American Psychiatric Association; 2012.

An update to prior treatment guidelines for the treatment of patients with eating disorders.

Nutritional Disorders, Alcohol and Drug Dependency

Brian J. Scott

43

Alcohol and Drug Abuse and Dependence

Kenneth Lakritz, Yuval Zabar, Brian J. Scott

CLINICAL VIGNETTE *A 73-year-old woman is seen in the emergency department after an unwitnessed fall at home in which her husband heard a crash and found her moments later on the ground in her bedroom. She was disoriented and bleeding from a head laceration that occurred when she fell and hit the corner of their bedroom dresser.*

She has a past medical history of anxiety, obesity, gastroesophageal reflux, and chronic low back pain. She underwent a lumbar discectomy 10 years earlier with minimal improvement in her symptoms. Her medications include citalopram, lorazepam, oxycodone, and pantoprazole. She retired early from her job as an office manager because it was exceedingly stressful for her and she lives with her husband, daughter, and infant grandson. She reports "social" alcohol use and denies tobacco or other drug use.

On examination, she is sleepy but readily arouses to voice. She does not participate in the history or examination and tells healthcare team members that she is "just here to get stitches." Her husband apologizes for her lack of cooperation. He explains that she tends to avoid medical care and is going through a lot of stress at home related to her daughter and grandchild. On mental status examination, she is oriented to year and city but not the name of the hospital or the date. She has moderate inattention but intact language and 3/5 recall at 5 min. Her remaining neurologic exam is significant for hyporeflexia, a distal, symmetric sensory neuropathy, and a slow, mildly ataxic gait with inability to tandem walk.

Urine toxicology screening was positive for benzodiazepines and opiates, and a blood alcohol concentration was 0.05%. A noncontrast head CT showed no hemorrhage or other sign of acute intracranial injury but was noted to have generalized mild atrophy.

Outside the room, the patient's husband expresses concern over his wife's use of pain and anxiety medications, noting that she frequently sleeps during the day. He has noticed that she has lost contact with her usual group of social contacts and that she gets extremely angry with him when he has asked her about cutting down on alcohol and pain killers. Upon further 1:1 questioning, the patient admits to drinking more than usual over the past several weeks and using higher doses of medication to treat "intolerable pain and anxiety."

Most physicians are intimately familiar with the protean manifestations of alcohol abuse and dependence (Fig. 43.1) and its characteristic clinical signs (Fig. 43.2). Incidence rates vary widely depending on geography and social and cultural dynamics. In North America and Europe, the lifetime rate of alcohol abuse is estimated at 5%–10%. Therefore physicians who assert that they *never see alcoholism* are likely not recognizing the diagnosis. When obtaining the substance use history, it is critical to ask nonjudgmental, open-ended questions. "How much alcohol do you drink?" or "What do you find helpful for your pain/anxiety?" is more likely to elicit an honest reply than "Do you ever drink excessive amounts of alcohol?" Asking in a comfortable, relaxed setting, phrasing similar questions differently, as well as interviewing an individual by themselves rather than in front of family members or friends are all helpful ways to obtain a more accurate alcohol and drug use history. Patient denial poses a significant barrier in identifying and treating substance overuse. This denial has several sources. Admitting to a problem with alcohol or other drugs may be humiliating for patients. Furthermore, alcohol use, even at dangerous levels, is a culturally embedded and accepted, often pleasurable part of social life.

The rubric of drug and alcohol abuse subsumes dozens of syndromes, but a few useful generalizations can be offered. Most drugs have safe and unsafe uses. Physicians routinely use opiates, sedative-hypnotics, psychostimulants, and dissociative anesthetics, all of which have abuse and addiction potential. Even over-the-counter drugs, including anticholinergics, pseudoephedrine, and dextromethorphan, can be abused.

Potentially *abusable drugs cause dopamine release* directly or indirectly in several forebrain structures. Beyond this, factors that may make a drug dangerous include the dosage, route of administration, and social context. High doses, routes of administration that rapidly deliver a drug to the brain (intranasal, injection, etc.), and ingestion beyond a stable social or religious context all predispose to abuse and addiction potential. These factors rather than, for example, the pharmacology of cocaine per se, explain why the Peruvian practice of chewing coca leaves rarely leads to addiction or neurologic injury, whereas smoking freebase cocaine is extremely addictive and risky.

ETIOLOGY

Liability to alcohol abuse and dependence, especially early-onset abuse, runs in families, but the mechanism of inheritance is not understood. Findings of a link between alcoholism and a particular dopamine DR-2 receptor allele remain controversial. Some Asian individuals are relatively protected from alcoholism because they possess a dysfunctional form of the enzyme alcohol dehydrogenase that leads to slow alcohol metabolism. This causes skin flushing and nausea with small amounts of alcohol ingestion. Conversely, young adults with a high alcohol tolerance, evaluated on measures of incoordination or subjectively, are at increased risk to develop alcoholism.

Alcohol is a central nervous system (CNS) depressant with cross-tolerance to benzodiazepines, barbiturates, and some other sedatives. It is distinguished within this group by its ease of manufacture, legal status, wide availability, rapid absorption, and exceptionally low therapeutic index. The lethal dose of alcohol is only a few times the intoxicating dose; one bottle of whiskey can be lethal to an individual who has not acquired tolerance. The dose at which tissue damage occurs is lower in this setting and falls within the range of commonly ingested

Criteria: Three distinct episodes in one year are indicative of alcohol abuse.

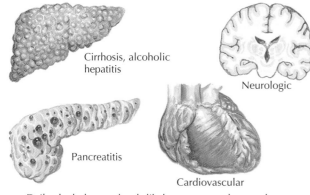

Failure to fulfill major obligations at work, school, or home

Continued use of alcohol despite interpersonal problems

JOHN A. CRAIG—MD
C. Machado
—M.D.

Recurrent use of alcohol in hazardous situations

Recurrent legal problems related to alcohol use

Other problem patterns of drinking

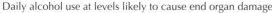

Mon	Tues	Wed	Thur	Fri	Sat	Sun	Mon	Tues	Wed	Thur	Fri	Sat	Sun

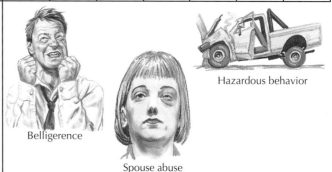

Cirrhosis, alcoholic hepatitis

Neurologic

Pancreatitis

Cardiovascular

Belligerence

Spouse abuse

Hazardous behavior

Daily alcohol use at levels likely to cause end organ damage

Intermittent abuse of alcohol at levels that result in dangerous and destructive behavior

Fig. 43.1 Alcohol Abuse.

doses. In adults, chemical signs of hepatic injury are detectable after consumption of three or more drinks within 24 hours. Alcohol is a potent fetal teratogen with no threshold dose and therefore contraindicated in pregnancy.

CLINICAL PRESENTATION

Acute alcohol intoxication at moderate doses causes disinhibition and incoordination. Even at socially acceptable doses, it impairs driving and is implicated in approximately half of all highway accidents and deaths. Alcohol is linked to a similar proportion of sexual assaults.

Patients with most major psychiatric illnesses have increased rates of alcohol abuse. Alcohol interacts with psychiatric illnesses and treatments. Many patients use alcohol to treat mood disorders, anxiety, or insomnia, but it is not a safe or effective treatment for any medical disorder. The toxicity and short duration of action of alcohol make it useless as an anxiolytic, and it disrupts sleep architecture and decreases sleep efficiency. The combination of alcohol abuse and depression is especially lethal. Alcohol use intensifies symptoms of depression and interferes with antidepressant response. Drinkers who are depressed

experience an approximately 10-fold increase in suicide rate compared with nondrinkers who are depressed.

Alcohol has direct toxic effects on multiple tissues, including the CNS, liver, pancreas, and heart. Patients may present with acute or chronic hepatitis, cirrhosis, esophageal varices, cardiomyopathy, and dementia. Acute withdrawal syndromes occur occasionally, leading to delirium tremens, Wernicke encephalopathy, and Korsakoff psychosis.

Alcoholics are especially at risk for *Wernicke encephalopathy,* an acute neurologic emergency resulting from acute thiamine and other B-vitamin depletion. It clinically manifests as gait ataxia and subsequently oculomotor abnormalities and delirium, developing during a period of days to weeks and presenting with confusion, ataxia, and ophthalmoplegia with diplopia and nystagmus. The delirium is characterized by disorientation, inattention, drowsiness, and indifference to surroundings. Conversation is sparse and tangential. Signs of alcohol withdrawal are seen in 15% of patients. When clinically suspected, Wernicke encephalopathy requires immediate administration of high-dose intravenous thiamine (100 mg or more), in a non–glucose-containing solution. This reverses the symptoms and can prevent irreversible brain injury. Intravenous thiamine is routinely provided in emergency departments for

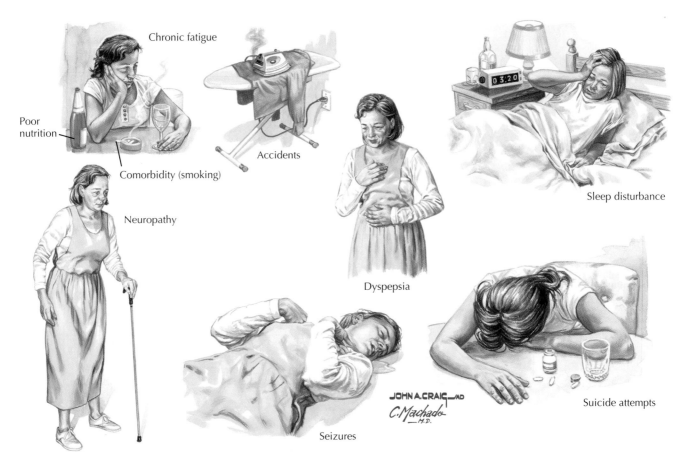

Chronic fatigue

Poor nutrition

Comorbidity (smoking)

Accidents

Neuropathy

Dyspepsia

Sleep disturbance

Suicide attempts

JOHN A. CRAIG _MD
C. Machado _M.D.

Seizures

Fig. 43.2 Signs Suggestive of Alcohol Abuse.

most patients presenting with an acute confusional state. Progressive stupor, coma, and death develop if the condition is left untreated. Thiamine and other B vitamins should be given parenterally to malnourished patients as supplements to replenish body stores.

Brain autopsy in Wernicke encephalopathy reveals symmetric necrosis of brainstem tegmentum nuclei, superior cerebellar vermis, and mammillary bodies. These findings resemble lesions produced by disorders of pyruvate metabolism.

Korsakoff psychosis is likely to develop without immediate repletion of thiamine in Wernicke encephalopathy patients. This disorder is mostly confined to alcoholics, with the only exception being individuals having bilateral hippocampal damage, typically from vertebrobasilar infarction. This condition is a nonprogressive devastating irretrievable disorder of memory affecting both acquisition of new information (anterograde amnesia) and memory (retrograde amnesia). The patient cannot make new memories because of poor encoding, which is similar to the memory impairment of Alzheimer disease. The retrograde amnesia may extend back many years, rendering the patient "stuck in time." Recollection of past events is usually disorganized and erratic. Additional cognitive impairment includes poor sequencing, arithmetic, and construction performance.

Hepatic encephalopathy (see Chapter 26) occurs in stages. Patients with liver failure experience confusion, with decreased psychomotor activity associated with accumulation of ammonia. Occasionally, hyperactivity and agitation occur. During this time, patients often have asterixis on clinical examination, which is not a sign specific to hepatic encephalopathy because it can occur in many other metabolic disturbances, such as uremic encephalopathy. Progressive stages of drowsiness, stupor, and coma follow, sometimes with seizures or status epilepticus. Significant motor abnormalities develop, including rigidity, bradykinesia, brisk reflexes, and

extensor plantar reflexes. The severity of hepatic encephalopathy tends to correlate with the degree of hepatic dysfunction and a higher Model for End-Stage Liver Disease (MELD) score and is an independent predictor of mortality. In some cases a chronic disorder of cognition and behavior occurs, with pyramidal and extrapyramidal dysfunction lasting months or years. This condition is seen in patients with repetitive bouts of hepatic encephalopathy. Electroencephalogram (EEG) shows generalized slowing of background rhythm with prominent triphasic waves. The purpose of treatment is to attempt to decrease NH_3 levels by reducing dietary protein, acidifying colonic contents with lactulose, and, occasionally, suppressing urease-producing colonic bacteria with antibiotics.

DIAGNOSIS

To avoid missing the diagnosis of a substance use disorder, physicians must maintain a high index of suspicion directed at eliciting classic historic signs of *substance overuse* (see Fig. 43.2). Similarly, asking about features suggestive of early *dependence* is important during routine screening in any patient (Fig. 43.3). Asking about average levels and patterns of alcohol and drug use should be part of every examination. Patients also need to be questioned about binge drinking, withdrawal signs, blackouts, and excessive tolerance. The four-question CAGE questionnaire is a good instrument to screen for alcohol overuse in adults and older adolescents (Box 43.1). One positive answer to a CAGE question is cause for concern; two positive answers are highly sensitive and moderately specific for excessive drinking or alcoholism.

Any individual who has had even one *driving while intoxicated* (DWI) conviction can be safely assumed to have a problem with alcohol, as can the occasional patient who presents in an intoxicated state for his or her appointment. In the latter case, the physician must take whatever

Three or more incidences during 1 year indicate pattern of physical dependence

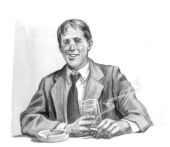

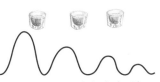

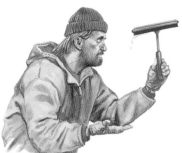

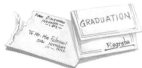

Increasing amounts of alcohol needed to achieve effect (tolerance)

Same amount of alcohol with decreasing effect

Great deal of time and effort spent on obtaining alcohol

Avoiding important social, occupational, or recreational events because of alcohol use

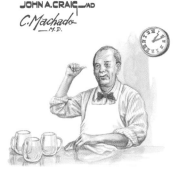

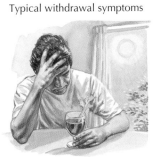

Typical withdrawal symptoms

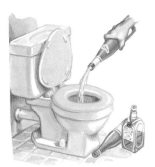

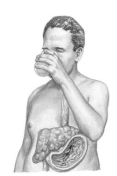

Drinking more or for longer periods

Similar substance used to avoid withdrawal symptoms

Persistent desire or unsuccessful efforts to curb abuse

Continued use of alcohol despite exacerbation of health problems

Fig. 43.3 Alcohol Dependence.

BOX 43.1   CAGE Questionnaire

Ask patients whether:
  They have felt a need to **C**ut down their intake
  Others have **A**nnoyed them by criticizing their drinking
  They have felt **G**uilty about their drinking
  They have ever needed an **E**ye-opener (a morning drink) to calm their nerves or treat a hangover

steps are immediately necessary to prevent this patient from driving away from the medical office.

When diagnostic uncertainty persists, interviewing family or friends is often informative; typically, they present a more accurate picture of the patient's substance use. Laboratory test results that reveal increased gamma-glutamyl-transpeptidase (GGTP) or transaminase levels, mild macrocytic anemia, or both can add confirmatory evidence.

TREATMENT

Withdrawal from alcohol and *other cross-tolerant sedative hypnotics* (barbiturates, benzodiazepines, methaqualone, etc.) is potentially hazardous (Figs. 43.4–43.6). Acute withdrawal can cause agitated delirium and seizures, with potentially dangerous or life-threatening complications including severe behavioral disturbances and status epilepticus. In contrast, most *other pharmacologic withdrawal* syndromes such as stimulant or opiate withdrawal are characterized by *dysphoria* but are not as medically dangerous; nevertheless, there can be serious secondary

effects such as withdrawal from cocaine and amphetamines leading to profound depression.

Addicted patients must remove themselves, as much as possible, from the routines and environment wherein they obtain and use drugs. Acute care or outpatient detoxification programs may be a helpful adjunct if the individual is willing to attend and participate. Twelve-step organizations such as Alcoholics Anonymous, Narcotics Anonymous, and other self-help groups are extremely valuable in overcoming denial of illness and in providing patients a culture of sobriety and social support. Similar support group resources (Alanon, Alateen, Adult Children of Alcoholics) are available worldwide for family members impacted by the deleterious effects of alcoholism or drug addiction. The treatment *goal* is total current and future *abstinence*. Although therapies incorporating a return to controlled substance use have been repeatedly proposed, these approaches are unsuccessful.

Pharmacologic treatments for addiction are adjunctive to psychotherapeutic and behavioral interventions. Long-term replacement of opiates with methadone or buprenorphine is effective in cases of overuse, as is the temporary use of nicotine administered by patch, gum, or inhalation to help smokers quit. The use of bupropion modestly increases the success rate of quitting cigarettes. Varenicline, a nicotine receptor partial agonist, is another pharmacologic adjunct to help with smoking cessation.

Disulfiram (Antabuse) is the oldest specific medicine to be prescribed to prevent use of alcohol. There is also limited evidence suggesting that disulfiram may be a useful therapy in those seeking to eliminate cocaine use. By blocking aldehyde dehydrogenase to inhibit the metabolic degradation of alcohol, disulfiram induces an unpleasant and potentially dangerous reaction within 10–30 minutes of alcohol ingestion. Disulfiram

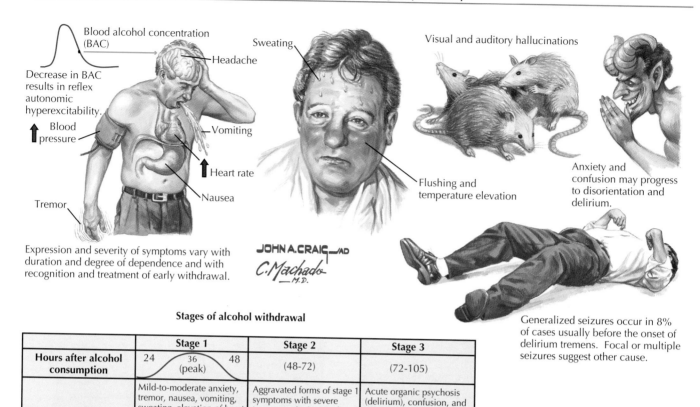

Blood alcohol concentration (BAC)

Decrease in BAC results in reflex autonomic hyperexcitability.

Blood pressure

Tremor

Headache

Vomiting

Heart rate

Nausea

Sweating

Visual and auditory hallucinations

Flushing and temperature elevation

Anxiety and confusion may progress to disorientation and delirium.

Expression and severity of symptoms vary with duration and degree of dependence and with recognition and treatment of early withdrawal.

JOHN A. CRAIG—AD
C. Machado—M.D.

Generalized seizures occur in 8% of cases usually before the onset of delirium tremens. Focal or multiple seizures suggest other cause.

Stages of alcohol withdrawal

	Stage 1	Stage 2	Stage 3
Hours after alcohol consumption	24 36 (peak) 48	(48-72)	(72-105)
Symptoms	Mild-to-moderate anxiety, tremor, nausea, vomiting, sweating, elevation of heart rate and blood pressure, sleep disturbance, hallucinations, illusions, seizures	Aggravated forms of stage 1 symptoms with severe tremors, agitation, and hallucinations	Acute organic psychosis (delirium), confusion, and disorientation with severe autonomic symptoms

Stage 1 withdrawal usually self-limited. Only small percentage of cases progress to stages 2 and 3. Progression prevented by prompt and adequate treatment.

Fig. 43.4 Alcohol Withdrawal.

Signs and Symptoms of Opioid Withdrawal

JOHN A. CRAIG—AD
C. Machado—M.D.

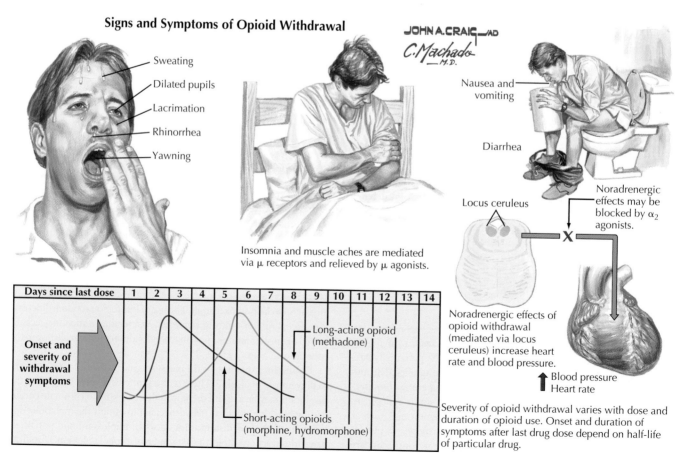

Sweating

Dilated pupils

Lacrimation

Rhinorrhea

Yawning

Insomnia and muscle aches are mediated via μ receptors and relieved by μ agonists.

Nausea and vomiting

Diarrhea

Locus ceruleus

Noradrenergic effects may be blocked by α₂ agonists.

Noradrenergic effects of opioid withdrawal (mediated via locus ceruleus) increase heart rate and blood pressure.

Blood pressure
Heart rate

Days since last dose	1	2	3	4	5	6	7	8	9	10	11	12	13	14
Onset and severity of withdrawal symptoms														

Long-acting opioid (methadone)

Short-acting opioids (morphine, hydromorphone)

Severity of opioid withdrawal varies with dose and duration of opioid use. Onset and duration of symptoms after last drug dose depend on half-life of particular drug.

Fig. 43.5 Opioid Withdrawal.

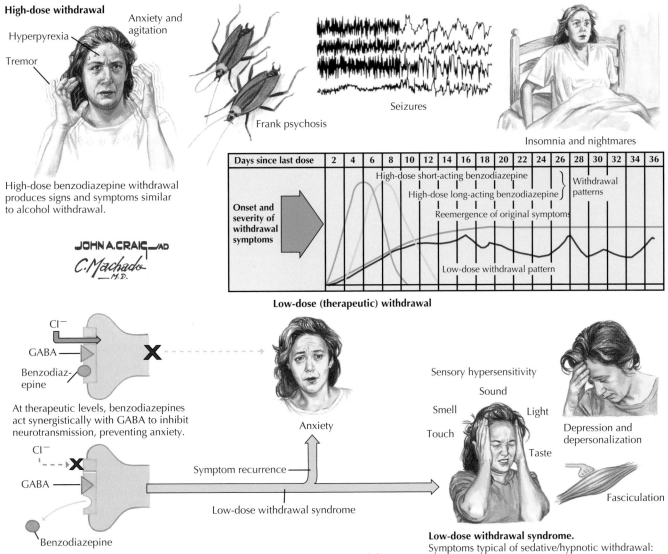

High-dose withdrawal

Hyperpyrexia

Tremor

Anxiety and agitation

Frank psychosis

Seizures

Insomnia and nightmares

High-dose benzodiazepine withdrawal produces signs and symptoms similar to alcohol withdrawal.

JOHN A. CRAIG—AD

C. Machado—M.D.

Days since last dose	2	4	6	8	10	12	14	16	18	20	22	24	26	28	30	32	34	36

Onset and severity of withdrawal symptoms

High-dose short-acting benzodiazepine
High-dose long-acting benzodiazepine } Withdrawal patterns
Reemergence of original symptoms
Low-dose withdrawal pattern

Low-dose (therapeutic) withdrawal

Cl⁻

GABA

Benzodiazepine

At therapeutic levels, benzodiazepines act synergistically with GABA to inhibit neurotransmission, preventing anxiety.

Cl⁻

GABA

Benzodiazepine

Withdrawing long-term benzodiazepine causes loss of synergism with GABA inhibition, resulting in recurrence of original symptoms and low-dose withdrawal syndrome.

Anxiety

Symptom recurrence

Low-dose withdrawal syndrome

Sensory hypersensitivity

Sound

Smell   Light

Touch

Taste

Depression and depersonalization

Fasciculation

Low-dose withdrawal syndrome.
Symptoms typical of sedative/hypnotic withdrawal: fluctuating hypersensitivity to sensory input, muscle twitching, depression, and depersonalization.

Fig. 43.6 Benzodiazepine Withdrawal.

treatment must be undertaken with medical oversight and works best in highly motivated but intermittently impulsive binge drinkers. However, this therapeutic approach is heavily dependent on patient motivation; it is easy for an alcoholic to simply choose to stop using the medicine.

Two other medications are approved for the treatment of alcoholism: *Naltrexone* is an opiate antagonist that also reduces alcohol intake, presumably by diminishing the rewarding effects of alcohol. *Acamprosate* is thought to subtly diminish protracted withdrawal systems by modulating glutamatergic activity. To date, there are no approved pharmacologic treatments for cocaine and other types of stimulant dependence. The most promising agents (topiramate, vigabatrin, etc.) increase γ-aminobutyric acid (GABA) activity.

Liability to alcoholism, especially early-onset alcoholism, is *partially inherited,* as may be the case with other addictions. Physiologic and epidemiologic evidence suggests that the adolescent brain is especially vulnerable to addiction, particularly to nicotine; few smoking habits begin after age 18. Persons with psychiatric illnesses, especially *bipolar disorder, attention-deficit hyperactivity disorder (ADHD), and personality disorders,* are at heightened risk for drug abuse and dependence. ADHD is diagnosable by age 8 and never starts in adulthood.

Some psychiatrists believe that many addicts are in fact "self-medicating" an underlying psychiatric disorder—this idea remains controversial. However, "dual diagnosis" patients are the rule rather than the exception. These individuals need simultaneous treatment for both addiction and psychiatric illness.

ADDITIONAL RESOURCES

Hays JT. Efficacy and safety of varenicline for smoking cessation. Am J Med 2008;121(4 Suppl. 1):S32–42.

Johnson BA, et al. Topiramate for treating alcohol dependence: a randomized controlled trial. JAMA 2007;298(14):1641–51.

Karila L, et al. New treatments for cocaine dependence: a focused review. Int J Neuropsychopharmacol 2008;11(3):425–38.

Khantzian EJ. The self-medication hypothesis of substance use disorders: a reconsideration and recent applications. Harv Rev Psychiatry 1997;4(5):231–44.

Krupitsky EM. Antiglutamatergic strategies for ethanol detoxification: comparison with placebo and diazepam. Alcohol 2007;31(4):604–11.

Spanagel R, Kiefer F. Drugs for relapse prevention of alcoholism: ten years of progress. Trends Pharmacol Sci 2008;29(3):109–15.

Infectious Diseases

Jayashri Srinivasan

44

Bacterial Diseases

Kenneth M. Wener, Winnie W. Ooi, Daniel P. McQuillen, Donald E. Craven,
Robert A. Duncan, Robert Peck, Samuel E. Kalluvya, Johannes B. Kataraihya

COMMON SYNDROMES

Bacterial Meningitis

> **CLINICAL VIGNETTE** *A 19-year-old woman presented to the emergency department with confusion, lethargy, and neck stiffness. Her dorm mates reported that she had experienced upper respiratory symptoms for 3 or 4 days before presentation. She had no significant past medical history. On physical examination, her findings were temperature, 98.6° F (37°C); pulse, 100 beats/ min; respirations, 20/min; and blood pressure, 110/70 mm Hg. Although her neck was stiff, Kernig and Brudzinski signs were absent. The pharynx was slightly injected without exudate. Heart and lung examination results were normal. No rash was present. Neurologic examination revealed a slightly obtunded, sleepy woman with otherwise intact mental status, intact cranial nerves, no motor or sensory deficits, and normal reflexes.*
>
> *The patient's white blood cell (WBC) count was 22,900/mm³, with a marked left shift, including 34% bands and 62% polymorphonuclear neutrophils (PMNs). Her platelet count was 120,000/mm³. Her electrolytes revealed a mild metabolic acidosis. Chest radiograph and brain computed tomography (CT) were normal.*
>
> *Initial cerebrospinal fluid (CSF) examination was normal. However, she was admitted for observation. Very soon thereafter, she complained of increasingly severe headache and neck pain. On examination, she was found to be in a confused state and now had a fever of 39.1°C (102.4° F). Repeat lumbar puncture demonstrated a cloudy CSF with 670 WBCs (90% PMNs), a glucose level of 1 mg/dL, and a protein level of 220 mg/dL. Gram stain revealed rare gram-negative diplococci that on culture grew Neisseria meningitidis. Blood cultures also grew N. meningitidis. She was treated with penicillin G 24 million U/d IV and recovered completely. Before discharge she was given rifampin to eliminate nasopharyngeal carriage of N. meningitidis.*

One of the most serious neurologic emergencies involves the evaluation and care of patients with bacterial meningitis. Usually, these individuals are previously healthy when they suddenly develop a severe headache, fever, and stiff neck. Despite more than 50 years of experience with antibiotic therapies, bacterial meningitis remains a very lethal disease. Expedient diagnosis is essential to prevent such an outcome. In the preceding vignette, typical for meningococcal meningitis, despite the history and findings suggestive of a meningeal infection, the initial CSF examination was normal. An emergency physician wisely admitted the patient for observation. When she experienced sudden deterioration, repeat CSF examination led to the diagnosis and appropriate therapy. Any delay in diagnosis and therapy of bacterial meningitis can be irretrievable, as death may occur unless appropriate antibiotic therapy is begun immediately.

Pathophysiology

Bacterial meningitis is defined as a microbial infection primarily involving the leptomeninges (Fig. 44.1). Typically, bacteria seed the leptomeninges via the bloodstream or from a contiguous site of infection, such as sinusitis, otitis media, or mastoiditis. Rarely a defect in the normal anatomic barriers, as with a perforating cranial or spinal injury or congenital dural defect, leads to a predisposition to recurrent bacterial meningitis.

The responsible microorganisms often differ between children and adult patients. Those commonly responsible for meningitis in adults include *Streptococcus pneumoniae*, *N. meningitidis*, and *Listeria monocytogenes*. *Haemophilus influenzae* still causes 20% to 50% of meningitis in developing countries, but in the United States this rate has been reduced by 90% with the *H. influenzae* type b vaccine. In neonates, *Escherichia coli* and group B β-hemolytic streptococci cause most cases. *L. monocytogenes* particularly leads to meningitis in immunocompromised patients and rarely in the newborn. *N. meningitidis* infection often occurs with a primary sepsis and a characteristic petechial and/or purpuric rash or disseminated intravascular coagulopathy. Conditions predisposing to pneumococcal meningitis in adults include sickle cell disease as well as conditions predisposing to immune deficiencies, including alcoholism, cirrhosis, splenectomy, and HIV/AIDS. Basilar skull fracture may also pose a risk for invasive pneumococcal meningitis.

Gram-negative bacilli (*E. coli*, *Proteus*, *Pseudomonas*, *Serratia*, *Klebsiella*, and *Citrobacter*) are rarely found in community-acquired meningitis but more commonly occur in association with head or spinal trauma or after neurosurgery. These organisms must always be considered in immunocompromised hosts. Meningitis due to *Staphylococcus aureus* may follow penetrating trauma, neurosurgery, or bacteremia. Coagulase-negative staphylococci (*Staphylococcus epidermidis*) or *S. aureus* and other organisms are associated with infected ventricular shunts.

Clinical Presentation and Diagnosis

The onset of acute bacterial meningitis is rapid: hours to a day or so. Classic clinical findings include signs of an acute cerebral disorder, with lethargy, seizures, and agitation as well as specific signs of meningeal involvement manifested by severe neck stiffness, called *meningismus*, and fever that may not be immediately present. The patient rapidly becomes confused, sleepy, obtunded, and often comatose.

The examining physician must carefully search for signs of nuchal rigidity in any febrile patient who presents with a headache or any changes in the level of alertness. Two clinical maneuvers are very important for identifying the presence of inflamed meningeal coverings involving the lumbosacral nerve roots: examination for the Kernig and Brudzinski signs (Fig. 44.2). The **Kernig sign** is elicited by flexing the patient's hip to a 90-degree angle and then attempting to passively

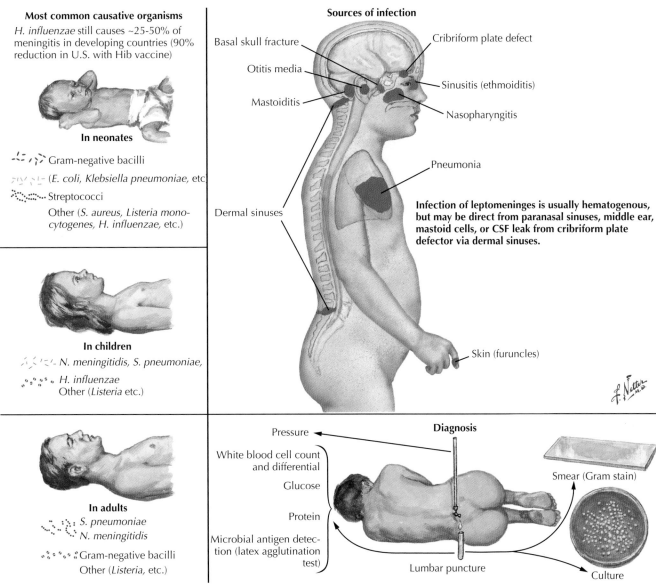

Most common causative organisms

H. influenzae still causes ~25-50% of meningitis in developing countries (90% reduction in U.S. with Hib vaccine)

In neonates

Gram-negative bacilli

(*E. coli, Klebsiella pneumoniae,* etc.)

Streptococci

Other (*S. aureus, Listeria monocytogenes, H. influenzae,* etc.)

In children

N. meningitidis, S. pneumoniae,

H. influenzae
Other (*Listeria* etc.)

In adults

S. pneumoniae
N. meningitidis

Gram-negative bacilli
Other (*Listeria,* etc.)

Sources of infection

Basal skull fracture

Otitis media

Mastoiditis

Dermal sinuses

Cribriform plate defect

Sinusitis (ethmoiditis)

Nasopharyngitis

Pneumonia

Infection of leptomeninges is usually hematogenous, but may be direct from paranasal sinuses, middle ear, mastoid cells, or CSF leak from cribriform plate defector via dermal sinuses.

Skin (furuncles)

Diagnosis

Pressure

White blood cell count and differential

Glucose

Protein

Microbial antigen detection (latex agglutination test)

Lumbar puncture

Smear (Gram stain)

Culture

Fig. 44.1 Bacterial Meningitis–I.

straighten the leg at the knee; pain and tightness in the hamstring muscles prevent completion of this maneuver. This sign should be present bilaterally to support a diagnosis of meningitis. The **Brudzinski sign** is positive if the patient's hips and knees flex automatically when the examiner flexes the patient's neck while the patient is supine. Because host responsiveness to the infection varies, these signs of meningeal irritation are not invariably present, especially in debilitated and elderly patients and infants. When the clinical picture is typical of meningitis, it is also very important to exclude the concomitant presence of a focal parameningeal source such as a brain abscess. Further history, careful neurologic examination, and various imaging studies are essential (Figs. 44.3 and 44.4). Frequently, concomitant dermatologic findings may be present. A maculopapular or petechial/purpuric rash usually indicates infection with *N. meningitidis* although an echovirus may mimic this. However, in viral meningitis, the CSF findings are significantly different, usually with predominant lymphocytosis, normal CSF sugar, and negative Gram stain. The dermatologic findings of *N. meningitidis* are usually secondary to an underlying vasculitis, concomitant coagulation defects, or a combination of the two. Meningococcal infection more commonly has a rash that affects the trunk and extremities, in contrast to the

echovirus exanthema, which usually involves the face and neck early in the infection. Purpuric lesions may also rarely be found in a fulminant pneumococcal bacteremia with meningitis as well as staphylococcal endocarditis, the latter primarily involving the finger pads.

Diagnostic Approach

CSF examination is essential to the diagnosis of bacterial and other microbial forms of meningitis. When there are signs of focal neurologic involvement or increased intracranial pressure in patients with suspected meningitis, a lumbar puncture (LP) may be contraindicated. These include papilledema, coma, and focal neurologic findings such as dilated pupils, hemiparesis, and aphasia. Accompanying signs of increased intracranial pressure may include bradycardia, Cheyne-Stoke respirations, and even projectile vomiting. When a patient is immunocompromised or has an altered level of consciousness, new-onset seizures, or focal neurologic deficits, a computed tomography (CT) scan must be obtained prior to LP to exclude brain abscess or a parameningeal focus with significant mass effect.

As soon as the diagnosis of meningitis is considered, even before proceeding with a CT scan and LP, administration of empiric antibiotics

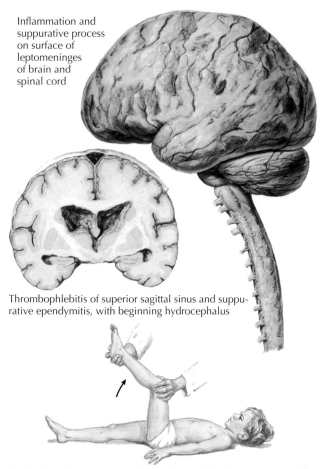

Inflammation and suppurative process on surface of leptomeninges of brain and spinal cord

Thrombophlebitis of superior sagittal sinus and suppurative ependymitis, with beginning hydrocephalus

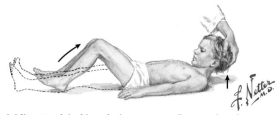

Kernig sign. Patient supine, with hip flexed 90°. Knee cannot be fully extended.

Neck rigidity (Brudzinski neck sign). Passive flexion of neck causes flexion of both legs and thighs.

Fig. 44.2 Bacterial Meningitis–II.

not need to await the results of Gram stain before immediate initiation of appropriate antibiotic therapy. Rapid detection of microbial antigens by immunochromatographic technique or latex agglutination tests can aid diagnosis when CSF Gram stain and cultures are not diagnostic. Newer polymerase chain reaction (PCR) technology has excellent sensitivity and specificity for the diagnosis of bacterial meningitis.

The initial CSF analysis needs to include measurement of the opening pressure, color (clear, turbid, or purulent), WBC count and differential, and levels of glucose and protein. Typically in bacterial meningitis, the CSF opening pressure is increased (>200 mm of water lying down and >35 mm water upright). The fluid is usually turbid or frankly purulent and contains predominantly (>80%) polymorphonuclear leukocytes. The CSF glucose level is very low, usually less than 40% of that found with measurement of concomitant serum glucose. A low glucose level (<40 mg/100 mL) is also found in some other types of microbial meningitides including *L. monocytogenes, Mycobacterium tuberculosis,* and *Cryptococcus neoformans.* Normal glucose levels are common in viral meningitis. Usually, CSF protein levels are increased, often greater than 100 mg/dL (reference range, <45 mg/dL). In patients with parameningeal foci such as a brain or epidural spinal abscess or with multiple septic emboli, CSF glucose may not be as low as with typical bacterial meningitis, even though in these instances, the CSF protein level is significantly increased.

Optimum Treatment

Bacterial meningitis is an extremely severe, life-threatening infection. Any delay in its diagnosis by not initially assessing the patient or not beginning therapy at the first consideration of this critical diagnosis will increase morbidity and mortality. Antibiotic treatment must be initiated as soon as possible and later guided by CSF examination results. When CSF examination cannot be performed promptly, empiric therapy must be instituted immediately. Patients must receive high-dose IV antibiotics that can easily cross the blood-brain barrier. Empiric IV therapy with a third-generation cephalosporin such as ceftriaxone or cefotaxime plus vancomycin must commence pending results of the bacterial cultures. High-dose corticosteroids, administered before antibiotic therapy, are recommended for all children and should be seriously considered for adults with community-acquired meningitis.

When culture and sensitivity data are available, a specific antimicrobial therapy can be determined. Penicillin G is recommended for documented meningococcal meningitis.

Antimicrobial therapy for meningitis caused by *S. pneumoniae* must be based on antibiotic sensitivity test results. If the strain is susceptible to penicillin, penicillin or ceftriaxone is recommended. Ceftriaxone or cefotaxime is recommended when the strain is not susceptible to penicillin and is susceptible to cephalosporins. If the strain is susceptible to neither cephalosporins nor penicillin, vancomycin must be added to a third-generation cephalosporin (cefotaxime or ceftriaxone). In patients older than 50 years of age, pregnant women, immunocompromised hosts, or alcoholics, empiric therapy with ampicillin must be added to vancomycin and a third-generation cephalosporin to provide coverage for *L. monocytogenes.*

Complications

Among patients with bacterial meningitis, approximately 15% experience acute and chronic complications, including various cranial nerve dysfunctions, particularly those affecting extraocular function (cranial nerves [CNs] III, IV, and VI), CN VII, and sometimes CN VIII, although this is less common today, with the antibiotics lacking specific ototoxicity or vestibular toxicity. However, permanent sensorineural hearing loss occurs occasionally, most commonly with pediatric meningococcal infections. Assorted cranial neuropathies are generally secondary to the

covering the broad spectrum of gram-positive and gram-negative organisms is essential. One can later adjust the treatment once CSF culture examination results are available. If CT examination confirms that there is no mass lesion suggestive of a parameningeal focus with potential for herniation, one can then safely proceed with a CSF examination. If a parameningeal mass lesion is identified as a source of the meningitis, its treatment is paramount. The precise identification of the pathogenic bacterium, per se, will then become possible at the time of surgical decompression, and the spinal tap as such will not be required.

CSF analysis provides the only conclusive proof of bacterial infection of the subarachnoid space. It must include a Gram-stained smear to define the causative organism morphology. Gram stain correlates with the precise microbial etiology, as defined by the more specific bacteriologic culture, in approximately 80% of patients. This is a simple technique that allows for better selection of appropriate antibiotic therapy before definitive culture and sensitivity data are available. However, one does

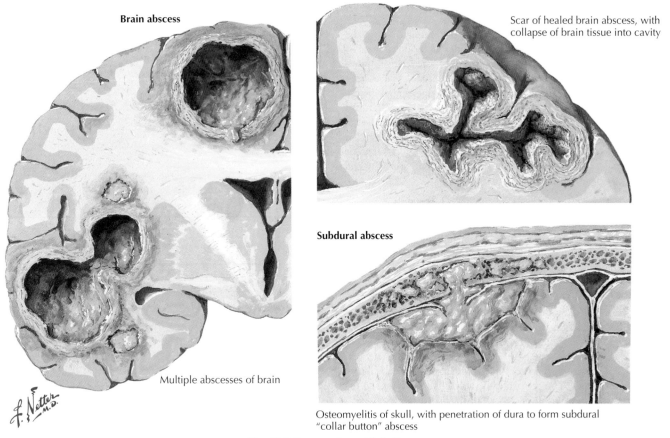

Brain abscess

Multiple abscesses of brain

Scar of healed brain abscess, with collapse of brain tissue into cavity

Subdural abscess

Osteomyelitis of skull, with penetration of dura to form subdural "collar button" abscess

Fig. 44.3 Parameningeal Infections.

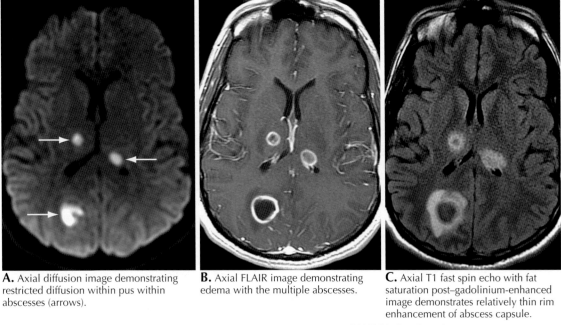

A. Axial diffusion image demonstrating restricted diffusion within pus within abscesses (arrows).

B. Axial FLAIR image demonstrating edema with the multiple abscesses.

C. Axial T1 fast spin echo with fat saturation post–gadolinium-enhanced image demonstrates relatively thin rim enhancement of abscess capsule.

Fig. 44.4 Multiple Brain Abscesses in a 32-Year-Old With Septicemia.

exudate that is common with the more purulent forms of bacterial and tuberculous meningitis.

Focal or generalized seizures, various focal cerebral signs, coma, and acute cerebral edema occasionally occur. Findings mimicking a stroke—such as a hemiparesis, aphasia, and hemianopsia—are relatively infrequent; persistence of such findings suggests secondary cerebral arteritis, cerebral venous thrombosis, or rarely a mass lesion, especially an abscess. Even with astute and early diagnosis, mortality rates are still at least 10% for meningococcal and 30% for pneumococcal meningitis, although the latter has very significantly decreased in frequency with the recent introduction of a pneumococcal immunization. Whenever any diagnostic delay occurs leading to less than immediate treatment, mortality and morbidity are significantly higher.

Chemoprophylaxis

Chemoprophylaxis is particularly recommended for persons in close contact with patients who have acquired meningococcal meningitis, especially in confined settings such as college dormitories and army barracks. Rifampin is preferred; ciprofloxacin is also effective.

Future Directions: Vaccines

Vaccines are available for three common organisms. *H. influenzae* type b protein-polysaccharide vaccine is highly effective in preventing meningitis in newborns and young infants. *N. meningitidis* (meningococcus) serogroups A, C, Y, and W135 polysaccharide vaccine is recommended for high-risk adults and contacts of persons with meningococcal disease. An additional monovalent serogroup B vaccine is recommended for individuals with complement deficiency, functional or acquired asplenia, and those exposed to *N. meningitidis* in an outbreak or laboratory setting. For *S. pneumoniae* (pneumococcus) infection, 13 valent protein conjugate vaccine is recommended for all children. Additionally, protein polysaccharide vaccine is given for those children who are at high risk for acquiring pneumococcal infections. Currently, 23 valent pneumococcal polysaccharide and 13 valent protein conjugate vaccines are recommended for adults based on age and risk.

PARAMENINGEAL INFECTIONS

CLINICAL VIGNETTE *A 76-year-old man presented with sinus headaches and underwent surgical drainage of the frontal sinuses. Postoperatively, he had headaches, seizures, and mild right-sided weakness, diagnosed as a mild cerebrovascular accident (CVA). He was discharged home, where he had some difficulty walking and his speech was "not quite normal." He gradually worsened and, 6 weeks after his surgery, could not hold anything in his right hand and became aphasic. He complained of chills but had no fever. On examination, he was awake and alert but globally aphasic, the cranial nerves were intact, gaze was conjugate, and there was a right hemiparesis. His WBC count was 9700/mm³ with a normal differential. Brain CT demonstrated a hypointense structural lesion with midline shift in the left frontal lobe. Brain magnetic resonance imaging (MRI) demonstrated a multiloculated lesion with marked ring enhancement and surrounding edema extending through the frontal lobe and posteriorly toward the left parietal lobe (see Fig. 44.3). There was 1.5-mm midline shift. The lesion was aspirated using a stereotactic technique; Gram staining revealed many polymorphonuclear leukocytes (PMNs), many gram-positive cocci, and rare gram-negative rods. Culture grew Proteus mirabilis and Bacillus species. He was treated for 4 months with ceftriaxone and metronidazole with full resolution of speech and recovery of ambulation with the assistance of a walker.*

Comment: Although parameningeal infections are relatively uncommon disorders, these lesions must always be considered in the differential diagnosis

of any acute cerebral or spinal lesion (see Fig. 44.3). These processes may not be suspected and thus go unrecognized until it is too late to prevent permanent neurologic deficits. CT and MRI scanning are useful tools to exclude such predisposing lesions. Although these abscesses are easily considered within the setting of an overt infection, a precise microbial source is not always defined by the character of the clinical presentation. It is essential always to consider whether any acute spinal or cerebral lesion possibly has an infectious basis. This is particularly important in the setting of a chronic illness such as diabetes mellitus, which often predisposes individuals to spinal epidural abscesses. The highest diagnostic and therapeutic priority is required in these settings. When they are identified, such processes are among the most urgent neurologic emergencies. These require immediate diagnostic and therapeutic attention. Even when appropriate diagnostic and therapeutic focus occurs, the patient's outcome may still be guarded, as in the preceding vignette.

Brain Abscess

CLINICAL VIGNETTE *A 26-year-old woman had a sudden onset of numbness in her right hand and face. This cleared within a few minutes, only to recur on two more occasions within the next 48 hours. She then suddenly became aphasic, with numbness and weakness of her right hand and face. Neurologic examination demonstrated a fluent aphasia with a right central facial and hand weakness. Her muscle stretch reflexes were enhanced in her right arm, associated with a right Babinski sign. She had a grade III/IV systolic murmur at the apex of her heart. Brain imaging demonstrated a left parietal temporal mass suggestive of a cerebritis or an abscess. Empiric antibiotics were begun. Within 36 hours, blood cultures demonstrated a gram-positive diplococcus. The antibiotics were adjusted appropriately. Within 48 hours, her condition had stabilized. Repeat imaging studies 1 week later showed improvement. Surgical decompression was considered early on; however, the antimicrobial therapy was sufficient. She gradually improved, having an almost complete recovery. Subsequently, when her speech improved, she recalled having had a dental hygiene appointment a few weeks before the onset of her illness. Previously, she had not been aware of having a mitral valve lesion. She was instructed that in the future, she would need antimicrobial therapy prior to any dental or other medically invasive procedure.*

Brain abscess, which may be indolent or fulminant, results from direct extension of a contiguous focus, such as middle ear or sinus infections, congenital heart disease with a right-to-left shunt, or very rarely a pulmonary arteriovenous malformation having similar shunt mechanisms. Hematogenous spread may occur from distant infection sites in the head and neck, heart (infectious endocarditis), lung, or abdomen, or from the direct introduction of bacteria after a penetrating head injury. Brain abscess can occur after surgical procedures, as in the vignette on p. 450. The cardinal symptom of brain abscess is relentless and progressive headache, usually followed by focal neurologic manifestations. Only two-thirds of patients have fever. Papilledema and other signs of increased intracranial pressure may occasionally develop; however, the availability of imaging studies makes it more likely that the abscess will be identified prior to its obtaining significant enough mass to create increased intracranial pressure.

Most cases of brain abscess are polymicrobial. Etiologic agents often include aerobic bacteria such as streptococci, Enterobacteriaceae, and staphylococci. *Streptococcus anginosus* group normally resides in the oral cavity, appendix, and female genital tract and has a proclivity for abscess formation. Anaerobic microorganisms such as *Bacteroides* and *Prevotella* species, are present in up to 40% of cases. Fungi are uncommon but increasingly recognized among immunosuppressed patients.

MRI is most helpful for making the initial diagnosis (see Fig. 44.3). The characteristic appearance is a focal cerebral lesion with a hypodense center and a peripheral uniform ring enhancement subsequent to the injection of contrast material. Sometimes, there is a concomitant area of surrounding edema. In these circumstances, if at all possible, lumbar puncture should be avoided to prevent abscess herniation or rupture into the ventricular system.

Therapeutically, the abscess may be directly aspirated. Empiric medical therapy is started with a third- or fourth-generation cephalosporin or penicillin plus metronidazole, depending on the setting. Surgery may not be necessary if follow-up CT demonstrates decreased abscess size. Brain edema associated with acute brain abscess necessitates the use of corticosteroids and mannitol as well as anticonvulsants to prevent seizures.

Subdural Abscess

This is another form of life-threatening neurologic infection. It is typically characterized by a purulent collection within the potential space between the dura mater and arachnoid membrane (see Fig. 44.3). An active paranasal sinusitis, particularly originating within the frontal sinuses or mastoid air cells, usually precedes extension of the infection into the subdural space. Occasionally, it is directly introduced through operative or traumatic wound sites.

Streptococci usually comprise 50% of cases; *S. aureus*, gram-negative bacteria, and anaerobic bacteria such as microaerophilic streptococci, *Bacteroides* species, and *Clostridium perfringens* are sometimes identified. Occasionally polymicrobial infections occur.

Localized swelling, erythema, headache, or tenderness of the site overlying the primary infection may occur. As the illness progresses, the headache becomes generalized and severe, with high fever, vomiting, and development of nuchal rigidity. Seizures, hemiparesis, visual field defects, and papilledema sometimes occur.

CSF contains 10 to 1000 WBCs; protein level is increased, and glucose level is usually normal, in contrast to bacterial meningitis; this is a particularly important clue if imaging studies have not been obtained previously. CT or MRI demonstrates a low-absorption extracerebral mass. A thin, moderately dense margin may be visualized with the contrast medium (see Fig. 44.3).

Treatment includes a combination of prompt surgical drainage and intensive antimicrobial therapy. The initial antibiotic choice requires intravenous third- or fourth-generation cephalosporin for aerobic bacteria and metronidazole for anaerobic bacteria. Prophylactic use of anticonvulsants and corticosteroids may also be required.

Spinal Epidural Abscess

CLINICAL VIGNETTE *A 52-year-old diabetic man experienced a non-specific upper respiratory tract syndrome thought of as influenza. Within a few days, he developed increasingly severe midthoracic spinal pain. He soon developed rigors, chills, and vomiting. His symptoms rapidly worsened over the subsequent 12 to 24 hours. He then suddenly noted numbness in both legs spreading up to his midback and had trouble climbing stairs; after lying down to regain his strength, he was unable to arise from bed even with his wife's attempted help. He could not urinate. His family called the local emergency ambulance and admitted him in the hospital.*

Neurologic examination demonstrated that he was paraplegic and had a T4 sensory level with marked loss of sensation below his nipple line. The patient required urinary catheterization. Spinal MRI demonstrated an epidural abscess extending between T4 and T10. Although an immediate neurosurgical decompression was carried out, the patient had only partial resolution of his neurologic deficit.

Patients with epidural spinal abscess typically present with fever and relatively severe back pain, sometimes with varying degrees of leg weakness. There are four clinical stages: (1) focal vertebral pain; (2) radicular pain corresponding to the dermatomal course of the specific involved nerve roots; (3) early signs of spinal cord compression, such as paresthesias, weakness, or delayed ability to urinate; and (4) paralysis below the lesion level.

A purulent or granulomatous collection within the spinal epidural space may overlie or encircle the spinal cord, nerve roots, and nerves (Fig. 44.5). Although the infection is usually localized within three to four vertebral segments, it rarely extends the length of the spinal canal.

S. aureus is the most common organism leading to a spinal epidural abscess, but aerobic or anaerobic streptococci and gram-negative organisms are occasionally isolated. Mixed anaerobic and aerobic organisms are sometimes responsible. When no organism is isolated or if granulomas are identified, *M. tuberculosis* infection of the spine—for example, Pott disease—also requires consideration. A skin infection, especially

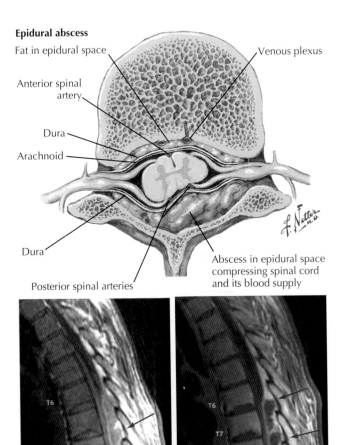

Epidural abscess

Fat in epidural space

Venous plexus

Anterior spinal artery

Dura

Arachnoid

Dura

Posterior spinal arteries

Abscess in epidural space compressing spinal cord and its blood supply

Epidural abscess. Sagittal T1-weighted images without (**A.**) and with (**B**) gadolinium enhancement demonstrate an extensive posterior epidural process from T6 to T11. Enhancement of the granulation tissue allows appreciation of nonenhancing focal pus collections.

Fig. 44.5 Spinal Epidural Abscess.

a furuncle, is the most common focus for a hematogenous spread to the epidural space. An antecedent vertebral osteomyelitis with a prior hematogenous source is responsible for approximately 40% of spinal epidural abscess. Dental and upper respiratory tract infections are other common predisposing factors.

Any patient presenting with back pain, fever, and localized tenderness or signs of cord compression requires immediate and complete spinal MRI. Surgical or CT-guided needle aspiration is necessary to define an accurate diagnosis and possible decompression. Blood cultures are recommended. Lumbar puncture should *not* be performed. Appropriate parenteral antibiotics are necessary for 3 to 4 weeks in uncomplicated cases and for up to 8 weeks or more if vertebral osteomyelitis is present.

SPECIFIC PATHOGENS

Lyme Disease *(Borrelia Burgdorferi)*

> **CLINICAL VIGNETTE** *A 39-year-old woman presented with complaints of fatigue progressing over a month, followed by aching in her back behind her right shoulder for 2 weeks. She developed severe headache with photophobia and nausea over the week before admission. On questioning, she remembered a bug bite followed by a 10-cm rash at about the time her fatigue began. She then developed upper back and neck stiffness, for which she sought chiropractic treatment. She was afebrile on examination, with no neck stiffness or neurologic deficits. A 10-cm oval area of erythema was noted near her left axilla. WBCs and metabolic profile were normal. CSF examination showed 129 WBCs (89% lymphocytes, 3% neutrophils) and 363 RBCs, glucose 48, and protein 54. CT scan of the brain was unremarkable. Serum Lyme enzyme-linked immunosorbent assay (ELISA) and confirmatory Western blot testing were positive. Lyme IgM was positive in the patient's CSF and Lyme PCR was negative. She was treated for 1 month with ceftriaxone 2 g IV daily, with complete resolution of symptoms.*
>
> *Comment: Lyme disease, which is caused by the tick-borne spirochete Borrelia burgdorferi, is endemic in parts of the United States, particularly the northeastern Atlantic coastal areas from Maine to Maryland, the upper Midwest, including Minnesota and Wisconsin, as well as the northern Pacific, including California and Oregon. Currently about 300 million cases per year are estimated to occur in the United States. The disease is also endemic in Europe and Asia in forested areas.*

Clinical Presentation

In 80% of patients in the United States, Lyme disease presents with a slowly expanding skin lesion called erythema migrans that occurs at the site of the tick bite (Fig. 44.6). Influenza-like symptoms—such as malaise, fatigue, fever, headache, arthralgias, myalgias, and regional lymphadenopathy—frequently accompany the rash and are often the presenting manifestation of Lyme disease. Early localized infection is followed within days to weeks by a systemic dissemination that variously affects the nervous system, heart, or joints. Untreated, late, or persistent Lyme infection ensues.

In the United States, 15% of untreated neuroborreliosis patients develop objective signs and symptoms of early disseminated infection. A variety of neurologic manifestations develop, including lymphocytic meningitis with episodic headache and mild neck stiffness, a subtle encephalitis with impaired memory, a cranial neuropathy (most commonly unilateral or bilateral facial palsy, sometimes an optic neuropathy), cerebellar ataxia, myelitis, motor or sensory radiculoneuritis, or a mononeuritis multiplex.

Untreated, acute neurologic abnormalities usually improve or resolve within weeks or months. However, 5% of untreated patients may develop a chronic neuroborreliosis with subtle cognitive changes. This is termed Lyme encephalopathy. Although the CSF in these patients shows no inflammatory changes, intrathecal antibody production against *B. burgdorferi* is often demonstrated. Sometimes, a chronic axonal polyradiculoneuropathy, presenting as spinal radicular pain or distal paresthesias, may develop. Diffuse involvement of proximal and distal nerve segments is found on electromyography (EMG).

Diagnosis

Culture of *B. burgdorferi* from specimens in Barboud-Stoenner-Kelly medium allows definitive microbiologic diagnosis but is possible only early in the illness and usually only from biopsies of erythema migrans lesions. In late infection, PCR detection of *B. burgdorferi* is superior to culture from joint fluid. In the United States, diagnosis of Lyme disease is usually made on the basis of characteristic clinical findings, history of exposure in an endemic area, and antibody response to *B. burgdorferi* by ELISA and Western blotting test interpreted according to Centers for Disease Control and Prevention (CDC) criteria. Serology is insensitive during the first weeks of infection (only 20%–30% positive and usually IgM alone), but by 4 weeks 70% to 80% are seropositive (generally IgM and IgG) even after antibiotic treatment. A positive IgM test alone after 1 month of illness is likely to represent a false-positive result. Patients with acute neuroborreliosis, especially meningitis, often demonstrate intrathecal production of IgM, IgG, or IgA antibody against *B. burgdorferi*.

MRI may demonstrate meningitic findings (Fig. 44.7AB) as well as cranial nerve involvement. Intraparenchymal white matter changes in the corpus callosum as well as centrum semiovale mimicking multiple sclerosis may be seen. Active enhancement is a good marker of active disease (see Fig. 44.7C–F).

Treatment

Evidence-based recommendations for Lyme disease have been developed by the Infectious Diseases Society of America. Early or localized disseminated infection can be successfully treated with 1 to 21 days of oral doxycycline. Children and pregnant women may be treated with amoxicillin. An advantage of doxycycline is its efficacy against *Anaplasma phagocytophilum*, a possible coinfecting pathogen that causes human granulocytic ehrlichiosis. Cefuroxime axetil is a third alternative in those allergic to the first options. Patients with objective neurologic abnormalities can be treated with 14 to 28 days of intravenous ceftriaxone (cefotaxime and penicillin G are possible alternatives). Manifestations of acute neuroborreliosis usually resolve within weeks, but chronic neuroborreliosis generally resolves over a period of months. Objective evidence of relapse is rare after 4 weeks of therapy.

Tuberculosis: Brain and Spine *(Mycobacterium Tuberculosis)*

> **CLINICAL VIGNETTE** *While visiting the United States, a 51-year-old Vietnamese woman presented with a history of 7 days of headache, vomiting, and episodic left facial and arm tingling and numbness. She reported diplopia, having fallen twice and fractured her nose. Some seizurelike activity was witnessed. The patient's temperature was mildly elevated. On neurologic examination, she was confused and only intermittently fluent. She had bilateral sixth cranial nerve palsies and early papilledema. Her neck was stiff and her lungs were clear.*
>
> *A lumbar puncture revealed a CSF opening pressure of 500 mm, protein of 218 mg/dL, glucose of 22 mg/dL (serum glucose level 137 mg/dL), an RBC count of 190/mm³, and a WBC count of 1390/mm³ (4% polymorphonuclear leukocytes, 94% lymphocytes). CSF acid-fast bacilli smear and PCR results were negative. Cranial CT and MRI results were normal. The patient was treated with isoniazid, rifampin, ethambutol, pyrazinamide, and methylprednisolone (Solu-Medrol). The CSF culture ultimately grew M. tuberculosis.*

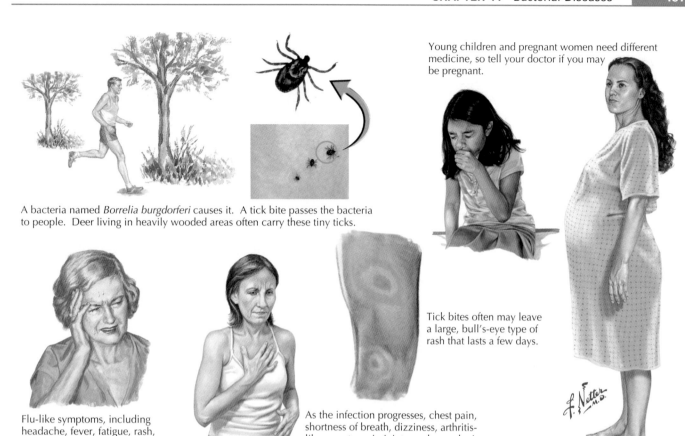

A bacteria named *Borrelia burgdorferi* causes it. A tick bite passes the bacteria to people. Deer living in heavily wooded areas often carry these tiny ticks.

Young children and pregnant women need different medicine, so tell your doctor if you may be pregnant.

Tick bites often may leave a large, bull's-eye type of rash that lasts a few days.

Flu-like symptoms, including headache, fever, fatigue, rash, and joint pain, are usually the first symptoms.

As the infection progresses, chest pain, shortness of breath, dizziness, arthritis-like symptoms in joints, and neurologic problems may occur.

Fig. 44.6 Lyme Disease—Clinical Settings.

The incidence of central nervous system (CNS) tuberculosis in the United States has markedly decreased; it most commonly occurs in foreign-born adults and those infected with HIV. Neurologically, it presents as a meningitis, mass lesion, or vertebral lesion. Because tuberculosis is still endemic in Southeast Asia, it must be considered in the differential diagnosis of patients immigrating from this area who present with a meningoencephalopathy, especially with cranial neuropathies; the vignette in this chapter is classic. It is important to make a clinical diagnosis and begin treatment while awaiting CSF culture results.

Tuberculous Meningitis

Tuberculous meningitis usually results from hematogenous meningeal seeding or contiguous spread from a tuberculoma or parameningeal granuloma, with subsequent rupture into the subarachnoid space (Fig. 44.8). Local foci of infection along the meninges, brain, or spinal cord, thought to be present from hematogenous seeding of the primary infection, also release bacilli directly into the subarachnoid space. Infection then spreads along the perivascular spaces into the brain. An intense inflammatory reaction at the brain base causes an occlusive arteritis, with small vessel thrombosis and resultant brain infarction. Direct cranial nerve compression and obstruction of CSF flow at the foramina of the fourth ventricle or the basal cisterns may result in subarachnoid block and cerebral edema.

Tuberculous meningitis progresses rapidly, with headache, fever, meningismus, and cranial nerve deficits, especially sixth nerve palsy. Focal cerebral or cerebellar deficits are followed by altered sensorium and coma.

CSF examination is critical in establishing the diagnosis. Classically, the CSF glucose level is less than two-thirds that of the serum glucose level; the CSF protein level is greater than 50 mg/dL; and the WBC count is increased, with lymphocyte predominance. PCR analysis and culture are the most sensitive diagnostic tools. PCR can detect fewer than 10 organisms in clinical specimens, compared with 10,000 necessary for smear positivity. False-negative PCR results have been reported (sensitivity in acid-fast smear-negative cases varies from 40% to 77%). Unfortunately, acid-fast (Ziehl-Neelsen) smears are positive only 25% of the time, and more commonly with concentrated CSF specimens.

It is imperative to initiate therapy at the slightest suspicion of CNS tuberculosis, as death may follow within a matter of weeks if this is left untreated. Isoniazid, rifampin, ethambutol, and pyrazinamide are the medications of choice until diagnostic identification and sensitivity testing are available. Both isoniazid and pyrazinamide achieve CSF concentrations equaling those in blood, and rifampin crosses the blood-brain barrier adequately. Corticosteroids are added when cerebral edema, subarachnoid block, or both occur. Mortality is greatest at the extremes of age (20% at <5 years and 60% at >50 years) or if the illness has been present for more than 2 months (80%).

Cerebral Tuberculomas

Cerebral tuberculomas are less common than tuberculous meningitis. These are often calcified and are usually located in the posterior fossa, particularly the cerebellum. Although most frequently multiple, tuberculomas can be single. Contrast-enhanced MRI is generally considered the modality of choice in detecting and assessing CNS tuberculosis (see Fig. 44.8). PCR and CSF culture or culture of biopsied lesional material confirms the diagnosis. Because standard medical therapy is usually successful, especially if multidrug resistance is not identified, antituberculous therapy must be attempted before surgery is contemplated.

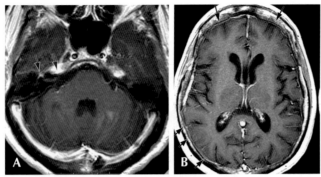

A and **B** Lyme meningitis with facial nerve involvement. (A) Axial T1-weighted fast spin echo following gadolinium enhancement demonstrates enhancement of right nerves VII and VIII complex (arrowheads). (B) Axial T1- weighted fast spin echo following gadolinium shows diffuse meningeal enhancement (arrows).

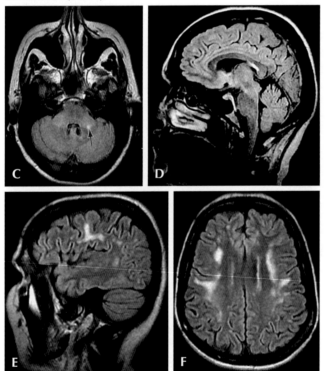

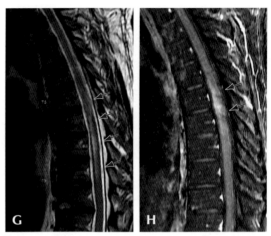

G and **H** Lyme myelitis. Varied manifestations of CNS Lyme disease. (G) Sagittal T2 weighted fast spin echo imaging of thoracic cord demonstrates patchy long segment ill-defined increased signal within a slightly expanded spinal cord (arrows). (H) Sagittal T1-weighted fast spin echo imaging with gadolinium enhancement shows patchy enhancement of portions of this abnormal cord (arrows).

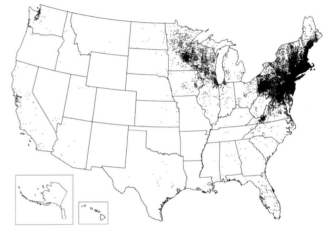

I Reported cases of Lyme Disease—United States, 2015. Each dot represents one case of Lyme disease and is placed randomly in the patient's county of residence. The presence of a dot in a state does not necessarily mean that Lyme disease was acquired in that state. People travel between states, and the place of residence is sometimes different from the place where the patient became infected

C–F Lyme CNS disease. Note primary demyelinating pattern as evidenced by the intraparenchymal brain lesions. Multiple FLAIR images demonstrate multiple regions of involvement, including left cerebellar peduncle (C), splenium of corpus callosum and posterior subfrontal region (D), and central white matter and subcortical involvement (E and F).

Fig. 44.7 **Lyme Disease.** Map of reported cases of Lyme Disease from https://www.cdc.gov/lyme/resources/reportedcasesoflymedisease_2016.pdf (Accessed April 2018).

Of course if there are signs of impending herniation, immediate surgery is indicated.

Vertebral Tuberculosis (Pott Disease)

> **CLINICAL VIGNETTE** *A 30-year-old man who emigrated from India to the United States 2 years previously to take a job with a software company presented with complaints of back pain, fever, and leg numbness. His examination was normal. Tuberculin skin testing elicited an 18-mm reaction. Chest radiograph demonstrated an infiltrate in the posterior apical segment of the right upper lobe. CT scan revealed a paraspinal abscess at the L5 level. Both the sputum and an aspirate of the abscess grew M. tuberculosis.*

Skeletal joints most subject to trauma are primarily affected. The spine—typically the disc space and adjacent vertebral bodies, the epidural space, or both—is involved in approximately 50% of tuberculosis cases. Back pain and fever are often followed by progressive spinal cord compression from unrecognized epidural infection or fracture, collapse, or angulation of vertebral segments.

Standard spinal radiographs reveal disc space infection with spread to adjacent vertebrae (see Fig. 44.8). MRI and/or CT myelography are the diagnostic procedures of choice. Bone biopsy or disc space aspiration is required for culture diagnosis before therapy.

A 9- to 12-month regimen of combination antituberculous medication is appropriate. Prolongation of therapy is indicated for tuberculosis in sites that are slow to respond.

TB with involvement of basal cisterns with vasculitis and ischemia

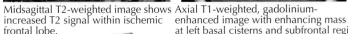

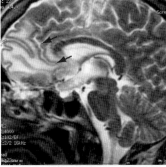

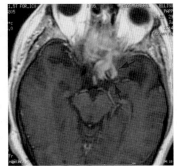

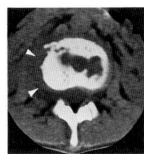

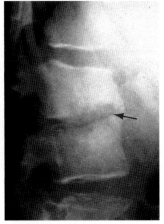

Midsagittal T2-weighted image shows increased T2 signal within ischemic frontal lobe.

Axial T1-weighted, gadolinium-enhanced image with enhancing mass at left basal cisterns and subfrontal region.

CT scan: paraspinous abscess in addition to bony destruction

X-ray film: destruction of disc space (arrow) and adjacent end plates of vertebrae

Tuberculous basilar meningitis

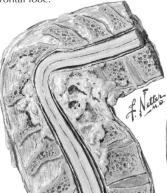

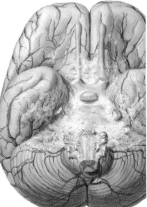

Tuberculosis of spine (Pott disease) with marked kyphosis

Tuberculoma. Axial T1-weighted fast spin echo post–gadolinium enhanced image demonstrates a rim enhancing inferior right cerebellar mass (arrow).

Fig. 44.8 Tuberculosis.

Hansen Disease (Leprosy—*Mycobacterium Leprae*)

> **CLINICAL VIGNETTE** *A 56-year-old woman from India was evaluated because she had been tripping on her left foot for 6 months. For the previous month, she noticed difficulty gripping objects with her right hand and had associated elbow and median forearm pain.*
>
> *Neurologic examination demonstrated weakness of finger abduction and adduction, mild clawing of the fourth and fifth digits, and sensory loss of the medial one and half fingers, consistent with a right ulnar neuropathy affecting ulnar-innervated structures in her right hand. Examination of the left leg revealed focal weakness of foot dorsiflexion and eversion with sensory loss on the lateral aspect of the left calf and the dorsum of the foot, indicating a left common peroneal neuropathy. Both ulnar and peroneal nerves were thickened and palpable. Two subtle hypopigmented anesthetic macules were found on her upper arm and trunk. Sensation was diminished on the ear pinna and tip of the nose.*
>
> *EMG confirmed moderately severe right ulnar and left peroneal axonal neuropathies. Skin biopsy revealed noncaseating granulomas with lymphocytic infiltration and giant cells; very rare acid-fast bacilli were seen on the modified Fite-Faraco stain. The diagnosis was tuberculoid (TT) leprosy; dapsone and rifampin were administered.*

Hansen disease is a chronic infectious granulomatous disease of the skin and peripheral nerves. The reader should understand that although leprosy has been the name of this disorder for many years, its use has led to unfortunate discrimination. Therefore Hansen disease, in recognition of the scientist who discovered the responsible mycobacterium,

is now the preferred nomenclature. However, these names are still interchangeably used in some circles.

Worldwide, Hansen disease is one of the most common infectious causes of neuropathy. Any patient from an area endemic for this disorder who has multiple mononeuropathies, particularly ulnar and peroneal, and has skin lesions, especially in superficial sensory areas that have cooler ambient temperatures, is most likely to have this disorder. The etiologic agent is *Mycobacterium leprae,* an acid-fast bacillus identified by Hansen in 1873. Today this disease occurs primarily in Asia, Africa, and Latin America. Since the World Health Organization (WHO) redefined Hansen disease as involving only cases under active treatment and the elimination of active case detection, the global registry of new cases has steadily declined since 2001, with 216,108 new cases registered globally in 2016. This represents a slight increase from the 211,973 new cases reported globally in 2015 (2.9 new cases per 100,000 people). Active case detection is now relegated to the primary care physician. However, these bureaucratic finesses create a false sense of security. Thus, we feel that the actual numbers of patients with Hansen disease is probably underestimated.

The existence of zoonotic infection with *M. leprae,* and possibly *M. lepromatosis* (see below), appears to constitute a major challenge to the WHO's paradigm for leprosy elimination, which is based entirely on the interruption of human-human transmission and does not address any kind of zoonotic transmission.

Bacteriology

The leprosy bacillus's genome demonstrates reductive evolution with extensive deletion and inactivation of genes and abundant pseudogenes; <50% of the genome contains functional genes. This may explain the unusually long generation time and the inability to culture *M. leprae* in artificial media. *M. lepromatosis*, a newly recognized species, is similar microbiologically and causes a disease that is clinically similar to that caused by *M. leprae.*

Hansen disease is transmitted by respiratory droplets and direct skin contact during frequent, close exposure to untreated patients. Other routes of infection include contact with armadillos (a reservoir in Texas and Louisiana), infected soil, and, rarely, direct dermal implantation during procedures such as tattooing. *M. lepromatosis* has also been reported in red squirrels in Scotland, suggesting the possibility that in addition to the well-documented *M. leprae* zoonosis in armadillos, there may be other natural reservoirs of organisms causing Hansen disease. The incubation period is usually 5 to 7 years. *M. leprae*/laminin-α_2 complexes bind to alpha/beta dystroglycan complexes expressed on Schwann cells and induce rapid demyelination by a contact-dependent mechanism. Myelinated Schwann cells are resistant to *M. leprae* invasion but undergo demyelination on bacterial attachment; Schwann cells proliferate and generate a nonmyelinated phenotype, whereas *M. leprae*

multiply intracellularly in large numbers. The clinical development of leprosy depends on host immune responses and genetic factors. The disease spectrum varies widely from limited TT forms (where few bacilli can be demonstrated) to an extensive lepromatous (LL) form (where more than 10 million organisms per high power field can be seen on skin biopsies).

Clinical Presentation and Diagnosis

The three cardinal diagnostic criteria are anesthetic skin patches, thickened nerves, and acid-fast bacilli in skin smears (Fig. 44.9). The WHO recommends classification based on clinical criteria: *paucibacillary* if less than five skin lesions and/or one nerve is involved or *multibacillary* if there are five or more skin lesions, more than two nerves involved, or both. This system determines the type and duration of therapy for patients evaluated in the field where laboratory help is not available. The commonly used classification is based on the disease's clinical spectrum, extending from TT to borderline tuberculoid (BT), borderline (BB), borderline lepromatous (BL), and LL. Indeterminate leprosy, seen

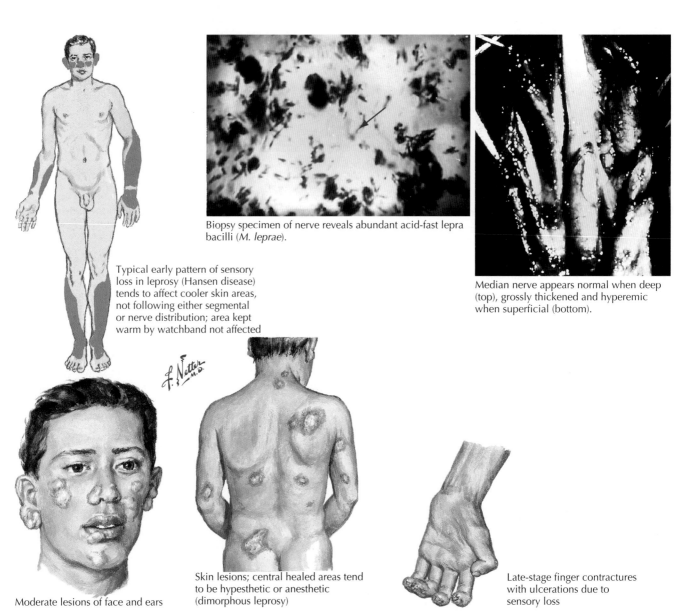

Biopsy specimen of nerve reveals abundant acid-fast lepra bacilli (*M. leprae*).

Typical early pattern of sensory loss in leprosy (Hansen disease) tends to affect cooler skin areas, not following either segmental or nerve distribution; area kept warm by watchband not affected

Median nerve appears normal when deep (top), grossly thickened and hyperemic when superficial (bottom).

Moderate lesions of face and ears

Skin lesions; central healed areas tend to be hypesthetic or anesthetic (dimorphous leprosy)

Late-stage finger contractures with ulcerations due to sensory loss

Fig. 44.9 Leprosy.

early in the infection, is diagnosed by the presence of a single or a few skin macules having variable sensory loss. A less common form of leprosy, known as primary neuritic leprosy, presents initially with a neuropathy of one or several large nerve trunks without the initial presence of skin lesions. This is more common in patients from India. If left untreated, the patient will develop skin lesions several years later.

In tuberculoid (TT and BT) Hansen disease, preserved cell-mediated immunity prevents significant dissemination of the bacillus, thus precluding more severe disease. Patients usually have asymmetrically distributed hypopigmented anesthetic lesions with erythematous margins and an associated asymmetric multifocal neuropathy (mononeuritis multiplex). Involved nerves are concomitantly enlarged, particularly the ulnar, posterior auricular, peroneal, and posterior tibial nerves. Skin or nerve biopsies demonstrate well-demarcated, noncaseating granulomas with many lymphocytes and Langerhans giant cells. Acid-fast bacilli are infrequently seen, especially in TT leprosy. Nerve biopsies are rarely needed to make this diagnosis.

BB leprosy stands between LL and TT leprosy in severity and disease manifestation. If treatment is delayed, patients with BB disease may progress toward more LL forms of disease.

Lepromatous Hansen disease (LL and BL) is the most severe form, with unrestricted bacterial multiplication and hematogenous dissemination. The organisms have a predilection for multiplying in cooler body areas such as the superficial nerves, nose, earlobes, skin, testes, and eyes. Nerve involvement is symmetric and more extensive than in TT leprosy but more frequently involves the superficial cutaneous nerves. Large nerves are less frequently affected than in TT leprosy. Cutaneous lesions are skin-colored nodules or papules that coalesce to form extensive symmetric raised plaques or more diffuse infiltration of the skin. On the face, they result in leonine facies. Skin biopsies demonstrate vacuolated foam cells within the dermis containing large numbers of *M. leprae* organisms with few inflammatory cells and rare granulomas.

The ulnar nerve is the most commonly affected peripheral nerve; when this condition is associated with median nerve involvement, the combination leads to clawing of the hand. Peroneal neuropathies are most common in the leg. At its extreme, patients with leprotic neuropathies develop autoamputation of digits, recurrent nonhealing ulcers that often result in osteomyelitis, and nasal bridge collapse.

Erythema Nodosum Leprosum and Reversal Reactions

Leprosy can be complicated by different reactional states, namely, erythema nodosum leprosum (ENL) and reversal reactions. ENL is thought to be an immune complex–mediated process and is characterized by the development of crops of new, small, tender subcutaneous nodules accompanied by fever, arthralgias or arthritis, adenopathy, and neuritis. Reversal reactions present as inflamed indurated skin plaques with neuritis and represent an upgrading of the cell-mediated response in the patient's immunity to the infection. Both ENL and reversal reactions can occur before, during, and after the completion of antimycobacterial treatment for leprosy. Tumor necrosis factor-alpha and other proinflammatory and antiinflammatory cytokines are considered key mediators in these reactional states.

Contrary to some initial reports, *M. lepromatosis* does not appear to be more pathogenic than its close relative, *M. leprae*. On the basis of limited reports about the treatment and follow-up of a small number of patients with this infection in the United States, Canada, and Mexico, it appears that infection with *M. lepromatosis* manifests clinically and histologically with a wide spectrum of lesions such as those described in leprosy. Similarly, the bacterial load in different patients ranges from low to high. Both infections respond to the same treatment and have the same prognosis—that is, some patients develop reactions and others do not.

Diagnostic Approach and Treatment

Other disorders that may present with similar skin lesions include sarcoidosis, leishmaniasis, lupus vulgaris, syphilis, yaws, and granuloma annulare. However, no other disease has hypopigmented anesthetic skin lesions associated with neuropathies. The diagnosis of Hansen disease depends on clinical findings and skin biopsy, a much less invasive procedure than nerve biopsy. Skin smears for Fite stains are infrequently done in developed countries. Nerve biopsies may often be needed to diagnose primary neuritic leprosy, especially when it presents outside of an endemic area.

Multidrug treatment (MDT) with the antibiotic combination of rifampin, dapsone, and clofazimine is highly effective for multibacillary disease. Clofazimine is omitted for paucibacillary leprosy. The risk of recurrence is increased with higher bacterial loads and may not be seen until 5 to 10 years after the completion of treatment. Severe neural damage is the major complication of reactional states and responds to oral prednisone. Thalidomide, the preferred medication for severe ENL, has significant teratogenic potential. Additionally, thalidomide usage can be complicated by a dose-dependent sensory polyneuropathy; electrophysiologic studies have shown that monitoring sural sensory amplitude may help in the early diagnosis of an emerging sensory neuropathy. Other treatments tried for peripheral neuropathies in other diseases have not been used much in leprotic neuropathies primarily due to the cost of the drugs. Management also includes injury prevention to anesthetic areas, hygiene maintenance, and reconstructive plastic surgery such as nasal reconstruction.

Future Directions

MDT has resulted in a 95% reduction in disease prevalence. The global Hansen disease elimination campaigns of early disease detection, prevention of deformity, and completion of predefined treatment regimens are now replaced by the integration of detection and treatment of cases into the less than adequate primary care framework of endemic countries.

The WHO definition of a case of leprosy includes only any patient who is on active MDT and therefore excludes the treatment of type 1 and 11 reactions (which may occur for up to 10 years after effective MDT) with the ensuing deforming neuropathies. Although specific preventive vaccines are not available, bacille Calmette-Guérin (BCG) is variably effective. The successful mapping of the genome for the *M. leprae* bacterium and a better understanding of disease pathogenesis have resulted in more effective detection of resistant strains and promise more effective differentiation between recurrence and resistance of disease caused by an organism that is not easily cultivable.

The main drawback in treating this eminently curable disease is the limited resource availability in countries where Hansen disease is endemic. Although the decrease in prevalence rates due to MDT is admirable, this has also led to decreased funding of leprosy research and treatment programs. Greater provision of funds and medical expertise by the international community would help to overcome this issue.

Tetanus *(Clostridium Tetani)*

Tetanus is caused by a potent neurotoxin, tetanospasmin, released by a gram-positive spore-forming obligate anaerobe, *Clostridium tetani*, which is typically found in occasional wound infections. This bacterial infection can be introduced at any site; contaminated wounds or retained foreign bodies are particularly dangerous. Although common in developing countries, tetanus occurs very uncommonly in North America and mostly after the age of 60 years. Rarely, patients contract tetanus despite adequate immunization.

Tetanus results from the release of tetanospasmin into the bloodstream from a focus of infection by *C. tetani;* subsequently, it binds to the neuromuscular junction and then attaches to peripheral motor neuron nerve endings. It travels centrally up the nerve, in retrograde fashion (antidromically), to the anterior horn cells, where it enters adjacent spinal inhibitory interneurons, exerting its primary pathophysiologic effect by blocking inhibitory neurotransmitter release to the anterior horn cell. This leads to the classic muscular hypertonia and muscle spasms as agonist and antagonist muscles simultaneously contract because reciprocal inhibition is blocked (Fig. 44.10).

Clinical Presentation

Generalized tetanus varies from mild to severe, depending on the incubation period, which is usually 2 to 14 days. It is occasionally delayed by weeks to months after the injury. A more severe clinical picture occurs when the incubation period is less than 8 days and the onset period is less than 48 hours.

In patients with partial or complete immunization, tetanus sometimes occurs in a mild form. It is often more severe in nonimmunized patients. Muscles close to the infection site are more severely affected initially. Typically trismus (lockjaw) and risus sardonicus (a spasmodic tetanic involuntary smile) are early and constant signs.

Subsequently, shocklike painful spasms of all muscles are provoked by the slightest disturbance, including sight, sound, or touch, or they may occur spontaneously. Between the intermittent severe spasms, continuous muscle rigidity is often characterized by the clenched jaw, risus sardonicus, and a stiff back, neck, abdominal wall, and limbs,

sometimes associated with laryngeal and respiratory muscle spasms that may cause airway obstruction.

Tetanus patients are fully conscious because this toxin does not affect cortical function or sensory nerves. They experience severe pain with every muscle contraction. The spasms become progressively severe in the first week after onset, gradually improving over 1 to 4 weeks. Sympathetic overactivity may occur with tachycardia, labile hypertension, and arrhythmias.

Focal tetanus is an unusual manifestation and is limited to muscles at the wound site. It is thought to occur when circulating antitoxin neutralizes the toxin, preventing systemic circulation of the toxin. However, this does not prevent the spread of the tetanus toxin regionally. Painful muscle spasms adjacent to the wound site may last a few weeks. Sometimes, focal tetanus proceeds to generalized tetanus. If generalization does not occur, there is eventually good recovery.

Diagnosis

Abdominal rigidity, generalized spasms, trismus, and risus sardonicus are highly characteristic clinical signs of tetanus. They may be mistaken for encephalitis, encephalomyelitis, meningitis, intracranial hemorrhage, or even stiff man syndrome. Normal CSF parameters and absence of an altered level of consciousness differentiate tetanus from primary CNS infections. Certain local conditions, including dental and peritonsillar abscesses, may also mimic tetanus. Hypocalcemic tetany is usually distinguished by carpopedal spasms and a positive Chvostek sign. Phenothiazine toxicity sometimes results in dystonia and opisthotonus mimicking tetanus; a prompt response to IV diphenhydramine

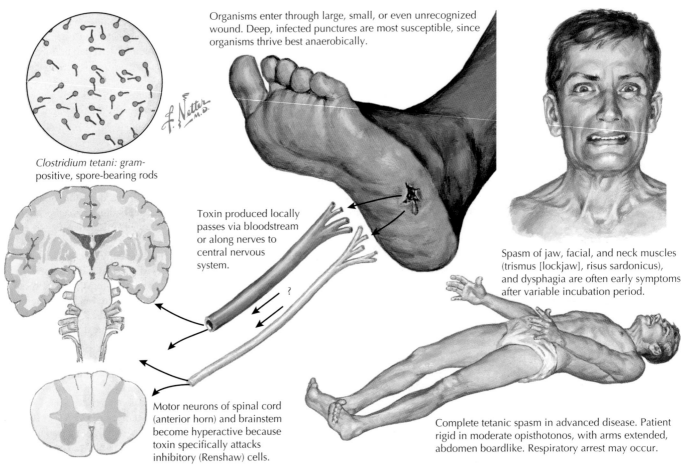

Organisms enter through large, small, or even unrecognized wound. Deep, infected punctures are most susceptible, since organisms thrive best anaerobically.

Clostridium tetani: gram-positive, spore-bearing rods

Toxin produced locally passes via bloodstream or along nerves to central nervous system.

Motor neurons of spinal cord (anterior horn) and brainstem become hyperactive because toxin specifically attacks inhibitory (Renshaw) cells.

Spasm of jaw, facial, and neck muscles (trismus [lockjaw], risus sardonicus), and dysphagia are often early symptoms after variable incubation period.

Complete tetanic spasm in advanced disease. Patient rigid in moderate opisthotonos, with arms extended, abdomen boardlike. Respiratory arrest may occur.

Fig. 44.10 Tetanus.

helps to distinguish this medication-induced partial mimic of tetanus. Epileptic seizures and drug withdrawal reactions also occur in the differential diagnosis.

Fortunately, tetanus has a characteristic clinical picture because *C. tetani* organisms are isolated from the wound in only one-third of affected patients. There are no specific confirmatory blood studies or CSF analyses for tetanus. Sometimes, EMG supports the diagnosis.

Treatment and Prognosis

Tetanus is entirely preventable with immunization. Treatment modalities include appropriate antibiotics and tetanus immunoglobulin, local wound care, control of spasms with muscle relaxants such as benzodiazepines and magnesium sulfate, anticonvulsants, ventilatory support, meticulous nursing care, and maintenance of adequate nutrition and hydration.

The incubation period and time to onset are important predictors of prognosis. If the incubation period is less than 8 days, the onset period is less than 48 hours, and reflex spasms have been present during more than 12 to 24 hours, the prognosis is generally poor. With multimodality treatment, mortality from tetanus may be substantially reduced in the coming years throughout the world.

Neurosyphilis *(Treponema Pallidum)*

> **CLINICAL VIGNETTE** *A 27-year-old man was brought to the hospital by his friends, who reported that he had been "acting strange" before complaining of headache, nausea, and vomiting. He was afebrile and his neurologic examination revealed anisocoria, palsies of the right seventh and eighth cranial nerves, and a Romberg sign. CSF examination revealed 10^5 WBCs (96% lymphocytes), protein 87, glucose 49. CSF VDRL (Venereal Disease Research Laboratory) was positive, as was serum rapid plasma reagin (RPR). HIV testing was negative. He was treated for 14 days with penicillin G 4 million units IV every 4 hours, with complete resolution of his symptoms.*

Syphilis, or lues, is an uncommon disorder occurring primarily within the immunocompromised population, particularly in those with AIDS. *Treponema pallidum*, a spiral bacterium that is difficult to culture in the laboratory, causes syphilis. The diagnosis is made by spirochete identification in material from primary lesions using dark-field microscopy or serologic methods. CNS syphilis occurs in less than 20% of patients with primary infection. Typically, in many patients with neurosyphilis, the diagnosis is made by clinical signs, particularly the disparate pupillary responses to light and accommodation, along with often subtle findings of posterior spinal cord column and dorsal root ganglion involvement.

If the infection remains untreated, *T. pallidum* causes chronic inflammation of CNS cellular and interstitial tissues, culminating in a granulomatous process that produces endarteritis and gummatous lesions. In the United States, syphilis occurs primarily in persons aged 20 to 39 years. Reported rates in men are one and a half times greater than those in women.

Cases of primary and secondary syphilis in the United States increased by 2% between 2000 and 2001 and by 12% between 2001 and 2002. Increase was observed only in men; several outbreaks, associated with high rates of HIV coinfection and high-risk sexual behavior, were seen among men who had sex with men. From 2005 to 2014, the overall number of reported primary and secondary syphilis cases increased further, from 8724 to 19,999. In 2015, a total of 23,872 cases of primary and secondary syphilis were reported, and the national rate increased by 19% to 7.5 cases per 100,000 population, which is the highest rate reported since 1994. Poverty, inadequate health care access, and lack of education are associated with the disproportionately high incidence of syphilis in certain populations.

Clinical Presentation

There are five classic neurologic presentations: meningitis, meningovascular syphilis, tabes dorsalis, general paresis, and gumma.

Syphilitic meningitis develops early on after primary infection, usually coinciding with the secondary-stage syphilis rash. Common symptoms are nocturnal headache, malaise, stiff neck, fever, and cranial nerve palsies. CSF examination demonstrates increased lymphocyte count and total protein; serum RPR test results are usually positive.

Meningovascular syphilis is a more chronic disorder. Usually evident 20 or more years after initial exposure, it rarely occurs as early as 2 years after the primary untreated infection. Chronic inflammation produces brain or spinal cord infarction, leading to cranial nerve palsies, cerebrovascular accidents, seizures, or paraplegia. Argyll Robertson pupils, which are small and irregular and accommodate to near vision but do not react to light or painful stimuli, are present.

Tabes dorsalis develops 10 to 20 years after primary infection, usually in persons aged 25 to 45 years. Both direct invasion by the spirochete and an immunologic reaction may occur, producing degenerative and sclerotic changes in the posterior nerve root fibers of the spinal cord, spinal ganglion cells, long fibers of the posterior columns of the spinal cord, optic nerves, and oculomotor nuclei. Symptoms may include lightning-like, very brief severe nerve root pains, gastric crisis, and spastic gait, failing vision, and urinary and sexual dysfunction. Optic nerves show progressive primary atrophy; Argyll Robertson pupils are small and irregular. Impaired vibration sense, ataxia, and a positive Romberg sign are present. Knee and ankle jerks are absent. In 54 patients with tabes dorsalis and positive serum VDRL, CSF VDRL and fluorescent treponemal antibody (FTA) tests were positive in only 18% and 73%, respectively.

General paresis (dementia paralytica) occurs most commonly in patients older than age 40 years due to direct spirochete invasion of neural tissue causing neuronal degeneration, astrocytic proliferation, and meningitis (Fig. 44.11). Resultant degenerative and sclerotic changes produce a thickened dura mater, chronic subdural hematoma, cortical atrophy, and astrocyte proliferation. The frontal lobes are disproportionately affected. Progressive dementia occurs in 60% of patients, but headaches, insomnia, personality change, impaired judgment, disturbed emotional responses, slurred speech, and tremors can also develop. Argyll Robertson pupils are characteristic. RPR test results in blood and VDRL test results in CSF are positive in more than 90% of patients.

Gumma of the brain and spinal cord are rare. Symptoms are consistent with expanding CNS lesions.

Diagnosis and Treatment

Diagnosis is based on serologic tests with blood syphilis IgG and CSF VDRL tests for screening and FTA absorption test or the microhemagglutination *T. pallidum* test for specific confirmation. The CSF usually demonstrates a modest increase primarily in lymphocytic cells, with a moderate protein increase and normal glucose level.

Penicillin is the treatment of choice for all forms of syphilis. Repeated CSF testing is necessary to see if it has normalized, as that will indicate successful treatment.

Future Directions

Although no large-scale randomized trial has compared azithromycin directly with benzathine penicillin, preliminary studies support the efficacy of azithromycin (a single oral dose of 1 or 2 g) in the treatment of early-stage syphilis. Evidence does not yet support its use in late- or tertiary-stage disease. Additional data support the use of ceftriaxone

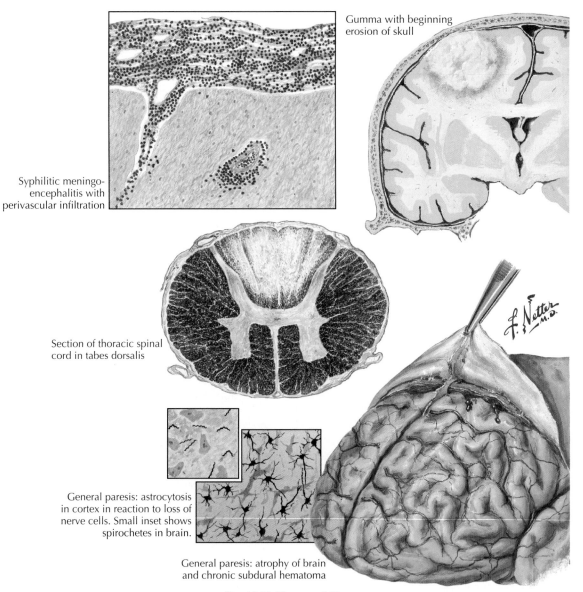

Gumma with beginning erosion of skull

Syphilitic meningo-encephalitis with perivascular infiltration

Section of thoracic spinal cord in tabes dorsalis

General paresis: astrocytosis in cortex in reaction to loss of nerve cells. Small inset shows spirochetes in brain.

General paresis: atrophy of brain and chronic subdural hematoma

Fig. 44.11 Neurosyphilis.

in early-stage disease. Ceftriaxone (2 g IM once daily for 10 days) produced similar CSF responses for the treatment of neurosyphilis in HIV-infected individuals. In aggregate, the data do not establish the equivalence or superiority of these agents to standard penicillin regimens but do support their use as alternatives when penicillin is not a therapeutic option. Concurrent HIV infection may modify the natural history of syphilis, but the overall response to standard therapy has been no different from that in HIV-seronegative individuals.

ACKNOWLEDGMENT

We gratefully acknowledge the contributions of Samuel Kalluvya and J. B. Kataraihya of Weill Bugando Medical Center, Mwanza, Tanzania.

ADDITIONAL RESOURCES

Halperin JJ, Shapiro ED, Logigian E, et al. Practice parameter: treatment of nervous system Lyme disease (an evidence-based review). Neurology 2007;69:91–102.

Hildenbrand P, Craven DE, Jones R, et al. Lyme neuroborreliosis: manifestations of a rapidly emerging zoonosis. AJNR Am J Neuroradiol 2009.

Wormser GP, Dattwyler RJ, Shapiro ED, et al. The clinical assessment, treatment, and prevention of Lyme disease, human granulocytic anaplasmosis, and babesiosis: clinical practice guidelines by the Infectious Diseases Society of America. Clin Infect Dis 2006;43:1089–134.

Evidence-based guidelines for the treatment of nervous system Lyme disease developed by the American Academy of Neurology.

Ooi WW, Moschella SL. Update on leprosy in immigrants in the United States: status in the year 2000. Clin Infect Dis 2001;32(6):930–7.

Ooi WW, Srinivasan J. Leprosy and the peripheral nervous system: basic and clinical aspects. Muscle Nerve 2004;30(4):393–409.

Practice Guidelines of the Infectious Diseases Society of America. Available from: http://www.idsociety.org/Content.aspx?id=9088. [Accessed 28 April 2011].

Evidence-based statements developed to assist practitioners and patients in making decisions about appropriate health care for specific clinical circumstances. Guidelines for treatment of infections by organ system and organism may be found here.

Sabin TD, Swift TR, Jacobson RR. Leprosy. In: Dyck PJ, Thomas PK, editors. Peripheral neuropathy. Philadelphia: WB Saunders; 2005. pp. 1354–79.

Sotiriou MC, Stryjewska BM, Hill C. Case report: two cases of leprosy in siblings caused by mycobacterium lepromatosis and review of the literature. Am J Trop Med Hyg 2016;95(3):522–7.

Evidence

Case records of the Massachusetts General Hospital. Weekly clinicopathological exercises. Case 12-2001: a 16-year-old boy with an altered mental status and muscle rigidity. N Engl J Med 2001;344:1232–9.

A classic description of a case of tetanus.

Dariouche RO. Spinal epidural abscess. N Engl J Med 2006;355: 2012–20.

This review addresses the pathogenesis, clinical features, diagnosis, treatment, common diagnostic and therapeutic pitfalls, and outcome of bacterial spinal epidural abscess.

Garcia-Monco JC. Central nervous system tuberculosis. Neurol Clin 1999;17:737–59.

A comprehensive review of diagnosis and treatment of central nervous system tuberculosis.

Heilpern KL, Lorber B. Focal intracranial infections. Infect Dis Clin North Am 1996;10:879–98.

Review of the diagnosis and management of focal intracranial infections including the use of magnetic imaging and magnetic resonance angiography as well as early surgical intervention.

Steere AC. Lyme disease. N Engl J Med 2001;345:115–25.

A comprehensive review of many manifestations of Lyme disease.

Stoner BP. Current controversies in the management of adult syphilis. Clin Infect Dis 2007;44:S130–46.

A review summarizing recent research on syphilis treatment—its efficacy and outcomes.

Tunkel AR, Hartman BJ, Kaplan SL, et al. Practice guidelines for the management of bacterial meningitis. Clin Infect Dis 2004;39:1267–84.

Evidence-based guidelines for the diagnosis, management, and treatment of bacterial meningitis developed by the Infectious Diseases Society of America.

van de Beek D, de Gans J, Tunkel AR, et al. Community-acquired bacterial meningitis in adults. N Engl J Med 2006;354:44–53.

This review summarizes the current concepts of the initial approach to the treatment of adults with bacterial meningitis, highlighting adjunctive dexamethasone therapy and focusing on the management of neurologic complications.

45

Viral Diseases

Daniel P. McQuillen, Donald E. Craven, H. Royden Jones, Jr.[†]

HERPES SIMPLEX ENCEPHALITIS

CLINICAL VIGNETTE *An independent 74-year-old man left a family wedding reception early because he did not feel well; he complained of mild nausea and general malaise. His daughter called the next day, and when he did not answer the phone, she went to his home to check on him, discovering him wandering in his backyard acutely confused. She convinced him to go to the emergency department, where he was found to be febrile with a temperature of 38.5°C (101.3°F). He soon became unresponsive to verbal stimuli, had conjugate eye deviation to the right, neck stiffness, and bilateral palmar grasps. He withdrew his extremities to noxious stimuli; plantar responses were flexor.*

A noncontrast head computed tomography (CT) was unremarkable. Cerebrospinal fluid (CSF) examination demonstrated a WBC count of 45/mm³, predominantly lymphocytes, protein of 110 mg/dL, and a normal glucose level. Intravenous (IV) acyclovir 10 mg/kg every 8 hours was begun. Magnetic resonance image (MRI) of the brain demonstrated T2-weighted hyperintensity with edematous changes in the left insular region of the inferior temporal lobe, the parahippocampal gyrus, and the hippocampus, extending into the subthalamic nucleus suggestive of herpes simplex virus (HSV) encephalitis. Electroencephalography (EEG) demonstrated periodic lateralized epileptiform discharges (PLEDs). This diagnosis was confirmed by HSV polymerase chain reaction (PCR) 4 days after symptom onset. The patient gradually improved and was treated with a 21-day course of acyclovir. After a short stay in a rehabilitation facility, he was discharged home.

Comment: This is an example of the rapidity with which herpes simplex encephalitis (HSE) will declare itself and the urgent need to consider this diagnosis in any acutely confused patient, initiating treatment based on clinical judgment alone without waiting for definitive diagnostic proof. Unless this type of decision-making takes place, HSE would have caused irreversible temporal lobe damage, particularly affecting memory and language function.

Etiology

A wide spectrum of viral agents may cause infectious encephalitis. Diagnosis and management are dependent on identifying the precise causative agent. Only a few viruses are amenable to specific antiviral therapy. Therefore, prevention strategies are particularly important, especially for arthropod-borne viruses such as West Nile virus (WNV) and Eastern Equine encephalitis (EEE).

HSE is the most common acute encephalitis in the United States, with an annual incidence of 1 in 250,000 to 1 in 500,000. It affects all ages and both sexes equally, without significant seasonal variation. Early antiviral treatment significantly reduces mortality, but morbidity remains unacceptably high. Most cases of HSE are caused by oral herpes virus (HSV-1); however, genital herpes virus (HSV-2) is more common among neonates with disseminated disease. HSE commonly develops as a recurrent infection, but occasionally may occur during primary infection. Animal data have verified the existence of retrograde viral transport into the brain via olfactory or trigeminal nerves. However, human disease pathogenic pathways are not fully clarified. There is a predilection for HSE, once established, to lead to a hemorrhagic necrosis with inflammatory infiltrates and cells containing intranuclear inclusions.

Clinical Presentation

The symptoms and signs of patients with subacute or acute focal encephalitis are generally nonspecific, with fever, headache, and altered consciousness being the most common. Focal manifestations often include seizures, typically complex partial in character because of the predisposition of the temporal lobe to develop herpes infection. It is common for these patients to also develop language difficulties, personality changes, hemiparesis, ataxia, cranial nerve defects, and papilledema (Fig. 45.1). The differential diagnosis includes stroke, brain tumors, other viral encephalitides, bacterial abscesses, tuberculosis, cryptococcal infections, and toxoplasmosis.

Diagnosis

One of the major issues in diagnosis is for the examining clinician to put HSE into the diagnostic spectrum very early on in the temporal profile of the patient's illness. If this is not applied, a major therapeutic window for successful treatment is lost. One unfortunate clinical scenario is failure to diagnose a patient with HSE who presents with confusion for 3 to 5 days that is wrongly attributed to medication or minor infection of the urinary or respiratory tracts.

For patients with suspected encephalitis, the initial diagnostic studies must include a CT scan (to rule out a mass effect) followed by immediate CSF examination. CT scan results are abnormal in 50% of cases early on and usually demonstrate localized edema, low-density lesions, mass effects, contrast enhancements, or hemorrhage. MRI and EEG may be subsequently obtained for further confirmation. These usually demonstrate temporal lobe damage (Fig. 45.2); however, normal studies do not exclude an HSE diagnosis. If this instance does occur, it is often wise to repeat the study within a few days, particularly if the patient continues to be confused.

CSF findings are nonspecific, often showing lymphocytic pleocytosis with a slight protein increase. Abnormal CSF findings are found in 96% of biopsy-proven HSE cases. EEG may show repetitive spike or

[†]Deceased.

Possible route of transmission in herpes simplex encephalitis

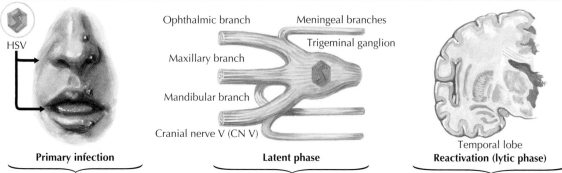

Primary infection

Virus enters via cutaneous or mucosal surfaces to infect sensory or autonomic nerve endings with transport to cell bodies in ganglia

Latent phase

Virus replicates in ganglia before establishing latent phase

Reactivation (lytic phase)

Reactivation of HSV in trigeminal ganglion can result in spread to brain (temporal lobe) via meningeal branches of CN V

Clinical features of HSV encephalitis

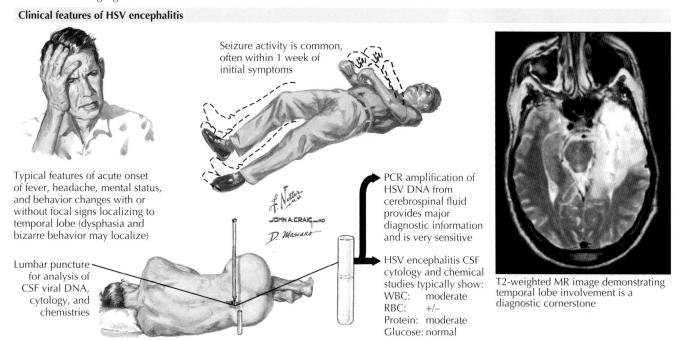

Typical features of acute onset of fever, headache, mental status, and behavior changes with or without focal signs localizing to temporal lobe (dysphasia and bizarre behavior may localize)

Seizure activity is common, often within 1 week of initial symptoms

Lumbar puncture for analysis of CSF viral DNA, cytology, and chemistries

PCR amplification of HSV DNA from cerebrospinal fluid provides major diagnostic information and is very sensitive

HSV encephalitis CSF cytology and chemical studies typically show:
WBC: moderate
RBC: +/−
Protein: moderate
Glucose: normal

T2-weighted MR image demonstrating temporal lobe involvement is a diagnostic cornerstone

Fig. 45.1 HSV Encephalitis.

sharp wave discharges, and slow waves localized to the involved area often as PLEDs.

The accuracy of PCR testing for HSV-DNA to detect HSV-1 and -2 in CSF compares favorably with the previous use of brain biopsy. This methodology provides excellent sensitivity and specificity (90%–98%). The viral sequence for HSV may be detected months after the acute episode and may be negative in early disease phases. PCR should not be used to monitor therapy success. Brain biopsy was previously the gold standard for specificity, but it is rarely indicated now with the widespread availability of HSV PCR testing. If used, biopsy specimens are examined for both histopathologic changes and HSV antigens by immunofluorescence testing and appropriate culture techniques.

Therapy

Immediate initiation of acyclovir is indicated after HSE is suspected. This relatively benign medication has the greatest chance of efficacy if it can be initiated very early on in the patient's clinical course. The excellent outcome of the patient in the initial vignette in this chapter emphasizes the absolute importance for primary care and emergency medicine physicians to immediately consider HSE in individuals of any age who experience relatively acute changes in mental status. Unfortunately, if therapy is not commenced immediately at presentation, the outcome is usually poor, with minimal chance of return to independent living.

Prognosis

Before the availability of IV acyclovir, mortality from HSE was approximately 70%. If one is able to initiate antiviral therapy within the first 24 hours of symptom onset, and if the patient is fully treated for 21 days, the prognosis for long-term outlook is much better. This approach has substantially reduced both mortality and morbidity. Overall, although morbidity remains high, with 60% to 70% of patients having significant neurologic deficits, the mortality is now at 10% to 20%.

On rare occasions, a patient seemingly doing well with initial therapy has a relapse. Inadequate early dosing of the acyclovir is the usual cause. Thus initial treatment regimens must include daily doses of 30 mg/kg intravenously, usually in three separate doses of 10 mg/kg.

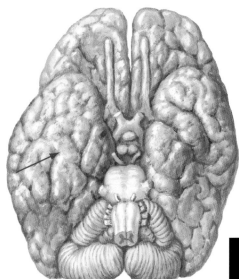

Swelling and patchy hemorrhagic areas, most marked in right temporal lobe

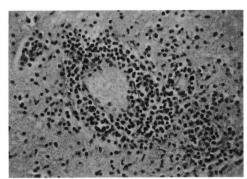

Perivascular infiltration with mononuclear cells in disrupted brain tissue

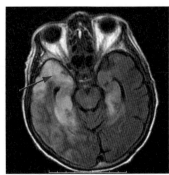

Axial FLAIR image with extensive intracranial signal in right temporal lobe and medial left temporal lobe

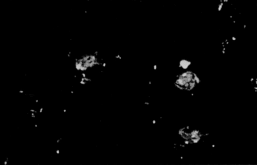

Immunofluorescent staining shows presence of herpesvirus antigen in neurons

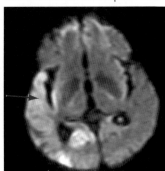

Diffusion with right temporal and insular changes

Fig. 45.2 Herpes Simplex Encephalitis.

EASTERN EQUINE ENCEPHALITIS

CLINICAL VIGNETTE *A 60-year-old New Hampshire man presented in mid-August with 2 weeks of headache, followed by dizziness, unsteady gait, and nausea and vomiting. He walked his dog past a local pond in the woods every day, sustaining multiple mosquito bites. He had type 2 diabetes mellitus and a history of a prior nephrectomy for renal cell cancer. At clinical presentation, he was febrile, 38.3°C (101°F), somnolent but arousable, answering questions inconsistently; there were fine tremors in his hands, and muscle stretch reflexes were globally depressed.*

Brain MRI revealed increased signal with mild mass effect in the left thalamus and basal ganglia. Spinal fluid examination demonstrated a WBC of 1860/mm³ (81% polymorphonuclear neutrophils [PMNs], 11% lymphocytes, 8% monocytes), 26 red blood cells/mm³, protein 106 mg/dL, glucose 98 mg/dL (serum 209), and negative Gram staining. He had continued fevers with progressive gait ataxia, upper extremity weakness, and memory loss. Bacterial cultures and studies for Borrelia burgdorferi, Treponema pallidum, HSV, and WNV were negative. CSF IgM and plaque assay were positive for EEE. He gradually recovered motor function over the next few months with supportive care, and 1 year later, he had minimal residual cognitive deficits.

Epidemiology

EEE virus is a member of the family Togaviridae, genus alphavirus, that is found in the eastern half of the United States. EEE is a mosquito-borne viral disease that causes disease in humans, horses, and some bird species. It generally takes 3 to 10 days to develop symptoms of EEE after being bitten by an infected mosquito. An average of five human cases occurs per year (approximately 220 confirmed cases in the United States between 1964 and 2004, most frequently in Florida, Georgia, Massachusetts, and New Jersey). EEE virus transmission is most common in and around freshwater hardwood swamps in the Atlantic and Gulf Coast states and the Great Lakes region. The main EEE virus transmission cycle is between birds and mosquitoes.

Clinical Presentation and Treatment

Most persons infected with EEE virus do not demonstrate a clearly discernible illness. In those individuals who do develop clinical illness, symptoms range from a mild flulike illness to fulminating encephalitis, eventually leading to coma and death. The mortality rate from EEE is approximately 33%, making it one of the most deadly mosquito-borne diseases in the United States.

Diagnosis

Laboratory diagnosis of EEE virus infection is based on serology, especially IgM testing of serum and CSF, and neutralizing antibody testing of acute- and convalescent-phase serum. MRI is the most sensitive imaging modality for the diagnosis of EEE (Fig. 45.3). The most commonly affected areas of the central nervous system (CNS) include the basal ganglia (unilateral or asymmetric, with occasional internal capsule involvement) and thalamic nuclei. Other areas include the brainstem (often the midbrain), periventricular white matter, and cortex (most often temporally). Affected areas appear as increased signal intensity on T2-weighted images.

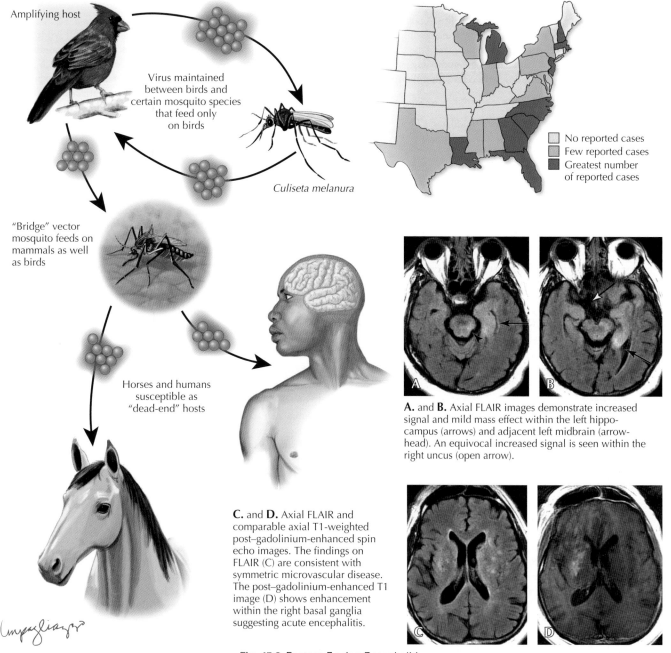

Amplifying host

Virus maintained between birds and certain mosquito species that feed only on birds

Culiseta melanura

"Bridge" vector mosquito feeds on mammals as well as birds

Horses and humans susceptible as "dead-end" hosts

No reported cases
Few reported cases
Greatest number of reported cases

A. and **B.** Axial FLAIR images demonstrate increased signal and mild mass effect within the left hippo-campus (arrows) and adjacent left midbrain (arrow-head). An equivocal increased signal is seen within the right uncus (open arrow).

C. and **D.** Axial FLAIR and comparable axial T1-weighted post–gadolinium-enhanced spin echo images. The findings on FLAIR (C) are consistent with symmetric microvascular disease. The post–gadolinium-enhanced T1 image (D) shows enhancement within the right basal ganglia suggesting acute encephalitis.

Fig. 45.3 Eastern Equine Encephalitis.

Therapy/Prognosis

There is no specific treatment for EEE; optimal medical care includes intensive hospitalization and supportive care.

Approximately half of those persons who survive EEE will have mild to severe permanent neurologic damage, usually with cognitive impairment. Those older than age 50 and younger than age 15 years appear to be at greatest risk for developing severe EEE.

WEST NILE VIRUS

Etiology/Epidemiology

WNV is a flavivirus usually found in Africa, West Asia, and the Middle East. The Middle Eastern strains are genetically closely related to the St. Louis encephalitis virus, found in the United States. There are many potential animal, ornithologic, and insect reservoirs, including humans, horses, other mammals, birds, and mosquitoes. The WNV was not documented in the Western Hemisphere until 1999. In the temperate zones of the world, West Nile encephalitis cases occur primarily in the late summer or early autumn. In southern climates, where temperatures are milder, WNV can be transmitted year-round.

Clinical Presentation

West Nile fever is typically a mild disease characterized by flulike symptoms that develop 3 to 15 days after the bite of an infected mosquito. West Nile fever usually lasts only a few days and does not seem to cause any long-term health effects. Mild fever, headache, body aches, occasional skin rash, and swollen glands are the most common symptoms.

However, there is a more severe disease spectrum that can manifest as encephalitis, meningitis, or meningoencephalitis. A poliomyelitis-like illness is also described, with an acute proximal and asymmetric flaccid paralysis, occasionally occurring during outbreaks in the United States. Neurophysiologic, radiologic, and pathologic studies suggest that WNV has a proclivity to damage anterior horn cells within the spinal cord.

Diagnosis

Diagnosis is made by serologic assays of blood and CSF.

Therapy

Treatment is entirely supportive; there is no specific drug treatment or vaccine available. In the rare instances of a polio-like illness, the long-term outcome hinges on the degree and distribution of anterior horn cell damage.

POWASSAN VIRUS

> **CLINICAL VIGNETTE** *A 52-year-old man from Massachusetts presented with 2 days of fever and myalgias. He lived outside of Boston but had recently traveled to Cape Cod, New York, Pennsylvania, and Wisconsin; at the time of symptom onset, he was camping in a lake area of New Hampshire. Although his initial neurologic examination was normal, several days later he developed inattention, somnolence, and left upper extremity dysmetria. Brain MRI showed evidence of bilateral basal ganglia and thalamic T2/fluid attenuation inversion recovery (FLAIR) hyperintensity and diffusion restriction in the dorsal midbrain. The patient improved incompletely and was discharged to an acute rehabilitation facility. Two years later, he had persistent headaches as well as cerebellar dysarthria, delayed motor function, and incoordination.*

Epidemiology

Powassan virus (POWV) encephalitis is an arthropod-borne infection caused by a flavivirus that, unlike most arboviruses, is transmitted by ticks rather than mosquitoes. It has been infrequently reported in North America, with approximately 100 cases since 1958. In the Great Lakes region, the traditional lineage of POWV is transmitted by *Ixodes cookei* ticks, which have a relatively high degree of specificity for their primary hosts, woodchucks and rodents. More recently, cases have been identified in the northeast, where POWV lineage II (also known as deer tick virus, DTV) is transmitted by *Ixodes scapularis*, which also transmits the causative agent of Lyme disease. Unlike other infectious agents transmitted by *Ixodes scapularis*, POWV can be transmitted within approximately 15 minutes of attachment to the host.

Clinical Presentation

The incubation period for POWV ranges from approximately 1 to 5 weeks. Like other arboviruses, presenting symptoms can include high fever and features of brain involvement, including confusion, depressed level of consciousness, seizures, and focal neurologic deficits. Rash and gastrointestinal symptoms are also fairly common. Some patients may have mild thrombocytopenia; otherwise, POWV encephalitis is not commonly associated with laboratory abnormalities. The reported mortality rate for POWV encephalitis is 10% to 15%, and even among survivors, memory loss and focal weakness can persist. At the other end of the spectrum, asymptomatic infection may occur, as serologic surveys have found an antibody prevalence of 1% to 4%.

CSF analysis usually shows pleocytosis (up to 200–700 WBCs/μL), which can be either lymphocyte or polymorphonuclear predominant. Most reported cases had elevated CSF protein and normal glucose; however, CSF findings can be nearly normal.

Diagnosis

POWV infection is diagnosed by a compatible clinical syndrome plus one of the following: virus isolation, detection of IgM antibodies by ELISA with a confirmatory plaque neutralization test (which measures the ability of patient serum to reduce virus infectivity in an experimental setting), detection of IgM in the CSF with negative studies for other causes of encephalitis, or documented fourfold rise in antibody titer. A recent report (Piantadosi et al., 2016) used metagenomic sequencing to detect POWV in CSF 4 weeks before the diagnosis was made by serology, demonstrating the utility of this method for timely pathogen detection in severe CNS infection.

Imaging

MRI in four of eight cases occurring in Massachusetts recently showed evidence of restricted diffusion acutely. In one patient who recovered fully, this finding was seen throughout the cortex and had completely resolved on follow-up imaging. Notably the other three patients that had diffusion restriction, including midbrain infarction in one and cerebellar findings in two others, had poor outcomes. Although MRI findings are nonspecific, they characteristically demonstrate extensive T2/FLAIR hyperintensities within the brainstem, extending to the deep gray structures and cortex. This suggests that diffusion restriction of the brainstem and posterior fossa may impart some negative prognostic significance.

Therapy

As with other arboviral encephalitides, treatment for POWV encephalitis is supportive. There is a reported fatality rate of 10% to 15%, with residual neurologic deficits in 50% of survivors. Anecdotally, high dose corticosteroids and/or intravenous immunoglobulin (IVIG) have been used with mixed outcomes.

ZIKA VIRUS

Zika virus is an arthropod-borne flavivirus transmitted by *Aedes* species mosquitoes (*Ae. aegypti* and *Ae. albopictus*) that is related to other flaviviruses, including dengue, yellow fever, and West Nile. These mosquitoes bite during the day and night. Clinical manifestations of Zika virus infection occur in approximately 20% to 25% of patients. These include acute onset of low-grade fever, maculopapular pruritic rash, arthralgias in small joints of the hands and feet, or nonpurulent conjunctivitis. Other commonly reported clinical manifestations include myalgia, headache, dysesthesia, retro-orbital pain, and asthenia. Zika virus infection has been associated with neurologic complications, including congenital microcephaly and other developmental problems among babies born to women infected during pregnancy, Guillain-Barré syndrome (GBS), myelitis, and meningoencephalitis. There is a current ongoing outbreak of Zika virus in the Americas, Caribbean, and the Pacific. Zika virus RNA has been detected in blood, urine, semen, saliva, female genital tract secretions, CSF, amniotic fluid, and breast milk. Zika virus RNA usually clears from semen after about 3 months, but has been detected in semen up to 188 days after onset of illness. Sexual transmission of Zika virus as late as 41 days after a partner's onset of symptoms has been described.

The diagnosis of Zika virus infection should be suspected in individuals with typical clinical manifestations and relevant epidemiologic exposure (residence in or travel to an area where mosquito-borne transmission of Zika virus infection has been reported, or unprotected sexual contact with a person who meets these criteria). The diagnostic approach depends on the timing of clinical presentation, with RT-PCR of serum (or whole blood) and urine for the detection of Zika virus RNA being the most useful tests within 14 days of exposure. For those presenting

≥14 days after onset of symptoms, diagnostic testing for Zika virus infection should consist of Zika virus serologic testing (Zika virus IgM and plaque reduction neutralization test [PRNT]). Of note, previous flavivirus exposure can alter serologic results via cross-reactivity. There is no specific treatment for Zika virus infection. Management consists of rest and symptomatic treatment.

CYTOMEGALOVIRUS

Cytomegalovirus (CMV) is a member of the Herpesvirus family and establishes latent infection after the resolution of acute (or primary) infection. Secondary, symptomatic disease may present later in life, either as reactivation of latent CMV or reinfection with a novel exogenous strain. Reactivation of CMV may occur at any time, although more commonly in the presence of systemic immunosuppression, either iatrogenic or secondary to underlying medical conditions, such as acquired immunodeficiency syndrome (AIDS) or systemic glucocorticoid administration. Notwithstanding, CMV encephalitis is relatively uncommon in patients with human immunodeficiency virus (HIV) and AIDS, occurring in less than 2% of clinical neurologic disorders. Acute onset and rapid progression help distinguish CMV from HIV encephalitis or progressive multifocal leukoencephalopathy (PML). CMV polyradiculitis can present as back pain, paresthesia, sciatica, sphincter dysfunction with urinary retention, distal sensory loss, or ascending paralysis.

Numerous neurologic manifestations occur in immunocompetent hosts. Encephalitis is a rare but potentially serious complication that should be considered in the differential diagnosis of unexplained encephalitis. GBS has been estimated to occur in approximately 0.6 to 2.2 per 1000 cases of primary CMV infection (compared with 0.25–0.65 per 1000 cases of *Campylobacter jejuni* infection). The median age of patients with CMV-related GBS is 32 years, and 85% of patients are women. CMV-related GBS is typically associated with the development of antibodies to ganglioside GM2, although the exact role of these antibodies remains unclear. Importantly, anti-GM2 IgM antibodies are often detected not only in patients with CMV-related GBS but also in patients with CMV infection who do not have GBS. Multiple focal neurologic deficits have been described in patients with CMV, including brachial plexus neuropathy, diffuse axonal peripheral neuropathy, transverse myelitis, Horner syndrome, and cranial nerve palsies.

In a prospective study of 506 patients with GBS over 10 years, with 12.4% having evidence of CMV by IgM and IgG avidity as well as CMV DNA PCR positivity in plasma, sensory defects (in 72% of cases) and facial palsy (49%) were frequent, and test results positive for CMV DNA in plasma at hospital admission (found in 62% of cases) tended to be associated with objective sensory defect ($P = 0.052$). The main factors associated with long-term neurologic sequelae (21%) were older age ($P < 0.001$) and assisted ventilation during hospitalization ($P = 0.005$).

Antibodies to ganglioside GM2 are often associated with GBS after CMV infection, but their relevance is not known. It is unlikely that CMV infection and antiganglioside GM2 antibodies are solely responsible, and an additional factor is required to elicit GBS.

HUMAN IMMUNODEFICIENCY VIRUS

CLINICAL VIGNETTE *A 31-year-old mother of a 13-month-old child presented to the emergency department with headache, vertigo, diplopia, and an unsteady gait. She had been treated with antibiotics for acute sinusitis during the preceding 8 days. Her neurologic examination demonstrated a lethargic, restless, febrile woman with meningismus, photophobia, horizontal nystagmus, and slight appendicular ataxia of her right arm and leg.*

Brain CT demonstrated signal changes bilaterally in both thalami and to a lesser degree in internal capsules, midbrain, pons, and right posterior temporal lobe. There were signs of maxillary and sphenoid sinusitis. Spinal tap demonstrated moderately increased opening pressure of 275 mm/CSF, cell count of 485 white blood cells (84% neutrophils), protein concentration of 106 mg/mL, and glucose of 66 mg/dL. IV antibiotics as well as acyclovir were begun. Gram staining and culture were negative.

During the first day of admission, she developed increased obtundation. Bilateral flexor posturing, and intermittent left-sided extensor posturing developed during her second day of hospitalization. Dexamethasone was administered every 6 hours. EEG demonstrated bilateral 3- to 5-Hz activity. Repeat imaging demonstrated extension of the low-density lesions into the basal ganglia and frontal lobe operculum. CSF was negative for HSV virus PCR. Three days after admission, all spontaneous movements ceased; her pupils became dilated, fixed, and nonreactive; she was now areflexic and did not respond to any form of sensory stimulation. EEGs were electrically silent on two occasions over the next 24 hours. She died on the 5th hospital day.

A history of marked sexual promiscuity became available during her hospitalization. CSF culture was eventually positive for HIV although no serum or CSF antibodies to HIV were defined; all other cultures for various microbes were negative. Pathologically, there was an encephalopathic demyelinating process affecting cerebral white matter, the thalamus, and brainstem with acute neuronal damage. There was no associated vasculitis.

Comment: This case, seen at Lahey in the mid-1980s, added further support to the proposal that HIV is a primary neurotropic virus. Our experience emphasized the importance of considering HIV in the differential diagnosis of any acute encephalitis, even if the patient is HIV antibody negative. Here the initial antibody negativity supported the concept that this patient's encephalitis represented the primary phase of her HIV. Today when one wishes to consider an acute HIV infection in the setting of a negative HIV antibody, one now has available an HIV viral load study. This will be positive, despite a negative HIV antibody study, if the patient has an active HIV infection. Thus, one does not need to depend on a viral culture to make the diagnosis, as occurred with this patient. This was not available at the time we evaluated this person.

Primary Neurologic HIV Infection

Acute aseptic meningitis is the most common neurologic disorder to develop among individuals presenting with primary neurologic HIV infection (PNHI; Fig. 45.4). These patients present with headache, meningismus, and sometimes myalgias and arthralgias. According to the above vignette, on rare occasions, a meningoencephalitis, an encephalopathy, an acute disseminated encephalomyelitis, a myelopathy, a meningoradiculitis, and a peripheral neuropathy, particularly a GBS, may be seen as the presenting clinical picture of HIV. Other systemic symptoms and signs seen with acute HIV infection include fever, night sweats, weight loss, rash, fatigue, lymphadenopathy, oral ulcers, thrush, pharyngitis, gastrointestinal upset, and genital ulcers. As HIV antibody testing may be negative in PNHI, laboratory clues to the presence of seroconversion include leucopenia, thrombocytopenia, and elevated transaminases. In such cases, the determination of serum HIV viral load may yield a positive result. A repeat HIV antibody study is often positive if the patient survives the initial neurologic illness. The primary infectious encephalitic forms have a significant morbidity and mortality, perhaps as high as 50%. Its importance in adolescents is illustrated by the finding that in the United States, HIV is the seventh leading cause of death among patients aged 15 to 24 years. Once seroconversion occurs, AIDS patients are at risk for a host of neurologic complications.

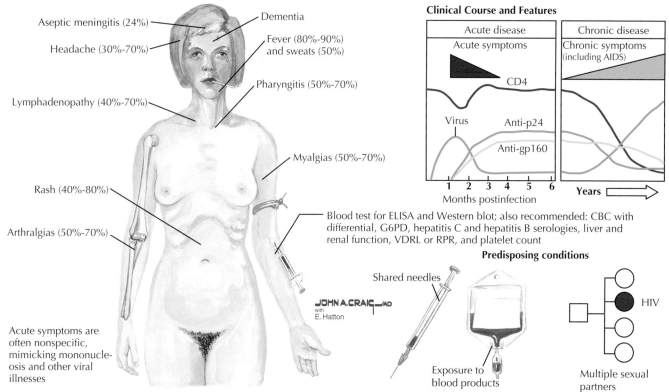

Aseptic meningitis (24%)

Dementia

Headache (30%-70%)

Fever (80%-90%) and sweats (50%)

Pharyngitis (50%-70%)

Lymphadenopathy (40%-70%)

Myalgias (50%-70%)

Rash (40%-80%)

Arthralgias (50%-70%)

Acute symptoms are often nonspecific, mimicking mononucleosis and other viral illnesses

JOHN A. CRAIG _AD with E. Hatton

Clinical Course and Features

Acute disease	Chronic disease
Acute symptoms	Chronic symptoms (including AIDS)

CD4
Virus   Anti-p24
Anti-gp160

1 2 3 4 5 6   Years
Months postinfection

Blood test for ELISA and Western blot; also recommended: CBC with differential, G6PD, hepatitis C and hepatitis B serologies, liver and renal function, VDRL or RPR, and platelet count

Predisposing conditions

Shared needles

Exposure to blood products

HIV

Multiple sexual partners

AIDS encephalopathy in a 39-year-old man with gait difficulties and cognitive decline. Brain MRI was normal 2 years ago.

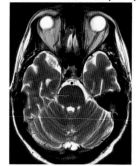

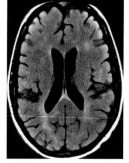

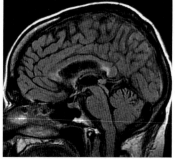

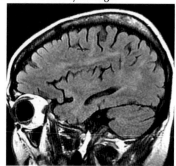

A. Axial T2 fast spin echo demonstrates ill-defined area of augmented T2 signal in upper left pons (arrow).

B. Axial FLAIR shows moderate sulcal and ventricular enlargement consistent with diffuse atrophy for age 39 in addition to paraventricular augmentation of T2 signal which in some regions extends to subcortical white matter and cortex (arrows).

C. Midsagittal FLAIR with ill-defined augmentation in both genu and splenium of corpus callosum (arrows).

D. FLAIR imaging more laterally again demonstrates paraventricular involvement extending to subcortical white matter (arrows).

Fig. 45.4 Primary HIV Infection of the Nervous System.

HIV Dementia

AIDS dementia complex (ADC) is the most important "primary" neurologic complication of HIV infection. It is almost universal for HIV-1 infection to occur within the CSF when AIDS is previously unrecognized and thus untreated. This was quite common early on in the AIDS epidemic prior to the availability of specific highly active antiretroviral therapy (HAART) protocols. These individuals presented with a varied dementia that was particularly characterized by early- to mid-adult-age changes in mental function. Such patients often were noted to have a relatively rapid to subacute change in personality with prominent apathy, inattention, inability to form new memory, and language dysfunction. ADC individuals were unable to carry out the basic requirements of normal activities of daily living. Although a number of AIDS patients develop a variety of opportunistic brain infections, as mentioned in

Chapter 48, at autopsy many proved to have a primary subacute demyelinating process with some mild cellular response, particularly characterized by clusters of foamy macrophages, microglial nodules, and multinucleated giant cells.

Once effective combinations of HAART became available in the mid-1990s, the prevalence of ADC declined dramatically. Because the brain is a viral sanctuary, further therapeutic effort to deal with long-term HIV effects is of importance. The prevalence of HIV-associated neurocognitive disorders (HANDs) is high, even in long-standing aviremic HIV-positive patients. However, from the practical viewpoint, HANDs does not usually have any daily functional repercussions. It is of concern, however, that as people with HIV live longer, the frequency of HIV-related neurologic impairment may be rising once again despite successful administration of life-prolonging HAART. There is little evidence that HAART per se leads to primary CNS toxicity. The benefits and risks of HAART in the preservation or enhancement of neurocognitive function in well, HIV-infected patients with more than 500 CD4+ cells/μL are unknown. Abnormal brain MRIs typified by both white matter (demyelination) and gray matter (atrophy) may be demonstrated in seemingly clinically asymptomatic persons living with HIV.

HIV Primary CNS Angiitis

CNS vascular involvement may develop in HIV infection. This is usually a result of associated opportunistic infections, including bacterial, viral (Epstein–Barr virus, CMV, hepatitis B), fungal, or parasitic organisms. Very rarely, neoplastic disease, or toxic drug abuse, may provide the mechanism for CNS angiitis in this setting. At autopsy, in some studies, perhaps a quarter of HIV-infected patients have cerebral infarcts.

HIV Myelopathy

Occasionally a primary vacuolar and inflammatory myelopathy is the presenting feature of AIDS. Its predisposition for the dorsal lateral spinal cord mimics the distribution and thus the clinical spectrum of B_{12} or copper deficiency syndromes (Chapter 44). There is no effective treatment for HIV-associated myelopathy. The introduction of HAART has made little difference to its natural history. Spinal cord pathology reveals vacuolization and inflammation.

HIV Anterior Horn Cell Myelopathy

Very rarely, one may see various forms of a motor neuron, anterior horn cell disorder with HIV infection. This is attributed to direct HIV damage to the motor neurons by neurotoxic HIV viral proteins, cytokines, and chemokines. Opportunistic viruses may also directly attack motor neurons in the AIDS clinical setting, mirroring those of progressive spinal muscular atrophy (Chapter 66). This may result in an inexorably progressive disorder of upper and lower motor neurons. One most unusual presentation has been the rare patient presenting with severe bilateral arm and hand weakness unassociated with either bulbar and/or leg weakness or any corticospinal tract findings. This is referred to as a neurogenic "man-in-the-barrel" syndrome or brachial amyotrophic diplegia.

HIV Peripheral Neuropathy

There are other HIV-related syndromes, primarily various polyneuropathies, that mimic motor neuron disease. These include chronic inflammatory polyradiculoneuropathy, a multifocal motor neuropathy with anti-GM1 antibodies, or a primary axonal motor polyradiculoneuropathy.

The most common HIV-related polyneuropathy is a distal symmetric primary sensory polyneuropathy (DSP). This occurs in more than one-third of infected patients but may occur in twice as many if asymptomatic patients are also considered. DSP patients develop slowly progressive symmetric numbness and burning sensations in their feet. The pathophysiologic mechanism underlying the development of HIV-associated DSP is not known. Possibilities include cytokine/HIV protein neurotoxicity or primary mitochondrial damage. In addition, several of the early nucleoside reverse transcriptase inhibitor (NRTI) drugs (zalcitabine [ddC], didanosine [ddI], and stavudine [d4T]) have been shown to produce a toxic neuropathy that resembles HIV peripheral neuropathy clinically and electrically. This neuropathy has been postulated to be due to mitochondrial toxicity of these agents, may be additive to HIV neuropathy, and has led these agents to be replaced by newer NRTIs in modern HAART regimens.

HIV Myopathy

Some AIDS patients develop proximal weakness and rarely rhabdomyolysis. Clinically these patients sometimes appear to have an inflammatory myopathy; some of these individuals may occasionally respond to corticosteroid therapy. At other times, the HIV virus has been primarily implicated as the cause of this myopathy. One of the original therapies, zidovudine, was also thought to be primarily myotoxic, although it is difficult to separate this from a primary viral mechanism.

SHINGLES (HERPES ZOSTER)

Etiology and Epidemiology

Shingles is the most common neurologic disease. In the United States, it is estimated that 15% of the population will experience shingles during their lifetime. An aging population, increasing prevalence of immunosuppressed hosts from myriad causes, and widespread adoption of varicella vaccination in children are causing these rates to rise. Advancing age is the most significant risk factor for acute herpes zoster reactivation and development of the chronic neuropathic pain of postherpetic neuralgia (PHN).

The growing use of varicella vaccine reduces the rates of chickenpox in children. As a consequence, fewer adults have experienced viral exposure. Waning varicella-specific immunity in older adults leads to higher rates of shingles. The precise breach of immune surveillance that allows for varicella reactivation remains unknown. Although most cases affect healthy adults, 10% of all patients with lymphoma will develop shingles. In addition to treatment of acute symptoms, further diagnostic evaluation for an underlying carcinoma or lymphoma needs to be considered. Other patients at high risk for herpes zoster include organ-transplant recipients and those receiving corticosteroid therapy. Immunocompromised persons can experience recurrent, multifocal, protracted bouts of acute neuralgia.

Pathophysiology

Focal reactivation of latent varicella-zoster virus (VZV) in sensory ganglia causes the distinctive rash known as shingles. This occurs in two discrete stages. VZV causes varicella (chickenpox), primarily during childhood. Once this disorder clears, this virus becomes inactive and remains latent within the peripheral nervous system sensory ganglia. Here, it persists in the host for many years, with the potential to be reactivated later in life. Reactivation is associated with a declining, virus-specific, cell-mediated immune response. If this dormant virus does regain virulence, it typically presents as shingles. In immunocompetent hosts, this is generally an isolated event, although with an increasingly aging population, some individuals may have more than one episode.

The dorsal root ganglion is the primary site of infection. The virus spreads transaxonally to the skin. Cellular level examination reveals hemorrhagic inflammation extending from the sensory ganglion to its projections in the nerve, skin, and adjacent soft tissue. Virions also spread centrally into the spinal cord, causing an occult focal myelitis in the anterior horn cells. The damage may also ascend into the CNS at the level of the dorsal columns and brainstem.

Clinical Presentation

The clinical onset is often heralded by a few days of relatively severe localized pain or nonspecific discomfort in the affected area. The acute pain of shingles is characterized by burning discomfort associated with volleys of a severe lancinating sensation. At times, this is so uncomfortable that it may mimic an acute to subacute intraabdominal or intrathoracic disorder such as an acute peptic ulcer or even a myocardial infarction. Nociceptive pain from soft tissue inflammation and itching may also be associated. Rarely, VZV produces pain without a rash (zoster sin herpete).

The eruption is unilateral and typically does not cross the midline. It overlaps adjacent dermatomes in 20% of cases. A vesicular skin rash, within a dermatomal distribution, forms the clinical signature of VZV reactivation in the dorsal root ganglion. Although any spinal segment or cranial nerve may be involved, the lower thoracic roots and the ophthalmic sensory ganglia are most commonly affected and thus a zoster rash is found frequently in these levels. Vesicles usually appear 72 to 96 hours later (Fig. 45.5). The lesions have an erythematous base, with a tight, clear bubble that becomes opaque and crusts after 5 to 10 days.

Persistence of neuropathic symptoms beyond 3 months fulfills diagnostic criteria for PHN. This chronic, devastating neuropathic pain of PHN, rather than the nociceptive pain, is the most common significant consequence of shingles. Patients experiencing neuropathic pain report the paradox of numbness and pain in the same region. Affected regions also commonly manifest motor and autonomic deficits. Age, rash severity, intensity of acute pain, and associated neurologic abnormalities are all risk factors for PHN. In most instances, PHN resolves within 6 months after the initial rash.

Ophthalmic herpes zoster with involvement of the first division of the trigeminal nerve is the most common cranial nerve affected. If the rash involves the tip of the nose, it is likely that ophthalmic herpes zoster is present (see Fig. 45.1). All patients with ophthalmic shingles require formal evaluation with a slit lamp and fluorescein study to assess any zoster dendrites and subsequent risk of corneal scarring. Surveillance is warranted because iritis and retinal necrosis may have delayed onset. Patients with this site of herpes zoster involvement are uniquely predisposed to developing a stroke from large vessel carotid vasculitis ipsilateral to the ophthalmic division involvement.

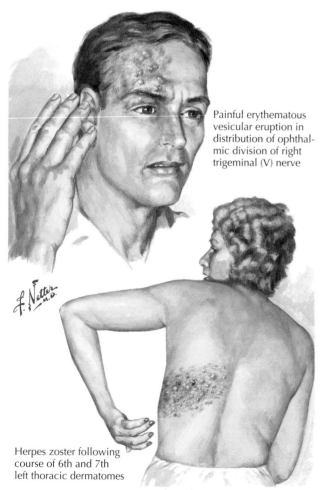

Painful erythematous vesicular eruption in distribution of ophthalmic division of right trigeminal (V) nerve

Herpes zoster following course of 6th and 7th left thoracic dermatomes

Fig. 45.5 Herpes Zoster.

Ramsay Hunt syndrome occurs when herpes zoster affects the geniculate ganglion and subsequently the facial nerve. This syndrome is usually associated with vesicles in the external ear; at times, these are easily overlooked. This lesion sometimes results in tinnitus, vertigo, and deafness.

Very uncommonly, patients whose zoster is characterized by radicular involvement of either the arm or leg may have concomitant loss of motor function. Rarely, severe spinal cord involvement may produce an acute meningoencephalitis mimicking a bacterial process with many polymorphonuclear leucocytes, with a variable prognosis. The telltale shingles rash may be delayed in onset for a few days.

Diagnosis

The rash in itself is sufficient to make the diagnosis. It is the delayed onset of the rash that leads to early diagnostic confusion. At times, the rash is rather subtle, with just a few vesicles developing. It may be easily missed, particularly in hirsute males, unless one carefully searches for its presence.

Treatment

Acute patient care combines treatment of the underlying viral infection, host inflammatory response, and accompanying neuropathic pain. Once the diagnosis of shingles is confirmed, early institution of appropriate antiviral therapy will have important ramifications for the risk of chronic pain symptoms. Formal assessment of pain quality and intensity is critical to analgesic decision making, especially in elderly patients who tend to minimize pain symptoms. Multiple validated verbal, numeric, and visual scales may be used to gauge pain intensity throughout the illness course.

Antiviral medications are the mainstay of acute herpes zoster treatment and need to be administered within 72 hours after rash onset. Acyclovir (800 mg 5 times daily for 1–1.5 weeks) is the treatment of choice for immunocompetent hosts. When treating an immunocompromised host, acyclovir needs to be administered intravenously to prevent generalized zoster rash dissemination. This medication accelerates cutaneous healing, shortens the duration of viral shedding, and reduces the risk of ophthalmic complications.

The effect of medications such as acyclovir on chronic pain is less clear. The potential benefit of combined treatment with corticosteroids is controversial with regard to cutaneous healing and alleviation of acute pain. To reduce the risk of bacterial superinfection, cutaneous lesions need to be kept clean and dry. Oral opioids are first-line therapy and have clearly proven efficacy in reducing neuropathic pain intensity in acute and chronic stages. Opioids are used in combination with a tricyclic drug or gabapentinoid (e.g., nortriptyline or gabapentin). Early use of low-dose tricyclic antidepressants (amitriptyline) for 90 days within the initial months after shingles reduces the likelihood of developing PHN. The most severe cases require IV opioids and regional anesthetic approaches, such as epidural catheter placement.

Because of the clearly defined clinical course and subsequent potential for onset of PHN, the efficacy of analgesics has been studied extensively. Research supports the use of four medication categories: tricyclic antidepressants, anticonvulsants, topical agents, and opioids. Tricyclic antidepressants were the initial medication that proved to have demonstrated efficacy in treatment of PHN. These therapies remain first-line agents. However, anticholinergic side effects and tolerability lead to limitations in the use of these medications.

Prompt trials with other medications may be required if moderate to severe pain persists. The anticonvulsant agent gabapentin and topical sodium channel blockers (lidocaine patches) are current standards of care. Adverse effects (most commonly somnolence and dizziness) are minimized, and patient adherence to treatment is improved when gabapentin is initiated at low doses. The opioid analgesics oxycodone and morphine provide very significant relief of neuropathic pain and often without the hangover associated with mild to increasing doses of gabapentin. Patients with PHN preferred controlled-release morphine in comparison to tricyclic antidepressants. This results in improved outcomes in pain relief and sleep improvement.

The current live attenuated virus shingles vaccine can be given in adults age 60 years and older. More recently, phase III clinical trials of an inactivated recombinant shingles vaccine in 38,000 adults showed 98% reduction in clinical disease and sustained efficacy over 4 years compared with the current live attenuated vaccine (51% reduction—69.8% in adults between the ages of 50 and 59 years to 37.6% in those ≥51 years of age). Reduction in PHN was similar (67%) between the two vaccines. The new vaccine was recently approved by the FDA for adults over 50 and may also be indicated for immunocompromised patients.

RABIES

This is an acute viral CNS disease caused by an RNA virus of the rhabdovirus family. Although usually transmitted to humans through wounds contaminated by the saliva of a rabid animal, rare airborne transmission has occurred in bat-infested caves. Transmission by corneal transplant is also rarely reported.

Etiology and Epidemiology

Animals predominantly infected and involved in rabies transmission vary by geographic area. During 2007 in the United States, 7258 cases of rabies were identified by the CDC in animals, representing a 4.6% increase. Approximately 93% of the cases were in wildlife, and 7% were in domestic animals. Relative contributions by the major animal groups included 2659 raccoons (36.6%), 1973 bats (27.2%), 1478 skunks (20.4%), 489 foxes (6.7%), 274 cats (3.8%), 93 dogs (1.3%), and 57 cattle (0.8%). This represents a significant increase in cases related to bats and foxes, with a diminution in the incidence of raccoon sources, whereas skunks maintain an important steady-state source (see Fig. 45.5). Among domestic sources, cats are three times more likely than dogs to be a potential human source. Cases of rabies in dogs and in sheep and goats increased 17.7% and 18.2% in 2007, respectively, whereas cases reported in cattle, cats, and horses decreased 30.5%, 13.8%, and 20.8%, respectively. These are unusual sources of animal rabies in the United States because of the prevalence of rabies vaccinations in farm animals and pets. Nevertheless, dog and cat bites continue to account for the vast majority of human rabies cases worldwide. Just one case of human rabies was reported in the United States in 2007.

After a rabid dog bite, the rabies virus may travel through the nerves to the spinal cord and into the brain, where it disseminates widely, traveling centrifugally along nerves to the retina, cornea, salivary glands, skin, and other organs. The incubation period ranges from 15 days to more than 1 year. If the virus involves the salivary glands, it usually manifests in 10 to 14 days. Quarantined animals always manifest the disease within 2 weeks if infected.

Clinical Presentation

There are two main "phenotypes": (1) encephalitic (furious) and (2) paralytic (dumb) rabies. There are often paresthesias at the bite site. A prodrome usually occurs with headache, anxiety, and fever. The *encephalitic form* predominates in occurrence (80%). Typically, these patients present with agitation, delirium, seizures, nuchal rigidity, severe pharyngeal spasms, stridor, autonomic instability, and sometimes hydrophobia or aerophobia. These symptoms occur approximately 2 to 10 days after the prodromal period. The *paralytic form* (20% of cases) presents with progressive paralysis until death. The clinical course is

more indolent, with a clear sensorium sometimes preserved until late in the course.

Diagnosis

This is made through demonstration of antirabies glycoprotein antibodies in serum or CSF or through immunofluorescence for glycoprotein antigens in the nuchal skin or brain biopsy. Molecular techniques detect the virus nucleoprotein in CSF, saliva, or biopsy samples.

Clinical manifestations contrast strikingly with neuropathologic findings. Only mild congestion and perivascular inflammation are noted. The Negri body, a neuronal cytoplasmic inclusion with a dark central inner body, is pathognomonic of rabies at autopsy (Fig. 45.6).

Therapy

Improvements in vaccine grown in human cells and human antirabies globulin have made early postexposure prophylaxis safe and effective. The Centers for Disease Control and Prevention's (CDC's) postexposure prophylaxis for rabies includes immediate and thorough wound cleansing with soap and water, administration of human rabies immune globulin around the wound, and rabies vaccine intramuscularly on days 0, 3, 7, 14, and 28. No effective treatment is available after clinical illness develops.

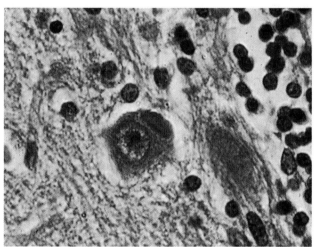

Negri inclusion body in Purkinje cell of brain

Common animal disseminators

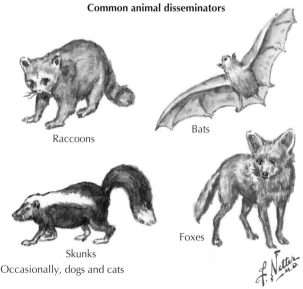

Raccoons

Bats

Skunks

Foxes

Occasionally, dogs and cats

Fig. 45.6 Rabies.

POLIOMYELITIS

> **CLINICAL VIGNETTE** *An 18-year-old man raised by parents who sought their medical care in faith and not from physicians, with no childhood immunizations, reported headache, fever, nausea, and general malaise 1 week after camping. Two days later, he felt better, but 48 hours after that, the general symptoms returned, with more headache, generalized muscle aching and pain, and some drowsiness. When weakness supervened a week after illness onset, he was brought to the emergency department.*
>
> *The patient's temperature was 39.5°C (103.1°F), his pulse was 100 beats/min, and his blood pressure 130/70 mm Hg. He had a stiff neck, generalized muscle tenderness, asymmetric weakness (right arm and left leg more than elsewhere), hypoactive muscle stretch reflexes, flexor plantar responses, normal sensation, and intact cranial nerves.*
>
> *His cough was weak, with a vital capacity of barely 1 L. His WBC count was 15,000/mm³ (40% lymphocytes). Lumbar puncture revealed somewhat cloudy fluid under increased pressure (220 mm water), 170/mm³ nucleated cells (60% polymorphonuclear leukocytes), 150 mg/dL protein, and 80 mg/dL glucose. Spinal MRI showed intramedullary enhancement of the cord, especially the right cervical region.*
>
> *Comment: This is a classic case of poliomyelitis as one would have experienced prior to the widespread utilization of oral and parenteral polio vaccines. In this instance, the patient was at high risk of developing polio from either exposure to a baby recently immunized with live vaccines or the more remote setting here, wherein this young man was inadvertently exposed to wild-type polio virus.*

Epidemiology and Etiology

Poliomyelitis is a word derived from the Greek polio (gray) and myelin (marrow), indicating inflammation of the gray matter of the spinal cord. Spinal cord infection with the poliomyelitis virus leads to the classic paralysis secondary to destruction of the anterior horn cells. The incidence of polio peaked in the United States in 1952, with more than 21,000 cases, but rapidly decreased after introduction of effective killed parenteral Salk vaccines in 1954 and the live Sabin vaccine a few years later.

The last case of wild-virus polio acquired in the United States was in 1979, and the Global Polio Eradication Program dramatically reduced transmission elsewhere. Polio is eradicated from most of the world but is still endemic in a few developing countries, particularly in Nigeria, Afghanistan, and Pakistan. Travelers to areas where naturally occurring poliovirus is endemic need to be vaccinated as follows: persons who have completed an adequate primary series during childhood should have a one-time booster dose of inactivated poliovirus vaccine (IPV); those who have not received a primary series should receive the whole series, although even a single dose prior to travel is of benefit.

Humans are the only known reservoir. Transmission occurs most frequently with an unapparent infection. An asymptomatic carrier state occurs only in those with immunodeficiency. Person-to-person spread occurs predominantly via the fecal–oral route. Infection typically peaks in summer in temperate climates, with no seasonality in the tropics. Poliovirus is highly infectious and may be present in stool up to 6 weeks; seroconversion in susceptible household contacts of children is nearly 100%, and that of adults is greater than 90%. Persons are most infectious from 7 to 10 days before and after symptom onset.

IPV, an inactive, killed vaccine, was licensed in 1955 and used until the early 1960s, when trivalent oral poliovirus vaccine (OPV), containing attenuated strains of all three serotypes of poliovirus in 10:1:3

ratios, largely replaced it. Enhanced potency IPV was introduced in 1988. The viruses are grown in monkey kidney (Vero) cells and are inactivated with formaldehyde. An occasional live vaccine–associated case of paralytic polio continued to occur in infants after their first immunization at approximately 3 months of age until the CDC mandated in the late 1990s that initial vaccinations must be with the Salk IPV. Since then, no such incidents have been reported. Between 1975 and 1992, 189 confirmed cases of paralytic poliomyelitis disease were reported in the United States. These included 10 epidemic cases, 152 vaccine-associated cases, 14 imported cases, and 13 cases of indeterminate origin. Since 1980, no epidemic or indigenously acquired cases of paralytic poliomyelitis caused by wild-type virus have been detected in the United States. Vaccine-associated paralytic polio is thought to occur from a reversion or mutation of the vaccine virus to a more neurotropic form. For this reason, in 2000, the recommendation was made to use IPV exclusively in the United States.

Live attenuated polioviruses replicate in the intestinal mucosa and lymphoid cells in lymph nodes. Vaccine viruses are excreted in stool for up to 6 weeks, with maximal shedding in the first 1 to 2 weeks after vaccination. IPV is highly effective in producing immunity (99% after three doses) and protection from paralytic poliomyelitis. IPV seems to produce less local gastrointestinal immunity than OPV. Thus, persons immunized with IPV could still become infected with wild-type poliovirus and shed it on return to the United States, with subsequent potential spread. Although most individuals in economically privileged countries are immunized, occasionally an instance such as described in the vignette in this chapter is seen. Asymmetric weakness, lack of sensory involvement, and CSF findings help differentiate polio from GBS.

Pathogenesis

Poliovirus is a member of the family Picornaviridae, enterovirus subgroup. Enteroviruses are transient inhabitants of the gastrointestinal tract and are stable at acidic pH. Picornaviruses have an RNA genome; the three poliovirus serotypes (P1, P2, and P3) have minimal heterotypic immunity among them. The virus enters through the mouth and multiplies primarily at the implantation site in the pharynx and gastrointestinal tract; usually, it is present in the throat and stool before clinical onset (Fig. 45.7). Within 1 week of clinical onset, little virus exists in the throat, but it continues to be excreted in the stool for several weeks. The virus invades local lymphoid tissue, enters the bloodstream, and then may infect CNS cells. Viral replication in anterior horn and brainstem motor neuron cells results in cell destruction and paralysis.

Clinical Presentation

The incubation period for poliomyelitis is usually 6 to 20 days, with a range of 3 to 35 days. Clinical response to poliovirus infection varies. Up to 95% of all polio infections are asymptomatic, even though infected persons shed virus in stool and are contagious.

Abortive poliomyelitis occurs in 4% to 8% of infections. It causes a minor illness, without evidence of CNS infection. Complete recovery characteristically occurs within 1 week. Upper respiratory infection (sore throat and fever), gastrointestinal disturbances (nausea, vomiting, abdominal pain, constipation, or rarely diarrhea), and influenza-like illness can all occur and are indistinguishable from other enteric viral illnesses.

Nonparalytic aseptic meningitis, usually occurring several days after a prodrome similar to the minor illness, occurs in a small percentage of infections. Increased or abnormal sensations may occur with stiffness in the neck, back, leg, or a combination of those areas, typically last 2 to 10 days, and are then followed by complete recovery.

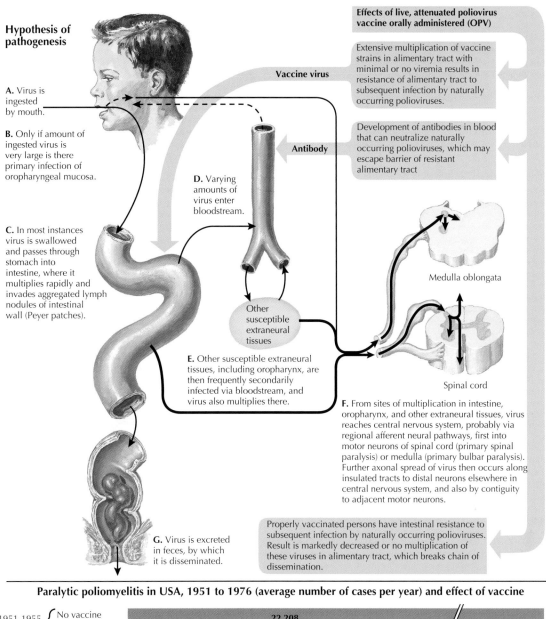

Hypothesis of pathogenesis

A. Virus is ingested by mouth.

B. Only if amount of ingested virus is very large is there primary infection of oropharyngeal mucosa.

C. In most instances virus is swallowed and passes through stomach into intestine, where it multiplies rapidly and invades aggregated lymph nodules of intestinal wall (Peyer patches).

Vaccine virus

D. Varying amounts of virus enter bloodstream.

Antibody

Other susceptible extraneural tissues

E. Other susceptible extraneural tissues, including oropharynx, are then frequently secondarily infected via bloodstream, and virus also multiplies there.

Effects of live, attenuated poliovirus vaccine orally administered (OPV)

Extensive multiplication of vaccine strains in alimentary tract with minimal or no viremia results in resistance of alimentary tract to subsequent infection by naturally occurring polioviruses.

Development of antibodies in blood that can neutralize naturally occurring polioviruses, which may escape barrier of resistant alimentary tract

Medulla oblongata

Spinal cord

F. From sites of multiplication in intestine, oropharynx, and other extraneural tissues, virus reaches central nervous system, probably via regional afferent neural pathways, first into motor neurons of spinal cord (primary spinal paralysis) or medulla (primary bulbar paralysis). Further axonal spread of virus then occurs along insulated tracts to distal neurons elsewhere in central nervous system, and also by contiguity to adjacent motor neurons.

Properly vaccinated persons have intestinal resistance to subsequent infection by naturally occurring polioviruses. Result is markedly decreased or no multiplication of these viruses in alimentary tract, which breaks chain of dissemination.

G. Virus is excreted in feces, by which it is disseminated.

Paralytic poliomyelitis in USA, 1951 to 1976 (average number of cases per year) and effect of vaccine

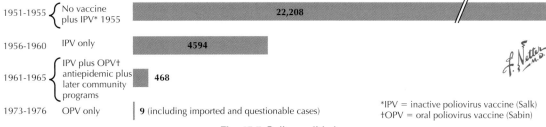

Period	Description	Cases
1951-1955	No vaccine plus IPV* 1955	22,208
1956-1960	IPV only	4594
1961-1965	IPV plus OPV† antiepidemic plus later community programs	468
1973-1976	OPV only	9 (including imported and questionable cases)

*IPV = inactive poliovirus vaccine (Salk)
†OPV = oral poliovirus vaccine (Sabin)

Fig. 45.7 Poliomyelitis-I.

Flaccid paralysis occurs in less than 1% of polio infections. Paralytic symptoms typically begin 1 to 10 days after the prodromal symptoms and evolve for 2 to 3 days. Paralysis does not usually progress after defervescence. In children, the prodrome may be biphasic, with initial minor symptoms separated by 1 to 7 days from major symptoms. Initially, severe muscle aches and spasms are typically seen with significant meningismus and a Kernig sign. The illness evolves into asymmetric flaccid paralysis with diminished muscle stretch reflexes, typically reaching a plateau within days or weeks. Some muscular strength gradually returns. No sensory or cognitive loss occurs. Most patients recover some function, and many recover completely; however, weakness or paralysis that is still discernible 12 months after onset is usually permanent.

Three types of paralytic polio are described. The most common is spinal polio (approximately 79% of cases in the 1970s), characterized by asymmetric paralysis usually involving the legs (Fig. 45.8). Bulbar polio (2%) causes weakness of muscles innervated by cranial nerves. Bulbospinal polio (19%) is a combination of the two. Mortality in paralytic polio cases is lower in children (2%–5%) than in adults (15%–30%) and highest (25%–75%) with bulbar involvement.

Stages in
destruction of
a motor neuron
by poliovirus

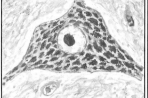

A. Normal motor neuron

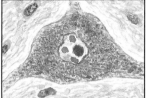

B. Diffuse chromatolysis; three acidophilic nuclear inclusions around nucleolus

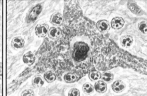

C. Polymorphonuclear cells invading necrotic neuron

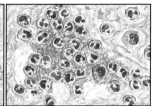

D. Complete neuronophagia

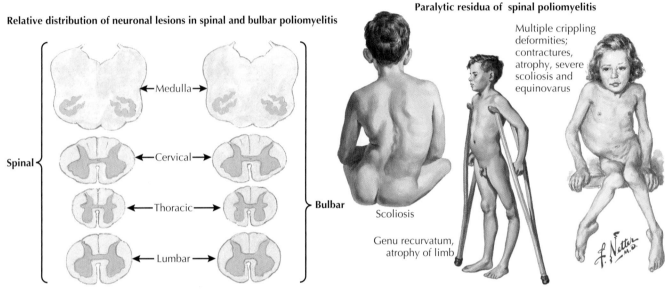

Relative distribution of neuronal lesions in spinal and bulbar poliomyelitis

Medulla

Spinal — Cervical

Thoracic

Lumbar

Bulbar

Paralytic residua of spinal poliomyelitis

Multiple crippling deformities; contractures, atrophy, severe scoliosis and equinovarus

Scoliosis

Genu recurvatum, atrophy of limb

Fig. 45.8 Poliomyelitis-II.

Postpolio Syndrome

This clinical picture usually presents 30 to 40 years after paralytic poliomyelitis early in life, especially during childhood; in these later, and often more advanced, years of life, 25% to 40% of previous acute polio patients note a seeming increased weakness. This, per se, does not constitute recurrence of a dormant infectious process likened to herpes zoster. Rather, it is thought to involve failure of oversized previously reinnervated motor units that developed during the recovery process from the initial paralytic syndrome.

Diagnostic Approach

Poliovirus can be isolated from the pharynx or stool; however, paradoxically this virus is rarely isolated from the CSF. Sequencing can distinguish wild-type from vaccine-type virus in acute flaccid paralysis. Neutralizing antibodies are often present early and at high levels. The CSF usually shows an increased WBC count (10–200 cells/mm^3, primarily lymphocytes) and a mildly increased protein level (generally 40–50 mg/dL).

Prognosis

At its most severe bulbospinal form, poliomyelitis often can be fatal. Today with very much enhanced intensive care support, the fatality rate more than likely would be significantly lessened if poliomyelitis reoccurred with the same incidence so typical of 50 years ago. Fortunately, this disease is now so rare that it is difficult to begin to predict what the outcome might be today. When WNV first appeared about 10 years ago, with its similar predilection for the anterior horn cell, those of us who lived through poliomyelitis as children and adolescents paused to wonder whether this terrible clinical disorder might once again appear in the mask of this virus previously unknown to the Western hemisphere. Very fortunately, our fears were not correct.

ADDITIONAL RESOURCES

Arboviral encephalitides. Available from: https://www.cdc.gov/ncezid/dvbd/index.html. Accessed 9 December 2017.

Comprehensive website maintained by the Centers for Disease Control and Prevention that includes basic fact sheets on the most common vector-borne diseases including arboviral encephalitides, along with information about transmission and life cycles, current global epidemiology, and information about clinical presentation.

CDC Shingles Vaccination. Available from: http://www.cdc.gov/vaccines/vpd-vac/shingles/default.htm. Accessed 9 December 2017.

Comprehensive resource on the herpes zoster vaccine, its use, and information about shingles.

Tunkel AR, Glaser CA, Bloch KC, et al. The management of encephalitis: clinical practice guidelines by the Infectious Diseases Society of America. Clin Infect Dis 2008;47:303–27. Available from: https://academic.oup.com/cid/article/47/3/303/313455. [Accessed 9 December 2017].

Guidelines for the diagnosis and treatment of patients with encephalitis prepared by an Expert Panel of the Infectious Diseases Society of America, intended for use by health care providers who care for patients with encephalitis. Includes data on the epidemiology; clinical features; diagnosis; and treatment of many viral, bacterial, fungal, protozoal, and helminthic etiologies of encephalitis, and provides information on when specific etiologic agents should be considered in individual patients with encephalitis.

CDC Powassan Virus web page: https://www.cdc.gov/powassan/index.html. Accessed 9 December 2017.

Comprehensive resource with up-to-date information on epidemiology, clinical findings, treatment, and prevention.

World Health Organization. Poliomyelitis. Available from: http://www.who.int/topics/poliomyelitis/en/. Accessed 9 December 2017.

Comprehensive resource with up-to-date information on global outbreaks, disease history and clinical findings, and current eradication efforts.

United States Centers for Disease Control and Prevention. Zika virus. Available from: https://www.cdc.gov/zika/.

Comprehensive information about symptoms of Zika virus infection, epidemiology of transmission, testing and treatment.

Pan American Health Organization/World Health Organization. Zika virus. Available from: https://www.paho.org/hq/index.php?option=com_content&view=article&id=11585&Itemid=41688&lang=en.

Comprehensive information with epidemiological alerts and general information about prevention strategies etc.

Centers for Disease Control. CMV infection. Available from: https://www.cdc.gov/cmv/.

Orlikowski D, Porcher R, Sivadon-Tardy V, et al. Guillain-Barré syndrome following primary cytomegalovirus infection: a prospective cohort study. Clin Infect Dis 2011;52(7):837.

Jacobs BC, Rothbarth PH, van der Meché FG, et al. The spectrum of antecedent infections in Guillain-Barré syndrome: a case-control study. Neurology 1998;51(4):1110.

Khalili-Shirazi A, Gregson N, Gray I, et al. Antiganglioside antibodies in Guillain-Barré syndrome after a recent cytomegalovirus infection. J Neurol Neurosurg Psychiatry 1999;66(3):376.

Evidence

Blanton JD, Palmer D, Christian KA, et al. Rabies surveillance in the United States during 2007. J Am Vet Med Assoc 2008;233(6):884–97.

An overview of the animal resources for the rabies virus in the United States.

Cikurel K, Schiff L, Simpson DM. Pilot study of intravenous immunoglobulin in HIV-associated myelopathy. AIDS Patient Care STDS 2009;23(2):75–8.

Dalakas MC, Sever JL, Madden DL, et al. Late postpoliomyelitis muscular atrophy: clinical, virologic, and immunologic studies. Rev Infect Dis 1984;6:S562–7.

Clinical description of 17 patients, ages 31 to 65 years (average, 45), with prior poliomyelitis, who after a number of years of stability had experienced new neuromuscular symptoms. Findings indicate that immunopathologic mechanisms may play a role in new motor-neuron disease that can occur in patients with prior poliomyelitis.

Gubler DJ. The continuing spread of West Nile virus in the western hemisphere. Clin Infect Dis 2007;45:1039–46.

Review article summarizing clinical and epidemiologic aspects of the West Nile virus in the Americas, with discussion and recommendations for vector control and potential vaccines.

Piantadosi A, Rubin DB, McQuillen DP, et al. Emerging cases of Powassan virus encephalitis in New England: clinical presentation, imaging, and review of the literature. Clin Infect Dis 2016;62(6):707–13.

Piantadosi A, Kanjilal S, Ganesh V, et al. Rapid detection of Powassan virus in a patient with encephalitis by metagenomic sequencing. Clin Infect Dis 2017.

Jones HR, Ho DD, Forgacs P, et al. Acute fulminating fatal leuko-encephalopathy as the only manifestation of HIV infection. Ann Neurol 1988;23:519–22.

Kaul M. HIV-1 associated dementia: update on pathological mechanisms and therapeutic approaches. Curr Opin Neurol 2009;22(3):315–20.

Noah DL, Drenzek CL, Smith JS, et al. Epidemiology of human rabies in the United States, 1980 to 1996. Ann Intern Med 1998;128:922–30.

Summary of epidemiologic, diagnostic, and clinical features of the 32 laboratory-confirmed cases of human rabies diagnosed in the United States from 1980 to 1996. Rabies should be included in the differential diagnosis of any case of acute, rapidly progressing encephalitis, even if the patient does not recall being bitten by an animal. Includes recommendations for postexposure prophylaxis.

Oxman MN, Levin MJ, Johnson GR, et al. A vaccine to prevent herpes zoster and postherpetic neuralgia in older adults. N Engl J Med 2005;352:2271–84.

Randomized, double-blind, placebo-controlled trial of live attenuated VZV vaccine in 38,546 adults ≥60 years of age. The vaccine markedly reduced morbidity from herpes zoster and postherpetic neuralgia in this population.

Lal H, Cunningham AL, Godeaux O, et al. Efficacy of an adjuvanted herpes zoster subunit vaccine in older adults. N Engl J Med 2015;372:2087–96.

Randomized, placebo-controlled, phase 3 study of 15,411 adults > 50 years old. During a mean follow-up of 3.2 years, herpes zoster was confirmed in 6 participants in the vaccine group and in 210 participants in the placebo group. Overall, vaccine efficacy against herpes zoster was 97.2% (95% confidence interval [CI], 93.7 to 99.0; P < 0.001). Vaccine efficacy was between 96.6% and 97.9% for all age groups.

Cunningham AL, Lal H, Kovac M, et al. Efficacy of the herpes zoster subunit vaccine in adults 70 years of age or older. N Engl J Med 2016;375:1019–32.

Randomized, placebo-controlled phase 3 study of 13,900 adults 70 years and older. During a mean follow-up period of 3.7 years, herpes zoster occurred in 23 vaccine recipients and in 223 placebo recipients. Vaccine efficacy against herpes zoster was 89.8% (95% confidence interval [CI], 84.2 to 93.7; P < 0.001).

In pooled analyses of data from participants 70 years of age or older in the previous study and the current study, vaccine efficacy against herpes zoster was 91.3% (95% CI, 86.8 to 94.5; P < 0.001), and vaccine efficacy against postherpetic neuralgia was 88.8% (95% CI, 68.7 to 97.1; P < 0.001).

Power C, Boissé L, Rourke S, et al. Neuro AIDS: an evolving epidemic. Can J Neurol Sci 2009;36(3):285-95. Prevention of herpes zoster. Available from: http://www.cdc.gov/mmwr/preview/mmwrhtml/rr5705a1.htm. Accessed 6 December 2017.

Morbidity and Mortality Weekly Report summary of the clinical trials supporting efficacy of herpes zoster vaccine and recommendations for its use in adults ≥60 years of age.

Whitley RJ, Gnann JW. Viral encephalitis: familiar infections and emerging pathogens. Lancet 2002;359:507–13.

Reviews current understanding of viral encephalitides with particular reference to emerging viral infections and the availability of existing treatment regimens, as well as vaccine prevention and vector control.

Wright EJ. Neurological disease: the effects of HIV and antiretroviral therapy and the implications for early antiretroviral therapy initiation. Curr Opin HIV AIDS 2009;4(5):447–52.

46

Parasitic and Fungal Disorders and Neurosarcoidosis

Winnie W. Ooi, Daniel P. McQuillen, H. Royden Jones, Jr.[†]

Parasitic infections of the nervous system range from acute syndromes such as diffuse cerebritis in cerebral malaria to more chronic mass lesions causing seizure disorders such as neurocysticercosis. This chapter will focus on the most common parasites causing central nervous system (CNS) infections.

CEREBRAL MALARIA

> **CLINICAL VIGNETTE** *A 45-year-old previously healthy Indian male working as an engineer in the United States returned from India in August after a 6-week stay visiting with his parents. One week after his return, he presented to the emergency ward with 4 days of fever to 102°F, headache, and diarrhea. His face was flushed; he had mild confusion, severe lethargy, a moderately stiff neck, and a temperature of 39.4°C (103°F). A lumbar puncture demonstrated a normal cerebrospinal fluid (CSF). His peripheral white blood cell (WBC) was 12,000/mm³, with a hemoglobin of 10 g and a platelet count of 40,000/mm³. His blood glucose level was 56 mg/dL. A peripheral blood smear demonstrated multiple intraerythrocytic ring forms consistent with the trophozoites of* Plasmodium falciparum *with a parasite count of 3%.*
>
> *The patient was treated with intravenous artesunate, obtained from the Centers for Disease Control and Prevention (CDC), and doxycycline. He became afebrile, alert, and oriented after 3 days of intravenous therapy. His oral treatment regimen was completed after 7 days of doxycycline.*
>
> *Comment: Malaria remains a major cause of morbidity and mortality in the developing world and the most important treatable cause of acute parasitic infection in travelers returning to their Westernized homelands. In the United States, 1564 imported cases were reported during 2006; 39% were attributable to* P. falciparum. *Immigrants who have recently visited with friends and relatives in their countries of origin often do not take antimalarial prophylaxis and are at higher risk of acquiring malaria.*

Malaria continues to have a global presence, primarily affecting individuals living in South and Central America, Africa, and Asia (Fig. 46.1). Close to a half billion individuals are affected annually with up to a million deaths each year. Previously endemic in the United States, public health measures have greatly decreased its incidence here. However, at least a thousand cases are reported annually here and are primarily related to *P. falciparum* affecting travelers to endemic geographic areas.

Epidemiology

Malaria is caused by four common species of parasites: *P. falciparum, P. vivax, P. ovale,* and *P. malariae.* Each form is transmitted to the human from the bites of infected Anopheles mosquitoes. Erythrocytes infected with mature parasites of *P. falciparum* adhere to endothelial cells in the microvasculature of many organs, including the brain, and undergo a complex interplay with host factors, leading to the manifestations of cerebral malaria.

Clinical Features

Cerebral malaria is the most life-threatening form, having an adult mortality rate of 20%–50%; this is even worse in children. It is caused by *P. falciparum,* with the rare exceptional instance of *P. vivax.* Its primary neurologic features range from irritability and confusion to seizures and coma. Early on there are usually several days of fever and other nonspecific symptoms indistinguishable from those of uncomplicated malaria. Patients may gradually develop coma or in contrast deteriorate suddenly and persistently after a generalized seizure. Grand mal convulsions occur in about half of adult patients. The seizures are often exacerbated by hypoglycemia and lactic acidosis metabolic features that often accompany severe malaria. Hypoglycemia is a common and important abnormality in patients with cerebral malaria and may not be suspected clinically because the symptoms (anxiety, restlessness, and tachycardia) are attributed to the infection itself.

Diagnosis

If malaria is suspected, peripheral blood smears need to be examined every 8–24 hours by an experienced microscopist. In a patient with fever and abnormal mental status who was potentially exposed to malaria, antimalarial chemotherapy must be started immediately even if blood smears are repeatedly negative. Microscopic examination and culture of CSF is also essential in patients with cerebral malaria to exclude other treatable CNS infections.

Therapy

Increased drug resistance has led to combination therapy for malaria. The treatment of cerebral malaria consists of either intravenous quinidine or artesunate accompanied by doxycycline (Fig. 46.2). Intravenous quinidine has to be administered in an intensive care unit (ICU) setting with electrocardiographic monitoring, as it may lead to severe arrhythmias. Exchange transfusion should be strongly considered for persons with a parasite density of more than 5%–10% or even with a lower level of parasitemia if the cerebral malaria is severe or other complications of the malaria occur, including non–volume overload pulmonary edema, or renal complications.

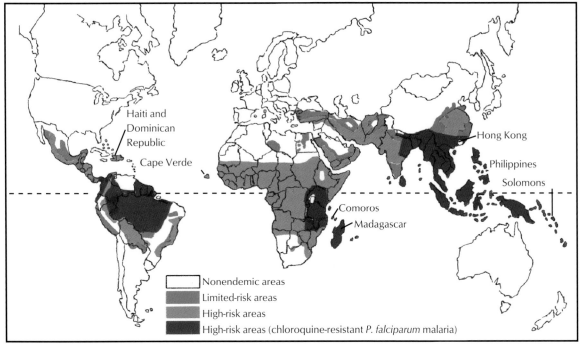

Fig. 46.1 Geographic Distribution of Malaria.

AFRICAN TRYPANOSOMIASIS (SLEEPING SICKNESS)

> **CLINICAL VIGNETTE** *A 38-year-old West African woman, who migrated from her native country 4 months ago, was evaluated in an emergency department for a few weeks of bizarre behavior. In the preceding months, she noted modest weight loss and progressive failure to thrive. She was referred to an inpatient psychiatric service, where she became more lethargic. Her physical examination revealed a low-grade fever with a suspicion of hepatomegaly but was otherwise normal.*
>
> *Laboratory tests demonstrated a white cell count of 6400/mm, hemoglobin 10 g, and normal platelets. Her liver function tests revealed a mild transaminitis. A careful exam of her peripheral blood smear showed a trypomastigote. HIV antibody was negative. The patient's basic CSF parameters were normal. However, both her indirect fluorescent antibody (IFA) and enzyme-linked immunosorbent assay (ELISA) to Trypanosoma gambiense in her CSF were positive. Treatment was started with melarsoprol but was stopped because of progressive encephalopathy. The patient's family signed her out of the hospital against medical advice and she was lost to follow-up.*
>
> *Comment: With the world becoming "smaller," previously "exotic" infectious diseases may now be seen anywhere, including economically highly developed countries. Cultural issues also arise, as illustrated here, where the family made a decision not to allow attempts at a second line of therapy such as intravenous eflornithine when the first medication trial was not successful.*

Epidemiology

After being brought under control for many years, ever since the 1970s, African trypanosomiasis has reemerged as a new epidemic of enormous proportions. This disease is divided into two different forms, each characterized by meningoencephalitis when it reaches more advanced stages. Both are transmitted by the bites of infected tsetse flies.

Clinical Features

West African sleeping sickness accounts for more than 90% of reported cases of sleeping sickness and causes a chronic infection primarily occurring in West and Central Africa. It is caused by *Trypanosoma brucei gambiense*. Individuals can be infected for months or even years without experiencing any major symptoms or signs. Initially, the systemic disease presents with fever, fatigue, weight loss, cervical lymphadenopathy, and hepatosplenomegaly.

Once the neurologic manifestations emerge, the patient often has developed an advanced stage of CNS infection. Personality changes are common; patients are frequently mistaken as having psychiatric disorders, as in the vignette. In the early phases of CNS disease, a disruption of the normal circadian sleep rhythm occurs (Fig. 46.3).

East African trypanosomiasis, caused by *Trypanosome brucei rhodesiense*, causes a more acute infection in contrast to the more chronic West African form. Neurologic symptoms develop rapidly after just a few months or weeks.

Diagnosis

An African sleeping sickness diagnosis is not an easy one to establish in the early phases of the disease when there may not be any CSF changes. Patients are classified as early- or late-stage disease based on CSF findings: those with a CSF WBC greater than 5/mm, often with mild lymphocytic pleocytosis (rarely above 400/mL) and an increased protein content accompanied by a high level of IGM or with trypanosomes demonstrated in CSF seen, are in late-stage disease. Electroencephalography (EEG) can aid in the diagnosis by demonstrating the characteristic impairment in vigilance.

Although visualization of the trypanosome on peripheral smear is the gold standard for diagnosis, immunologic tests such as the ELISA and IFA for antibody levels in the CSF are relatively sensitive and specific for the diagnosis of West African trypanosomiasis. However, no reliable serologic tests for East African trypanosomiasis are currently available for practical diagnostic use.

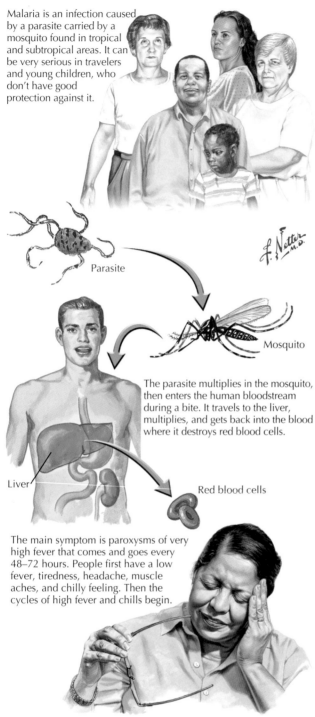

Malaria is an infection caused by a parasite carried by a mosquito found in tropical and subtropical areas. It can be very serious in travelers and young children, who don't have good protection against it.

Parasite

Mosquito

The parasite multiplies in the mosquito, then enters the human bloodstream during a bite. It travels to the liver, multiplies, and gets back into the blood where it destroys red blood cells.

Liver

Red blood cells

The main symptom is paroxysms of very high fever that comes and goes every 48–72 hours. People first have a low fever, tiredness, headache, muscle aches, and chilly feeling. Then the cycles of high fever and chills begin.

Fig. 46.2 Treatment of Malaria.

Therapy

Treatment of African trypanosomiasis is handicapped by the lack of effective nontoxic drugs. Drugs used for early-stage *T. rhodesiense* infection, such as suramin, do not cross the blood-brain barrier. Therefore the risk of disease progression to the neurologic stage exists despite therapy of earlier disease. The most widely used drug is melarsoprol; this is highly toxic because of its own predisposition to cause an encephalopathy. There are also reports of high relapse rates with standard treatment with melarsoprol.

Intravenous eflornithine is an alternative, less toxic drug recommended in areas where the resistance to melarsoprol is greater than

15%. However, it is more expensive and more difficult to administer because it requires longer intravenous injection as opposed to melarsoprol, which requires five intramuscular injections. However, concerns about the development of resistance to monotherapy have prompted clinical trials using combination eflornithine and nifurtimox. Other drugs such as suramin do not cross the blood-brain barrier, and therefore the risk of progression of the disease to the neurologic stage exists despite therapy of earlier disease.

CYSTICERCOSIS

CLINICAL VIGNETTE *A 29-year-old Asian man, a native Chinese previously living in northern India before he immigrated to the United States 10 years ago, presented to the emergency department after having several witnessed tonic-clonic seizures. He had complained of intermittent mild headaches over the prior week and had no significant past medical history.*

On presentation he was postictal; his temperature was 38.5°C (101.3°F). His right pupil was minimally larger than the left, and there was no papilledema. He was intubated during a subsequent seizure for airway protection.

Brain computed tomography (CT) revealed a single hypodense area lateral to the right lateral ventricle. Spinal fluid analysis indicated normal results, including a negative Gram stain. Plain radiographs of his extremities showed multiple small calcific densities in the soft tissues, and a serum cysticercosis immunoblot was positive. He was treated with albendazole and dexamethasone, and his seizures resolved.

Epidemiology

Cysticercosis is a relatively common cause of seizure disorders, particularly in individuals from Central and South America, including those who have immigrated to the United States. It may occur in both immunocompromised and nonimmunocompromised individuals. It results from infection with the larval form of the porcine tapeworm *Taenia solium*. Humans acquire the adult tapeworm by eating undercooked pork and become infected with the larval stage (cysticercus) by ingesting tapeworm eggs. Eggs hatch within the small intestine, burrow into venules, and are carried to distant sites, including the CNS and muscle. Because the larvae are relatively large, they may lodge in the subarachnoid space, ventricles, or brain tissue (Fig. 46.4).

Clinical Presentation

Symptoms may not occur for 4–5 years, when larvae die and provoke an inflammatory response. Cysts within the cerebrum may mimic brain tumors, leading to a variety of focal symptoms. Intraventricular cysts may lead to CSF obstruction with signs of hydrocephalus. On other occasions, subarachnoid space cysts may lead to symptoms of a chronic meningitis and arachnoiditis.

Diagnosis

Old nonviable cysts eventually calcify, simplifying detection. Magnetic resonance imaging (MRI) or contrast-enhanced CT may reveal signs of CNS infection. Serum or CSF serologic study and biopsy of subcutaneous cysts or skeletal muscle calcifications support the diagnosis.

Therapy

Albendazole or praziquantel is the therapy of choice for cysticercosis. Steroids are used to decrease inflammation. Traditional anticonvulsants are indicated to control seizures.

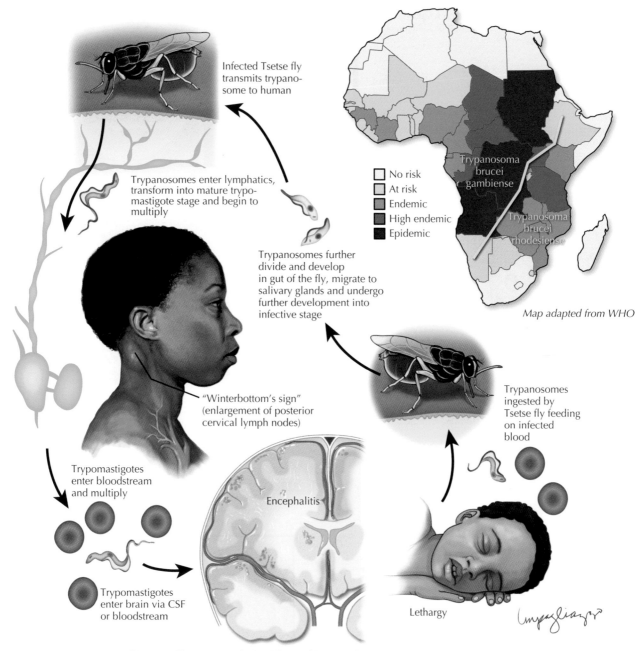

Infected Tsetse fly transmits trypano-some to human

Trypanosomes enter lymphatics, transform into mature trypo-mastigote stage and begin to multiply

Trypanosomes further divide and develop in gut of the fly, migrate to salivary glands and undergo further development into infective stage

Trypanosoma brucei gambiense

Trypanosoma brucei rhodesiense

☐ No risk
☐ At risk
☐ Endemic
☐ High endemic
☐ Epidemic

Map adapted from WHO

"Winterbottom's sign" (enlargement of posterior cervical lymph nodes)

Trypanosomes ingested by Tsetse fly feeding on infected blood

Trypomastigotes enter bloodstream and multiply

Encephalitis

Trypomastigotes enter brain via CSF or bloodstream

Lethargy

Fig. 46.3 Trypanosomiasis (African Sleeping Sickness). *CSF*, Cerebrospinal fluid.

EOSINOPHILIC MENINGITIS

The two major helminths causing acute eosinophilic meningoencephalitis are *Angiostrongylus cantonensis* and *Gnathostoma spinigerum*. These two pathogens are widespread in the tropics, especially Southeast Asia and Central America, and are contracted from the ingestion of contaminated food substances. Other common parasitic pathogens that may rarely cause meningoencephalitis are *Trichinella spiralis*, *Toxocara canis*, and filarial species (including loa loa and *Mansonella perstans*).

TRICHINOSIS

Trichinosis occurs secondary to *Trichinella spiralis*, an intestinal nematode. Human disease most typically occurs after ingestion of contaminated meats, particularly homemade pork sausage or, rarely, bear. These meats contain cysts that harbor the *T. spiralis* larvae that were originally liberated within the stomach by action of gastric enzymes. Subsequently the females are fertilized and then burrow into the intestinal mucosa, eventually reaching the blood supply after traversing the lymphatic system. These larvae have a propensity to survive only in skeletal or cardiac muscle tissue, where they become encysted and eventually calcify. These are passed on from animals to humans after the latter's consumption of the infected tissue.

Shortly after ingestion, one may develop significant upper gastrointestinal distress with nausea and vomiting (Fig. 46.5). Periorbital edema may develop but may be relatively transient, disappearing in few days. If heavily infested pork is ingested, this is soon followed by severe generalized myalgia and sometimes an overwhelming encephalomyelitis and fever not unlike acute bacterial meningitis. Cardiac and diaphragmatic muscle is also at risk and may lead to a fatal outcome

Ovum of *Taenia solium* (pork tapeworm); indistinguishable from that of *T. saginata* (beef tapeworm)

Cysticercus (larval stage) of pork tapeworm; fluid-filled sac (bladder) containing scolex (head) of worm

T. solium ova hatch after ingestion by hogs; embryos migrate to hog tissues and form cysticerci. When humans eat infested pork, intestinal tapeworms develop. However, if humans ingest ova instead of larvae, or if ova reach stomach by reverse peristalsis from intestinal worm, human cysticercosis may occur.

Cysticercosis of brain

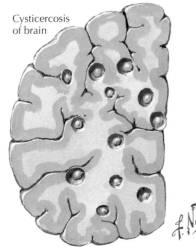

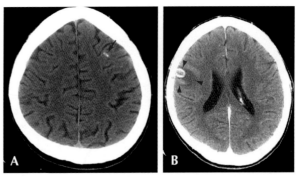

A, Focal calcified cortical mass in left frontal convexity (arrow).
B, Axial post-enhanced cranial CT image demonstrates rim enhancing lesion with surrounding edema in right frontal convexity (arrowheads).

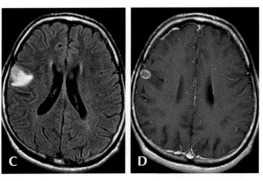

C and **D** Axial FLAIR image demonstrates considerable edema associated with the right frontal convexity mass (arrows), and rim enhancement is noted on the T1-weighted fast spin echo post–gadolinium-enhanced image (arrowheads).

Fig. 46.4 Cysticerosis. *FLAIR,* Fluid-attenuated inversion recovery.

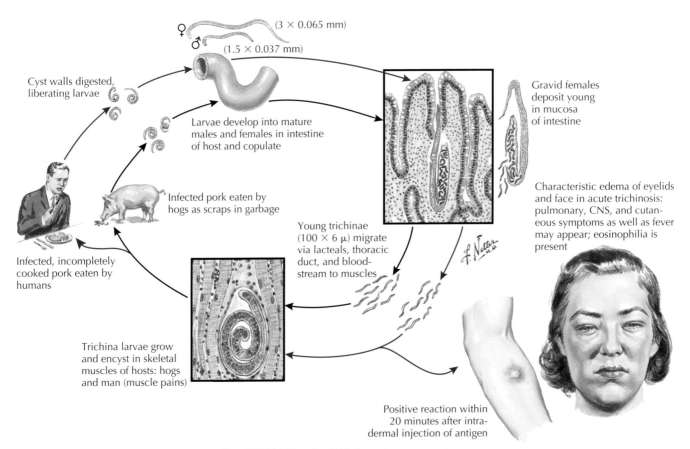

♀ (3 × 0.065 mm)
♂ (1.5 × 0.037 mm)

Cyst walls digested, liberating larvae

Larvae develop into mature males and females in intestine of host and copulate

Gravid females deposit young in mucosa of intestine

Infected pork eaten by hogs as scraps in garbage

Young trichinae (100 × 6 μ) migrate via lacteals, thoracic duct, and bloodstream to muscles

Characteristic edema of eyelids and face in acute trichinosis: pulmonary, CNS, and cutaneous symptoms as well as fever may appear; eosinophilia is present

Infected, incompletely cooked pork eaten by humans

Trichina larvae grow and encyst in skeletal muscles of hosts: hogs and man (muscle pains)

Positive reaction within 20 minutes after intradermal injection of antigen

Fig. 46.5 Trichinosis. *CNS,* Central nervous system.

when severely infested by the trichinella organism. Very rarely there may be cerebral infestation leading to seizures. Major clinical clues to diagnosis include history of periorbital edema, overwhelming myalgia, and a blood count demonstrating a marked leukocytosis with a very marked degree of eosinophilia (>700 cells/mm³).

A more chronic form of trichinosis typically presents with a modest low-grade myalgia. There is also a predilection to involvement of cranial nerve–innervated muscles. This may lead to diplopia, difficulty chewing and swallowing, and dysarthria. Although any extremity muscle may be affected, usually there is a maximal proximal involvement. Initial biopsy may demonstrate an inflammatory myopathy. Once diagnosis is confirmed, usually by skeletal muscle biopsy—sometimes requiring a half gram of tissue to isolate a cyst—treatment is initiated. Corticosteroids, at 40–60 mg of prednisone daily, combined with thiabendazole is the treatment of choice. This leads to recovery in most patients. However, specific therapy is not necessary per se in less severely affected patients, particularly those presenting with only mild myalgia.

SCHISTOSOMIASIS

Schistosoma japonicum and *S. mansoni* are the most common trematodes to affect the nervous system. Schistosomiasis has a global distribution within tropical areas such as the Nile and Amazon river basins. Unwary bathers, particularly those from Europe or North America, become infected when bathing in inviting local rivers and lakes. (One might think that the crocodile population would dissuade these individuals from enjoying these otherwise cooling and inviting waters!)

The host snails are in plentiful supply; the parasite enters the body through the skin, leading to "swimmer's itch." Neurologic symptoms may occur a few months later in about 5% of the exposed population. Typically this leads to an acute myelopathy near the conus medullaris. Cerebral infestation results in seizures.

Complement fixation or liver/rectal mucosa biopsy provide the best diagnostic methodology.

Treatment with praziquantel is often very efficacious. However, it must be expeditiously initiated with acute myelopathy patients; if not, a permanent paraplegia may result. In contrast, cerebral schistosomiasis patients may become seizure free.

OVERVIEW OF FUNGAL INFECTIONS

Cryptococcus neoformans and *Coccidioides immitis* are the most common fungi responsible for CNS fungal disease. These two fungi together with *Histoplasma capsulatum* are capable of causing disease in both healthy individuals and immunocompromised hosts. As cryptococcal disease is discussed in Chapter 50, this section primarily discusses CNS disease caused by *H. capsulatum* and *C. immitis*.

HISTOPLASMOSIS

CLINICAL VIGNETTE *A 30-year-old, right-handed male insurance agent was evaluated for intermittent twitching of his right hand for 3 months. The patient was currently in good health; however, 3 years earlier he experienced an episode of disseminated histoplasmosis when he was working in Ohio trapping rodents in the outdoors. He was treated with itraconazole for 9 months, with apparent cure of his disease. On a recent routine medical examination, a mild neutropenia with a WBC count of 2800/mm and borderline thrombocytopenia were noted. A bone marrow biopsy revealed rare granulomas but negative culture for H. capsulatum.*

Neurologic examination demonstrated a slight intention tremor of his right hand with difficulty writing. His general physical examination was completely

normal. Brain MRI revealed two brain abscesses: a large one in the cerebellum causing a mild midline shift and another in the right frontal cerebral cortex. His urine Histoplasma antigen was positive at 4.6 ELISA units. HIV antibody was negative.

He underwent a biopsy and debulking of his cerebellar lesion, and the fungal smear showed many yeast forms of Histoplasma. The patient was treated for 12 months with voriconazole. He responded well with a rapid normalization in his urinary Histoplasma antigen; however, he had a persistent neutropenia.

Epidemiology

In the United States, histoplasmosis is primarily acquired in the endemic areas of the Ohio and Mississippi river valleys. This occurs from the inhalation of spores of *H. capsulatum* found in the soil contaminated by fecal material from chickens, starlings, and bats. Travelers to other countries where histoplasmosis is also found have acquired it after exposure in caves inhabited by infected bats or from inhalation from spores found in the soil. Most infections are asymptomatic, but symptomatic disease may occur even in the normal host. Disseminated disease tends to occur in infants, the elderly, and patients with hematologic malignancies and HIV infection (where disseminated disease is usually diagnosed in patients with CD4 counts less than 200 cells/mm³).

CNS histoplasmosis is a manifestation of disseminated disease and is uncommon in North America. It mimics tuberculosis with parenchymal involvement occurring as single or multiple focal granulomas (Fig. 46.6). Granulomatous basilar meningitis may also occur. Abscess formation is rare except in immunocompromised hosts. Patients usually present with signs and symptoms of subacute meningitis with fever, stiff neck, and photophobia. Focal neurologic deficits are more common in CNS histoplasmosis than either cryptococcosis or coccidioidomycosis.

Diagnosis

Isolation of *H. capsulatum* is difficult from the CSF; cultures of bone marrow, blood, and urine are more likely to be positive. The more rapid detection of Histoplasma antigen in blood, urine, or CSF is often diagnostic of disseminated histoplasmosis and can be followed to negativity with antifungal therapy. A false-positive test for serum Histoplasma antigen may be present in disseminated coccidioidomycosis.

Therapy

There is no clearly defined therapy that is most effective for CNS histoplasmosis. Initial therapy with liposomal amphotericin followed by itraconazole for at least 1 year is suggested. High rates of relapse of up to 40% occur with shorter periods of therapy. The newer azoles, such as voriconazole and posaconazole, are also effective in vitro and may obviate the unreliable blood levels achieved by itraconazole. HIV-positive patients with histoplasmosis need to stay on suppressive itraconazole therapy unless their CD4 count exceeds 150 cells/mm³.

COCCIDIOIDOMYCOSIS

CLINICAL VIGNETTE *A 68-year-old California woman developed intermittent fever, weight loss, and occasional confusion a few months after a trip around the world that included traveling to West Africa and Brazil. She subsequently had headache and stiff neck and saw her local doctor, who found her with a temperature of 37.7°C (99.8°F), minimally confused but no meningismus, that is, a stiff neck. There were no other significant physical findings.*

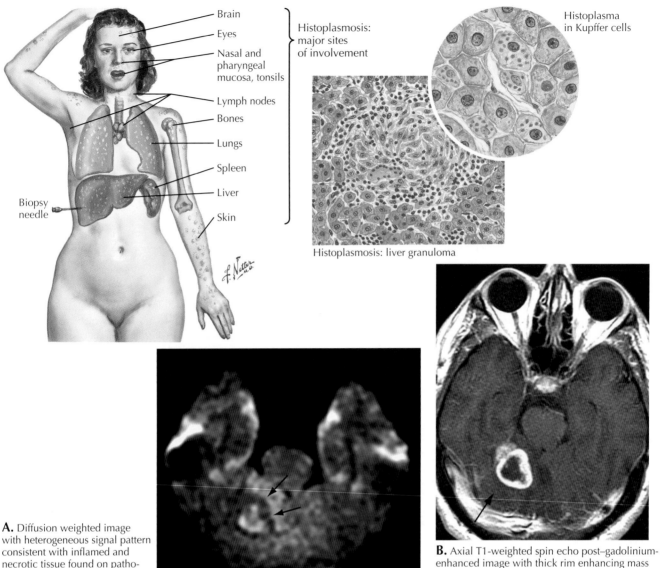

Brain
Eyes
Nasal and pharyngeal mucosa, tonsils
Lymph nodes
Bones
Lungs
Spleen
Liver
Skin

Histoplasmosis: major sites of involvement

Histoplasma in Kupffer cells

Biopsy needle

Histoplasmosis: liver granuloma

A. Diffusion weighted image with heterogeneous signal pattern consistent with inflamed and necrotic tissue found on pathologic examination (arrows).

B. Axial T1-weighted spin echo post–gadolinium-enhanced image with thick rim enhancing mass (arrow).

Fig. 46.6 Histoplasmosis.

Chest radiograph revealed mediastinal lymphadenopathy with some fibrosis in the right upper lobe. Her tuberculin skin test, purified protein derivative (PPD) was negative. A lumbar puncture demonstrated a CSF WBC count of 112/mm³, a protein of 80 mg/dL, and glucose of 45 mg/dL. Brain MRI showed basilar meningitis. Her complement fixation titer to C. immitis was 1:8 in the CSF. Her CSF culture did not grow any fungal organisms.

She was started on 800 mg of intravenous fluconazole and intrathecal amphotericin. Mild right-sided hydrocephalus developed but it did not progress with continued therapy. Her symptoms cleared over the next several months with improvement of her MRI. She completed a course of 6 months of intrathecal amphotericin until her CSF parameters normalized and her complement fixation titer became negative. She is being continued on 400 mg of oral fluconazole. It is anticipated that because of her advanced age, she would require this drug lifelong.

Epidemiology

C. immitis is found in soil only in the Western Hemisphere, particularly in the southwestern United States, the northern Pacific coast of Mexico, Guatemala, Honduras, and Venezuela. Aerosolized arthroconidia are inhaled and frequently infect individuals asymptomatically in endemic areas. About 0.5% of exposed patients will develop disseminated disease via lymphatic or vascular spread to the skin, bone, meninges, and genitourinary tract. CNS involvement develops in 33%–50% of patients with disseminated disease. Sometimes the neuraxis is the only site of symptomatic disease. Risk factors for dissemination include older age, pregnancy, and immunosuppression (including HIV infection).

Clinical Features

When there is CNS involvement, this infection causes a subacute to chronic meningitis with a predilection for the basilar meninges. Here a progressive fibrosing granulomatous reaction occurs. This may result in hydrocephalus that eventually requires shunting. Focal space-occupying lesions are rare. *C. immitis* is recovered in CSF in only 50% of patients with known meningitis.

Diagnosis

Confirmation of the presence of coccidiomycosis is presumptively made in patients with chronic meningitis if the complement fixing antibody to *C. immitis* is positive in the CSF and any titer or the serum complement fixation titer to *C. immitis* is positive at 1:16.

Therapy

Treatment with high-dose fluconazole (400–800 mg/day) in uncomplicated cases is preferred by many physicians. In patients with high antibody titers in the CSF or who are immunosuppressed, this is often best accompanied by intrathecal administration of amphotericin. Patients who respond to oral fluconazole should probably continue on this regimen indefinitely. Those who do not respond initially to the azoles should be started on intrathecal amphotericin. CNS vasculitis is another complication of coccidioidal meningitis. This may respond to the addition of high-dose steroids.

EVIDENCE

Bos MM, Dvereem S, van Engelen BGM, et al. A case of neuromuscular mimicry. Neuromuscul Disord 2006;16:510–13.

Galgiani JN, Ampel NM, Blair JE, et al. Practice guidelines for the management of coccidioidomycosis. Clin Infect Dis 2005;41:1217–23.

Kaiboriboon K, Olsen TJ, Hayat GR. Cauda equina and conus medullaris syndrome in sarcoidosis. Neurologist 2005;11:179–83.

Kellinghaus C, Schilling M. Lüdemann P. Neurosarcoidosis: clinical experience and diagnostic pitfalls. Eur Neurol 2004;51:84–8.

Lejon V, Buscher P. Cerebrospinal fluid in human African trypanosomiasis: a key to diagnosis, therapeutic decision and post-treatment follow-up. Trop Med Int Health 2005;10(5):395–403.

Neurologic involvement in falciparum malaria. J Watch Neurol 2007;2007:3.

Stitch A, Abel PM, Krishna S. Clinical review of human African trypanosomiasis. Br Med J 2002;325:203–6.

Terushkin V, Stern BJ, Judson MA, et al. Neurosarcoidosis: presentations and management. Neurologist 2010;16(1):2–15. Review.

Wheat LJ, Musial CE, Jenny-Avital E. Diagnosis and management of central nervous system histoplasmosis. Clin Infect Dis 2005;40:844–53.

ADDITIONAL RESOURCES

Centers for Disease Control Division of Parasitic Disease—African trypanosomiasis. Available from: http://www.cdc.gov/ncidod/dpd/parasites/trypanosomiasis/default.htm. [Accessed 5 February 2009].

Coccidioidomycosis. Available from: http://www.idsociety.org/content.aspx?id=9200#cocc.

Evidence-based statements developed to assist practitioners and patients in making decisions about appropriate health care for specific clinical circumstances. Guidelines for treatment of infections by organ system and organism may be found here.

Fungal infections. Available from: http://www.idsociety.org/content.aspx?id=9200.

Histoplasmosis. Available from: http://www.idsociety.org/content.aspx?id=9200#hist.

Practice guidelines of the Infectious Diseases Society of America. Available from: http://www.idsociety.org/Content.aspx?id=9088. [Accessed 5 February 2009].

World Health Organization—African trypanosomiasis. Available from: http://www.who.int/topics/trypanosomiasis_african/en/. [Accessed 5 February 2009]. www.medicalecology.org/diseases/d_african_trypano.htm.

47

Neurosarcoidosis

Pooja Raibagkar, Haatem M. Reda

Sarcoidosis is a multisystem granulomatous autoinflammatory disorder that typically affects lungs, lymph nodes, and skin. The nervous system is involved in 5% to 20% of patients with sarcoidosis. Neurosarcoidosis (NS) has a predilection for the meninges (resulting in cranial neuropathies and radiculopathies), pituitary gland, hypothalamus, and orbital apex but can involve any level of the neuraxis including the brain parenchyma, cerebellum, spinal cord, peripheral nerves, and muscle. Given its protean manifestations, a high clinical suspicion is necessary to identify NS as a diagnostic possibility, not least for its potential to cause long-term disability if untreated.

CLINICAL VIGNETTE *A 31-year-old man experienced gradually progressive tingling and numbness from the nipples down to his feet on both sides accompanied by weakness in the lower limbs and symptoms of urinary retention. He experienced shocklike paresthesias in his back and lower limbs with neck flexion (Lhermitte sign). A week later he developed painless lumpy swellings in the cheeks and anterior neck that gradually decreased in size over the subsequent several weeks. During this time, he developed a chronic nonproductive cough and shortness of breath. He did not have a rash or difficulty with vision. On examination, he had mild asymmetric spastic paraparesis with extensor plantar responses. He had a spastic gait and a truncal sensory level at approximately T5.*

The patient underwent magnetic resonance imaging (MRI) of the cervical and thoracic spine, which revealed an intramedullary, expansile, T2-hyperintense lesion extending from the level of the C4 vertebral body to just above the conus medullaris with nodular enhancement along the ventral aspect of the lesion between the T2 and T8 levels (Fig. 47.1). Computed tomography (CT) of the chest, abdomen, and pelvis revealed extensive mediastinal and hilar lymphadenopathy as well as multiple small pulmonary nodules. A transbronchial lung biopsy was performed showing noncaseating granulomatous inflammation in the lung parenchyma. Acid-fast, periodic acid–Schiff, and Gomori methenamine silver stains were negative for acid-fast and fungal organisms. In retrospect, it was thought that he had also had parotitis based upon the history of transient cheek swelling.

Treatment was started with oral prednisone 1 mg/kg for 4 weeks followed by a gradual taper over 6 months. The patient's symptoms ceased progressing soon after the initiation of treatment, and over the ensuing months he experienced modest improvement but not complete resolution of symptoms, signs, or radiographic abnormalities.

EPIDEMIOLOGY

Isolated nervous system involvement is uncommon (observed in 5%–17% of patients with NS). The worldwide prevalence of sarcoidosis is 1 to 40 per 100,000, with a relatively higher rate in women and in people of African or Scandinavian descent. Onset is typically in the third to fifth decades of life.

CLINICAL PRESENTATION

The most common presenting features are cranial nerve palsies (reported in 55%) and headache (30%). The facial and optic nerves are preferentially affected, with occasional involvement of the trigeminal and vestibulocochlear nerves. Bilateral facial nerve palsy is seen in about one-third of cases. Cranial nerve involvement can be related to nuclear and/or nerve involvement at any level or to subacute leptomeningitis, which is a characteristic clinical manifestation of NS that most commonly causes headache with or without focal neurologic deficits.

Hypothalamic and pituitary involvement may result from extension of inflammation along the perivascular Virchow-Robin spaces from the basal meninges. Inflammation of the ependyma and arachnoid villi disrupts cerebrospinal fluid (CSF) outflow and predisposes to communicating hydrocephalus. Other forms of cerebral involvement occur from masslike lesions in the supratentorial or infratentorial parenchyma, resulting in headache, seizures, focal neurologic deficits, and cognitive dysfunction. Rare cerebral manifestations include vasculitis and ischemic stroke.

Spinal cord, peripheral nerve, and muscle involvement is seen in 15% to 20% of NS cases. Although the cranial nerve palsies of NS can be self-limiting, spinal cord and spinal nerve root involvement usually causes lifelong disability. Pathologic evidence of small-fiber peripheral neuropathy can be found in nearly 50% and may result in burning pain and paresthesias in a nonlength-dependent pattern (that is, in the limbs, trunk, and/or face, often asymmetrically). Autonomic dysfunction—including gastroparesis, orthostatic hypotension, and hypohidrosis—may accompany cutaneous small-fiber peripheral neuropathy. Nonlength-dependent demyelinating or axonal polyneuropathy and polyradiculoneuropathy have also been reported. Myopathy is usually subclinical but may present as myositis or chronic progressive nodular myopathy, occasionally with palpable intramuscular nodules.

Because the neurologic and neuroendocrine manifestations are nonspecific, the general examination may provide additional clues, such as lymphadenopathy, parotitis, uveitis, erythema nodosum, and hepatomegaly.

DIAGNOSIS

The diagnosis of NS can be challenging in cases of isolated nervous system disease, as definitive diagnosis requires histopathologic confirmation. In such cases, a tissue specimen is essential prior to starting immunomodulatory therapy. When the diagnosis of sarcoidosis has been established by systemic involvement, the focus of management

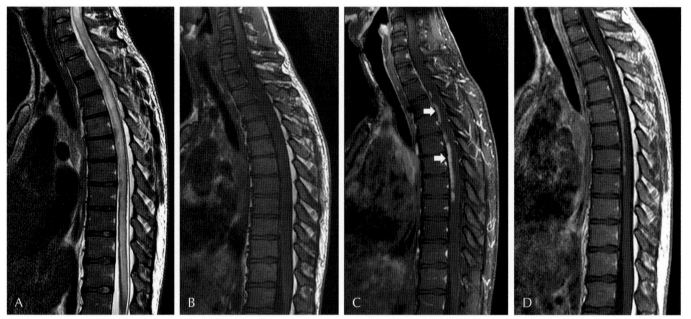

Fig. 47.1 Imaging Findings of Neurosarcoidosis Affecting the Spinal Cord. (A) T2-weighted (T2W) sagittal magnetic resonance imaging (MRI) showing intramedullary T2-hyperintensity extending from the level of the C4 vertebral body to just above the conus medullaris. T1W precontrast (B) and postcontrast (C) sagittal MRI showing nodular enhancement along ventral cord from the T2–T8 vertebral levels *(arrows)*. (D) T1W sagittal postcontrast MRI at 6 months after initiation of treatment showing improvement in a nodular enhancing lesion from the T2–T8 vertebral levels.

becomes excluding other etiologies with neuroimaging, spinal fluid analysis, and laboratory testing.

Diagnostic criteria have been proposed that simplify the classification of NS as definite, probable, or possible. Patients with definite NS have histopathologic confirmation by nervous system biopsy. Patients with probable NS have compatible evidence for nervous system inflammation in the setting of known systemic sarcoidosis. Patients with possible NS have a typical clinical and radiographic presentation without pathologic confirmation. In practice, typical evidence for granulomatous inflammation (either by gadolinium-enhanced magnetic resonance imaging [MRI] or CSF analysis) in patients with confirmed systemic disease may suffice to initiate treatment for presumed NS.

Contrast-enhanced MRI is sensitive but not specific for NS. In the brain, special attention should be paid to abnormalities of the basal meninges, including focal or widespread nodular leptomeningeal or pachymeningeal thickening and enhancement along with involvement of the pituitary stalk, hypothalamus, and cranial nerves. Although enhancing lesions indicate active disease, the converse is not the rule—enhancement patterns are quite variable. Nonspecific imaging features include hydrocephalus and periventricular white matter abnormalities. In the spine, the range of abnormalities on MRI is equally broad but typically includes infiltrative intramedullary lesions spanning multiple levels with nodular enhancement and meningeal involvement. Spinal nerve root thickening and enhancement, including of the cauda equina, are also within the spectrum of NS. Sarcoid nodules are metabolically active and avidly take up fluorodeoxyglucose (FDG) on positron emission tomography (PET).

Elevated protein with or without pleocytosis, oligoclonal bands, elevated immunoglobulin G (IgG) index, and hypoglycorrhachia are typical CSF findings in at least two-thirds of patients with NS. The CSF angiotensin converting enzyme (ACE) level has poor diagnostic accuracy and correlation with clinical activity. There is likewise no specific serum marker for the diagnosis of sarcoidosis. Serum ACE, erythrocyte sedimentation rate (ESR), and/or C-reactive protein (CRP) may be elevated in less than half of these patients. Detailed evaluation for extraneural sarcoidosis is especially important when only neural involvement is suspected. Lymphadenopathy on examination or body computerized tomography (CT) may identify targets for biopsy. Elevated liver enzyme levels and hypercalcemia may also be seen in patients with sarcoidosis.

THERAPY

The mainstay of treatment of NS is suppression of granulomatous inflammation. Induction is achieved with high-dose corticosteroid therapy followed by prevention of recurrence with steroid-sparing immunomodulatory treatment. To date there have been no randomized controlled trials comparing steroid-sparing agents, durations of treatment, or monitoring of disease activity by ancillary investigations. However, tumor necrosis factor-α (TNF-α) inhibitors have been considered more effective at maintaining remission than mycophenolate mofetil, azathioprine, or methotrexate.

Initial treatment is typically with corticosteroids, usually oral prednisone 1 mg/kg/day. Intravenous methylprednisolone 1000 mg/day for 3 to 5 days followed by an oral corticosteroid is favored by some centers for severe brain or spinal cord disease. A gradual taper of the corticosteroid over 3 to 6 months may be considered after resolution and/or stability of the inflammatory process has been established. A second-line steroid-sparing agent is usually required to taper down steroids and prevent steroid-related side complications. Patients should be monitored closely for disease relapse during a corticosteroid taper in a multidisciplinary setting. About one-third of patients may not achieve complete remission and mortality is about 5%.

FUTURE DIRECTIONS

NS is an idiopathic autoimmune disorder capable of causing disease at every level of the nervous system. It has a broad spectrum of clinical presentations and a paucity of definitive tests. However, once the diagnosis is made with either histopathologic confirmation or the ancillary investigations described earlier, complete remission can be achieved in about one-third of patients. Despite the availability of multiple immunomodulatory agents with promising results, mostly from TNF-α inhibitors, there is a need for more evidence-based guidelines regarding the duration of treatment and monitoring of disease activity.

ADDITIONAL RESOURCES

Fritz D, van de Beek D, Brouwer MC. Clinical features, treatment and outcome in neurosarcoidosis: systematic review and meta-analysis. BMC Neurol 2016;16(1):220.

Hebel R, Dubaniewicz-Wybieralska M, Dubaniewicz A. Overview of neurosarcoidosis: recent advances. J Neurol 2015;262(2):258–67.

Kellinghaus C, Schilling M, Lüdemann P. Neurosarcoidosis: clinical experience and diagnostic pitfalls. Eur Neurol 2004;51:84–8.

Tana C, Wegener S, Borys E, et al. Challenges in the diagnosis and treatment of neurosarcoidosis. Ann Med 2015;47(7):576–91.

Tavee JO, Stern BJ. Neurosarcoidosis. Continuum (Minneap Minn) 2014;20(3 Neurology of Systemic Disease):545–59.

Infections in the Immunocompromised Host

Sujit Suchindran, Daniel P. McQuillen, Donald E. Craven

Immunocompromised hosts are susceptible to a wide range of neurologic infections, which include both opportunistic infections and those typically found in normal hosts. The risk for particular infections is related to a number of factors including the type of immune suppression, the duration of immune compromise, and geographic or epidemiologic risk factors. For example, the infection risk profile of a human immunodeficiency virus and acquired immunodeficiency syndrome (HIV/AIDS) patient with CD4 (cluster of differentiation 4) T cell count less than 100 cells/μL is different from the risk profile of a patient taking low-dose chronic corticosteroids. Immunocompromised patients often have more blunted clinical presentations based on the degree of immunosuppression, but remain at risk for more severe manifestations compared to nonimmunocompromised hosts. They are also more likely to have multiple infections, which can make diagnosis difficult.

LISTERIOSIS

Microbiology and Epidemiology

Listeria monocytogenes is a gram-positive rod that is found widespread in the environment, but primarily in soil and decaying food. It is transmitted via oral consumption and has pathologic connotations in the immunocompromised, pregnant women, neonates, and the elderly.

Clinical Presentation

This organism must always be suspected in patients with epidemiologic risk factors such as long-term corticosteroid use who develop acute meningoencephalitis. Neurologic presentation can be variable, with a significant portion of those with central nervous system (CNS) infection not displaying classic meningeal signs. In addition to headache, fever, and meningismus, listeriosis can lead to focal neurologic signs, ataxia, cranial nerve palsies, and seizure. Brain abscesses are less common, but have been noted. Apart from CNS manifestations, listeriosis causes gastroenteritis and a sepsis syndrome of unclear etiology.

Diagnostic Approach

Cerebrospinal fluid (CSF) identification of gram-positive rods in association with a polymorphonuclear leukocytosis and a concomitant low CSF glucose level are the cornerstones to recognition of this uncommon form of bacterial meningitis (Fig. 48.1). Frequently, blood cultures will also be positive. MRI findings of isolated rhombencephalitis in the appropriate clinical scenario are suggestive of listeriosis.

Treatment

Ampicillin or penicillin and synergistic gentamicin are the treatments of choice. In penicillin-allergic patients, trimethoprim-sulfamethoxazole is an alternative, although penicillin desensitization is preferable.

NOCARDIOSIS

Microbiology and Epidemiology

Nocardia species are filamentous, gram-positive branching rods in the actinomycetes group. The most common species found to cause infection are in the *Nocardia asteroides* group. They are normally present in soil and water environments. Infection is more associated with chronic glucocorticoid use and organ transplantation than HIV/AIDS.

Clinical Presentation

Primary nocardiosis usually involves the lung, which is the route of inoculation. Due to specific affinity for neural tissue, infection can spread to the CNS where it can lead to brain abscess without any predilection for specific location. Predominant symptoms include fever, headache, and seizure, rather than meningeal signs. Pulmonary disease even in the absence of neurologic symptoms should prompt CNS imaging in immunocompromised patients.

Diagnostic Approach

Brain biopsy is the most reliable diagnostic technique if the diagnosis cannot be made by evaluation of pulmonary or skin lesions (Fig. 48.2). Nocardia are weakly acid-fast and can be stained with the modified Ziehl-Neelsen method. They may be isolated on Sabouraud medium or brain-heart infusion agar, but growth may not be visible for 2 to 4 weeks.

Treatment

Trimethoprim-sulfamethoxazole is the drug of choice for nocardiosis, although combination therapy may be warranted empirically until drug susceptibility data are known. Initial drug regimens can also include a carbapenem or an aminoglycoside such as amikacin. Therapy should continue for at least 3 months or for several weeks after clinical resolution of the lesion. The latter part of treatment can be on oral antibiotics.

CRYPTOCOCCOSIS

CLINICAL VIGNETTE *A 34-year-old man presented with a month-long history of constant increasingly intense headaches having recently been evaluated for the same complaint at two other hospitals. The headache was accompanied by intermittent photophobia, nausea, and vomiting. Two weeks previously, an ulcerating lesion on his cheek was unsuccessfully treated with doxycycline for possible rickettsial infection. He also had a 20-pound weight loss. Previously, he had helped his father raise homing pigeons.*

He was lethargic but able to answer simple questions. Temperature was 39.4°C (102.9°F). Mild nuchal rigidity was present. No focal neurologic findings were present. His CSF was hazy in color with an elevated opening pressure, white blood cell (WBC) 29 (22% neutrophils, 54% lymphocytes, and 20% monocytes), a protein of 50 mg/dL, and glucose of 9 mg/dL (concomitant serum glucose 125). India ink staining of his CSF demonstrated multiple encapsulated yeast forms. Cryptococcal antigen was positive at 1:1024. HIV testing was negative; however, his CD4 count was low (100 cells/μL).

Despite intravenous amphotericin B and flucytosine, and daily spinal taps, he suffered some loss of vision because of effects of increased intracranial pressure. He was subsequently discovered to have a B-cell lymphoma.

Cryptococcosis

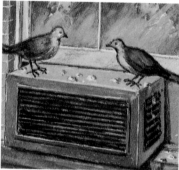

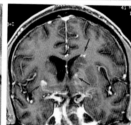

Infection is by respiratory route. Pigeon dung and air conditioners may be factors in dissemination.

Coronal SPGR T1-weighted image post–gadolinium enhanced demonstrates multiple small enhancing lesions in bilateral basal ganglia (arrows).

f. Netter
M.D.

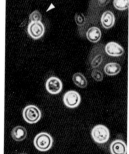

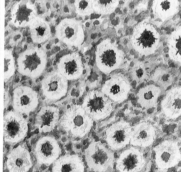

India ink preparation showing budding and capsule

Accumulation of encapsulated cryptococci in subarachnoid space (PAS or methenamine-silver stain)

Listeriosis

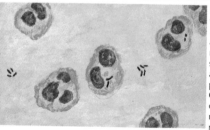

Smear of CSF showing white blood cells and *Listeria* organisms, which appear as gram-positive rods. They may be very short, to resemble cocci, and they often orient in palisades suggestive of Chinese characters. They cause severe purulent meningitis, most commonly in immunocompromised patients or newborns.

Fig. 48.1 Cryptococcosis and Listeriosis. *CSF,* Cerebrospinal fluid; *PAS,* periodic acid-Schiff.

Microbiology and Epidemiology

This chronic, subacute, and, rarely, acute CNS infection is caused by *Cryptococcus neoformans,* a yeastlike fungus. Distributed worldwide in soil, fruits, and matter contaminated by pigeon excreta, this organism probably enters the body through the lungs and then disseminates to all organs (see Fig. 48.1). Mild, self-limited infections are common. It is considered an AIDS-defining illness among those with HIV, and is typically associated with CD4 cell count less than 100 cells/μL.

Clinical Presentation

Cryptococcal disease can develop in both healthy and immunocompromised patients. Chronic meningitis is the most common presentation. These patients are often afebrile and have no more than minimal nuchal rigidity. Clinically this disorder usually presents insidiously over a matter of months with symptoms of low-grade headache, nausea, irritability, somnolence, and clumsiness. Cranial nerve involvement occurs in 20% of patients characterized by diminished visual acuity sometimes with papilledema, diplopia, and facial numbness. Dementia may occur in some secondary to direct cerebral involvement. Skin lesions can indicate disseminated infection.

Diagnostic Approach

Examination of the CSF demonstrates an elevated opening pressure, often greater than 200 mm H$_2$O in HIV/AIDS patients, a lymphocytic leukocytosis with a WBC count of 40 to 400/mm^3, increased CSF protein concentration, and a decreased glucose level. Although India ink preparations can define the organism, isolation in culture of *C. neoformans* is the best diagnostic test. Latex agglutination for detection of cryptococcal capsular antigen (in serum and CSF) is also available as a rapid test that is often replacing India ink staining.

Treatment

Treatment is best carried out with at least a 2-week course of intravenous amphotericin B or liposomal amphotericin B with or without flucytosine. Neurologic complications including ocular manifestations or focal infection known as cryptococcoma should prompt longer induction treatment. Thereafter, oral fluconazole is administered for at least 6 weeks. Maintenance therapy is recommended for patients with HIV/AIDS until immune reconstitution occurs with combination antiretroviral therapy (ART), with ultimate duration typically at least 1 year. In HIV/AIDS patients diagnosed with cryptococcal infection, initiation of ART typically occurs weeks after antifungal treatment has started due to the risks posed by immune reconstitution inflammatory syndrome (IRIS).

TOXOPLASMOSIS

CLINICAL VIGNETTE *A 49-year-old male with a history of genital herpes presented with neurologic deficits after a motor vehicle accident. In the weeks prior to admission, he noted severe frontal headache with right-sided weakness. In the field after the accident, he had a witnessed seizure with urinary incontinence. He was brought to the hospital in a postictal state.*

Brain computed tomography (CT) showed left-sided vasogenic edema with midline shift and magnetic resonance imaging (MRI) revealed four heterogeneously enhancing lesions, measuring up to 2.0 cm. HIV test was positive and CD4 count was 66 cells/μL with HIV viral load 258,000 copies/mL. Toxoplasma immunoglobulin G (IgG) titer was 232.0 IU/mL. Biopsy was deferred and treatment was initiated with pyrimethamine, sulfadiazine, and leucovorin along with antiepileptics. He started ART as an outpatient with dolutegravir, tenofovir, and emtricitabine. Repeat MRI 6 weeks later showed marked improvement of the enhancing lesions, surrounding edema, and associated mass effect. There were no new lesions seen.

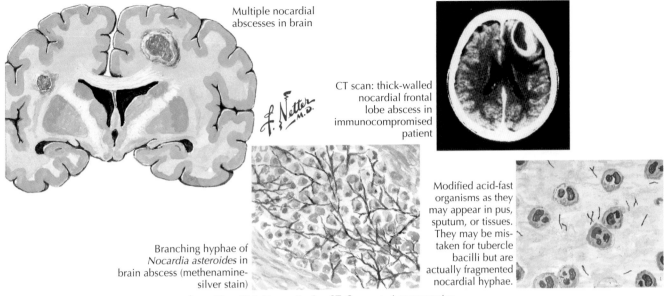

Multiple nocardial abscesses in brain

CT scan: thick-walled nocardial frontal lobe abscess in immunocompromised patient

Branching hyphae of *Nocardia asteroides* in brain abscess (methenamine-silver stain)

Modified acid-fast organisms as they may appear in pus, sputum, or tissues. They may be mistaken for tubercle bacilli but are actually fragmented nocardial hyphae.

Fig. 48.2 Nocardiosis. *CT,* Computed tomography.

Microbiology and Epidemiology

Toxoplasma gondii is a parasite that infects most mammalian species (Fig. 48.3). Humans may acquire *T. gondii* infections by ingestion, transplacental transmission, blood transfusion, or organ transplantation. Oral route infection results from ingestion of *T. gondii* cysts in undercooked food (pork, lamb) or *T. gondii* oocysts found in the feces of cats. Human intestinal tract enzymes liberate *T. gondii* trophozoites, which cause clinical toxoplasmosis. Serologic evidence of toxoplasma infection is present in 50% of the US population. In most instances, *T. gondii* is a subclinical infection primarily manifested by cervical lymphadenopathy.

Clinical Presentation

In immunocompetent hosts, the major manifestations of *T. gondii* infection are a congenital infection, nonspecific febrile syndrome, ocular infection, or lymphadenopathy. Diffuse encephalitis, meningoencephalitis, or cerebral mass lesions due to reactivation of infection are the predominant neurologic abnormalities in advanced AIDS patients having toxoplasmosis. Common symptoms are fever, headache, focal deficits, or seizure. Focal masses are often multiple, leading potentially to multifocal symptoms depending on the clinical sites of involvement.

Diagnostic Approach

The diagnosis of toxoplasma encephalitis is typically based on clinical grounds, rather than by direct sampling. Invariably, the CD4 count among AIDS patients is less than 100 cells/μL. Brain MRI with gadolinium is the most sensitive radiologic diagnostic technique, and typically shows multiple ring-enhancing lesions. If the clinical symptoms and radiographic findings are consistent, positive serologic testing of *T. gondii* IgG is then sufficient to make the diagnosis. Consideration should also be given to a diagnosis of primary CNS lymphoma particularly in the setting of a solitary lesion.

Treatment

Pyrimethamine and sulfadiazine are the most effective antibiotic agents; they are coadministered with leucovorin to prevent hematologic suppression associated with pyrimethamine. Due to limited availability of pyrimethamine in the United States, trimethoprim-sulfamethoxazole alone can be an alternative regimen. Treatment is continued for 4 to 6 weeks. In patients with AIDS, maintenance therapy is often needed until immune reconstitution occurs with combination ART.

PROGRESSIVE MULTIFOCAL LEUKOENCEPHALOPATHY (JOHN CUNNINGHAM [JC] VIRUS)

CLINICAL VIGNETTE *A 65-year-old man with a history of follicular lymphoma initially treated with conventional chemotherapy 4 years previously was given three courses of rituximab for maintenance therapy because of persistence of clonal changes in his bone marrow. He developed confusion, dysarthria, and aphasia after the third course. MRI revealed nonenhancing lesions in the posterior and frontal lobes and left centrum semiovale. Peripheral blood polymerase chain reaction (PCR) was positive for JC virus, but CSF was negative.*

Brain biopsy demonstrated changes characteristic of progressive multifocal leukoencephalopathy (PML). His peripheral blood demonstrated a CD4 count of 100. Treatment with cidofovir was ineffective as the patient's clinical condition worsened with progressive aphasia and confusion, urinary and fecal incontinence, flaccid paralysis of the left arm, accompanied by radiologic progression with mass effect. He died 3 months after presentation.

Microbiology and Epidemiology

JC virus is a human polyomavirus, a small nonenveloped virus with a circular, double-stranded DNA genome. Infection is acquired during childhood and persists in the kidney or lymph tissue. JC virus is the cause of PML, a rare demyelinating disease of immunosuppressed patients. PML is most often an AIDS-defining illness but its incidence in HIV-infected patients has decreased after the introduction of effective ART. It also occurs in other immunocompromised settings such as hematologic malignancies, long-term corticosteroid or methotrexate (MTX) therapy, and natalizumab treatment. The latter is a monoclonal antibody used for the treatment of multiple sclerosis or inflammatory bowel disease.

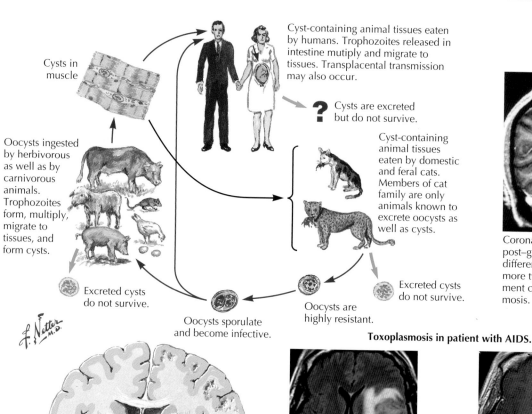

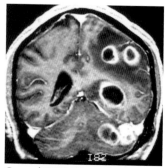

Coronal SPGR T1-weighted image post–gadolinium enhanced in a different patient demonstrates the more typical thick-rimmed enhancement commonly seen with toxoplasmosis.

Toxoplasmosis in patient with AIDS.

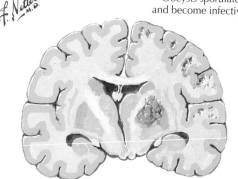

Brain section with nodule of *Toxoplasma gondii* in basal ganglia and necrotizing encephalitis in left frontal and temporal corticomedullary zones

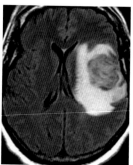

Axial FLAIR MR image demonstrates mixed intensity heterogeneous mass surrounded by a broad band of edema.

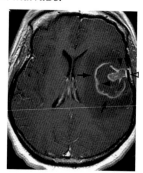

Comparable axial T1-weighted fast spin echo post–gadolinium-enhanced MR image shows a thin rim of enhancement (arrows) as well as a more lateral enhancing nodule (arrowheads) and adjacent dural enhancement (open arrowhead).

Fig. 48.3 Toxoplasmosis.

Clinical Presentation

PML has a variable presentation depending on which part of the brain is initially infected. The temporal profile and clinical symptomatology are no different in HIV patients from those with other immunodeficiencies. Common neurologic scenarios include a progressive hemiparesis, visual field deficits, aphasia, and cognitive impairment. Occasionally patients present with a pure cerebellar truncal and/or appendicular ataxia or cranial nerve deficits. Late in the course of PML, affected patients develop severe neurologic deficits, including cortical blindness, quadriparesis, profound dementia, and coma. Lesions may be primarily located in the cerebral white matter or sometimes in the cerebellum and brainstem (Fig. 48.4). Spinal cord involvement is rare but is reported. However, survival remains poor once PML is diagnosed.

Diagnostic Approach

MRI scans reveal hypodense, nonenhancing lesions of the cerebral white matter. The severity of clinical findings is often greater than is suggested by the extent of involvement on CT scan. The latter may even be normal.

MRI typically helps to differentiate brain tumors, especially lymphoma, or abscesses in the immunocompromised. PCR has been used to amplify JC virus DNA in CSF samples (sensitivities range from 60% to 100%). CSF cell count and chemistry results are usually normal. Electroencephalogram (EEG) may reveal focal slowing or may be normal early in the course of PML.

A definitive diagnosis of PML requires identification of the characteristic pathologic changes on brain biopsy: multiple asymmetric foci of demyelination at various stages of evolution in the cerebral white matter. Oligodendrocytes demonstrate characteristic cytopathic effects, including nuclear enlargement, loss of normal chromatin pattern, and intranuclear accumulation of deeply basophilic homogenous staining material. Electron microscopy reveals polyomavirus particles in enlarged oligodendrocyte nuclei (see Fig. 48.4).

Treatment

There is no specific antiviral therapy effective for PML. Although there were initial studies suggesting that cidofovir, a nucleoside analog, or cytarabine might have therapeutic potential, further studies have not shown clinical benefit. Marked clinical and radiographic improvement

Progressive multifocal leukoencephalopathy

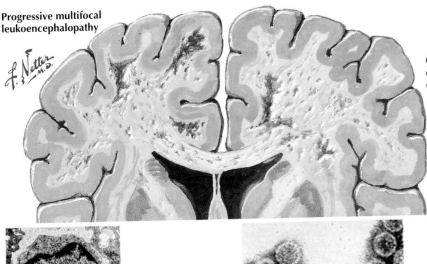

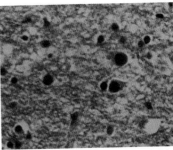

Coronal section of brain showing many minute demyelinating lesions in white matter, which have coalesced in some areas to form irregular cavitations

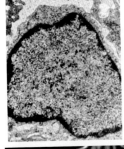

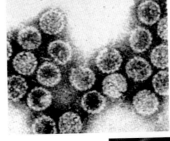

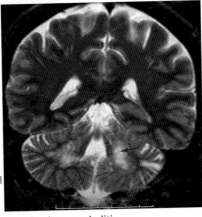

Section from edge of demyelinated focus showing abnormal oligodendrocytes with large hyperchromatic nuclei (H and E stain)

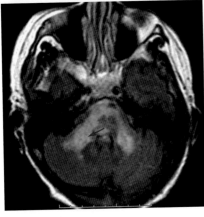

Electron micrograph showing giant glial nucleus with inclusion bodies

Electron micrograph showing papovavirus virions isolated from brain

Axial FLAIR image demonstrates increased signal in pons and bilateral cerebellar peduncles

Coronal T2-weighted image with increased signal in central cerebellar white matter

Fig. 48.4 Progressive Multifocal Leukoencephalitis.

in HIV-infected patients with PML has been seen after treatment with effective ART regimens. In immunosuppressed patients without HIV infection, discontinuation or decreasing doses of immunosuppressive agents is recommended if feasible. Opportunity for treatment may be better with the natalizumab-induced PML patient as plasma exchange and steroid pulse therapy are shown to provide some clinical benefit. In most patients, unless the accompanying underlying immune deficit can be reversed, PML typically progresses to death fairly rapidly.

ADDITIONAL RESOURCES

Anagnostou T, Arvanitis M, Kourkoumpetis TK, et al. Nocardiosis of the central nervous system: experience from a general hospital and review of 84 cases from the literature. Medicine (Baltimore) 2014;93:19–32.
Review of cases of CNS nocardiosis showing chronic corticosteroid use as the most common predisposing factor, followed by organ transplantation.
Cohen BA. Neurologic manifestations of toxoplasmosis in AIDS. Semin Neurol 1999;19:201–11.
Examination of characteristic presentations of cerebral toxoplasmosis in AIDS along with therapeutic options.

Cunha BA. Central nervous system infections in the compromised host: a diagnostic approach. Infect Dis Clin North Am 2001;15:567–90.
Comprehensive guidelines for the diagnostic approach to the compromised host with CNS infection. Discussion focuses on an analysis of the patient's clinical manifestations of CNS disease, the acuteness or subacuteness of the clinical presentation, and an analysis of the type of immune defect compromising the patient's host defenses.
Engsig FN, Hansen AB, Omland LH, et al. Incidence, clinical presentation, and outcome of progressive multifocal leukoencephalopathy in HIV-infected patients during the highly active antiretroviral therapy era: a nationwide cohort study. J Infect Dis 2009;199(1):77–83.
Population-based series of HIV-infected patients analyzing incidence rates, survival times, and clinical features associated with PML diagnosis. Disease incidence decreased with the introduction of effective ART.
Mylonakis E, Hohmann EL, Calderwood SB. Central nervous system infection with Listeria monocytogenes: 33 years' experience at a general hospital and review of 776 episodes from the literature. Medicine (Baltimore) 1998;77:313–36.
Review of cases of CNS listeriosis outside of pregnancy and neonates. One-third of patients had focal neurologic findings, and approximately one-fourth developed seizures.

Panel on Opportunistic Infections in HIV-Infected Adults and Adolescents. Guidelines for the prevention and treatment of opportunistic infections in HIV-infected adults and adolescents: recommendations from the Centers for Disease Control and Prevention, the National Institutes of Health, and the HIV Medicine Association of the Infectious Diseases Society of America. Available from http://aidsinfo.nih.gov/contentfiles/lvguidelines/adult_oi.pdf. Accessed 1 August 2017.

Comprehensive guidelines on the treatment of opportunistic infections in HIV patients, with specific updates on toxoplasma encephalitis and PML diagnosis.

Perfect JR, Dismukes WE, Dromer F, et al. Clinical practice guidelines for the management of cryptococcal disease: 2010 update by the Infectious Diseases Society of America. Clin Infect Dis 2010;50(3):291–322.

Expert consensus guidelines on the treatment of central nervous system cryptococcal disease.

Sahraian MA, Radue EW, Eshaghi A, et al. Progressive multifocal leukoencephalopathy: a review of the neuroimaging features and differential diagnosis. Eur J Neurol 2012;19(8):1060–9.

A review of the clinical characteristics of PML with extensive discussion of imaging features using various modalities. Comparison is made to other conditions which may have similar radiologic features.

Neuro-Oncology

Brian J. Scott

49

Brain Tumors

Lloyd M. Alderson, Peter K. Dempsey, G. Rees Cosgrove

CLINICAL VIGNETTE *A 47-year-old self-employed father presented to the emergency department having difficulty discriminating coins in his pocket. He had been skiing that day and was concerned enough to seek medical attention on his way home. His general health was excellent. The only abnormality on his neurologic examination was confined to his right hand. Here he demonstrated loss of two-point discrimination in his fingers as well as an inability to identify numbers traced on his right palm and to identify common objects such as a safety pin, paper clip, or various coins with these fingers. All of these maneuvers were normal for his left hand.*

Magnetic resonance imaging (MRI) demonstrated a 4- by 6-cm heterogeneously gadolinium-enhancing, vascular tumor with a large amount of peritumor edema high in his left parietal lobe. Stereotactic needle biopsy demonstrated a glioblastoma (GBM). Radiation and chemotherapy were given. He ultimately died as a result of local tumor recurrence that did not respond to treatment 15 months after presentation.

Brain tumors are a relatively common neurologic disorder particularly when one combines primary central nervous system (CNS) lesions and those metastatic to the brain and its leptomeninges. Taken together, these tumors are among the most common cerebral disorders in adults, second only to Alzheimer disease, stroke, and multiple sclerosis. With the exception of leukemia in children, primary brain tumors are the most common malignancy. GBM arising from within the glial cell matrix occurs in all age groups but is most prevalent after age 65 years. A higher age at onset is the most significant predictor of poor outcome. GBM is the most devastating of CNS malignancies; there are very few 2-year survivors. Glial cell tumors comprise more than two-thirds of all primary brain tumors.

Although one might think that the temporal profile of a patient's illness may sometimes suggest either a benign or malignant process, one cannot depend on this history to make a differential diagnosis. Brain tumors typically present with one of four clinical scenarios: (1) focal cerebral or cranial nerve (CN) deficits that are gradually progressive over a few weeks to many months, (2) seizures, (3) headache and signs of increased intracranial pressure primarily demonstrating papilledema and sixth-nerve palsies, or (4) stroke mimic—that is, involving an apocalyptic onset. Personality changes, evolving language dysfunction, focal loss of sensory discrimination, or motor limitation such as a clumsy hand, and ataxic gait are focal signs that usually define the site of the tumor accurately. However, there are certain *false localizing* signs that may lead to initial confusion.

When a slowly enlarging, previously asymptomatic cerebral tumor decompensates, certain *false localizing signs* may cause diagnostic confusion. Transtentorial uncal-parahippocampal herniation occurs, with the offending hemisphere herniating medially through the tentorium cerebri, compressing the contralateral corticospinal tract carrying motor fibers. These fibers originating in the opposite motor cortex control movement on the same side of the body as the site of the tumor. For example, a very large right-sided tumor affects the left corticospinal tract carrying right-sided motor fibers, leading paradoxically to a hemiparesis ipsilateral to the tumor. Another false localizing sign occurs when a large herniating tumor compresses the opposite third nerve, thus leading to pupillary dilation contralateral to the side of the lesion. Today these clinically confusing signs are less likely to occur with earlier MRI diagnosis of these tumors before they reach a critical mass that could cause these herniation syndromes.

The occurrence of a new-onset seizure in an adult must always lead to diagnostic consideration of a brain tumor. It is estimated that 30% of brain tumors present in this fashion. The tumor types and their locations are essential determinants significantly influencing seizure characteristics. Brain tumors with a high risk for epilepsy include diffuse gliomas, brain metastases, and various developmental tumors.

The availability of MRI makes the differentiation relatively simple for those occasional brain tumors that present so acutely that they mimic a stroke. MRI primarily provides morphologic and functional information, including tumor localization, vascular permeability, cell density, and tumor perfusion. The concurrent employment of positron emission tomography (PET) enables the assessment of molecular processes, such as glucose consumption, expression of nucleoside and amino acid transporters, as well as alterations of DNA and protein synthesis. Perhaps multimodal diagnostic imaging will eventually allow one to differentiate a "tumefactive" demyelinating lesion from the much more common glioma. At present, however it is necessary to establish a tissue diagnosis to determine an appropriate therapeutic plan.

Despite tremendous advances in both the understanding of the biology of malignant gliomas and new neuro-oncologic therapies, the prognosis remains very poor. However, antiangiogenic agents, immune therapies, and checkpoint inhibitors are demonstrating some therapeutic promise for malignant gliomas.

MALIGNANT BRAIN TUMORS

When considering a new brain tumor diagnosis, it is important to determine whether the lesion has arisen from within the brain itself (primary), or whether it has spread to the brain from a cancer elsewhere in the body (metastatic). Primary brain tumors are commonly solitary

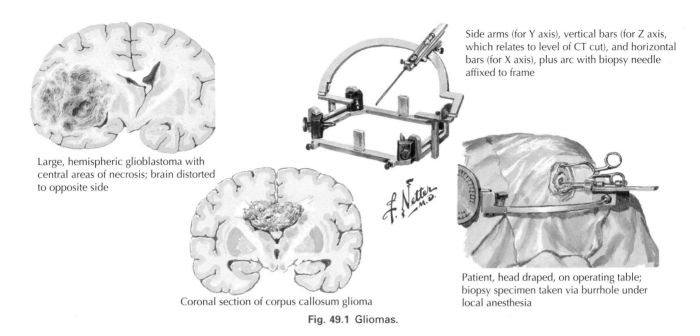

Large, hemispheric glioblastoma with central areas of necrosis; brain distorted to opposite side

Side arms (for Y axis), vertical bars (for Z axis, which relates to level of CT cut), and horizontal bars (for X axis), plus arc with biopsy needle affixed to frame

Coronal section of corpus callosum glioma

Patient, head draped, on operating table; biopsy specimen taken via burrhole under local anesthesia

Fig. 49.1 Gliomas.

and frequently have irregular margins. They may arise from glial, ependymal, or lymphoid cells. Gliomas are the most common tumors of glial origin; however, both astrocytes and oligodendrocytes can also form tumors. In contradistinction, primary neuronal tumors are very rare, particularly in adults. Metastatic tumors are often multiple, with gadolinium enhancement on MRI and sharply defined borders. The most common systemic cancers that metastasize to the brain are lung, breast, melanoma, and kidney.

Traditionally microscopic features have been the primary means of glial cell tumor classification. However, an emerging understanding of the molecular events responsible for the genesis of gliomas is having an impact not only on the diagnostic classification of these tumors but also on treatment selection as well as survival for specific glioma types. Small-molecule inhibitors and monoclonal antibodies may eventually provide targeted therapies that selectively block newly appreciated aberrant growth-signaling pathways within gliomas.

Gliomas
Epidemiology

The chance of developing a primary malignant brain tumor in the United States is small relative to the chance of developing a tumor of the lung, breast, colon, or prostate. The majority of these primary malignant brain tumors are gliomas. Data collected by the Central Brain Tumor Registry of the United States (CBTRUS) and Surveillance, Epidemiology, and End Results consortia demonstrate an adult incidence of 5.1 gliomas per 100,000 person-years; almost 50% of these are glioblastomas. Brain cancer incidence rises with age, peaking at 65–70 years. For glioblastoma the highest incidence is at age 62 years. Men are significantly more likely to develop a glioma (M:F = 1.8). Brain cancer incidence also varies regionally; the incidence in Hawaii is roughly half that in New England, and globally the incidence of brain tumors in Israel is roughly eight times that in Japan. Although some studies suggest that Caucasians are more predisposed to gliomas than African or Asian populations, variable access to healthcare and diagnostic imaging across regions and cultures may be the primary mechanism explaining this discrepancy rather than genetic susceptibility differences. Gliomas, like

most cancers, are usually a random event and rarely have a familial predisposition. However, having a first-degree relative with a glioma doubles a patient's risk. Rarely, gliomas occur as part of an inherited disorder such as neurofibromatosis types 1 or 2 or tuberous sclerosis. There are no well-defined environmental risk factors with the exception of previous brain irradiation that predispose patients to glioma.

Pathology

Gliomas typically exhibit features of astrocytes, oligodendrocytes, or both (mixed glioma) (Fig. 49.1). Microscopically, gliomas appear as diffusely infiltrating cancers of three types: astrocytic, oligodendroglial, and oligoastrocytic (combining the morphologic features of both oligodendroglioma and astrocytoma).

The World Health Organization (WHO) uses a three-tiered classification system based on histologic criteria that divide gliomas into infiltrating (WHO grade II), anaplastic (WHO grade III), and GBM (WHO grade IV). WHO grade II tumors may contain a high proportion of cells that appear histologically normal. Here the percentage of cells that are dividing (as determined by mib-1 or KI-67 staining) is often 2% or less. Anaplastic gliomas exhibit more atypical cells, with pleomorphic nuclei having growth rates in the range of 5%–10% but no evidence of necrosis. High growth rates (>10% mitotic figures) and necrosis are characteristic for GBM. Pilocytic astrocytomas (WHO grade I) are a separate category of glioma that are histologically characterized by Rosenthal fibers; they usually occur in children and often have a good prognosis if surgical resection can be achieved.

Gliomas are not staged as other cancers are because they rarely metastasize outside the CNS. Analysis of tumor samples for genetic abnormalities can help to predict response to therapy and will likely lead to a better classification system for gliomas. This classification is valuable prognostically; diffuse glioma (WHO grade II) has a median survival of 5–15 years; anaplastic glioma 2–5 years; and GBM 12–18 months.

Glioblastoma

These malignant tumors frequently present with seizures, aphasia, or other focal symptomatology, pointing to the specific areas of pathologic origin. Very infrequently, a glioma may manifest itself more globally, as *gliomatosis cerebri*, wherein there is widespread dissemination of neoplastic cells globally through a hemisphere or even the entire brain. These relatively rare patients may present with cognitive or personality changes. On other occasions, even though the patient presents relatively acutely with focal findings, the clinician is surprised to find a diffusely invasive malignant tumor despite a clinical presentation compatible with an acute focal brain pathology. This is the very common, most aggressive, and least likely of the gliomas to respond to therapy. The historical descriptor *multiforme* refers to the tumor's heterogeneous gross pathologic appearance. Often areas of necrosis, hemorrhage, and fleshy tumor exist within the same tumor focus.

Two types of GBM (WHO grade IV astrocytomas) are distinguished by molecular features. *Primary GBM* arises without evolving from a lower grade tumor with a median age at diagnosis of 62. Characteristically, primary GBMs have an amplification and overexpression of the epidermal growth factor receptor (EGFR) and ligand (EGF). *Primary GBM* is characterized by the presence of the wild-type isocitrate dehydrogenase 1 (IDH-1) gene and is associated with a shorter overall survival (15 months). *Secondary GBM* arises from a low-grade astrocytoma in a younger adult (median age at diagnosis mid-40's). It is characterized by the presence of IDH-1 mutation and more commonly harbors a *p53* mutation. As it undergoes anaplastic transformation, the secondary GBM accumulates other genetic derangements, most notably, mutation of the Rb gene, deletion of the tumor suppressor gene p16/ *cyclin-dependent kinase inhibitor 2A (CDKN2A)*, and amplification of *cyclin-dependent kinase 4 (CDK4)*.

When the clinical behavior and genetic abnormalities of GBM tumors are reviewed, a developmental dichotomy emerges. Younger patients with GBM sometimes have a longer history of symptoms or a history of a lower-grade glioma, suggesting that the tumor developed from a lower-grade precursor, whereas older patients with GBM tend to have relatively sudden symptom onset, suggesting that the malignancy did not evolve from a less aggressive tumor. Genetic analysis of GBM samples from older patients frequently reveals overexpression of the EGFR and loss of 10q. Tumor samples from younger patients are more likely to show mutations in *p53* and *RB*, overexpression of the platelet-derived growth factor receptor, and loss of 19q—changes often seen in lower-grade gliomas.

Diagnosis, Treatment, and Prognosis

MRI is the most specific diagnostic modality (Fig. 49.2). On most occasions, one sees focal heterogeneous and irregularly margined cystic mass lesions with perilesion edema, gadolinium rim enhancement. In contrast, occasional patients with gliomatosis cerebri have a characteristic diffusely abnormal MRI picture characterized by multiple areas of subtle white matter enhancement with extension into the cortical mantle, extending far beyond what their clinical presentation usually dictates (Fig. 49.3).

Even with early diagnosis, the prognosis for individuals with glioblastoma remains grim and most patients will fail therapy within 12 months of diagnosis. The first treatment step is to perform as wide a surgical resection as is functionally tolerable. Younger patients with a normal examination who have had a gross total resection have the best prognosis. Postoperative radiation therapy (RT) clearly benefits many patients, as those GBM patients who receive RT have a median survival twice that of those who did not.

Combining RT with concomitant and adjuvant chemotherapy is now the standard of care for patients with GBM. RT plus temozolomide leads to a modest benefit in overall survival (14.6 vs. 12.1 months). However, more importantly, there is a significant increase in the percentage of those surviving 2 or more years (26.5% vs. 10.4%).

Bevacizumab, an antagonist of vascular endothelial growth factor, has been approved by the US Food and Drug Administration for patients with recurrent GBM.

With the limited efficacy of standard treatments, there is an imperative to develop better therapies through translational science and clinical trials. Molecular research is defining a number of potential glioma cell targets. These are mostly second messenger molecules involved in pathways that enhance cell proliferation or inhibit programmed cell death. The goal is to treat a selected group of patients whose tumors overexpress the specific target of the treatment drug.

Diffuse Astrocytic and Oligodendroglial Glioma

CLINICAL VIGNETTE *A 34-year-old right-handed woman presented with generalized seizures. Several months earlier, she had noted episodes of an unusual smell, but these did not cause her immediate concern. Brain MRI demonstrated a right temporal lobe lesion, bright on T2 and fluid-attenuated inversion recovery (FLAIR) imaging but hypointense on T1, with no evidence of enhancement after gadolinium (Fig. 49.4). The patient was treated with oxcarbazepine and admitted to the hospital. Open biopsy was nondiagnostic but subsequent temporal lobectomy revealed an oligodendroglioma with a Ki-67 index of 3.8%. Postoperatively, the patient was treated with monthly temozolomide for 1 year. She is now receiving no treatment and has been clinically and radiographically stable for 2 years.*

Clinical Presentation/Pathology

Diffuse gliomas are slow-growing tumors with a symptom history that can extend from months to years. Although easily defined by MRI (see Fig. 49.4), diffuse gliomas often do not enhance with gadolinium. Their course is usually relatively stable for several years before eventually progressing. At the time of diagnosis, diffuse glioma has a more favorable overall survival than glioblastoma. However, eventually some diffuse gliomas may progress to become GBM, with its inherently poor prognosis. Histologically, diffuse gliomas may be described as infiltrating astrocytoma, oligodendroglioma, or oligoastrocytoma (mixed glioma). A low mitotic index, younger patient age, and a supratentorial non-elegant locus (i.e., not affecting language function) that is amenable to resection predict a longer progression-free survival.

Treatment and Prognosis

The choice of therapeutic modalities is always an issue. Retrospective studies suggest that gross total resection for gliomas that can be safely removed provides longer progression-free survival. However, the surgeon can never remove all tumor tissue when dealing with infiltrative gliomas. These lesions harbor an innate, almost serpiginous invasion of what appears to be grossly normal brain tissue to the surgeon's eye. At the time of resection, these characteristics prevent appreciation of the full microscopic extent of the entire tumor mass. Therefore gliomas will eventually demonstrate progression even after what appears initially to be a gross "total resection." In this setting, so-called disabling resections in patients with astrocytomas or oligodendrogliomas are neither wise nor helpful. This is especially true when dealing with tumors in eloquent cerebrocortical areas—including language, memory, and function—as well as those portions essential to the use of extremities, particularly motor structures within the dominant hemisphere, where preservation of functional mobility is particularly important.

Subtotal resection is indicated for most gliomas remediable by decompression without leaving a significant disability (such as aphasia) and especially when the tumor's mass effect is causing disability. In patients with pilocytic astrocytoma, surgical indications differ slightly;

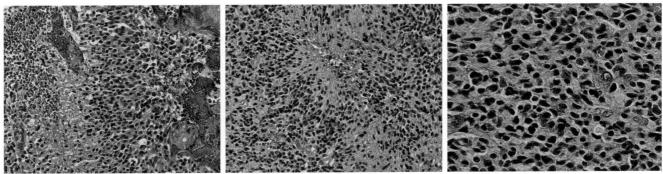

Glioblastoma. Dense population of astrocytes with malignant nuclear features, palisaded around area of necrosis

Glioblastoma

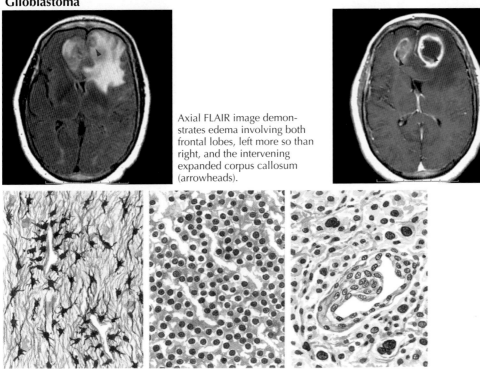

Axial FLAIR image demonstrates edema involving both frontal lobes, left more so than right, and the intervening expanded corpus callosum (arrowheads).

T1-weighted, post–gadolinium-enhanced image shows rim-enhancing lesions with irregular margins and central hypointensity. This central hypointensity represents necrosis, and the enhancing region represents the more active regions within this butterfly glioma.

Astrocytoma   Oligodendroglioma   Glioblastoma

Fig. 49.2 Glioma: Magnetic Resonance Imaging and Pathology.

a complete resection may provide a cure; therefore a more aggressive surgical approach may be appropriate.

The next therapeutic decision is whether to recommend external beam RT. Although RT does not prolong overall survival, there is a significant increase in progression-free survival in the treated group. Unfortunately this benefit may be offset by a higher incidence of long-term cognitive impairment in the RT-treated group. Survival is not the only factor when RT is being considered, since some clinical predictors suggest which patients will benefit from RT. If more than two answers to the five following questions are yes, the patient is likely to benefit from RT: (1) Is the patient older than age 40 years? (2) Is the tumor symptomatic (other than seizures)? (3) Does the tumor cross the midline? (4) Is the tumor an astrocytoma (as opposed to an oligodendroglioma)? (5) Is the tumor larger than 5 cm?

The dose of RT for diffuse glioma is usually 54 Gy given in 30 fractions. Higher doses have not shown a clear benefit and should not be used.

Until recently chemotherapy has not been employed for the treatment of diffuse glioma. However, the recent widespread use of temozolomide, an oral alkylating agent for GBM, raises the question of whether there are a selected group of patients with diffuse glioma who potentially may also benefit from this therapy. Temozolomide is currently used in patients who do not meet the criteria for RT, as listed earlier, but whose tumors have a mitotic index of greater than 3%. Although patients with low-grade tumors have a much better prognosis than those with anaplastic glioma and GBM, diffuse glioma is still usually fatal. The median survival is 5–7 years for astrocytoma and 7–10 years for oligodendroglioma.

Anaplastic Glioma

CLINICAL VIGNETTE *A 49-year-old right-handed man presented with 5 weeks of numbness and weakness in the left leg. Examination revealed decreased strength and slowed rapid movements of his left foot. There was*

Gliomatosis cerebri in 46-year-old with 3-day history of headache and left facial droop

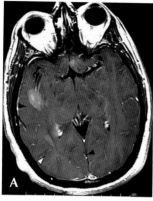

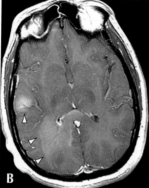

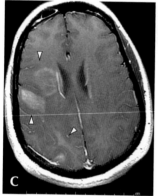

A.-C. Multiple axial post–gadolinium-enhanced T1-weighted fast spin echoes images demonstrate multiple areas of subtle enhancement involving white matter with extension into cortex. These same regions were subtly T2 bright on FLAIR (arrowheads).

Fig. 49.3 Gliomatosis Cerebri.

extinction to touch and loss of joint position sense. Brain MRI revealed a 3-by-4-cm cystic mass centered in the medial aspect of the right parietal lobe and heterogeneous enhancement with gadolinium (Fig. 49.5).

Lesion resection revealed an anaplastic astrocytoma (AA) (see Fig. 49.5). Postoperatively, the patient was treated with a combination of RT and concomitant temozolomide. He is neurologically intact and radiographically stable 3 years after diagnosis.

Pathology

Anaplastic gliomas are WHO grade III tumors with a higher mitotic index than diffuse gliomas but lack the necrosis and endothelial proliferation of glioblastomas. They commonly affect patients in the age range of 35–50 years who often present with symptoms dating back just a few weeks or months. As in diffuse glioma, anaplastic gliomas can be composed of astrocytes (AAs), oligodendrocytes (anaplastic oligodendroglioma [AO]), or a mixture of the two (anaplastic oligoastrocytoma [AOA]). The presence of an oligodendroglial component and especially co-deletion of chromosome 1p and 19q confers a better prognosis.

Oligodendroglioma in a 34-year-old woman with recent uncinate seizures

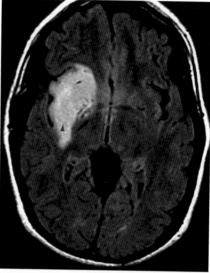

A. Axial FLAIR MR image demonstrates T2 hyperintensity that involves the right basal ganglia, insula, and intervening subinsular region with subtle expansion when compared with the opposite side.

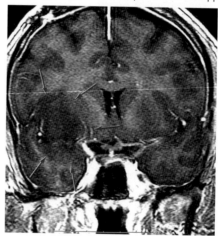

B. Coronal T1-weighted fast spin-echo MR image following gadolinium enhancement shows ill-defined T1 hypointensity within the insula, subinsular region, and adjacent basal ganglia with uncinate fasciculus extension into the superior medial anterior left temporal lobe (arrows). Note absence of enhancement.

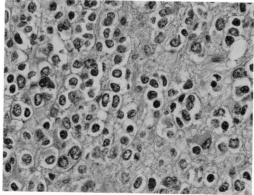

C. Oligodendroglioma. Uniform population of round cells, many with clear cytoplasm—so-called "fried egg" appearance.

Fig. 49.4 Oligodendroglioma.

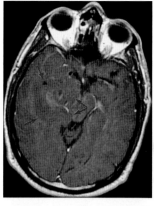

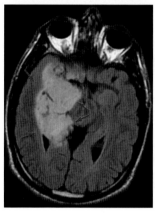

A. Axial FLAIR image demonstrates slight expansion and increased T2 signal involving the medial aspect of the right temporal lobe with the insula and posterior temporal expansion slightly distorting midbrain (arrows).

B. T1-weighted fast spin echo image following gadolinium enhancement shows some slight heterogeneity with medial hypointensity which may represent small cystic or degenerative regions with equivocal surrounding enhancement (arrows).

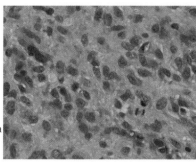

C. A low-power image of anaplastic astrocytoma shows a tumor with high cellularity, but no areas of necrosis or endothelial proliferation are present. (H&E, original magnification 100x)

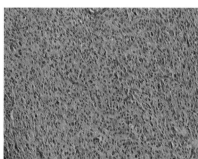

D. A high-power image shows crowded atypical astrocytic cells with irregular nuclei and frequent mitotic figures. (H&E, original magnification 400x)

Fig. 49.5 Glioma, Anaplastic Astrocytoma.

Treatment and Prognosis

Theoretically, complete surgical resection is the best initial intervention; however, a heroic but neurologically disabling procedure is not indicated, as noted in the section on diffuse astrocytic and oligodendroglial tumors. Most patients with anaplastic gliomas should be treated with radiation. It is not clear whether adding a chemotherapy drug such as temozolomide at the time of diagnosis is beneficial. Previous studies have shown a high rate of response to temozolomide in patients with recurrent AAs. AA has a median survival of approximately 3 years.

Anaplastic Oligodendrogliomas

These are a special subset of tumors where the optimal treatment remains controversial. They frequently (70%) respond to procarbazine, lomustine, and vincristine (PCV) chemotherapy. Genetic analysis demonstrates that the vast majority of the responders have a specific genetic profile (loss of 1p and 19q). This group has a median survival of 10 years; in contrast, other AO patients lacking this profile have a median survival much closer to the 3 years of AA patients. The addition of alkylating chemotherapy to radiation improves long-term survival in co-deleted anaplastic oligodendroglioma. Aggressive chemotherapy (with bone marrow transplant), even in patients with AO, has not significantly prolonged survival.

Primary Central Nervous System Lymphoma

Previously a relatively rare tumor, primary CNS lymphoma (PCNSL) has risen dramatically in incidence over the past 30 years. There are two clinical subtypes of this disease. In *immunocompetent* patients,

PCNSL occurs in an older population. This is similar to other non-Hodgkin lymphomas. Pathologic evaluation typically demonstrates *monoclonal B cells.* Patients with human immunodeficiency virus, organ transplantation, or other intrinsic or medication-induced immunosuppression are much more likely to develop PCNSL than non-immunosuppressed individuals. Histologically, this is a *polyclonal B-cell* tumor that is associated with the activation of Epstein-Barr virus.

MRI in PCNSL patients usually demonstrates a homogeneously enhancing lesion or lesions often adjacent to a ventricle (Fig. 49.6). A positive cerebrospinal fluid (CSF) cytology is found in 25%–50% of these individuals. Biopsy is essential to make the diagnosis. A large resection is usually not indicated, as most of these tumors respond well to chemotherapy and/or RT. In some immunocompetent patients these enhancing brain lesions can disappear either spontaneously or with corticosteroid therapy. For this reason, if PCNSL is suspected, biopsy should be performed prior to treatment with corticosteroids.

PCNSL is markedly sensitive to therapy in *immunocompetent patients;* median survival is often in excess of 3 years. There are two approaches to treatment. The first involves high-dose intravenous (IV) methotrexate as a single agent or in combination with rituximab and temozolomide. The second combines a lower dose of IV methotrexate with ara-C, intrathecal methotrexate, and whole-brain RT. This approach is well tolerated in younger patients; however, significant cognitive toxicity occurs in patients older than age 60 years. *Immunosuppressed patients* are less likely to benefit from chemotherapy and treatment with RT alone. If possible, consideration should be given to reversing the immunosuppression.

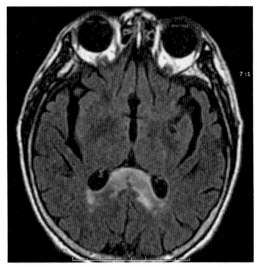

A. Axial FLAIR image demonstrates increased signal within a diffusely expanded splenium of the corpus callosum.

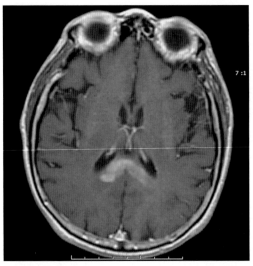

B. Axial T1-weighted, post–gadolinium-enhanced image shows enhancement within the same region.

Fig. 49.6 Primary Central Nervous System Lymphoma. *Arrow* in A is pointing to the area of abnormal signal in the corpus callosum.

Other Primary Brain Tumors
Ependymoma

These are unusual tumors of glial origin that can arise anywhere within the neuraxis. The floor of the fourth ventricle is the most common intracranial site for an ependymoma to develop. Histologically, ependymomas often have a cellular appearance characterized by a pseudo-rosette perivascular pattern. There is also a more malignant version with an anaplastic appearance; although unlike the case in gliomas, anaplasia may not confer poor prognosis. Myxopapillary ependymoma is a variant that occurs within the filum terminale at the end of the spinal cord.

MRI is the study of choice (Fig. 49.7). Surgical resection is the primary treatment; however, tumor location determines whether a complete resection is achievable. The extent of tumor resection is the most important indicator of the eventual clinical course. Surgical resection of a myxopapillary ependymoma frequently results in a cure. Indicators of poor prognosis include incomplete resection and CSF spread. Such

patients require either local or craniospinal RT. Chemotherapy is seldom used at the time of diagnosis.

Medulloblastoma

These are a class of uncommon primitive neuroectodermal tumors that usually occur in the posterior fossa, often in the midline. Typically these patients present with double vision, ataxia, hydrocephalus, nausea, and vomiting (Fig. 49.8). These tumors comprise 3% of all primary brain tumors and are significantly more prominent in children. Brain MRI usually reveals a homogeneously enhancing mass situated in the roof of the fourth ventricle, often with some degree of hydrocephalus. Pathologically medulloblastomas are characterized by sheets of small, poorly differentiated cells with minimal cytoplasm.

Medulloblastomas require both surgery and RT. When one is able to surgically remove more than 90% of the tumor mass, there is usually an improved survival. Because of this tumor's propensity to spread along the leptomeninges and throughout the CSF, patients must undergo evaluation of the entire craniospinal axis to establish the extent of disease. If such has occurred, additional treatment is usually required. External beam RT is directed at the areas identified, often the entire brain and spine. Chemotherapy is then given. This combination therapy is associated with improved survival.

Cerebellar Astrocytoma

Most childhood primary brain tumors are in the glioma family, and many of these occur within the cerebellum (Fig. 49.9). Pilocytic astrocytomas are the most common posterior fossa variant. These tend to arise within the cerebellar hemisphere. A second form of cerebellar astrocytoma, the diffuse or fibrillary form, often arises in the midline and produces obstruction of the fourth ventricle and hydrocephalus. Cerebellar astrocytomas are often cystic in appearance, with an enhancing mural nodule.

Surgical resection can sometimes be curative, particularly with pilocytic astrocytomas. Incompletely resected tumors often require post-surgical irradiation. The survival rate of patients with cerebellar astrocytomas is often very significantly better than that of those with supratentorial glial tumors.

Pontine Glioma

These serious tumors primarily occur in childhood but are on rare occasions found in adults. They tend to be higher-grade tumors that expand the pons and infiltrate into the surrounding tissue (Fig. 49.10). Presenting symptoms are consistent with their location—namely, hydrocephalus from fourth ventricle obstruction or long tract signs from impairment of corticospinal axonal pathways. Isolated cranial neuropathies, particularly sixth and seventh nerve lesions, may also occur from compression of brainstem nuclei. The infiltrative nature of these tumors often precludes any degree of significant surgical resection. Unfortunately RT is usually ineffective at achieving long-term growth control.

Metastatic Brain Tumors

CLINICAL VIGNETTE *A 52-year-old right-handed physician had a 2-week history of clumsiness using her right hand, which was particularly noticeable while she was performing electromyographies. Neurologic evaluation revealed moderate weakness and clumsiness of her right hand and a hint of a right central facial weakness. She had a 30-pack-year history of tobacco abuse but had discontinued this habit 8 years earlier.*

Gadolinium-enhanced brain MRI demonstrated multiple round ring-enhancing lesions consistent with metastases. As she had no known primary lesion identified during this evaluation, a stereotactic biopsy of a lesion close to the surface

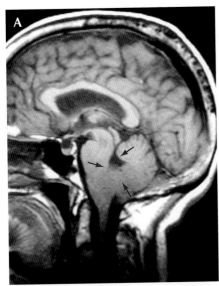

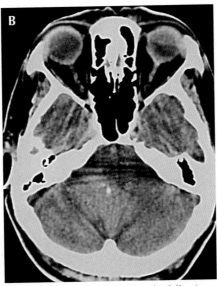

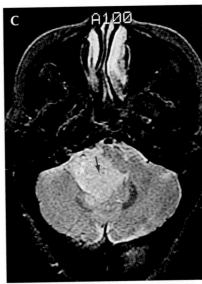

A. Sagittal T1-weighted fast spin echo shows mass within the posterior fourth ventricle and somewhat ill-defined extending into the vallecula and adjacent brainstem (arrows).

B. Axial T1-weighted fast spin echo following intravenous gadolinium shows modest diffuse enhancement. An area of increased signal is associated with a small calcification (arrow).

C. Axial FLAIR shows this central right-sided mass, moderately T2-weighted bright extending into right lateral recess.

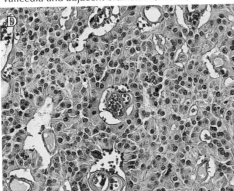

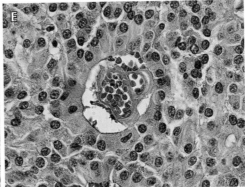

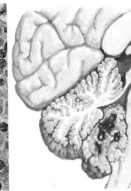

D.-E. Uniform population of epithelioid cells, palisaded around a central blood vessel.

Ependymoma of 4th ventricle protruding into cisterna magna

Fig. 49.7 Ependymoma.

demonstrated small-cell carcinoma consistent with lung cancer. It took another 4 months for the presumed primary lung lesion to be identified with chest CT. She was treated with whole-brain RT followed by systemic chemotherapy. Although she had initial symptomatic improvement, her difficulties returned and focal motor seizures developed followed by a dense hemiparesis. She died within 18 months despite three attempts to achieve remission with focused beam radiosurgery.

For the medical oncologist and internist, metastatic brain tumors represent the most common neuro-oncologic challenge. Of all cancer patients, 25% develop CNS metastases, usually after the primary tumor has been diagnosed but occasionally as the initial sign as noted in this vignette. Typically CNS metastases are either single or multiple solid tumors compressing the brain and spinal cord or appear more diffusely with leptomeningeal infiltration of cancer cells throughout the CSF and neuraxis, especially involving spinal and CN roots.

Lung cancer is the most common primary tumor that metastasizes to the CNS (50%), followed by breast (33%), colon (9%), and melanoma (7%) (Fig. 49.11). The interval between the primary diagnosis and

presentation of a CNS metastasis depends on the tumor type. For lung cancer, the median interval is 4 months; for breast cancer, 3 years. CNS metastasis is an indicator of poor prognosis and portends a survival of less than 6 months for most patients.

Clinical Presentation and Diagnosis

As with primary CNS malignancies, clinical presentation depends on the tumor site. The onset can be almost precipitous, mimicking a stroke, or can be indolent, with gradual development of focal neurologic deficit: motor, sensory, language, visual, gait, or coordination. In other instances, patients may have focal or generalized seizures or present with nonspecific symptoms, perhaps suggesting increased intracranial pressure, such as positional headaches, cranial neuropathies, and rarely nausea, vomiting, or both.

Gadolinium-enhanced MRI typically demonstrates the presence of focal metastases. Meningeal gadolinium enhancement portends the presence of carcinomatous leptomeningeal invasion with the important exception of the low-pressure syndrome (see further on). The malignant enhancement usually has a very irregular character, in contrast to the very smooth enhancement seen with the very benign low-pressure syndrome (see Fig. 49.23). CSF cytologic analysis, in most instances of leptomeningeal

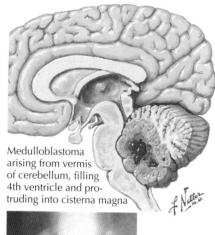

Medulloblastoma arising from vermis of cerebellum, filling 4th ventricle and protruding into cisterna magna

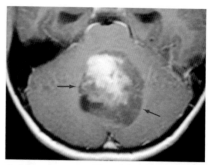

CT scan showing enhancing medulloblastoma in region of 4th ventricle; obstructive hydrocephalus indicated by dilated temporal horn (arrows)

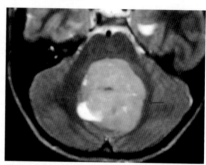

Axial post contrast T1-weighted brain MR: Large, hetero-geneously enhancing intra-fourth ventricular mass lesion (arrows).

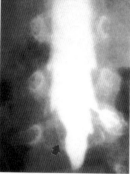

Postoperative lumbar metrizamide myelogram showing lumbar seeding of tumor evidenced by nonfilling of S1 root on right side (arrow)

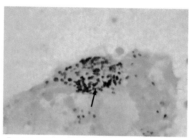

Positive CSF cytologic findings in patient with medulloblastoma; malignant tumor cells clumped on Millipore filter

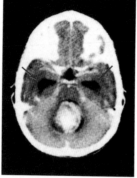

T2-weighted axial brain MR: Gray matter isointense large intraventricular mass lesion (arrows).

Diagnostic images courtesy Tina Young Poussaint, MD, Children's Hospital, Boston.

Fig. 49.8 Medulloblastoma.

cancer, demonstrates an increased number of malignant cells, thus confirming the diagnosis. Sometimes the initial CSF in this setting is negative. Here, if there is a high clinical suspicion, one must make repeated spinal taps. On one occasion we had a patient who required six different CSF cytologic examinations before a specific diagnosis could be made.

Treatment

Although treatment is clearly palliative, most metastatic brain cancer patients benefit to some degree from CNS-directed therapy. Whole-brain RT is indicated for most of these individuals. The patient with an isolated, single brain lesion who has no evidence of systemic recurrence is a candidate for surgical resection. On occasion the pathology is totally unexpected in that some resected solitary lesions, initially thought to be metastases, prove to have an entirely different pathology, including benign tumors such as meningiomas. Focal radiation is helpful in patients with one to two lesions who are otherwise stable. In the occasional patient having a solitary brain metastasis who has received surgery or focal RT, it is reasonable to withhold whole-brain RT until there is evidence of tumor progression in the brain. Rarely there is a symptom-free interlude of a number of years after the initial resection of an isolated metastasis.

Treatment of carcinomatous meningitis involves the direct infusion of chemotherapeutic agents, either methotrexate or cytarabine, directly into the CSF via lumbar puncture or preferably a ventricular reservoir. This is a palliative treatment at best; the overall prognosis is usually survival for only a matter of months once malignant leptomeningeal invasion has been confirmed.

Therapy and Future Directions

Treatment of malignant brain tumors remains challenging and often unsuccessful. Advances in therapy are being made in the field of imaging, where PET and MR spectroscopy are used to distinguish recurrent tumors from necrotic posttreatment change. Image guidance in the operating room allows for smaller, more precisely located incisions and provides real-time information on the extent of tumor resection.

Perhaps the greatest improvements in treating gliomas are the novel chemotherapy treatments, such as temozolomide, that are showing promise in controlling tumor growth. Gene therapy and other targeted, biochemically based treatments are also showing promise.

BENIGN BRAIN TUMORS

Meningiomas

CLINICAL VIGNETTE *A 48-year-old healthy woman, mother of two young adult children and a respected schoolteacher, had a history of chronic intermittent low-grade generalized headaches with a family history of migraine. Recently she noted that her headaches were occurring more frequently. These were not responding to the modest simple analgesics that she had previously used. She was unaware of any precipitating factors. Her family physician evaluated her; she also reported that recently her marriage had fallen apart when it became widely acknowledged in her small local community that her husband was having multiple affairs. She was very embarrassed and had become socially withdrawn. Her practitioner requested a neurologic consultation. Subsequently this neurologic*

and the olfactory groove along the anterior skull base. Meningioma is typically a benign lesion arising from arachnoid meningeal cells.

Classically these are slow-growing tumors that attain a large size before becoming symptomatic; however, occasionally they seem to grow much more rapidly, especially during pregnancy. Meningiomas arising adjacent to the frontal lobe are particularly prone to being clinically silent because of the disproportionately large size of this part of the brain, where there is much more tissue to be "forgiving." Such a slowly enlarging lesion can gradually compress brain tissue without producing definitive symptoms in this "clinically silent" part of the brain. A good example occurs when a meningioma affects the prefrontal cortex. Subtle personality changes gradually develop that are appreciated only in retrospect. However, if the tumor lies adjacent to overtly functional brain tissue, such as the motor cortex, symptoms may present relatively early (Fig. 49.12).

Clinical Presentation

Meningiomas usually have an ingravescent course, presenting with a variety of symptoms such as long-standing headache, personality change, particularly disinhibition when they involve the prefrontal cortex, various types of focal seizures, gait difficulties, or varied CN palsies as simple as unilateral loss of smell with olfactory groove lesions. On rare occasions, meningiomas may have a precipitous onset, mimicking a stroke or even a brief transient ischemic attack. Today many relatively small and clinically silent meningiomas are first identified incidentally on CT and MRI during the evaluation of unrelated events, such as a posttraumatic injury. Presumed meningiomas located at the base of the skull near blood vessels must be differentiated from cerebral aneurysms. These lesions are best evaluated with magnetic resonance angiography (MRA) to distinguish them prior to consideration for possible neurosurgery.

Treatment

A decision to treat a meningioma rests on several factors. Because many are initially asymptomatic, it is important to determine that subsequently appearing neurologic symptoms arise from the lesion per se. Given the typically slow growth of these benign tumors while the patient continues to be asymptomatic, radiographic follow-up is recommended on an annual to biannual basis. No treatment is necessary for those individuals who remain asymptomatic when follow-up CT and MRI demonstrate no change in tumor size or configuration. When the patient develops progressive symptoms or follow-up imaging indicates increasing size of the tumor, surgical resection is in order.

The surgical complexity is directly related to tumor site; those on the brain convexity or along the falx cerebri are often easily resected. Skull base tumors located near blood vessels and CNs often present a surgical challenge when the meningioma becomes entwined with these structures. RT, chemotherapy, or both are rarely used to treat typical benign meningiomas. Antiprogesterone agents to slow the growth of the meningiomas are being investigated.

Pituitary Adenoma

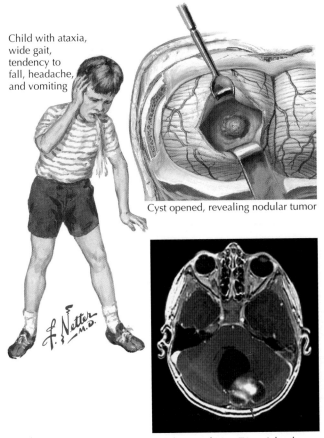

Child with ataxia, wide gait, tendency to fall, headache, and vomiting

Cyst opened, revealing nodular tumor

Axial post infusion T1-weighted brain MR: Cyst (arrowheads) and enhancing nodule (arrow)

Fig. 49.9 Cystic Astrocytoma of Cerebellum.

consultant determined that her examination was normal. A diagnosis of tension stress headache was made. Amitriptyline was prescribed prophylactically. She was referred to a marriage counselor.

The headaches became increasingly bothersome, at times awakening her from sleep; she had periods of helplessness and spells of crying. She was switched to a selective serotonin reuptake inhibitor for presumed increasing depression. However, she was not convinced of the diagnosis and sought another neurologic opinion. Her history remained unchanged. The only possible abnormal finding on neurologic examination was a subtle suggestion of a left central facial weakness. When this was called to her attention and she was asked whether this finding was new or just a normal asymmetry, neither she nor her accompanying sister had previously noted it, suggesting that it was a significant observation. Contrast-enhanced brain CT demonstrated a homogeneously enhancing mass overlying the right frontal cortex. Brain MRI confirmed its superficial location. There was concomitant dura mater enhancement within the area immediately adjacent to the tumor. A meningioma was identified at surgery; a complete surgical resection was successfully performed. Postoperatively her headaches ceased.

Demographics

Meningiomas typically occur in middle-aged and older individuals, especially women, but can occur at any age. Approximately 15%–20% of intracranial tumors are meningiomas. These tumors may present at any level of the neuraxis; they are primarily located intracranially, typically at the parasagittal falx cerebri separating the two hemispheres, the meninges covering the hemispheres, along the sphenoid ridge medial skull base,

CLINICAL VIGNETTE Bilateral galactorrhea developed in a 32-year-old woman. Her menses had stopped a few months earlier and she thought she was pregnant; however, pregnancy testing was negative. Otherwise, she was in excellent health. Three years earlier, she had given birth to a healthy child. Her neurologic examination was normal.

Endocrinologic evaluation demonstrated a significantly elevated serum prolactin with decreased follicle-stimulating hormone (FSH) and luteinizing hormone (LH) levels in her blood. With MRI of her sella turcica, a mass became evident. This was consistent with a pituitary adenoma.

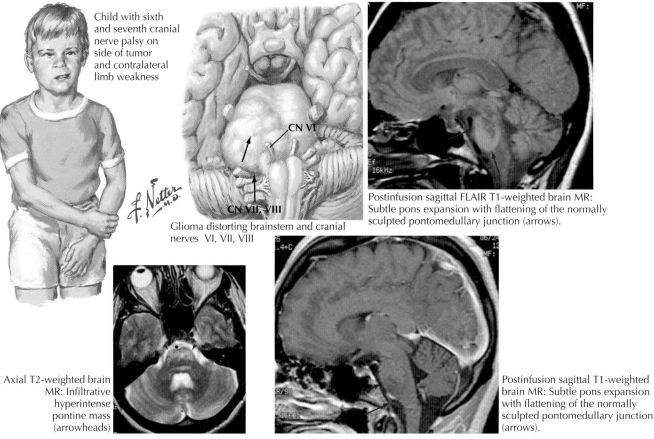

Child with sixth and seventh cranial nerve palsy on side of tumor and contralateral limb weakness

CN VI

CN VII, VIII

Glioma distorting brainstem and cranial nerves VI, VII, VIII

Postinfusion sagittal FLAIR T1-weighted brain MR: Subtle pons expansion with flattening of the normally sculpted pontomedullary junction (arrows).

Axial T2-weighted brain MR: Infiltrative hyperintense pontine mass (arrowheads)

Postinfusion sagittal T1-weighted brain MR: Subtle pons expansion with flattening of the normally sculpted pontomedullary junction (arrows).

Fig. 49.10 Brainstem Glioma.

Demographics

Pituitary adenomas are the second most common of the various benign brain tumors. Intrinsic pituitary lesions represent approximately 10% of all intracranial tumors; these are classified according to whether they are endocrinologically active. The majority of pituitary adenomas arise from the anterior portion of the pituitary gland (adenohypophysis).

Clinical Presentation

Endocrinologically active tumors secrete hormones, often resulting in symptoms appropriate to the target glands to which the specific active cell type is directed. The clinical picture characteristic of a pituitary tumor depends on its primary cell type of origin (Fig. 49.13). For example, in the preceding vignette, abnormal galactorrhea was directly related to the production of increased amounts of prolactin-secreting tumor cells. These are among the most common endocrinologically active pituitary tumors. Pituitary acidophil adenomas that primarily secrete growth hormone lead to the clinical syndrome of acromegaly with gigantism and/or enlarged bony features in the face, skull, and hands. Cushing disease with truncal obesity, cervical buffalo hump, moonlike flushed facies, proximal muscle weakness, hypokalemia, and glucose intolerance occurs when pituitary adenomas primarily secrete adrenocorticotropic hormone, leading to increased circulating serum cortisol (Fig. 49.14).

Chromophobe adenomas are not endocrinologically productive; however when an adenoma develops here initially, these tumors may be clinically silent. Although histologically benign, pituitary adenomas may have serious consequences when they remain undiagnosed early on because their proximity to the optic nerves, the optic tracts, the

cavernous sinus, and the temporal lobe tip may lead to significant neurologic consequences. The nonendocrinologically active tumors frequently reach a large size before symptoms develop (Fig. 49.15). Typically their diagnosis depends on the presentation of mass effect symptoms. Bitemporal visual field cuts result when pituitary macroadenomas extend above the sella and compress the overlying optic chiasm.

Pituitary apoplexy is a relatively rare clinical presentation for pituitary adenomas. Classically, this is an acute-onset severe headache associated with significant visual impairment and decreased mental status. Sometimes this may well mimic a ruptured intracranial aneurysm. The cause is often a hemorrhage into a preexisting pituitary adenoma (Fig. 49.16).

Diagnostic Approach

Patients with suspected pituitary adenomas are evaluated with a combination of imaging and endocrinologic studies. Brain MRI is the best radiographic modality to identify pituitary tumors. Expansion of the sella, diminished enhancement within it, and shifting of the pituitary stalk to one side are all clues for a possible pituitary microadenoma. In contrast, macroadenomas (measuring >25 mm) extend above the sella or into the cavernous sinus on either side of the sella and are easily identified with MRI (see Fig. 49.16). A thorough endocrine evaluation includes serum levels of prolactin, FSH and LH, cortisol, and growth hormone as well as thyroid function parameters.

Treatment

Initially many patients with pituitary adenomas primarily require medical therapy. Prolactin-secreting tumors are often successfully controlled with bromocriptine, a dopamine agonist that suppresses prolactin

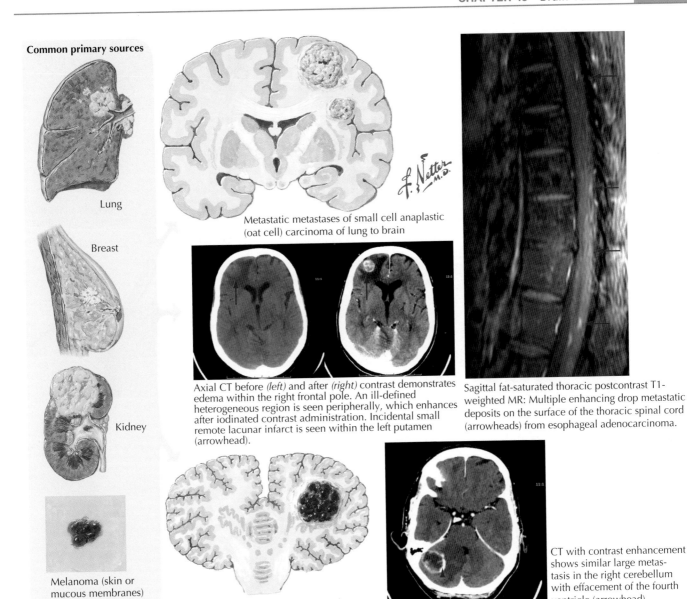

Common primary sources

Lung

Breast

Kidney

Melanoma (skin or mucous membranes)

Metastatic metastases of small cell anaplastic (oat cell) carcinoma of lung to brain

Axial CT before (left) and after (right) contrast demonstrates edema within the right frontal pole. An ill-defined heterogeneous region is seen peripherally, which enhances after iodinated contrast administration. Incidental small remote lacunar infarct is seen within the left putamen (arrowhead).

Sagittal fat-saturated thoracic postcontrast T1-weighted MR: Multiple enhancing drop metastatic deposits on the surface of the thoracic spinal cord (arrowheads) from esophageal adenocarcinoma.

Cerebellar metastasis of cutaneous melanoma

CT with contrast enhancement shows similar large metastasis in the right cerebellum with effacement of the fourth ventricle (arrowhead).

Fig. 49.11 Tumors Metastatic to Brain.

production and concomitantly decreases tumor volume. Growth hormone–secreting tumors are often controlled with octreotide, a somatostatin analog. Small nonsecreting pituitary tumors may often be observed for endocrine dysfunction or signs of growth with combined clinical and MRI modalities.

Endocrinologically active tumors that cannot be controlled with medication are a prime indication for surgical treatment, as are patients who harbor a macroadenoma producing mass effect. The surgery is primarily performed using a transsphenoidal approach through the nasal cavity and the sphenoid sinus, wherein the contents of the sella can be visualized and the tumor can be removed, often sparing the pituitary gland.

Postoperatively, these patients require follow-up for signs of hypopituitarism. This is particularly important for those individuals presenting with Cushing disease. Subsequent to surgery, their adrenocorticotropic hormone secretion is diminished. These patients usually require postoperative and sometimes lifelong steroid replacement. Pituitary adenoma surgery is associated with concomitant problems of sodium balance and fluid intake, leading to hyponatremia with polydipsia and polyuria. This necessitates careful follow-up and sometimes treatment with

desmopressin acetate 1-deamino-8-D-arginine vasopressin [DDAVP] to replace the naturally occurring antidiuretic hormone (ADH). This is a synthetic analog of the natural pituitary hormone 8-arginine vasopressin, an ADH affecting renal water conservation.

Craniopharyngioma

Craniopharyngiomas are uncommon tumors thought to arise from a remnant of the brain's embryologic development, namely the Rathke pouch. These histologically benign cystic lesions—often occurring in the region of the sella, hypothalamus, or third ventricle—comprise 2%–3% of all intracranial tumors. There is a greater incidence in children. Typically the presenting symptoms include visual impairment, pituitary dysfunction, and hydrocephalus.

The radiographic features of craniopharyngiomas distinguish them from other tumors of the suprasellar region (Fig. 49.17). Cystic changes, variable contrast enhancement, and calcification seen on CT occur frequently.

Surgery is the treatment of choice for symptomatic craniopharyngiomas. The suprasellar location limits tumor access, making incomplete

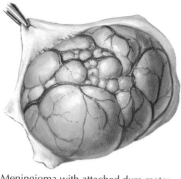

Meningioma with attached dura mater removed from brain, leaving depressed bed

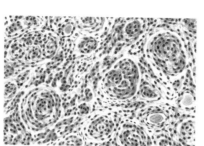

Histologic section showing whorl formation

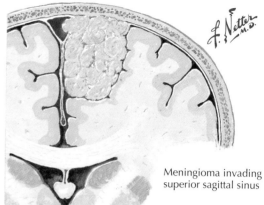

Meningioma invading superior sagittal sinus

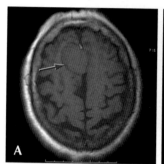
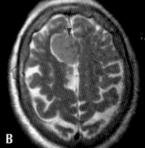
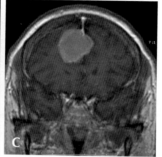

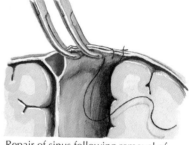

Repair of sinus following removal of tumor

Meningioma of falx. Axial T1-weighted FLAIR (A) and coronal post–gadolinium-enhanced T1-weighted images with fat saturation demonstrate an extraaxial, right falx-based mass (B), which extends through the falx to the left (C). The lesion is isointense to brain on T1- weighted sequences and enhances homogeneously.

Fig. 49.12 Meningiomas.

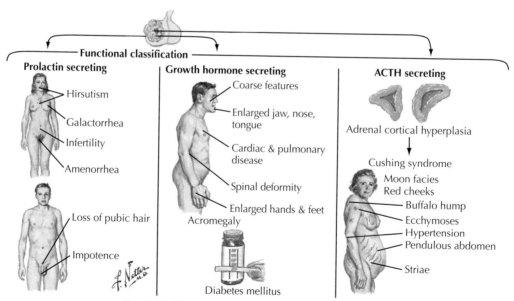

Functional classification

Prolactin secreting
- Hirsutism
- Galactorrhea
- Infertility
- Amenorrhea
- Loss of pubic hair
- Impotence

Growth hormone secreting
- Coarse features
- Enlarged jaw, nose, tongue
- Cardiac & pulmonary disease
- Spinal deformity
- Enlarged hands & feet

Acromegaly

Diabetes mellitus

ACTH secreting

Adrenal cortical hyperplasia

↓

Cushing syndrome
- Moon facies
- Red cheeks
- Buffalo hump
- Ecchymoses
- Hypertension
- Pendulous abdomen
- Striae

Fig. 49.13 Pituitary Adenoma: Clinical Manifestations.

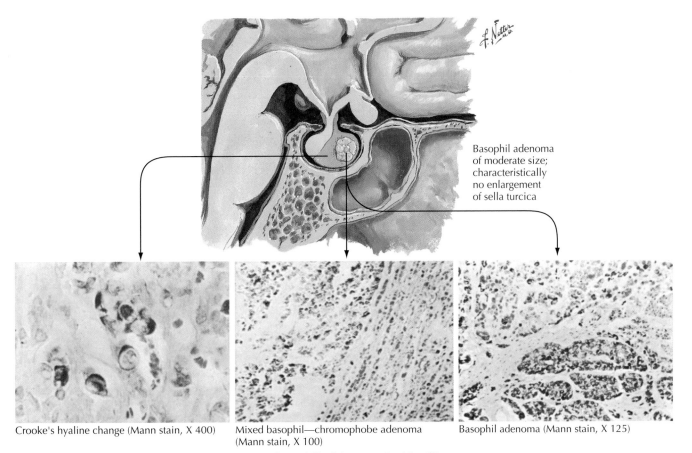

Crooke's hyaline change (Mann stain, X 400)

Mixed basophil—chromophobe adenoma (Mann stain, X 100)

Basophil adenoma (Mann stain, X 125)

Basophil adenoma of moderate size; characteristically no enlargement of sella turcica

Fig. 49.14 Basophilic Adenoma: Cushing Disease.

resections common. Resection is also difficult because of the intense glial reaction of the surrounding brain, causing adherence to critical brain structures and nearby blood vessels. As with pituitary surgery, craniopharyngioma resection may also have a difficult postoperative course, particularly with endocrine dysfunction. Although RT and possibly radiosurgery can decrease recurrence rates, craniopharyngiomas have a high rate of local recurrence.

Acoustic Neuroma/Vestibular Schwannoma

CLINICAL VIGNETTE *A previously healthy 42-year-old Army chaplain noted that he could no longer hear well on the telephone using his left ear or understand a colleague when there was much ambient noise, particularly from other conversations. In retrospect, he had experienced mild progressive ringing in this ear. Initially this was attributed to chronic exposure to loud noises while he was assigned to an artillery brigade. Although the hearing loss gradually worsened over several years, it was not until his telephone difficulties led him to test himself that he found he could no longer appreciate the sound of a watch ticking. He was otherwise totally well. The only abnormal finding on his neurologic examination was grossly diminished hearing in his left ear.*

Audiometric examination revealed markedly decreased high-frequency appreciation and diminished speech discrimination in his left ear. Gadolinium MRI demonstrated a homogeneously enhancing 2- by 1.5-cm mass within the left cerebellopontine angle. This emanated from his internal auditory canal and was associated with mild pontine distortion.

Demographics

Acoustic neuromas are the second most common of the benign brain tumors. These comprise approximately 6%–8% of all primary intracranial neoplasms. There is a 2% incidence within the general population. Most commonly, acoustic neuromas present between ages 40 and 60 years. With the exception of patients who have genetically determined neurofibromatosis type II, it is unusual for an acoustic neuroma to be recognized clinically in a patient younger than 20 years of age. The non–genetically determined acoustic neuromas predominantly develop unilaterally. In contrast, those occasional patients with type II neurofibromatosis often have bilateral acoustic neuromas. These benign tumors arise from the Schwann cells of the vestibular nerve within the eighth CN complex (Fig. 49.18).

Clinical Presentation

The classic history is illustrated in the earlier clinical vignette. Patients typically report a slowly progressive unilateral hearing loss associated with tinnitus. This is consistent with the innate slow growth of a benign acoustic neuroma (also referred to as a vestibular schwannoma).

Although acoustic neuromas arise from the vestibular portion of CN VIII, hearing loss is usually the most prominent symptom. Anatomically, CN-VII (facial) is closely related to CN-VIII; however, it is almost unheard of for an acute facial nerve palsy to be the initial presenting symptom of an acoustic neuroma. Because of the eighth nerve's relation to the vestibular nerve within the cerebellopontine angle, adjacent to the brainstem and cerebellum, patients with very large acoustic neuromas may also have gait instability and sometimes associated headaches;

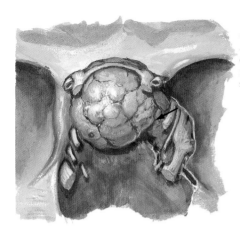

Invasive (malignant) adenoma; extension into right cavernous sinus

Large acidophil adenoma; extensive destruction of pituitary substance, compression of optic chiasm, invasion of third ventricle and floor of sella

f. Netter M.D.

Nonfunctioning

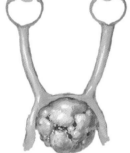

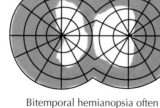

May grow large due to lack of early endocrine symptoms; optic chiasm compressed

Bitemporal hemianopsia often initial symptom

Fig. 49.15 Pituitary Macroadenoma.

however, these individuals do not present with acute vertigo. Later on an acoustic neuroma may sometimes lead to pressure on either the trigeminal (fifth) CN or its adjacent brainstem, affecting CN-V function, with a resultant ipsilateral facial sensory loss and a diminished corneal reflex. Occasionally very large tumors may impair the CSF circulation near the fourth ventricle, leading to hydrocephalus.

During clinical examination, CN evaluation is the key to this diagnosis and of utmost importance. Hearing loss from CN-VIII involvement

is the hallmark finding for acoustic neuromas. Lateral gaze nystagmus is occasionally noted when extraocular movements are tested. Larger tumors may cause CN-VII and CN-V impairment as previously summarized. It is most unusual to have any lower CN involvement or clinically significant enough brainstem compression to lead to either a hemiparesis or hemisensory loss.

Diagnostic Studies

MRI is the primary diagnostic modality. Its clarity, resolution, and ability to scan in multiple planes allow for three-dimensional assessment. Because the size of the lesion and its relation to adjacent neurologic structures, such as the pons and various CNs, often determine treatment, MRI is also a therapeutically very crucial investigational modality. Typically these well-demarcated, homogeneously enhancing tumors arise within the cerebellopontine angle and extend into the internal auditory canal (see Fig. 49.18).

Treatment

Surgery is the traditional and primary therapeutic modality; stereotactic radiosurgery is occasionally used. Acoustic neuromas often grow slowly. It is reasonable to observe some tumors temporally, if clinically warranted, particularly with elderly patients presenting with unilateral hearing loss who also have multiple other medical issues. Often the better part of valor here is simply to follow the patient with serial imaging. When MRI evidence demonstrates significant tumor growth or patients have progressively worsening symptoms, especially in addition to hearing loss, surgical intervention is indicated.

Surgical resection of acoustic neuromas is often performed using both neurosurgery and otorhinolaryngology specialists concomitantly. The surgical goal is tumor resection and preservation of CN-VII and CN-VIII function when at all possible. This approach is particularly important with large-volume tumors exhibiting brainstem compression. Hearing preservation in patients with these large acoustic neuromas is often impossible because the cochlear nerve becomes indistinguishable from the tumor. Success rates for hearing preservation vary directly with tumor volume. When CN-VII is densely adherent to the tumor capsule, a subtotal resection is often indicated because preservation of the facial nerve is more important than complete surgical removal.

Stereotactic radiosurgery involves a single nonsurgical treatment using high-dose radiation to a precisely localized three-dimensional volume. This modality can control approximately 80%–85% of acoustic tumors. It involves many of the same risks as conventional surgery but is an excellent option for patients with small tumors (2–3 cm) who have no useful hearing. Control of tumor growth is achieved and operative risks are avoided. With improved imaging, acoustic neuromas are being detected earlier; therefore a greater potential for a complete cure exists early on in the natural history of the acoustic neuroma.

Other Benign Intracranial Tumors
Chordoma

These are very rare, usually benign tumors that have embryologic elements similar to those of intervertebral disks. Typically chordomas develop either on the clivus of the skull base or the sacrum (Fig. 49.19). Intracranial chordomas arise from within the skull bone and cause local destruction. Concomitantly these tumors enter the intradural space, where they sometimes affect the brainstem and CNs.

The histology of typical chordomas is characterized by large, mucus-filled cells called physaliferous cells. Very uncommonly, a few chordomas demonstrate features of frank malignancy. Additionally, their aggressive local invasion of bone mimics a locally malignant process. The tumors that lead to significant bony destruction often recur locally at a high rate, thus making a surgical cure difficult to achieve. Nevertheless,

A. Grade of sella turcica enlargement and/or erosion

Enclosed adenomas ───────── ───────── Invasive adenomas

I. Sella normal, floor may be indented

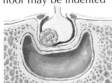

II. Sella enlarged, but floor intact

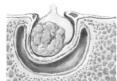

III. Localized erosion of floor

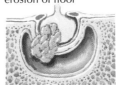

IV. Entire floor diffusely eroded

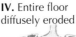
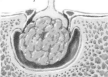

B. Type of suprasellar extension

A. No suprasellar extension of tumor

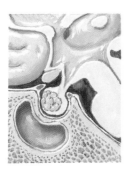

B. Suprasellar bulge does not reach floor of 3rd ventricle

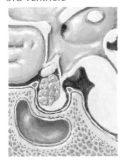

C. Tumor reaches 3rd ventricle, distorting its chiasmatic recess

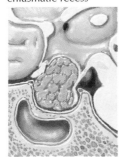

D. Tumor fills 3rd ventricle almost to interventricular foramen (of Monro)

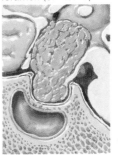

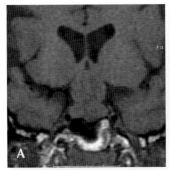
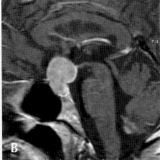

Large pituitary tumor. (**A**) Coronal T1-weighted and (**B**) sagittal T1-weighted post–gadolinium-enhanced images show a dumbbell-shaped tumor within a moderately enlarged sella with a larger component protruding above and posterior to the sella with elevation and distortion of the optic chiasm.

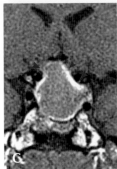
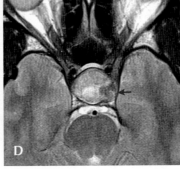

Pituitary apoplexy in a 44-year-old man presenting with severe headache, diplopia, photophobia, nausea and vomiting. (**C**) Coronal T1-weighted post gadolinium-enhanced fast spin echo imaging demonstrates a large intrasellar mass with peripheral enhancement (arrowheads) and upward displacement of the optic chiasm. (**D**) The central nonenhanced component shows a very heterogeneous signal pattern on axial T2-weighted imaging with more compression of the left cavernous sinus (arrow) and represents a hemorrhagic necrotic pituitary adenoma.

Fig. 49.16 Pituitary Adenoma Gradation Vis-à-Vis Enlargement of the Sella.

surgical resection is often used initially, although complete resection is often impossible because of local anatomic constraints. Although RT is generally used, the role of this modality for the treatment of residual tumor is unclear. Radiosurgery and proton beam irradiation have been proposed, but their benefit is also uncertain. Chemotherapy is not of value in the treatment of chordomas.

Pineal Region Tumors

Tumors occurring in the region of the pineal gland are uncommon, comprising approximately 1% of intracranial tumors. These neoplasms, having a histologically mixed benignancy, include germ cell tumors, glial neoplasms, and pineal parenchyma tumors (Fig. 49.20). Tumors of germ cell origin are the most common, usually occurring in younger

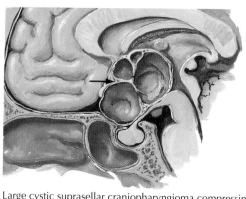

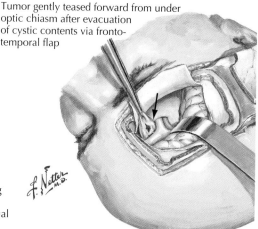

Tumor gently teased forward from under optic chiasm after evacuation of cystic contents via fronto-temporal flap

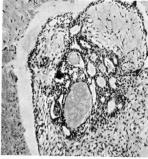

Large cystic suprasellar craniopharyngioma compressing optic chiasm and hypothalamus, filling 3rd ventricle up to interventricular foramen (of Monro), thus causing visual impairment, diabetes insipidus, and hydrocephalus

Histologic section: craniopharyngioma (H and E stain, ×125)

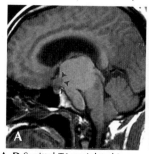
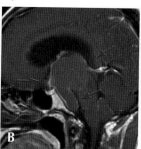
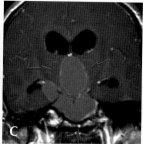
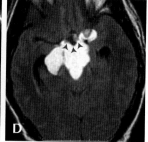

A–D Sagittal T1-weighted images without **A** and after **B** gadolinium enhancement and **C** coronal T1-weighted gadolinium-enhanced images demonstrate a multilobulated mass above the sella and normal pituitary extending into the interpeduncular cistern and into the prepontine cistern. The posterior portion above the sella is solid (arrowheads in Figure A), whereas the remainder is cystic with faint rim enhancement (indicated by the arrows in Figure B and C). The T2-weighted axial image **D** shows the darker solid component (arrowheads) and the T2-bright cystic portions.

Fig. 49.17 Craniopharyngioma.

patients. Gliomas can arise from within the pineal gland itself or from the glial cells in the surrounding tissue. In this region, glial tumors tend to be of lower grade. Tumors arising from the pineal parenchyma comprise approximately 20% of pineal region tumors.

These neoplasms are further classified into pineoblastomas and pineocytomas. *Pineoblastomas* are poorly differentiated tumors that can spread throughout the CSF pathways or directly into adjacent brain parenchyma. *Pineocytomas* are usually well-encapsulated cellular tumors that do not invade surrounding tissue. A mixed form of pineal parenchymal tumor contains features of both pineocytoma and pineoblastoma. Teratomas, embryonal carcinomas, endodermal sinus tumors, and choriocarcinomas are also found in the pineal region.

With the increasing use of MRI, asymptomatic pineal region cysts are identified more commonly. These cysts are usually incidental findings and rarely require any treatment. Serial MRI scans are used to track any growth over time.

Colloid Cysts

These are histologically benign third ventricle tumors that arise from remnants of embryologic development. The cells lining the walls of the cyst are ciliated. Third ventricular lesions of this type typically become symptomatic during adulthood, but they can also be seen in children. Posturally precipitated headaches, with concomitant symptoms and signs of hydrocephalus, are the most common clinical presentations for colloid cysts. Because of their inherent intraventricular location, these cysts lead to CSF obstruction at the foramina of Monro (Fig. 49.21).

Colloid cysts are occasionally associated with sudden death, presumably from an acute hydrocephalus; however, most patients present with a more gradual temporal profile. Although the diagnosis is typi-

cally suggested by recurrent posturally triggered headaches, MRI or CT is ideal for confirming the presence of a cystic-appearing intraventricular mass.

Treatment of symptomatic colloid cysts is usually surgical, and complete resection is often possible. Care must be exercised during surgical resection because the fornix, adjacent to the tumor, can be injured, resulting in severe memory impairment. If surgery for resection is not possible, CSF diversion through shunting can often relieve the symptoms of hydrocephalus.

With the increased use of MRI, many more cystic tumors within the third ventricle are being described. These asymptomatic lesions are followed with serial scans; treatment is reserved for those patients whose cysts increase in size.

Differential Diagnosis
Pseudotumor Cerebri/Idiopathic Intracranial Hypotension, Intracranial Hypotension, and Other Brain Lesions

> **CLINICAL VIGNETTE** *An obese 42-year-old woman presented with a 2-month history of increasingly severe headaches and intermittent double vision. Her headaches were exacerbated by postural changes, particularly bending forward or jarring in the car. Bilateral limitation of adduction of her eyes, compatible with sixth CN paresis and modest papilledema (Fig. 49.22), were noted on neurologic examination. Brain imaging demonstrated diminished size of her lateral ventricles. CSF pressure was 350 mm (normal is <180 mm); it was otherwise normal.*

This case is representative of a rather uncommon syndrome known as idiopathic intracranial hypertension (i.e., pseudotumor cerebri [PTC]).

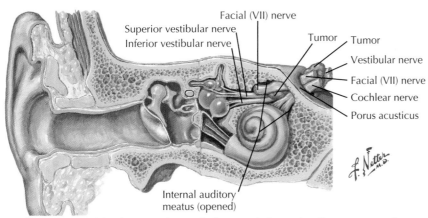

Small neurinoma arising from superior vestibular nerve in internal auditory meatus and protruding into posterior fossa

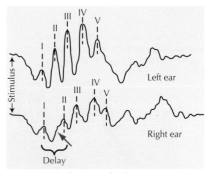

Brainstem auditory evoked response (BAER) in patient with acoustic neurinoma on right side. There is delay in action potentials of cochlear nerve (wave I) and cochlear nuclei (wave II) on affected side.

Neurofibromatosis, Type II

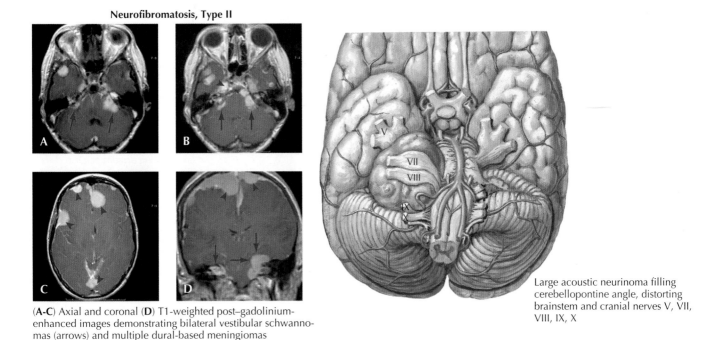

(A-C) Axial and coronal (D) T1-weighted post–gadolinium-enhanced images demonstrating bilateral vestibular schwannomas (arrows) and multiple dural-based meningiomas (arrowheads). Both types of tumors enhance avidly.

Large acoustic neurinoma filling cerebellopontine angle, distorting brainstem and cranial nerves V, VII, VIII, IX, X

Fig. 49.18 Acoustic Neuroma.

This usually occurs in obese young women who are otherwise healthy. Clinically PTC is primarily characterized by progressively severe poorly defined headaches, often with diplopia. Transient visual obscurations and pulsatile tinnitus may also occur. On neurologic examination these patients are typically awake, alert, have papilledema, sometimes a lateral rectus muscle weakness, but no focal neurologic deficits. By definition MRI is normal or demonstrates small lateral ventricles. PTC, again by definition, is associated with increased CSF pressure (250–500 mm).

Although idiopathic PTC has no identifiable etiology, certain predisposing factors must be considered, including oral contraceptives, corticosteroids, estrogen and progestational therapies, non-steroidal anti-inflammatory drugs [NSAIDs], hypervitaminosis A, various antibiotics (tetracycline, minocycline, nitrofurantoin, ampicillin, or nalidixic acid), and anesthetic agents (ketamine and nitrous oxide), amiodarone, and perhexiline.

Other neurologic disorders may occasionally present with a PTC clinical picture. These include leptomeningeal diseases such as chronic

infectious or granulomatous processes—that is, tuberculosis, metastatic cancer or lymphoma seeding, cerebral venous sinus obstruction, and various endocrinologic disorders such as, for example, myxedema, hypoparathyroidism, and Addison and Cushing diseases. There are very rare reports of a PTC picture presumed to be related to extremely elevated CSF protein levels, particularly with Guillain-Barré syndrome or primary spinal cord malignancies.

Treatment

Discontinuation of an offending medication will reverse the PTC syndrome on the rare occasion that such is identified. Most importantly, one needs to be concerned by the fact that chronically increased intracranial pressure will lead to loss of visual acuity. This is secondary to swelling of the optic nerve head, that is, papilledema. It is measured by frequent and formal visual field testing to identify increasing size of the blind spots. This is essential to prevent permanent visual loss with PTC. Potential treatments include weight loss, low-salt diet, diuretics, and symptomatic headache control. When PTC continues to evolve

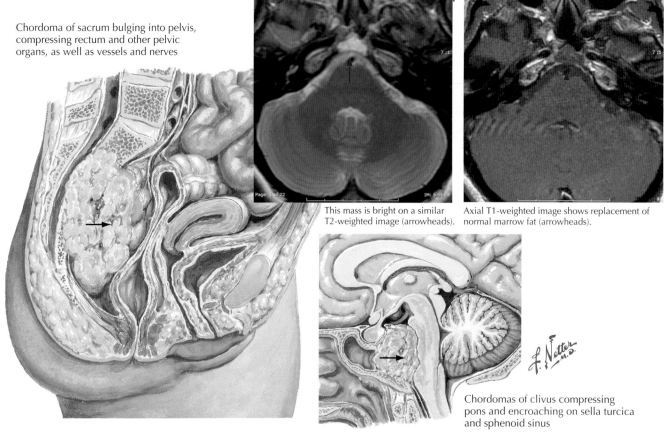

Chordoma of sacrum bulging into pelvis, compressing rectum and other pelvic organs, as well as vessels and nerves

This mass is bright on a similar T2-weighted image (arrowheads).

Axial T1-weighted image shows replacement of normal marrow fat (arrowheads).

Chordomas of clivus compressing pons and encroaching on sella turcica and sphenoid sinus

Fig. 49.19 Chordomas.

with progressive visual compromise, more aggressive therapy is indicated, including fenestration of the optic nerve sheath or one of the various CSF shunting procedures.

Intracranial Hypotension (Syndrome of Low Cerebrospinal Fluid Pressure)

CLINICAL VIGNETTE *A vigorous, previously healthy 60-year-old physician who had recently developed severe depression, requiring both a serotonin reuptake inhibitor and unilateral electroshock therapy (EST), developed increasingly severe posturally exacerbated headaches. When these were greatly exacerbated while he was a passenger in a small float plane as it landed bouncing over the water, he went to a neurologist. His examination was normal. Postgadolinium MRI demonstrated leptomeningeal enhancement but no mass lesions. CSF pressure was too low to measure. No known relation with the EST was identified. He then recalled having a relatively severe closed head injury 3 weeks earlier when he forcefully struck his forehead on the unexpectedly low-set frame of a barn door. As a result, 20-mL extradural blood patch was empirically injected at his midlumbar spine. The headaches gradually and totally cleared within 2 weeks.*

Classic low-CSF-pressure headaches are severe, exacerbated by postural factors; they often mimic the ball-valve effect seen in some intraventricular brain tumors. Most commonly, these occur subsequent to a diagnostic lumbar puncture, spinal anesthesia, or a seemingly benign closed head injury. MRI with gadolinium is essential to the diagnosis (Fig. 49.23). When there is no history of a spinal tap or significant head trauma, this clinical setting, as well as the MRI, somewhat mimics various leptomeningeal neoplastic or inflammatory lesions. The MR imaging

with low-pressure headache syndrome has a smooth enhancement, in contrast to the serpiginous irregular enhancement seen with neoplastic infiltration. The CSF analysis primarily helps make this differentiation. Occasionally introduction of a radioisotope into the CSF will identify a source of CSF leak that may require surgical repair. In many of these instances, no site of potential spinal fluid leak is identified. As in the earlier vignette, a spinal blood patch can provide relief and a therapeutic diagnosis; however, it is not universally successful and in rare instances the patient may have permanent incapacitation (e.g., not being able to raise his or her head, being unable to pursue one's occupation, or even to maintain many routine activities of daily living).

Other Intracranial Lesions

Subdural hematomas, herpes encephalitis, brain abscess, and arteriovenous malformations may all have a clinical presentation similar to that of a brain tumor. There are other rare disorders of a demyelinating nature that require consideration in the differential diagnosis of brain tumors. Occasional patients have MRI findings mimicking a malignant glioma, but stereotactic biopsy demonstrates a primary monofocal acute inflammatory demyelination (see Chapter 39). These lesions are usually self-limited and occur in a setting where there is no prior clinical or MRI evidence of multiple sclerosis. Fortunately these are often responsive to corticosteroids. Subsequently, new lesions may appear in different portions of the cerebral cortex. Acute disseminated encephalomyelitis (ADEM) and acute hemorrhagic leukoencephalopathy (AHL) are two acute postinfectious demyelinating disorders; the former is more likely to respond to corticosteroids and the latter frequently has a fulminate course (see Chapter 40).

Progressive multifocal leukoencephalopathy (PML) may also present in a fashion similar to a brain tumor in immunocompromised hosts

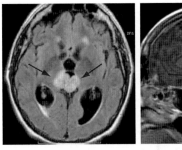

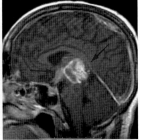

Pineoblastoma. Axial FLAIR and sagittal T1-weighted gadolinium-enhanced images show a large mass in the pineal region, bright on FLAIR imaging, heterogeneous after gadolinium enhancement, compressing the aqueduct with enlargement of the third and lateral ventricles.

Tumor compressing mesencephalic tectum and corpora quadrigemina, occluding cerebral aqueduct (of Sylvius), and invading 3rd ventricle

Parinaud syndrome: paresis of upward gaze, unequal pupils, loss of convergence

Diabetes insipidus in some patients

Sexual precocity in boys may occur

Anatomic aspects of exposure

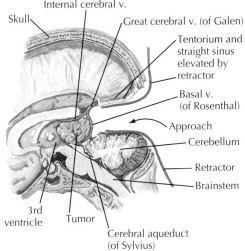

Skull

Internal cerebral v.

Great cerebral v. (of Galen)

Tentorium and straight sinus elevated by retractor

Basal v. (of Rosenthal)

Approach

Cerebellum

Retractor

Brainstem

3rd ventricle

Tumor

Cerebral aqueduct (of Sylvius)

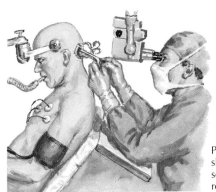

Position of patient (undraped to show detail), surgeon, and microscope for resection of pineal region tumors

Fig. 49.20 Pineal Region Tumors.

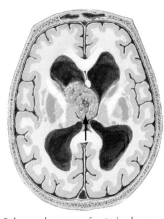

Subependymoma of anterior horn of left lateral ventricle obstructing interventricular foramen (of Monro), thus producing marked hydrocephalus

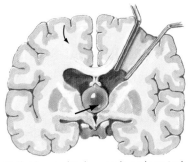

Colloid cyst of 3rd ventricle and surgical approach via right prefrontal (silent) cerebral cortex. May also be approached through corpus callosum (arrow). Note enlarged lateral ventricles (posterior view).

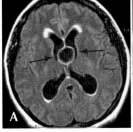

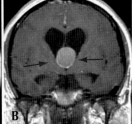

Colloid cyst. (**A**) Axial, FLAIR and (**B**) coronal, T1-weighted gadolinium-enhanced images demonstrate a round cystic mass in the region of the foramina of Monro, with dilatation of the lateral ventricles. The signal characteristics are variable. This cyst is hypointense on T2-weighted images and bright on T1-weighted imaging, with minimal peripheral enhancement.

Fig. 49.21 Intraventricular Tumors.

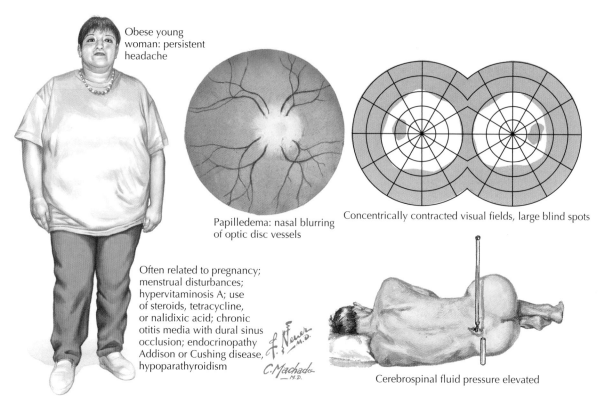

Obese young woman: persistent headache

Papilledema: nasal blurring of optic disc vessels

Concentrically contracted visual fields, large blind spots

Often related to pregnancy; menstrual disturbances; hypervitaminosis A; use of steroids, tetracycline, or nalidixic acid; chronic otitis media with dural sinus occlusion; endocrinopathy Addison or Cushing disease, hypoparathyroidism

Cerebrospinal fluid pressure elevated

Fig. 49.22 Pseudotumor Cerebri.

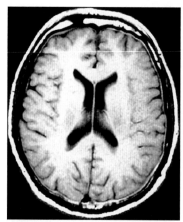

A. Axial FLAIR image with dural thickening.

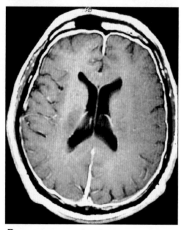

B. Axial T1-weighted, gadolinium-enhanced image with striking enhancement of the thickened dura.

Fig. 49.23 Intracranial Hypotension.

receiving long-term immunosuppressive therapy or in patients with human immunodeficiency virus (HIV) infection (see Chapter 48).

Future Directions

Treatment of benign intracranial tumors has improved with better MR imaging and the development of new surgical techniques that exploit bone removal rather than brain manipulation. These skull base techniques allow for exposure and resection of tumors in previously inaccessible locations within the skull. Intraoperative monitoring of CN function is being used more frequently to limit the morbidity of these operations.

Improvements in stereotactic radiosurgery continue to allow for the control of tumor growth while causing fewer radiation adverse effects. Further research into the relation of hormonal receptors in meningiomas may someday allow for a medical means of controlling these tumors.

ADDITIONAL RESOURCES

Ahsan H, Neugut AI, Bruce JN. Trends in incidence of primary malignant brain tumors in USA, 1981-1990. Int J Epidemiol 1995;24(6):1078–85.

Berger MS, Hadjipanayis CG. Surgery of intrinsic cerebral tumors. Neurosurgery 2007;61(Suppl. 1):279–304.

Binder DK, Horton JC, Lawton MT, et al. Idiopathic intracranial hypertension. Neurosurgery 2004;54:538–51.

Black PM. Meningiomas. Neurosurgery 1993;32:643–57.

Castrucci WA, Knisely JP. An update on the treatment of CNS metastases in small cell lung cancer. Cancer J 2008;14(3):138–46.

Ciric I. Long-term management and outcome for pituitary tumors. Neurosurg Clin N Am 2003;14:167–71.

Daumas-Duport C, Scheithauer BW, O'Fallon J, et al. Grading of astrocytomas: a simple and reproducible method. Cancer 1988;62:2152–65.

Dietrich J, Norden AD, Wen PY. Emerging antiangiogenic treatments for gliomas—efficacy and safety issues. Curr Opin Neurol 2008;21(6):736–44.

Gutrecht JA, Berger JR, Jones HR, et al. Monofocal acute inflammatory demyelination (MAID): a unique disorder simulating brain neoplasm. South Med J 2002;95:1180–6.

Karim AB, Afra D, Cornu P, et al. Randomized trial on the efficacy of radiotherapy for cerebral low-grade glioma in the adult: European Organization for Research and Treatment of Cancer Study 22845 with the Medical Research Council study BRO4: an interim analysis. Int J Radiat Oncol Biol Phys 2002;52(2):316–24.

Kennedy PG. Viral encephalitis: causes, differential diagnosis, and management. J Neurol Neurosurg Psychiatry 2004;75(Suppl. 1):i10–15.

Koss SA, Ulmer JL, Hacein-Bey L. Angiographic features of spontaneous intracranial hypotension. AJNR Am J Neuroradiol 2003;24:704–6.

Larijani B, Bastanhagh MH, Pajouhi M, et al. Presentation and outcome of 93 cases of craniopharyngioma. Eur J Cancer Care (Engl) 2004;13:11–15.

Maarouf M, Kuchta J, Miletic H, et al. Acute demyelination: diagnostic difficulties and the need for brain biopsy. Acta Neurochir (Wien) 2003;145:961–9.

MacFarlane R, King TT. Acoustic neurinoma: vestibular schwannoma. In: Kaye AH, Larz ER Jr, editors. Brain tumors. Philadelphia, PA: Churchill Livingstone; 1995. p. 577–622.

Mason WP, Cairncross JG. Invited article: the expanding impact of molecular biology on the diagnosis and treatment of gliomas. Neurology 2008;71(5):365–73.

Mathiesen T, Grane P, Lindgren L, et al. Third ventricle colloid cysts: a consecutive 12-year series. J Neurosurg 1997;86:5–12.

Menezes AH, Gantz BJ, Traynelis VC, et al. Cranial base chordomas. Clin Neurosurg 1997;44:491–509.

Mokri B. Headaches caused by decreased intracranial pressure: diagnosis and management. Curr Opin Neurol 2003;16:319–26.

Ohgaki H. Epidemiology of brain tumors. Methods Mol Biol 2009;472:323–42.

Prados MD, Scott C, Curran WJ Jr, et al. Procarbazine, lomustine, and vincristine (PCV) chemotherapy for anaplastic astrocytoma: a retrospective review of radiation therapy oncology group protocols comparing survival with carmustine or PCV adjuvant chemotherapy. J Clin Oncol 1999;17(11):3389–95.

Rapport RL, Hillier D, Scearce T, et al. Spontaneous intracranial hypotension from intradural thoracic disc herniation: case report. J Neurosurg 2003;98(Suppl.):282–4.

Raschilas F, Wolff M, Delatour F, et al. Outcome of and prognostic factors for herpes simplex encephalitis in adult patients: results of a multicenter study. Clin Infect Dis 2002;35:254–60.

Tentori L, Graziani G. Recent approaches to improve the antitumor efficacy of temozolomide. Curr Med Chem 2009;16(2):245–57.

Ullrich RT, Kracht LW, Jacobs AH. Neuroimaging in patients with gliomas. Semin Neurol 2008;28(4):484–94.

50

Spinal Cord Tumors

Peter K. Dempsey, Lloyd M. Alderson

The most common spinal cord tumors are metastatic extradural lesions most commonly occurring in patients with already identified systemic cancers. Their presentation is often relatively acute, usually associated with focal back and/or radicular pain. On occasion, these lesions are the initial clinical manifestation of a heretofore unsuspected systemic malignancy. In contrast, primary intradural spinal cord tumors occur infrequently; typically their presentation is a relatively subtle one, ingravescent in temporal profile. Spinal cord and spinal column tumors are best classified within two categories: *extradural*, occurring outside of the dura, and *intradural*, contained within the dura mater (Table 50.1; Fig. 50.1).

Intradural tumors are further categorized as *extramedullary* or *intramedullary*, depending on their relationship to the spinal cord. *Intradural extramedullary* tumors, usually meningiomas or schwannomas, arise outside the spinal cord parenchyma. These are initially clinically silent; however, with time these tumors surreptitiously enlarge. Once a critical mass is reached, spinal cord compression occurs and symptoms develop. In contrast, *intradural intramedullary* tumors, such as gliomas and ependymomas, originate within parenchyma of the spinal cord. As these intramedullary malignancies primarily expand, important neurologic pathways and cell populations are subsequently compromised and eventually destroyed.

Extradural tumors generally are derived from metastatic lesions to vertebral bodies with extension into the epidural space, causing external compression of the thecal sac and its contents. Primary bony vertebral tumors also occur, both malignant (i.e., myeloma) and benign (i.e., hemangioma or osteoid osteoma).

EXTRADURAL SPINAL TUMORS

CLINICAL VIGNETTE *A 62-year-old postal carrier presented with midthoracic pain, rapidly progressive weakness and numbness in both legs and difficulty initiating his urine stream. During the preceding 6 weeks, he intermittently awakened with midthoracic vertebral pain that increasingly radiated to his epigastrium. This was particularly precipitated by lifting, bending, or straining at stool. An initial gastrointestinal evaluation was normal. Twenty-four hours before admission, he began to experience progressive difficulty standing, walking, and voiding. The morning of this evaluation, he was unable to get out of bed on his own and was totally unable to void. During the past 3 months, he had noted an increasingly irritating cough; he was a 60-pack-year smoker.*

Neurologic examination demonstrated a T9 "cord level" to both pinprick and temperature. Muscle stretch reflexes were absent at the knees and ankles, and plantar stimulation was flexor. There was mild tenderness to palpation over the lower thoracic spine. He became incontinent of urine. Rectal sphincter tone was reduced.

Spinal radiographs revealed destruction of the T9 vertebral body. Magnetic resonance imaging (MRI) demonstrated a soft tissue mass involving most of the T9 vertebral body, extending into the pedicle, with epidural extension of the tumor into the spinal canal leading to marked compression of the spinal cord. Immediate dexamethasone therapy and subsequent radiation therapy were unsuccessful in reversing his clinical course. Chest radiograph (Fig. 50.2) demonstrated a left main stem bronchus tumor that on biopsy proved to be a primary small cell lung cancer.

Spinal neoplasms are predominantly secondary to metastatic cancer. This occurs in up to one-third of cancer patients. Lung, breast, prostate, and lymphoma are the most common metastatic lesions leading to spinal cord compression.

Clinical Presentation

Severe focal vertebral pain is frequently the presenting symptom of a metastatic spinal cancer (see Fig. 50.2). Unfortunately, back pain is such a ubiquitous complaint that the serious nature of a newly occurring pain is often not appreciated even when there is no history of recent trauma. Sometimes, it is difficult to distinguish pain of a metastatic spinal tumor from the much more common mechanical, degenerative, or osteoarthritic musculoskeletal lower back and/or nerve root disorders. However, pain of metastatic spinal cancer origin is often persistent, frequently unrelated to posture, and tends to increase at night. In contrast to more common mechanical back pain, this pain can be of more recent origin.

Progressive neurologic symptoms often vary and are related to the precise level of spinal column involvement; typically the temporal profile is relatively rapid. Tumors at the cervical and thoracic spinal cord levels present with progressive weakness, numbness, and sphincter dysfunction at levels below the tumor. Sphincter difficulties are nonspecific symptoms per se that may develop with tumors at any spinal level. On occasion, bladder and bowel dysfunction per se may be the initial presenting symptom related to a conus medullaris tumor at the distal tip of the spinal cord. The essential message is that whenever sphincter problems develop in a patient with a known cancer, one needs to be alert to the potential of a spinal metastasis. Examination usually reveals hyperreflexia, Babinski signs, and other long tract signs at spinal levels below the tumor involvement.

When evaluating patients with recent-onset sphincter difficulties and suspicion for a metastatic lesion, it is important to recognize that differentiation of conus medullaris lesions at the spinal cord tip versus those within the cauda equina may be difficult. Classically when the clinical findings are symmetric and relatively equally involving both lower extremities, the conus medullaris is much more likely the site of the specific pathology. In contrast, cauda equina lesions often lead to

TABLE 50.1   Classification of Magnetic Resonance Imaging Abnormalities[a]

Extradural Extramedullary	Intradural Extramedullary	Intradural Intramedullary
Intervertebral disc disease	Neurinoma	Syringomyelia
Metastasis	Meningioma	Ependymoma
Lymphoma	Ependymoma	Glioma
Sarcoma	Medulloblastoma	Hemangioblastoma
Plasmacytoma	Cauda equina lesions	Myelitis
Primary bone tumor	Scarring	Edema
Scarring	Hypertrophic neuropathy	Lipoma
Abscess	Lymphoma	Abscess
Hemangioma	Metastasis	Hematoma
Hemorrhage	Hemangioblastoma	Varix with arteriovenous malformation
Neurilemmoma	Lipoma	Lymphoma
Chordoma	Dermoid	Neuroblastoma
	Epidermoid cyst	Metastasis
	Hemorrhage	

[a]Dermoid or epidermoid, teratoma, lipoma, and cysts are often associated with spinal dysraphism. In this setting, many tumors are intradural, although they may involve all three areas.

Extradural tumors

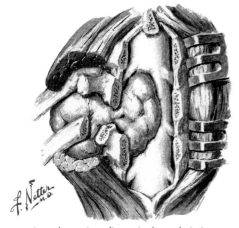

Lymphoma invading spinal canal via intervertebral foramen, compressing dura mater
and spinal cord

Intradural extramedullary tumors

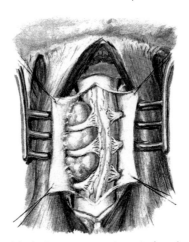

Meningioma compressing spinal cord
and distorting nerve roots

Intramedullary tumors

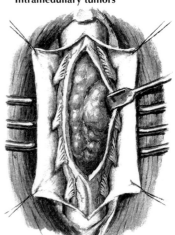

Astrocytoma exposed by longitudinal
incision in bulging spinal cord

Fig. 50.1 Classification of Spinal Tumors.

an asymmetric distribution of signs and symptoms because not all nerve roots within the cauda equina are equally affected.

Typically, the course of extradural metastatic spinal tumors is more rapid than intradural tumors. It is not unusual for these lesions to have an almost precipitous onset, often producing rapidly evolving motor and sensory deficits within just a few hours to a day or so (Fig. 50.3). A prior diagnosis of either a cancer or a lymphoma will alert the astute clinician to the precise pathophysiologic nature of the spinal lesion. However, occasionally a spinal metastasis may be the initial presentation of a metastatic malignancy.

Diagnostic Approach

MRI is the standard for evaluating potential metastatic spine lesions, especially those with evolving cord compression. When an MRI is contraindicated, such as with a patient who has a pacemaker, computed tomography (CT) myelogram is still indicated and potentially diagnostic. An initial preliminary spinal tap is best avoided in these patients because it can change pressure dynamics when there is an obstructing focal cord lesion. If a spinal tap is performed, this study can precipitate a rapid worsening of the patient's neurologic deficits.

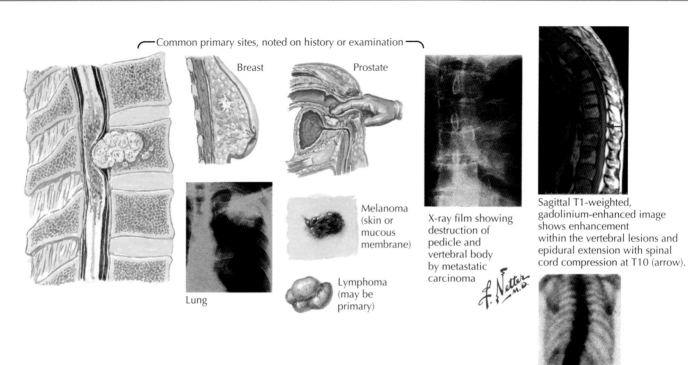

Common primary sites, noted on history or examination

Breast

Prostate

Melanoma (skin or mucous membrane)

Lung

Lymphoma (may be primary)

X-ray film showing destruction of pedicle and vertebral body by metastatic carcinoma

Sagittal T1-weighted, gadolinium-enhanced image shows enhancement within the vertebral lesions and epidural extension with spinal cord compression at T10 (arrow).

Bone scan showing multiple metastases

Fig. 50.2 Extradural Metastatic Spinal Tumors.

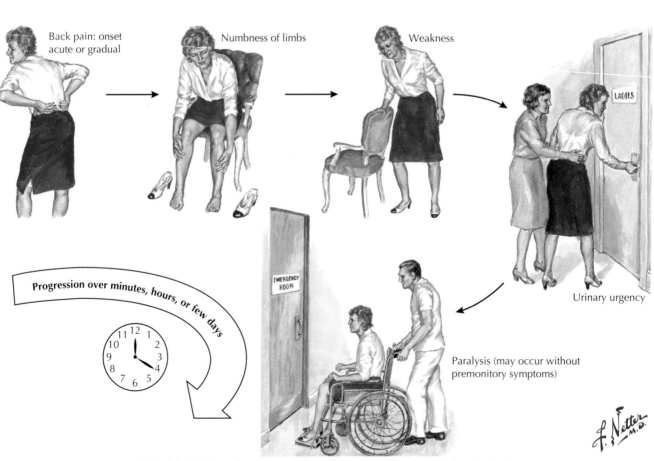

Back pain: onset acute or gradual

Numbness of limbs

Weakness

Urinary urgency

Progression over minutes, hours, or few days

Paralysis (may occur without premonitory symptoms)

Fig. 50.3 Clinical Profile: Acute Spinal Cord Decompensation With an Epidural Tumor.

If a primary cancer has not been previously found, a histologic diagnosis becomes mandatory to confirm the nature of the lesion. In some instances, there is a primary bony malignancy such as multiple myeloma originating within the vertebrae (Fig. 50.4). Currently, percutaneous CT-guided needle biopsy is often the most useful procedure if no primary is immediately apparent, such as occurred in this chapter's opening vignette, where a routine chest radiograph led to a diagnostic lung biopsy. When there is no evidence of a primary lesion identified on body CT, an image-guided biopsy by interventional radiology or an open surgical procedure, such as neurosurgical spinal cord decompression with a conjoint biopsy, is very important.

Treatment and Prognosis

There are three primary indications for treatment of spinal column metastatic disease: (1) to prevent further spinal cord destruction, (2) to prevent progression of the neurologic deficits, and (3) to control pain. Typically, large-dose corticosteroids (i.e., 10–20 mg of dexamethasone, followed by 4–6 mg every 4–6 hours) are administered at the time epidural spinal cord compression is identified, and continued throughout the initial treatment stages for their protective effect on the neural elements.

Focused radiation therapy and/or surgical decompression are the two primary treatment modalities for epidural metastases. When the patient's neurologic examination demonstrates serious neurologic compromise, radiation therapy may be the initial treatment of choice, particularly depending on the identification of the specific pathology. This is administered locally in multiple fractions that are precisely directed to the involved vertebrae. Pain relief often occurs relatively rapidly

within just a few days after commencement of the radiation therapy. Unfortunately, some tumors such as renal cell cancer are radiotherapy-resistant tumors. Here the symptoms typically evolve progressively despite radiation therapy.

On occasion, patients who present with specific neurologic symptoms and signs are best treated with surgery. This provides for rapid decompression of the neural elements and preserves previously unaffected neurologic function. Surgical intervention generally requires removal of as much tumor as possible. In many instances, when spinal column destruction has caused significant spinal instability, fusion and/or grafting is initially required followed by radiotherapy to the area to slow local tumor growth and recurrence of symptoms.

Prognosis for patients with metastatic disease to the spine depends on their clinical status upon presentation. Individuals who have presented with a severe neurologic deficit such as inability to ambulate due to paraplegia existing at least 24–36 hours often do not regain significant neurologic function. However, many patients who present with acute deterioration, still retaining some distal neurologic function, who undergo rapid evaluation and treatment may experience improvement.

Very occasionally, one finds a few types of primary benign bony vertebral tumors. Although histologically these are not malignant (as are most extradural tumors), these lesions may reach a critical mass, causing vertebral collapse and spinal cord compression (Fig. 50.5). Usually these benign tumors have a less aggressive clinical course; however, once they reach a critical mass, they may portend a serious threat to spinal cord function. In cases of spinal cord compression or vertebral instability, surgical decompression is indicated.

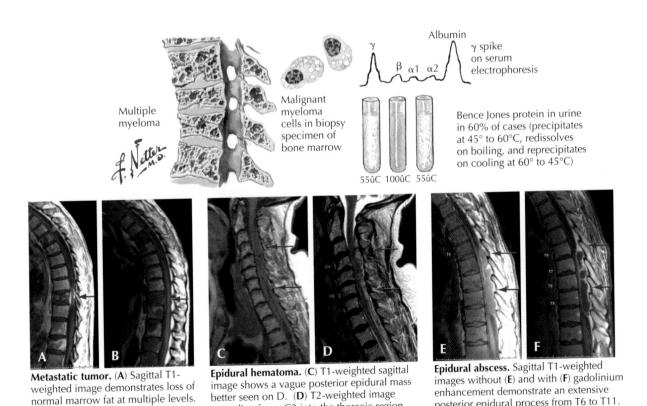

Multiple myeloma

Malignant myeloma cells in biopsy specimen of bone marrow

γ spike on serum electrophoresis

Bence Jones protein in urine in 60% of cases (precipitates at 45° to 60°C, redissolves on boiling, and reprecipitates on cooling at 60° to 45°C)

55ûC 100ûC 55ûC

Metastatic tumor. (**A**) Sagittal T1-weighted image demonstrates loss of normal marrow fat at multiple levels. (**B**) Sagittal T1-weighted, gadolinium-enhanced image shows enhancement within the vertebral lesions and epidural extension with spinal cord compression at T10 (arrow).

Epidural hematoma. (**C**) T1-weighted sagittal image shows a vague posterior epidural mass better seen on D. (**D**) T2-weighted image extending from C2 into the thoracic region.

Epidural abscess. Sagittal T1-weighted images without (**E**) and with (**F**) gadolinium enhancement demonstrate an extensive posterior epidural process from T6 to T11. Enhancement of the granulation tissue allows appreciation of nonenhancing focal pus collections.

Fig. 50.4 Extradural Primary Malignant Spinal Tumors.

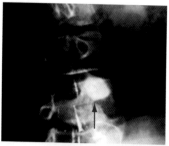
Osteoid
osteoma

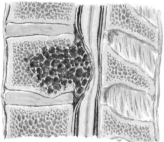
Hemangioma

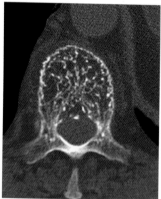
Axial CT demonstrates coarsened trabeculae interspersed with fat lucency. Intraosseous hemangioma involving whole vertebral body with small epidural extension

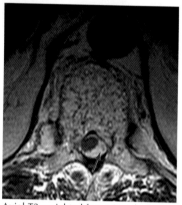
Axial T2-weighted fast spin echo image demonstrates mixed intensity pattern within vertebral body with left anterolateral epidural extension (arrow). Intraosseous hemangioma with small epidural extension (arrow)

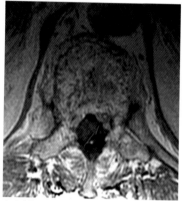
Axial T1-weighted fast spin echo post–gadolinium-enhanced image shows a heterogeneous but generally bright signal pattern within the vertebral body similar to the nonenhanced T1 image; however there is enhancement of the epidural component (arrow). Intraosseous hemangioma with small epidural extension (arrow)

Fig. 50.5 Extradural Primary Benign Spinal Tumors.

INTRADURAL EXTRAMEDULLARY TUMORS

Intradural extramedullary tumors originate within the dural sleeve of the spinal column but outside the spinal cord. These lesions primarily arise within the leptomeninges or the nerve roots.

> **CLINICAL VIGNETTE** *A 41-year-old woman noted the occasional appearance of tingling in her right leg that was particularly prominent when she played tennis. She had no significant back pain. Her initial detailed neurologic examination was perfect. MRI of the lumbosacral spine was normal. A follow-up appointment was scheduled for 2 months. However, within just a few weeks, she noted persistent right leg numbness particularly present when she shaved her leg. On self-testing, she became cognizant of diminished touch sensation in a pretibial distribution. Lumbar spine MRI was normal. Subsequently, her walking began to be limited as her left foot seemed to turn in after walking a few blocks.*
>
> *Repeat neurologic examination demonstrated a slightly spastic gait, subtle weakness of the left iliopsoas, more brisk muscle stretch reflexes on the left, a left Babinski sign, and a subtle cord level to pin and temperature sensation at T6 on the right.*
>
> *MRI confirmed the presence of a large intradural extramedullary tumor compressing the spinal cord. An encapsulated well-circumscribed tumor was surgically removed and histopathology revealed a meningioma (WHO grade I). She had an excellent recovery with no clinical residua.*

There was a seeming paradox here in that even when the patient developed clinical symptoms, her neurologic examination was initially normal. And then as her symptoms became more specific and subtle

abnormalities appeared on neurologic examination, her MRI demonstrated very marked spinal cord compression with a very significant-sized tumor. The clinical temporal profile of meningiomas is to gradually enlarge, subtly compressing the spinal cord. This tissue is amazingly resilient when the pathologic process is a very ingravescent one. Here the initial symptoms were relatively benign, with intermittent leg numbness precipitated by exercise and body heat. Such a setting, in the face of a normal lumbar MRI, suggested the possibility of early multiple sclerosis.

Continued observation was therefore important, as were patient instructions to call with any new symptomatology and return for follow-up within a few months. On this occasion, subsequent neurologic examination demonstrated a subtle sensory cord level and contralateral corticospinal dysfunction, typical of a classic *Brown-Séquard syndrome*, indicating a specific level of spinal cord dysfunction (see Chapter 55). Focused spinal MRI at a higher level led to the diagnosis of this treatable lesion.

Intradural extramedullary tumors are most commonly meningiomas (Fig. 50.6A) or nerve sheath tumors. The latter are classified into two main groups: schwannomas (~65%) (see Fig. 50.6B), and neurofibromas. Both often have a similar gross appearance and require microscopic analysis for differentiation. Neurofibromas have less dense cellular structure (Antoni B pattern) and often contain nerve elements. Usually benign, these lesions occur as a solitary finding or as multiple nodules throughout the body. Type I neurofibromatosis (von Recklinghausen disease) is a familial condition with two or more neurofibromas, associated neurocutaneous findings such as café au lait spots, and axillary freckling. Nerve sheath tumors such as schwannomas typically develop in middle-aged women. These lesions are slow-growing tumors that gradually lead to significant

Intradural extramedullary tumor (meningioma) compressing spinal cord and deforming nerve roots

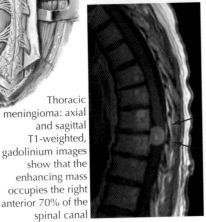

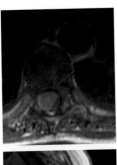

Dumbbell tumor (neurilemmoma) growing out along spinal nerve through intervertebral foramen (neurofibromas of von Recklinghausen disease may act similarly)

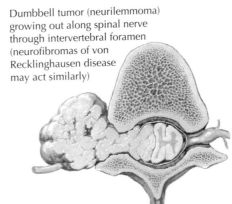

Foraminal neurolemmoma seen on axial T1-weighted, gadolinium-enhanced image (arrowheads)

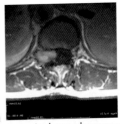

Thoracic meningioma: axial and sagittal T1-weighted, gadolinium images show that the enhancing mass occupies the right anterior 70% of the spinal canal

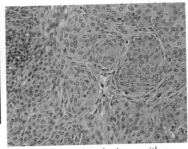

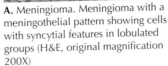

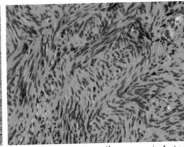

A. Meningioma. Meningioma with a meningothelial pattern showing cells with syncytial features in lobulated groups (H&E, original magnification 200X)

B. Schwannoma (neurilemmoma). Antoni B pattern in a schwannoma showing spindle cells arranged in fascicles (H&E, original magnification 200X)

Fig. 50.6 Intradural Extramedullary Primary Spinal Tumors.

clinical symptomatology, especially when these originate near the spinal cord. Type I neurofibromatosis (von Recklinghausen disease) is an autosomal dominant disorder often associated with optic gliomas and Lisch nodules of the iris, along with certain skeletal abnormalities. Type II neurofibromatosis is most frequently associated with bilateral hearing loss due to neurofibromas of the eighth cranial nerve and are not associated with spinal cord compression. Schwannomas have a dense pattern on microscopic analysis and may be found at the level of the nerve root.

CLINICAL VIGNETTE *A 36-year-old man reported a several-month history of progressive numbness on the lateral left foot. There was no associated back or leg pain, leg weakness, contralateral leg symptoms, or sphincter dysfunction. Neurologic examination demonstrated sensory loss to light touch and pinprick in the left S1 dermatome. He had full strength in both lower extremities. Muscle stretch reflexes were notable for an absent left Achilles reflex.*

An intradural mass was demonstrated at the left S1 level with MRI. There was no bony destruction, but the nerve root foramen was widened compared with the contralateral side. Given the progressive evolution of his clinical difficulties, he underwent surgical resection. Histologic analysis revealed a schwannoma (i.e., a nerve sheath tumor).

Clinical Presentation

If a single nerve root is involved without invasion of the spinal cord or cauda equina, symptoms mimic a radiculopathy but often without

the typical pain such as seen with either sciatica or herpes zoster (i.e., shingles). When these intradural extramedullary tumors develop, their initial symptoms are not always associated with significant neurologic signs at the first clinical evaluation. The evanescent symptoms may lead the clinician to consider the possibility of multiple sclerosis. Eventually, patients with a spinal lesion develop neurologic signs reflecting posterior column, spinothalamic, and corticospinal tract dysfunction.

Treatment

The management of intradural, extramedullary nerve sheath tumors is dictated by the clinical scenario. Patients presenting with neurologic deficits are best managed by surgical resection. Often, intradural extramedullary nerve sheath tumors can be completely resected without a resultant neurologic deficit. The nerve fascicle upon which the tumor arises can usually be separated from other fascicles, avoiding nerve root injury. Although the fascicle is amputated when the tumor is resected, the patient often has no deficit. Radiation and chemotherapy are not required for these benign tumors. If an intradural extramedullary tumor is incidentally discovered, having no associated symptoms or signs, observation is often appropriate because many of these lesions have benign courses.

INTRADURAL INTRAAXIAL TUMORS

Tumors that originate and grow within the substance of the spinal cord are designated as intraaxial lesions (i.e., "intradural, *intramedullary*" neoplasms) (Fig. 50.7). These account for approximately 15% of all primary intradural tumors occurring in both children and adults.

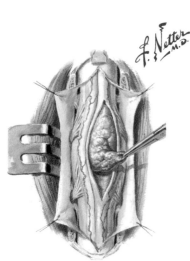

Intramedullary tumor and myelogram showing widening of spinal cord

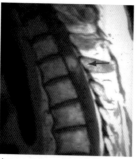

Astrocytoma on gadolinium-enhanced T1-weighted image with diffuse cord enlargement and focal enhancement (arrow)

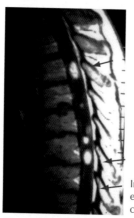

Intramedullary metastases: multiple enhancing masses within the spinal cord (arrows)

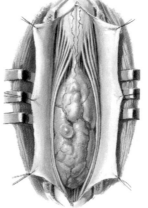

Tumor of filum terminale compressing cauda equina: enlarged vessels feed tumor

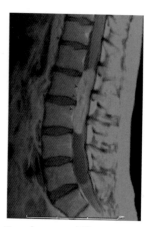

Ependymoma of filum with cyst: sagittal T1-weighted, gadolinium-enhanced image with large, moderately enhancing mass (arrowheads) and cyst distal to it (thin arrows)

Fig. 50.7 Intradural Intramedullary Primary Spinal Cord Tumors.

CLINICAL VIGNETTE *A young woman, known to be an avid athlete, noted a few months' history of right leg clumsiness; difficulty walking, often catching her foot; losing her balance; and experiencing some associated numbness. Her symptoms gradually increased. Subsequently, similar but milder symptoms developed in her left leg. There were no other associated symptoms and particularly no back or neck pain.*

Neurologic examination demonstrated mild right leg weakness, increased muscle stretch reflexes, a right Babinski sign, with loss of position and vibratory sensation in the right leg, and diminished pinprick and temperature sensation on the left up to a T7 level.

A T6 intraaxial spinal cord mass lesion was demonstrated with thoracic spine MRI. There was extensive T2 signal change within the cord, extending rostrally and caudally to the lesion. Furthermore, similar imaging of the brain and distal spinal cord was normal, as were visual evoked potentials. A lumbar puncture was performed to further exclude a primary central nervous system demyelinating process such as multiple sclerosis demonstrated an elevated protein level (96 mg/dL). However, there were no oligoclonal bands present. Cell counts were normal.

At surgical exploration, an anaplastic spinal cord astrocytoma was found. A complete resection was not attempted because of the infiltrative nature of these tumors. Unfortunately, her symptoms continued to progress postoperatively, leaving her paraplegic and incontinent. These tumors do not respond to other treatment modalities such as radiation or chemotherapy.

Although relatively quite rare, primary intradural intramedullary tumors always need to be considered in the differential diagnosis of any patient with possible primary spinal forms of multiple sclerosis and a progressive clinical course. The majority of intramedullary spinal cord malignancies have a primary glial cell source: either an ependymoma or

astrocytoma. Spinal cord astrocytomas are more infiltrative and nonencapsulated. Hemangioblastomas, lipomas, and dermoid, epidermoid, and metastatic tumors are among the other extremely rare intramedullary spinal cord tumors.

Clinical Presentation

Intramedullary tumors often present with progressive painless neurologic decline over several weeks. The previous vignette demonstrated a classic Brown-Séquard syndrome characterized by unilateral hemimotor weakness, diminished position and vibratory sensation ipsilateral to the lesion, and loss of pain and temperature in the contralateral lower extremity. This classic presentation is typically seen in tumors predominantly occupying one side of the spinal cord. A "pure" Brown-Séquard syndrome is rare, because most patients with intradural intramedullary lesions have a mixed clinical presentation affecting both sides of the spinal cord (see Fig. 50.7).

Treatment

Total resection of ependymomas is occasionally a possibility because the surgeon may find that a tissue plane exists between the tumor and the normal spinal cord, allowing precise removal of the tumor. In contrast, astrocytoma cells have a tendency to more diffusely infiltrate other previously normal tissue, making any thought of a clean surgical extraction totally impossible. In addition, the highly organized architecture of the spinal cord makes manipulation and resection of the malignant tissue extremely difficult, if not impossible. Therefore the current recommendation is to perform a primary biopsy and possibly a limited resection when dealing with presumed astrocytomas. Recent technologic developments in the operating room, including ultrasound, intraoperative MRI, and ultrasonic aspirators, may eventually lead to improved surgical outcomes.

Although both chemotherapy and radiation therapy are advocated for treatment of spinal cord astrocytomas, the results are no more than equivocal. In contrast, ependymomas that are thought to have been completely resected do not require radiation and chemotherapy. Often the best course for such a patient is a period of careful observation with clinical and MRI follow-up.

Future Directions

The major issue and challenge relate to finding medically successful treatment modalities for the primary glial cell spinal tumor groups, particularly the astrocytomas. Advances in their treatment are occurring in several areas. Imaging, such as MRI, is being used earlier as a screening tool in many patients with spine-related symptoms. Minimally invasive techniques and advances in instrumentation are improving surgical treatment. Intraoperative monitoring procedures provide improved outcomes for patients undergoing surgical resection of intramedullary and extramedullary tumors. Stereotactic radiosurgery, usually confined to treating intracranial pathology, is now being developed to administer high-dose radiation with surgical precision to lesions within the spine.

ADDITIONAL RESOURCES

Albanese V, Platania N. Spinal intradural extramedullary tumors. Personal experience. J Neurosurg Sci 2002;46(1):18–24.

Avanzo M, Romanelli P. Spinal radiosurgery: technology and clinical outcomes. Neurosurg Rev 2009;32(1):1–13.

Bowers DC, Weprin BE. Intramedullary spinal cord tumors. Curr Treat Options Neurol 2003;5(3):207–12.

Cole JS, Patchell RA. Metastatic epidural spinal cord compression. Lancet Neurol 2008;7(5):459–66. Review.

Conti P, Pansini G, Mouchaty H, et al. Spinal neurinomas: retrospective analysis and long-term outcome of 179 consecutively operated cases and review of the literature. Surg Neurol 2004;61(1):34–44.

George R, Jeba J, Ramkumar G, et al. Interventions for the treatment of metastatic extradural spinal cord compression in adults. Cochrane Database Syst Rev 2008;(4):CD006716.

Gibson CJ, Parry NM, Jakowski RM, et al. Anaplastic astrocytoma in the spinal cord of an African pygmy hedgehog (Atelerix albiventris). Vet Pathol 2008;45(6):934–8.

Minehan KJ, Brown PD, Scheithauer BW, et al. Prognosis and treatment of spinal cord astrocytoma. Int J Radiat Oncol Biol Phys 2008.
This consecutive series of patients with spinal cord astrocytoma were treated at Mayo Clinic Rochester between 1962 and 2005. RESULTS: A total of 136 consecutive patients were identified. Of these 136 patients, 69 had pilocytic and 67 had infiltrative astrocytoma. The median follow-up for living patients was 8.2 years (range, 0.08–37.6), and the median survival for deceased patients was 1.15 years (range, 0.01–39.9). The extent of surgery included incisional biopsy only (59%), subtotal resection (25%), and gross total resection (16%). The results of our study have shown that histologic type is the most important prognostic variable affecting the outcome of spinal cord astrocytomas. Surgical resection was associated with shorter survival and thus remains an unproven treatment. Postoperative radiotherapy significantly improved survival for patients with infiltrative astrocytomas but not for those with pilocytic tumors.

White BD, Stirling AJ, Paterson E, et al. Diagnosis and management of patients at risk of or with metastatic spinal cord compression: summary of NICE guidance. Guideline development group. BMJ 2008;337:a2538.

51

Paraneoplastic Neurologic Disorders

Pooja Raibagkar

Paraneoplastic neurologic disorders are seen when antitumor immunologic responses, primarily antibodies, directed against antigens expressed in the cancer, attack neural cells (neurons or glia) also expressing these antigens. Based on the neurologic presentation and the antibody profile, there are numerous well-defined paraneoplastic syndromes such as limbic encephalitis with small cell lung cancer (SCLC) and seropositivity for ANNA-1 (anti–neuronal nuclear antibody type-1 [Hu]); stiff person syndrome with breast cancer and amphiphysin–immunoglobulin (Ig) G); Lambert-Eaton syndrome with SCLC and P/Q-type voltage-gated calcium channel (VGCC) antibodies. Early recognition of these disorders is of paramount importance due to the need to begin appropriate treatment before there is irreversible neurologic injury.

EPIDEMIOLOGY

Overall, paraneoplastic neurologic disorders are rare; they are present in up to 0.01% of the cancer patients; exceptions exist, for example myasthenia gravis (MG) is seen in 30%–40% of patients with thymoma. The commonest cancers associated with paraneoplastic neurologic disorder include SCLC, adenocarcinoma of the breast and ovary, and thymoma.

PATHOGENESIS

Paraneoplastic autoimmunity is initiated by onconeural proteins expressed in the plasma membrane, cytoplasm, nucleus, or nucleolus of certain tumor cells; neural cell populations are coincidental targets. Depending on the location of antigen, cell surface versus intracellular, the consequent neural damage and response to immunotherapy may differ. It is thought that antibodies directed toward intracellular antigens are probably not causative of neural injury, because the antibodies do not come in direct contact with the intracellular epitopes. The immune response in these disorders with intracellular antigens involves cytotoxic T cell–mediated cytotoxicity. In contrast, antibodies against cell surface antigens have access to epitopes on cell surfaces resulting in immune-mediated attack on the function and structure of neurons; these disorders are usually more amenable to immunotherapy treatments (Table 51.1).

DIAGNOSTIC PRINCIPLES

- Key indicators of paraneoplastic autoimmunity-related neurologic disorders include acute to subacute course of disease, multifocal and broad range of neurologic signs and symptoms, and positive family and/or personal history of autoimmunity.
- Identification of specific antibodies in serum and/or cerebrospinal fluid (CSF) targeting neural (neuronal and glial) cells may provide clues to the specific cancer type; however, one cannot extrapolate definitively from these data to the neurologic presentation, because one specific antibody may be associated with different phenotypes, and different antibodies may cause the same clinical syndrome.
- It is not unusual to find more than one serum antibody on testing for paraneoplastic syndromes, because cancer cells often express multiple antigens with resulting activation of an immune response. These antibody clusters allow prediction of the associated cancer. For example, thymoma is present in 85% of patients, younger than 50 years, who have a combination of muscarinic acetylcholine receptor (AChR) antibody and striational antibody.
- Antibody testing should be done both in CSF and serum, where indicated, because this will increase the diagnostic yield. CSF has higher sensitivity compared with serum in detection of N-methyl-D-aspartate receptor (NMDAR) antibodies; in contrast, serum is more sensitive for detection of aquaporin-4 (AQP4) IgG.
- Low titers of paraneoplastic antibodies may be seen in patients with autoimmune disorders, and these may not be pathogenic. Patients prone to autoimmunity may show incidental seropositivity for voltage-gated potassium channel (VGKC) complex or ganglionic AChR without evidence of corresponding neurologic disorders. Therefore the clinical syndrome must match the disease profile of the detected antibody; if it does not, then alternative causes should be sought for the patient's symptoms.
- Monitoring for relapses primarily consists of serial clinical assessment. Usually, antibody titers are not monitored. In some instances, significant elevation in antibody titers may portend return of the underlying cancer.
- CSF analysis in paraneoplastic neurologic disorders may show additional abnormalities such as elevated protein, pleocytosis, oligoclonal bands, elevated IgG, IgG index, and/or kappa chains.

IDENTIFICATION OF TUMOR IN PARANEOPLASTIC DISORDERS

Screening for cancer should be done promptly when a paraneoplastic neurologic disorder is a consideration. Eliciting risk factors for cancer such as smoking and family history of cancer can help to narrow down the differential. The paraneoplastic neurologic presentation and the identified antibody will help to strategize cancer screening. Computed tomography (CT) chest, abdomen, and pelvis with contrast is the preferred initial step. Often, the initial test may not reveal any systemic malignancy, in which case, if clinical suspicion for an underlying cancer is high, a positron emission tomography (PET)-CT scan can be performed. PET-CT scan increases the diagnostic yield of cancer by 39%–56%. Additional testing for specific organ-related cancer such as testicular ultrasound, mammogram, pelvic ultrasound, or magnetic resonance imaging (MRI) for gynecologic cancer can be performed if indicated.

TABLE 51.1 Comparison of Features of Neural Antibodies Directed Against Intracellular Proteins Versus Antibodies Against Cell Surface Epitopes

	Antibodies Against Intracellular Protein	Antibodies Against Cell Surface Epitopes
Examples of antibody targets	Nuclear or intracytoplasmic enzymes, transcription factors, RNA binding proteins	Neurotransmitter receptors, ion channels, water channels, channel-complex proteins
Pathogenicity	Not pathogenic; serves as a biomarker	Pathogenic effector
Type of injury	Neural-peptide specific cytotoxic effector T cell–mediated injury	Antibody-mediated injury
Response to treatment	Poorly responsive to immunotherapy	Highly responsive to immunotherapy
Tumor association	Highly predictive of cancer	Not necessarily associated with tumor
Examples	ANNA-1 (Hu), ANNA-2 (Ri), GAD65	NMDAR, AMPAR, muscle AChR

AChR, Acetylcholine receptor; *AMPAR,* alpha-amino-3-hydroxy-5-methyl-4-isoxazole-propionic acid receptor; *ANNA,* anti–neuronal nuclear antibody; *GAD65,* 65-kDa isoform of glutamic acid decarboxylase; *NMDAR, N*-methyl-D-aspartate receptor.

In spite of extensive screening, cancer may not be identified on initial search. Follow-up screening every 3–6 months for several years may be necessary.

CLINICAL VIGNETTE *A 61-year-old woman presented with paresthesias in hands and feet for 3 months. She had difficulty walking and using her hands for 2 months. In addition, she noted excessive fatigue, loss of appetite, and change in taste sensation for a few weeks. Her neurologic examination was notable for mild to moderate symmetric weakness in distal extremities with loss of all sensory modalities in hands and feet. Reflexes were 1+ in upper extremities and absent in lower extremities. She had intention tremor on right and dysmetria on left with finger-nose-finger testing.*

Her laboratory investigation was notable for hyponatremia. Electrophysiologic evaluation, a month after initial symptoms, showed moderate chronic axonal, length-dependent generalized, symmetric polyneuropathy with superimposed bilateral median and ulnar mononeuropathies.

Brain MRI showed a 6-mm lesion in the left cerebellar hemisphere with contrast enhancement (Fig. 51.1). MRI of the cervical and thoracic spinal cord showed diffuse nerve root enhancement in the lower cervical and upper thoracic region (Fig. 51.2). PET-CT showed increased uptake in multiple mediastinal lymph nodes (Fig. 51.3). Biopsy of one of the lymph nodes showed SCLC. She had elevated anti-Hu (1:61,440) and anti-striational antibodies (1:960).

Patient was diagnosed as having paraneoplastic ANNA-1 (Hu) antibody-mediated sensorimotor polyneuropathy related to SCLC. She started chemotherapy followed by radiation for metastatic lung cancer, with no further progression of neuropathy.

Comment: Paraneoplastic neurologic syndromes are heralded by subacute progressive neurologic syndrome with systemic manifestations of cancer. Because anti-Hu antibodies serve as the biomarker of T cell–mediated nerve injury, the goal of treatment is appropriate management of primary cancer with close monitoring for symptom/sign progression, in which case immunotherapy can be considered.

PARANEOPLASTIC DISORDERS WITH ANTIBODIES TO INTRACELLULAR ANTIGENS

These disorders are associated with antibodies directed toward intracellular antigens and are characterized by a high risk for an underlying cancer and less responsiveness to immunotherapy, leading to significant disability. The most important treatment for this group is treatment of the primary cancer with integrated immunotherapy for the associated neurologic syndrome. Immunotherapy for neurologic syndrome includes

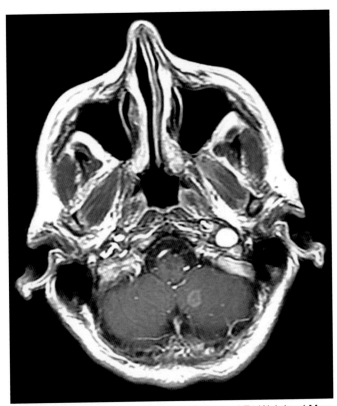

Fig. 51.1 Axial, Gadolinium Contrast–Enhanced T1-Weighted Magnetic Resonance Image Shows 6-mm Enhancing Metastasis in Left Cerebellar Hemisphere.

corticosteroids, rituximab, and cyclophosphamide. One of the prototypic antibodies is ANNA-1 (Hu), which can cause a broad spectrum of neurologic involvement, including sensory neuronopathy, sensorimotor neuropathy, gastric dysmotility, limbic encephalitis, encephalomyelitis, and cerebellar degeneration. Involvement of multiple levels of neuroaxis is not unusual. Diagnosis of incidental positivity of anti-Hu antibody carries a very high risk of underlying lung cancer (>85%) even without a well-defined paraneoplastic neurologic disorder. At the same time, only a few patients (0.1%) with incidental anti-Hu antibodies and SCLC end up having well-defined neurologic paraneoplastic disorder. ANNA-2 (Ri) antibodies may cause opsoclonus/myoclonus, laryngospasm, and/or trismus in addition to other usual manifestation described in Table 51.2. Anti-Ma (paraneoplastic Ma antigen family-like 1 [PNMA-1]) and

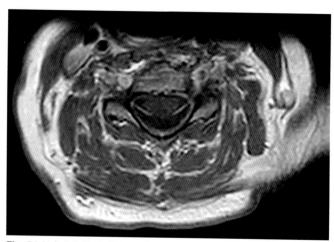

Fig. 51.2 Axial, Gadolinium Contrast–Enhanced T1-Weighted Magnetic Resonance Image of Lower Cervical Spine Shows Enhancing Anterior and Posterior Nerve Roots.

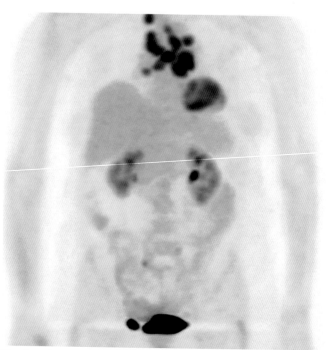

Fig. 51.3 Positron Emission Tomography–Computed Tomography Scan Shows Intense Fluorodeoxyglucose Uptake in Bilateral Mediastinal, Hilar, and Subcarinal Lymph Nodes.

anti-Ta (paraneoplastic Ma antigen family-like 2 [PNMA-2]) antibodies cause a neurologic disorder of the brainstem. Young men with anti-Ta antibodies should undergo thorough evaluation for germ cell tumors. Anti-Yo (Purkinje cell antibody type 1 [PCA-1]) antibodies are usually associated with severe, irreversible, cerebellar degeneration, with strong association with female-specific tumors of breast, ovaries, or reproductive tract. Collapsin Response-Mediator Protein-5 (CRMP-5) antibodies are usually observed in elderly men and women, with diverse clinical phenotypes including paraneoplastic cranial neuropathy, chorea, uveitis, and retinitis. GAD65 (65-kDa isoform of glutamic acid decarboxylase) antibodies have female predominance with broad spectrum of manifestations, including stiff person syndrome, cerebellar degeneration, epilepsy, and limbic encephalitis, and are not usually associated

with a tumor. Amphiphysin is involved in the recycling of synaptic vesicles and antibodies to it often coexist with other autoantibodies. The neurologic syndrome with amphiphysin antibodies is quite variable and includes stiff person syndrome, encephalitis, encephalomyelitis, myoclonus, cerebellar syndrome, and neuropathy.

PARANEOPLASTIC DISORDERS WITH ANTIBODIES TO CELL SURFACE ANTIGENS

This group of immune-mediated brain disorders includes some of the commonest forms of autoimmune encephalitis in young and elderly population, anti-NMDAR encephalitis and anti–leucine-rich glioma-inactivated 1 (LGI 1) encephalitis, respectively. Antibody detection in CSF is more sensitive than serum in the majority of these disorders. They are often treatable with the aim of treatment being removal of the circulating pathogenic antibodies and deactivation of B cells involved in producing these antibodies. Treatment of the underlying cancer, if one is present, is the first step, followed by first-line immunotherapy (corticosteroids, intravenous immunoglobulin, and plasma exchange) and/or second-line immunotherapy (rituximab, cyclophosphamide). Neurologic disorders associated with autoantibodies to alpha-amino-3-hydroxy-5-methyl-4-isoxazole-propionic acid receptors (AMPAR), gamma-aminobutyric acid (GABA) receptors and few others are described further in Table 51.3.

Anti-NMDAR encephalitis is considered to be the second most common cause of autoimmune encephalitis after acute demyelinating encephalomyelitis. The clinical syndrome begins with a viral-like prodrome in more than 50% of patients. Anti-NMDAR encephalitis may begin with behavioral changes, memory difficulties, and other psychiatric manifestations, often prompting initial psychiatric evaluation. However, approximately 85%–90% of patients develop other neurologic dysfunction within 2–4 weeks; these consist of confusion, disorientation, movement disorders, and seizures. Autonomic instability may be seen and presents as rapid changes in heart rate, blood pressure, and core temperature, with fluctuating levels of consciousness; this may require neurologic intensive care. Although MRI of brain may initially be normal in up to 70% of patients, it will eventually show findings of increased FLAIR/T2 signal in hippocampal area in more than 50% of patients. Testing of anti-NMDAR antibody in CSF is more sensitive than serum. Electroencephalogram (EEG) may show delta brush pattern in approximately 30% of patients. Early immunotherapy is associated with improved prognosis. The relapse rate in the first 2 years is 12%. This disorder specifically has predominance for females (80%), with approximately one-third of them being younger than 18 years. There is a strong association with ovarian teratoma. Pelvic tumors may be undetected initially, and periodic pelvic MRI or transvaginal ultrasound for 4 years after initial diagnosis is recommended.

VGKC antibody-complex targets LGI 1 and contactin-associated protein 2 (CASPR2). Anti-LGI 1 antibodies mainly affect elderly men. Faciobrachial dystonic seizures are a characteristic feature; in addition, limbic encephalopathy features such as psychiatric disturbance, amnesia, and disorientation are also seen. Although seizures may be hard to control with antiepileptic medications alone, they often respond promptly to steroids. A very slow taper of steroids over months is recommended to reduce the incidence of relapse seen in 35%. No specific tumor association has been found with potassium channel antibodies. Antibodies against the GABA receptor family have two subtypes: A and B; both present with limbic encephalitis and seizures. Seizures are the most common initial manifestation in a majority of patients; approximately 10% present with cerebellar ataxia. GABA-B receptor encephalitis is strongly associated with lung cancer. MRI of the brain may show multifocal cortical and subcortical areas of increased T2 signal

TABLE 51.2 Characteristics of Neural Antibodies Targeting Intracellular Antigens

Antibody (Alternative Name)	Neurologic Manifestations	Patient Demographics	Tumor Association
ANNA-1 (Hu)	Neuropathies (80%; sensory, and autonomic), GI dysmotility (25%), limbic encephalitis, cerebellar degeneration, myelopathy, radiculopathy	75% males, median 63 years	SCLC, rarely thymoma
ANNA-2 (Ri)	Brainstem syndrome (opsoclonus/myoclonus, cranial neuropathy, laryngospasm, and trismus), cerebellar degeneration, encephalomyelitis, neuropathy, movement disorder, seizures	66% female, mean age 65 years	Lung and breast
ANNA-3	Neuropathies, cerebellar ataxia, myelopathy, brainstem and limbic encephalopathy	Male and female, ages 8–83 years	SCLC
PNMA-1 (Ma)	Cerebellar/brainstem syndrome, limbic encephalitis, ophthalmoplegia, extrapyramidal symptoms, myelopathy	Females > males, middle aged	Breast, lung, colon, renal, NHL
PNMA-2 (Ma2 or Ta)	Brainstem/cerebellar syndrome, diencephalic (narcolepsy/cataplexy), polyneuropathy, limbic encephalitis, myelopathy	Males (median age 34 years) > females (median age 64 years)	Testicular or extragonadal germ cell, breast, lung, NHL, ovary
PCA-1 (Yo)	Cerebellar degeneration (90%), polyneuropathy (10%)	Almost all females (young adult to elderly)	Breast, ovarian, or female reproductive tract cancers
PCA-2	Cerebellar ataxia, brainstem/limbic encephalitis, neuropathy	Limited cases reported	SCLC
PCR-Tr	Cerebellar dysfunction	Limited cases reported	Hodgkin lymphoma
CRMP-5-IgG	Peripheral/autonomic/cranial neuropathies, movement disorder, myelopathy, radiculoplexopathy, neuromuscular junction disorder, retinopathy	Males and females, older adults	Lung cancer, thymoma
GAD65	Stiff-person syndrome, limbic encephalitis, cerebellar ataxia, palatal tremor, downbeat or periodic alternating nystagmus, myelopathy, brainstem disorder	33–80 years, 82% females	Uncommon, thymoma, breast
Amphiphysin	Neuropathy, encephalopathy, myelopathy, encephalomyelitis with rigidity, cerebellar syndrome, myoclonus, stiff person syndrome	Males > females, mean age 64 years	Breast, ovarian

ANNA, Anti–neuronal nuclear antibody; *CRMP-5*, collapsin response-mediator protein-5; *GAD65*, 65-kDa isoform of glutamic acid decarboxylase; *GI*, gastrointestinal; *IgG*, immunoglobulin G; *NHL*, non-Hodgkin lymphoma; *PCA*, Purkinje cell antibody; *PNMA*, paraneoplastic Ma antigens; *SCLC*, small cell lung cancer.
Modified from Pittock SJ, Palace J. Paraneoplastic and idiopathic autoimmune neurologic disorders: approach to diagnosis and treatment. *Handb Clin Neurol.* 2016;133:165–183; Lancaster E. Paraneoplastic disorders. *Continuum (Minneap Minn).* 2017;23(6, Neuro-oncology):1653–1679.

abnormality. Two-thirds of patients respond well to immunotherapy. AMPAR encephalitis is associated with cancer in 50% of patients. The presentation is of limbic encephalitis in an older patient. Metabotropic glutamate receptor 1 (mGluR1) antibodies are associated with paraneoplastic cerebellar degeneration usually in the setting of Hodgkin lymphoma. Ophelia syndrome is named after a 15-year-old girl who exhibited symptoms of encephalitis in the setting of newly diagnosed Hodgkin lymphoma; this syndrome is associated with mGluR5 antibodies and has a good outcome with immunotherapy. Glycine receptor (GlyR) antibodies are associated with progressive encephalomyelitis with rigidity and myoclonus (PERM) syndrome. Dopamine receptor (D2) antibodies are associated with basal ganglia encephalitis.

PARANEOPLASTIC NEUROMUSCULAR JUNCTION DISORDERS

MG, a disorder of postsynaptic neuromuscular transmission, is associated with thymoma in up to 10%–15% of patients. It is characterized by fatigable weakness affecting bulbar and proximal limb muscles. Nearly all patients with paraneoplastic MG have AChR antibodies, especially receptor modulating with striational antibodies. Muscle-specific tyrosine kinase (MuSK) antibody–associated myasthenia is usually not associated with thymomas. Lambert-Eaton myasthenic syndrome (LEMS) is a disorder of presynaptic neuromuscular transmission characterized by presence of P/Q-type VGCC. More than half of the patients with LEMS have SCLC; rarely leukemia and prostate cancer are associated with this syndrome. Patients usually present with generalized weakness, fatigue, dry mouth, and dysarthria (Fig. 51.4). Autoimmune neuromyotonia (Isaac syndrome) is a disorder of motor nerve terminal hyperexcitability. Common manifestations include muscle cramps, twitches, rippling, weight loss, sweating, and weakness. It is associated with thymoma, SCLC, lymphoma, and thyroid cancer. CASPR2 antibodies can be found in up to 50% of patients. When additional symptoms (cognitive changes, delirium, sleep disturbance, and autonomic instability) are present along with peripheral nerve hyperexcitability and potassium channel antibodies, Morvan syndrome is a consideration.

Subacute sensory neuropathy

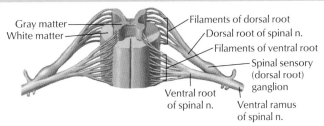

Gray matter
White matter

Filaments of dorsal root
Dorsal root of spinal n.
Filaments of ventral root
Spinal sensory (dorsal root) ganglion
Ventral root of spinal n.
Ventral ramus of spinal n.

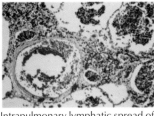

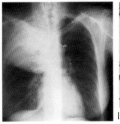

Intrapulmonary lymphatic spread of neoplasm

Lambert-Eaton in bronchogenic small cell carcinoma

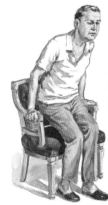

Lambert-Eaton syndrome; weakness of proximal muscle groups (often manifested by difficulty in rising from chair); compound muscle action potential facilitation with high frequency motor nerve stimulation

Electromyography with voluntary exercise
Each tracing represents 3 superimposed action potentials evoked by stimulation at 3/second

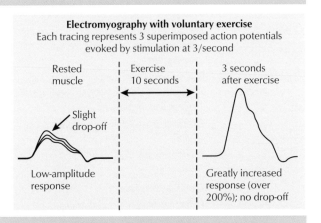

Rested muscle

Slight drop-off

Low-amplitude response

Exercise 10 seconds

3 seconds after exercise

Greatly increased response (over 200%); no drop-off

Myasthenia gravis thymoma

Thymus gland abnormality in myasthenia gravis

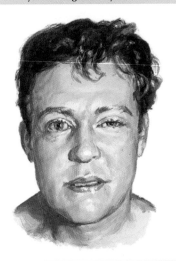

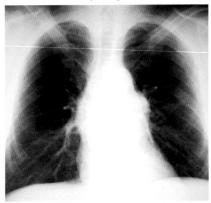

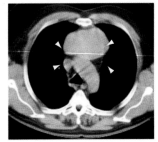

CT scan clearly demonstrates same large tumor anterior to aortic arch (arrowheads)

X-ray film shows large mediastinal tumor, which localized to anterior compartment (view not shown)

Dermatomyositis and typical rash

Difficulty in arising from chair, often early complaint

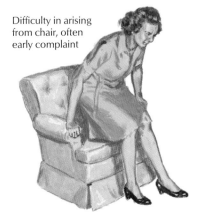

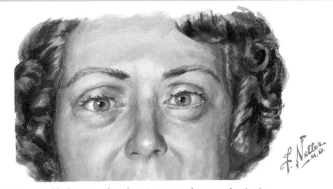

Edema and heliotrope discoloration around eyes a classic sign. More widespread erythematous rash may also be present.

Fig. 51.4 Paraneoplastic Disorder of Peripheral Nervous System.

TABLE 51.3 Characteristics of Neural Antibodies Targeting Cell Surface Proteins and Ion Channels

Antibody (Alternative Name)	Neurologic Manifestations	Patient Demographics	Tumor Association
NMDA receptor	Limbic encephalitis, autonomic instability, opsoclonus-myoclonus	80% females, mostly young adults	Ovarian teratoma
VGKC-complex (anti-LGI 1, anti-CASPR2 antibodies)	Limbic encephalitis, frontotemporal dementia-like presentation, brainstem encephalitis, cerebellar ataxia, extrapyramidal disorders, peripheral/autonomic neuropathy, neuromyotonia, chronic pain	Male > females, median age 60 years	Rare thymoma, SCLC, adenocarcinoma of breast or prostate
AMPA receptor	Limbic encephalitis, nystagmus, seizures	90% female adult to elderly	Lung, breast, thymoma
GABA-B receptor	Limbic encephalitis, orolingual dyskinesias	Males > females, mean age 62 years, but younger in nonparaneoplastic cases	SCLC
GABA-A receptor	Refractory status epilepticus	Males >> females, median age 22 years	Hodgkin lymphoma
Glycine receptor	Stiff person syndrome, PERM	5–69 years	Hodgkin lymphoma
mGluR1	Cerebellar degeneration	19–69 years	Hodgkin lymphoma, prostate cancer
mGluR5	Limbic encephalitis (Ophelia syndrome)	15–46 years	Hodgkin lymphoma
DPPX	Encephalitis with CNS hyperexcitability (tremor, seizures, myoclonus, agitation), PERM, dysautonomia (GI tract, bladder, cardiac conduction system, and thermoregulation)	50% male, age 45–76 years	Hematologic malignancies (<20%)

AMPA, Alpha-amino-3-hydroxy-5-methyl-4-isoxazole-propionic acid; *CASPR,* contactin-associated protein; *GABA,* gamma-aminobutyric acid; *GI,* gastrointestinal; *mGluR,* metabotropic glutamate receptor; *NMDA,* N-methyl-D-aspartate; *SCLC,* small cell lung cancer; *PERM,* progressive encephalomyelitis with rigidity and myoclonus; *VGKC,* voltage-gated potassium channel.
Modified from Pittock SJ, Palace J. Paraneoplastic and idiopathic autoimmune neurologic disorders: approach to diagnosis and treatment. *Handb Clin Neurol.* 2016;133:165–183; Lancaster E. Paraneoplastic disorders. *Continuum (Minneap Minn).* 2017;23(6, Neuro-oncology):1653–1679.

PARANEOPLASTIC NEUROPATHY

Paraneoplastic peripheral polyneuropathy may account for 5% of axonal, length-dependent sensorimotor polyneuropathy. One of the distinguishing features includes a rapidly progressive course. Multitudes of cancers and antibodies are associated with paraneoplastic sensorimotor polyneuropathy. A subset of patients with demyelinating features on electrophysiologic evaluation have osteosclerotic myeloma as part of the POEMS syndrome: polyneuropathy, organomegaly, endocrinopathy, monoclonal protein, and skin changes. The neuropathy of POEMS syndrome is often poorly responsive to immunotherapy; treatment of the underlying myeloma results in improvement of the neuropathy. Paraneoplastic sensory ganglionopathy is characterized by the development of rapidly progressive pain and numbness in an asymmetric distribution, preferentially affecting upper limbs, resulting in sensory ataxia and gait unsteadiness. Cancer may account for 20% of cases, the most common associated cancer being SCLC. Many antibodies are found to be associated with sensory ganglionopathy, with the commonest being anti-Hu and anti CV-2/CRMP-5 antibody. Predominant involvement of autonomic fibers either alone, or in combination with other symptoms, can result in disabling paraneoplastic pandysautonomia. Unifocal (isolated gastrointestinal dysautonomia causing abdominal pain, bloating, early satiety, nausea, constipation) or multifocal (dry mouth, dry eyes, anhidrosis, erectile dysfunction, pupillary abnormality, orthostasis, and fixed heart rate) involvement can be seen. Anti-Hu antibodies in the context of SCLC and ganglionic (g)AChR antibodies (typically in high titers) in the context of adenocarcinoma of lung are typically seen in paraneoplastic pandysautonomia. Up to 10% of patients may have thymoma, and these patients often have overlapping MG.

PARANEOPLASTIC MYOPATHY

Paraneoplastic myopathy encompasses inflammatory myopathies such as dermatomyositis and polymyositis, which are, respectively, associated in up to 30% and 15% of patients with cancer. Dermatomyositis is typically associated with ovarian, lung, pancreatic, gastric, and colorectal cancers, and lymphoma. Polymyositis is most commonly associated with non-Hodgkin lymphoma, lung cancer, and bladder cancer. Rarely, a rapidly progressive proximal weakness with elevated creatine kinase (CK) and necrotizing features on skeletal muscle biopsy with little inflammation is found, which is called paraneoplastic necrotizing myopathy in the context of SCLC and breast and prostate cancer. It is typically responsive to steroids that are initiated after treatment of primary tumor.

ADDITIONAL RESOURCES

Dalmau J, Graus F. Antibody-mediated encephalitis. N Engl J Med 2018;378(9):840–51.

Höftberger R, Rosenfeld MR, Dalmau J. Update on neurological paraneoplastic syndromes. Curr Opin Oncol 2015;27(6):489–95.

Lancaster E. Paraneoplastic disorders. Continuum (Minneap Minn) 2017;23(6, Neuro–oncology):1653–79.

Pittock SJ, Palace J. Paraneoplastic and idiopathic autoimmune neurologic disorders: approach to diagnosis and treatment. Handb Clin Neurol 2016;133:165–83.

Rosenfeld MR, Dalmau J. Paraneoplastic neurologic syndromes. Neurol Clin 2018;36(3):675–85.

Sharp L, Vernino S. Paraneoplastic neuromuscular disorders. Muscle Nerve 2012;46(6):841–50.

Disorders of the Autonomic Nervous System

Jayashri Srinivasan

52

Autonomic Disorders

Jayashri Srinivasan, Jose A. Gutrecht

CLINICAL VIGNETTE *A 65-year-old man presented with subacute onset of severe, unexplained orthostatic dizziness and light-headedness. Over the next 2 months, he developed dry mouth, dry eyes, urinary hesitancy, erectile dysfunction, and severe constipation. His previous medical history was unremarkable. His only medication was aspirin. He smoked one pack per day and drank sparingly. His family history was noncontributory. The patient's blood pressure was 124/76 mm Hg supine and 66/40 mm Hg standing at 2 minutes, with normal heart rates of 72 and 76 beats/minute while supine and standing, respectively. His remaining general examination was normal. There were impaired pupillary responses to light and accommodation and dry mucous membranes. Sensory examination revealed distal sensory loss to proprioception in both hands and feet.*

Tilt-table testing revealed orthostatic hypotension. Sweat testing demonstrated profound anhidrosis. Paraneoplastic autoantibody studies revealed positive anti-HU (antineuronal) antibodies. Chest computed tomography demonstrated left hilar mass. Small-cell lung carcinoma was diagnosed after bronchoscopic biopsy. The patient's orthostatic intolerance improved after the third course of chemotherapy. Remission has persisted.

Comment: Development of signs and symptoms related to parasympathetic and sympathetic dysfunction in the absence of central nervous system abnormalities was compatible with an autonomic neuropathy.

ANATOMY OF THE AUTONOMIC SYSTEM

The primary role of the autonomic system is the maintenance of homeostasis and this is done by two separate but complementary systems: the sympathetic and the parasympathetic systems. The central regulation of the autonomic system is mediated by neurons in the frontal lobe, limbic system, and the hypothalamus.

The preganglionic neurons of the sympathetic nervous system arise from the intermediolateral column of the thoracic spinal cord. These axons form the white communicating rami that synapse with the neurons of the sympathetic ganglia in the paravertebral chain; postganglionic fibers form the gray communicating rami that travel along with the spinal nerves to blood vessels and sweat glands (Fig. 52.1). Sympathetic innervation of the adrenal medulla is the exception as it receives preganglionic sympathetic fibers; the adrenal medulla is considered the equivalent of a sympathetic ganglion and it secretes epinephrine and norepinephrine directly into the blood stream (see Fig. 52.1).

The parasympathetic system consists of cranial and sacral output; the cranial output arises in the brainstem in visceral nuclei of the cranial nerves III, VII, IX, and X, and the axons travel along with the respective cranial nerves to innervate target organs. Preganglionic fibers from the Edinger-Westphal nucleus travel in the oculomotor nerve (III) and synapse in the ciliary ganglion; postganglionic fibers innervate the ciliary and pupillary muscles (Fig. 52.2). Preganglionic fibers from the superior salivatory nuclei travel with the facial nerve (VII) as the greater petrosal nerve and the chorda tympani, synapse in the sphenopalatine and submandibular ganglion, and innervate the lacrimal, submandibular, and sublingual glands (Fig. 52.3). Preganglionic fibers from the inferior salivatory nuclei travel with the glossopharyngeal nerve (IX) and synapse in the otic ganglion, and innervate the parotid gland (Fig. 52.4). Preganglionic fibers from the dorsal motor nucleus of the vagus travel with the vagal nerve (X) and synapse in ganglia in the walls of the viscera, and innervate the visceral organs of the gastrointestinal, cardiac, and renal systems (Fig. 52.5). The sacral part of the parasympathetic system arises from the sacral spinal cord, synapses in ganglia in the walls of the organs, and innervates the colon, bladder, and pelvic organs (Fig. 52.6).

Autonomic functions are mediated through neurotransmitters released by the sympathetic and parasympathetic neurons. *Acetylcholine* is the most important neurotransmitter. This is released by preganglionic sympathetic and parasympathetic neurons, as well as all postganglionic parasympathetic neurons and some postganglionic sympathetic neurons (e.g., sweat glands). *Norepinephrine* is the other important autonomic neurotransmitter. It is secreted by the remaining postganglionic sympathetic neurons directing its action on both α- and β-adrenergic receptors.

DIAGNOSTIC APPROACH

Patients with dysautonomic symptoms require careful, and complete, neurologic examinations to find concomitant features of central and peripheral nervous system involvement. Electromyography is often valuable in patients who have concomitant sensorimotor neuropathy findings.

Formal autonomic testing done in specialized laboratories is also recommended to confirm the diagnosis of autonomic dysfunction. Commonly used parameters to assess sympathetic competency include blood pressure responses to standing and to Valsalva maneuvers and quantitative measurements of sweat production in response to cholinergic stimuli. The latter is typically done at four standardized locations to detect the abnormality pattern. Heart rate responses to Valsalva maneuvers and deep breathing are used to assess cardiovagal parasympathetic function. Quantitative sensory testing, comparing thresholds for vibration to cold- and heat-pain thresholds, is helpful for detecting small myelinated and unmyelinated somatic peripheral nerve dysfunction. Quantitation of intraepidermal nerve fiber density by skin punch biopsy and subsequent immunostaining directed at axons is performed to assess the severity of small-fiber loss. Comprehensive screening for all recognized

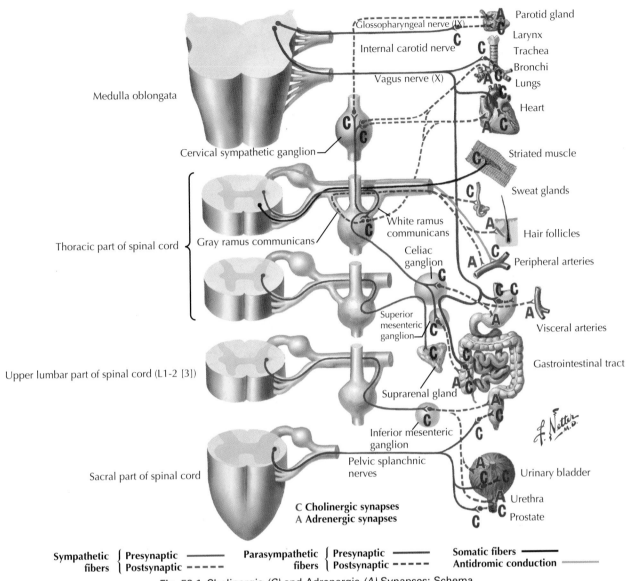

Striated muscle
Sweat glands
Hair follicles
Peripheral arteries

Visceral arteries

Gastrointestinal tract

Urinary bladder
Urethra
Prostate

Parotid gland
Larynx
Trachea
Bronchi
Lungs

Heart

Glossopharyngeal nerve (IX)
Internal carotid nerve
Vagus nerve (X)

Medulla oblongata

Cervical sympathetic ganglion

Thoracic part of spinal cord
Gray ramus communicans

White ramus communicans
Celiac ganglion

Superior mesenteric ganglion

Upper lumbar part of spinal cord (L1-2 [3])

Suprarenal gland

Inferior mesenteric ganglion

Sacral part of spinal cord

Pelvic splanchnic nerves

C Cholinergic synapses
A Adrenergic synapses

| Sympathetic fibers | Presynaptic ——— Postsynaptic - - - - - | Parasympathetic fibers | Presynaptic ——— Postsynaptic - - - - - | Somatic fibers ——— Antidromic conduction ——— |

Fig. 52.1 Cholinergic *(C)* and Adrenergic *(A)* Synapses: Schema.

paraneoplastic antibodies is recommended in acute to subacute cases where paraneoplastic autonomic neuropathy is possible.

CLINICAL PRESENTATIONS

Typically, patients have combinations of both parasympathetic and sympathetic dysfunction (Fig. 52.7). The former is characterized by dry mucous membranes, particularly noticeable in the eyes and mouth, with varying gastrointestinal involvement manifested as early satiety, nausea, vomiting, constipation, diarrhea, urinary bladder dysmotility, and erectile dysfunction.

Abnormal sweating and sudden feelings of severe light-headedness or syncope when assuming an upright posture are usual symptoms of impaired sympathetic function. Combinations of parasympathetic (erection) and sympathetic (ejaculation) disorders affect male sexual function. Signs of autonomic dysfunction include fixed heart rate, tonic pupils, and orthostatic hypotension, with normal strength and sensory examination (i.e., sparing the somatic nerves). Autonomic disorders may be classified as peripheral or central autonomic disorders and may present acutely or in a chronic fashion.

Acute Peripheral Autonomic Disorders

Acute or subacute autonomic neuropathies are usually related to toxic, metabolic, or autoimmune disorders. In the absence of toxic or metabolic influences, autoimmune and paraneoplastic disorders should be considered the primary mechanism. Primary autonomic polyneuropathies represent an uncommon subgroup of disorders. However, many length-dependent polyneuropathies have various degrees of autonomic involvement, occasionally with important implications. Impotence is a prime example in young male patients with diabetic polyneuropathies.

Antecedent viral infections occur in more than half of patients with *autoimmune autonomic neuropathy,* suggesting that it may be a Guillain-Barré syndrome variant. The rare patient with acute pandysautonomic neuropathy presents with rapid onset of sympathetic and parasympathetic dysfunction. They most often have severe generalized disorders, but restricted milder forms also occur. Orthostatic intolerance and

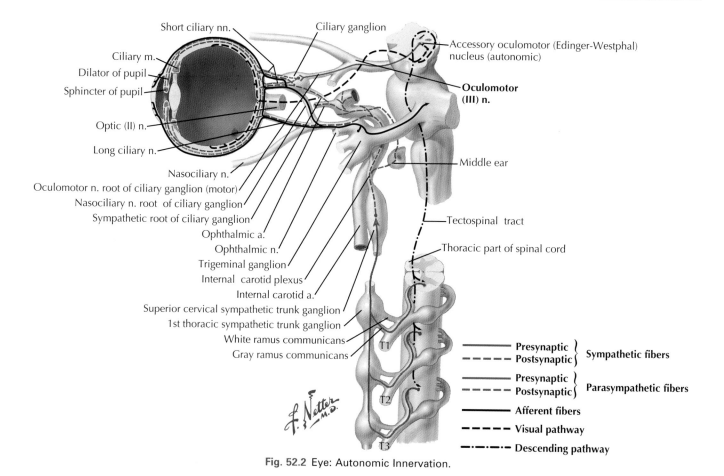

Short ciliary nn.
Ciliary ganglion
Accessory oculomotor (Edinger-Westphal) nucleus (autonomic)
Ciliary m.
Dilator of pupil
Sphincter of pupil
Oculomotor (III) n.
Optic (II) n.
Long ciliary n.
Middle ear
Nasociliary n.
Oculomotor n. root of ciliary ganglion (motor)
Nasociliary n. root of ciliary ganglion
Sympathetic root of ciliary ganglion
Tectospinal tract
Ophthalmic a.
Ophthalmic n.
Thoracic part of spinal cord
Trigeminal ganglion
Internal carotid plexus
Internal carotid a.
Superior cervical sympathetic trunk ganglion
1st thoracic sympathetic trunk ganglion
White ramus communicans
Gray ramus communicans
T1

Presynaptic } Postsynaptic } **Sympathetic fibers**
Presynaptic } Postsynaptic } **Parasympathetic fibers**
Afferent fibers
Visual pathway
Descending pathway
T2
T3

Fig. 52.2 Eye: Autonomic Innervation.

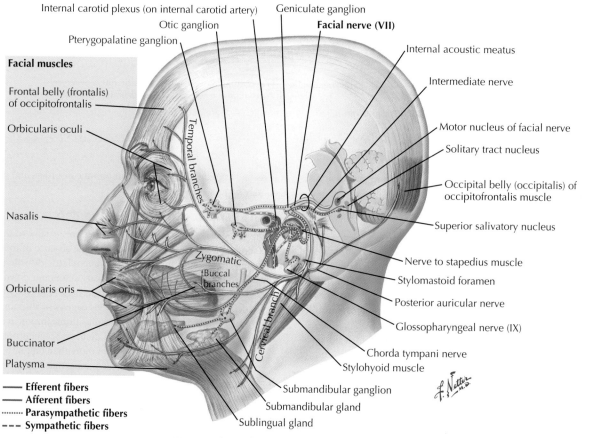

Internal carotid plexus (on internal carotid artery)
Geniculate ganglion
Otic ganglion
Facial nerve (VII)
Pterygopalatine ganglion
Internal acoustic meatus
Facial muscles
Intermediate nerve
Frontal belly (frontalis) of occipitofrontalis
Orbicularis oculi
Motor nucleus of facial nerve
Solitary tract nucleus
Temporal branches
Occipital belly (occipitalis) of occipitofrontalis muscle
Nasalis
Superior salivatory nucleus
Zygomatic
Nerve to stapedius muscle
Buccal branches
Stylomastoid foramen
Orbicularis oris
Posterior auricular nerve
Cervical branch
Glossopharyngeal nerve (IX)
Buccinator
Chorda tympani nerve
Platysma
Stylohyoid muscle
Efferent fibers
Afferent fibers
Parasympathetic fibers
Sympathetic fibers
Submandibular ganglion
Submandibular gland
Sublingual gland

Fig. 52.3 Facial Nerve: Autonomic Innervation.

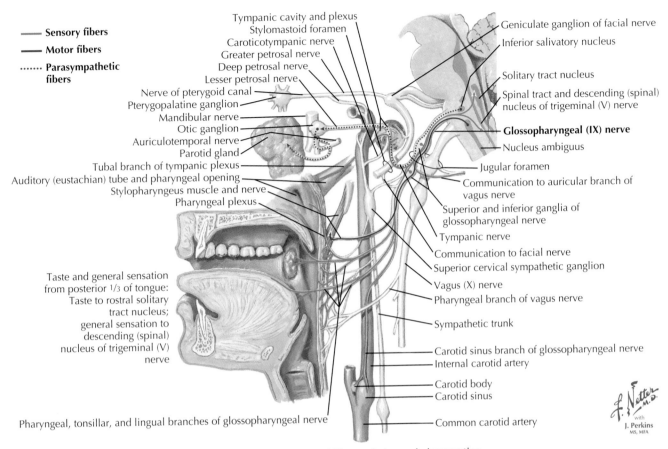

— Sensory fibers
— Motor fibers
······ Parasympathetic fibers

Tympanic cavity and plexus
Stylomastoid foramen
Caroticotympanic nerve
Greater petrosal nerve
Deep petrosal nerve
Lesser petrosal nerve
Nerve of pterygoid canal
Pterygopalatine ganglion
Mandibular nerve
Otic ganglion
Auriculotemporal nerve
Parotid gland
Tubal branch of tympanic plexus
Auditory (eustachian) tube and pharyngeal opening
Stylopharyngeus muscle and nerve
Pharyngeal plexus

Geniculate ganglion of facial nerve
Inferior salivatory nucleus
Solitary tract nucleus
Spinal tract and descending (spinal) nucleus of trigeminal (V) nerve
Glossopharyngeal (IX) nerve
Nucleus ambiguus
Jugular foramen
Communication to auricular branch of vagus nerve
Superior and inferior ganglia of glossopharyngeal nerve
Tympanic nerve
Communication to facial nerve
Superior cervical sympathetic ganglion
Vagus (X) nerve
Pharyngeal branch of vagus nerve
Sympathetic trunk
Carotid sinus branch of glossopharyngeal nerve
Internal carotid artery
Carotid body
Carotid sinus
Common carotid artery

Taste and general sensation from posterior 1/3 of tongue: Taste to rostral solitary tract nucleus; general sensation to descending (spinal) nucleus of trigeminal (V) nerve

Pharyngeal, tonsillar, and lingual branches of glossopharyngeal nerve

Fig. 52.4 Glossopharyngeal Nerve: Autonomic Innervation.

gastrointestinal dysmotility are common presentations. Autonomic tests are almost always abnormal. Nerve biopsies demonstrate inflammatory infiltrates supporting an immune-mediated hypothesis. Recovery is slow and often incomplete. High titers of ganglionic nicotinic acetylcholine receptor antibodies are reported in approximately half of these patients, supporting the presumed autoimmune basis.

Guillain-Barré syndrome preferentially involves somatic motor fibers but also causes dysautonomia in two-thirds of cases, especially affecting the cardiovascular and gastrointestinal systems. Bladder dysfunction is less common. Autonomic complications may be life threatening; patients must be monitored in the intensive care unit (ICU).

Paraneoplastic autonomic neuropathy is often indistinguishable from primary autoimmune autonomic neuropathy. Gastrointestinal dysmotility is a common presenting manifestation. Antineuronal nuclear antibody type 1 is associated with small-cell lung cancer. It is the most frequently demonstrated abnormal paraneoplastic neurologic antibody. Less frequently anti-collapsin response-mediator protein-5 (CRMP5) antibody is present, also associated with small-cell lung cancer. Other malignancies associated with paraneoplastic autonomic dysfunction include cancers of pancreas, colon, and thyroid.

Hereditary porphyria presents with acute attacks of dysautonomic symptoms (abdominal pain, vomiting, constipation, hypertension, and tachycardia) in addition to predominantly motor polyneuropathies. Diagnosis requires demonstration of increased urinary excretion of porphobilinogen.

Toxins: Chemicals, including various medications, particularly cisplatinum and vinca alkaloids, cause peripheral neuropathies with autonomic features. Other specific nerve toxins such as organophosphates, heavy metals (e.g., thallium and arsenic), hexacarbons, and acrylamide may produce acute autonomic peripheral neuropathies.

Chronic Peripheral Autonomic Disorders

Diabetic autonomic neuropathies are common accompaniments of diabetic peripheral neuropathies and often correlate with the duration and control of diabetes. Early clinical autonomic testing often reveals evidence of cardiovagal dysfunction manifested by impairment of heart rate response to Valsalva maneuver or to deep breathing. Autonomic dysfunction due to uncontrolled diabetes can cause considerable morbidity.

Postural orthostatic tachycardia syndrome (POTS) is seen predominantly in young women. It is characterized by orthostatic symptoms associated with significant rise in heart rate on standing without orthostatic hypotension or other clinical or laboratory evidence of autonomic neuropathy, except for distal sweat loss. The pathophysiology of POTS is heterogeneous. It may include findings seen in limited autonomic neuropathies, hypovolemia, and deconditioning and often there may be an associated anxiety or depressive disorder.

Amyloidosis is a multisystem disorder that may be sporadic or familial. Autonomic neuropathy often occurs presenting with symptoms of somatic small-fiber dysfunction, orthostatic intolerance, and constipation alternating with diarrhea.

Pure autonomic failure is also known as idiopathic autonomic hypotension. It is an insidious process with typical signs of disordered autonomic function. The absence of parkinsonian features helps differentiate this disorder from multiple systems atrophy. It results from postganglionic sympathetic neuron degeneration.

Hereditary autonomic neuropathies are rare disorders. Hereditary sensory and autonomic neuropathy type III, also known as Riley Day syndrome, is an autosomal recessive disorder, presenting with defective

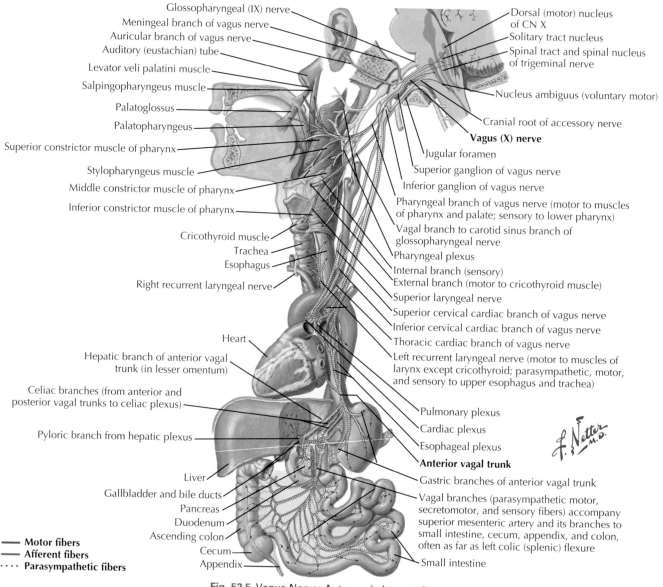

Fig. 52.5 Vagus Nerve: Autonomic Innervation.

control of blood pressure, sweating, temperature, and lacrimation in children. Dysautonomic manifestations are less pronounced in the other hereditary sensory and autonomic neuropathies.

Central Disorders

Parkinson disease is associated with significant autonomic dysfunction, particularly in long-standing disease. There is a loss of pigmented substantia nigra dopaminergic cells and other pigmented nuclei, including the locus ceruleus and the dorsal vagal nucleus, and this may partially explain the autonomic symptoms. Peripheral sympathetic heart denervation is common, resulting in orthostatic hypotension in severe cases.

Multiple systems atrophy is a degenerative disorder characterized by parkinsonian features with autonomic, cerebellar, and corticospinal involvement. When autonomic symptoms predominate, the disorder is called *Shy-Drager syndrome*. Depletion of catecholaminergic neurons in the brainstem contributes to development of orthostatic hypotension. Other autonomic symptoms include bladder dysfunction, constipation, sexual dysfunction, and laryngeal stridor.

Spinal cord disorders of various etiologies may also have autonomic symptoms. Common disorders include trauma, syringomyelia, and multiple sclerosis. They usually manifest with arrhythmias, blood pressure lability, and bladder atony.

THERAPY

Primary treatment consists of specific therapies for the underlying disorders, when these are identified, and, when possible, symptomatic relief per se. Nonpharmacologic treatments of orthostatic hypotension include increasing intake of dietary salt and water, eating smaller and more frequent meals, avoiding alcohol, and wearing elastic stockings or abdominal binders. Medications include sympathetic agents such as midodrine and fluid- and salt-conserving agents such as fludrocortisone. Orthostatic symptoms typically seen in POTS may respond to low-dose β-blockers or low-dose midodrine. Other medications that can be used include the acetylcholine esterase inhibitor pyridostigmine, this improves ganglionic neurotransmission and increases the release of norepinephrine by postganglionic sympathetic neurons; unlike

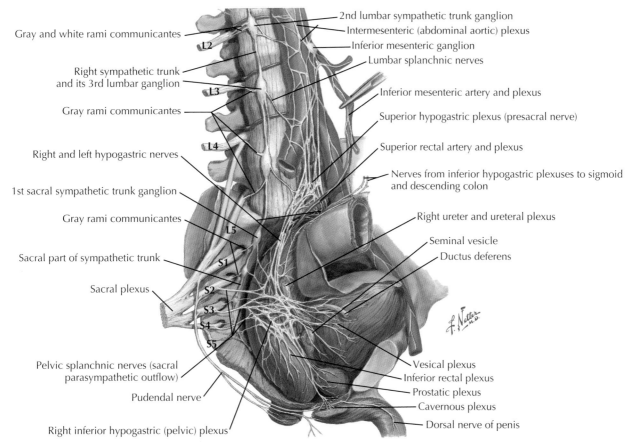

Gray and white rami communicantes

L2

Right sympathetic trunk and its 3rd lumbar ganglion

L3

Gray rami communicantes

L4

Right and left hypogastric nerves

1st sacral sympathetic trunk ganglion

Gray rami communicantes

L5

Sacral part of sympathetic trunk

S1

Sacral plexus

S2

S3

S4

S5

Pelvic splanchnic nerves (sacral parasympathetic outflow)

Pudendal nerve

Right inferior hypogastric (pelvic) plexus

2nd lumbar sympathetic trunk ganglion

Intermesenteric (abdominal aortic) plexus

Inferior mesenteric ganglion

Lumbar splanchnic nerves

Inferior mesenteric artery and plexus

Superior hypogastric plexus (presacral nerve)

Superior rectal artery and plexus

Nerves from inferior hypogastric plexuses to sigmoid and descending colon

Right ureter and ureteral plexus

Seminal vesicle

Ductus deferens

Vesical plexus

Inferior rectal plexus

Prostatic plexus

Cavernous plexus

Dorsal nerve of penis

Fig. 52.6 Pelvic Organs: Autonomic Innervation.

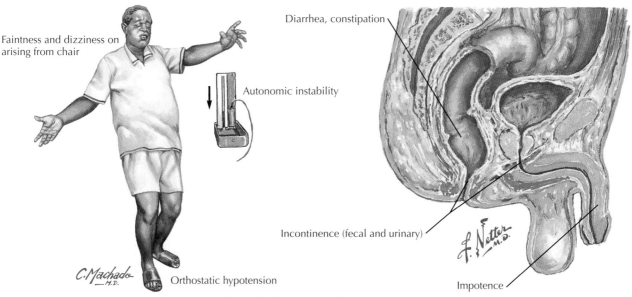

Faintness and dizziness on arising from chair

Autonomic instability

Orthostatic hypotension

Diarrhea, constipation

Incontinence (fecal and urinary)

Impotence

Fig. 52.7 Symptoms of Dysautonomia.

other agents used in orthostatic hypotension it does not cause supine hypertension. Droxidopa is a synthetic norepinephrine precursor that is approved for use in Parkinson disease, multiple systems atrophy, and pure autonomic failure; it can cause supine hypertension.

Bladder dysfunction in most dysautonomic conditions is characterized by failure to empty. Treatments include timed voiding, intermittent catheterizations, and, rarely, indwelling catheters. Pharmacologic agents that promote bladder emptying, such as bethanechol, have limited efficacy. Bladder pacemakers and botulinum toxin injections may benefit select patients.

Treatment of erectile dysfunction includes agents such as phosphodiesterase-5 inhibitors such as sildenafil and its analogs, yohimbine, topical nitroglycerin or minoxidil, injections of prostaglandins, or penile implants.

Gastrointestinal dysfunction is best aided by strategies to maintain hydration and nutrition. Gastroparesis is treated with prokinetic agents such as metoclopramide; constipation is treated with increased fiber intake and laxatives.

Plasma exchange and intravenous immunoglobulin are used for the treatment of suspected immune-mediated autonomic neuropathy with variable success.

PROGNOSIS

This depends on the etiology, severity, and overall degree of autonomic dysfunction. Autoimmune autonomic neuropathies often have a limited, unsatisfactory improvement. Patients with Guillain-Barré syndrome usually experience complete resolution of autonomic dysfunction in parallel with clinical recovery of strength. Prognosis for chronic peripheral and central autonomic disorders is less favorable.

ADDITIONAL RESOURCES

Benarroch EE, Smithson IL, Low PA, et al. Depletion of catecholaminergic neurons in the rostral ventrolateral medulla in multiple system atrophy with autonomic failure. Ann Neurol 1998;43:56–163.

Cohen J, Low P, Fealey R, et al. Somatic and autonomic function in progressive autonomic failure and multiple system atrophy. Ann Neurol 1987;22:692–9.

Lipp A, Sandroni P, Ahlskog JE, et al. Prospective differentiation of multiple system atrophy from parkinson disease, with and without autonomic failure. Arch Neurol 2009;66(6):742–50.

Low PA, Vernino S, Suarez G. Autonomic dysfunction in peripheral nerve disease. Muscle Nerve 2003;27:646–61.

Vernino S, Low PA, Fealey RD, et al. Autoantibodies to ganglionic acetylcholine receptors in autoimmune autonomic neuropathies. N Engl J Med 2000;343:847–55.

Winston N, Vernino S. Autoimmune autonomic ganglionopathy. Front Neurol Neurosci 2009;26:85–93.

53

Syncope

Jayashri Srinivasan, Jose A. Gutrecht

CLINICAL VIGNETTE *A 24-year-old man was at work on his first day as a laboratory technical assistant. He was assisting the phlebotomist with a difficult blood draw when he went pale and sweaty and fell to the ground. There was no tonic–clonic activity, tongue biting, or urinary incontinence. He came around and was alert in a few seconds. His only symptom when he came around was "embarrassment." His general physical examination including blood pressure and pulse and neurologic examination was normal.*

Syncope is defined as a brief and transient loss of consciousness from cerebral hypoperfusion. Lightheadedness, visual dimming, paleness, cold sweating, nausea, and a feeling of warmth are common premonitory symptoms (Fig. 53.1). These are followed by loss of consciousness and postural muscle tone, and, if the patient is standing, he or she will usually fall. Significant trauma and fractures occur in approximately 5% of these patients. In contrast to patients who lose consciousness from a convulsion, individuals who have syncope generally have no confusion after the episode. Typically, they have good recollection of premonitory symptoms. Loss of consciousness lasts just a few seconds. Occasionally, a few clonic twitches or a brief generalized seizure-like activity occurs at the end of the episode. Electroencephalogram (EEG) recorded during syncope demonstrates early depression of activity followed by slow wave activity in the theta and delta ranges. Transient EEG voltage depression may follow. Elderly patients may be amnestic for the event. Almost 20% of people have had a syncopal episode in their lifetime.

Syncope may be classified as having cardiac or noncardiac origin. Cardiac syncope may be due to cardiac disease (arrhythmias or valvular disease) or may be cardiac reflex syncope from orthostatic hypotension. Noncardiac syncope is subclassified as neurologic, metabolic, or idiopathic.

The most common type, cardiac reflex syncope, has three subtypes: vasovagal (called neurocardiogenic or vasodepressor), situational (e.g., micturition, Valsalva, ocular compression, venipuncture, fear, exertion), and carotid hypersensitivity.

Vasovagal cardiac reflex syncope is the most commonly seen syncope in neurologic practice. Its pathophysiology is unresolved. The reflex is initiated by an intense sympathetic activation (e.g., a painful stimulus or fear) with increase of blood pressure, tachycardia, decreased cardiac filling ("empty heart"), and powerful cardiac contractions that stimulate heart mechanoreceptors. Subsequently, cardiac inhibitor pathway activation causes a short-term increase of vagal activity and withdrawal of sympathetic activity, known as the Bezold-Jarisch reflex. The loss of consciousness, secondary to cerebral hypoperfusion, is primarily from a combination of profound bradycardia and arterial pressure collapse. Vasovagal syncope often occurs while assuming the upright posture; in these instances, diminished blood return from the lower limbs and viscera and a subsequent pooling of blood in the lower body result in decreased cardiac filling and initiation of the cascade of events.

Orthostatic hypotension is another common cause of syncope. A tilt-table test is essential to the evaluation of these patients and in the investigation of syncope of unclear origin. The causes of orthostatic hypotension vary and merit further evaluation. Medications of many classes are common causes of hypotension leading to syncope. Dehydration and hypovolemia are other, easily excluded, common pathophysiologic mechanisms.

Hyperventilation with associated hypocapnia is a rare cause of syncope. Metabolic causes of syncope include hypoglycemia and hypoxia. *Psychogenic syncope* sometimes can be difficult to document. It is best excluded by a careful history, witnessing the event, or both.

Primary neurologic causes of syncope are uncommon and usually have other associated symptoms. *Peripheral neuropathies* are the most common neurologic causes of syncope associated with orthostatic hypotension, particularly in patients with neuropathies secondary to diabetes and rarely primary amyloidosis. *Central nervous system disorders* such as multiple system atrophy with parkinsonian, cerebellar, or mixed features, previously called Shy-Drager disease, and pure autonomic failure must be considered despite their rare occurrence. Transient ischemic attacks in the vertebrobasilar system or basilar migraine are conditions that rarely produce syncopal episodes. There is no evidence that unilateral or bilateral critical carotid stenosis can cause syncope. The drop attacks of epileptic seizures are infrequently confused with syncope; although these patients lose postural tone and "drop," they do not lose consciousness.

The clinical examination of a patient with presumed syncope aims first to exclude serious illnesses, including structural heart disease, such as valvular aortic stenosis, cardiac rhythm disturbances, such as brady-arrhythmias, coronary artery disease, and cardiomyopathies with compromised cardiac output. Patients with syncope from heart disease have a higher mortality rate than individuals with other causes of syncope. Evaluation must include a detailed history and physical examination with particular attention to the heart, an electrocardiogram (ECG), Holter monitor, other forms of cardiac event monitoring, echocardiography, stress test, and occasionally invasive electrophysiologic testing. Autonomic testing including quantitative sweat testing, heart rate responses to deep breathing and Valsalva maneuver, and tilt-table tests are indicated in patients where autonomic dysfunction is suspected.

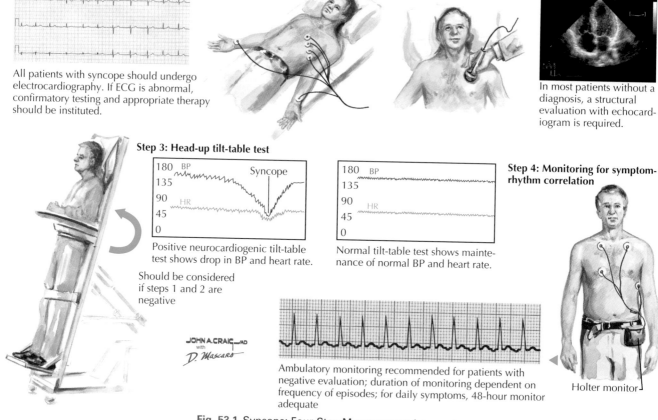

Step 1: Electrocardiogram

All patients with syncope should undergo electrocardiography. If ECG is abnormal, confirmatory testing and appropriate therapy should be instituted.

Step 2: Echocardiography

In most patients without a diagnosis, a structural evaluation with echocardiogram is required.

Step 3: Head-up tilt-table test

Positive neurocardiogenic tilt-table test shows drop in BP and heart rate.

Should be considered if steps 1 and 2 are negative

Normal tilt-table test shows maintenance of normal BP and heart rate.

Step 4: Monitoring for symptom-rhythm correlation

Ambulatory monitoring recommended for patients with negative evaluation; duration of monitoring dependent on frequency of episodes; for daily symptoms, 48-hour monitor adequate

Holter monitor

JOHN A. CRAIG—AD
with
D. Mascaro

Fig. 53.1 Syncope: Four-Step Management Approach.

The management of syncope focuses on the underlying disease process, often requiring specialized medical or surgical treatments. Cardiac, neurologic, and situational mechanisms must be addressed. The therapy of reflex vasovagal syncope is problematic. Analysis of whether syncope is primarily from cardiac inhibition or hypotension is sometimes difficult because these often occur together. Education, increased salt and fluid intake, β-blockers, blood volume expanders such as mineralocorticoids (fludrocortisone), α-adrenergic agonists such as midodrine, and serotonin reuptake inhibitors are recommended. Antiarrhythmic agents and pacemakers are also sometimes indicated.

Spinal Cord Disorders

Claudia J. Chaves

54

Anatomic Aspects of Spinal Cord Disorders

Ann Camac, H. Royden Jones, Jr.[†], Jose A. Gutrecht

Knowledge of spinal cord neuroanatomy is integral to the understanding, diagnosis, and management of spinal cord disorders. The spinal cord syndrome depends on site, process, and extent of spinal cord damage. A myelopathy is defined as any disorder that impairs spinal cord function. Myelopathies will be presented in the next chapter.

SPINAL CORD ANATOMY

External Structure

The spinal cord has major functional importance, despite representing only 2% of the entire central nervous system volume. The spinal cord is a cylindrical elongated structure flattened dorsoventrally, having a length of 42–45 cm (Fig. 54.1). It lies within the vertebral canal extending from the atlas, continuous with the medulla through the foramen magnum, to the level of the first and second lumbar vertebra. Here it tapers into the conus medullaris and terminates as the cauda equina (see Fig. 54.1). The spinal canal dimensions are slightly larger, allowing the cord to move freely within the canal during neck and back flexion/extension as its perspective changes with movement. When performing a lumbar puncture, the spinal needle can be inserted safely below the L3 vertebra, which is well below spinal cord termination.

The cervical and lumbar enlargements of the spinal cord provide the nerve roots innervating, respectively, the upper and lower limbs. There are 31 pairs of spinal nerves, each having dorsal sensory and ventral motor roots that exit the cord (8 cervical, 12 thoracic, 5 lumbar, 5 sacral, and 1 coccygeal). Although there are 7 cervical vertebrae, there are 8 cervical nerve roots (Fig. 54.2). The C1–C7 roots exit above their respective vertebrae whereas C8 exits below the seventh cervical vertebra and all thoracic, lumbar, and sacral roots exit below their specific vertebrae.

Three protective membranes, the meninges including the dura mater, being the outer layer; then the arachnoid; and the most inner one, the pia, surround the cord (see Fig. 54.2). Cerebrospinal fluid flows between the arachnoid and pia. Epidural fat is present in the epidural space between the spinal canal and dura mater. When clinical myelopathies develop, these various disorders are classically categorized as *intramedullary*, that is, intrinsic to the cord; or *extramedullary*, occurring secondary to disorders extrinsic to the cord. Extramedullary disorders are further subdivided into those with either an *intradural* extramedullary locus or a purely *extradural* site of pathology.

Internal Structure

White matter, consisting of myelinated fibers, surrounds the butterfly or H-shaped gray matter that contains cell bodies and their processes within the cord's center. These include both primary ascending sensory fibers and descending motor fibers. The sensory pathways are most superficial, while the motor fibers such as the corticospinal fibers are more deeply situated but still superficial and superior to the ventral horn containing the anterior horn cells that are the primary receptors for the corticospinal tract fibers. Longitudinal furrows on the cord's surface divide the white matter into columns or funiculi that are large bundles of nerve fibers having diverse functions. The anterior median fissure, posterior median, posterior intermediate, and the anterolateral sulci divide the dorsal or posterior, lateral, and anterior columns. The posterior columns are further divided into two fasciculi: gracilis medially (present at all spinal levels) and cuneatus laterally (T6 and above).

Specific Spinal Tracts

Ascending and descending tracts within the cord are interrupted at sites of cord damage (Figs. 54.3–54.5). The subsequent clinical sequelae develop based on the specific tracts that are affected.

Ascending Sensory Tracts (See Fig. 54.4)

- **Dorsal columns** subserving *touch, pressure, position,* and *movement* sensations arise from dorsal root fibers and ascend posteriorly. Their fibers do not decussate (i.e., cross) until within the medulla. They then travel to the ventral posterolateral thalamic nuclei.
- **Lateral spinothalamic tracts** arise from secondary *pain and temperature* neurons within the spinal cord, cross into the anterior commissure, and ascend in the lateral funiculus to the reticular formation and ventral posterolateral thalamic nuclei.
- **Anterior spinothalamic tracts** arise from dorsal horn neurons within the spinal cord, cross in the anterior commissure, and ascend anterolaterally to the posterior thalamic and ventral posterolateral thalamic nuclei. The anterior spinothalamic tract provides *light touch* sensation.
- **Dorsal spinocerebellar tracts** are uncrossed, ascending in the lateral funiculus to the cerebellar vermis. At subconscious levels, they provide fine coordination of posture and limb muscle movement.
- **Anterior (ventral) spinocerebellar tracts** are dedicated to lower extremity movement and posture, initially cross and then ascend the lateral funiculus to the cerebellum.
- **Cuneocerebellar tracts** contribute to upper extremity coordination and movement, are uncrossed, and ascend to the cerebellum.

Descending Motor Tracts

Corticospinal tracts are responsible for *voluntary, skilled movement.* They originate in the motor cortex (precentral and premotor areas 4 and 6), postcentral gyrus, and adjacent parietal cortex (see Fig. 54.5). These primary motor fibers descend via the corona radiata, posterior limb of internal capsule, pons, and into the medulla where most distally

---

[†]Deceased.

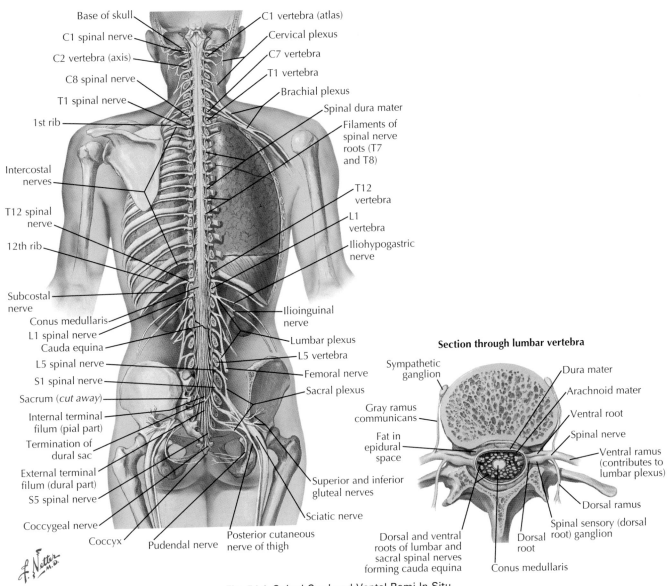

Section through lumbar vertebra

Fig. 54.1 Spinal Cord and Vental Rami In Situ.

they then divide into three separate motor tracts (see Fig. 54.3). Up to 90% of these fibers descend in the lateral funiculus as the *lateral corticospinal tract.* Most decussate within the distal medulla; the *uncrossed lateral corticospinal tract* is much smaller. The **anterior corticospinal tract** travels in the anterior funiculus, crossing within the cord.

Tectospinal, rubrospinal, and vestibulospinal tracts (see Fig. 54.3) originate in the superior colliculus, red nucleus, and the lateral vestibular nucleus, respectively. These tracts variously affect reflex postural movements, tone in flexor muscles, and facilitate antigravity and extensor muscles.

Spinal Gray Matter

The gray matter within the central cord from dorsal to ventral, respectively, includes the dorsal horn, the medial commissure, and the anterior horn. Various types of sensory fibers end in different layers of the dorsal horn. The high-threshold, very thin, and unmyelinated A delta and C fibers, conducting impulses from the nociceptors, end almost exclusively in the substantia gelatinosa (lamina I and II). In contrast, nerves

carrying the low-threshold mechanoreceptors subserving A beta fibers terminate in the deeper layers of the dorsal horn Rexed layers III–V. Lastly the largest, A alpha joint position sensory nerves, end in the deepest layer VI of the dorsal horn (see Fig. 54.4).

Motor neurons are primarily contained within the anterior horn. The preponderant numbers of these somatic efferent neurons are primarily located within the cervical and lumbosacral enlargements (see Fig. 54.5). Here these provide the motor innervation for their respective extremities. In contrast, the ventral horn areas subsume a much smaller portion of the thoracic cord. Here the lateral horn of the gray matter becomes preeminent, where it includes the **intermediolateral nucleus.** Here the preganglionic sympathetic neuron perikarya are located; similar neurons are also found within the brainstem (Fig. 54.6).

Vascular Supply
Arterial

One anterior and two posterior spinal arteries course the length of the cord supplying the anterior two-thirds and posterior one-third of the cord, respectively (Fig. 54.7). Sulcal or central branches of the anterior

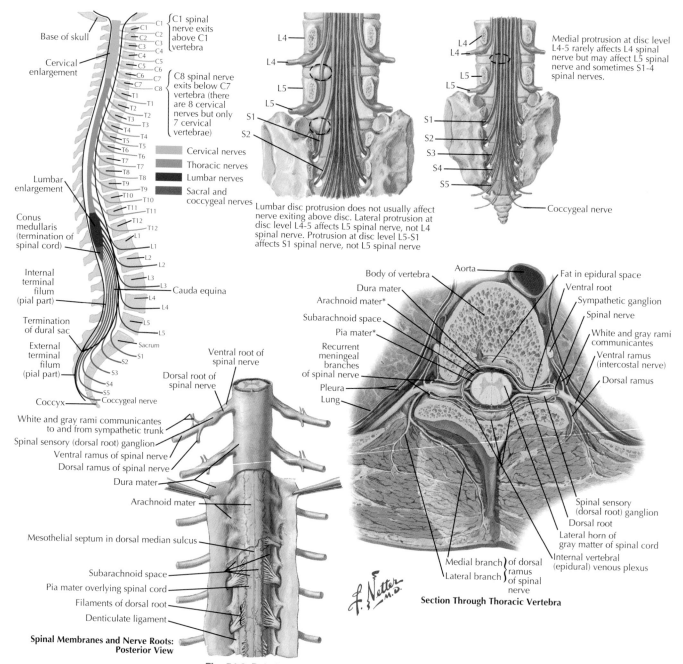

Fig. 54.2 Relation of Spinal Nerve Roots to Vertebrae.

spinal artery supply the central cord, whereas coronal or circumferential branches supply the ventral and lateral columns (Fig. 54.8).

- **Anterior spinal artery** supplies the anterior horn, spinothalamic tract, and corticospinal tract.
- **Posterior spinal artery** supplies the dorsal column, dorsal gray matter, and superficial dorsal aspect of lateral columns.
- **Vertebral artery medullary branches** join the anterior and posterior spinal arteries to supply the cervical cord.
- **Aortic segmental arteries** provide the supply for the remainder of the cord by branching into dural arteries that supply the dura and nerve root sleeve. *Radicular* branches supply the anterior and posterior nerve roots, and *medullary* branches join the anterior and posterior spinal arteries to supply the cord. Adamkiewicz artery, at

the lumbar enlargement, usually arises from the left side between T6 and L4. It provides the major arterial supply to the lower cord. The cord levels of C1–T2 and T9 caudally have excellent vascular supplies. In contrast, the T3–T8 arterial vasculature is more limited in number of vessels. Thus this is usually considered a watershed area that is quite vulnerable to ischemic events.

Venous

The anteromedial cord (anterior horns and white matter) is drained by the central or sulcal veins into the anterior median spinal vein that extends the length of the cord. The anterolateral, peripheral, and dorsal cord capillary plexus drain into the radial veins. The radial veins subsequently drain into the coronal venous plexus on the spinal cord surface

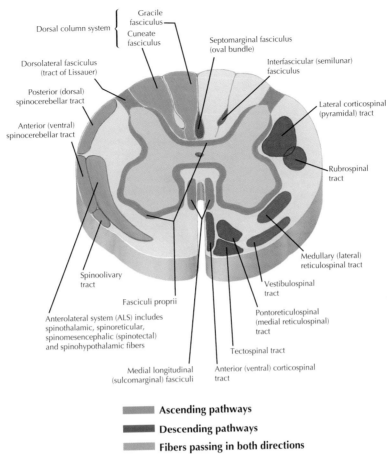

Fig. 54.3 Principal Fiber Tracts of Spinal Cord.

(Fig. 54.9). This plexus, with superficial spinal cord veins (anterior median, anterolateral, posterior median, posterior intermediate), drains into medullary veins. These are anatomically linked to the nerve roots traveling through the intervertebral foramen forming the epidural venous plexus. Subsequent drainage is to the inferior vena cava, azygous, and hemizygous veins.

PATHOANATOMY

Although a magnetic resonance image often expeditiously demonstrates the site and type of spinal cord abnormality, an appreciation of the anatomy and clinical temporal profile of the precise spinal cord disorder is fundamental to the care of every patient presenting with a myelopathy. Focal spinal cord lesions lead to degeneration of ascending tracts above the pathoanatomic site and descending tracts below the lesions. The key to localizing the site of spinal cord involvement is identifying the exact distribution of the various motor, reflex, and sensory deficits. The motor and sensory symptoms often correspond to the motor and sensory segmental levels (Fig. 54.10). In addition, knowledge of the somatotopic organization of the different motor and sensory tracts can help with the localization of the lesion; in the corticospinal and spinothalamic tracts, the sacral fibers are located more laterally and cervical fibers situated medially, while the opposite is true for the dorsal columns.

Muscle stretch reflex examination can point to a precise site when there is loss of a specific reflex; for example, a diminished or absent triceps reflex pointing to a lesion at C7 or loss of the quadriceps (knee jerk) pointing to an L3/L4 lesion. Total loss of muscle stretch reflexes may occur with an acute spinal cord lesion (spinal shock), such as a traumatic severance. More traditionally, muscle stretch reflexes are increased with a central nervous system lesion; often Babinski signs and clonus are also identified.

Lastly a very precise sensory evaluation is essential to the proper investigation of any potential myelopathy (Fig. 54.11). When the pathology affects the spinothalamic tract, assessment of pain and temperature sensation often provide the best evidence of a distinct *spinal level* of sensory loss. Often a *"cord level"* is a dramatic and distinct finding that can be elicited by using variable sensory modalities: a cold stimulus, such as the handle of a tuning fork; a safety pin; or just touching the skin (Fig. 54.12). Here the examiner takes one of these sensory tools and starting proximally or distally looks to see if there is a dramatic loss of appreciation if coming from the neck to the buttocks, or significant increased appreciation if one moves proximally in a reverse fashion. The patient's trunk must be examined both anteriorly and posteriorly. It is also vital to examine sensation in the extremities. Modalities such as position sense are best evaluated by moving the great toe or a finger subtly up or down and asking the patient to report its direction of movement from its prior position.

CLINICO-ANATOMICAL CORRELATION

Utilizing the data obtained from the patient's history as well as careful motor, sensory, and reflex examinations, one can make a clinical prediction as to the location of the lesion, whether it is intramedullary,

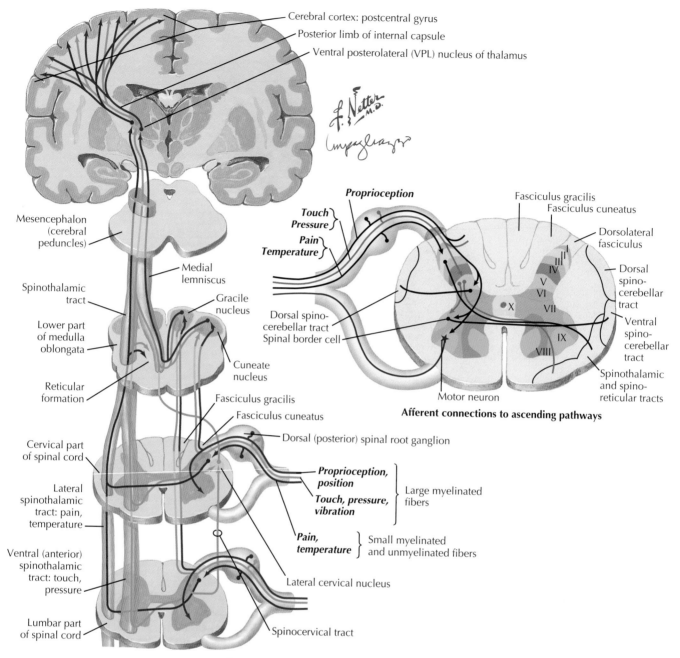

Fig. 54.4 Spinal Cerebral Afferent Systems.

intradural extramedullary, and extradural extramedullary as well as its potential etiologies.

There are some very classic patterns of myelopathies (Fig. 54.13) that we will summarize below:

1. **Central cord syndrome:** As the name implies, this syndrome is the result of damage to the central portions of the spinal cord, such as seen in patients with syringomyelia, but also with intramedullary cord tumor or a central hemorrhagic spinal necrosis. These patients present with a classic dissociated sensory syndrome characterized by a "cape loss" of pain and temperature modalities. That is, the patient may note loss of temperature and pain sensation limited to their hands, arms, and shoulders with preservation of the same on the trunk and lower extremities. For example, in a patient with a cervical syringomyelia, the decussating pain and temperature fibers,

such as C5–C8 fibers, are damaged as they pass under the spinal cord's expanding central canal. Normally, these fibers join the ascending spinothalamic tracts from the legs and trunk to ascend to the brain (Fig. 54.14). Here temperature and pain sensation are intact distal to the site of the intramedullary lesion; thus there is a dissociation in the patient's ability to perceive these basic modalities proximally at the midcervical levels but preserving the same modalities below the affected areas. Light touch and proprioception are typically preserved. Extension of the lesion into the anterior horn cells leads to segmental neurogenic atrophy, paresis, and areflexia. As the corticospinal tracts become involved, a spastic paresis develops below the level of the syrinx.

2. **Anterior spinal artery syndrome:** In this instance, the patient experiences damage to the lateral corticospinal and anterior and

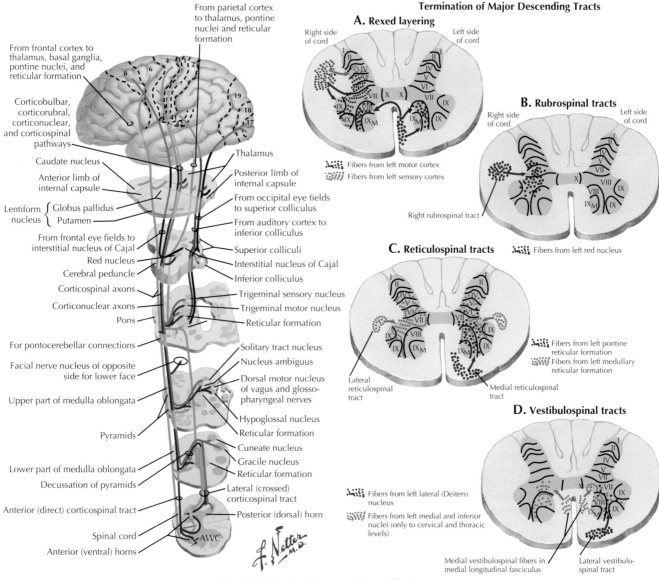

Fig. 54.5 Cerebral Cortex: Efferent Pathways.

lateral spinothalamic tracts, as well as the relevant anterior horn cells (see Fig. 54.12), due to interruption of the blood flow from the anterior spinal artery, the primary supply of the anterior two-thirds of the cord. Typically, these patients become paraparetic or paraplegic, with a complete pain and temperature sensory loss below the level of the lesion. These patients characteristically have preservation of proprioception modalities as the posterior columns remain intact. Very rarely, weakness occurs in all four extremities when the cervical cord is infarcted; however, the abundance of collateral circulation at this level makes this an exceedingly rare clinical scenario.

3. **Brown-Séquard syndrome:** This syndrome occurs due to damage of one-half of the spinal cord secondary to local trauma, tumor, infection, or inflammation. It is characterized by weakness and loss of proprioception ipsilateral to the lesion, due to involvement of the corticospinal tract and dorsal columns, respectively, and contralateral loss of pain and temperature, as the fibers composing the damaged spinothalamic tract have already decussated as it ascends within the cord. Thus a patient with a left-sided hemicord lesion should

present with left-sided weakness and impaired proprioception as well as inability to perceive pain and temperature on the right side of the body, below the lesion level.

4. **Posterior column syndrome:** A posterior one-third myelopathy would be expected to lead to a sensory ataxia, with preserved pain and temperature and corticospinal tract function; however, this clinical picture is extremely rare.

5. **Transverse myelopathy:** When a lesion extensively damages the entire transverse section of the spinal cord, the resultant clinical picture is characterized by total interruption of all sensory and motor functions below the damaged level. An acute insult causes flaccid paralysis and areflexia secondary to "spinal shock"; subsequently, spasticity and hyperreflexia develop. More gradual cord disruption will present with a slowly evolving weakness. If the anterior horn cells, ventral roots, or both are also involved, lower motor neuron signs, including fasciculations, atrophy, areflexia, and weakness, occur at the lesion level. An extensive cord insult is necessary to completely affect touch sensation as both the posterior columns and spinothalamic tracts

Text continued on p. 556

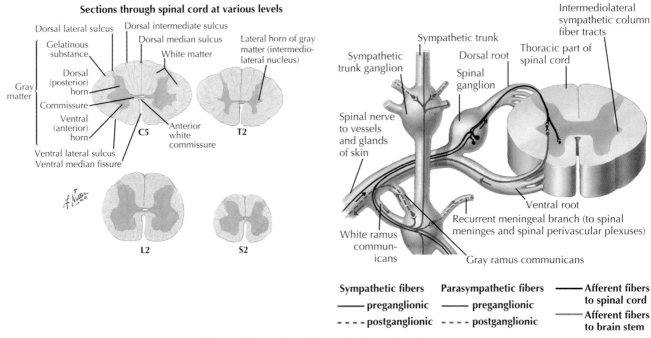

Sections through spinal cord at various levels

Dorsal lateral sulcus
Dorsal intermediate sulcus
Gelatinous substance
Dorsal median sulcus
White matter
Lateral horn of gray matter (intermediolateral nucleus)
Dorsal (posterior) horn
Gray matter
Commissure
Ventral (anterior) horn
Anterior white commissure
Ventral lateral sulcus
Ventral median fissure

C5   T2   L2   S2

Intermediolateral sympathetic column fiber tracts
Sympathetic trunk
Sympathetic trunk ganglion
Dorsal root
Spinal ganglion
Thoracic part of spinal cord
Spinal nerve to vessels and glands of skin
Ventral root
Recurrent meningeal branch (to spinal meninges and spinal perivascular plexuses)
White ramus communicans
Gray ramus communicans

Sympathetic fibers	Parasympathetic fibers	Afferent fibers to spinal cord
——— preganglionic	——— preganglionic	
- - - - postganglionic	- - - - postganglionic	Afferent fibers to brain stem

Fig. 54.6 Spinal Cord Cross Sections: Fiber Tracts.

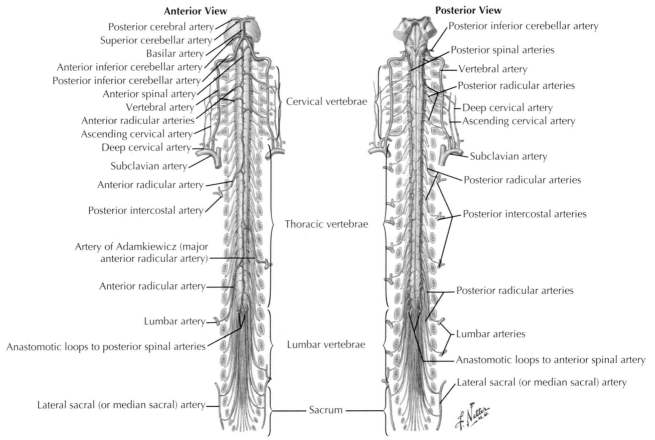

Anterior View

Posterior cerebral artery
Superior cerebellar artery
Basilar artery
Anterior inferior cerebellar artery
Posterior inferior cerebellar artery
Anterior spinal artery
Vertebral artery
Anterior radicular arteries
Ascending cervical artery
Deep cervical artery
Subclavian artery
Anterior radicular artery
Posterior intercostal artery
Artery of Adamkiewicz (major anterior radicular artery)
Anterior radicular artery
Lumbar artery
Anastomotic loops to posterior spinal arteries
Lateral sacral (or median sacral) artery

Cervical vertebrae
Thoracic vertebrae
Lumbar vertebrae
Sacrum

Posterior View

Posterior inferior cerebellar artery
Posterior spinal arteries
Vertebral artery
Posterior radicular arteries
Deep cervical artery
Ascending cervical artery
Subclavian artery
Posterior radicular arteries
Posterior intercostal arteries
Posterior radicular arteries
Lumbar arteries
Anastomotic loops to anterior spinal artery
Lateral sacral (or median sacral) artery

Fig. 54.7 Arteries of Spinal Cord: Schema.

Section through Thoracic Spine

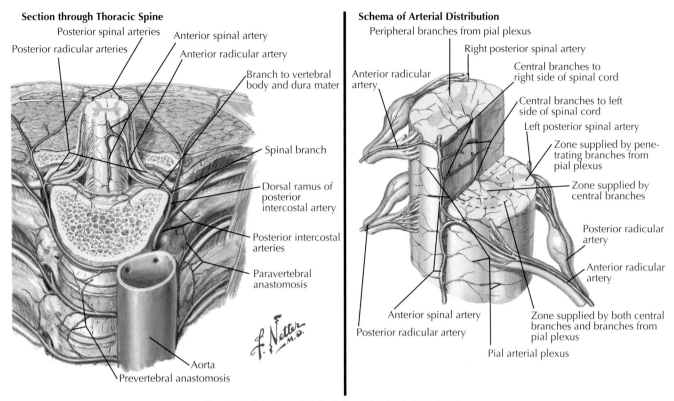

Posterior spinal arteries

Anterior spinal artery

Posterior radicular arteries

Anterior radicular artery

Branch to vertebral body and dura mater

Spinal branch

Dorsal ramus of posterior intercostal artery

Posterior intercostal arteries

Paravertebral anastomosis

Aorta

Prevertebral anastomosis

Schema of Arterial Distribution

Peripheral branches from pial plexus

Right posterior spinal artery

Anterior radicular artery

Central branches to right side of spinal cord

Central branches to left side of spinal cord

Left posterior spinal artery

Zone supplied by penetrating branches from pial plexus

Zone supplied by central branches

Posterior radicular artery

Anterior radicular artery

Anterior spinal artery

Posterior radicular artery

Zone supplied by both central branches and branches from pial plexus

Pial arterial plexus

Fig. 54.8 Arteries of Spinal Cord: Intrinsic Distribution.

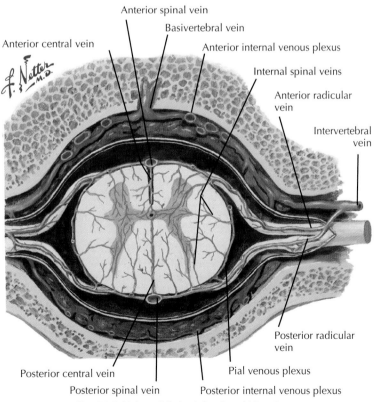

Anterior spinal vein

Basivertebral vein

Anterior central vein

Anterior internal venous plexus

Internal spinal veins

Anterior radicular vein

Intervertebral vein

Posterior radicular vein

Posterior central vein

Pial venous plexus

Posterior spinal vein

Posterior internal venous plexus

Fig. 54.9 Veins of Spinal Cord and Vertebrae.

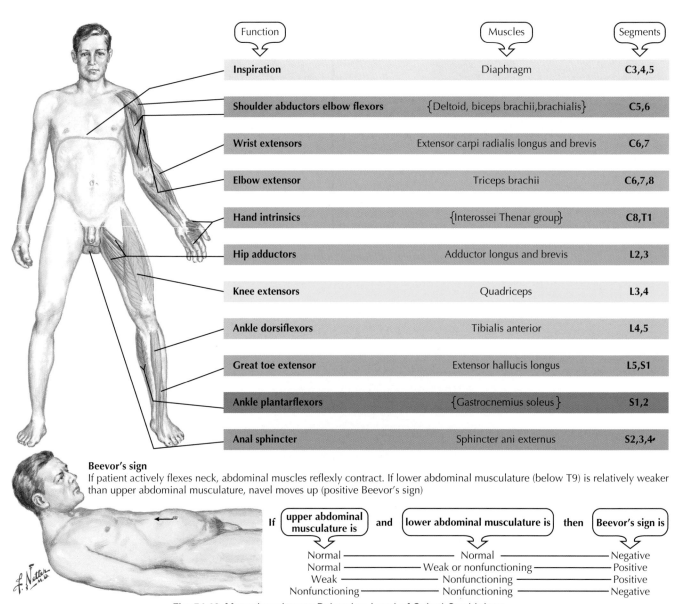

Function	Muscles	Segments
Inspiration	Diaphragm	**C3,4,5**
Shoulder abductors elbow flexors	{Deltoid, biceps brachii, brachialis}	**C5,6**
Wrist extensors	Extensor carpi radialis longus and brevis	**C6,7**
Elbow extensor	Triceps brachii	**C6,7,8**
Hand intrinsics	{Interossei Thenar group}	**C8,T1**
Hip adductors	Adductor longus and brevis	**L2,3**
Knee extensors	Quadriceps	**L3,4**
Ankle dorsiflexors	Tibialis anterior	**L4,5**
Great toe extensor	Extensor hallucis longus	**L5,S1**
Ankle plantarflexors	{Gastrocnemius soleus}	**S1,2**
Anal sphincter	Sphincter ani externus	**S2,3,4**

Beevor's sign

If patient actively flexes neck, abdominal muscles reflexly contract. If lower abdominal musculature (below T9) is relatively weaker than upper abdominal musculature, navel moves up (positive Beevor's sign)

If upper abdominal musculature is	and lower abdominal musculature is	then Beevor's sign is
Normal	Normal	Negative
Normal	Weak or nonfunctioning	Positive
Weak	Nonfunctioning	Positive
Nonfunctioning	Nonfunctioning	Negative

Fig. 54.10 Motor Impairment Related to Level of Spinal Cord Injury.

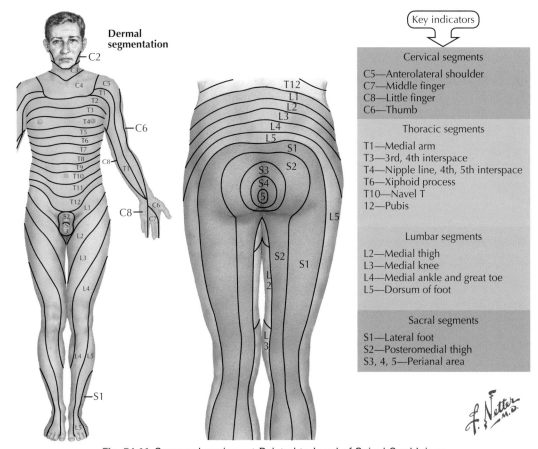

Dermal segmentation

Key indicators

Cervical segments

C5—Anterolateral shoulder
C7—Middle finger
C8—Little finger
C6—Thumb

Thoracic segments

T1—Medial arm
T3—3rd, 4th interspace
T4—Nipple line, 4th, 5th interspace
T6—Xiphoid process
T10—Navel T
12—Pubis

Lumbar segments

L2—Medial thigh
L3—Medial knee
L4—Medial ankle and great toe
L5—Dorsum of foot

Sacral segments

S1—Lateral foot
S2—Posteromedial thigh
S3, 4, 5—Perianal area

Fig. 54.11 Sensory Impairment Related to Level of Spinal Cord Injury.

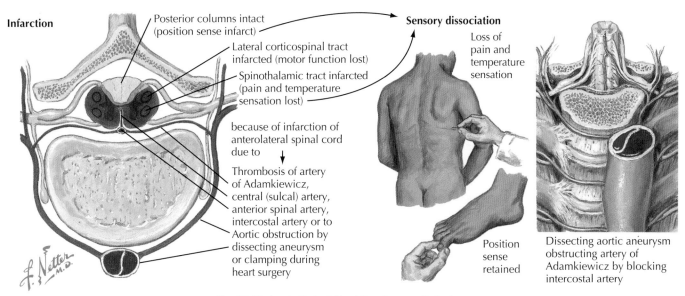

Infarction

Posterior columns intact (position sense infarct)

Lateral corticospinal tract infarcted (motor function lost)

Spinothalamic tract infarcted (pain and temperature sensation lost)

because of infarction of anterolateral spinal cord due to

↓

Thrombosis of artery of Adamkiewicz, central (sulcal) artery, anterior spinal artery, intercostal artery or to Aortic obstruction by dissecting aneurysm or clamping during heart surgery

Sensory dissociation

Loss of pain and temperature sensation

Position sense retained

Dissecting aortic aneurysm obstructing artery of Adamkiewicz by blocking intercostal artery

Fig. 54.12 Acute Spinal Cord Syndromes Pathology.

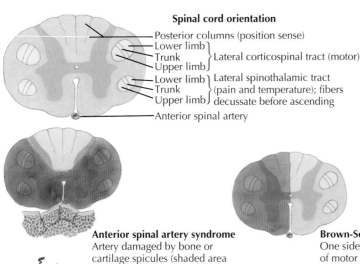

Spinal cord orientation

Posterior columns (position sense)

Lower limb
Trunk }Lateral corticospinal tract (motor)
Upper limb

Lower limb
Trunk }Lateral spinothalamic tract
Upper limb }(pain and temperature); fibers decussate before ascending

Anterior spinal artery

Central cord syndrome
Central cord hemorrhage and edema. Parts of 3 main tracts involved on both sides. Upper limbs more affected than lower limbs.

Anterior spinal artery syndrome
Artery damaged by bone or cartilage spicules (shaded area affected). Bilateral loss of motor function and pain sensation below injured segment; position sense preserved.

Brown-Séquard syndrome
One side of cord affected. Loss of motor function and position sense on same side and of pain sensation on opposite side.

Posterior column syndrome
(uncommon)
Position sense lost below lesion; motor function and pain sensation preserved.

Fig. 54.13 Incomplete Spinal Cord Syndromes.

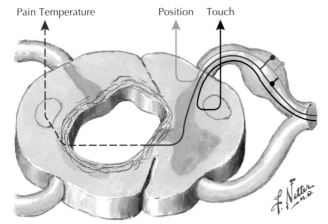

Pain Temperature   Position   Touch

Diagram demonstrating interruption of crossed pain and temperature fibers by syrinx; uncrossed light touch and proprioception fibers preserved

Fig. 54.14 Syringomyelia.

provide touch. The demonstration of a sensory level, assessed by testing pain and temperature (spinothalamic tract), segmental paresthesia, or radicular pain, often helps to localize the spinal cord level.

For details about different intramedullary and extramedullary pathologies, including intradural and extradural, please see Chapter 55.

ADDITIONAL RESOURCES

Brazis PW, Masdeu JC, Biller J. Localization in clinical neurology. 7th ed. Wolters Kluwer; 2017.

Brodal P. The central nervous system. 5th ed. Oxford, UK: Oxford University Press; 2016.

Kandel ER, Schwartz JH, Jessel TM, et al. Principles of neural science. 5th ed. New York: McGraw-Hill; 2013.

Louis ED, Mayer SA, Rowland LP. Merritt's neurology. 13th ed. Wolters Kluwer; 2016.

Ropper AH, Samuels MA, Klein JP. Adams and Victor's principles of neurology. 10th ed. New York: McGraw-Hill; 2014.

55

Myelopathies

Claudia J. Chaves, H. Royden Jones, Jr.[†]

The spinal cord may be affected by a broad spectrum of disorders, some of them directly damaging the cord (intramedullary), others affecting the cord indirectly due to pathologies involving the extramedullary region, including the intradural and extradural spaces. Some of these conditions present acutely, whereas others have a more progressive course. A careful history and detailed neurologic exam are extremely important to help localize where the lesion may be as well as identify its potential etiologies. Neuroimaging studies, most often magnetic resonance imaging (MRI) of the spine, are frequently required to confirm the diagnosis. On occasion, blood work, spinal fluid analysis, and spinal angiogram are also needed to clarify the etiology.

INTRAMEDULLARY DISORDERS

Intramedullary diseases frequently present with widespread lower motor neuron signs, occurring due to involvement of the anterior horn cells, while upper motor neuron signs tend to occur later in the course of these disorders. Dissociative sensory loss with preserved sacral sensation is common. Pain, if present, is reported as an uncomfortable feeling in the extremities and occurs due to involvement of the spinothalamic tracts (funicular pain). Intramedullary pathologies can be divided according to the mode of presentation into acute and chronic disorders (Table 55.1).

ACUTE INTRAMEDULLARY MYELOPATHIES

Vascular–Spinal Cord Infarction

> **CLINICAL VIGNETTE** *A 70-year-old man with past medical history significant for diabetes, hypertension, and high cholesterol reported bilateral leg weakness associated with decreased sensation from his waist down shortly after waking up from an extensive surgery for a thoracic-abdominal aneurysm repair. Neurologic examination demonstrated the patient to be paraplegic but with preserved strength in his upper body, loss of temperature, and pain sensation with a T10 level, and preserved position and vibratory sensation. No hypotension during the surgical procedure was noted. Stat MRI of the spine revealed subtle patchy areas of T2 hyperintensity involving the anterior spinal cord from T9 to T12. The patient was treated with induced hypertension and a lumbar drain with a goal intracranial pressure (ICP) from 8 to 12 mm Hg for the first 24 h with some improvement of his neurologic function.*
>
> *Comment: This is a typical case of spinal cord ischemia involving the thoracic cord in the territory of the anterior spinal artery, after an extensive thoracic-abdominal aneurysm repair. While the use of the induced systemic hypertension combined with lumbar drainage is not the standard of care, it has shown to be beneficial in some patients and can be considered.*

Spinal cord infarction is rare, with an estimated incidence of 1%–2% of all stroke cases. It typically occurs in adults and can be caused by a broad spectrum of conditions, including iatrogenic after thoracic or thoraco-abdominal aortic aneurysm surgeries, dissection of the descending thoracic or upper abdominal aorta, atherosclerosis of the aorta or its branches, and systemic hypotension. Less commonly, emboli (atheromatous, cardioembolic, septic or fibrocartilaginous), hypercoagulable conditions, and vasculitis may be responsible for a spinal cord infarct.

Spinal cord infarction typically occurs due to inadequate blood supply through the anterior spinal artery. This artery supplies the anterior two-thirds of the spinal cord, including the anterior horns of the gray matter and corticospinal and spinothalamic tracts. The lower thoracic and lumbar spinal levels are the most commonly affected regions. In contrast, infarction involving the posterior spinal artery territory is quite rare, due to the presence of well-developed collaterals supplying the dorsal cord.

Patients usually present with an acute onset of weakness involving lower and/or upper extremities, depending on the site of the arterial occlusion, associated with bowel and bladder dysfunction as well as impaired pain and temperature sensation below the lesion level, with relative sparing of proprioception and vibratory sense (Fig. 55.1). Radicular pain can occur at the infarct level.

MRI of the spine is the procedure of choice to confirm the diagnosis of spinal cord infarction as well as rule out other etiologies that can present in a similar fashion such a transverse myelitis (TM) and compressive myelopathy secondary to an abscess, epidural or subdural hematoma, or less frequently a neoplasm. A spinal cord infarction is usually seen as a "pencil-like" hyperintensity on sagittal T2-weighted images. On axial images, T2 hyperintense signal conforms to the arterial territory involved. If spinal cord infarction is specifically suspected prior to imaging, diffusion-weighted imaging (DWI) of the spinal cord can help confirm the diagnosis with the presence of restricted diffusion. Although not frequently present, the finding of hemi-vertebral body infarction at the level of the cord signal abnormality may be a helpful confirmatory sign for spinal cord infarction.

Other tests, such as echocardiogram to rule out an embolic source, vascular imaging to rule out aortic dissection, and hypercoagulable and rheumatologic screens, are required to assess for other potential etiologies for the cord infarction. Spinal fluid analysis is sometimes needed in cases where infection or inflammatory conditions are being entertained in the differential.

Treatment of spinal cord infarctions is generally supportive in nature. There are no proven treatments so far to reverse or decrease cord ischemia. Thrombolytic therapy has been used with success in a few patients, where the diagnosis of cord ischemia was made shortly after symptom onset, but further confirmatory studies are needed. In patients with

[†]Deceased.

TABLE 55.1 Intramedullary Pathologies According to Their Mode of Presentation

	Acute	Chronic
Vascular	Anterior spinal cord infarct	Cavernous malformation, AVM
Inflammatory	RRMS NMOSD Sarcoidosis Connective tissue disorders	PPMS
Infectious	Enterovirus, flavivirus, herpesvirus, HIV (rarely) Syphilis, Tuberculosis Schistosomiasis	HIV, HTLV-1 Syphilis, Tuberculosis
Trauma	Hematomyelia	
Genetic		Hereditary spastic paraparesis Friedreich ataxia Adrenomyeloneuropathy
Congenital/acquired		Syringomyelia, hydromyelia
Degenerative		ALS, PLS
Toxic		Lathyrism Konzo Radiation, intrathecal chemotherapy
Nutritional		B12 deficiency Copper deficiency Vitamin E deficiency
Neoplasm		Ependymoma Astrocytoma Hemangioblastoma Metastasis

ALS, Amyotrophic lateral sclerosis; *AVM,* arterio-venous malformation; *NMOSD,* neuromyelitis optica spectrum disorder; *PLS,* primary lateral sclerosis; *PPMS,* primary progressive multiple sclerosis; *RRMS,* relapsing remitting multiple sclerosis.

spinal cord ischemia after aortic surgery of thoracic endovascular aortic repair, a combination of induced hypertension and reduced spinal cord pressure with a lumbar drain has been shown to be of benefit in some cases and can be considered in the appropriate setting. Treatment of the underlying cause, if found, is recommended, usually with the goal of preventing further events.

The prognosis of spinal cord infarction depends on the extent and location of the cord ischemia as well as of the underlying etiology. In general, lack of improvement within the first 24 hours of symptom onset is a predictor of poor recovery.

Inflammatory

Inflammatory disorders of the spinal cord are commonly referred to as transverse myelitis (TM). They can be idiopathic or secondary to multiple sclerosis (MS), neuromyelitis optica spectrum disorder (NMOSD), sarcoidosis, and connective tissue disorders, such as systemic lupus erythematosus and Sjögren syndrome. Many of the patients with idiopathic form have a history of a previous infection and are presumably autoimmune.

Differently from MS and NMOSD, patients with sarcoidosis and collagen disorders usually have clinical manifestations of systemic involvement in addition to the acute myelitis.

In both MS and NMOSD, the spinal cord involvement can be the first manifestation of the disease. While in patients with MS, the involvement of the cord is usually incomplete, affecting mostly sensory fibers and involving less than one vertebral body segment (Fig. 55.2), in NMOSD, the myelitis is more extensive, affecting more than three vertebral body segments as well as the central cord (Fig. 55.3). For more details regarding differences between MS and NMOSD, see Chapters 39 and 40.

Infectious

The spinal cord may be affected by a wide spectrum of microorganisms, including viruses, bacteria, fungi, and parasites.

Many viruses can affect the spinal cord and cause an acute myelitis, including enterovirus, flavivirus, and herpesvirus. Rarely an acute transverse myelopathy can occur during the time of seroconversion in HIV patients.

Enterovirus, such as poliovirus, coxsackie, and enterovirus 71, can affect the spinal cord and cause myelitis. Poliovirus has a unique predilection to the anterior horn cells of the spinal cord, causing a paralytic poliomyelitis characterized by an asymmetric flaccid weakness, associated with decreased reflexes and fasciculation, with preservation of sensation and bowel and bladder functions. Fortunately, this entity has become very rare in the Western world due to the widespread use of vaccination. Flaviviruses, such as West Nile virus, are also associated with a poliomyelitis-like presentation. MRI in those cases may show abnormal T2 hyperintensity involving the anterior horns, and moderate pleocytosis is usually seen in the cerebrospinal fluid (CSF). Treatment is symptomatic.

Herpesviruses, including herpes simplex type 2, varicella-zoster, Epstein-Barr, and cytomegalovirus, can affect the spinal cord acutely. Herpes simplex type 2 can cause a sacral radiculitis or an ascending myelitis, usually at the time of the primary infection, and may be recurrent. Varicella-zoster on rare occasions can cause a necrotizing myelitis, usually in immunosuppressed patients. Epstein-Barr and cytomegalovirus may also cause TM at the time of the initial infection, with cytomegalovirus myelitis being more commonly seen in immunocompromised patients. Antiviral therapy is commonly used; however, the response is not as robust with cytomegalovirus myelitis as compared with the other herpesviruses.

A number of bacterial infections can be associated with myelitis, often through direct spread from adjacent infections or hematogenous dissemination; however, epidural bacterial infections are far more common than a direct involvement of the cord. Syphilis and tuberculosis can affect the spinal cord acutely through arteritis and formation of intramedullary granulomas, respectively.

Fungal myelopathies are not common, but can occur by extension or compression from lesions involving the vertebral bodies. Spinal cord infarction due to meningovascular inflammation and intraspinal granulomas are other ways that the spinal cord can be affected in those patients.

Parasites can also infect the spinal cord, with *Schistosoma mansoni* and *Schistosoma haematobium* being the most common offenders. These parasites are only seen in certain areas of the globe, such as South America, Africa, and the Far East. A history of traveling to these areas and swimming or bathing in potentially contaminated rivers and lakes may suggest the diagnosis. The patients usually present with an acute or subacute low cord syndrome with associated cauda equina involvement. MRI of the cord may demonstrate enlargement of the conus medullaris and thickening of the cauda equina with a heterogeneous

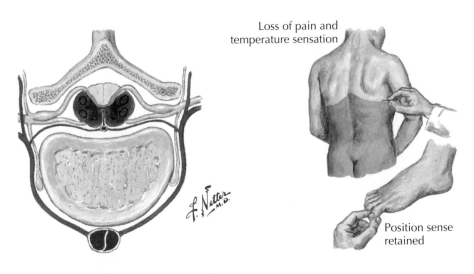

Loss of pain and temperature sensation

Position sense retained

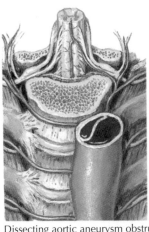

Dissecting aortic aneurysm obstructing artery of Adamkiewicz by blocking intercostal artery

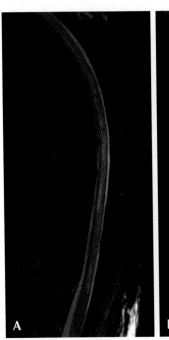

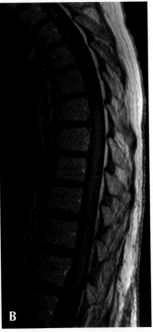

A. Sagittal T2-weighted MR image showing slightly enlarged spinal cord with patchy increased T2 signal representing edema. **B.** Sagittal T1-weighted MR image with only minimal enhancement within the spinal cord.

Fig. 55.1 Spinal Cord Infarction.

pattern of enhancement while the spinal fluid frequently shows pleocytosis with increased protein. Increases in eosinophils can be seen in both serum and spinal fluid. Treatments include praziquantel and steroids.

Trauma

Spinal hematomyelia secondary to direct trauma is not common. Patients present with an acute myelopathy after sustaining a direct trauma to the spine, with signs and symptoms varying according to the location of the injury. Often there is some associated neck or back pain and sometimes radicular pain. MRI is the preferred imaging modality for diagnosis and should include T2* (T2 star)-weighted sequences, such as gradient echo or susceptibility weighted imaging, since they are more sensitive for hemorrhage detection. There are no clinical trials to guide the management of hematomyelia, and in general conservative treatment is used for small cord hemorrhages, while surgical intervention is often pursued in cases with large expanding cord hematomas and in patients with associated spinal fractures. The use of corticosteroids is controversial.

CHRONIC INTRAMEDULLARY MYELOPATHIES

Genetic

Hereditary Spastic Paraplegia

CLINICAL VIGNETTE *A 25-year-old man who jogged short distances daily began to trip over pavement and uneven surfaces. His jogging became slower and more labored over the course of a year. Eventually, he completely stopped running. On examination, he had a slightly broad based, spastic gait, hyperreflexia with pronounced ankle clonus, and bilateral Babinski signs. He was adopted and had no knowledge of family medical history. MRI of the cervical and thoracic spine reported some mild diffuse cord atrophy without other spinal cord abnormalities. DNA testing was performed and showed the presence of a mutation in the SPG4 gene encoding spastin.*

Hereditary spastic paraplegia (HSP) is a genetically and clinically heterogeneous condition characterized by progressive spastic weakness of

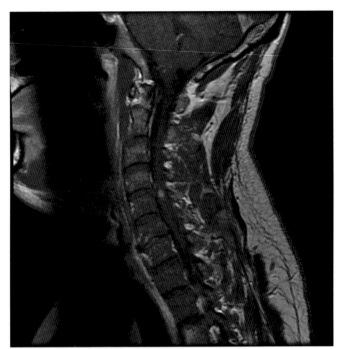

Fig. 55.2 Acute Cervical Spinal Demyelinating Plaque in a Patient With Multiple Sclerosis.

the lower extremities, often accompanied by subtle decreased vibration in toes, caused by involvement of the corticospinal tract and dorsal column, respectively. There are more than 70 different genetic types with autosomal dominant, autosomal recessive, and X-linked forms. The most common type of autosomal dominant HSP is due to spastin gene mutation (*SPG4* gene), while the most common childhood-onset autosomal dominant HSP is due to atlastin gene mutation (*SPG3A*). Age of onset and the severity of symptoms may vary widely within a given family.

HSP has an "uncomplicated" form characterized by spastic gait with increased muscle tone in the legs, hyperreflexia with presence of clonus, and Babinski signs. Vibratory sensation is sometimes mildly decreased, and occasionally patients experience sphincter disturbances manifested by a spastic bladder with urgency and frequency. The "complicated" form has in addition to the provided signs systemic and/or other neurologic manifestations such as cataracts, mental retardation, ataxia, muscle wasting, and peripheral neuropathy.

Having a positive family history is important for the diagnosis of HSP, but it may be absent. Currently genetic testing helps confirm the diagnosis in many of these patients. MRI of the spine usually shows severe spinal atrophy, a nonspecific finding, but it helps rule out other causes of spastic paraparesis.

The differential diagnoses of HSP include primary progressive MS, primary lateral sclerosis, B_{12} deficiency, human T-lymphotropic virus (HTLV)-I myelopathy, leukodystrophies, intrinsic or extrinsic cord tumor, syringomyelia, and dural arteriovenous malformations (AVMs).

Treatment is primarily symptomatic, including bladder training, and measures to help the gait and spasticity, including intensive physical therapy, antispastic drugs, Botox treatment, and baclofen pump. Eventually most of these individuals require ambulatory aids, including canes, walkers, or wheelchairs.

Friedreich Ataxia

Friedreich ataxia (FA) is an autosomal recessive neurodegenerative condition characterized by progressive ataxia. The disease affects the

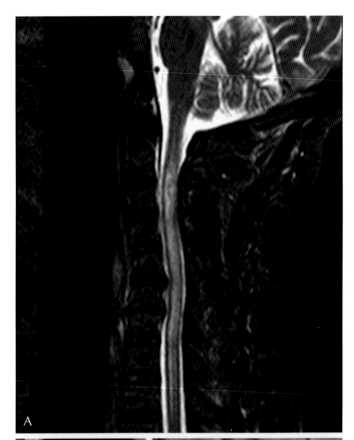

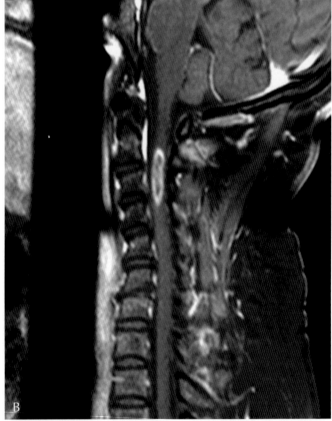

Fig. 55.3 Acute Myelitis in a Patient With Neuromyelitis Optica Spectrum Disorder.

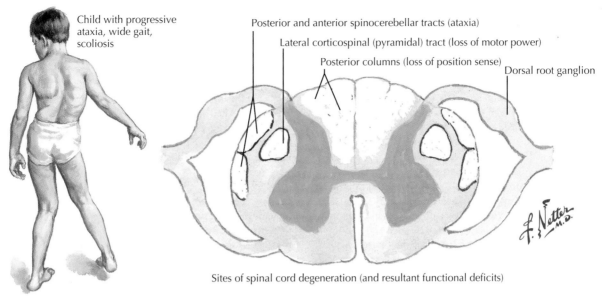

Child with progressive ataxia, wide gait, scoliosis

Posterior and anterior spinocerebellar tracts (ataxia)

Lateral corticospinal (pyramidal) tract (loss of motor power)

Posterior columns (loss of position sense)

Dorsal root ganglion

Sites of spinal cord degeneration (and resultant functional deficits)

Fig. 55.4 Friedreich Ataxia.

posterior columns, lateral corticospinal tracts, dorsal and ventral spinocerebellar tracts, dorsal roots and ganglia, and peripheral nerves, causing a combined sensory and cerebellar ataxia (Fig. 55.4). This disease is caused by a hyperexpansion of a GAA trinucleotide repeat in the first intron of the frataxin gene on the long arm of chromosome 9, interfering with gene transcription and leading to deficiency of frataxin, a nuclear-encoded mitochondrial protein. Frataxin is important for iron homeostasis, and its deficiency leads to increased mitochondrial iron accumulation, sensitivity to oxidative stress, and free radical–mediated cell death, particularly to neurons and cardiomyocytes. The larger the size of the expanded repeat, the greater the severity of the specific phenotype. Longer repeats are associated with earlier onset and more severe disease.

FA commonly presents in mid-childhood and adolescence. Gait ataxia is the earliest symptom and tends to progress overtime.'Vibration and position sense are also compromised early. Hand clumsiness and dysarthria may occur months or years later. Areflexia results from peripheral nerve damage; however, in what initially seems to be a paradox, plantar responses are extensor, because of concomitant corticospinal tract damage. Nystagmus, tremor, athetoid, and choreiform movements, along with visual and hearing loss, can also occur.

High arched feet and hammer toes may present at birth or later, or can be a forme fruste in individuals who do not develop full-blown disease. Scoliosis often develops later on (see Fig. 55.4). A very serious cardiomyopathy with potential for the development of various serious arrhythmias develops in most affected individuals. Carbohydrate intolerance and diabetes can occur in 20% and 10% of FA patients, respectively.

Diagnosis is made on clinical grounds and can be confirmed by genetic testing. The differential diagnoses include MS, HSP, tabes dorsalis, ataxia telangiectasia, peroneal muscular atrophy, and olivopontocerebellar and spinocerebellar degenerations. Treatment includes balance training and muscle strengthening. If bracing is inadequate, orthopedic surgery for scoliosis may be necessary. Regular orthopedic and cardiology follow-up is important. Over time, individuals may become wheelchair-dependent or bed-bound. Death is usually secondary to cardiac arrhythmia, infection, or restrictive pulmonary disease. Investigational therapies for FA have focused on increasing frataxin expression with gene therapy and improving mitochondrial function with the use

of antioxidants such as idebenone (a free radical scavenger), coenzyme Q10, or vitamin E; however, to date there is still no proven specific treatment available.

Adrenomyeloneuropathy

Adrenomyeloneuropathy (AMN) is an X-linked recessive inherited disorder with the gene located on the long arm of the chromosome X (Xq28) causing impairment of very long chain fatty acid (VLCFA) peroxisomal oxidation and its accumulation in the nervous system, adrenal glands, plasma, and testes. It usually affects adult males between 20 and 40 years of age or female carriers, presenting with a progressive spastic paraparesis, sensory changes, and sphincter dysfunction. Adrenal and gonadal dysfunction can be seen in over 60% of the males with AMN and less commonly seen in women carriers who tend to have a milder involvement. Cerebral involvement with cognitive and behavior abnormalities as well as visual and auditory impairments can occur in some of the patients with AMN. Those patients tend to have a more rapidly progressive disease.

Diagnosis is made by measurement of serum VLCFA, including the level of hexacosanoic acid (C26:0) and the ratio of hexacosanoic acid to tetracosanoic acid (C26:0/C24:0) and to docosanoic acid (C26:0/C22:0). This is elevated in nearly all males and in approximately 85% of female carriers. The diagnosis should be confirmed by molecular genetic testing. Elevated plasma ACTH with impaired cortisol response to stimulation test can be seen in affected males as well as low testosterone, luteinizing, and follicle-stimulating hormones. Females usually have normal adrenal function. MRI of the spine usually demonstrates spinal cord intramedullary T2 hyperintensities, while the brain is usually normal. The only exceptions are patients with AMN with cerebral involvement, where T2 hyperintensities are also detected in the brain. Unfortunately, there is no specific drug treatment available for AMN, and current therapy is mostly symptomatic. Use of a low-fat diet to decrease exogenous VLCFA or of Lorenzo's oil, a mixture of glyceroltrioleate and glyceroltrierucate, that decreases the endogenous VLCFA synthesis, is often recommended in these patients; however, there is little information about its effects on disease progression. In patients with a cerebral form of AMN, hematopoietic stem cell transplantation can be considered, but outcomes have not been studied.

Congenital/Acquired
Syringomyelia/Hydromyelia

Syringomyelia is a fluid-filled cavity within the spinal cord. It can represent a focal dilation of the central canal, in this case called hydromyelia, or it can occur separately within the spinal cord parenchyma. It often occurs between C2 and T9, but it can ascend and involve the brainstem (syringobulbia) or descend to the lower thoracic levels.

Syringomyelia can be congenital and associated with a Chiari malformation type 1, Klippel-Feil syndrome, and tethered spinal cord or acquired and secondary to trauma, tumors, inflammation, or infection of the cord. Patients with syringomyelia can be asymptomatic or present with dissociated sensory loss in upper extremities, worsening spasticity in lower extremities, and atrophy and fasciculations due to involvement of the crossing spinothalamic tracts, descending corticospinal tract, and anterior horn cells, respectively. Neuropathic pain is also common. MRI of the spine is the most reliable method to diagnosis syringomyelia (Fig. 55.5). Surgical treatment with drainage of the cavity is usually performed in patients with progressive neurologic deterioration or with associated structural abnormalities, such as in patients with spinal cord tumors.

Degenerative
Amyotrophic Lateral Sclerosis

Amyotrophic lateral sclerosis (ALS) is a neurodegenerative disease that affects both upper and lower motor neuron causing progressive muscle weakness, leading to disability and eventually death. ALS is more common in the seventh and eighth decades of life and most often sporadic. Weakness, spasticity, and hyperreflexia occur as a result of degeneration of the frontal motor neurons and atrophy and fasciculations as a consequence of lower motor neuron degeneration in the spinal cord and brainstem. Diagnosis of ALS is suggested by the clinical history and exam, and supported by the EMG findings. MRIs of the neuraxis are often performed in patients with ALS mostly to exclude other pathologies. Currently there are only two disease-modifying agents available to treat ALS, riluzole, and edaravone, both with a modest impact in the disease progression. Symptomatic treatment of the multiple ALS related issues, such as respiratory and speech difficulties, dysphagia, functional decline, and psychosocial problems, is of extreme importance and often better addressed in a multidisciplinary ALS clinic. For more details, see Chapter 62.

Primary Lateral Sclerosis

Primary lateral sclerosis (PLS) is a rare progressive disorder involving only the upper motor neurons. Patients present with progressive spasticity without any associated weakness or atrophy. This disease tends to progress slower than ALS. The diagnosis is one of exclusion, since there is no specific positive test finding. No specific treatment is available to date.

Toxic

Lathyrism and Konzo are disorders caused by the ingestion of plants with potential neurotoxicity; overconsumption of grass pea (*Lathyrus sativus*) and consumption of improperly processed cassava (*Manihot esculenta*), respectively. The neuroexcitatory amino acid β-N-oxalyl-l-α, β-diaminopropionic acid (β-ODAP) in grass pea and cyanogenic glycosides in cassava are the substances incriminated in the causation of Lathyrism and Konzo, and to be involved in the depletion of sulfur amino acids (methionine and cysteine) contributing to oxidative stress.

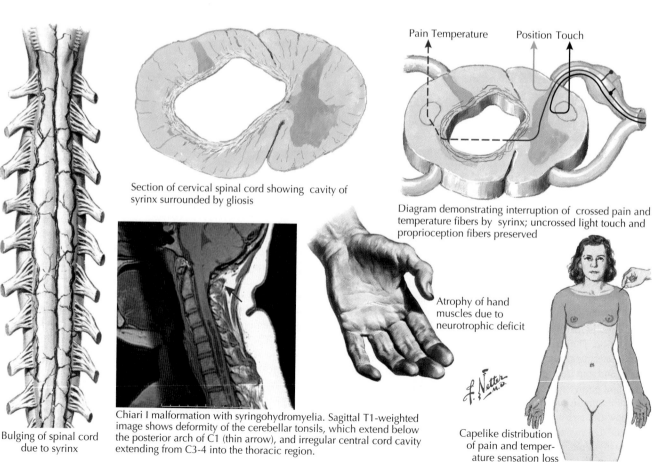

Section of cervical spinal cord showing cavity of syrinx surrounded by gliosis

Diagram demonstrating interruption of crossed pain and temperature fibers by syrinx; uncrossed light touch and proprioception fibers preserved

Atrophy of hand muscles due to neurotrophic deficit

Bulging of spinal cord due to syrinx

Chiari I malformation with syringohydromyelia. Sagittal T1-weighted image shows deformity of the cerebellar tonsils, which extend below the posterior arch of C1 (thin arrow), and irregular central cord cavity extending from C3-4 into the thoracic region.

Capelike distribution of pain and temperature sensation loss

Fig. 55.5 Syringomyelia.

These two conditions affect thousands of people in Africa and Asia, especially during periods of drought and famine, and both present with a progressive spastic paraparesis. No specific treatment is available, but both conditions can be preventable by a balanced diet.

Other toxic etiologies include radiation and intrathecal chemotherapy. In radiation myelopathy, symptoms can occur shortly after exposure and are due to spinal cord edema, often treated with steroids. An early delayed postradiation myelopathy can occur after a few months of radiation, and a later delayed myelopathy can develop after several months of exposure. The early delayed form tends to be mild and reversible while the later has a more progressive course. MRI of the spine usually demonstrates T2 hyperintensity in the affected cord. Currently no effective treatment is available, but frequently steroids are used. Any type of intrathecal chemotherapy can potentially cause an acute transient chemical meningitis; however, cytarabine liposome is associated with a later neurotoxicity, most commonly a cauda equine syndrome.

Nutritional

The most frequent nutritional deficiency is the subacute combined degeneration (SCD) of the spinal cord due to B12 deficiency. Low B12 can occur due to decrease oral intake as seen in patients with a strict vegetarian diet or malnutrition, or be secondary to pernicious anemia and gastrointestinal diseases, as well as chronic use of H2 blockers and proton pump inhibitors. It is characterized by a slowly progressing vacuolar myelopathy affecting the lateral and posterior columns of the cord. Many of these patients may also have a concomitant neuropathy, cognitive decline, as well as psychiatric symptoms. In addition, hematologic abnormalities with a megaloblastic anemia can be seen. Diagnosis is made by showing decreased B12 levels and/or increased levels of methylmalonic acid and homocysteine. MRI of the spine often demonstrates symmetric bilateral posterior column T2 hyperintensity, most commonly along the cervical and upper thoracic spine, often described as the "inverted V sign" (Fig. 55.6). The lateral corticospinal tracts, and sometimes lateral spinothalamic tract, may be involved. In addition, cerebral white matter T2 changes are often seen on brain MRI. Treatment consists of high doses of intramuscular cyanocobalamin. Folate supplementation, if needed, should be delayed by at least 2 weeks after starting the B12 replacement, since it can lead to potential worsening of the neurologic syndrome.

Other nutritional myelopathies are associated with copper and vitamin E deficiency. Copper deficiency causes a clinical and radiologic syndrome similar to the SCD of vitamin B12 deficiency, and can be seen in patients with malnutrition, nephrotic syndrome, excess zinc intake, and treatment with penicillamine or alkali agents. Evaluation of serum cooper, ceruloplasmin, and urinary copper excretion is the primary means to make this diagnosis. Zinc levels may be normal or elevated. Treatment includes oral or parenteral copper supplementation, as well as discontinuation of zinc supplements in patients with high serum levels. Vitamin E deficiency is most commonly seen in patients with malabsorption and often clinically resembles spinocerebellar degeneration and is treated with high doses of vitamin E.

Prognosis for a neurologic recovery in all the above nutritional deficiencies is best with early treatment, reinforcing the importance of prompt diagnosis of these conditions.

Neoplasm

Gliomas (astrocytomas and ependymomas) are the most common intramedullary spinal cord neoplasms representing 80%–90% of the intramedullary tumors, followed by hemangioblastomas (3%–8%) and intramedullary metastasis (0.1%–2%).

The most common intramedullary gliomas in adults are ependymomas (60%–70%) and astrocytomas (30%–40%). In pediatric patients, astrocytomas are more common than ependymomas. Ependymomas and astrocytomas are intramedullary lesions, which may be located anywhere in the spinal cord. Myxopapillary ependymomas (an ependymoma variant) occur almost exclusively along the conus or filum terminale. Hemangioblastomas of the cord are usually sporadic tumors, but are a recognized component of a von Hippel-Lindau syndrome. Intramedullary metastasis is quite rare and is most often observed in patients with already widespread metastatic disease. Approximately half of the cases are secondary to lung cancer, followed by breast cancer, renal cell carcinoma, lymphoma, and melanoma (Fig. 55.7).

Patients with intramedullary tumors usually present with a picture of a progressive myelopathy frequently with central cord features (see Chapter 54). Rarely, spinal hemangioblastomas can present more acutely, when there is associated subarachnoid hemorrhage or hematomyelia. MRI of the spine with gadolinium is the best imaging technique to demonstrate spinal cord tumors, and usually shows spinal cord enlargement that is hyperintense on T2, hypo or isointense on T1. The degree and pattern of enhancement may vary with the specific neoplastic entity. In addition, syringomyelia may be present, although it is more common with ependymomas than astrocytomas. Although not always present, disproportionately large syrinxes may be associated with small hemangioblastomas. In addition, focal flow voids on T2W can be seen in large hemangioblastomas as a clue to diagnosis. Biopsy is usually needed for the final diagnosis of intramedullary tumors, as their imaging characteristics often overlap. Surgery with maximal resection of the tumor is the most common initial treatment step. Preoperatively, endovascular embolization is sometimes used in patients with hemangioblastoma to reduce blood loss during the procedure. For patients in whom the resection is incomplete or not possible or have recurrent disease following initial resection, radiation therapy may be useful. See Chapter 50 for more details.

Vascular

Cavernous angioma or cavernomas of the spinal cord are rare vascular malformations of the central nervous system (CNS) characterized by abnormally dilated blood vessels lined by a thin endothelium with little or no interviewing nervous tissue. There is no sex predilection, and symptoms usually present during the fourth decade of life. They are more commonly located in the thoracic cord. Patients often present with a slowly progressive myelopathy; however, sometimes patients can present more acutely, in cases associated with larger hemorrhages. Symptoms include weakness and paresthesias of lower extremities, often associated with acute dorsal pain. MRI of the spine with and without contrast is the best modality to diagnose cavernomas of the spine. Due to the fact that blood flow through the cavernous malformation is minimal, this can be missed by conventional angiography. In cases that have not had any associated bleeding, the abnormalities are quite discrete showing minimal cord expansion sometimes with mild enhancement. However, in patients who have had prior hemorrhages, lobulated heterogeneous signal intensity on T1 and T2 may demonstrate the classic "popcorn" appearance. In particular, a T2 hypointense rim along the margins of the lesion may be a valuable clue to imaging diagnosis. Surgical resection is usually considered in symptomatic patients.

Intramedullary AVM of the spine often presents in the third decade of life and is more frequently located in the thoracic and lumbar regions. Its clinical picture can vary from a chronic myelopathy with gradual neurologic symptoms caused by mass effect or ischemia from vascular steal or venous congestion; or patients can have a more acute presentation in cases associated with intraparenchymal or subarachnoid hemorrhage. MRI of the spine shows a cluster of serpiginous low intensity sign signal correlating with the nidus, and magnetic resonance angiogram (MRA) of the spine may help identify its vascular supply. However, often

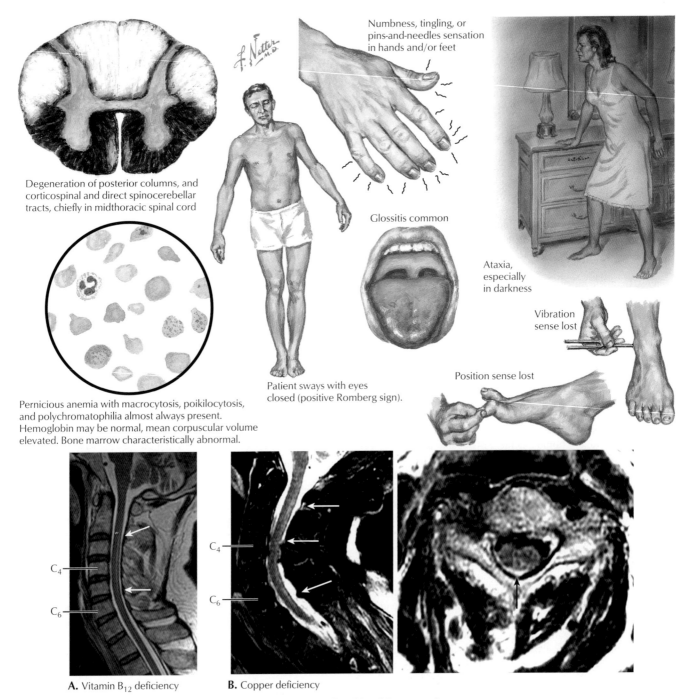

Degeneration of posterior columns, and corticospinal and direct spinocerebellar tracts, chiefly in midthoracic spinal cord

Pernicious anemia with macrocytosis, poikilocytosis, and polychromatophilia almost always present. Hemoglobin may be normal, mean corpuscular volume elevated. Bone marrow characteristically abnormal.

Numbness, tingling, or pins-and-needles sensation in hands and/or feet

Glossitis common

Patient sways with eyes closed (positive Romberg sign).

Ataxia, especially in darkness

Vibration sense lost

Position sense lost

C_4

C_6

C_4

C_6

A. Vitamin B_{12} deficiency

B. Copper deficiency

Fig. 55.6 Subacute Combined Degeneration.

conventional angiography of the spine is needed. Treatment includes surgical resection and/or endovascular occlusion.

Inflammatory

The primary progressive form of multiple sclerosis (PPMS) is characterized by an evolving myelopathy with patients presenting with an increasing gait impairment early on in the course of the disease. Over time, patients develop a spastic paraparesis or tetraparesis associated with sphincter disturbances and sensory abnormalities. Differently from relapsing remitting multiple sclerosis (RRMS), PPMS is usually diagnosed in the fifth to sixth decades of life, and men are affected as commonly as women. In addition, there is no history of preceding relapses. Diagnosis criteria include the presence of 1 year of disease

progression and two of the following: evidence of dissemination in space in the brain, evidence of dissemination in space in the spinal cord, or presence of oligoclonal bands/high immunoglobulin G (IGG) index in the spinal fluid. PPMS therapy includes symptomatic treatment of the spasticity, neurogenic bladder, fatigue, and neuropathic pain, as well as the use of the disease modifying agent ocrelizumab, a recent FDA-approved monoclonal antibody that has shown a 24% reduction of the risk of disability progression in those patients as compared with placebo. See Chapter 39 for more detailed information

Infectious

The spinal cord involvement by HIV usually presents as a vacuolar myelopathy affecting the lateral and posterior columns of the thoracic

Common primary sites

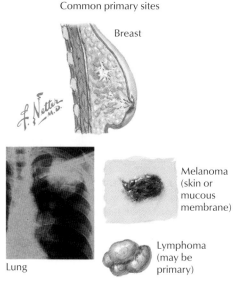

Fig. 55.7 Metastatic Malignancies.

Breast

Melanoma (skin or mucous membrane)

Lymphoma (may be primary)

Lung

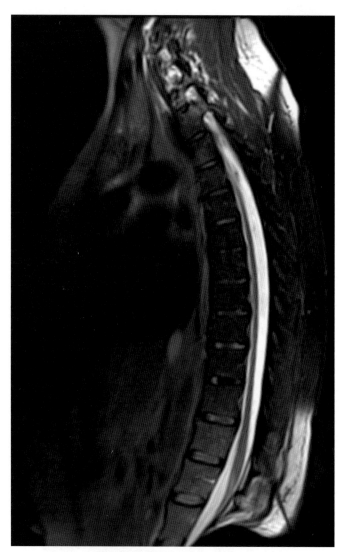

Fig. 55.8 HTLV-1 Myelopathy.

cord. The vacuolar myelopathy is more commonly recognized at autopsy than clinically, and the cases diagnosed in vivo are typically in patients with advanced AIDS. Patients often present with leg weakness and gait unsteadiness, followed by bowel and bladder incontinence. Paresthesias of the lower extremities are also common. Exam usually shows spastic paraparesis associated with impaired sensation, usually with a greater impairment of vibratory and position sense than with temperature and pinprick. The diagnosis of HIV myelopathy is one of exclusion. Common opportunistic infections (herpes, cytomegalovirus, syphilis, tuberculosis, toxoplasmosis) and tumors (CNS lymphoma) in this population should be considered in the differential diagnosis, as well as B12 deficiency. Therefore investigation in those patients usually includes various serologies, B12 level, MRI of the spine, and spinal fluid studies. The MRI of the cord is usually normal, and spinal fluid may show mild pleocytosis and protein elevation. Treatment is mostly symptomatic and includes antispasticity drugs, neurogenic bladder management, and physical therapy (PT). Antiretroviral regimen should also be maximized.

HTLV-1 can cause a chronic progressive myelopathy also referred to as tropical spastic paraparesis (TSP). It is estimated that 1 in 250 individuals infected with HTLV-1 will develop TSP. This condition is characterized by chronic involvement of the pyramidal tracts, mostly at the thoracic level, causing spastic paraparesis and a spastic bladder. Some sensory disturbances and cerebellar ataxia can also occur. HTLV-1 is endemic within the Caribbean, eastern South America, equatorial Africa, and southern Japan. Transmission can occur via semen, blood or blood products, breast milk, or by sharing needles. Therefore a detailed history including prior travel to endemic areas is of utmost importance. HTLV-1 is usually positive in both serum and spinal fluid of most patients, with spinal fluid also showing a mild leukocytosis with increased protein and IGG, as well as the presence of oligoclonal bands. MRI can sometimes show cord atrophy (Fig. 55.8), whereas nonspecific T2 hyperintensities in the white matter can be detected in the brain. Primary progressive MS and B12 deficiency should be considered in the differential. There is no effective treatment for HTLV-1 myelopathy; therefore, most of the treatment is symptomatic. Glucocorticoids can potentially help in some patients, often when used early in the course of the disease.

Tabes dorsalis is a form of tertiary neurosyphilis, with a latent period between primary infection and onset of symptoms of approximately 20 years. It is characterized by a progressive sensory ataxia and severe pain due to involvement of the posterior columns of the cord and dorsal nerve roots, respectively. MRI of the spine may demonstrate longitudinal T2 hyperintense signal abnormality involving the posterior columns of the spinal cord. CSF examination may be normal or show increased lymphocytes, elevated protein, and/or a reactive Venereal Disease Research Laboratory (VDRL). Antibiotic treatment with intravenous penicillin is the treatment of choice.

EXTRAMEDULLARY DISORDERS

In extramedullary disorders, upper motor neuron signs are common early in its presentation, and lower motor neuron signs tend to be localized to one or two segments. Dissociated sensory loss is usually absent, while altered sacral sensation and radicular pain are common. Autonomic involvement with bowel and bladder dysfunction usually occurs late in the course of these diseases.

Extradural extramedullary involvement has a more symmetrical mode of onset, while intradural extramedullary pathologies tend to be asymmetric. Vertebral body pain and/or deformity are typical of extradural involvement.

EXTRAMEDULLARY INTRADURAL DISORDERS

Acute

Vascular

Subdural spinal hematoma. Subdural spinal hematoma (SSH) is rare, may occur at any age, and has a female predominance. It is most commonly seen in the thoracic and lumbar regions, and is commonly associated with spinal trauma, spinal taps, vascular malformations, and hemorrhagic diatheses. Patients usually present with back pain followed by sensorimotor impairment secondary to compression of the cord or cauda equina. MRI of the spine is the imaging of choice to diagnose SSH. Treatment includes clot evacuation to relieve the local pressure and repair of any underlying AVM.

Chronic

Tumor

Extramedullary intradural spinal tumors include meningiomas, schwannomas, and neurofibromas (Fig. 55.9).

Meningiomas of the spinal cord correspond to approximately one-quarter of all the primary spinal cord tumors. They are most commonly located in the thoracic cord (~80% of cases); however, occasionally they can occur in the high cervical cord at the level of the foramen magnum and rarely at the lumbar level. Almost any age group may present with a meningioma; individuals in their fourth to seventh decades are most vulnerable, particularly women. Patients usually present with progressive weakness, sensory loss, bladder and bowel dysfunction, and gait difficulty. Radicular pain may antedate other symptoms, as the nerve root is affected early on. Ipsilateral spasticity, hyperreflexia, and Babinski sign, due to the involvement of the corticospinal tract, are prominent initial signs. As the tumor enlarges, ipsilateral loss of proprioception due to involvement of the dorsal column and contralateral pain and temperature loss due to involvement of the spinothalamic tract become evident (Brown-Séquard syndrome). MRI of the spine is the best method to diagnose extramedullary intradural lesions with noncalcified meningiomas, usually demonstrating homogeneous enhancement with gadolinium. CT myelogram is also a valuable diagnostic tool that can demonstrate a partial or complete block and also assess for tumor calcification, but is primarily used when MRI cannot be performed. Plain spine films may demonstrate erosion of a pedicle or articular process by the meningioma and intraspinal calcification. Most meningiomas are benign, slow growing, and well circumscribed; the majority are successfully resected. Radiation therapy may be administered in cases of early recurrence or limited surgical resection. Prognosis is often very good, with improved motor, sensory, and sphincter function after surgical removal, particularly when the tumor is diagnosed at an early stage. Postoperative mortality is low. The tumor recurs in only a minority of patients. Negative prognostic factors include elderly age, severe neurologic deficits, long duration of symptoms before diagnosis, subtotal tumor resection, and extradural extension.

Schwannomas and neurofibromas are nerve sheath tumors that occur sporadically or associated with neurofibromatosis type 1 or 2. They typically grow slowly, and their manifestations depend on the level of the tumor and the degree of spinal compression. They can present initially with pain and radicular sensory symptoms, followed by signs of a progressive myelopathy. MRI of the spine with contrast is the best

Intradural extramedullary tumor (meningioma) compressing spinal cord and deforming nerve roots

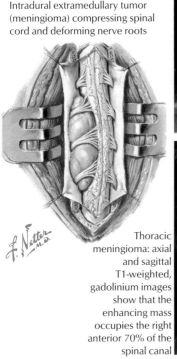

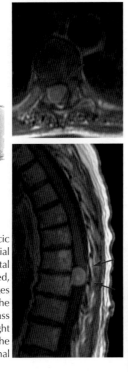

Thoracic meningioma: axial and sagittal T1-weighted, gadolinium images show that the enhancing mass occupies the right anterior 70% of the spinal canal

Dumbbell tumor (neurilemmoma) growing out along spinal nerve through intervertebral foramen (neurofibromas of von Recklinghausen disease may act similarly)

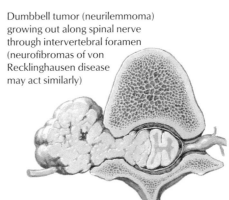

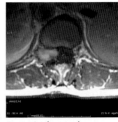

Foraminal neurolemmoma seen on axial T1-weighted, gadolinium-enhanced image (arrowheads)

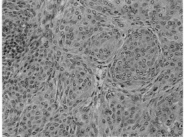

A. Meningioma. Meningioma with a meningothelial pattern showing cells with syncytial features in lobulated groups (H&E, original magnification 200X)

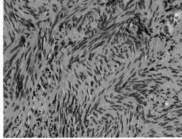

B. Schwannoma (neurilemmoma). Antoni B pattern in a schwannoma showing spindle cells arranged in fascicles (H&E, original magnification 200X)

Fig. 55.9 Extramedullary Intradural Spinal Tumors.

diagnostic modality to identify those tumors and usually shows an enhancing extramedullary mass. Sometimes the enhancement is heterogeneous due to the presence of intratumor necrosis, cyst, or hemorrhage. In some patients, the tumors can have an intradural and extradural component, with a "dumbbell" appearance. The treatment of choice for those tumors is surgery.

Dural Arteriovenous (AV) Fistula

> **CLINICAL VIGNETTE** *A 55-year-old man presented with a 1-year history of progressive weakness in his legs, left worse than right, associated with gait difficulties. He also complained of numbness in his legs and pain in his lower thoracic region. He recalled that symptoms tended to get worse with exercise and has had a stepwise progression worsening over the past 2 months, prompting a neurologic evaluation. His neuro exam was remarkable for weakness in both legs, left slightly weaker than the right, patchy decreased pinprick in both legs, and impaired vibration in toes and knees. There is a presence of hyperreflexia in legs, with a left Babinski. The right toe was mute. Gait was broad-based and ataxic. MRI of the thoracic spine showed cord edema from the T10 thoracic level to the conus, with suggestion of increased vasculature in the intradural space. A selective intercostal angiogram showed a dural fistula with its feeder vessel nidus at T10 on the left. The patient underwent a successful endovascular treatment with significant improvement of his symptoms.*

Dural arteriovenous fistulas are the most frequent vascular malformation of the cord representing more than 70% of all AVMs. They are more common in men after the fifth decade of life and more frequently located in the mid-lower thoracic to upper lumbar level. The fistulas are located in the dural sleeve of the nerve roots and directly connect a radicular artery and vein, leading to arterialization of the coronal plexus around the cord and development of venous congestion with increased venous pressure. Cord perfusion decreases, leading to prolonged hypoxia/ischemia and a progressive, usually stepwise, myelopathy. The most common initial presentation is the development of weakness and decreased sensation in lower extremities, at times asymmetrically initially. Symptoms tend to get worse with exercise and improve with rest. Pain in the legs or back can occur, and sphincter issues are more common later in the course of the disease. MRI of the spine may show intramedullary T2 hyperintense signal abnormality, as well as subtle serpiginous flow voids dorsal to the cord representing dilated venous collaterals overwhelmed by the arterialized flow. MRA of the spine with contrast can also be helpful in identifying the abnormal intradural vessels. However, spinal angiogram is still the gold standard for diagnosis (Fig. 55.10). Treatment includes surgical or endovascular occlusion of the fistula.

EXTRAMEDULLARY EXTRADURAL DISORDERS
(Table 55.2)

Acute

Trauma
Central herniated disc.

> **CLINICAL VIGNETTE** *A 68-year-old part-time musician suddenly fell as he was reaching for his morning newspaper while standing on an icy, hilly driveway. He was paralyzed from his neck down, and he noted numbness in all extremities. He recalled a brief involuntary ballistic movement of his right arm. A diagnosis of a brainstem stroke was made at the local hospital, as it*

was presumed that the stroke led to his fall. Brain computed tomography (CT) was normal. Within a few days, he recovered some right-sided motor function.

The family sought a second opinion at The Lahey Clinic. Here he had a left > right quadriparesis, bilaterally brisk muscle stretch reflexes, left Babinski sign, and a midcervical right-sided sensory level for pain and temperature with preserved position sense. MRI demonstrated a centrally herniated nucleus pulposus at C3–C4 with spinal cord compression, contusion, and a severe stenotic spondylotic lesion at that level. Emergency surgical decompression was performed. He had a gradual increase in function; within 1 year he could perform most activities of daily living independently, although his finger dexterity for clarinet playing was not back to his preinjury level.

In retrospect, he had sustained a syncopal event secondary to a cardiac arrhythmia. The fall led to the spinal column injury, the extruded central disc and cord injury. A careful neurologic examination sorted out the site of pathology and led to the diagnostic and therapeutic success.

Comment: Initially this patient was thought to have a basically untreatable brainstem stroke—that is, a lesion in an entirely different part of the neuraxis. A more careful subsequent clinical examination, lying the patient on his side and examining for a specific sensory level, was the key to diagnosis, as patients with brainstem stroke rarely have total loss of sensory function in a spinal cord–level distribution.

Acute spinal cord injuries, with subsequent paraplegia or quadriplegia, are among the most dreaded sequelae to a serious bodily injury. There is a tragic propensity for traumatic myelopathies to occur among vigorous and healthy young persons. Automobile and motorcycle accidents as well as sports injuries are the most common etiologies. Gunshot wounds, whether resulting from war, accident, or assault, are another source of traumatic spinal cord injury.

Cervical spinal fracture dislocation with resultant ligamentous tear, allowing bony fragments to directly tear or transect the spinal cord, is the common denominator in this setting (Fig. 55.11). Sometimes there is concomitant compromise of the spinal arteries, causing an associated spinal cord infarction, hematomyelia, or both. Typically, in the acute setting, *spinal shock* results with complete paralysis, loss of sensation, areflexia distal to the trauma site, and loss of bladder and bowel function (Fig. 55.12).

Occasionally these traumatic spinal lesions are amenable to immediate surgical correction or external traction. Prognosis is always guarded. Once emergent management is completed, these patients are cared for at specialized spinal rehabilitation centers. Treatment of autonomic and sphincter dysfunction has greatly improved the long-term survival for many patients. Spinal cord repair, leading to functional recovery, is one of the greatest challenges for 21st-century neuroscientists.

Among senior citizens, unexpected falls at home, as in the above vignette, may lead to an acute central disc protrusion. Their inherent gait instability secondary to chronic neurologic or orthopedic handicaps

TABLE 55.2 Extramedullary Extradural Pathologies According to Their Mode of Presentation

	Acute	Chronic
Vascular	Central herniated disc Epidural hematoma	Cervical spondylosis AVM
Infectious	Epidural abscess	Pott disease (TB)
Neoplasm	Metastasis, lymphoma	Metastasis, lymphoma Primary bone tumor with secondary invasion of the epidural space

AVM, Arteriovenous malformation.

Normal Spinal Segment

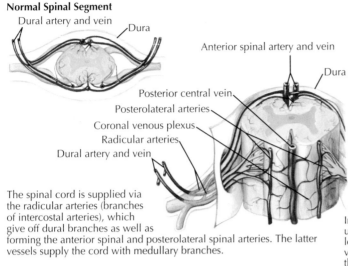

Dural artery and vein

Dura

Anterior spinal artery and vein

Dura

Posterior central vein

Posterolateral arteries

Coronal venous plexus

Radicular arteries

Dural artery and vein

The spinal cord is supplied via the radicular arteries (branches of intercostal arteries), which give off dural branches as well as forming the anterior spinal and posterolateral spinal arteries. The latter vessels supply the cord with medullary branches.

Dural Arteriovenous Malformation

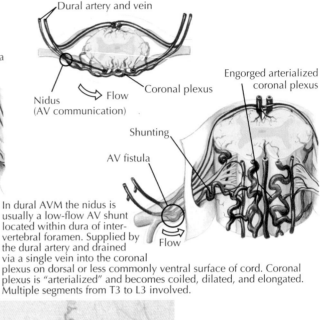

Dural artery and vein

Engorged arterialized coronal plexus

Flow

Coronal plexus

Nidus (AV communication)

Shunting

AV fistula

Flow

In dural AVM the nidus is usually a low-flow AV shunt located within dura of inter-vertebral foramen. Supplied by the dural artery and drained via a single vein into the coronal plexus on dorsal or less commonly ventral surface of cord. Coronal plexus is "arterialized" and becomes coiled, dilated, and elongated. Multiple segments from T3 to L3 involved.

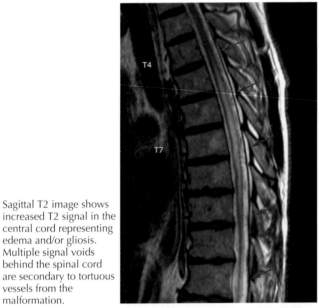

Sagittal T2 image shows increased T2 signal in the central cord representing edema and/or gliosis. Multiple signal voids behind the spinal cord are secondary to tortuous vessels from the malformation.

Spinal angiogram of radicular artery, left T6, with arterio-venous fistula filling multiple draining veins at the dural level. These join to form a complex medullary venous plexus.

Fig. 55.10 Dural AV Fistula.

makes them susceptible to tripping on stairs, rugs, or door jams. Cardiac bradyarrhythmias leading to syncope, or epileptic seizure, with sudden loss of consciousness have a similar risk of serious spinal cord injury.

As these lesions are eminently treatable with neurosurgical intervention, consideration of these less common lesions is vital in patients who have sudden unexplained falls leading to immediate paralysis. Anatomically the extruded disc compressed the anterior spinal cord between two vertebral bodies. Occasionally these lesions present subacutely or chronically. Because associated bony pain or tenderness may be present, these lesions often mimic metastatic or primary tumors. However, if the patient does not have a history of malignancy, a benign mechanism, such as a central disc, must be sought (Fig. 55.13). Rarely, a dural AVM or spinal epidural hematoma (SEH) mimics this clinical picture.

Surgery is the treatment of choice. Prognosis depends on the degree of cord compromise before surgery, the acuity of the event, the patient's general health status, and the disc location. Cervical lesions are treated by a neurosurgeon, although a combined approach with an orthopedic surgeon is sometimes indicated. When the central disc is in the thoracic cord area, a combined neurologic and thoracic surgical approach is required.

Vascular

Epidural hematoma. SEH rarely occurs spontaneously. It can complicate procedures that involve dural puncture often in patients who have a bleeding diathesis, low platelets, or are anticoagulated. At times it can occur after a local trauma. Patients usually present with back or radicular pain, followed by weakness, numbness, and bowel and bladder dysfunction that can present acutely or over days. Epidural hematomas are usually secondary to venous rather than arterial bleeding. Diagnosis is confirmed by MRI of the spinal cord, with a hemorrhagic epidural collection present (Fig. 55.14). Treatment varies from conservative, in case with mild deficits, to prompt surgical intervention with evacuation of the blood, for patients with significant and progressive neurologic deficits.

Infectious

Epidural abscess. Epidural spinal abscess is a rare clinical process occurring in 2–20 cases per 100,000 hospital admissions, more often seen in middle-aged men. Despite its rarity, the potential for an epidural abscess to cause permanent paraplegia makes it one of the most urgent spinal cord emergencies (see Fig. 55.14). The epidural space in the posterior thoracic cord is the primary site for an epidural spinal abscess to develop. These may extend to the cervical cord and rarely into the lumbar spine. The most common microorganism leading to epidural spinal abscesses is *Staphylococcus aureus*. Usually a distant septic focus provides bacterial seeding via the bloodstream—for example, skin furuncles, dental abscesses, simple pharyngitis, or a recently infected traumatic site (see Fig. 55.14). Often there is a concomitant history of diabetes mellitus, alcoholism, drug abuse, or recent spinal or extraspinal trauma. Less commonly, epidural spinal abscesses develop subsequent to vertebral osteomyelitis, pulmonary or urinary infection, sepsis, or extremely rarely bacterial endocarditis. Invasive procedures, including epidural anesthesia, spinal surgery, vascular access lines, and paravertebral injections, also provide potential mechanisms for bacterial seeding. Corticosteroid therapy may contribute to immune suppression and the possibility of secondary nosocomial infections.

Percussion tenderness over the posterior spinal processes, as well as fever, are important diagnostic clues compatible with an epidural spinal abscess. Some of these individuals also develop signs of meningeal irritation, such as a Kernig sign. A rapidly developing combination of motor, sensory, and sphincter dysfunction then occurs. Often the patient becomes paraplegic and demonstrates a spinal cord sensory level.

A contrast-enhanced MRI of the spine easily identifies the epidural abscess. Concomitantly, there may be an elevated C-reactive protein and erythrocyte sedimentation rate, with a modestly elevated WBC count. Emergency surgical decompression with systemic antibiotics is the treatment of choice. Occasionally, when no significant neurologic compromise exists, antibiotics are the primary treatment. However, careful follow-up is indicated, as the patient's clinical picture may rapidly evolve with motor and sensory loss, leading to the need for another MRI and surgical intervention.

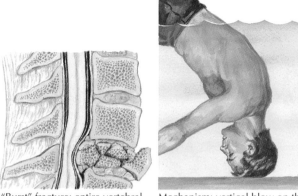

"Burst" fracture: entire vertebral body crushed, with intraspinal bone fragments

Mechanism: vertical blow on the head as in diving or surfing accident, being thrown from car, or football injury

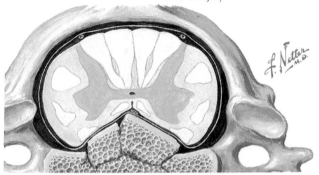

Dislocated bone fragments compressing spinal cord and spinal artery: blood supply to anterior two thirds of spinal cord is impaired

Fig. 55.11 Trauma.

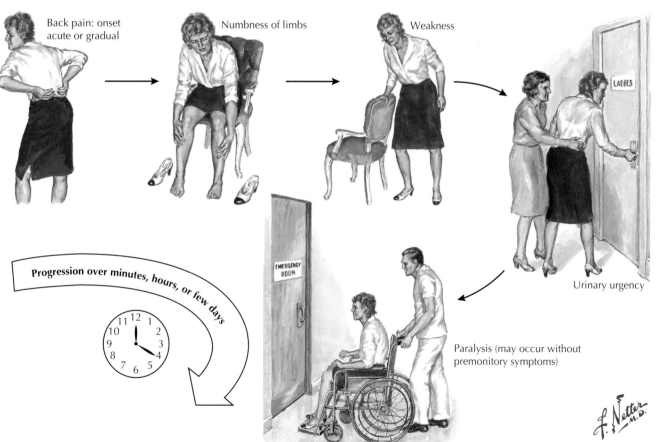

Back pain: onset acute or gradual

Numbness of limbs

Weakness

Urinary urgency

Progression over minutes, hours, or few days

Paralysis (may occur without premonitory symptoms)

Fig. 55.12 Acute Spinal Cord Syndromes: Evolution of Symptoms.

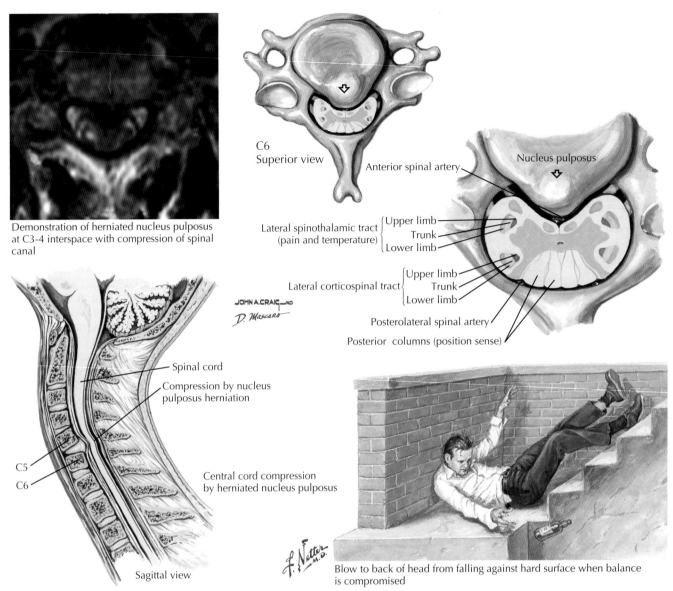

Demonstration of herniated nucleus pulposus at C3-4 interspace with compression of spinal canal

C6
Superior view

Nucleus pulposus

Anterior spinal artery

Lateral spinothalamic tract
(pain and temperature)
{
Upper limb
Trunk
Lower limb
}

Lateral corticospinal tract
{
Upper limb
Trunk
Lower limb
}

Posterolateral spinal artery

Posterior columns (position sense)

JOHN A. CRAIG—MD
D. Mascaro

Spinal cord

Compression by nucleus pulposus herniation

C5

C6

Central cord compression by herniated nucleus pulposus

Sagittal view

Blow to back of head from falling against hard surface when balance is compromised

Fig. 55.13 Cervical Disc Herniation.

Prognosis depends entirely on the patient's expeditious presentation to a medical facility and the clinician's level of suspicion, leading to relatively early diagnosis of the epidural spinal abscess. If treatment is not initiated until after the patient becomes paraplegic, prognosis is extremely guarded.

Tumor

Metastatic malignancies. One of the most common etiologies for a nontraumatic extradural myelopathy occurs with various forms of metastatic carcinoma (breast, lung, prostate) or lymphoma (Fig. 55.15). These can have an acute presentation, but also a more protracted course with the presence of spinal pain for weeks or months. Neurologic symptoms can begin as a radiculopathy and are followed by symptoms and signs of spinal cord compromise, usually with a spastic gait or bladder. Once these symptoms appear, the progression to paraplegia may be very rapid, due to vascular compression and consequent cord ischemia. On occasion, the spinal metastasis may be the presenting sign of a previously undiagnosed lung cancer. Metastases can be osteoblastic, such as with prostate carcinoma, or osteolytic, for example from lung cancer. Lymphoma and breast cancer metastases are predominantly osteolytic, but can rarely become osteoblastic. Urgent MRI is indicated. Treatment of metastatic extradural tumors should be prompt and include high-dose corticosteroids with radiotherapy and/or surgical decompression.

Chronic Cervical Spondylosis

CLINICAL VIGNETTE *An obese septuagenarian, with previously diagnosed diabetic polyneuropathy manifested by burning discomfort in his feet, presented with a 4- to 6-month history of increasing leg numbness. These new symptoms were totally different from the mild tingling and burning that had been chronically present for the past 10 years. He began to require a cane to maintain his equilibrium when walking. Although he initially tolerated the newer symptoms, he began to be concerned that he could not walk safely without relying on a walker. He sought further medical opinion. He previously had a myocardial infarction. Neurologic examination demonstrated a broad-based, spastic gait, brisk muscle stretch reflexes, and bilateral Babinski signs. Pinprick and temperature sensation were reduced in a stocking-glove distribution*

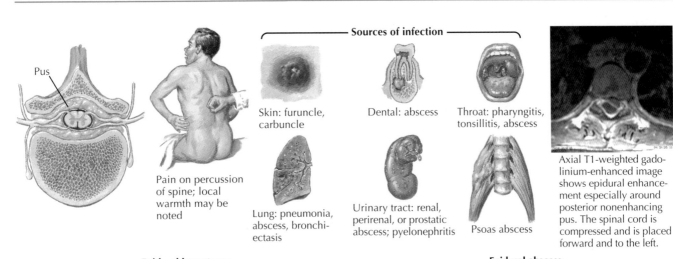

Sources of infection

Pus

Pain on percussion of spine; local warmth may be noted

Skin: furuncle, carbuncle

Lung: pneumonia, abscess, bronchiectasis

Dental: abscess

Urinary tract: renal, perirenal, or prostatic abscess; pyelonephritis

Throat: pharyngitis, tonsillitis, abscess

Psoas abscess

Axial T1-weighted gadolinium-enhanced image shows epidural enhancement especially around posterior nonenhancing pus. The spinal cord is compressed and is placed forward and to the left.

Epidural hematoma

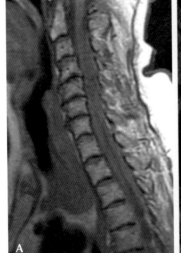

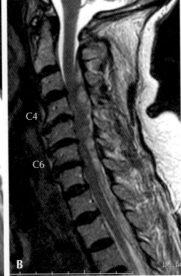

Epidural abscess

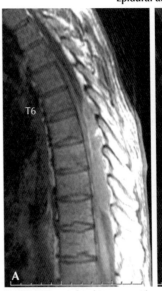

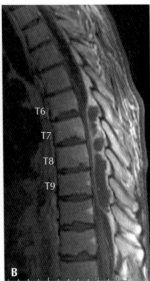

C4

C6

T6

T6
T7
T8
T9

A. T1-weighted sagittal image shows a vague posterior epidural mass.

B. T2-weighted image shows heterogeneous collection posterior to spinal cord.

Sagittal T1-weighted images without (**A**) and with (**B**) gadolinium enhancement demonstrate an extensive posterior epidural process from T6 to T11. Enhancement of the granulation tissue allows appreciation of nonenhancing focal pus collections.

Fig. 55.14 Epidural Abscess and Epidural Hematoma.

in his legs. There was a question of a bilateral cord level to pin sensation at C7. Position sense was absent at the toes, and vibratory sense was lost at the ankles. MRI revealed spinal stenosis and cord edema at C5–C6. He had severe spinal stenosis with multilevel spondylosis, disc protrusion, and endplate osteophytes. After a 3-month period of observation, his gait difficulties increased. A cervical posterior laminectomy was performed. Subsequently, after a period of rehabilitation hospitalization, he gradually regained the ability to walk independently.

Comment: One needs to always carefully evaluate the patient with a chronic primary sensory polyneuropathy who begins to develop disproportionately increased gait difficulty. Cervical spinal stenosis is a common chronic disorder. As occurred in this instance, one may define a quite remediable condition.

Spondylosis, a normal aging process, is the most common cause of a cervical myelopathy (Fig. 55.16). This results from disc degeneration followed by reactive osteophyte formation, fibrocartilaginous bars, spondylotic transverse bars, articular facet hypertrophy, and thickening of the ligamentum flavum causing spinal canal narrowing. Subsequently,

gradual spinal cord compression may occur; it is particularly likely in patients having congenitally narrowed spinal canals. In its simplest form, a chronically herniated central nucleus pulposus in patients with congenital stenosis can produce a cervical myelopathy. Although many senior individuals have radiographic signs of cervical spondylosis, most are asymptomatic. Sometimes both a cervical myelopathy and adjacent radiculopathy may occur in the same spondylotic patient.

Typically the diameter of the spinal canal is 17–18 mm between C3 and C7, and diameter of the cervical cord varies from 8.5 to 11.5 mm. A narrower cervical spinal canal may range from 9 to 15 mm; however, a compressive spondylitic myelopathy rarely occurs when the canal diameter is greater than 13 mm. Normally the spinal cord moves cephalad and posteriorly within the canal during neck flexion and caudally and anteriorly during neck extension. If osteophytes, discs, and hypertrophied ligaments make contact with the cord, the cord sustains additive trauma, leading to development of a clinical myelopathy. The disc levels affected are C5–C6, C6–C7, and C3–C4, in order of their clinical frequency. In this setting, the spinal cord may become pathologically grossly flattened, distorted, or indented. Demyelination of the lateral columns occurs at the lesion site with consequent lateral column degeneration below the

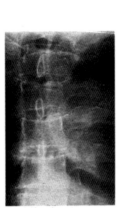

X-ray film showing destruction of pedicle and vertebral body by metastatic carcinoma

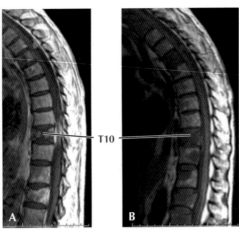

Metastatic tumor. A. Sagittal T1-weighted image demonstrates loss of normal marrow fat at multiple levels. **B.** Sagittal T1-weighted, gadolinium-enhanced image shows enhancement within the vertebral lesions and epidural extension with spinal cord compression at T10.

Fig. 55.15 Metastatic Malignances.

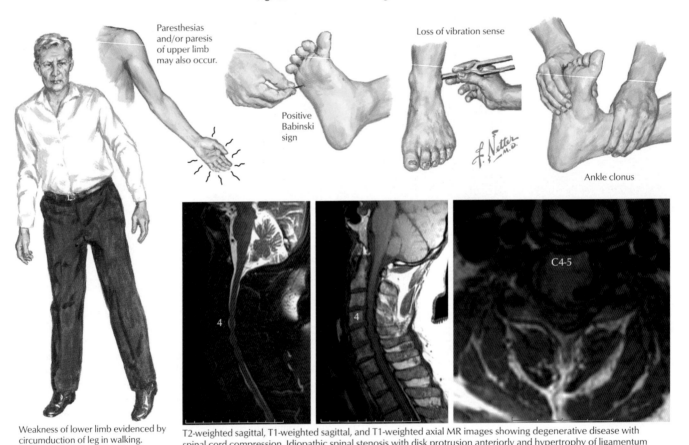

Weakness of lower limb evidenced by circumduction of leg in walking.

T2-weighted sagittal, T1-weighted sagittal, and T1-weighted axial MR images showing degenerative disease with spinal cord compression. Idiopathic spinal stenosis with disk protrusion anteriorly and hypertrophy of ligamentum flavum posteriorly, most extreme at C4-5.

Fig. 55.16 Cervical Spondylosis.

lesion. Concomitant dorsal column degeneration occurs at and above the damaged segment(s). There may also be damage and loss of nerve cells in gray matter. Ischemic changes, gliosis, demyelination, and even cavitation necrosis sometimes also result.

Patients with cervical spondylosis can present with a variety of neurologic symptoms and signs, including neck pain with radiation to the upper extremities, Lhermitte sign, gait difficulties, upper motor neuron

pattern of weakness in lower extremities, lower motor neuron pattern weakness in upper extremities mostly involving C5–C7 myotomes, altered sensation in upper extremities, and sphincter dysfunction. A radicular syndrome can occasionally accompany the myelopathy signs.

Most commonly, patients present with an insidious course characterized by progressive gait disorder attributed to leg weakness, stiffness, and/or unsteadiness, followed by altered sensation in upper extremities and sphincter dysfunction. Sometimes patients can have a subacute presentation progressing over a few months to a relatively severe disability. Infrequently, these patients are prone to acute cord compression secondary to a fall, as the compromised spinal canal diameter makes it more likely that the cord will be contused with sudden hyperextension or flexion. This may even mimic a stroke, as noted in the initial vignette in this chapter. Rarely, sudden neck hyperextension leads to a temporary "person in the barrel" syndrome. Here there is an acute compression of the anterior spinal cord. This transiently impairs the segmental anterior horn cells innervating the arm musculature. The clinical picture of isolated arm and hand weakness relates to the preserved lateral column corticospinal tract function; thus the legs are unaffected.

MRI is the diagnostic imaging of choice to evaluate cervical spondylosis and can show not only the abnormalities in the spine but also any associated compressive spinal cord abnormalities, including cord deformation, edema, and/or myelomalacia. CT/myelogram is an alternative when MRI is contraindicated because of cardiac pacemakers or severe claustrophobia. CT can provide additional information about the bony structure regarding the foramen, facets, and uncovertebral joints. Electromyography/nerve conduction can be of help when there is a suspicious for concomitant nerve root compression.

Epidemiologic data regarding the natural history of cervical spondylosis are lacking. In patients with mild deficits from cervical myelopathy, it is unclear whether surgical decompression is superior to conservative management. Some patients remain stable or improve without treatment. For patients with evolving symptoms and deficits, surgical decompression is the treatment of choice to arrest progression of the myelopathy. Functional recovery may not occur if the deficit is already severe, possibly because of chronic ischemic cord damage from spinal artery compression.

Surgical approaches include the posterior approach, which allows for generous decompressive laminectomies, and the anterior approach, which enables operation on bars and spurs anterior to the cord and fusion when instability or subluxation is present. Discectomy, corpectomy, laminectomy, and laminoplasty are other surgical options.

Significant variations exist in the degree of postsurgical clinical improvement. Duration and severity of the myelopathy before surgery are key determinants for clinical outcome. Cord atrophy, irreversible signal change within the cord on T2-weighted MRI (gliosis rather than cord edema), superimposed trauma, and advanced age are negative prognostic factors. Maintaining spinal stability and treating anterior compression improve outcome.

Vascular

Arteriovenous malformation. AVMs located exclusively in the extradural space are rare and can present as a radiculopathy. AVMs with a nidus in the extradural space and draining veins to the intradural region mainly via the coronal plexus can also occur and present with a subarachnoid or intraparenchymal hemorrhage, steal phenomena, or mass effect. MRI and MRA of the spine followed by a conventional angiogram are usually necessary for the diagnosis. Treatment consists of surgical resection and/or endovascular occlusion.

Infectious

Pott disease. Tuberculosis can infect the vertebral body causing a tuberculous spondylitis also known as Pott disease, most commonly seen in the lower thoracic and upper lumbar regions, which can potentially lead to a spinal cord compression. Patients usually present with low grade fever and weight loss, associated with localized back pain and signs of a compressive myelopathy. MRI of the spine with and without contrast is the modality of choice for the evaluation of

tuberculous involvement of the spine. As compared with bacterial discitis-osteomyelitis, tuberculosis tends to spread under the anterior longitudinal ligament, and therefore signal abnormality is most salient anterior to the disc space and vertebral bodies. Late-stage tuberculous involvement of the spine may demonstrate prominent vertebral body destruction with a Gibb deformity. Diagnosis of certainty is usually established by microscopy and culture of the infected tissue. Treatment includes antituberculosis therapy and surgery for patients with cord compression or severe kyphosis.

Tumors

Primary spine tumors are rare. Plasmacytoma/multiple myeloma and lymphoproliferative tumors are the most common malignant tumors, while hemangioma is the most common benign one. The clinical picture can vary from asymptomatic lesions, as for example in patients with hemangiomas, to progressive development of localized spine pain, followed by spinal cord compression and associated myelopathy in patients with malignant tumors. CT of the spine is helpful to assess the tumor matrix and osseous changes, while MRI provides helpful information regarding soft tissue extension, marrow infiltration, and intraspinal compromise. The tumors often have characteristic imaging features. In addition, age, sex, tumor location, and presentation can help with the differential diagnosis. Preoperative biopsy is reserved for cases in which diagnosis is doubtful and surgery is not being entertained. Treatment is usually surgical and aimed at removal of the local disease, with preservation of the mechanical functions of the spine. Adjuvant radiotherapy and chemotherapy are also used, depending on the histologic type.

ADDITIONAL RESOURCES

Robertson CE, Brown RD, Wijdicks EFM, et al. Recovery after spinal cord infarcts—long-term outcome in 115 patients. Neurology 2012;78:114–21.
Retrospective review of 115 patients with spinal cord infarcts with emphasis on outcome.

Augoustides JG, Stone ME, Drenger B. Novel approaches to spinal cord protection during thoracoabdominal interventions. Curr Opin Anaesthesiol 2014;27(1):98–105.
Review of therapeutic approaches for spinal cord protection during thoraco-abdominal aortic procedures.

Fink JK. Hereditary spastic paraplegia: clinical principles and genetic advances. Semin Neurol 2014;34(03):293–305.
Review highlighting the clinical and genetic features of HSP.

Delatycki MB, Corben LA. Clinical features of Friedreich ataxia. J Child Neurol 2012;27(9):1133–7.
Overview of the clinical features of Friedreich ataxia and differential diagnosis.

Hardiman O, Van der Berg LH. Edaravone: a new treatment for ALS on the horizon? Lancet Neurol 2017;16(7):490–1.
Editorial reviewing the benefits and limitations of Edaravone as a treatment for ALS.

Román GC. Tropical myelopathies. Handb Clin Neurol 2014;121:1521–48.
Review of the most common causes of myelopathy in the tropics, including etiologies that are specific to those regions, such as nutritional, toxic, bacterial, and parasitic.

Chamberlain MC. Neoplastic myelopathies. Continuum (N Y) 2015;21:132–45.
Review of the different myelopathies secondary to neoplasms.

Marcus J, Schwarz J, Singh IP, et al. Spinal dural arteriovenous fistulas: a review. Curr Atheroscler Rep 2013;15(7):335.
Review of clinical features, pathogenesis, imaging, and treatment of dural fistulas.

Tavee JO, Levin KH. Myelopathy due to degenerative and structural spine diseases. Continuum (N Y) 2015;21:52–66.
Review of the current evaluation and treatment of patients with myelopathy due to cervical spondylotic disease and other structural disorders of the spine.

Radiculopathies and Plexopathies

Jayashri Srinivasan

56

Cervical Radiculopathy

Subu N. Magge, Robert G. Whitmore, Stephen R. Freidberg

> **CLINICAL VIGNETTE** *A 42-year-old woman presented with a 2-week history of increasingly severe neck pain with radiation to the back of her right upper arm. In retrospect she had developed acute right medial scapular pain 4 weeks earlier after carrying a heavy briefcase to a meeting; this discomfort improved within 10 days. However, she then developed the neck and right arm discomfort; this was associated with numbness and tingling in her second and third fingers. She was an active tennis player and tried to play despite her discomfort but noted difficulty serving as she could not fully extend her arm. Her family physician initially treated her for "bursitis" and suggested that she might also have an emerging carpal tunnel syndrome because of the hand paresthesias. However, when the pain suddenly worsened, she consulted a neurologist. The neurologist elicited a 2-year history of similar but milder intermittent pain and numbness, especially after the patient had been driving long distances. Neurologic examination demonstrated modest right triceps weakness with an absent right triceps muscle stretch reflex. A trial of physical therapy was ineffective, and her symptoms significantly worsened after an afternoon of raking leaves. Further neurologic evaluation demonstrated more severe triceps weakness. Magnetic resonance imaging (MRI) of the cervical spine demonstrated a herniated disc at C6–C7. A neurosurgeon performed a posterior laminoforaminotomy and microdiscectomy. This provided immediate relief of her radicular pain. Her triceps strength improved to normal in the ensuing 3 months.*

This vignette illustrates the classic history of a C7 nerve root irritation. More than 80% of these radiculopathies resolve spontaneously with conservative therapy. However, on occasion the patient experiences increasing pain and progressive weakness. Unresolved pain and significant weakness are the two primary indications for cervical spine surgery.

Cervical radiculopathy, due to compression of a cervical nerve root, is a common clinical problem. It affects most adult age groups but is uncommon in adolescents and children. The symptoms may be relatively minor and chronic or acute and may be associated with weakness and sensory disturbance. On most occasions the cervical root symptoms have a spontaneous onset; not infrequently, however, the symptoms begin with a specific precipitating incident, such as trauma.

CLINICAL PRESENTATION

The clinical presentations of cervical radiculopathy depend on the specific root involved. It is unusual to have multiple nerve roots compressed at one time. The usual symptoms are pain, weakness, and sensory disturbance. Neck and/or medial scapular pain commonly occur with cervical root compression; shoulder or arm pain is also often present. Typical clinical findings include both arm weakness and sensory disturbance appropriate to the affected nerve root (Fig. 56.1). Neck movement often exacerbates the radicular pain and may result in an electric shock–like sensation (Fig. 56.2). Very rarely, pressure on the spinal cord as well as the nerve root may result in concomitant evidence of myelopathy. In any patient with cervical radiculopathy, clinical examination requires careful evaluation for evidence of a myelopathy by making certain the neurologic examination does not demonstrate a spastic gait with enhanced muscle stretch reflexes, a Babinski sign, and/or evidence of a spinal cord sensory level.

As a result of the incongruence between the cervical vertebrae (seven vertebrae) and the cervical nerve roots (eight roots), the root that exits is numbered after the vertebra inferior to it. For example the C6 root exits between the C5 and C6 vertebral bodies and the C7 between the C6 and C7 vertebral bodies. However, the C8 root exits between the C7 and T1 vertebral bodies and T1 between the T1 and T2 vertebral bodies. Of the various cervical radiculopathies, the C7 nerve root is the most commonly affected. It exits the spinal canal between C6 and C7. Typically compression leads to pain in the posterior arm. Unlike C5 and C6 lesions, C7 has little functional overlap with other roots. C7 innervates the triceps muscle, which extends the elbow (see Fig. 56.2). Unless patients perform activities that demand extension of the elbow— such as hammering, serving in tennis, rowing, or performing pushups— many individuals with a C7 radiculopathy are unaware of significant triceps weakness. To best ascertain the presence of triceps weakness, the examiner must ask the patient to flex his or her arm at the elbow to 90 degrees and then have the patient try to extend against resistance. In contrast, if one first asks the patient to extend his arm fully, relatively subtle degrees of weakness will be missed. In repose, gravity extends the elbow in most cases. Sensory loss in C7 radiculopathy usually extends to the index and middle fingers (Table 56.1).

The C6 nerve root exits the spine between C5 and C6 vertebrae. Compression here leads to pain in the medial scapula and into the arm, frequently to the lateral side of the forearm, as well as to the hand and into the thumb. Motor loss overlaps with C5 root and there is weakness in the proximal arm muscles, particularly the biceps, with difficulty flexing the arm at the elbow and abducting the arm at the shoulder. Sensory changes affect the thumb and index finger.

C8 is the lowest of the cervical roots, exiting the spinal column between the C7 and T1 vertebrae. When this nerve root is compressed, the pain radiates from the neck into the medial forearm and into the medial hand. If there is significant C8 compromise, patients develop weakness of their intrinsic hand muscle function. They also often complain of numbness and demonstrate sensory change in the medial hand as well as the fourth and fifth digits.

C5 is the least frequent level for radiculopathy. The C5 nerve root exits the spine between the C4 and C5 vertebral bodies. Compression of the C5 root produces pain within the medial scapula and into the

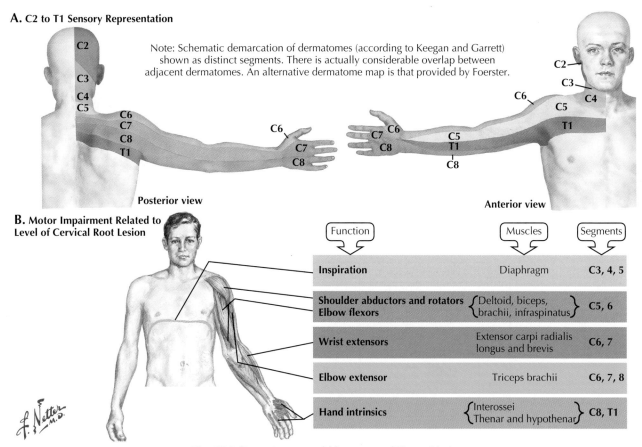

A. C2 to T1 Sensory Representation

Note: Schematic demarcation of dermatomes (according to Keegan and Garrett) shown as distinct segments. There is actually considerable overlap between adjacent dermatomes. An alternative dermatome map is that provided by Foerster.

Posterior view

Anterior view

B. Motor Impairment Related to Level of Cervical Root Lesion

Function	Muscles	Segments
Inspiration	Diaphragm	**C3, 4, 5**
Shoulder abductors and rotators Elbow flexors	Deltoid, biceps, brachii, infraspinatus	**C5, 6**
Wrist extensors	Extensor carpi radialis longus and brevis	**C6, 7**
Elbow extensor	Triceps brachii	**C6, 7, 8**
Hand intrinsics	Interossei Thenar and hypothenar	**C8, T1**

Fig. 56.1 Dermatomes and Myotomes of Upper Limb.

TABLE 56.1 Cervical Nerve Roots and Primary Clinical Findings

Root	Motor Weakness	Sensory Loss	Reflex Loss
C5	Deltoid	Around shoulder	None
C6	Biceps	Thumb and index finger	Biceps and brachioradialis
C7	Triceps	Index and middle finger	Triceps
C8	Intrinsic muscles of hand	Fourth and fifth fingers	None

upper arm; the pain rarely radiates below the elbow. There may be weakness of the deltoid resulting in difficulty carrying out tasks with the arm elevated (see Fig. 56.2). Sensory loss will be over the shoulder and upper arm and is often minimal (see Table 56.1).

When evaluating a patient with a suspected radiculopathy, it is important to define the temporal profile as well as the degree of progression of the symptoms. Has there been slow progression or rapid worsening? Has there been a plateau or improvement in the condition? How long have the symptoms persisted? The severity and quality of the pain and its provocative factors provide other useful information. In particular, does the arm pain worsen with movement of the neck? Is the pain of an electric quality? It is important to palpate the axilla or supraclavicular fossa, as a mass there could suggest the presence of an extraspinal tumor (Fig. 56.3) or a tumor of the brachial plexus (Fig. 56.4).

DIFFERENTIAL DIAGNOSIS

A modest number of pathologic conditions affect the cervical spine and require consideration in the evaluation of the individual with neck pain associated with limb muscle weakness and sensory loss. Radiculopathy secondary to a ruptured cervical disc is the most common cause (Fig. 56.5). Degenerative encroachment of the neural foramen from cervical spondylitic disease is another common cause. Primary or secondary neoplastic tumors of the cervical spine or vertebral infection can mimic disc herniation. Metastatic extradural tumor is the most common neoplasm within the cervical spine; the common sites of origin are breast, lung, prostate, and myeloma. The intradural extramedullary tumors, that is, schwannoma and meningioma, are also considerations. In contrast, intramedullary lesions, including a tumor or syrinx, usually present with symptoms of myelopathy. Spinal infection, especially epidural abscess, has increased in frequency; this may be due to sepsis associated with infection in the skin, wounds, or urinary tract or as a result of dental manipulation; there is a higher incidence in drug abusers and immune-suppressed patients. Patients with spinal infection usually have significant spine and root pain and may have a myelopathy. The presence of myelopathic signs in this clinical setting demands urgent surgical decompression. Furthermore, these patients may have significant spinal instability, which must be a consideration in planning surgery.

On occasion a lesion in the brachial plexus may be confused with a cervical radiculopathy. Neoplasms, either cancers or lymphoma invading the medial brachial plexus, may mimic a C8 radiculopathy; this also occurs with occult superior sulcus apical lung tumors (Pancoast syndrome). Schwannomas are the most common primary nerve tumors arising from the brachial plexus. Brachial plexitis (Parsonage-Turner

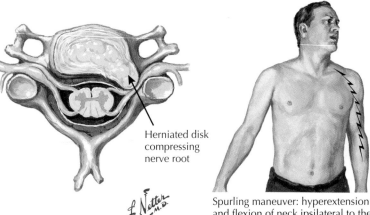

Herniated disk compressing nerve root

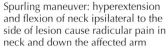

Spurling maneuver: hyperextension and flexion of neck ipsilateral to the side of lesion cause radicular pain in neck and down the affected arm

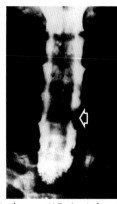

Myelogram (AP view) showing prominent extradural defect *(open arrow)* at C6-7

Level	Motor signs (weakness)	Reflex signs	Sensory loss
C5	Deltoid	0	
C6	Biceps brachii	Biceps brachii — Weak or absent reflex	
C7	Triceps brachii	Triceps brachii — Weak or absent reflex	
C8	Interossei	0	

Fig. 56.2 Cervical Disc Herniation: Clinical Manifestations.

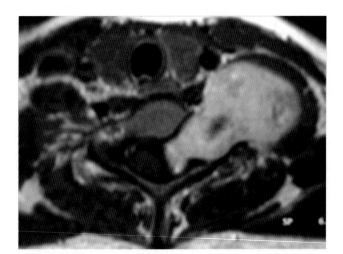

Axial T1-weighted post-gadolinium MR image demonstrating a dumbbell-shaped tumor, a schwannoma, exiting the spine through the left enlarged C6-7 foramen. This mass was palpable in the supraclavicular fossa.

Fig. 56.3 Extraspinal Tumor. *MR*, Magnetic resonance.

syndrome) may mimic a C5 radiculopathy. Other diagnostic considerations include ulnar neuropathy and the rare neurogenic thoracic outlet syndrome.

DIAGNOSTIC APPROACH

Approximately 80% of patients with cervical radiculopathy improve spontaneously; therefore imaging is often unnecessary. MRI studies of the spine are important in patients with unusual presentations or those who do not improve. To ensure there is no mismatch between symptoms and imaging findings, the studies should be evaluated carefully. It is not uncommon for asymptomatic patients to have significant abnormalities on imaging that are of no consequence. The clinical findings must correlate with imaging abnormalities if surgical treatment is to be considered.

It is common practice to omit standard cervical radiographs, but these may have some clinical value. Such images provide excellent visualization of the degree of spondylosis and disc degeneration and are of great importance to detect the presence of kyphosis. Flexion and extension lateral views of the spine are important whenever abnormal movement between the vertebrae is suspected.

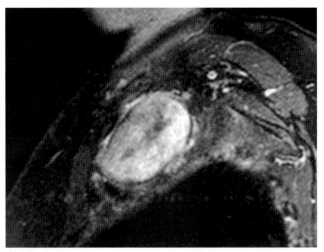

A. T1-weighted post-gadolinium MR image of the brachial plexus demonstrating a large enhancing mass.

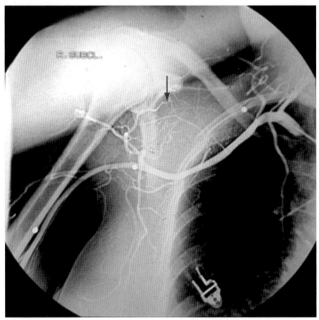

B. Angiogram demonstrating downward displacement of the sub-clavian artery.

Fig. 56.4 Desmoid Tumor. *MR,* Magnetic resonance.

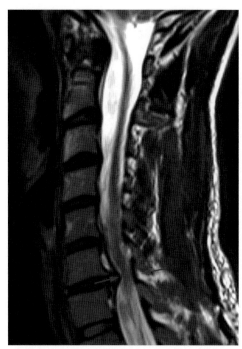

A. Far right lateral sagittal T2-weighted MR image demonstrates large disc herniation at C6-C7 (arrows).

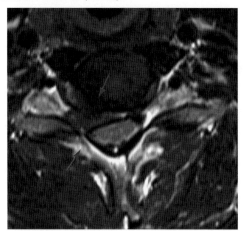

B. Axial T2-weighted MR image at C6-C7 shows the disc herniation extending from the left side across into the right lateral recess with slight deformity of the anterior aspect of the cervical spinal cord (arrows).

Fig. 56.5 Large Right Lateral C6–C7 Disc Herniation. *MR,* Magnetic resonance.

MRI is the imaging modality of choice for evaluating the spine and spinal cord. Occasionally open MRI or computed tomography (CT) myelography are good options for claustrophobic patients. Imaging studies will demonstrate the nerve root compression caused by disc herniation or spondylosis. A bright signal in the spinal cord on the T2-weighted image is indicative of an injury to the cord (Fig. 56.6). Additionally, it is possible to visualize tumors within the vertebrae or epidural space. Intradural tumors have a well-defined relationship to both the nerve root and spinal cord; MRI clearly demonstrates these lesions. Extramedullary tumors usually readily enhance with gadolinium; in contrast, intramedullary tumors are often difficult to differentiate from intrinsic spinal cord demyelinating lesions such as those of multiple sclerosis.

Spinal CT has limited value when used as a stand-alone diagnostic modality. However, CT used in conjunction with myelography is particularly useful in patients unable to have an MRI (e.g., because of cardiac pacemakers). Standard myelography followed by postmyelography CT will show nonfilling of nerve root sleeves or direct compression of the nerve roots (see Fig. 56.2). It may also demonstrate pressure on the spinal cord (extramedullary lesions) as well as pathology within the cord (intramedullary lesions). CT is particularly effective for demonstration of ossification of the posterior longitudinal ligament (OPLL). Additionally, reconstructed spinal CT is an excellent study when attempting to understand complex spinal deformities. We recommend electrodiagnostic studies if there is a conflict between the clinical presentation and imaging findings or if a diagnosis other than radiculopathy is suspected—for example, brachial plexopathy.

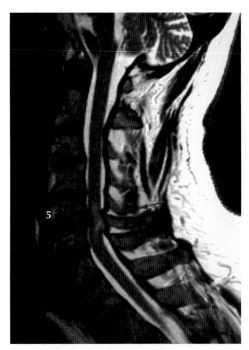

Sagittal T2-weighted MR image demonstrating marked stenosis at C5-6. There is an altered bright signal at that level within the spinal cord (arrow).

Fig. 56.6 Cervical Spinal Stenosis. *MR,* Magnetic resonance.

TREATMENT AND PROGNOSIS

The choice of therapy for a cervical radiculopathy depends on the patient's clinical presentation. Because most individuals improve spontaneously, early imaging and active treatment are rarely necessary unless there is significant weakness or signs of a concomitant myelopathy. Approximately 80% of patients with cervical radiculopathy secondary to either disc herniation or foraminal narrowing will improve spontaneously within 3 months. Heavy activity is restricted in individuals with acute nerve root compression. This particularly applies to activity that exerts tension on the cervical nerve roots leading to protective muscle spasm, with consequent worsening of the pain. Examples include

carrying a heavy briefcase, heavy lifting, or making a bed, etc. These patients are reexamined within few weeks. Occasionally muscle relaxants, simple analgesics, or antiinflammatory agents will be helpful adjuncts. Narcotics are used for severe pain, usually only for a limited period. Usually these modalities are successful. The good results of these conservative treatments and similarly of treatments such as traction, acupuncture, chiropractic manipulation, and massage probably owe their therapeutic success to the natural history of the condition.

For those patients with unremitting severe pain, with significant neurologic deficit, or with evidence of myelopathy, MRI is mandatory. If there is evidence of cervical disc herniation and the finding is appropriate to the clinical examination, surgery is an option.

For a ruptured lateral cervical disc, either an anterior or posterior approach is feasible. One approach involves anterior neck dissection, complete removal of the disc, and reconstruction with spinal fusion or an artificial disc implant. Arthroplasty may prevent the late development of stress-related degenerative changes that can occur at levels adjacent to a fusion. Alternatively, for a lateral disc herniation, a posteromedial facetectomy with elevation of the nerve root and removal of the ruptured disc fragment is a good option. The posterior approach is more uncomfortable for the patient than the anterior approach, but the patient does not have the potential long-term problems associated with fusion, including reduced mobility and end-fusion degeneration. An anterior approach is also best for midline disc herniations causing cord and/or root symptoms. If imaging demonstrates a diagnosis such as tumor or infection, treatment must be appropriately tailored.

ADDITIONAL RESOURCES

Albert TJ, Murrell SE. Surgical management of cervical radiculopathy. J Am Acad Orthop Surg 1999;7(6):368–76.

Freidberg SR, Pfeifer BA, Dempsey PK, et al. Intraoperative computerized tomography scanning to assess the adequacy of decompression in anterior cervical spine surgery. J Neurosurg (Spine 1) 2001;94:8–11.

Guzman J, Haldeman S, Carroll LJ, et al. Clinical practice implications of the bone and joint decade 2000-2010. Task force on neck pain and its associated disorders: from concepts and findings to recommendations. Spine 2008;33(Suppl. 4):S199–213. Review.

Levine MJ, Albert TJ, Smith MD. Cervical radiculopathy: diagnosis and nonoperative management. J Am Acad Orthop Surg 1996;4(6):305–16.

Wirth FP, Dowd GC, Sanders HF, et al. Cervical discectomy. A prospective analysis of three operative techniques. Surg Neurol 2000;53(4):340–6.

57

Lumbar Radiculopathy

Subu N. Magge, Robert G. Whitmore, Stephen R. Freidberg

CLINICAL VIGNETTE *A 53-year-old man had a history of occasional severe episodes of low back pain radiating down his buttock and posterior left thigh; it had begun with an athletic injury at age 17. Typically he experienced exacerbations, which lasted for a few days, every few years. Precipitating factors included sitting for prolonged periods and activities such as jogging or playing hockey. In general he "toughed out" these exacerbations by forcing himself out of bed in the morning despite the pain and continuing with his usual activities while being careful not to suddenly bend over. If his symptoms persisted, he found it necessary to use simple analgesics, low-dose muscle relaxants, and to "take it easy." After a weekend of skiing, he developed severe left sciatica that worsened progressively over a 3-day period. The pain was excruciating; it kept him up at night and did not respond to the usual medications. Getting out of bed in the morning was very painful, and he had to force himself up despite the "paralyzing" pain. He noticed left foot drop with paresthesia over his great toe. Straining or coughing further exacerbated the discomfort. He went to see a neurosurgeon; on the way, routine jolting of the car significantly exacerbated the pain. Neurologic exam demonstrated a left foot drop, marked lumbosacral paravertebral muscle spasm, diminished lumbar lordosis, and an inability to tolerate straight leg raising on the left. Magnetic resonance imaging (MRI) demonstrated an extruded disc fragment at the L4–L5 interspace with compression of the left L5 root. A micro-hemilaminectomy was performed, the disc fragment removed, and the nerve root decompressed. The sciatic pain was relieved the next morning.*

Comment: This patient's course was typical for an intermittent, recurrent, subacute lumbosacral radiculopathy; his intermittent symptoms had always improved with conservative therapy. The sudden onset of an acute severe radiculopathy secondary to disc extrusion with excruciating pain and the rapid development of a foot drop over a few days led to successful surgical intervention.

Lumbosacral radiculopathy, frequently called "sciatica," is one of the most common neurologic afflictions, typically affecting 1% of the population per year. Most individuals with sciatica experience some degree of chronic low back pain. These symptoms are a major cause of disability and are the primary cause of workers' compensation disability in the United States.

CLINICAL PRESENTATION

Sciatic pain may occur acutely or evolve more gradually; when the onset is sudden, it may be spontaneous or related to a specific incident, sometimes a seemingly trivial event, such as bending over to make a bed. The symptoms may be minor and clinically inconsequential or significant, requiring urgent evaluation and treatment (Fig. 57.1). Depending on the specific nerve root involved, the pain may be classic "sciatica"

with radiation down the posterior aspect of the leg into the foot, as seen with compression of the L5 or S1 roots (Figs. 57.2 and 57.3). At higher levels, with L3 or L4 root compression, the pain may radiate to the anterior thigh. The clinical signs of lumbar radiculopathy are due to the specific level of involvement (Table 57.1), and the most common levels of nerve root irritation are the L5 and S1 roots, followed less commonly by the L4 and L3 roots. It is very rare to have involvement of the higher roots (L1 and L2).

In the adult, the spinal cord ends between L1 and L2; therefore the nerve root compressed by disc herniation depends on whether the lesion is medial in the spinal canal or lateral in the neural foramen. The exiting root passes around the pedicle cephalad to the disc space. Therefore a lesion occurring at the disc space within the spinal canal compresses the passing root, the root with the next lower number. For example, a medial disc rupture in the spinal canal at L4–L5 will compress the L5 root, whereas less commonly the disc rupturing laterally in the neural foramen will compress the L4 root.

ETIOLOGY

The most frequent cause of lumbar radiculopathy is a herniated lumbar disc, due to herniation of the nucleus pulposus, usually occurring with an equal frequency at the lowest two levels, L4–L5 and L5–S1 (Figs. 57.4 and 57.5; see Fig. 57.1). Only some 5% of lumbar disc herniations occur at higher levels. Herniation is the last manifestation of disc degeneration, which is an ongoing process in all humans. Hence disc herniation is uncommon in youth, although occasionally teenagers and rarely toddlers have symptomatic herniations. Disc herniation occasionally occurs with spinal stenosis and may be the cause of rapid deterioration in an older person with mild chronic back pain. Most lumbar radiculopathies are unilateral; bilateral sciatica has an ominous significance, suggesting compression of the cauda equina; these patients are at risk for loss of sphincter function and in males of sexual function. Early recognition is essential, as even after expeditious decompression, sphincter control and potency may not always return. Rarely spondylosis with foraminal encroachment resulting from disc degeneration may cause radiculopathy.

DIFFERENTIAL DIAGNOSIS

Spinal stenosis is becoming more prevalent with the increase in the aging population. It rarely occurs before age 60 years, although individuals with achondroplasia or other congenital processes, with narrow spinal canals caused by shortened pedicles, are predisposed to premature spinal stenosis. Spondylosis is the primary pathologic process, characterized by hypertrophy of the ligaments and facet joints (Fig. 57.6). Patients may develop single or multilevel spinal canal compression of

Peripheral annulus fibrosus and posterior longitudinal ligament supplied with nociceptors (small unmyelinated nerve fibers with free or small capsular-type nerve endings). Nociceptors connect to sinu-vertebral nerve and/or to somatic afferent nerves carried within the sympathetic chain to the upper lumbar levels, which lead to dorsal root ganglion in spinal nerve root.

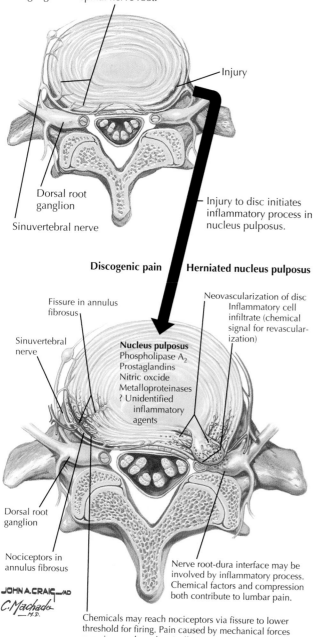

Injury

Dorsal root ganglion

Sinuvertebral nerve

Injury to disc initiates inflammatory process in nucleus pulposus.

Discogenic pain   **Herniated nucleus pulposus**

Fissure in annulus fibrosus

Sinuvertebral nerve

Neovascularization of disc
Inflammatory cell infiltrate (chemical signal for revascular-ization)

Nucleus pulposus
Phospholipase A₂
Prostaglandins
Nitric oxcide
Metalloproteinases
? Unidentified inflammatory agents

Dorsal root ganglion

Nociceptors in annulus fibrosus

Nerve root-dura interface may be involved by inflammatory process. Chemical factors and compression both contribute to lumbar pain.

JOHN A.CRAIG—MD
C.Machado—M.D.

Chemicals may reach nociceptors via fissure to lower threshold for firing. Pain caused by mechanical forces superimposed on chemically activated nociceptors.

Fig. 57.1 L4–L5 Role of Inflammation in Lumbar Pain.

the lumbosacral nerve roots; the L3–L4 and L4–L5 interspaces are the most commonly affected; it is rare at L5–S1 unless there is subluxation of the vertebral bodies. Characteristically the patient has a neurogenic claudication pain pattern mimicking arteriosclerotic occlusive (ASO) disease of the legs. Most individuals become symptomatic with standing or ambulating (see Fig. 57.6). They are able to walk a set distance and then feel the need to sit; relief is usually rapid with sitting. Character-istically patients are more comfortable flexed at the waist; thus walking uphill may be easier than walking downhill, as spinal hyperextension associated with walking downhill may precipitate symptomatology. Patients may also be more comfortable leaning forward on a walker or grocery cart. Often the patient has a normal neurologic exam; occasion-ally, with long-standing symptomatic spinal stenosis, there may be neurologic deficits.

The primary issue is often the differentiation of spinal stenosis from vascular claudication. The demographic population for both condi-tions is similar. Individuals with spinal stenosis tend to have pain of a more dysesthetic burning character in contrast to the squeezing tight discomfort typical for ASO. Another useful differentiating point on history is that those with spinal stenosis can ride a bicycle long distances, whereas arteriosclerotic patients are as limited as if they were walking. Unlike patients with disc herniations, patients with spinal stenosis are typically comfortable at rest, showing no signs of paraspinal spasm, difficulty with straight leg raise testing, or problems bending forward. Plain radiographs provide a good inexpensive means to recognize severe spondylotic changes. MRI is the diagnostic modality of choice. Com-puted tomographic (CT) myelography is helpful if the patient cannot tolerate MRI. For individuals who have relatively modest symptom-atology, there is no urgency to proceed with surgery. However, once patients are limited in walking or uncomfortable even when seated, a wide decompressive laminectomy and foraminotomy at appropriate spinal levels brings significant relief for a high percentage. For patients whose stenosis may be associated with spondylolisthesis, spinal fusion is indicated.

Spondylolisthesis, the anterior slippage of the superior vertebral body with respect to the inferior, is another common cause of lumbar root compression, resulting in low back pain (see Figs. 57.6A and B), radiculopathy symptoms, and sometimes cauda equina syndrome. The two common causes of spondylolisthesis involve spinal degenerative (spondylotic) changes and congenital defects of the vertebral pars inter-articularis. Patients with degenerative spondylolisthesis tend to be older, whereas those with a pars defect usually present in their third or fourth decade with significant lumbar and root pain usually related to postural change.

Although relatively uncommon, synovial cysts may produce symp-toms identical to disc herniation. The cysts develop from hypertrophy of synovial tissue in the facet joint. Neurosurgeons may encounter these cysts pushing into the paraspinal muscles while reflecting them for exposure of the spine. In this location, they indicate degenerative joint disease, but by themselves they are not symptomatic. When cysts become

TABLE 57.1	Nerve Root Signs of Lumbar Radiculopathy		
Root	Motor Weakness	Sensory Loss	Muscle Stretch Reflexes
L3	Iliopsoas/quadriceps	Anterior thigh	KJ diminished but still present
L4	Quadriceps	Anterior thigh to below knee	KJ absent
L5	Tibialis anterior	Dorsum and medial foot	Internal hamstring
S1	Gastrocnemius	Lateral aspect of foot, sole, and heel	AJ absent

AJ, Ankle jerk; *KJ*, knee jerk.

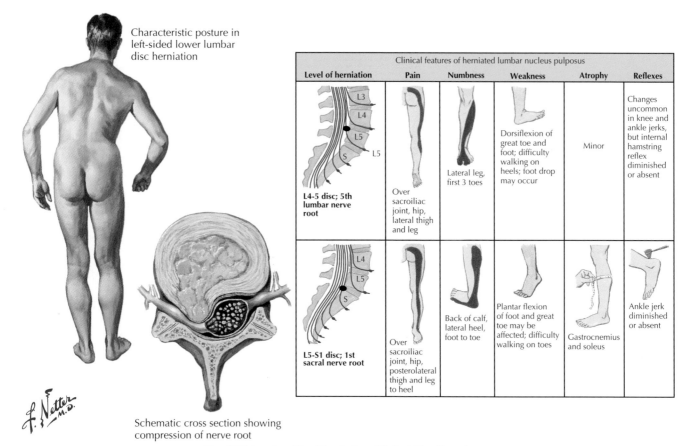

Characteristic posture in left-sided lower lumbar disc herniation

Schematic cross section showing compression of nerve root

Fig. 57.2 Lumbar Disc Herniation: Clinical Manifestations.

intraspinal, they may compress the nerve root; synovial cysts create a surrounding inflammatory reaction and therefore must be carefully dissected from the dura of the nerve roots. Resection of lumbar epidural synovial cysts usually relieves patients' pain.

Epidural infections can occur secondary to disc surgery, epidural injections, or via hematogenous spread. Unlike metastatic tumors that primarily involve the vertebral bodies, abscess involves the disc space, with secondary spread to the adjacent vertebral bodies. Back pain from disc space and vertebral body involvement and secondary nerve root pain are usually very severe. Common causative organisms in the United States are coagulase-positive and coagulase-negative *Staphylococcus* from surgical or hematogenous spread. Gram-negative organisms from urinary sepsis may also be causative agents. Intravenous drug users and immuno-compromised patients have higher incidences of epidural abscess. Worldwide, the most common cause of spinal infection is tuberculosis (TB). The incidence of spinal TB appears to be increasing with the increasing incidence of human immunodeficiency virus (HIV) positivity in susceptible populations.

Neoplasms may be a cause of lumbosacral pain. Metastatic extradural cancers of the spine are the most common tumors. Primary bone tumors and intradural primary and metastatic tumors may also mimic disco-genic disorders. The common cancers that metastasize include prostate, breast, lung, melanoma, and myeloma. Usually symptoms begin with spine pain that worsens gradually; root pain starts once neural elements become involved and may worsen rapidly. Evaluation and treatment in this situation are urgent, as recovery after treatment may not be complete. Schwannoma, meningioma, myxopapillary ependymoma, and lipoma are the common lumbar spinal intradural tumors (Fig. 57.7). The symptoms of schwannoma, meningioma, and ependymoma are

gradually progressive. Patients with a lipoma, a congenital tumor, may have a history of baseline neurologic deficits with a slow later progression.

DIAGNOSTIC APPROACH

The evaluation of patients having their initial bout of acute sciatica or low back pain does not routinely require any diagnostic testing. Most individuals recover spontaneously. However, for those who do not fit the classic pattern of nerve root compression or acute low back strain and for patients who do not improve, neurodiagnostic testing is necessary.

Plain radiographs of the lumbar spine, including lateral flexion and extension views, serve two purposes: the anatomy of the spine with its degenerative changes is demonstrated, as are subluxations and instability, and destructive lesions in the vertebral bodies and disc space can be seen. MRI is the primary spinal imaging modality (see Figs. 57.5 and 57.6). Good-quality MRI demonstrates disc herniation or spinal stenosis and identifies the rare tumor or infection. However, on occasion, for technical reasons, MRI may not be successful; for example, the patient may have moved during imaging, pacemaker or other hardware may preclude MRI, and obesity or claustrophobia may be other impediments. CT myelography continues to be a valuable adjunct to the diagnostic repertoire, especially when MRI is contraindicated or not tolerated. Myelography with water-soluble contrast followed by axial CT scanning can demonstrate nerve root filling or lack thereof with more clarity than MRI. Sagittal and coronal reconstructions of CT data give excellent additional information. Electrodiagnostic studies are invaluable in those situations where data from imaging are difficult to interpret or where other superimposed conditions, such as polyneuropathy, coexist.

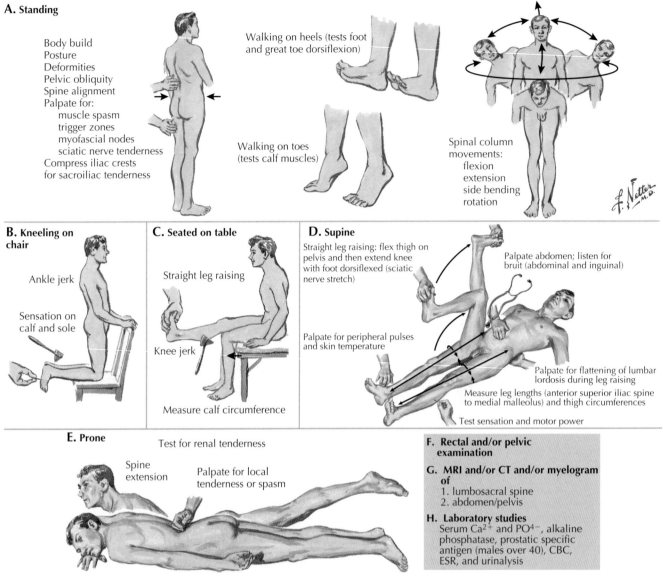

A. Standing

Body build
Posture
Deformities
Pelvic obliquity
Spine alignment
Palpate for:
   muscle spasm
   trigger zones
   myofascial nodes
   sciatic nerve tenderness
Compress iliac crests
for sacroiliac tenderness

Walking on heels (tests foot
and great toe dorsiflexion)

Walking on toes
(tests calf muscles)

Spinal column
movements:
   flexion
   extension
   side bending
   rotation

B. Kneeling on chair

Ankle jerk

Sensation on
calf and sole

C. Seated on table

Straight leg raising

Knee jerk

Measure calf circumference

D. Supine

Straight leg raising: flex thigh on
pelvis and then extend knee
with foot dorsiflexed (sciatic
nerve stretch)

Palpate for peripheral pulses
and skin temperature

Palpate abdomen; listen for
bruit (abdominal and inguinal)

Palpate for flattening of lumbar
lordosis during leg raising

Measure leg lengths (anterior superior iliac spine
to medial malleolus) and thigh circumferences

Test sensation and motor power

E. Prone

Test for renal tenderness

Spine
extension

Palpate for local
tenderness or spasm

F. Rectal and/or pelvic examination

G. MRI and/or CT and/or myelogram of
   1. lumbosacral spine
   2. abdomen/pelvis

H. Laboratory studies
Serum Ca^{2+} and PO^{4-}, alkaline
phosphatase, prostatic specific
antigen (males over 40), CBC,
ESR, and urinalysis

Fig. 57.3 Examination of Patient With Low Back Pain. *CBC,* Complete blood count; *CT,* computed tomography; *ESR,* erythrocyte sedimentation rate; *MRI,* magnetic resonance imaging.

TREATMENT

Treatment of lumbar radiculopathy is usually successful if the history, physical examination, and imaging correlate. Most acute episodes of back pain or nerve root pain without significant neurologic deficit require only judicious rest and simple analgesics. Strict bed rest is not necessary because it may lead to rapid deconditioning; it may also predispose to more serious complications, such as deep venous thrombosis, pulmonary embolism, and rarely fatal paradoxical cerebral emboli. Patients must be encouraged to get up as much as possible but to avoid activities that exacerbate their symptoms. When patients have recovered from their acute symptoms, they can begin a judicious exercise program, graduating to a full fitness program. Analgesics and antiinflammatory medications including occasional use of steroids may help patients. With this approach, 80% of patients improve within 3 months. This is the natural history of discogenic nerve root compression, and care is advised when evaluating therapeutic claims for other treatment modalities such as chiropractic manipulations or acupuncture. For patients with more chronic nondisabling pain, lifestyle changes with weight loss

and health club membership constitute the best approach, although, unfortunately, few patients successfully change their behavior patterns.

When acute symptoms do not improve or the chronic degenerative disc-related pain persists, surgery is an option (Fig. 57.8). An important indication for surgery is the presence of a significant persistent neurologic deficit such as foot drop. However, severe or chronic unrelenting nerve root pain that disrupts a patient's life is a common reason to proceed with nerve root decompression. When advising patients who are making decisions about surgery, the physician should make it clear that postponing surgery would not place them in neurologic jeopardy although the discomfort would likely persist. Surgical goals for patients with degenerative disease or disc rupture relate to the pain's origin. If the patient has root pain with corresponding root compression on imaging, the root or roots should be decompressed and the herniated disc or synovial cyst removed. Surgery for an extruded disc requires removal of the extruded fragment with freeing of the compressed nerve root. With this technique, more than 90% of patients obtain symptomatic relief.

If posture-related lumbar pain is the primary symptom, root decompression alone will not resolve the symptoms. Spinal segmental instability,

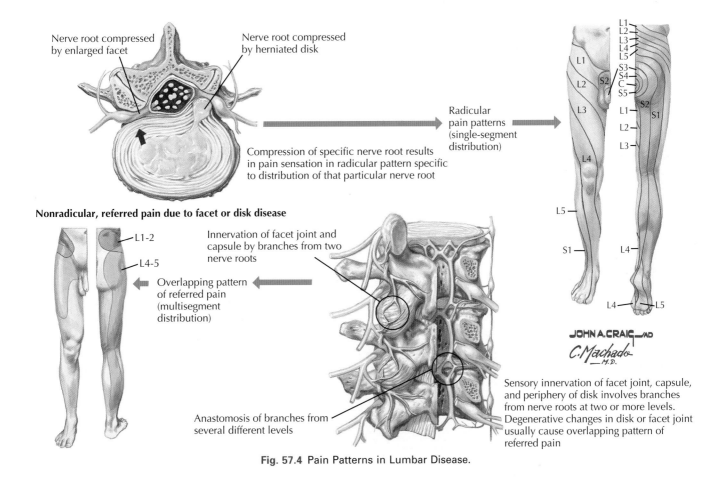

Nerve root compressed by enlarged facet

Nerve root compressed by herniated disk

Compression of specific nerve root results in pain sensation in radicular pattern specific to distribution of that particular nerve root

Radicular pain patterns (single-segment distribution)

Nonradicular, referred pain due to facet or disk disease

L1-2

L4-5

Innervation of facet joint and capsule by branches from two nerve roots

Overlapping pattern of referred pain (multisegment distribution)

Anastomosis of branches from several different levels

Sensory innervation of facet joint, capsule, and periphery of disk involves branches from nerve roots at two or more levels. Degenerative changes in disk or facet joint usually cause overlapping pattern of referred pain

JOHN A. CRAIG—MD

C. Machado —M.D.

Fig. 57.4 Pain Patterns in Lumbar Disease.

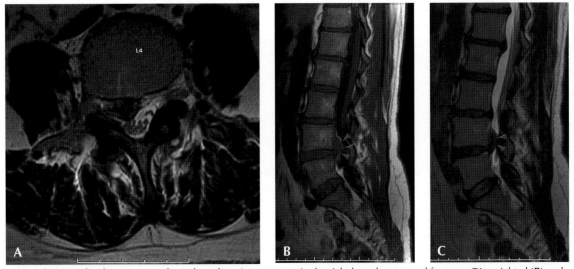

(A) Axial T2-weighted image at L4 shows large hypointense mass in the right lateral recess and foramen. T1-weighted **(B)** and T2-weighted **(C)** sagittal MR images show mass extending cephalad from the L4-5 disc (arrowheads).

Fig. 57.5 Disc Extrusion.

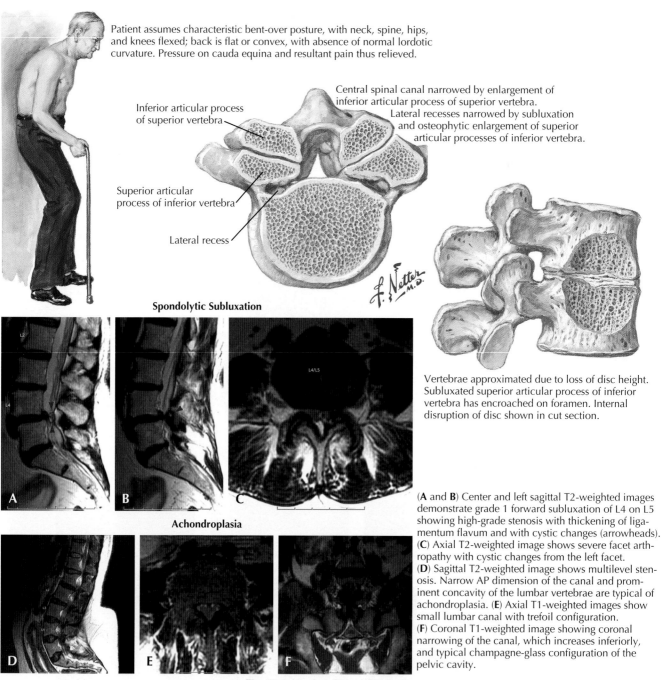

Patient assumes characteristic bent-over posture, with neck, spine, hips, and knees flexed; back is flat or convex, with absence of normal lordotic curvature. Pressure on cauda equina and resultant pain thus relieved.

Inferior articular process of superior vertebra

Superior articular process of inferior vertebra

Lateral recess

Central spinal canal narrowed by enlargement of inferior articular process of superior vertebra.
Lateral recesses narrowed by subluxation and osteophytic enlargement of superior articular processes of inferior vertebra.

Spondolytic Subluxation

Vertebrae approximated due to loss of disc height. Subluxated superior articular process of inferior vertebra has encroached on foramen. Internal disruption of disc shown in cut section.

Achondroplasia

(**A** and **B**) Center and left sagittal T2-weighted images demonstrate grade 1 forward subluxation of L4 on L5 showing high-grade stenosis with thickening of ligamentum flavum and with cystic changes (arrowheads). (**C**) Axial T2-weighted image shows severe facet arthropathy with cystic changes from the left facet. (**D**) Sagittal T2-weighted image shows multilevel stenosis. Narrow AP dimension of the canal and prominent concavity of the lumbar vertebrae are typical of achondroplasia. (**E**) Axial T1-weighted images show small lumbar canal with trefoil configuration. (**F**) Coronal T1-weighted image showing coronal narrowing of the canal, which increases inferiorly, and typical champagne-glass configuration of the pelvic cavity.

Fig. 57.6 Lumbar Spinal Stenosis.

with abnormal spinal motion, can also cause significant pain secondary to intermittent compression of nerve roots. It can also increase degeneration around the facet joints and disc annulus, causing primary back pain. In these uncommon instances, spinal fusion is a reasonable consideration.

The treatment of a patient with a tumor depends on the tumor's histology and the extent of neurologic involvement. If the initial presentation of a metastatic tumor is in the spine, needle biopsy of the spinal tumor or biopsy of an obvious tumor demonstrated in the lung, breast, prostate, or skin can provide the diagnosis. Radiotherapy is appropriate when the tumor is radiosensitive, the spine is stable, and there is relatively minimal neural compression. However, if these considerations are not met, surgery is indicated. A major destructive lesion

involving most of the vertebral body and both pedicles usually requires a 360-degree decompression and fusion. Neurologic deterioration can be rapid, and once paresis has occurred, the patient may not recover, even after emergency surgery.

Appropriate therapy of an epidural infection is controversial. Some reports demonstrate good results with antibiotic treatment. This approach is best for patients who are not overtly septic and have no significant mass effect on the neural structures. However, because of the potential for rapid loss of neurologic function, surgical drainage of large purulent collections is advisable to reduce pain and prevent paraplegia. Rapid deterioration can occur in patients treated nonoperatively with antibiotics, and such patients should be observed very closely.

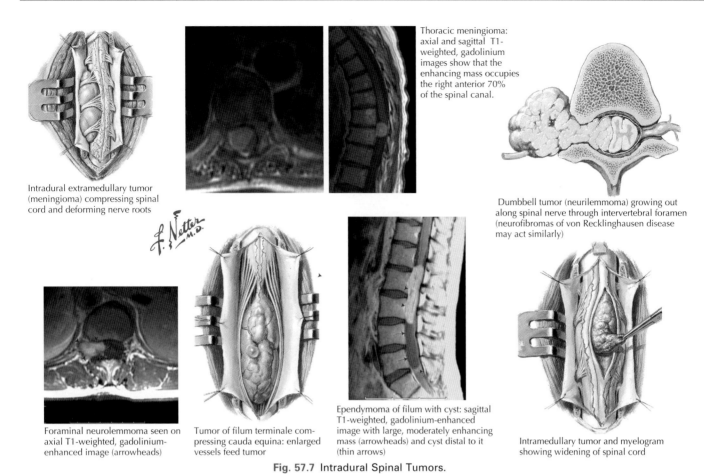

Intradural extramedullary tumor (meningioma) compressing spinal cord and deforming nerve roots
Thoracic meningioma: axial and sagittal T1-weighted, gadolinium images show that the enhancing mass occupies the right anterior 70% of the spinal canal.
Dumbbell tumor (neurilemmoma) growing out along spinal nerve through intervertebral foramen (neurofibromas of von Recklinghausen disease may act similarly)
F. Netter M.D.
Foraminal neurolemmoma seen on axial T1-weighted, gadolinium-enhanced image (arrowheads)
Tumor of filum terminale compressing cauda equina: enlarged vessels feed tumor
Ependymoma of filum with cyst: sagittal T1-weighted, gadolinium-enhanced image with large, moderately enhancing mass (arrowheads) and cyst distal to it (thin arrows)
Intramedullary tumor and myelogram showing widening of spinal cord

Fig. 57.7 Intradural Spinal Tumors.

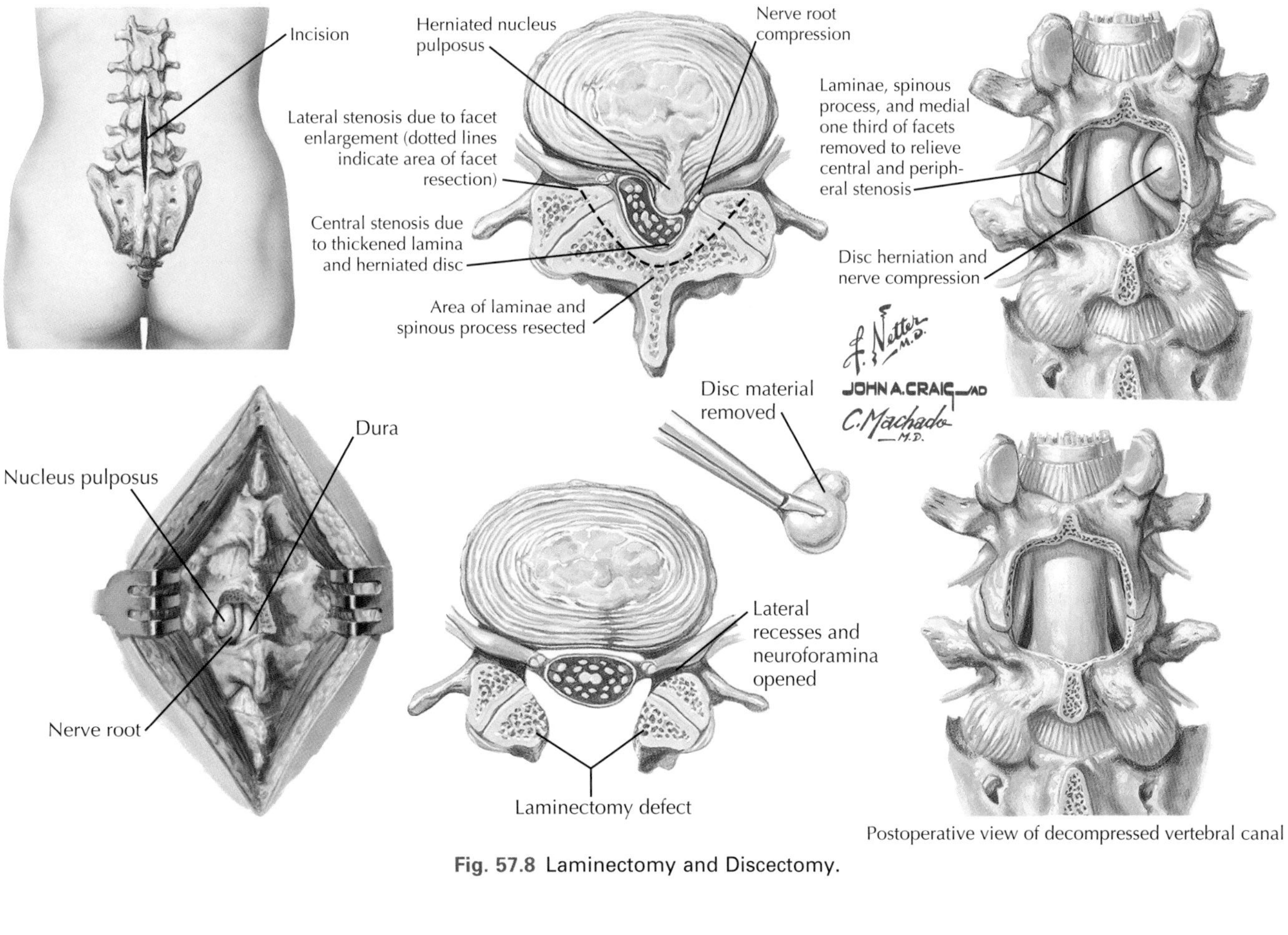

Incision
Herniated nucleus pulposus
Nerve root compression
Lateral stenosis due to facet enlargement (dotted lines indicate area of facet resection)
Central stenosis due to thickened lamina and herniated disc
Area of laminae and spinous process resected
Laminae, spinous process, and medial one third of facets removed to relieve central and peripheral stenosis
Disc herniation and nerve compression
F. Netter M.D.
JOHN A.CRAIG MD
C.Machado M.D.
Disc material removed
Dura
Nucleus pulposus
Nerve root
Lateral recesses and neuroforamina opened
Laminectomy defect
Postoperative view of decompressed vertebral canal

Fig. 57.8 Laminectomy and Discectomy.

ADDITIONAL RESOURCES

Berven S, Tay BB, Colman W, et al. The lumbar zygapophyseal (facet) joints: a role in the pathogenesis of spinal pain syndromes and degenerative spondylolisthesis. Semin Neurol 2002;22(2):187–96.

Binder DK, Schmidt MH, Weinstein PR. Lumbar spinal stenosis. Semin Neurol 2002;22(2):157–66.

Katz JN, Dalgas M, Stucki G, et al. Degenerative lumbar spinal stenosis. Diagnostic value of the history and physical examination. Arthritis Rheum 1995;38(9):1236–41.

Minamide A, Yoshida M, et al. Minimally invasive spinal decompression for degenerative lumbar spondylolisthesis and stenosis maintains stability and may avoid the need for fusion. Bone Joint J 2018;100-B(4):499–506.

Schultz IZ, Crook JM, Berkowitz J, et al. Biopsychosocial multivariate predictive model of occupational low back disability. Spine 2002;27(23):2720–5.

Shah AA, Paulino Pereira NR, et al. Modified en bloc spondylectomy for tumors of the thoracic and lumbar spine: surgical technique and outcomes. J Bone Joint Surg Am 2017;99(17):1476–84.

Stochkendahl MJ, Kjaer P, et al. National clinical guidelines for non-surgical treatment of patients with recent onset low back pain or lumbar radiculopathy. Eur Spine J 2018;27(1):60–75.

Storm PB, Chou D, Tamargo RJ. Lumbar spinal stenosis, cauda equina syndrome, and multiple lumbosacral radiculopathies. Phys Med Rehabil Clin N Am 2002;13(3):713–33, ix.

Tang HJ, Lin HJ, et al. Spinal epidural abscess—experience with 46 patients and evaluation of prognostic factors. J Infect 2002;45(2):76–81.

Williams MG, Wafai AM, Podmore MD. Functional outcomes of laminectomy and laminotomy for the surgical management lumbar spine stenosis. J Spine Surg 2017;3(4):580–6.

Winstein JN, Lurie JD, Tosteson TD, et al. Surgical vs nonoperative treatment for lumbar disk herniation: the spine patient outcomes research trial (SPORT) a randomized trial. JAMA 2006;296(20):2441–50.

58

Back Pain

Daniel Vardeh

EPIDEMIOLOGY

Low back pain is an extremely common condition; according to the World Health Organization's Global Burden of Disease Study, of 291 studied conditions, it is the greatest contributor to global disability. As the leading cause of activity limitation and work disability, low back pain is responsible for tremendous costs by way of healthcare expenditure, disability insurance, and lost productivity. Chronic low back pain, defined typically as lasting more than 3 months, affects both men and women equally; its onset is typically between age 30 and 50, and the incidence of low back pain increases steadily with age.

PATHOPHYSIOLOGY

Despite the very high prevalence of chronic low back pain, its underlying etiology often remains uncertain. As a first step, it is important to distinguish a defined underlying disease process from nonspecific benign conditions. Specific conditions include rheumatologic disorders such as rheumatoid arthritis of the lumbar facet joints or ankylosing spondylitis, bone disease such as diffuse idiopathic skeletal hyperostosis (DISH), spondylolisthesis, vertebral body fractures due to trauma, or spontaneous fractures in the setting of osteoporosis, neoplastic disease (either as a primary tumor or more commonly vertebral body metastases), infectious disease such as an epidural abscess or osteomyelitis, or herniation of an intervertebral disc. It is important to remember that referred pain from visceral structures can present as back pain, as is seen with the rupture or dissection of an aortic aneurysm, fibroid uterus, retroperitoneal bleed, or kidney stones. "Red flags" in the history can often give a clue to a more serious underlying condition. For spinal fractures, red flags with the highest predictive value include older age, prolonged use of steroids, severe trauma, and the presence of contusion.

In most cases no specific underlying disease can be found and the underlying pain mechanisms remain uncertain. Conceptually these conditions can be categorized in anatomic or pathologic etiologies. Anatomically the low back contains a large number of potential pain generators, including the intervertebral discs, multiple pairs of facet joints, vertebral end plates, nerve roots, ligaments, and spinal muscles (Fig. 58.1). Any or all of these structures may be involved in generation of low back pain, and there is often interplay between them. For example, in the healthy spine, the two facet joints carry approximately 30% of the total load at a given spinal level. In the setting of disc herniation and a decrease of disc height, this load can increase to 70%, causing both discogenic pain from the disc rupture itself as well as facetogenic pain from the increased pressure load. The extruded disc material can cause both nerve root compression and inflammation as well as a local inflammatory response, resulting in focal muscle spasms (Fig. 58.2).

Pathophysiologically, in concordance with any other chronic pain state, pain generation can be divided into nociceptive, inflammatory, and neuropathic conditions. Nociceptive pain is caused by direct activation of C and A-δ fibers—for instance by an intervertebral disc rupture, increased pressure or destruction of the facet joint, or muscle spasm. Inflammatory pain is the result of infectious (e.g., bacterial abscess) or noninfectious conditions (e.g., autoimmune-mediated synovitis in rheumatoid arthritis). For both cases, multiple inflammatory mediators activate and sensitize peripheral nociceptors. Neuropathic pain is the direct result of injury to the peripheral nerve (e.g., compression of the nerve root from a herniated disc) or injury to the central nervous system (e.g., compressive spinal myelopathy). Often, several pathologic states coexist, as is shown in the example (see Fig. 58.2). In addition, ongoing peripheral nociceptive input often results in structural and functional changes of the central nervous system termed *central sensitization*, resulting in more widespread pain beyond the initial site of injury (secondary hyperalgesia), which makes precise diagnosis or targeted treatment even more challenging.

Beyond the neurobiologic process of nociception, the interplay of psychological and social aspects (biopsychosocial model) eventually results in a complex "pain" phenotype of an unpleasant sensory and emotional experience as well as disability. Although the nociceptive component often cannot be cured, the affective reaction and subsequent behavior can be modulated using psychologic interventions, and this often results in a meaningful reduction of disability. Examples of counterproductive patient beliefs and emotions (pain catastrophizing) include that activity-induced pain causes more damage (causing avoidance of any activity), that pain controls one's life (helplessness), or that a serious illness is the cause of pain despite a negative workup. In addition, secondary gain—in the form, for example, of financial compensation for a work-related injury, the attestation of disability status, or the settlement of a lawsuit—will typically prevent any improvement in the patient's condition until the case is settled and the gain achieved.

DIAGNOSIS

History and a thorough physical examination are important to exclude a specific underlying condition for the patient's low back pain. The musculoskeletal clinical exam for low back pain (Fig. 58.3) has poor localizing value and little interindividual reliability. However, the straight leg raise test shows high sensitivity, and the crossed straight leg raise test shows high specificity for lumbar radiculopathy or sciatic nerve disease. Numbness in a dermatomal distribution is often an early sign of radiculopathy, and weakness in a myotomal distribution with reflex loss typically indicates more severe nerve root compression. Neuraxial signs and symptoms are important to note in order to detect potentially reversible spinal cord disease; signs include a sensory trunk level, increased

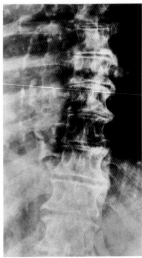

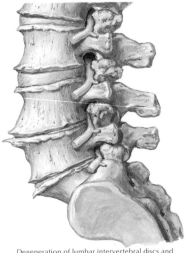

Radiograph of thoracic spine shows narrowing of intervertebral spaces and spur formation

Degeneration of lumbar intervertebral discs and hypertrophic changes at vertebral margins with spur formation. Osteophytic encroachment on intervertebral foramina compresses spinal nerves

Lumbar Disc Herniation

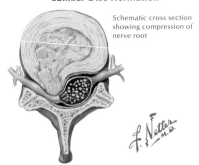

Schematic cross section showing compression of nerve root

Fig. 58.1 Structural Causes of Low Back Pain.

leg tone/spasticity, a Babinski sign (typically occurs in a subacute and chronic condition) or decreased tone and loss of reflexes (hyperacute condition), loss of the anal reflex, the Beevor sign (weakness of the lower half of the abdominal muscles), and incontinence. Saddle anesthesia in the perineal region can be indicative of a cauda equina syndrome, and early bowel and bladder dysfunction can herald a conus medullaris syndrome. Transient loss of ankle reflexes and leg weakness after walking are indicative of neurogenic claudication typically caused by lumbar spinal stenosis.

In clinical practice, imaging plays a major role in trying to define anatomic pathology in the patient with chronic pain and is often viewed as the most objective way to establish a diagnosis. However, in spite of great advances in imaging technology, correlation between symptoms and objective radiologic findings (e.g., magnetic resonance imaging [MRI]) remain poor, underscoring the importance of functional changes in the nervous system over anatomic alterations. Additionally, there is evidence that radiologic abnormalities on spine imaging can be seen in asymptomatic patients; for example, of 98 pain-free, healthy volunteers, about half had evidence of a bulging disc, 38% had pathology at more than one level, 8% had facet arthropathy, and only about one-third had an entirely normal MRI. The reverse is also common in clinical practice, where patients with chronic back pain are overtreated or undergo surgery based on a non-significant radiographic abnormality such as a bulging disc. Nevertheless, imaging of the lumber spine has increased by more than 300% between 1994 and 2005 without any sign of improved outcomes. However, imaging should be obtained, starting with a lumbar x-ray, in any patient with concern for systemic disease, a history of "red flags," or concerning exam findings.

Fluoroscopy-guided injections of local anesthetics are often used to elucidate the underlying anatomic pain driver. For example, resolution of pain shortly after an injection into the sacroiliac (SI) joint or around the lumbar facet joint is indicative of SI joint and facetogenic pain, respectively. Likewise selective nerve root blocks are often used by neurosurgeons to determine the symptomatic nerve roots. Whether this results in improved outcomes remains uncertain.

TREATMENT AND PROGNOSIS

For acute back pain, prognosis is overall favorable, and most patients improve regardless of treatment. Therefore first-line treatment consists of easy and safe measures, including superficial heat, massage, spinal manipulation or acupuncture. Mild physical activity is recommended, bed rest is often counterproductive. If pharmacologic treatment is desired, a short course of nonsteroidal antiinflammatory drugs

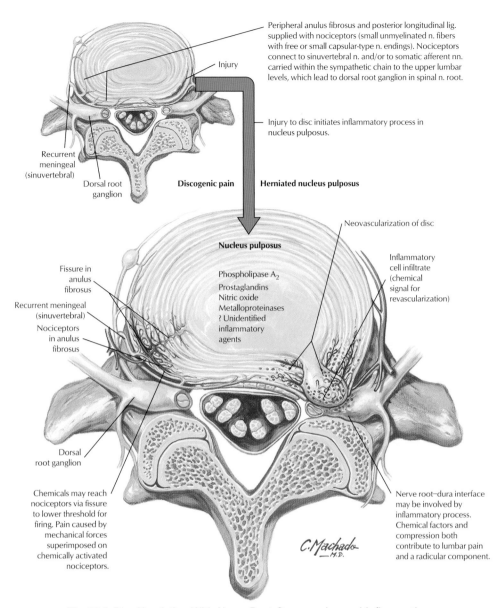

Fig. 58.2 Disc Herniation With Nerve Root Compression and Inflammation.

(NSAIDs) and sometimes a short course of muscle relaxants are first-line treatments; however, sedation often occurs with many muscle relaxants. The majority of acute low back pain resolves within a few weeks; however, recurrence of symptoms within a year, often of lower intensity, is common. About 20% to 50% of patients develop chronic low back pain at 1 year, and identifying these patients for early intervention remains an unresolved major challenge. Genetic factors, the occupational environment, psychosocial factors, preexisting chronic pain conditions, and preexisting psychiatric disease such as depression are all risk factors for chronicity.

Treatment of chronic low back pain remains extremely challenging, as shown by the high prevalence of the condition and its associated disability. For proven treatments, the clinical effect is typically small and useful only for the short term. Therefore, a biopsychosocial rehabilitation program—involving a combination of medical, physical, psychological, educational, and work-related components—is recommend to address the many facets of the biopsychosocial pain model. Unfortunately limited availability and high cost remain major hurdles

to implement these treatments, and most patients receive only small fractions of this broader approach.

According to the American College of Physicians 2017 practice guidelines, nonpharmacologic treatments should be considered first, including exercise, multidisciplinary rehabilitation, acupuncture, mindfulness-based stress reduction (moderate-quality evidence), tai chi, yoga, motor control exercise, progressive relaxation, electromyography biofeedback, low-level laser therapy, operant therapy, cognitive behavioral therapy, or spinal manipulation (all having low-quality evidence). If these measures are unsuccessful, first-line pharmacologic treatment consists of NSAIDs; second-line treatment consists of tramadol and duloxetine. The use of stronger opioids has been shown to have only small short-term benefit and must be carefully weighed against their side effects and risks of dependence and misuse. Gabapentin and amitriptyline have been shown to have no benefit for chronic low back pain.

Fluoroscopy-guided interventions are sometimes used to treat patients with refractory low back pain. Procedures include epidural steroid injections, lumbar facet blocks, SI joint injections, and radiofrequency

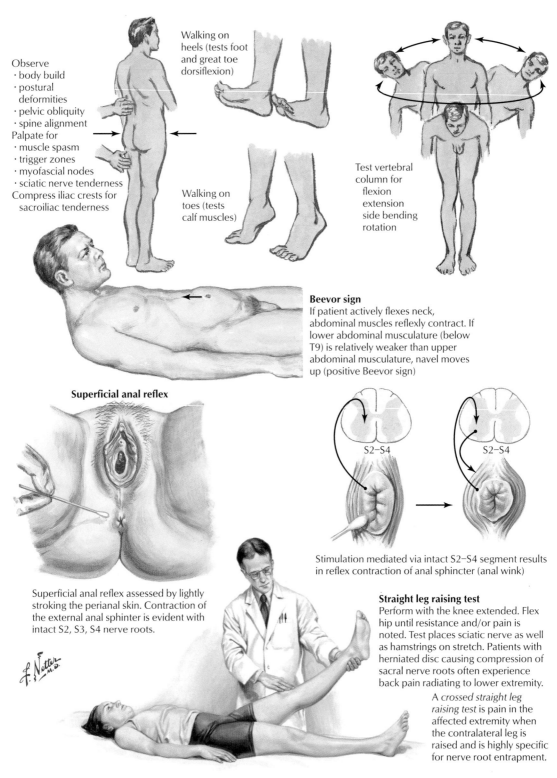

Observe
· body build
· postural deformities
· pelvic obliquity
· spine alignment

Palpate for
· muscle spasm
· trigger zones
· myofascial nodes
· sciatic nerve tenderness

Compress iliac crests for sacroiliac tenderness

Walking on heels (tests foot and great toe dorsiflexion)

Walking on toes (tests calf muscles)

Test vertebral column for flexion extension side bending rotation

Beevor sign
If patient actively flexes neck, abdominal muscles reflexly contract. If lower abdominal musculature (below T9) is relatively weaker than upper abdominal musculature, navel moves up (positive Beevor sign)

Superficial anal reflex

S2–S4

S2–S4

Stimulation mediated via intact S2–S4 segment results in reflex contraction of anal sphincter (anal wink)

Superficial anal reflex assessed by lightly stroking the perianal skin. Contraction of the external anal sphinter is evident with intact S2, S3, S4 nerve roots.

Straight leg raising test
Perform with the knee extended. Flex hip until resistance and/or pain is noted. Test places sciatic nerve as well as hamstrings on stretch. Patients with herniated disc causing compression of sacral nerve roots often experience back pain radiating to lower extremity.

A *crossed straight leg raising test* is pain in the affected extremity when the contralateral leg is raised and is highly specific for nerve root entrapment.

Fig. 58.3 Physical Exam for Low Back Pain.

ablations of sensory nerve fibers innervating lumbar facet and SI joints. Although short-term improvement from these procedures is common, evidence for long-term benefit is contradictory. Neurosurgical procedures for benign low back pain—including disc replacement, decompressive surgery, and lumbar fusion—have outcomes similar to those of intensive rehabilitation programs; moreover, they run the risk of creating a chronic "failed back syndrome." However, for significant compressive pathology such as spinal myelopathy, cauda equina syndrome, radiculopathy with significant neurologic deficits, or spinal instability, prompt neurosurgical intervention can be curative. Spinal cord stimulation therapy has recently emerged as a promising albeit invasive treatment option for longer-term improvement in patients with refractory low back pain; however, long-term studies are needed to ensure that this is an efficacious and well-tolerated option.

ADDITIONAL RESOURCES

Koes BW, van Tulder MW, Thomas S. Diagnosis and treatment of low back pain. BMJ 2006;332(7555):1430–4.

Question-and-answer format for the diagnosis, treatment, and prognosis of low back pain.

Vardeh D, Mannion RJ, Woolf CJ. Toward a mechanism-based approach to pain diagnosis. J Pain 2016;17.

Overview of mechanisms contributing to low back pain.

Froud R, Patterson S, Eldridge S, et al. A systematic review and meta-synthesis of the impact of low back pain on people's lives. BMC Musculoskelet Disord 2014;15:50.

Impact of low back pain on social function.

Kamper SJ, Apeldoorn AT, Chiarotto A, et al. Multidisciplinary biopsychosocial rehabilitation for chronic low back pain: Cochrane systematic review and meta-analysis. BMJ 2015;350:h444.

Evaluation of biopsychosocial rehabilitation for chronic low back pain.

Jensen MC, Brant-Zawadzki MN, Obuchowski N, et al. Magnetic resonance imaging of the lumbar spine in people without back pain. N Engl J Med 1994;331(2):69–73.

Description of lumbar MRI findings in asymptomatic patients.

Qaseem A, Wilt TJ, McLean RM, et al. Clinical Guidelines Committee of the American College of Physicians. Noninvasive treatments for acute, subacute, and chronic low back pain: a clinical practice guideline from the American College of Physicians. Ann Intern Med 2017;166(7):514–30.

Treatment guidelines by the American College of Physicians for noninvasive treatments for low back pain.

Chou R, Deyo R, Friedly J, et al. Nonpharmacologic therapies for low back pain: a systematic review for an American College of Physicians clinical practice guideline. Ann Intern Med 2017;166(7):493–505.

Treatment guidelines by the American College of Physicians for nonpharmacologic treatments for low back pain.

59

Brachial and Lumbosacral Plexopathies

Sui Li, Ted M. Burns, Monique M. Ryan, H. Royden Jones, Jr.[†]

CLINICAL VIGNETTE *A 54-year-old man developed acute-onset right thigh, hip, and buttock pain. He reported right knee "buckling" when he stepped off a curb, resulting in a fall. He also noted right foot drop. Paresthesias developed over the right thigh, shin, and foot. He required oral narcotics for pain relief.*

His past medical history was remarkable for type II diabetes mellitus, for which he took an oral hypoglycemic. His blood sugars had been under fair control. His review of systems was remarkable for a 30-pound weight loss over the past 3 months, which he attributed to renewed efforts at dieting. He did not smoke or drink heavily. He was an attorney. Family history was negative.

His general examination was unremarkable. His neurologic examination was notable for moderate weakness of right hip flexion, hip extension, knee extension, and ankle dorsiflexion. He had an absent right knee and ankle reflex, but reflexes were normal on the left lower extremity and upper extremities. Sensory testing demonstrated reduced vibration sensation at the right great toe and ankle. His gait was hesitant and revealed a right foot drop.

Electromyography (EMG) demonstrated borderline right peroneal and tibial compound motor action potentials with normal velocities and distal latencies. The sural and superficial peroneal sensory nerve action potentials were absent on the right and normal on the left. Active denervation was present in right femoral- and sciatic-innervated muscles, and to a lesser extent in lumbosacral paraspinals and gluteal muscles.

Magnetic resonance imaging (MRI) of the lumbosacral spine and pelvis was unremarkable, except for signal changes in denervating muscles. A lumbar puncture demonstrated an elevated cerebrospinal fluid (CSF) protein with a normal cell count. Glycosylated hemoglobin was slightly elevated but otherwise his laboratory studies were normal.

He was diagnosed with diabetic lumbosacral radiculoplexus neuropathy (also known as diabetic amyotrophy). After discussion of the pros and cons he was prescribed an empiric trial of intravenous methylprednisolone.

The most important diagnostic tool for the evaluation of a possible plexopathy is a thorough and accurate history. The history-taking must be aided by a solid understanding of the risk factors for brachial or lumbosacral plexopathy. The most common etiologies of plexopathy are trauma, surgery (e.g., related to arm or leg positioning, injury with regional anesthetic block), injury at birth, inherited genetic mutations (e.g., hereditary neuralgic amyotrophy), primary autoimmune processes (e.g., Parsonage–Turner, also known as neuralgic amyotrophy), previous radiotherapy, and neoplastic invasion (Fig. 59.1; Table 59.1). Systemic vasculitis and peripheral nerve sarcoidosis are other uncommon etiologies. Diabetes mellitus is a risk factor for an immune-mediated lumbosacral (and less often, brachial) plexopathy, known as diabetic lumbosacral radiculoplexus neuropathy (DLRPN). Thus, if a prior or concomitant history of any of these risk factors (e.g., previous surgery, trauma, diabetes, or family history of plexopathy) is present, the clinician must take that into consideration. It is also helpful to remember that recent infection, vaccination, and parturition are triggers for the immune-mediated plexopathies, especially brachial plexopathies. There are often other clues about etiology found in the presenting symptoms. For example, the abrupt, spontaneous onset of shoulder and upper extremity symptoms favors an immune-mediated mechanism, such as that seen with hereditary neuralgic amyotrophy, neuralgic amyotrophy, and diabetic cervical radiculoplexus neuropathy (diabetic CRPN). A more gradual or insidious onset of symptoms would point toward neoplastic invasion or postradiotherapy plexopathy. Immune-mediated plexopathies (e.g., DLRPN, CRPN, or neuralgic amyotrophy) usually begin with severe pain, lasting days to weeks, followed by the development of weakness a few days to weeks later. Radiation-associated plexopathy usually presents with less pain and has a more gradual onset, often months to decades after radiotherapy. Recurrent, painful brachial plexopathy is most typical of hereditary neuralgic amyotrophy. The recognition of accompanying symptoms is also important. For example, weight loss is a common accompaniment of DLRPN or CRPN, as well as plexopathies secondary to neoplasm or a systemic vasculitis.

In the case presented earlier, the temporal evolution was of an abrupt-onset neuropathic process in one lower extremity. The pain was so severe that the patient required narcotics. The patient had not experienced antecedent trauma, surgery, or radiotherapy. There was no family history of plexopathy. These factors suggested that an immune-mediated plexopathy was likely. Furthermore, the clinical setting was remarkable for diabetes mellitus and weight loss. Diabetes mellitus is believed to be a significant risk factor for immune-mediated plexopathy. Many of these patients experience contemporaneous weight loss. Additional evaluation, including examination, electrodiagnostic testing, and imaging, further supported the diagnosis of DLRPN (Fig. 59.2).

CLINICAL PRESENTATION

Plexus lesions commonly result in unilateral or asymmetric extremity muscle weakness and sensory complaints that do not conform to the distributions of single roots or nerves. Brachial plexopathies cause shoulder girdle weakness if the upper plexus is involved and hand weakness if the lower or medial plexus is principally involved. Sensory loss is usually variable but follows a similar pattern; for example, a medial plexus lesion causes numbness of the fourth and fifth fingers. Autonomic disturbances, caused by disruption of the sympathetic fibers traversing the lower trunk to the superior cervical ganglia of the brachial plexus,

---

[†]Deceased.

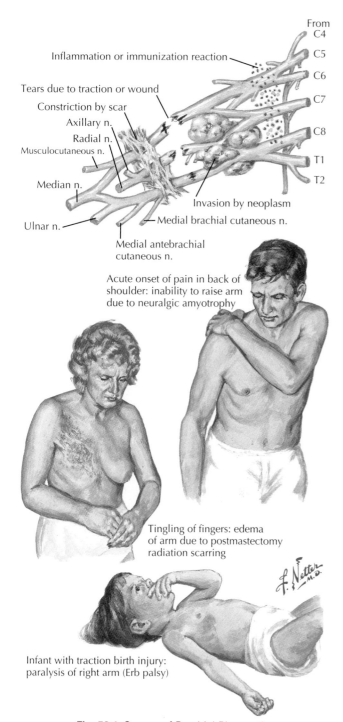

Inflammation or immunization reaction

From
C4
C5
C6
C7
C8
T1
T2

Tears due to traction or wound

Constriction by scar

Axillary n.

Radial n.

Musculocutaneous n.

Median n.

Ulnar n.

Medial antebrachial cutaneous n.

Invasion by neoplasm

Medial brachial cutaneous n.

Acute onset of pain in back of shoulder: inability to raise arm due to neuralgic amyotrophy

Tingling of fingers: edema of arm due to postmastectomy radiation scarring

Infant with traction birth injury: paralysis of right arm (Erb palsy)

Fig. 59.1 Causes of Brachial Plexopathy.

reasonably exclude pure motor processes, such as motor neuronopathies (e.g., amyotrophic lateral sclerosis), disorders of neuromuscular junction transmission (e.g., myasthenia gravis), and myopathies. Orthopedic injuries can sometimes mimic plexopathy; electrodiagnostic testing may rule out underlying nerve damage. The most important mimic of plexopathy is polyradiculopathy; nerve root lesions also present with both weakness and pain. The mechanism of nerve root injury may be structural (e.g., neural foraminal stenosis or disk herniation), infectious (e.g., Lyme neuroborreliosis), or neoplastic (e.g., carcinomatous meningitis).

ANATOMY

Brachial Plexus

The brachial plexus is formed from the ventral rami of cervical roots 5 to 8 and thoracic root 1 (Fig. 59.3). The ventral rami of the fifth and sixth cervical roots together form the upper trunk, the ventral ramus of the seventh cervical root becomes the middle trunk, and the ventral rami of the eighth cervical and first thoracic root join to form the lower trunk. The trunks of the brachial plexus are located above the clavicle between the scalenus anterior and scalenus medius muscles, in the posterior triangle of the neck, posterior and lateral to the sternocleidomastoid muscle. The dorsal scapular, long thoracic, and suprascapular nerves originate from the brachial plexus above the clavicle. Behind the clavicle and in front of the first rib, each trunk separates into anterior and posterior divisions. The anterior divisions of the upper and middle trunks unite to become the lateral cord, whereas the anterior division of the lower trunk forms the medial cord. The posterior divisions of all three trunks unite to become the posterior cord. The three cords are named for their positions relative to the axillary artery. Below the clavicle, the upper extremity nerves arise from the cords. The musculocutaneous, the lateral head of the median, and the lateral pectoral nerves arise from the lateral cord. The ulnar, the medial head of the median, the medial pectoral, and the medial brachial and medial antebrachial nerves come from the medial cord. The radial, axillary, subscapular, and thoracodorsal nerves arise from the posterior cord.

Lumbosacral Plexus

The femoral nerve, innervating the iliopsoas and the quadriceps femoris muscles, is the predominant derivative of the lumbar portion of the lumbosacral plexus (Fig. 59.4). Its sensory supply includes the anterior and lateral thigh. The femoral nerve terminates into the saphenous nerve, which is a pure sensory nerve of the medial foreleg. The obturator nerve innervating the adductor magnus also originates from the lumbar plexus. The sacral portion of the lumbosacral plexus innervates the remainder of the lower extremity muscles, including posterior thigh and buttocks muscles and all leg musculature below the knee. The superior and inferior gluteal nerves, the most proximal nerves originating from the sacral derivative of the lumbosacral plexus, innervate the gluteal muscles (medius, minimus, and maximus). The sciatic nerve innervates the hamstring group and bifurcates into the peroneal (fibular) and tibial nerves, providing all motor innervation below the knee. The sciatic nerve provides sensory innervation to the posterior thigh and the entire leg below the knee, with the exception of the medial foreleg, which is supplied only by the saphenous nerve. The peroneal (fibular) nerve is derived from the lateral portion of the sciatic nerve within the thigh; it supplies only one muscle above the knee, the short head of the biceps femoris. This site provides a means to differentiate proximal peroneal or sciatic nerve lesions from common peroneal nerve compression or entrapment syndromes at the fibular head. The peroneal nerve bifurcates into the superficial and deep peroneal nerves, the latter innervating all anterior compartment muscles. The superficial peroneal

may be present and include trophic skin changes, edema, reflex sympathetic dystrophy (complex regional pain syndrome), and Horner syndrome (miosis, ptosis, ipsilateral facial anhidrosis).

Upper plexus lesions of the lumbar plexus cause weakness of thigh flexion, adduction, and knee extension. Lower sacral plexus lesions result in weakness of thigh extension, knee flexion, foot dorsiflexion, and plantar flexion. Sensory changes are seen in both lesions. Complete lumbosacral plexopathy produces weakness and muscle atrophy throughout the lower extremity, with total areflexia and anesthesia. Concurrent autonomic loss results in warm, dry skin and peripheral edema.

In addition to differentiating etiologies for plexopathy, the clinician needs to consider mimickers. The presence of neuropathic pain can

TABLE 59.1	**Brachial Plexus Etiologies**	
Mechanism	**Examples**	**Comments**
Trauma, traction	Motorcycle injury, cardiothoracic surgery	Often severe degree, poor prognosis
Stinger	Football, etc.	Good prognosis
Perinatal	Mixed mechanisms	Generally good prognosis
Idiopathic	Autoimmune?	Self-limited
Hereditary	Genetically determined	Recurrent, benign
Malignancy	Infiltration of tumor cells	Poor prognosis
Radiation	RoRx-induced ischemia	Prognosis guarded but not suggestive of recurrent tumor
Knapsack, rucksack, etc.	Compression	Usually self-limited
Thoracic outlet	Entrapment	Rare, confused with CTS
Heroin induced	Indeterminate	

CTS, Carpal tunnel syndrome; *RoRx,* radiation therapy.

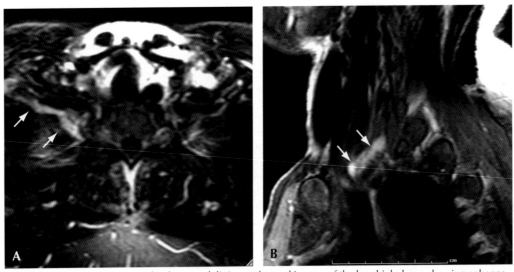

Axial (**A**) and sagittal (**B**) T1-weighted post gadolinium-enhanced images of the brachial plexus showing enhancement around the right brachial plexus (arrows).

Fig. 59.2 Parsonage-Turner Brachial Plexitis.

motor nerve supplies the lateral compartment. The tibial nerve, the other primary sciatic nerve derivative, supplies the calf. In addition to the saphenous nerve, the superficial peroneal sensory, the sural, and the medial and lateral plantar nerves are the primary superficial sensory nerves below the knee.

DIAGNOSTIC APPROACH

The neurologic examination should focus on identifying any motor, sensory, and reflex impairment referable to the different components of the plexus. For example, a diminished or absent biceps reflex would be expected for a brachial plexopathy involving the upper trunk. Weakness involving the hand and wrist would point toward lower trunk/ medial cord brachial plexus involvement. In addition to localizing a lesion to particular trunks and cords, the examination can sometimes help determine whether lesions are preganglionic (e.g., root avulsion) or postganglionic (e.g., upper trunk plexopathy). Weakness of the rhomboid muscles (from C4 and C5 roots) and the serratus anterior muscle (from C5, C6, and C7 roots) would suggest involvement as proximal as the cervical root. Needle examination of these muscles and cervical paraspinal muscles, discussed below, will be helpful also in determining where the lesions are along the length of the nerve.

Electrodiagnostic (EDX) testing helps confirm the diagnosis and localization of a suspected plexopathy. Rarely, nonneuropathic processes (e.g., rotator cuff tendinitis, hip fracture) can mimic plexopathy, in which case EDX testing will be normal. More commonly, EDX testing serves to confirm the localization of a neuropathic process to the plexus. Lesions may also be proximal to the dorsal root ganglia (DRG). These are classified as preganglionic lesions, whereas those distal to the DRG are labeled as postganglionic lesions. Assessment of sensory nerve action potentials (SNAPs) is very helpful with this localization because the preservation of SNAPs favors a preganglionic lesion (e.g., radiculopathy), whereas the diminution or loss of SNAPs favors a postganglionic lesion (e.g., plexopathy). For a unilateral plexopathy, the SNAP abnormality should be on the side of the lesion, and for bilateral, asymmetric plexopathies, the SNAP abnormalities should theoretically be more severe on the more affected side. Side-to-side differences in SNAP amplitude of greater than 50% are typically considered significant. Differentiating preganglionic radiculopathy from postganglionic plexopathy is important when trying to evaluate for structural (e.g., spinal stenosis), infectious (e.g., Lyme), or neoplastic etiologies. Determining whether a traumatic plexus injury is preganglionic or postganglionic is also important for surgical management. For instance, preganglionic lesions (e.g., root avulsions) are generally not amenable to direct plexus repair with nerve grafting and

Comparison of Embryonic Limb Organization to the Plan of the Brachial Plexus

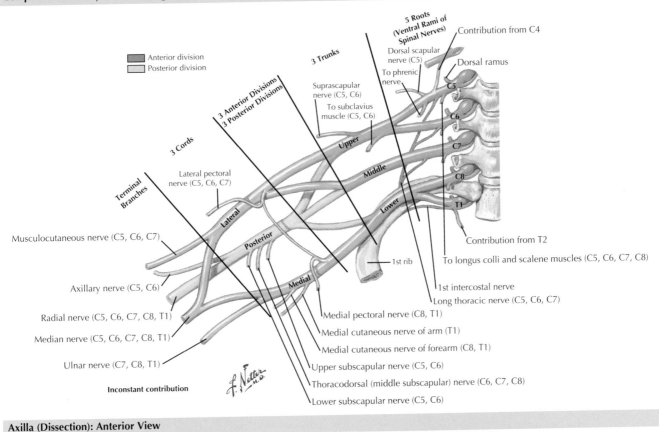

Axilla (Dissection): Anterior View

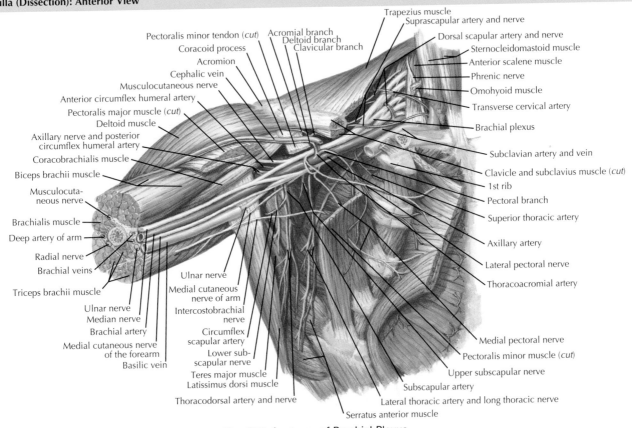

Fig. 59.3 Anatomy of Brachial Plexus.

Lumbar Plexus

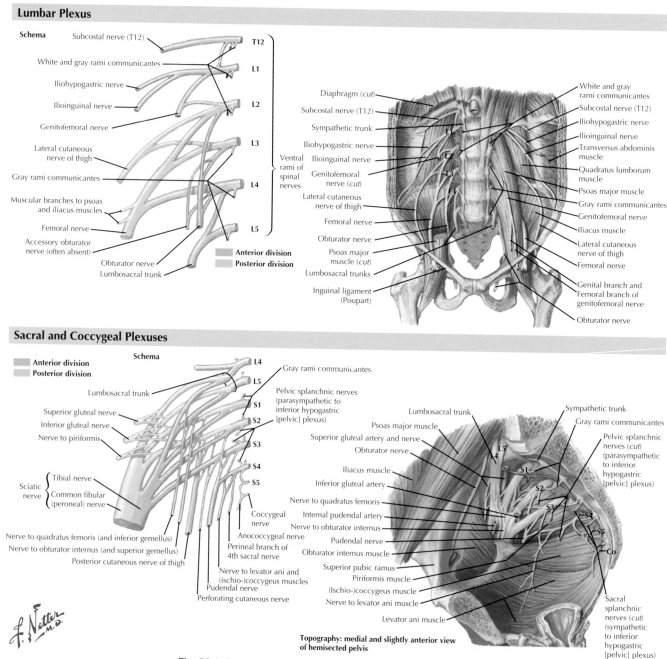

Fig. 59.4 Anatomy of Lumbar, Sacral, and Coccygeal Plexuses.

hence would more likely be surgically treated with a nerve transfer (e.g., spinal accessory nerve to suprascapular nerve in order to allow shoulder abduction, ulnar nerve fascicle innervating the flexor carpi ulnaris to the musculocutaneous nerve in order to allow elbow flexion). On the other hand, postganglionic lesions may be directly repaired at the plexus with nerve grafting or internal neurolysis. In the case presented earlier, the absent sural sensory and superficial peroneal sensory responses were consistent with a postganglionic plexopathy. Motor nerve conduction studies should also be performed, particularly to look for low compound motor action potential amplitudes over muscles innervated by affected nerves. Needle examination should *ideally* be performed at least 2 to 3 weeks after onset in order to maximize yield, but it still can be helpful to perform a study earlier because reduced recruitment of motor unit potentials of weak muscles can help with localization. The presence of fibrillation potentials in paraspinal muscles would point to involvement of the roots; however, the absence of fibrillation potentials in the

paraspinals does not exclude radiculopathy because needle examination of paraspinal muscles will be normal in about half of the patients with radiculopathy. It is important also to note that patients with radiculoplexus neuropathies will demonstrate evidence of both preganglionic and postganglionic damage. Needle examination can also sometimes assist in determining etiology. For example, plexopathies secondary to radiotherapy are sometimes associated with myokymic discharges on needle study.

Routine radiographs, computed tomography (CT), and MRI of the lumbosacral spine and pelvis are often required to exclude inflammatory or mass lesions within the spine or pelvis. CSF examination may be indicated to exclude infection. CSF protein is increased in approximately 50% of patients with idiopathic lumbosacral plexopathy. In vasculitic lumbosacral plexopathy, nerve biopsy may reveal ischemic nerve injury caused by vasculitis. Histopathologic evidence of vasculitis is frequently seen on biopsy of patients with DLRPN.

DIFFERENTIAL DIAGNOSIS

Trauma is the most common pathophysiologic mechanism for a brachial plexopathy. The superficial anatomic location of the brachial plexus with close proximity to bony and vascular structures within the shoulder and neck predisposes it to this risk. Traumatic mechanisms for brachial plexopathy include compression, traction, ischemia, or laceration. Motor vehicle accidents, high-speed cycling accidents, gunshot or knife wounds, and falls can be the inciting cause. Some events may be iatrogenic; for example, positioning during cardiothoracic surgery that maximally abducts the arm may cause stretching of the lateral brachial plexus. Sporting activities causing "burners" or "stingers" are common mechanisms for brachial plexopathy; despite their relative frequency, the pathophysiology is unclear. These injuries are likely caused by compression, traction, or both, usually of the C5–6 cervical nerve roots and upper trunk of the brachial plexus. Trauma to the lumbosacral plexus, on the other hand, is uncommon because the nerves are relatively immobile and protected by the vertebrae, psoas muscle, and pelvis. Most traumatic injuries are associated with pelvic or acetabular fractures, as well as with soft-tissue injuries to other pelvic organs.

Neuralgic amyotrophy (also known as idiopathic brachial plexus neuropathy or Parsonage–Turner syndrome) and DLRPN (also known as diabetic amyotrophy) are thought to be autoimmune in origin. Both conditions are likely caused by microvasculitis, in which case the autoimmune attack is directed at small vessels within and near the nerves of the roots and plexus. Neuralgic amyotrophy of the brachial plexus sometimes occurs after a viral illness, vaccination, mild trauma, or during the immediate postpartum period. Usually, these patients present with relatively acute shoulder pain and partial loss of brachial plexus function. Typically, neuralgic amyotrophy predominantly affects nerves of the shoulder girdle muscles, although other portions of the plexus and its terminal branches are occasionally involved, especially the anterior interosseous segment of the median nerve. Approximately one-third of patients with neuralgic amyotrophy have bilateral, asymmetric involvement.

DLRPN is the most common cause of lumbosacral plexopathy (Fig. 59.5). DLRPN typically presents in older patients who have type 2 diabetes mellitus, with abrupt or subacute onset of hip and thigh severe pain (see case presentation earlier). Weakness and muscle atrophy occur within a week or two, often at the time the pain begins to improve. Muscle stretch reflexes may be lost, especially at the knee. DLRPN often begins unilaterally but frequently progresses to bilateral involvement. This monophasic disorder is usually disabling and is commonly associated with unexplained weight loss. Like neuralgic amyotrophy, DLRPN is thought to originate from peripheral nerve microvasculitis. Idiopathic LRPN is a rare primary plexopathy that occurs in nondiabetics. It is also manifested by rapid onset of pain, leg weakness, and atrophy. Patients often experience a viral illness 1 to 2 weeks before symptoms begin. Lumbar plexus involvement often affects the most proximal musculature, causing weakness of the iliopsoas, quadriceps, and adductor muscles. Often, significant recovery occurs within 3 months.

Hereditary neuralgic amyotrophy (also known as hereditary brachial plexus neuropathy [HBPN]) is an autosomal dominant disorder characterized by periodic, often recurrent, episodes of unilateral or asymmetric pain, weakness, atrophy, and sensory alterations in the shoulder girdle and upper extremity. Genetically, many cases of HBPN are caused by mutations in the *SEPT9* gene. Hereditary neuralgic amyotrophy is also believed to be an immune-mediated disorder and likely a microvasculitis with a strong genetic predisposition caused by an inherited *SEPT9* mutation.

Malignant tumors, particularly apical lung or postradiation breast cancer, are common causes of brachial plexus lesions (Fig. 59.6). With

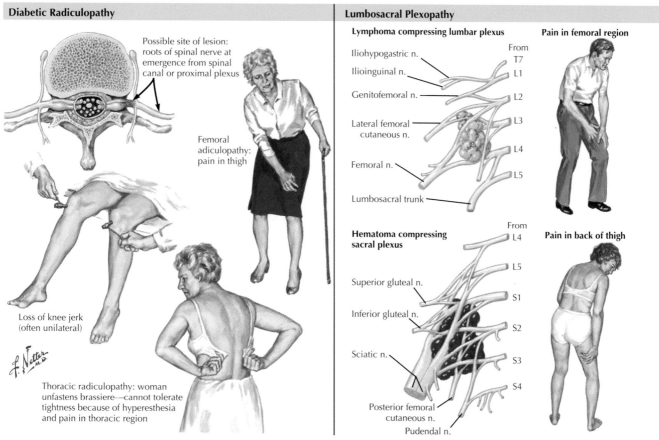

Diabetic Radiculopathy

Possible site of lesion: roots of spinal nerve at emergence from spinal canal or proximal plexus

Femoral adiculopathy: pain in thigh

Loss of knee jerk (often unilateral)

Thoracic radiculopathy: woman unfastens brassiere—cannot tolerate tightness because of hyperesthesia and pain in thoracic region

Lumbosacral Plexopathy

Lymphoma compressing lumbar plexus

Iliohypogastric n.
Ilioinguinal n.
Genitofemoral n.
Lateral femoral cutaneous n.
Femoral n.
Lumbosacral trunk

From T7
L1
L2
L3
L4
L5

Pain in femoral region

Hematoma compressing sacral plexus

Superior gluteal n.
Inferior gluteal n.
Sciatic n.
Posterior femoral cutaneous n.
Pudendal n.

From L4
L5
S1
S2
S3
S4

Pain in back of thigh

Fig. 59.5 Causes of Lumbosacral Radiculoplexopathies.

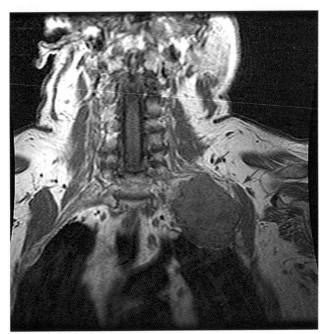

Coronal T1-weighted image demonstrates large left apical lung mass extending into brachial plexus (arrows).

Fig. 59.6 Apical Lung Tumor Invading Left Brachial Plexus.

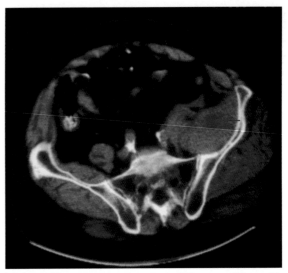

Fig. 59.7 Large Hematoma Involves the Left Iliacus and Psoas Muscles *(Arrow)* and Adjacent Region, Likely Involving the Lumbar Plexus and Femoral Nerve.

apical lung tumors (Pancoast tumor), the lesion may insidiously cause compression, leading to numbness in the fourth and fifth fingers, weakness in the ulnar and median hand intrinsic muscles, and Horner syndrome (Pancoast tumor). Often, pain is significant, secondary to neoplastic infiltration of the brachial plexus. This clinical constellation sometimes precedes recognition of the lung tumor. Every patient who smokes and presents in this fashion requires a chest CT or MRI. Tumors occasionally invade the lumbosacral plexus by primary extension from pelvic, abdominal, or retroperitoneal malignancies (see Fig. 59.5). Pain in the distribution of the affected nerves is the cardinal symptom. Late symptoms and signs may include numbness and paresthesias, weakness and gait abnormalities, and lower extremity edema. Retroperitoneal hematomas can compress the lumbar or sacral plexuses or both. Patients present with unilateral pelvic or groin pain; the patient preferentially has the hip flexed to minimize pressure on the plexus (Fig. 59.7). This condition is typically a complication of anticoagulation therapy—or less commonly bleeding diatheses—and immediate surgical decompression can be beneficial.

Compressive lumbosacral plexopathies may also occur from other mechanisms, including late pregnancy or childbirth and abdominal aortic aneurysms. A retroperitoneal infection, such as a psoas abscess, rarely affects the lumbosacral plexus. Radiation-induced lumbosacral plexopathies develop months to years after radiotherapy to pelvic malignancies. The lumbar plexus is more commonly affected in radiation-induced lesions, whereas the sacral plexus is more frequently affected by neoplastic plexopathies. Painless weakness develops at a variable rate, ultimately causing asymmetric but significant weakness of both lower extremities. Paresthesias and pain are common but usually mild. Sphincter involvement is rare.

TREATMENT AND PROGNOSIS

Treatment of plexus lesions involves management of the primary condition. Careful glucose control may hasten DLRPN recovery and improve outcome. The efficacy of steroids or intravenous immunoglobulin in the acute or subacute phase of DLRPN is not proven, although anecdotal reports suggest clinical benefit. Some evidence is emerging that the pain and other neuropathic symptoms may respond to these treatment options. Most traumatic lesions are treated conservatively, although some may necessitate surgery. No effective treatment exists for radiation-induced brachial or lumbosacral plexopathy. Oncologic intervention is necessary for neoplastic brachial or lumbosacral plexopathy. Pain control with narcotics is often necessary in the acute phase of DLRPN, LRPN, neuralgic amyotrophy, hereditary neuralgic amyotrophy, traumatic plexopathy, and neoplastic plexopathies.

ADDITIONAL RESOURCES

Dyck PJ, Norell JE, Dyck PJ. Microvasculitis and ischemia in diabetic lumbosacral radiculoplexus neuropathy. Neurology 1999;53:2113–21.

Dyck PJ, Norell JE, Dyck PJ. Non-diabetic lumbosacral radiculoplexus neuropathy: natural history, outcome and comparison with the diabetic variety. Brain 2001;124:1197–207.

Ferrante MA. Brachial plexopathies: classification, causes, and consequences. Muscle Nerve 2004;30:547–68.

Lederman RJ, Wilbourn AJ. Postpartum neuralgic amyotrophy. Neurology 1996;47:1213–19.

Moghekar AR, Moghekar AB, Karli N, et al. Brachial plexopathies. Etiology, frequency and electrodiagnostic localization. J Clin Neuromuscul Dis 2007;9:243–7.

Parsonage MJ, Turner JWA. Neuralgic amyotrophy. The shoulder-girdle syndrome. Lancet 1948;973–8.

Rubin DI. Diseases of the plexus. Continuum (N Y) 2008;14:156–81.

Suarez GA, Giannini C, Bosch EP, et al. Immune brachial plexus neuropathy: suggestive evidence for an inflammatory immune pathogenesis. Neurology 1996;46:559–61.

Triggs W, Young MS, Eskin T, et al. Treatment of idiopathic lumbosacral plexopathy with intravenous immunoglobulin. Muscle Nerve 1997;20:244–6.

Tsairis P, Dyck PJ, Mulder DW. Natural history of brachial plexus neuropathy. Report on 99 patients. Arch Neurol 1972;27:109–17.

Van Alfen N. The neuralgic amyotrophy consultation. J Neurol 2007;254:695–704.

Van Alfen N, van Engelen BGM. The clinical spectrum of neuralgic amyotrophy in 246 cases. Brain 2006;129:438–50.

Verma A, Bradley WB. High dose intravenous immunoglobulin therapy in chronic progressive lumbosacral plexopathy. Neurology 1994;44:248–50.

Mononeuropathies

Jayashri Srinivasan

60

Mononeuropathies of the Upper Extremities

Gisela Held

MONONEUROPATHIES OF THE SHOULDER GIRDLE

Mononeuropathies of the shoulder girdle are relatively uncommon and can be challenging to diagnose. Unlike other mononeuropathies, pain is often the cardinal symptom. Shoulder pain and weakness can originate not only from mononeuropathies, but also from cervical disc disease, disorders of the musculoskeletal system, or vascular causes. True weakness can be difficult to separate from impaired effort due to pain. Shoulder muscles might appear weak in rotator cuff or other tendon tears in the absence of nerve injury.

Shoulder girdle mononeuropathies are caused by the following mechanisms: stretch, transecting injury, brachial plexus neuritis with patchy involvement of isolated nerves, direct compression, or entrapment. The history should help define the precise location of the pain, the positions and activities that provoke pain, the time of day of maximal discomfort, and any precipitating injury. Paresthesias or sensory loss, particularly if defined within a recognized single nerve distribution, usually indicates peripheral nerve pathology. Atrophy can be related to axon loss or occasionally prolonged disuse; sometimes the clinical distinction is difficult. Shoulder motion is evaluated for abnormal dynamics of the glenohumeral, acromioclavicular, and scapulothoracic joints.

Long Thoracic Neuropathies

> **CLINICAL VIGNETTE** *A 57-year-old left-handed woman underwent a left mastectomy for breast cancer. Immediately following the surgery, she noted an aching pain in the left posterior shoulder area. After discharge from the hospital, she had difficulty using her left arm. In particular, she complained of being unable to get dishes from the kitchen cabinets. She was not aware of sensory loss. Electrodiagnostic testing 3 weeks later showed evidence of acute denervation changes in the left serratus anterior muscle, consistent with a mononeuropathy of the long thoracic nerve.*

The long thoracic nerve originates directly from C5–C7 roots, before the formation of the brachial plexus. It innervates the serratus anterior muscle and has no cutaneous sensory representation (Fig. 60.1). Weakness of the serratus anterior is debilitating because it stabilizes the scapula for pushing movements and elevates the arm above 90 degrees. This is the most common cause of scapular winging; it is best recognized by having the patient push against a wall. The inferior medial border is the most prominently projected away from the body wall. A dull shoulder ache may accompany this neuropathy. When severe acute pain occurs with the onset of scapular winging, brachial plexus neuritis should be considered.

The long thoracic nerve may be damaged by mechanical factors, including repetitive or particularly forceful injuries to the shoulder or lateral thoracic wall, and by surgical procedures including first rib resection, mastectomy, or thoracotomy. It is one of the most common nerves to be affected by acute brachial neuritis, solely or in combination with others.

Scapular winging also can be related to scapular fracture and avulsion. Because they are surgically correctable, it is important to distinguish them from a primary long thoracic nerve injury. Furthermore, scapular winging can be caused by weakness of the trapezius (resulting from injury of the spinal accessory nerve) or the rhomboid muscles (resulting from a dorsal scapular nerve lesion). Inspection of the posterior shoulder region can provide diagnostic clues. Although the scapula is typically displaced medially in long thoracic nerve lesions, lateral deviation points to weakness of the trapezius or rhomboids. Scapular winging is a predominant feature in patients with facioscapulohumeral muscular dystrophy, where its bilateral representation and the other associated clinical features distinguish it from long thoracic nerve palsy.

Dorsal Scapular Neuropathies

> **CLINICAL VIGNETTE** *A 27-year-old professional weight lifter complained of difficulty exercising. He had trouble getting his wallet out of the right back pocket of his pants. Examination revealed weakness of the right rhomboid muscles without noticeable muscle atrophy. There was scapular winging with lateral displacement of the scapula, which was most pronounced during elevation of the arm. Electrophysiologic testing disclosed active and chronic denervation-reinnervation changes in the right rhomboids. Testing of other arm and shoulder muscles was normal.*

The dorsal scapular nerve receives fibers from the C5 nerve root. It innervates the levator scapulae and the rhomboideus major and minor muscles, which assist in the stabilization of the scapula, the rotation of the scapula in a medial-inferior direction, and the elevation of the arm (Fig. 60.2). Rhomboid weakness can lead to scapular winging, which is most prominent when the patient raises the arm overhead. Possible etiologies of injury to this nerve include shoulder dislocation, weightlifting, and entrapment by the scalenus medius muscle.

Suprascapular Neuropathies

> **CLINICAL VIGNETTE** *A 25-year-old right-handed woman was evaluated for dull right shoulder pain and weakness. The symptoms were most noticeable during overhead activities. She had no sensory loss, and no injury had preceded the onset of her symptoms. Examination disclosed tenderness to palpation at the spinoglenoid notch. Shoulder position was normal; range*

Suprascapular Nerve

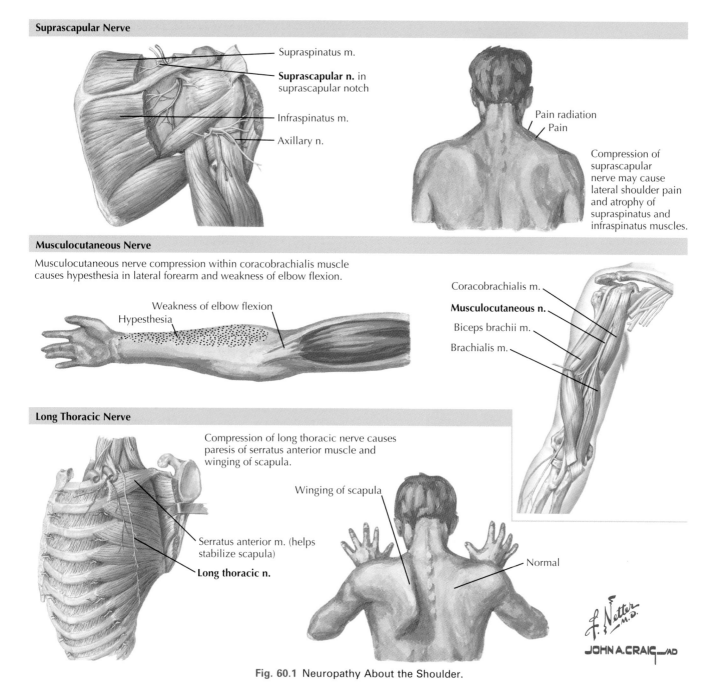

Supraspinatus m.

Suprascapular n. in suprascapular notch

Infraspinatus m.

Axillary n.

Pain radiation
Pain

Compression of suprascapular nerve may cause lateral shoulder pain and atrophy of supraspinatus and infraspinatus muscles.

Musculocutaneous Nerve

Musculocutaneous nerve compression within coracobrachialis muscle causes hypesthesia in lateral forearm and weakness of elbow flexion.

Weakness of elbow flexion
Hypesthesia

Coracobrachialis m.

Musculocutaneous n.

Biceps brachii m.

Brachialis m.

Long Thoracic Nerve

Compression of long thoracic nerve causes paresis of serratus anterior muscle and winging of scapula.

Winging of scapula

Serratus anterior m. (helps stabilize scapula)

Long thoracic n.

Normal

JOHN A. CRAIG—AD

Fig. 60.1 Neuropathy About the Shoulder.

of motion was full. Motor examination was significant for weakness of external shoulder rotation and mild atrophy of the infraspinatus muscle overlying the scapula. Reflexes and sensory examination were normal. These findings of infraspinatus atrophy, weak external rotation of the shoulder, and point tenderness over the spinoglenoid notch were consistent with a focal suprascapular neuropathy. Electromyography (EMG) demonstrated active denervation changes confined to the infraspinatus muscle, consistent with the clinical diagnosis. A magnetic resonance image (MRI) of the right shoulder revealed a cystic lesion at the spinoglenoid notch, which was confirmed by surgical exploration.

The suprascapular nerve emerges from the upper trunk of the brachial plexus, receiving fibers from C5 and C6 roots. It does not have any cutaneous innervation. The suprascapular nerve first provides innervation to the supraspinatus muscle, a shoulder abductor, and then to the infraspinatus, a shoulder external rotator (see Fig. 60.1). The suprascapular nerve may be injured at the suprascapular notch, before the innervation of the supraspinatus muscle, or distally at the spinoglenoid notch, affecting the infraspinatus alone. The most common site of entrapment is at the suprascapular notch, under the transverse scapular ligament. Acute-onset cases result from blunt shoulder trauma, with or without scapular fracture, or from forceful anterior rotation of the scapula. The suprascapular nerve may also be affected by brachial plexus neuritis in isolation or with other nerves. Suprascapular neuropathies of insidious

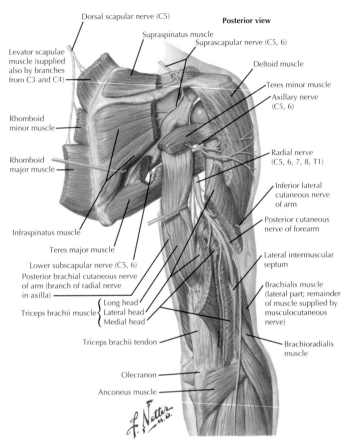

Fig. 60.2 Radial Nerve in the Arm and Nerves of the Posterior Shoulder.

onset often occur subsequent to callous formation after fractures, from entrapment at the suprascapular or spinoglenoid notch, by compression from a ganglion or other soft tissue mass, or by traction caused by repetitive overhead activities, such as volleyball or tennis.

Axillary Neuropathies

> **CLINICAL VIGNETTE** *A 72-year-old man had pain and weakness of the right arm following a fall. Evaluation in the emergency room disclosed an anterior dislocation of the right shoulder, which was reduced. Despite treatment, the patient continued to have difficulty raising the arm above the head. Electrodiagnostic testing several weeks later showed a reduced recruitment pattern of motor unit action potentials in the right deltoid and teres minor muscles. The EMG was suggestive of stretch injury with demyelinating nerve injury without evidence of axon loss. The patient recovered spontaneously over the course of the following month.*

The axillary nerve, along with the radial nerve, is a terminal branch of the posterior cord of the brachial plexus. It innervates the deltoid and the teres minor and provides sensory innervation to the lateral upper part of the shoulder via the superior lateral brachial cutaneous nerve of the arm (Fig. 60.3, see also Fig. 60.2). In lesions of the axillary nerve, shoulder abduction is weakened and cutaneous sensibility of the lateral shoulder diminishes, overlapping the C5 dermatome. Because the teres minor is not the predominant external rotator of the shoulder, clinical isolation and testing are difficult. EMG may be necessary to define neurogenic injury to this muscle. Most axillary neuropathies are traumatic, related to anterior shoulder dislocations, humerus fractures, or both. Recognition of nerve injury may be delayed because of the shoulder injury. Acute axillary neuropathies can result from blunt trauma or as a component or sole manifestation of brachial plexus neuritis.

Musculocutaneous Neuropathies

> **CLINICAL VIGNETTE** *A 43-year-old woman presented to the laboratory for routine blood work after her annual physical examination. During phlebotomy in the right antecubital fossa, she experienced a sharp pain, radiating from the elbow to the wrist, which persisted for several days. She then developed numbness of the right lateral forearm. She had no weakness. Nerve conduction studies showed an absent sensory nerve action potential of the lateral antebrachial cutaneous nerve. The needle examination was normal.*

The musculocutaneous nerve originates directly from the lateral cord of the brachial plexus. It innervates the coracobrachialis, biceps brachii, and brachialis muscles, and terminates in its cutaneous branch, the lateral antebrachial cutaneous nerve. Isolated musculocutaneous neuropathies are rare. They have been reported in weight lifters, after biceps tendon rupture, after surgery, and after prolonged pressure during sleep. Damage to the musculocutaneous nerve results in weakness of forearm flexion and supination and sensory loss of the lateral volar forearm (see Fig. 60.1). The biceps reflex is diminished, but the brachioradialis reflex (same myotome, different nerve) is preserved. More commonly, injury to this nerve occurs as part of a more widespread traumatic injury, usually involving the proximal humerus. The musculocutaneous nerve can also be preferentially involved in acute brachial plexus neuritis. Distal lesions of the lateral antebrachial cutaneous nerve may result from attempted cannulation of the basilic vein in the antecubital fossa. Rupture of the biceps tendon is a significant differential diagnostic consideration of musculocutaneous neuropathy.

Differential Diagnosis of Shoulder Mononeuropathies

The most common etiologies of shoulder pain are injuries to glenohumeral, subacromial, and acromioclavicular regions. Pain often may be reproduced by local pressure or provocative movements and positions. Rotator cuff tears can mimic nerve injury because of apparent weakness of shoulder abduction (supraspinatus) and external rotation (teres minor and infraspinatus). Motor neuron disease may begin in the shoulder region. It must be considered in the differential diagnosis of weakness without associated pain or sensory signs and symptoms. C5 radiculopathy also enters the differential diagnosis in patients reporting shoulder pain, sometimes extending into the upper arm with weakness and numbness. This pain might originate within the scapular region and not the neck. Having patients flex their neck laterally in the direction of the symptomatic limb may reproduce the pain. Patients with C5 weakness have problems with shoulder abduction (deltoid and supraspinatus muscles), external rotation (infraspinatus), and arm flexion (biceps brachii). The biceps stretch reflex is often diminished. Paresthesias or sensory loss occurs in a discrete patch on the lateral proximal arm overlying the deltoid muscle.

Diagnostic Approach

EMG is the primary diagnostic tool in the evaluation of suspected shoulder mononeuropathies. It is particularly helpful to identify mononeuropathies affecting the shoulder girdle for several reasons. Neurogenic injury may go unsuspected, because pain is the predominant symptom. Weakness may be hidden by the observation of normal strength within unaffected muscles performing similar functions; for example,

Anterior (palmar) view

Posterior (dorsal) view

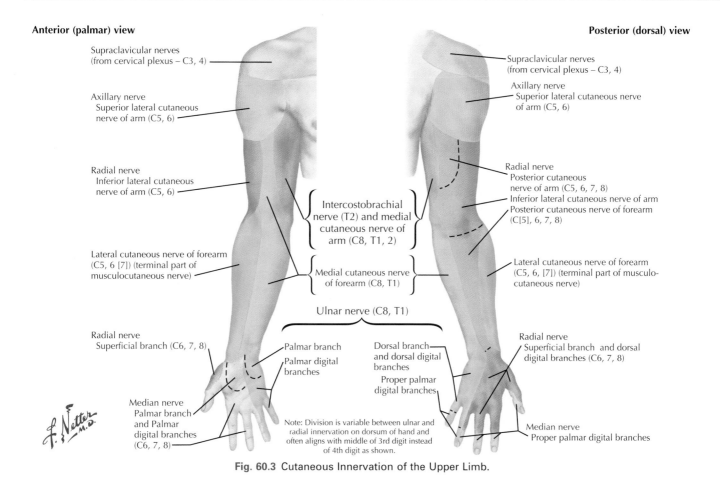

Supraclavicular nerves
(from cervical plexus – C3, 4)

Axillary nerve
Superior lateral cutaneous
nerve of arm (C5, 6)

Radial nerve
Inferior lateral cutaneous
nerve of arm (C5, 6)

Intercostobrachial
nerve (T2) and medial
cutaneous nerve of
arm (C8, T1, 2)

Lateral cutaneous nerve of forearm
(C5, 6 [7]) (terminal part of
musculocutaneous nerve)

Medial cutaneous nerve
of forearm (C8, T1)

Ulnar nerve (C8, T1)

Radial nerve
Superficial branch (C6, 7, 8)

Palmar branch
Palmar digital
branches

Dorsal branch
and dorsal digital
branches

Proper palmar
digital branches

Median nerve
Palmar branch
and Palmar
digital branches
(C6, 7, 8)

Note: Division is variable between ulnar and
radial innervation on dorsum of hand and
often aligns with middle of 3rd digit instead
of 4th digit as shown.

Supraclavicular nerves
(from cervical plexus – C3, 4)

Axillary nerve
Superior lateral cutaneous nerve
of arm (C5, 6)

Radial nerve
Posterior cutaneous
nerve of arm (C5, 6, 7, 8)
Inferior lateral cutaneous nerve of arm
Posterior cutaneous nerve of forearm
(C[5], 6, 7, 8)

Lateral cutaneous nerve of forearm
(C5, 6, [7]) (terminal part of musculocutaneous nerve)

Radial nerve
Superficial branch and dorsal
digital branches (C6, 7, 8)

Median nerve
Proper palmar digital branches

Fig. 60.3 Cutaneous Innervation of the Upper Limb.

supraspinatus weakness obscured by normal deltoid function. Conversely, nerve injury may be suspected because of apparent weakness caused by tendon rupture, only to be refuted by the absence of denervation on needle EMG. Although theoretically nerve conduction studies can be performed on the musculocutaneous and axillary nerves, their value is limited by technical factors. These nerves are typically accessible at only one stimulation site, precluding the determination of conduction velocities and accurate identification of conduction block. However, demyelination with conduction block may be suspected when a normal compound muscle action potential is obtained from a weak muscle; often, this finding portends an excellent prognosis. This conclusion should be reached cautiously because the same pattern may result from axon loss when the study is performed within the first week after injury, before wallerian degeneration has taken place.

Needle EMG can identify even subtle axon loss by the detection of fibrillation potentials. The evaluating physician and the electromyographer should always examine the patient and consider every potential neuropathic cause of shoulder pain. Otherwise, uncommon neuropathies can easily be overlooked.

A common clinical dilemma occurs with patients who have nontraumatic shoulder girdle mononeuropathies. It is difficult to differentiate a primary idiopathic lesion from a limited form of brachial plexus neuritis and to determine whether entrapment or a related process necessitating surgical exploration is involved. A thorough clinical and electrodiagnostic examination is thus required. Subtle clinical or electrodiagnostic evidence of involvement of muscles innervated by a different nerve usually suggests that a conservative approach is indicated, as this constellation of findings speaks against compression of a single nerve.

Routine radiographs are useful to detect scapular fractures secondary to acute injuries, which sometimes predispose patients to suprascapular neuropathies or serratus anterior dehiscence from the scapula. MRI can define insidious-onset neuropathies that may be caused by expanding masses, for example a ganglion cyst in the spinoglenoid notch.

Management and Prognosis

Unfortunately, shoulder bracing provides little benefit to patients with shoulder girdle weakness. Exercises to strengthen other shoulder girdle muscles may provide partial functional compensation. If nerve transection from acute penetrating injury is suspected, surgical exploration and primary anastomosis should be considered, although results are mixed. In acute nonpenetrating injury, exploration can be considered after 3–6 months, provided no clinical or electrodiagnostic evidence of reinnervation exists. Nerve grafting is an option if unanticipated nerve transection is found. For insidious-onset neuropathies without a defined cause, imaging can exclude ganglion cysts or other masses. If no mass is demonstrable and the patient shows no evidence of improvement, exploration may be considered, particularly at potential sites of entrapment such as the suprascapular or spinoglenoid notches.

Despite apparent axonal injury in brachial plexus neuritis, the prognosis is good for functional recovery, which may take 6 months to 2 years. The prognosis for direct compressive injury is less predictable and probably depends on reinnervating distance, patient age, and comorbidities. Stretch injuries and entrapment have the highest likelihood of a significant demyelinating component, with excellent outcome being the rule, particularly if entrapment is recognized and removed before significant axon loss occurs.

MEDIAN MONONEUROPATHIES

The anatomy of the median nerve is important in understanding the signs and symptoms of entrapment lesions at the level of the wrist, versus the more proximal lesions. The median nerve provides essential motor and sensory function to the lateral aspect of the hand (Fig. 60.4). It supplies the intrinsic hand muscles of most of the thenar eminence and innervates several forearm muscles. Its major sensory role is to provide innervation for the thumb, index, and middle fingers, and the lateral half of the ring finger.

The median nerve is formed by lateral and medial cord fibers of the brachial plexus. The lateral cord carries median sensory fibers from C6–C7 roots and provides the sensory innervation to the thumb and the first two and a half fingers. It also contains median motor fibers from the C6–C7 roots, which contribute to the innervation of the forearm muscles. The medial cord carries motor fibers from the C8–T1 roots that innervate the thenar eminence. The distal median nerve at the wrist is the primary site of clinical involvement in carpal tunnel syndrome. More proximal lesions at the elbow are far less common.

Distal Median Entrapment

CLINICAL VIGNETTE *A 45-year-old factory worker presented with a 3-year history of intermittent right-hand tingling. Initially, this had occurred only in the morning on awakening. In recent months, his symptoms had awoken him at night, interfering with his sleep. He felt that all digits were affected. The paresthesias were sometimes accompanied by aching of the wrist and forearm. Shaking of the hand relieved the discomfort. There was no decline of hand strength. Neurologic examination disclosed minimal weakness of right thumb abduction without loss of thenar eminence bulk. Results of reflex and sensory examinations were normal, including 2-point discrimination and graded monofilament touch. The symptoms were reproduced by nerve percussion over the median nerve at the wrist (Tinel sign).*

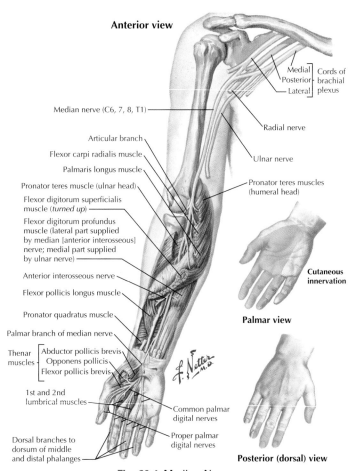

Fig. 60.4 Median Nerve.

Etiology and Epidemiology

Carpal tunnel syndrome (CTS) is common and associated with high economic costs. The lifetime risk of acquiring CTS might be as high as 10%, with an approximate annual incidence of 0.3% and a peak in the sixth decade. CTS is more than three times more prevalent in women than in men and often affects both hands. The incidence is substantially increased in the working population, particularly blue-collar workers, and it appears to be more common in patients with Charcot-Marie-Tooth disease. Carpal tunnel syndrome has been associated with numerous other conditions, such as pregnancy, endocrine disorders (hypothyroidism, acromegaly, and diabetes), rheumatoid arthritis, sarcoid, hemodialysis, and amyloidosis. However, most of the cases are idiopathic, related to repeated stress to the nerve, followed by edema, ischemia, and demyelination of the median nerve at the wrist. If the compression is severe or prolonged enough, axonal loss ensues.

Clinical Presentation and Testing

Median nerve entrapment at the wrist commonly presents with intermittent symptoms, including pain and paresthesias in the hand and forearm. The symptoms tend to occur on awakening or at night, and they are often provoked by certain postures or activities such as reading or driving (Fig. 60.5). The perception that paresthesias affect all digits (rather than just the lateral three and a half innervated by the median nerve) is likely related to the greater cortical representation of the thumb and first two fingers. As CTS progresses, persistent numbness ensues, alerting the patient that the precise sensory distribution involves predominantly the volar surface of the first three and a half digits. The

neurologic examination, particularly in mild CTS cases, may offer few clues. It is helpful in severe cases in which atrophy of the thenar eminence is common. Median hand functions, primarily thumb abduction and opposition, are weak. Having the patient supinate the forearm so the palm is flat, and then raise the thumb vertically against resistance, tests the abductor pollicis brevis muscle. Forearm muscles supplied by the median nerve proximal to the flexor retinaculum are spared in CTS.

Provocative tests offer supportive but not diagnostic evidence in suspected CTS (Fig. 60.6). A positive Tinel sign consists of an electric, shooting sensation (not just local discomfort) radiating into the appropriate digits with wrist percussion. Tinel and Phalen (reproduction of paresthesias on forceful flexion of the wrist) maneuvers should be performed with nonleading questions to improve response credibility. It is recommended that the Phalen maneuver be maintained for at least 1 minute before determining that the result is negative. The pressure test may be the most reliable of the three maneuvers; pressure is placed over the carpal tunnel (proximal palm, not wrist) for 20–30 seconds, attempting to reproduce paresthesias in a median nerve distribution.

Differential Diagnosis

Diagnosis of CTS is usually straightforward, although other conditions may mimic CTS. The assessment of the patient needs to incorporate clinical and electrophysiologic data, as more than 10% of the asymptomatic general population might have abnormal nerve conduction parameters suggestive of CTS. The most common differential diagnosis is a C6–C7 radiculopathy, in which numbness occurs in a similar distribution. Patients with a radiculopathy usually have neck or radicular

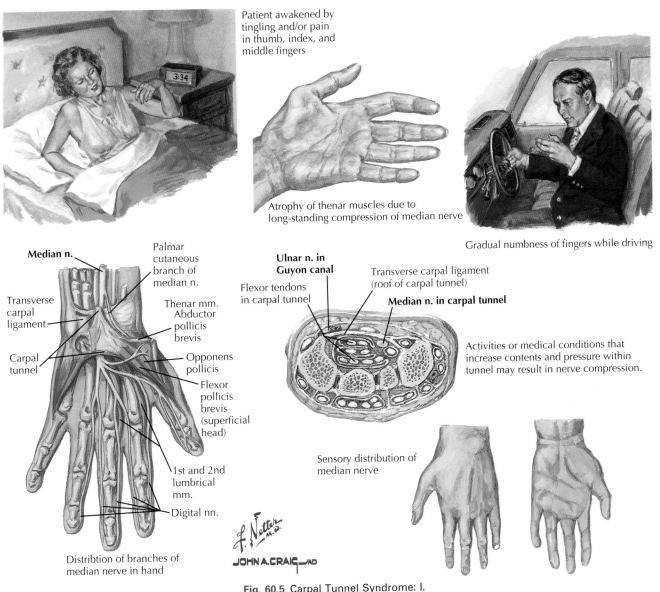

Patient awakened by tingling and/or pain in thumb, index, and middle fingers

Atrophy of thenar muscles due to long-standing compression of median nerve

Gradual numbness of fingers while driving

Median n.

Palmar cutaneous branch of median n.

Transverse carpal ligament

Carpal tunnel

Thenar mm. Abductor pollicis brevis

Opponens pollicis

Flexor pollicis brevis (superficial head)

1st and 2nd lumbrical mm.

Digital nn.

Distribtion of branches of median nerve in hand

Ulnar n. in Guyon canal

Flexor tendons in carpal tunnel

Transverse carpal ligament (roof of carpal tunnel)

Median n. in carpal tunnel

Activities or medical conditions that increase contents and pressure within tunnel may result in nerve compression.

Sensory distribution of median nerve

Fig. 60.5 Carpal Tunnel Syndrome: I.

pain. Nerve conduction studies and needle EMG can differentiate these entities. Although the muscles of both thenar and hypothenar eminence originate from the C8 root, its sensory territory is confined to the medial aspect of the hand and arm. The C8 root also innervates the flexor digitorum profundus of digits 4 and 5 and the extensor indicis proprius muscles via the ulnar and radial nerves, respectively. Ulnar neuropathies have an entirely different pattern of motor and sensory loss.

Carpal tunnel syndrome virtually never presents with predominant motor symptoms. If thumb abduction is weak, evidence of other motor involvement should be sought to confirm a different lesion. Weakness and atrophy of the median forearm muscles suggest a proximal median nerve lesion, particularly at the elbow (pronator syndrome). If more widespread weakness is demonstrated in the absence of sensory signs or symptoms, motor neuron diseases or multifocal motor neuropathy require diagnostic consideration.

Polyneuropathy should be excluded; this can occur particularly in patients with diabetes, who may not be as aware of sensory loss in their feet compared with their hands. Clinical examination and EMG usually clarify this issue. Plexopathies typically produce motor and sensory dysfunction within multiple nerve distributions in a single extremity

and pain in the shoulder region. They rarely enter the CTS differential diagnosis. Although it is uncommon for central nervous system disorders to produce sensory signs and symptoms within the distribution of a single peripheral nerve, occasionally cervical spinal cord lesions (e.g., cervical spinal stenosis or intrinsic cord tumors), and very rarely focal frontoparietal brain lesions, may mimic CTS. Vitamin B$_{12}$ deficiency and syringomyelia are considerations in patients with bilateral hand numbness.

Management

Data regarding the natural history of CTS are scarce. Over 1 to 2 years, 20%–30% of hands appear to improve spontaneously, but in part this might be due to lifestyle changes, and long-term follow-up is not available. There are few randomized controlled trials comparing different treatment modalities. Treatment recommendations are further complicated by conflicting data as to whether clinical features or electrophysiological parameters can predict treatment outcome.

Conservative therapies should be considered first, as carpal tunnel release surgery carries a risk of potentially serious complications, such as reflex sympathetic dystrophy (complex regional pain syndrome),

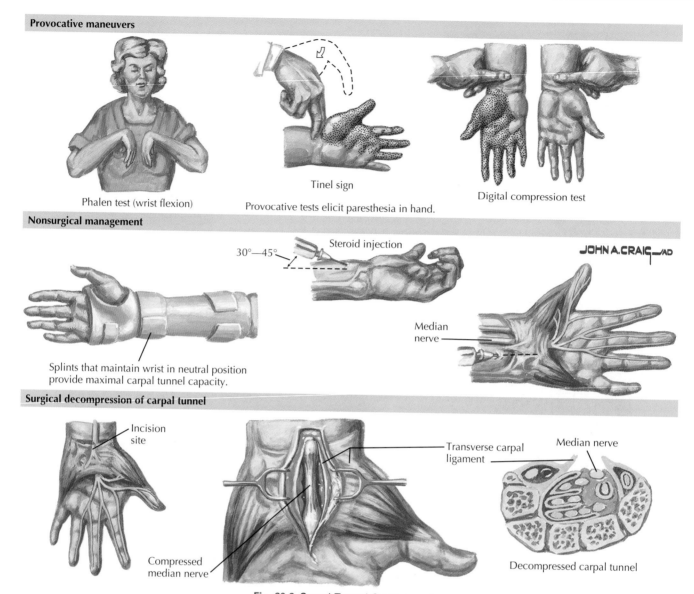

Provocative maneuvers

Phalen test (wrist flexion)

Tinel sign

Provocative tests elicit paresthesia in hand.

Digital compression test

Nonsurgical management

30°—45°   Steroid injection

JOHN A. CRAIG ᴀᴅ

Median nerve

Splints that maintain wrist in neutral position provide maximal carpal tunnel capacity.

Surgical decompression of carpal tunnel

Incision site

Transverse carpal ligament

Median nerve

Compressed median nerve

Decompressed carpal tunnel

Fig. 60.6 Carpal Tunnel Syndrome: II.

injury to the median palmar cutaneous branch, and hypertrophic scar. Ergonomic workplace alterations and avoidance of offending activities or positions are generally recommended, but data regarding the efficacy of these interventions are limited. Neutral wrist splints, typically worn at night, initially help more than 50% of patients by maximizing the carpal tunnel diameter and minimizing nerve pressure, which is better than the natural remission rate. Local steroid injections may provide temporary pain relief. However, this is rarely a permanent solution, as there are frequent relapses requiring repeated injections, and there is the possible risk of flexor tendon rupture. Some patients improve with nerve gliding exercises.

Surgical decompression is offered to patients with increasingly annoying sensory symptoms and progressive abnormalities on neurologic examination and electrophysiological testing (see Fig. 60.6). Although published success rates vary significantly, the average surgical success rate is 75%; after surgery 8% of patients may worsen. Long duration of symptoms, increasing age, and the presence of workers compensation claims may be associated with poorer outcome. Patients with moderate electrophysiological abnormalities appear to do best, and the success rate of surgery in the absence of nerve conduction abnormalities is

only 51%. Occasionally, patients present with end-stage CTS and absent motor responses on nerve conduction studies. Meaningful return of thenar strength is less likely this late in the course of the neuropathy, and resolution of pain may be a more realistic goal of surgical intervention for these patients. Endoscopic techniques of carpal tunnel decompression are associated with fewer minor, but not major complications compared with open carpal tunnel release. There is limited evidence guiding postoperative management.

Proximal Median Neuropathies

CLINICAL VIGNETTE *A 36-year-old secretary complained of difficulty holding a pen and snapping her fingers to music for 6 months. The onset of weakness had been preceded by an aching pain in the volar forearm. There was no sensory loss. The patient had delivered healthy twins 3 months prior to presentation. Neurologic evaluation demonstrated weakness of the flexor pollicis longus muscle and the median-innervated portion of the flexor digitorum profundus, manifested by the inability to flex the distal phalanx of the thumb and the index and long fingers.*

EMG confirmed active and chronic denervation in the flexor pollicis longus, flexor digitorum profundus 2 and 3, and pronator quadratus muscles. MRI of the forearm showed evidence of atrophy in the muscles supplied by the anterior interosseous nerve, but no other abnormalities were detected. Surgical exploration revealed entrapment of the anterior interosseous nerve by the deep head of the pronator teres muscle.

Median neuropathies arising rostral to the most proximal muscle innervated by the median nerve (the pronator teres) occur at a frequency of less than 1% of that of CTS. In a very small proportion of the population, there is a bony spur that originates from the shaft of the medial humerus, proximal to the medial epicondyle. A tendinous band called the ligament of Struthers stretches between these two structures and may represent a site of compression for the median nerve. More distally, in the antecubital fossa, the median nerve may become entrapped beneath the lacertus fibrosus, a fibrous band that runs between the tendon of the biceps and the proximal flexors of the forearm. Even more distally, the nerve can become entrapped in the substance of the pronator teres muscle or beneath the sublimis bridge of the flexor digitorum superficialis muscle (pronator teres syndrome).

The clinical and electrophysiologic recognition of weakness in the distribution of the forearm muscles innervated by the median nerve is the diagnostic key (Fig. 60.7). When the median nerve lesion is most proximal, the pronator teres muscle is involved and may be atrophied. Clinical features also include pain in the volar forearm exacerbated by physical activity. There is weakness of thenar muscles and sensory loss in the thumb, index finger, long finger, and lateral aspect of the ring finger.

Mechanical lesions within the axilla, secondary to shoulder dislocation or penetrating injury, also may affect the proximal median nerve, although concomitant injury of other nerves often exists. More distal lesions of the proximal median nerve include humeral fractures, elbow dislocations, tourniquet compression, and forms of penetrating trauma such as catheterization of the antecubital veins.

EMG is the crucial initial study. Imaging studies, particularly MRI of the elbow region, are indicated when EMG results are positive. Focal lesions, such as the bony origin of a ligament of Struthers or a venous infarction secondary to tourniquet compression, may be defined on neuroimaging.

Conservative treatment consists of rest and antiinflammatory medications. In patients with severe symptoms and electrodiagnostic evidence of axonal loss, surgical exploration of the median nerve in the proximal forearm should be considered.

Anterior Interosseous Neuropathies

The anterior interosseous nerve is the largest motor branch of the median nerve. It does not supply any sensory innervation to the skin, but does carry sensory fibers to the muscles of the forearm and interosseous membrane. It arises about 5 to 6 cm below the elbow. The muscles supplied by the anterior interosseous nerve are flexor pollicis longus, flexor digitorum profundus to the second and third digits, and the pronator quadratus. Possible etiologies for anterior interosseous neuropathy are aberrant fibrous bands, fractures, compression by the deep head of the pronator teres muscle, pregnancy, brachial plexus neuritis (which might present as a multifocal neuropathy), or idiopathic.

Anterior interosseous neuropathy usually presents with nonspecific pain in the proximal forearm. The motor symptoms include weakness

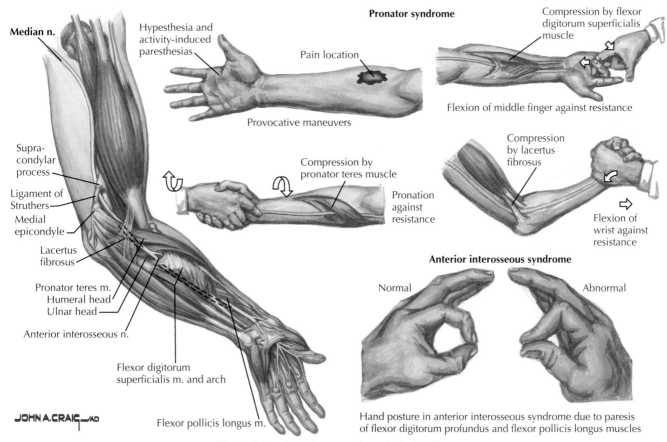

Fig. 60.7 Proximal Compression of Median Nerve.

of forearm pronation with the elbow flexed and weakness of distal phalanx flexion of the thumb, the index finger, and the long finger. Affected persons cannot form a circle by pinching their thumb and index finger. This presentation is similar to more proximal median neuropathies but without involvement of the pronator teres. Furthermore, there is no sensory involvement.

The treatment, depending on etiology, may be nonsurgical or surgical. Rest, antiinflammatory medications, and splints can help. Surgical treatment includes exploration of the nerve.

ULNAR MONONEUROPATHIES

The ulnar nerve primarily innervates intrinsic hand muscles, including all hypothenar muscles (Fig. 60.8). The muscles of the thenar eminence supplied by the ulnar nerve are the adductor pollicis and part of the flexor pollicis brevis. Only two forearm muscles have ulnar innervation: the flexor carpi ulnaris and the medial part of the flexor digitorum profundus. The ulnar nerve also supplies sensation to the medial one-and-a-half fingers (digit 5 and the medial aspect of digit 4), on the dorsal surface sometimes the medial two-and-a-half fingers (see Figs. 60.3 and 60.8). Manifestations of ulnar neuropathies vary with location and severity. Progressive motor deficits lead to the classic "claw hand," with hyperextension of the fourth and fifth metacarpophalangeal joints and flexion of the proximal and distal interphalangeal joints (Fig. 60.9). This is most pronounced when the patient is asked to open the hand because of the unopposed action of radial nerve-innervated muscles. Similar to its median counterpart, the ulnar nerve is typically affected at two anatomic loci, the elbow and wrist, however, in reverse frequency. The majority of ulnar nerve lesions occur at the elbow (Fig. 60.10).

Proximal Lesions

> **CLINICAL VIGNETTE** *A 55-year-old man presented to the emergency room afraid he was having a heart attack. He had suddenly experienced sharp, shooting pain radiating from the left elbow distally, associated with tingling of the hand. Upon further questioning, the patient mentioned occasional tingling of digits 4 and 5 of the left hand for several years. He was an avid reader and frequently read with his elbows resting on his desk.*
>
> *The neurologic examination revealed decreased light touch in the left ring finger and little finger, splitting the ring finger. There was minimal weakness of finger abduction, and a Tinel sign at the left elbow was present.*
>
> *Electrodiagnostic testing showed a demyelinating left ulnar neuropathy at the elbow.*

Proximal ulnar neuropathies are second only to CTS in frequency. Etiologies include external compression or entrapment at the elbow after remote elbow trauma (tardy ulnar palsy) and entrapment just distal to the elbow joint (cubital tunnel syndrome, Fig. 60.11).

Numbness and paresthesias of the fifth and sometimes half of the fourth digit are the rule, and may be provoked by having the patient maintain a fully flexed elbow posture for 30 to 60 seconds. Sensory signs or symptoms should not extend proximal to the wrist, in which case a C8 radiculopathy has to be considered in the differential diagnosis. Weakness of the intrinsic muscles of the hand is more common in ulnar neuropathies than in CTS. Clinically apparent involvement of ulnar forearm muscles is rarely detected. Sometimes, there is associated aching of the elbow or forearm pain. The diagnosis is confirmed by EMG. High-resolution sonography can be helpful when precise localization of the lesion by EMG is difficult, but it is not routinely performed.

Distal Lesions

> **CLINICAL VIGNETTE** *A 40-year-old jackhammer operator noted progressive wasting of muscle bulk in the right hand. He had no pain or sensory loss. He had read about his symptoms on the Internet, and he became concerned he might have Lou Gehrig disease.*
>
> *On neurologic examination, the patient had difficulty holding a piece of paper between the right thumb and index finger. While attempting to do so, he flexed the distal phalanx of the thumb (Froment sign). There was atrophy of the first dorsal interosseous muscle, and fasciculations were observed within this muscle. Abduction of the little finger was of normal strength, and no sensory deficits were demonstrated.*
>
> *Electrodiagnostic testing was consistent with a distal left ulnar neuropathy involving only the deep motor branch. The patient regained some strength after switching jobs.*

Ulnar neuropathies at the level of the wrist or palm are less common than proximal lesions. The nerve might become entrapped at the level of the ulnar tunnel or the Guyon canal. Common causes are trauma, ganglion cysts, rheumatoid arthritis, and wrist fractures. Depending on the exact site of injury, there may or may not be associated sensory symptoms (see Fig. 60.9). Sensory loss on the dorsal aspect of the medial hand points to a more proximal ulnar neuropathy with involvement of the dorsal ulnar cutaneous nerve.

Ulnar neuropathies in the palm distal to the Guyon canal present with weakness confined to the ulnar muscles on the lateral aspect of the hand, particularly thumb adduction. This is secondary to weakness of the adductor pollicis, the only thenar muscle not primarily innervated

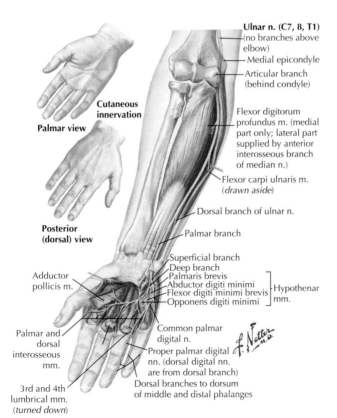

Palmar view

Posterior (dorsal) view

Cutaneous innervation

Ulnar n. (C7, 8, T1) (no branches above elbow)

Medial epicondyle

Articular branch (behind condyle)

Flexor digitorum profundus m. (medial part only; lateral part supplied by anterior interosseous branch of median n.)

Flexor carpi ulnaris m. (*drawn aside*)

Dorsal branch of ulnar n.

Palmar branch

Superficial branch
Deep branch
Palmaris brevis
Abductor digiti minimi
Flexor digiti minimi brevis } Hypothenar mm.
Opponens digiti minimi

Adductor pollicis m.

Palmar and dorsal interosseous mm.

3rd and 4th lumbrical mm. (*turned down*)

Common palmar digital n.

Proper palmar digital nn. (dorsal digital nn. are from dorsal branch)

Dorsal branches to dorsum of middle and distal phalanges

Fig. 60.8 Ulnar Nerve.

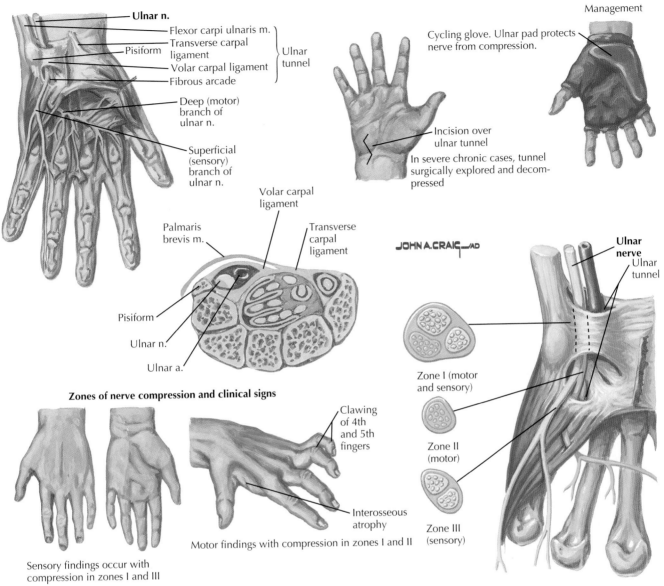

Zones of nerve compression and clinical signs

Sensory findings occur with compression in zones I and III

Motor findings with compression in zones I and II

Fig. 60.9 Ulnar Tunnel Syndrome.

by the median nerve. The first dorsal interosseous muscle is also affected, whereas abduction of the little finger may be preserved. The accompanying intrinsic muscle atrophy and the lack of sensory deficits sometimes prompt consideration of motor neuron disease. Lesions in the palm usually result from local trauma and repetitive injury; for example, from bicycling or from occupations that use tools requiring significant intermittent pressure over the distal ulnar motor fibers (i.e., electricians, clam or oyster shuckers, and pizza cutters). EMG is essential for diagnosis. When the pressure is discontinued, significant recovery of function can occur.

Differential Diagnosis

Motor neuron disease is a primary consideration in patients presenting with asymmetric painless atrophy of the intrinsic hand muscles. One key differentiating feature between motor neuron disease and an ulnar nerve lesion is the frequent involvement of the abductor pollicis brevis muscle in motor neuron disease; this is innervated by the median nerve.

Lower brachial plexus injuries are accompanied by motor and sensory dysfunction in the distribution of multiple peripheral nerve territories within a single extremity. Historically, thoracic outlet syndrome, a distal T1 radiculopathy or proximal lower trunk brachial plexopathy, was considered a common cause of upper extremity neurologic symptoms. Thoracic outlet syndrome is now recognized as a rare condition that is more likely to mimic an ulnar neuropathy than CTS. Perhaps many cases of CTS were erroneously diagnosed and treated as thoracic outlet syndrome before the recognition of the frequency of CTS in the late 1950s and early 1960s. EMG defined the relative frequency of these lesions.

C8 radiculopathies are less common than C7 or C6 radiculopathies but can easily be confused with an ulnar neuropathy because of their overlapping sensory territory. Medial forearm numbness and weakness of nonulnar innervated C8 muscles (i.e., the thenar eminence, the flexor pollicis longus, and the extensor indicis proprius) provide the major diagnostic distinctions.

Management

Conservative treatment consists of avoiding the stretch produced by a fully flexed elbow via a padded splint that prevents further direct nerve

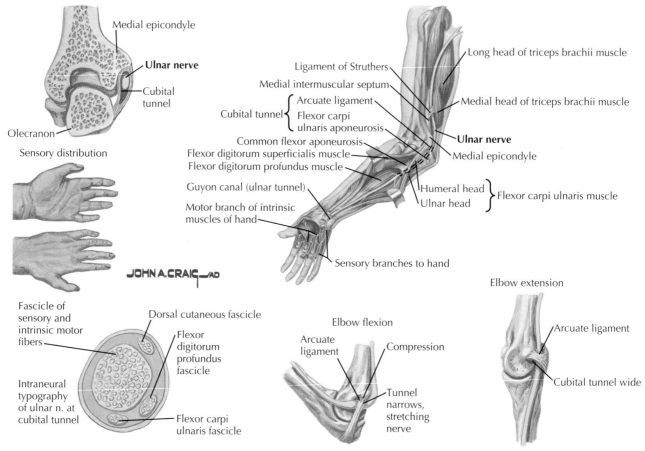

Fig. 60.10 Compression of Ulnar Nerve.

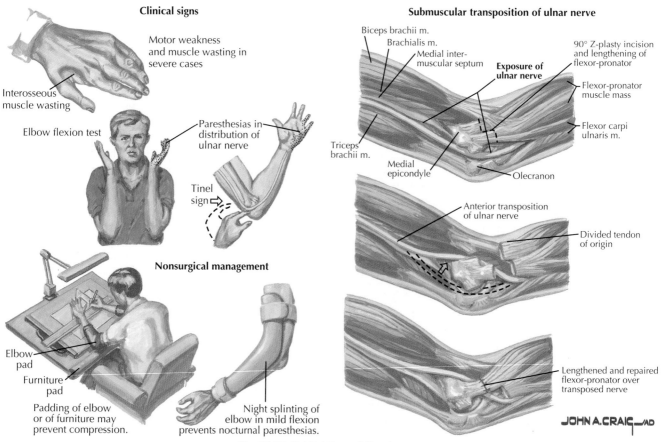

Fig. 60.11 Cubital Tunnel Syndrome.

pressure. More than 50% of patients with mild nerve compression might recover with conservative therapy, although data on long-term outcome are limited. Surgical management of ulnar lesions is not as well defined as with CTS. It is even less clear who is likely to benefit from surgery, and there is no consensus on which surgical procedure is appropriate. Persistent pain, progressive motor deficits, and to a lesser extent failure to improve after 3–6 months of conservative management are reasons to consider surgery. For cubital tunnel lesions in the absence of trauma or prior surgical procedure involving the elbow, anterior transposition seems to offer no advantage over simple decompression of the nerve.

RADIAL NEUROPATHIES

CLINICAL VIGNETTE *An 82-year-old man was seen in urgent consultation for a possible stroke. He had awoken in his chair during the late morning with weakness of the right arm. The night prior, he had taken a sleeping pill for the first time in his life.*

The neurologic examination revealed weakness of elbow flexion in the semipronated position (brachioradialis muscle), wrist extension, and finger extension. The brachioradialis reflex was absent, whereas the triceps reflex and triceps strength were preserved. There was sensory loss to light touch and pinprick on the dorsal aspect of the forearm and dorsolateral hand.

Electrodiagnostic testing performed on the day of presentation was suggestive of an acute right radial neuropathy at the spiral groove. At the time of his follow-up visit 4 weeks later, the patient had completely recovered.

The radial nerve is formed by fibers from all three trunks of the brachial plexus, hence from roots C5 to T1. It primarily supplies the extensor muscles of the arm, forearm, and fingers, and one flexor of the arm—the brachioradialis (see Fig. 60.2). It also provides the sensory innervation to the dorsal arm, the dorsolateral aspect of the hand, and the dorsum of the first three-and-a-half, sometimes two-and-a-half fingers (Fig. 60.12).

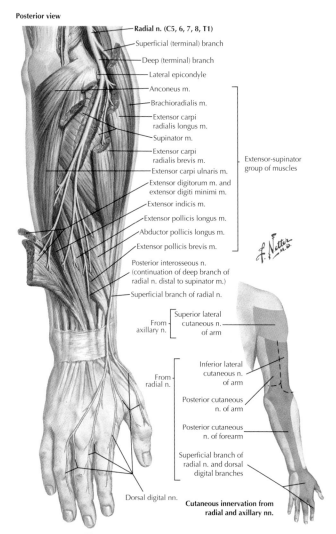

Fig. 60.12 Radial Nerve in Forearm.

Predominant Motor Radial Neuropathies

Radial neuropathies most commonly occur at the midhumeral level near the spiral groove, secondary to external compression (Fig. 60.13). This can occur as a result of impaired consciousness during anesthesia or due to drug or alcohol intoxication ("Saturday night palsy"). These lesions primarily present with wrist and finger drop but little or no pain. Sensory signs and symptoms are often elusive. Elbow extension is spared because the branches of the triceps originate proximal to the spiral groove. The brachioradialis reflex is typically diminished or lost, whereas the triceps and biceps reflexes are unaffected. A potentially confounding examination feature is apparent weakness of ulnar-innervated finger abduction that appears concomitant with wrist drop. The full strength of these ulnar muscles requires at least partial wrist extension. Testing the strength of finger abduction while placing the hand and forearm flat on a hard and flat surface circumvents this problem and prevents false localization.

The posterior interosseous nerve is analogous to the anterior interosseous nerve because it is a distal, predominantly motor branch, of a major peripheral nerve trunk. Posterior interosseous neuropathies commonly occur with fractures of the proximal radius and sometimes have a delayed onset. The posterior interosseous nerve also can be compromised by soft tissue masses. A syndrome of pain and weakness in the muscles innervated by the posterior interosseous nerve may occur in patients who perform repetitive and strenuous pronation/supination movements, which, in some instances, leads to intermittent posterior

interosseous nerve compression by the fibrous edge of the arcade of Frohse (the proximal aspect of the supinator muscle). Entrapment may also develop secondary to a hypertrophied or anomalous supinator muscle. The extensor carpi radialis longus and brevis and the brachioradialis muscles are innervated by branches exiting the radial nerve before the origin of the posterior interosseous nerve; therefore, finger drop, rather than wrist drop—as with a more proximal radial nerve lesion—is the dominant manifestation. However, the extensor carpi ulnaris is weak, which leads to radial deviation of the hand during wrist extension (see Fig. 60.13). There is no sensory loss. Pain near the lateral epicondyle of the humerus, extending distally, may occur, as the posterior interosseous nerve gives off sensory fibers supplying the interosseous membrane and joints of the forearm. Partial fascicular involvement of the radial nerve in the proximal arm with a similar clinical presentation has been described. Magnetic resonance neurography can be helpful for localization.

Predominant Sensory Radial Neuropathies

The superficial radial nerve, a primary distal sensory branch, may be injured in isolation with external pressure at the wrist; for example, with handcuff injuries. These lesions are readily recognized by the distribution of sensory symptoms on the dorsolateral portion of the hand. Weakness does not occur.

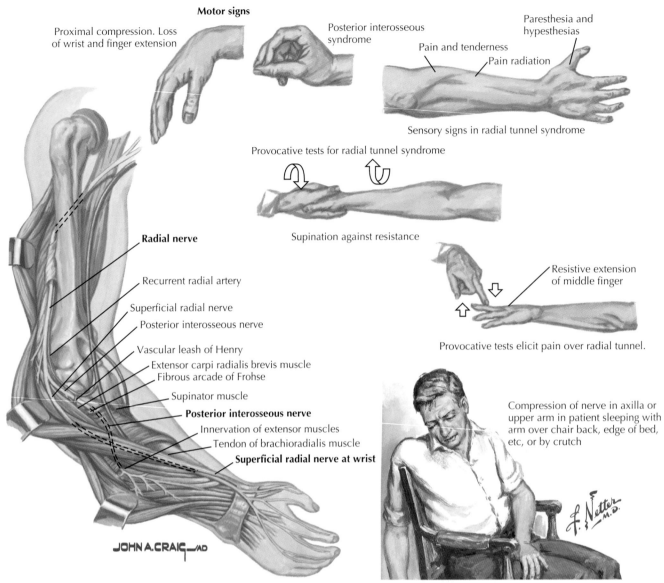

Fig. 60.13 Radial Nerve Compression.

Management

Radial neuropathies usually result from monophasic external compression. They are almost always treated conservatively and successfully.

MONONEUROPATHIES OF THE MEDIAL AND POSTERIOR CUTANEOUS NERVES OF THE FOREARM

Isolated injuries of the medial cutaneous nerve of the forearm are rare (see Fig. 60.3). Sensory symptoms in the medial volar forearm are more commonly a result of more proximal injuries to the lower trunk or medial cord of the brachial plexus or to the C8 nerve root. Nerve injuries at these levels are associated with additional clinical findings, particularly hand weakness. Sensory symptoms on the posterior forearm from isolated injuries to the posterior cutaneous nerve of the forearm are equally rare.

Diagnostic Approach to Mononeuropathies
Electromyography and Nerve Conduction Studies

Myelin loss manifests electrodiagnostically in three ways: focal slowing, differential slowing (also known as temporal dispersion), and conduction block. Focal slowing occurs when all nerve fibers are affected, approximately to the same extent, in one precise anatomic area. Impulse transmission is slowed uniformly in all fibers at that location. When patients have evidence of differential slowing (i.e., temporal dispersion), demyelination is typically multifocal, varying in severity in different fibers within the same nerve. Temporal dispersion is the EMG hallmark of acquired demyelinating polyneuropathies, such as Guillain-Barré syndrome, and is not typically seen in focal mononeuropathies. Primary conduction block is consistent with a demyelinating process in one or more locations that is sufficient to prohibit impulse transmission across involved sections of affected nerve fibers, and this causes clinical weakness. Because axonal integrity is not compromised, muscle wasting does not occur. Since unmyelinated fibers are also not affected, pain and thermal sensation are relatively spared. Conduction block commonly occurs with ulnar neuropathies at the elbow, radial neuropathies at the spiral groove, and peroneal neuropathies at the fibular head.

With motor axonal disruption, the axon is separated from the anterior horn cell and degenerates. Myofibers are deprived of the trophic influence provided by that axon, with resultant atrophy greater than that produced by disuse. Abnormal spontaneous activity characterized by fibrillation potentials and positive sharp waves appears on needle examination, and the number of activated motor unit potentials decreases. Similarly, the loss of unmyelinated axons mediating nociceptive, thermal, and autonomic functions usually produces clinical features different from primary demyelinating insults. These are characterized by loss of pain and thermal perception, hypersensitivity to touch, changes in sweat production, and sometimes vasomotor changes secondary to focal dysautonomia. Clinical features of axon loss can be superimposed upon those associated with the demyelinating component of the nerve injury.

The various mononeuropathies do not have identical pathophysiologic signatures. Some, such as CTS, are initially characterized by focal slowing (Fig. 60.14), whereas others may preferentially produce a demyelinating conduction block, such as an ulnar neuropathy at the elbow, or axon loss as with a primary laceration, or a combination of the above.

EMG and nerve conduction studies provide the means to confirm the existence, location, pathophysiology, and severity of most mononeuropathies. However, electrodiagnosis has important limitations. Ideally, the injured nerve needs to be accessible to stimulation at multiple levels, including at least one site proximal to the site of a demyelinating lesion. This can be technically difficult, even impossible, with proximal nerve segments that are deep and in close proximity to other nerve elements. Localization also can be predicted by the pattern of muscles demonstrating changes of denervation on needle examination. However, the major limitation of this methodology is anatomic as nerve branching is erratic. For example, the ulnar nerve has no branches in the upper arm, two near the elbow, and then none until the hand. The other limitation is selective fascicular involvement, whereby a nerve injury at a given location may not result in denervation of all muscles innervated distal to that injury. Understandably, a false estimate of nerve injury location may result.

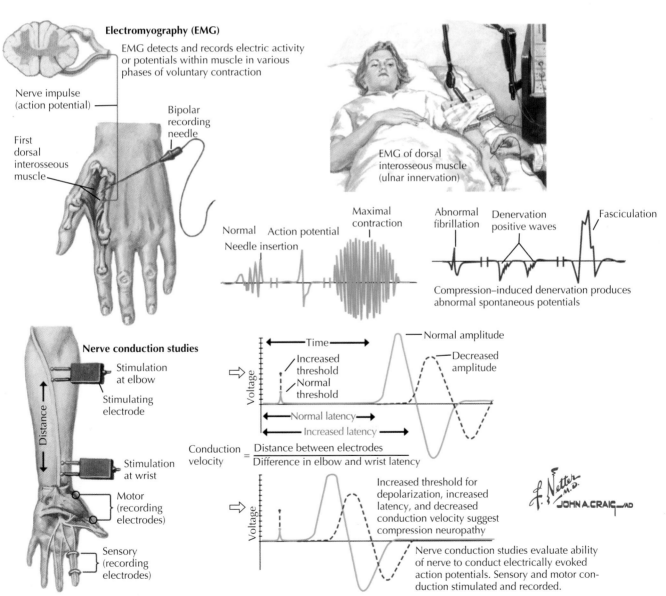

Electromyography (EMG)

EMG detects and records electric activity or potentials within muscle in various phases of voluntary contraction

Nerve impulse (action potential)

First dorsal interosseous muscle

Bipolar recording needle

EMG of dorsal interosseous muscle (ulnar innervation)

Normal Needle insertion

Action potential

Maximal contraction

Abnormal fibrillation

Denervation positive waves

Fasciculation

Compression–induced denervation produces abnormal spontaneous potentials

Nerve conduction studies

Stimulation at elbow

Stimulating electrode

Distance

Stimulation at wrist

Motor (recording electrodes)

Sensory (recording electrodes)

Time

Normal amplitude

Increased threshold

Normal threshold

Decreased amplitude

Normal latency

Increased latency

$$\text{Conduction velocity} = \frac{\text{Distance between electrodes}}{\text{Difference in elbow and wrist latency}}$$

Increased threshold for depolarization, increased latency, and decreased conduction velocity suggest compression neuropathy

Nerve conduction studies evaluate ability of nerve to conduct electrically evoked action potentials. Sensory and motor conduction stimulated and recorded.

Fig. 60.14 Electrodiagnostic Studies in Compression Neuropathy.

False-positive results can result from cold limb temperature, failure to recognize normal anatomic variants, or poor technique. Caution is required not to overcall on the basis of borderline data. Ideally, the presence of abnormalities in two concordant parameters enables conclusive diagnosis. False-negative results also occur. Approximately 10% of patients with clinical histories strongly suggestive of CTS might have normal electrodiagnostic evaluations.

Other Testing Modalities

Although most mononeuropathies occur secondary to recognizable compression, stretch, or entrapment mechanisms, some seem to be idiopathic. Additional testing, such as MRI or ultrasound, may be diagnostic when mononeuropathies develop in atypical locations or under unusual circumstances.

PROGNOSIS OF MONONEUROPATHIES

Prognosis primarily depends on whether the injury has a demyelinating or axonal pathophysiologic mechanism or both. If axonal, recovery depends on the number of axons damaged, the persistence or resolution of the causative insult, the distance between the site of injury and the innervated muscle or cutaneous region, and the patient's age and comorbidities. Demyelinating lesions usually resolve spontaneously after removal of focal compression or entrapment.

ADDITIONAL RESOURCES

American Association of Neuromuscular and Electrodiagnostic Medicine. Available from: http://www.aanem.org. [Accessed 25 March 2018].
The information on this website includes a list of suggested reading for physicians as well as educational material for patients with various neuromuscular disorders.
Bland JDP. Do nerve conduction studies predict the outcome of carpal tunnel syndrome? Muscle Nerve 2001;24:935–40.
This study examines factors influencing the outcome of surgical carpal tunnel decompression.
Bland JDP. Treatment of carpal tunnel syndrome. Muscle Nerve 2007;36:167–71.
This review article summarizes different treatment modalities for carpal tunnel syndrome.
Caliandro P, La Torre G, Padua R, et al. Treatment for ulnar neuropathy at the elbow. Cochrane Database Syst Rev 2016;(11):CD006839.
This is an update of previously reported reviews summarizing the data of nine randomized controlled trials comparing treatment modalities for ulnar neuropathy at the elbow.

Dumitru D, Amato A, Zwarts M. Electrodiagnostic medicine. 2nd ed. Philadelphia, PA: Hanley & Belfus; 2001.
This textbook is an excellent reference for physicians interested in disorders of the peripheral nervous system and electrophysiological techniques.
Knutsen E, Calfee R. Uncommon upper extremity compression neuropathies. Hand Clin 2013;29:443–53.
The authors review the anatomy, presentation, and treatment of rarely encountered compression neuropathies of the upper extremity and offer their experience from the perspective of the orthopedic surgeon.
Marshall S, Tardif G, Ashworth N. Local corticosteroid injection for carpal tunnel syndrome. Cochrane Database Syst Rev 2007;(2):CD001554.
This article reviews data from 12 randomized or quasi-randomized studies regarding the effectiveness of local corticosteroid injection for carpal tunnel syndrome.
O'Connor D, Marshall S, Massy-Westropp N. Non-surgical treatment (other than steroid injection) for carpal tunnel syndrome. Cochrane Database Syst Rev 2003;(1):CD003219.
This review article evaluates the effectiveness of conservative treatment options (other than corticosteroid injection) for carpal tunnel syndrome based on data from 21 randomized or quasi-randomized studies.
Padua L, Padua R, Aprile I, et al. Multiperspective follow-up of untreated carpal tunnel syndrome. A multicenter study. Neurology 2001;56:1459–66.
The authors evaluate the natural history of untreated carpal tunnel syndrome over a 10- to 15-month follow-up period.
Scholten RJPM, Mink van der Molen A, Uitdehaag BMJ, et al. Surgical treatment options for carpal tunnel syndrome. Cochrane Database Syst Rev 2007;(4):CD003905.
The authors compare the outcome of various surgical techniques for carpal tunnel syndrome, including data from 33 randomized controlled trials.
Choi Soo-Jung, Ahn Jae Hong, Kang Chae Hoon, et al. Ultrasonography for nerve compression syndromes of the upper extremity. Ultrasonography 2015;34:275–91.
The authors describe the ultrasound findings in common compression neuropathies of the upper extremity and provide helpful illustrations and images.
Sunderland S. Nerves and nerve injuries. 2nd ed. Edinburgh, Scotland: Churchill Livingstone; 1978.
This outstanding textbook provides a detailed description of the anatomy and physiology of peripheral nerves and outlines the various mechanisms of nerve injury in great depth.
Verdugo RJ, Salinas RS, Castillo JL, et al. Surgical versus non-surgical treatment for carpal tunnel syndrome. Cochrane Database Syst Rev 2008;(4):CD001552.
This is an update of a prior review of randomized controlled trials evaluating surgical versus conservative management of carpal tunnel syndrome.

61

Mononeuropathies of the Lower Extremities

Gisela Held

SCIATIC NEUROPATHIES

> **CLINICAL VIGNETTE** *An 82-year-old frail woman fell in her home. She sustained a hip fracture, which necessitated surgical repair. Postoperatively, she received anticoagulation. Two days later, she had discomfort in her right buttock and foot weakness. Within 24 hours, marked buttock pain, and numbness and paralysis of all muscles below the right knee developed. Computed tomographic (CT) scan revealed a pelvic hematoma. Electromyography (EMG) confirmed a right sciatic neuropathy.*

The sciatic nerve is the body's largest nerve, receiving contributions primarily from the L5, S1, and S2 nerve roots, but also carrying L4 and S3 fibers (Fig. 61.1). It has two major divisions: the laterally situated more superficial, peroneal (fibular) nerve and the medially placed tibial nerve (see Fig. 61.1). These separate into two distinct nerves in the mid- to distal thigh. The sciatic nerve and its branches innervate the hamstrings (biceps femoris, semimembranosus, and semitendinosus muscles), distal adductor magnus, anterior and posterior lower leg compartments, and intrinsic foot musculature. Through sensory branches of the tibial nerve (sural, medial and lateral plantar, and calcaneal) and the superficial peroneal nerve, the sciatic nerve also supplies sensation to the skin of the entire foot and the lateral and posterior lower leg.

Etiology

Sciatic neuropathies can be due to hip arthroplasty, pelvic or femoral fractures, or posterior dislocation of the hip. Like femoral neuropathies, they are sometimes caused by prolonged lithotomy positioning, presumably from stretching of the nerve in individuals who are anatomically predisposed. Occasionally, sciatic neuropathies develop from external pressure in patients who are comatose or immobilized for protracted periods such as with drug overdose. They may result from traumatic mechanisms including misplaced intramuscular injections into the inferior medial quadrant of the buttock. Mass lesions including nerve sheath tumors and external compression from hematoma, aneurysm, endometriosis; other mechanisms also have been described. Sciatic neuropathies due to nerve infarcts may occur in patients with systemic vasculitis.

Clinical Presentation

Acute sciatic neuropathies typically present with distal leg weakness, pain, and sensory loss. Foot pain is a frequent complaint. Because of predominant affliction of the peroneal division, the weakness often manifests itself as foot drop and needs to be differentiated from a common peroneal neuropathy at the fibular head. Weakness of the more proximal muscles (hamstrings) and of foot plantar flexion and inversion (gastrocnemius, tibialis posterior) help differentiate the two entities. The ankle and internal hamstring reflexes are usually depressed or absent. Sensory loss and dysesthesia of the sole, dorsum of the foot, and posterolateral lower leg are common.

Differential Diagnosis

A lumbosacral plexus lesion is the other primary consideration in most patients with sciatic neuropathies, especially when findings clearly encompass a territory outside the peroneal nerve. Diminished sensation on the posterior thigh points to a concomitant neuropathy of the posterior femoral cutaneous nerve, which exits the greater sciatic foramen in proximity to the sciatic nerve. Injury to the perineal branches of this nerve leads to sensory loss on the scrotum or labia majora. Hip extension and abduction should be preserved in sciatic neuropathies. When clinical or EMG evidence suggests gluteal muscle involvement, a primary lesion within the pelvis is a consideration. Examples include benign tumors, such as schwannoma, or malignant processes, particularly lymphoma.

Piriformis syndrome is a poorly understood disorder that is phenomenologically similar to the thoracic outlet and tarsal tunnel syndromes. The piriformis muscle lies deep to the gluteal muscles; it originates from the sacral spine and attaches to the greater trochanter of the femur. The sciatic nerve usually exits inferior to the piriformis muscle but anatomical variations with the nerve piercing through the muscle have been described. It is postulated that acute or chronic injury of the muscle may cause irritation of the sciatic nerve, resulting in posterior thigh and gluteal pain. Objective clinical or electrodiagnostic evidence of sciatic neuropathy is not seen in most patients in whom piriformis syndrome is suspected. Patients may benefit from intramuscular injections with botulinum toxin, or steroids and lidocaine.

PERONEAL NEUROPATHIES

> **CLINICAL VIGNETTE** *A 44-year-old woman presented with right foot drop and numbness of the dorsum of the right foot. She had first noted difficulty walking 7 weeks earlier, when she had tripped over a curb and fallen down. She had intentionally lost 70 pounds over the past year. To accomplish this, she had done frequent exercises in a squatting position on the floor. There was no history of recent trauma to the back or buttock or of radicular leg pain.*
>
> *On examination, there was tenderness to palpation at the proximal lateral knee, but there was no discrete mass. She had weakness in right toe extension, foot dorsiflexion, and foot eversion. Plantar flexion and inversion of the foot, knee flexion, and hip abduction were preserved. Sensory examination was notable for reduced pinprick and light touch on the dorsum and first web space of the right foot. Muscle stretch reflexes were normal. Nerve conduction studies revealed motor conduction block on peroneal motor studies across the*

Sciatic Nerve (L4, L5; S1, S2, S3)

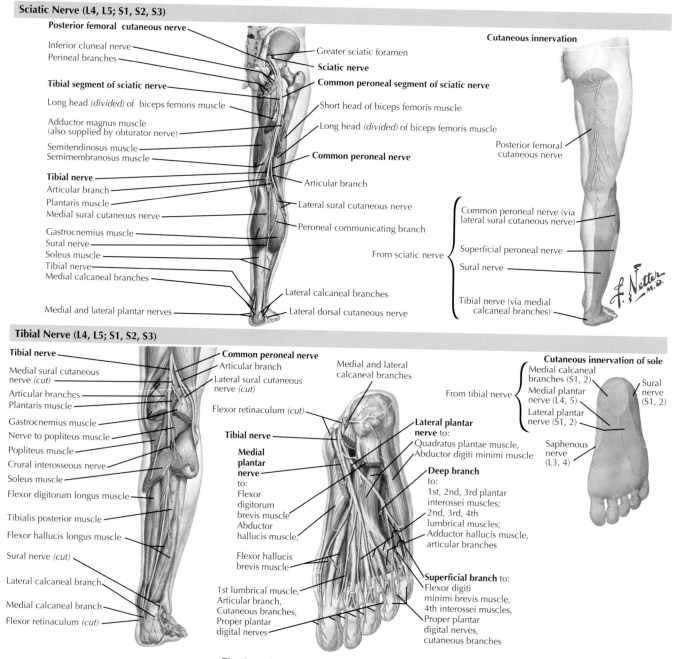

Fig. 61.1 Sciatic, Peroneal, and Tibial Nerves.

fibular head; needle electromyography showed reduced recruitment pattern in peroneal muscles with sparing of the short head of the biceps femoris, consistent with a demyelinating peroneal neuropathy. Her weakness improved significantly over the following weeks, and 3 months later she had recovered completely.

Axons originating from the L4, L5, S1, and S2 roots, primarily L5 nerve root fibers, come together to form the common peroneal nerve. It is one of the two major divisions of the sciatic nerve and separates from it as a distinct nerve in the mid- to distal thigh. It travels through the popliteal fossa and gives off the lateral sural cutaneous nerve, which unites with the medial sural cutaneous nerve (a branch of the tibial nerve) to form the sural nerve. The lateral cutaneous nerve of the calf also branches off in the popliteal fossa. It provides sensation to the skin of the lateral leg just below the knee. On its course around the fibular head, the common peroneal nerve is very superficial and covered only by skin and subcutaneous tissue. It then pierces through a fibrous, sometimes tight opening in the peroneus longus muscle (fibular tunnel) and divides into superficial and deep branches.

Etiology

Common peroneal neuropathy is the most frequent lower extremity mononeuropathy. The common peroneal nerve is most susceptible to external compression at the fibular head, where it is very superficial (Fig. 61.2). Predisposing causes include recent substantial weight loss, habitual leg crossing, or prolonged squatting. External devices, such as

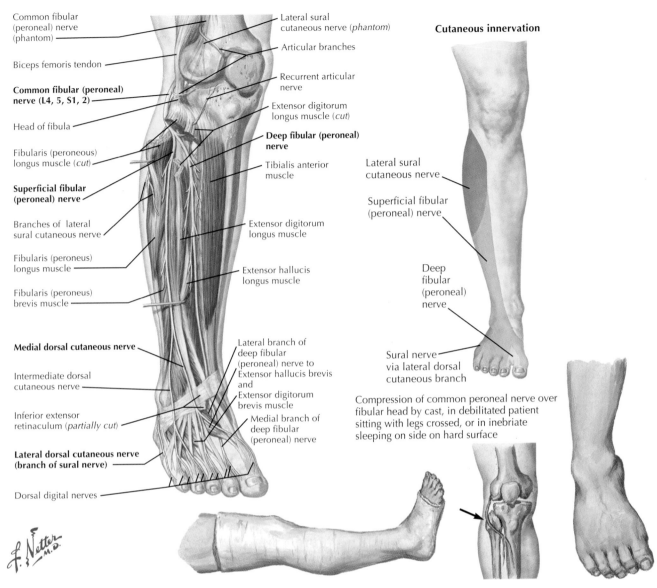

Fig. 61.2 Peroneal Nerve.

casts, braces, and tight bandages, can cause peroneal neuropathy. Diabetes mellitus, vasculitis, and rarely hereditary tendency to pressure palsy (HNPP) are other etiologic conditions. An acute anterior or lateral compartment syndrome below the knee can also lead to acute common, deep, or superficial peroneal neuropathies. Patients with insidious onset and progressive course require evaluation for mass lesions, including a Baker cyst or ganglion, osteoma, or schwannoma (Fig. 61.3). The common peroneal nerve is sometimes injured iatrogenically, such as during arthroscopic knee repair.

Isolated superficial peroneal neuropathies are uncommon but can result from lateral compartment syndrome, local trauma, or rarely an isolated schwannoma.

Clinical Presentation

Most peroneal neuropathies involve the common peroneal nerve at the fibular head causing weakness of foot dorsiflexion and eversion (see Fig. 61.2). Ambulation reveals a "steppage gait" with compensatory hip and knee flexion in order to lift the foot off the floor. The foot might hit the floor with a slap, as the patient has poor control over its

movements. With the less frequently occurring deep peroneal neuropathies, there is weakness of the tibialis anterior, extensor hallucis, extensor digitorum longus, and extensor digitorum brevis. Primary superficial peroneal neuropathies cause weakness of the peroneus longus and brevis muscles, which are mainly responsible for foot eversion.

Sensory symptoms are limited to the web space between the first and second toes with deep peroneal neuropathies. Superficial peroneal neuropathies can diminish sensation on the dorsum of the foot and lateral distal half of the leg.

EMG involvement of the short head of the biceps femoris is the major distinguishing feature with proximal peroneal division sciatic neuropathies, but function of this muscle cannot always be isolated clinically. Therefore, EMG is crucial in establishing this diagnosis.

Differential Diagnosis

Differential diagnoses of peroneal neuropathies include anterior horn cell disease, L5 radiculopathy, lumbosacral trunk or plexus lesions, sciatic neuropathy, or rarely neuromuscular junction disorders. Sciatic neuropathies are sometimes mistakenly diagnosed as peroneal neuropathies.

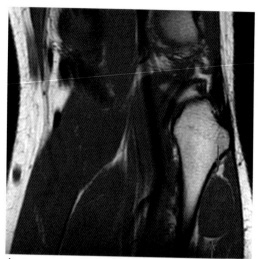

A. Coronal T1-weighted MRI demonstrates an oval mass of left peroneal nerve (arrows)

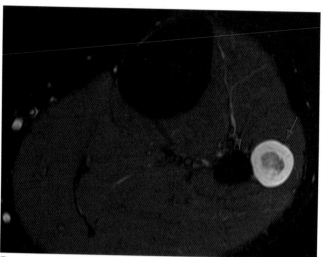

B. Axial T1-weighted post gadolinium-enhanced fat-saturated MRI demonstrating enhancing peroneal nerve schwannoma with central myxoid degeneration (arrow) near fibula (arrowhead).

Fig. 61.3 Peroneal Nerve Schwannoma.

The peroneal division of the sciatic nerve is more superficial than its tibial division; therefore external compressive proximal lesions of the sciatic nerve involve the common peroneal more than the tibial divisions. Most sciatic neuropathies also affect some tibial nerve functions with weakness of knee flexion, foot plantar flexion, and foot inversion. The ankle jerk is characteristically depressed or absent if there is involvement of the tibial component of the sciatic nerve, whereas it is typically unaffected in primary peroneal neuropathies. Sensory loss involves the common peroneal territory described above and the plantar and lateral foot surface. L5 radiculopathy remains a consideration in any patient with a foot drop. Back pain is common with nerve root lesions and is uncommon in peroneal neuropathies; the pain is typically radicular, with buttock, thigh, and leg components sometimes aggravated by positional change. The distribution of weakness is very important; involvement of muscles outside the peroneal nerve territory innervated by the L5 root, such as the tibialis posterior or gluteus medius, is critical. Isolated weakness of great toe extension occurs with mild L5 radiculopathy but is uncommon in peroneal neuropathy. In moderate to severe L5 radiculopathies, foot inversion will be weak because of the involvement of the tibial nerve-innervated tibialis posterior muscle. Uncommonly, hip abduction weakness due to the involvement of the gluteus medius, an L5 muscle supplied by the superior gluteal nerve, is noticeable. The distribution of sensory symptoms in L5 radiculopathies overlaps significantly with peroneal neuropathies, although L5 nerve root sensory loss may extend more proximally onto the lateral leg. Lumbosacral plexus lesions rarely enter the differential diagnosis of peroneal neuropathies, but are a consideration in patients who have a foot drop, proximal lower extremity pain, and motor and sensory findings extending beyond a single peripheral nerve or root distribution. Involvement of hip abduction and extension, clinically and/or by EMG, suggests plexus localization. Polyneuropathy is easily distinguished from peroneal neuropathy. The clinical examination and EMG usually reveal bilateral widespread motor and sensory abnormalities, not confined to a particular nerve or root distribution, and muscle tendon reflexes are depressed or absent. The possibility of motor neuron disease or amyotrophic lateral sclerosis exists with insidious onset of a foot drop without pain or sensory findings. In these instances, there may be evidence of upper motor neuron dysfunction. In patients with myasthenia, a disorder of neuromuscular transmission, unilateral foot drop is not seen. Distal

myopathies may produce foot drop, but usually do so bilaterally, and there is often evidence of weakness elsewhere. Unilateral foot drop with or without sensory symptoms can occur with disorders of the spinal cord or parasagittal frontal lobe. These conditions are usually associated with hyperreflexia, and magnetic resonance imaging (MRI) is useful to diagnose them.

TIBIAL NEUROPATHIES

CLINICAL VIGNETTE *A 39-year-old man presented to the emergency room for severe pain and swelling of the right leg associated with difficulty walking. On neurologic examination, there was weakness of right foot plantar flexion and inversion and flexion of the toes. The ankle jerk was absent. Doppler ultrasound and an MRI of the right knee revealed a ruptured Baker cyst in the popliteal fossa. Surgical removal of the synovial cyst resulted in resolution of the pain and foot weakness.*

Tibial nerve fibers arise primarily from L5, S1, and S2 nerve roots with some contributions from L4 and S3. The tibial nerve leaves the sciatic nerve in the mid- to distal thigh (see Fig. 61.1). The medial sural cutaneous nerve comes off in the popliteal fossa and joins the lateral sural cutaneous nerve (a branch of the common peroneal nerve) in the distal calf to form the sural nerve, which supplies the skin of the lateral aspect of the foot and the posterior lower leg to a variable degree. After innervating the gastrocnemius and soleus muscles, the tibial nerve travels distally between the tibialis posterior and gastrocnemius muscles. It sends branches to the tibialis posterior, flexor digitorum longus, and flexor hallucis longus before entering the tarsal tunnel under the flexor retinaculum. Here, it divides into the medial plantar, lateral plantar, and medial calcaneal nerves. While the medial calcaneal nerve is a purely sensory branch to the medial heel, the medial and lateral plantar nerves are mixed nerves innervating the intrinsic foot muscles as well as the skin of the sole.

Proximal Lesions

Proximal tibial neuropathies may result from Baker cysts, ganglia, tumors (Fig. 61.4), or rarely indirectly from severe ankle strains, the latter

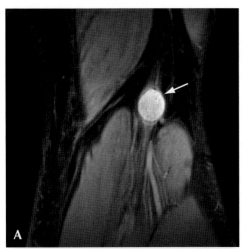

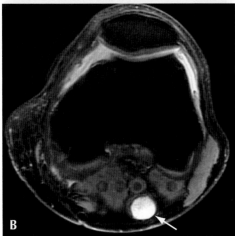

Coronal **(A)** and axial **(B)** proton density fat-saturated MR images demonstrate discrete T2 bright tumor that enlarges the nerve sheath (arrow).

Fig. 61.4 Tibial Neurofibroma.

presumably resulting from traction injury. They rarely occur in isolation. They are characterized by weakness of foot plantar flexion and inversion; although flexion, abduction, and adduction of the toes may be affected, these latter functions are difficult to evaluate clinically. The ankle jerk is absent if the nerve injury occurs proximal to the branch points of the gastrocnemius–soleus complex. Sensory loss occurs on the heel and plantar foot surface.

Tarsal Tunnel Syndrome

Tarsal tunnel syndrome (TTS), a distal tibial neuropathy, presents primarily with sensory symptoms. It is classified as an entrapment neuropathy of the posterior tibial nerve and of its primary branches, the medial and lateral plantar nerves, at the ankle (see Fig. 61.1). Although well described, there is controversy regarding its prevalence as electrophysiologic documentation is infrequent. Whether this reflects its uncommon occurrence or the inadequate sensitivity of diagnostic procedures is unclear. Fractures, ankle sprain, foot deformities due to rheumatoid arthritis or other conditions, varicose veins, tenosynovitis, and fluid retention have been implicated as possible etiologies. Patients typically present with burning pain and numbness on the sole of one or both feet. Symptoms may occur while weight bearing and are often exacerbated at night. In well-established instances, examination may disclose intrinsic plantar surface muscle atrophy. However, weakness of these muscles

is difficult to appreciate because the more proximal long toe flexors in the leg mask weakness from the involved short toe flexors within the foot. Toe abduction weakness occurs early but is difficult to assess even in healthy individuals. Sensory loss is confined to the sole of the foot; there is sparing of the lateral foot (sural distribution), the dorsum of the foot (peroneal territory), and the instep (saphenous nerve). Muscle stretch reflexes are unaffected. A Tinel sign elicited from the tibial nerve at the ankle is supportive, although not confirmatory.

If TTS results from nerve entrapment, simulating carpal tunnel syndrome, EMG should demonstrate demyelination via prolongation of the distal latencies. However, prolonged tibial motor and mixed nerve distal latencies from the medial and lateral plantar nerves are rarely seen in patients with suspected TTS. Absent mixed nerve responses from the plantar nerves may be seen, but have limited localizing value because they also occur in some seemingly healthy elderly individuals and in those with an underlying polyneuropathy. Fibrillation potentials in tibial innervated foot muscles must be interpreted with similar caution. Imaging in suspected TTS includes radiographs to detect osseous abnormalities involving the tarsal tunnel region, and CT or MRI.

Initial treatment of TTS is nonoperative, consisting of footwear modification, particularly the avoidance of high-heeled and poorly fitting footwear. Antiinflammatory medications may help. Steroid injections, augmented with lidocaine, can be helpful if flexor tenosynovitis is suspected. Care is taken to avoid an intraneural injection with the unlikely possibility of causing local nerve sclerosis. Hind foot valgus deformities can benefit from orthoses. When nonoperative measures fail in TTS, surgical intervention may be considered.

FEMORAL NEUROPATHIES

> **CLINICAL VIGNETTE** *A 63-year-old man with hemophilia presented with right knee buckling a week after a motor vehicle accident. He also complained of dull pain in the right flank radiating into the thigh and knee. He could not raise his right leg off the bed. There was no back pain or sphincter dysfunction. The neurologic examination revealed weakness of the right iliopsoas and quadriceps muscles, an absent right quadriceps muscle stretch reflex, and diminished sensation to touch and pinprick over the anterior thigh and medial leg below the knee. Pelvic CT demonstrated a hemorrhage of the right iliacus and psoas muscles in the pelvis. Surgery revealed a large hematoma compressing the femoral nerve. This was successfully drained. Postoperatively, the patient gradually improved, regaining significant function within a week.*

The femoral nerve comes off the lumbar plexus and is formed by the posterior divisions of the L2–L4 roots (Fig. 61.5). It travels between two important hip flexors, the iliopsoas and iliacus muscles, which it innervates. Approximately 4 cm proximal to the inguinal ligament, the femoral nerve is covered by a tight fascia at the iliopsoas groove. It exits the pelvis by passing beneath the medial inguinal ligament to enter the femoral triangle just lateral to the femoral artery and vein. Here, the nerve separates into the anterior and posterior divisions. The anterior division innervates the sartorius muscle and the anteromedial skin of the thigh via the medial cutaneous nerve of the thigh. The posterior division gives off muscular branches to the pectineus and quadriceps femoris muscles as well as the saphenous nerve, a cutaneous branch to the skin of the inner calf. The nerve can be compressed anywhere along its course, but it is particularly susceptible within the body of the psoas muscle, at the iliopsoas groove, and at the inguinal ligament.

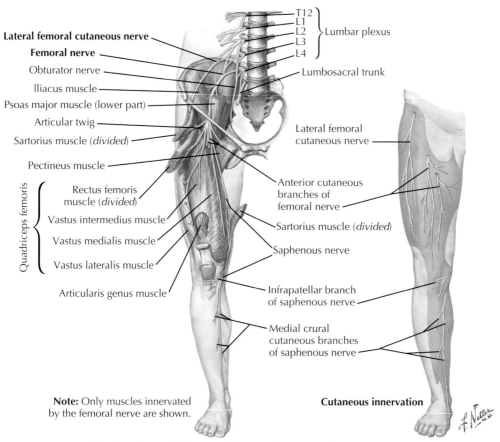

Fig. 61.5 Femoral Nerve and Lateral Cutaneous Nerve of Thigh.

Etiology

Femoral mononeuropathies are infrequent. Historically, diabetic femoral neuropathies were considered common, although most of these probably represented diabetic radiculoplexusneuropathies in which the femoral component dominated. Vasculitis may present as mononeuritis multiplex with acute involvement of the femoral nerve.

Femoral neuropathies occasionally follow prolonged surgeries or childbirth in the lithotomy position, presumably from anatomic predisposition to kinking beneath the inguinal ligament. Iliacus hematoma or abscess, misplaced attempts at femoral artery or vein puncture, or iatrogenic injury after nephrectomy or hip arthroplasty are other recognized causes. Tumors, benign and malignant, can rarely cause femoral neuropathy (Fig. 61.6). Isolated saphenous nerve injuries may result from knee arthroscopy, femoral–popliteal artery bypass surgery, and in the course of coronary artery bypass graft surgery.

Clinical Presentation

When the more proximal femoral nerve is involved, weakness of the iliopsoas manifests as limited hip flexion. Mild hip flexion weakness may also occur with more distal femoral nerve involvement from poor function of the rectus femoris, the only head of the quadriceps muscle originating within the pelvis and contributing to hip flexion. Patients with severe quadriceps weakness are unable to extend the leg or lock the knee; when severe, this often interferes with walking. Initially, mild femoral neuropathies may present with difficulty descending stairs because the knee buckles from mild quadriceps weakness. Eversion of the thigh might be impaired because of sartorius weakness. The patellar muscle stretch reflex is almost always diminished or absent in femoral

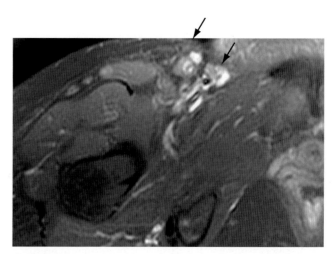

Fig. 61.6 Femoral Nerve Neurofibromas in Neurofibromatosis (*Arrows*).

neuropathies. Groin and thigh pain are frequent presenting symptoms. When patients experience sensory symptoms, these typically involve the anteromedial thigh and medial lower leg. A pure motor syndrome with quadriceps weakness and atrophy can result from lesions distal to the branching of the saphenous nerve in the thigh.

Differential Diagnosis

A nerve root lesion at L3–L4 is the most common consideration, but a herniated nucleus pulposus infrequently involves the level L3–L4.

Lumbosacral plexus lesions primarily affecting the lumbar nerves may also mimic femoral neuropathies.

LATERAL FEMORAL CUTANEOUS NEUROPATHY

CLINICAL VIGNETTE *A 38-year-old woman presented with pain and numbness of the left thigh in her seventh month of pregnancy. She described a burning discomfort extending from the hip to the lateral aspect of the thigh, intensified by standing or walking. There was associated cutaneous hypersensitivity with an aversion to having clothes or bed sheets rub against her. She was unaware of any other precipitating events. Examination demonstrated an elliptically shaped area of sensory loss on the distal half of the left anterolateral thigh. She had no atrophy, weakness, or reflex loss. The symptoms gradually improved in the months following the delivery of a healthy baby.*

The lateral femoral cutaneous nerve (LFCN) arises from the second and third lumbar roots and travels through the retroperitoneum. After traversing the psoas muscle, the nerve reaches the iliacus muscle (see Fig. 61.5). Medial to the anterior superior iliac spine, it exits the pelvis under or through the inguinal ligament, the presumed usual site of entrapment. Subsequently, it supplies sensation to the anterolateral thigh.

Etiology

Meralgia paresthetica is an entrapment mononeuropathy of the lateral femoral cutaneous nerve (Fig. 61.7). It is usually unilateral. Certain anatomical variations of its inguinal course might predispose to injury. Like many mononeuropathies, it is more common in people with diabetes. Meralgia paresthetica often occurs in overweight individuals, especially after sudden gain in weight, or in individuals wearing tight belts and garments. It can be iatrogenic, for example, secondary to iliac bone graft harvesting or inguinal herniorrhaphy. Occasionally, the nerve

is injured within the thigh secondary to blunt or penetrating trauma (e.g., a misplaced injection), or rarely by a soft tissue sarcoma within the thigh.

Clinical Presentation

Often aggravated by standing or walking, symptoms include an uncomfortable positive component (burning, hypersensitivity) and negative features (numbness). Typically, the area of demonstrable sensory loss on examination is smaller than the lateral femoral cutaneous nerve territory in most anatomic diagrams, likely due to significant overlap with adjacent nerves. Because the LCFN is a purely sensory nerve, there are no associated reflex or motor abnormalities, helping to distinguish meralgia from other disorders that deserve diagnostic consideration.

Differential Diagnosis

Although uncommon, L2 radiculopathy of any etiology, evidenced as weakness and denervation of L2-innervated hip flexors and adductors, is a differential consideration. Sensory symptoms and signs extend over the anterior and medial aspects of the thigh. Lumbar spinal stenosis also tends to be exacerbated by prolonged standing or walking, although it does not cause numbness in this specific distribution.

Disorders of the lumbosacral plexus may mimic meralgia, particularly in patients having insidious onset of invasive or compressive disorders, in which pain and other sensory symptoms have no obvious motor component. Retroperitoneal neoplasms or hematomas and abdominal surgery might affect the LCFN; however, they are unlikely to cause isolated meralgia. Instead, concomitant involvement of adjacent nerves usually leads to widespread motor, reflex, and sensory loss, indicating that there may be a plexus lesion rather than a single nerve problem.

Isolated femoral neuropathies are uncommon and unlikely to be confused with meralgia because of the type and distribution of abnormalities. Sensory symptoms involve the anterior and medial thigh and extend to the medial surface of the lower leg. Weakness of the quadriceps muscle and loss of its stretch reflex are other objective and distinguishing features.

Although the LFCN can be tested by nerve conduction studies in the thigh distal to the inguinal ligament, technical difficulties interfere with the detection of mild demyelinating injuries. A response cannot be obtained from all individuals and is particularly difficult to record in overweight individuals who are most susceptible to this syndrome. Nerve conduction studies of the LFCN are of greatest value when a normal response is readily obtained from the asymptomatic side and a low-amplitude or absent response is obtained from the symptomatic side. In patients with atypical symptoms, thigh MRI is indicated to exclude primary lesions, such as soft tissue sarcoma. MRI and CT of the retroperitoneum and pelvis should be considered in patients with unexplained LFCN neuropathy. Fasting blood glucose measurement is appropriate in acute-onset, painful LFCN neuropathies without alternative explanation.

Management

The natural history of meralgia varies, but most patients become asymptomatic within 2 years. Others have a more protracted and chronic course, but data on the natural history of this neuropathy are limited. Conservative management includes weight loss and avoidance of tight garments. Medications, such as gabapentin and amitriptyline, might alleviate neuropathic pain. Injections of local anesthetics and steroids near the anterior superior iliac spine may serve diagnostic and therapeutic roles and are sometimes "curative." Patients with intractable symptoms may benefit from nerve release or transection. The chance of success of surgical treatments decreases with prolonged duration of symptoms and direct injury to the nerve.

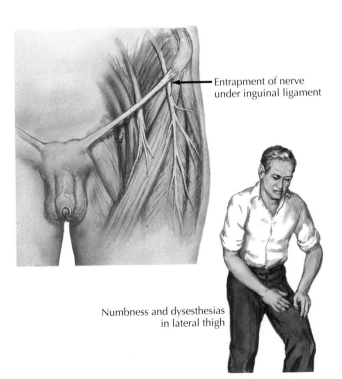

Entrapment of nerve under inguinal ligament

Numbness and dysesthesias in lateral thigh

Fig. 61.7 Lateral Femoral Cutaneous Nerve.

OBTURATOR NEUROPATHIES

> **CLINICAL VIGNETTE** *A 35-year-old woman presented with pain in the right medial thigh and difficulty walking. This had begun 6 months prior, immediately after the delivery of her son. After 8 hours of labor complicated by fetal failure to progress, she had eventually undergone an emergency cesarean section. On neurologic examination, she had weakness of the right thigh adductors and a patch of numbness and dysesthesia on the medial surface of the thigh.*

The obturator nerve originates from the anterior rami of the L2, L3, and L4 nerve roots (Fig. 61.8). After its course through the pelvis, the nerve exits through the obturator canal and separates into the anterior and posterior divisions. The anterior division supplies the adductor longus, adductor brevis, and gracilis muscles, whereas its terminal branch provides sensation to the distal medial thigh. The posterior division innervates the obturator externus, the superior portion of the adductor magnus, and sometimes the adductor brevis.

Etiology

Obturator neuropathies may be caused by pelvic masses, difficult parturition, or obturator hernias, or may be complications of hip arthroplasty or pelvic surgery.

Clinical Presentation

Obturator neuropathies are exceedingly uncommon focal nerve lesions that typically present with hip instability. Weakness and denervation are confined to the large hip adductors. Occasionally, they present with pain and sensory symptoms in the medial thigh without obvious weakness.

ILIOHYPOGASTRIC, ILIOINGUINAL, AND GENITOFEMORAL NEUROPATHIES

These mononeuropathies should be considered in the differential diagnosis of dysesthesias of the pelvis and groin without apparent motor deficits.

Iliohypogastric Nerve

The iliohypogastric nerve arises from the T12–L1 nerve roots. Like the ilioinguinal nerve, it supplies the internal oblique and transversus abdominis muscles. However, weakness of these muscles is difficult to demonstrate on physical examination. The iliohypogastric nerve divides in lateral and anterior cutaneous branches. Iliohypogastric neuropathies thus produce sensory symptoms in two distinct areas: the lateral aspect of the iliac crest and the suprapubic region. The anterior branch is most commonly injured by lower abdominal surgery with a lateral incision site extending to the internal oblique muscle, and the lateral branch is most commonly injured by major pelvic surgery. The prognosis for recovery is generally good in both.

Ilioinguinal Nerve

This nerve arises from the L1 nerve root. Loss of sensation along the inguinal ligament, over the pubic symphysis and the anterior scrotum or mons pubis, with or without associated pain, characterizes ilioinguinal neuropathies. Ilioinguinal neuropathies most frequently

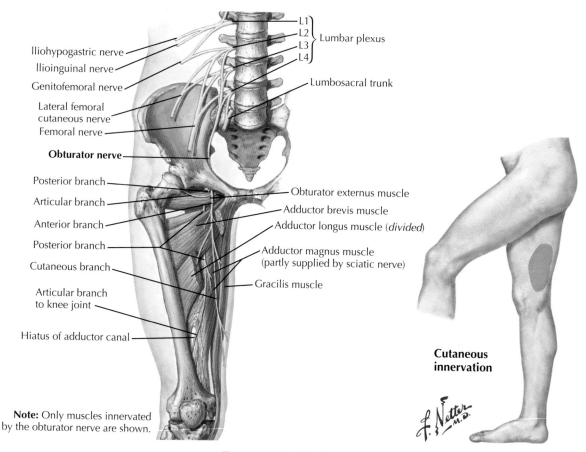

Fig. 61.8 Obturator Nerve.

result from lower abdominal surgeries, bone graft harvesting from the iliac crest, and parturition. Rarely, nerve entrapment occurs as it passes through the abdominal wall, causing groin pain relieved by hip flexion.

Genitofemoral Nerve

The genitofemoral nerve is supplied by fibers originating from the L1 and L2 nerve roots. It separates into genital and femoral branches. Genitofemoral neuropathy presents with pain, numbness, and paresthesias of the labia majora or scrotum as well as the proximal anterior thigh, lateral to the sensory territory of the ilioinguinal nerve. Standing or hip extension may exaggerate symptoms. Surgical procedures, such as inguinal herniorrhaphies or appendectomies, are causes of genitofemoral neuropathy. The genitofemoral nerve has a motor branch innervating the cremaster muscle. Unfortunately, the cremasteric reflex is not a reliable diagnostic clue.

Diagnosis

As the sensory territories of these three nerves overlap, their mononeuropathies are difficult to distinguish by clinical examination alone. The ilioinguinal, iliohypogastric, and genitofemoral nerves are inaccessible to nerve conduction techniques. Therefore, EMG is of limited value and mainly serves the purpose to rule out differential diagnoses, such as proximal lumbar radiculopathies or plexopathies. Local injections of anesthetics not only provide symptomatic relief but also may be diagnostically helpful. Retroperitoneal and pelvic MRI and CT are indicated when a progressive ilioinguinal, iliohypogastric, or genitofemoral neuropathy develops without obvious cause.

Management

Most patients with postoperative neuropathies experience full recovery; persistent symptoms can be seen in those with unrepaired nerve transection. Medications, such as amitriptyline, carbamazepine, gabapentin, and venlafaxine, may diminish pain intensity.

Diagnostic Approach to Mononeuropathies

Electrodiagnosis is a primary means of assessing a suspected mononeuropathy. EMG may differentiate other lesions that mimic mononeuropathies, particularly at the respective plexus or nerve root level. Besides providing anatomic localization, EMG helps to assess prognosis. A specific etiology is rarely revealed, even with abnormal EMG. Demonstration of a predominantly demyelinating lesion provides the primary basis for localization, but this is generally not possible in sciatic, femoral, and obturator neuropathies, as conduction studies of these nerves are limited by technical factors.

Further testing is sometimes indicated, depending on the index of suspicion regarding causation. Plain radiographs can assess possible bone spurs or exostoses, arthritides, congenital deformities, fractures, or bony tumors that may contribute to nerve injury. MRI and occasionally ultrasonography are useful in assessing soft tissue lesions, localizing areas of entrapment, and providing a spatial image of the nerve and its surrounding structures. However, when EMG indicates a defined localization without clinical or imaging evidence of a specific mechanism, surgical exploration is an important diagnostic tool that sometimes also offers a therapeutic option. Acute axonal nerve lesions are characterized by a hyperintense signal on T2-weighted MRI. Thus, MRI can demonstrate the site of nerve injury when localization by EMG is difficult. Occasionally, elevated C-reactive protein provides a clue to an underlying vasculitis. Rarely, cerebrospinal fluid examination is indicated to distinguish an inflammatory or carcinomatous polyradiculopathy from a mononeuropathy.

Management and Prognosis of Mononeuropathies

When a definable mechanism exists, such as a mass causing nerve compression, surgery is indicated. If the neuropathy resulted from nerve traction from excessive squatting or compression from habitual leg crossing, the primary treatment is discontinuation of these activities. If a cast or brace is compressing the nerve (e.g., the peroneal nerve at the fibular head) it must be modified to protect the nerve. Nerve injury from an acute compartment syndrome is a surgical emergency and necessitates fasciotomy.

Foot drop can be symptomatically treated by an ankle–foot orthosis, its primary goal being the prevention of falls. Patients also state that their walking endurance improves with this device. An ankle–foot orthosis should be prescribed cautiously in patients with significant quadriceps weakness; it may destabilize a patient's marginally compensated technique of "knee locking" and weight bearing, thus increasing the risk of falling.

Recovery depends on the nature, location, severity, and persistence of the injury and the patient's underlying health and age. An optimistic prognosis can be expected with a primary demyelinating lesion. Demyelinating lesions secondary to monophasic external compression or stretch typically recover within weeks to months. However, when evidence of significant axonal damage exists, reinnervation must occur, a process that progresses at a rate of 1 mm/day or approximately 1 inch/month. A longer period (months to years) is thus required for recovery. The degree of axon loss and distance from the site of injury to the target site of reinnervation also influence the eventual outcome.

Future Directions

More sensitive neurophysiologic and neuroimaging techniques are needed to improve the diagnosis of mononeuropathies and their etiologies and to guide research into the treatment of these often-disabling disorders. Improvements in the management of neuropathic pain related to mononeuropathy, a chronic problem for many patients, are particularly desired.

Functional outcome after severe traumatic nerve injuries is often unsatisfactory. Autografts serve to bridge nerve gaps with variable success. Nerve conduits manufactured from synthetic or natural materials are used as scaffolds in lieu of nerve grafts. These conduits can be engineered to deliver nerve growth factors. A more detailed understanding of the molecular mechanisms of axonal regeneration including the role of Schwann cells, growth factors, and the extracellular environment is essential for the development of better treatment options. The role of microRNAs as well as macrophages in functional nerve recovery is being studied. Stem cell therapy, particularly using mesenchymal stem cells that can differentiate into various cell types, might also offer treatment options in the future.

ADDITIONAL RESOURCES

American Association of Neuromuscular and Electrodiagnostic Medicine. Available from: http://www.aanem.org. Accessed March 25, 2018.
The information on this website includes a list of suggested reading for physicians as well as educational material for patients with various neuromuscular disorders.
Benezis I, Boutaud B, Leclerc J, Fabre T, Durandeau A. Lateral femoral cutaneous neuropathy and its surgical treatment: a report of 167 cases. Muscle Nerve 2007;36:659-63.
The authors retrospectively evaluate the clinical response to nerve release or transection in patients with meralgia paresthetica.
Dumitru D, Amato A, Zwarts M. Electrodiagnostic medicine. 2nd ed. Philadelphia, PA: Hanley & Belfus; 2002.

This textbook is an excellent reference for physicians interested in disorders of the peripheral nervous system and electrophysiological techniques.

Katirji B. Peroneal neuropathy. Neurol Clin 1999;17:567-91.

The author provides a good review of the clinical presentation and electrophysiology of peroneal nerve lesions.

Kuntzer T, van Melle G, Regli F. Clinical and prognostic features in unilateral femoral neuropathies. Muscle Nerve 1997;20:205-11.

This article studies the clinical and electrodiagnostic features influencing outcome in 32 patients with femoral neuropathy.

Sorenson EJ, Chen JJ, Daube JR. Obturator neuropathy: causes and outcome. Muscle Nerve 2002;25:605-7.

The authors retrospectively examine the causes and prognosis of obturator neuropathy in 22 patients.

Sunderland S. Nerves and nerve injuries. 2nd ed. Edinburgh, Scotland: Churchill Livingstone; 1978.

This outstanding textbook provides a detailed description of the anatomy and physiology of peripheral nerves and outlines the various mechanisms of nerve injury in great depth.

Motor Neuron Disorders

Jayashri Srinivasan

62

Amyotrophic Lateral Sclerosis

Doreen T. Ho, James A. Russell

CLINICAL VIGNETTE *A 54-year-old man reported painless left arm weakness for 6 months. While exercising at the gym, he noticed difficulty lifting weights with his left arm. Progressively he had difficulty cutting food and opening jars with his left hand. He reported cramps in both arms and visible muscle twitching in his left arm and occasionally in other regions of the body. He denied neck pain, numbness, or tingling. His examination revealed normal cognitive function. Mental status and cranial nerves were normal. He was weak in every muscle in his left arm with continuous fasciculations observed in many of these muscles. Reflexes were brisk throughout with a Hoffman sign present on the left.*

In 1874, Jean-Martin Charcot described a disorder that he named amyotrophic lateral sclerosis (ALS). In France, it is referred to as Charcot disease, whereas motor neuron disease (MND) is the preferred name for the disorder in the United Kingdom. In the United States, ALS is better known as Lou Gehrig disease.

Charcot described a disorder characterized by loss of voluntary motor function, resulting from degeneration of anterior horn cells, corticospinal tracts, select motor cranial nerve nuclei, and cortical motor neurons (Figs. 62.1 and 62.2). ALS is a sporadic disorder (sALS) of unknown cause in the majority of cases. In approximately 5%–21% of cases, patients have a clear family history and are characterized as having familial ALS (fALS), typically with an autosomal dominant pattern of inheritance. In individual cases, fALS and sALS are phenotypically indistinguishable although the average age of onset in familial cases may be 10 years younger than in sporadic counterparts.

The incidence of ALS approximates 1.8 in 100,000. Men are affected nearly twice as often as women, although this ratio becomes closer to 1:1 postmenopause. The median age at onset in sALS is 55 years; however, this disease may afflict patients in their late teens or their 90s. The average life expectancy is between 2 and 3 years; in less than 10% of patients, ventilator-independent survival of less than 1 year or greater than 10 years is seen. Half of the affected individuals die within 3 years and only a quarter survive 5 years without dependency on invasive mechanical ventilation. Young males and patients with restricted upper motor neuron (UMN) or lower motor neuron (LMN) presentations tend to have a slower course. Primary bulbar (disordered speech and swallowing) presentations tend to disproportionately affect older women and appear to have a more rapid course.

In the United States, it is estimated that at any given time 25,000 patients are diagnosed with ALS. The prevalence of ALS appears to be increasing, perhaps because of an aging population. Other than historical observations identifying an increased incidence among inhabitants of Guam and the Kii peninsula of Japan, there does not appear to be any particular geographic location or ethnic group that has a significantly higher risk of developing ALS.

CLINICAL PRESENTATIONS

The presenting features of ALS are variable but can be characterized as painless weakness typically presenting focally in limb, bulbar, or axial muscles, and then progressing both within, and outside of the originally involved region. Typically, the patient seeks medical care when his or her weakness begins to affect activities of daily living (Fig. 62.3). It is not uncommon for ALS to be misdiagnosed initially and the time between symptom onset and diagnosis is usually months. Unfortunately, there is a tendency to misdiagnose ALS as a potentially treatable nerve, nerve root, or spinal cord compressive syndrome or orthopedic condition. A significant percentage of ALS patients may undergo unnecessary surgeries. It should be emphasized that progressive weakness and atrophy in the absence of pain and sensory symptoms rarely represent a surgically treatable condition.

The exclusive motor involvement and the chronologic course distinguish ALS from other neurologic diseases. Simultaneous involvement of both UMNs and LMNs and progression both within and outside of the originally involved regions is necessary for a definite clinical diagnosis. LMN involvement may be documented by clinical, electrodiagnostic, or pathologic (muscle biopsy) means, although muscle biopsy is used occasionally. UMN involvement is currently defined by clinical criteria alone. Classic ALS is usually an easy diagnosis for an experienced neurologist. Diagnosis may be delayed in patients with limited clinical evidence of the LMN or UMN component, slow disease progression, and confounding neurologic signs from unrelated problems such as sensory loss from mononeuropathies, radiculopathies, and polyneuropathies.

The signature of anterior horn cell loss is painless weakness and atrophy, hypoactive or absent deep tendon reflexes, and fasciculations. Atrophy is best appreciated when it is focal, in contrast to normal muscle bulk elsewhere. It may be difficult to distinguish atrophy from LMN disease resulting from the atrophy of disuse, particularly in the elderly. Suppressed deep tendon reflexes may also be difficult to interpret as they may represent a normal variant. In ALS, muscle weakness due to LMN dysfunction occurs in a segmental (myotomal) distribution and spreads in a regional fashion. As an example, a patient with ALS and hand weakness may have all hand muscles innervated by C8–T1 roots affected. Weakness occurring in a nerve distribution should lead to consideration of a different disorder (e.g., multifocal motor neuropathy).

Fasciculations seen in many muscles in multiple limbs are ominous and are strongly suggestive of motor neuron disease. Fasciculations that occur infrequently, or repetitively in one spot in one muscle, are more

Cerebral Cortex: Efferent Pathways

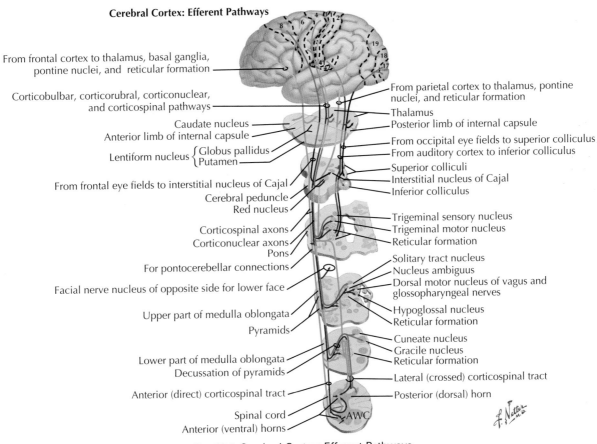

From frontal cortex to thalamus, basal ganglia, pontine nuclei, and reticular formation

From parietal cortex to thalamus, pontine nuclei, and reticular formation

Corticobulbar, corticorubral, corticonuclear, and corticospinal pathways

Thalamus

Caudate nucleus
Anterior limb of internal capsule

Posterior limb of internal capsule

Lentiform nucleus { Globus pallidus / Putamen

From occipital eye fields to superior colliculus
From auditory cortex to inferior colliculus

From frontal eye fields to interstitial nucleus of Cajal
Cerebral peduncle
Red nucleus

Superior colliculi
Interstitial nucleus of Cajal
Inferior colliculus

Corticospinal axons
Corticonuclear axons
Pons

Trigeminal sensory nucleus
Trigeminal motor nucleus
Reticular formation

For pontocerebellar connections

Facial nerve nucleus of opposite side for lower face

Solitary tract nucleus
Nucleus ambiguus
Dorsal motor nucleus of vagus and glossopharyngeal nerves

Upper part of medulla oblongata

Pyramids

Hypoglossal nucleus
Reticular formation

Lower part of medulla oblongata
Decussation of pyramids

Cuneate nucleus
Gracile nucleus
Reticular formation

Anterior (direct) corticospinal tract

Lateral (crossed) corticospinal tract
Posterior (dorsal) horn

Spinal cord
Anterior (ventral) horns

AWC

Fig. 62.1 Cerebral Cortex: Efferent Pathways.

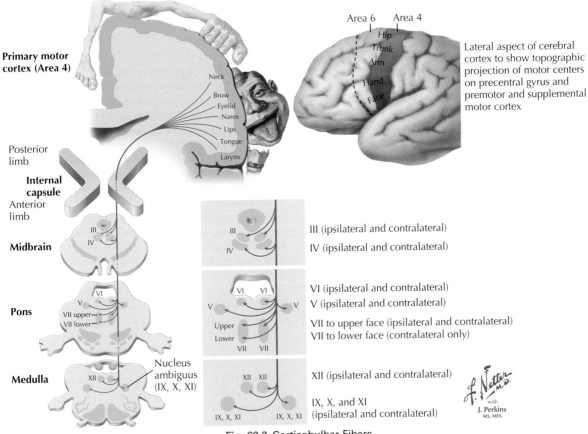

Primary motor cortex (Area 4)

Neck
Brow
Eyelid
Nares
Lips
Tongue
Larynx

Posterior limb

Internal capsule
Anterior limb

Midbrain

III
IV

Pons

VI
V
VII upper
VII lower

Medulla

XII

Nucleus ambiguus (IX, X, XI)

Area 6   Area 4

Hip
Trunk
Arm
Hand
Face

Lateral aspect of cerebral cortex to show topographic projection of motor centers on precentral gyrus and premotor and supplemental motor cortex

III (ipsilateral and contralateral)

IV (ipsilateral and contralateral)

VI (ipsilateral and contralateral)

V (ipsilateral and contralateral)

VII to upper face (ipsilateral and contralateral)
VII to lower face (contralateral only)

XII (ipsilateral and contralateral)

IX, X, and XI (ipsilateral and contralateral)

Fig. 62.2 Corticobulbar Fibers.

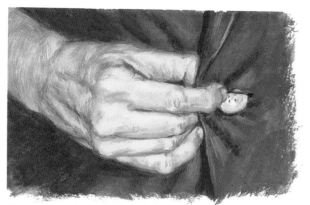

Fine movements of hand impaired; prominent metacarpal bones indicate atrophy of interossei muscles

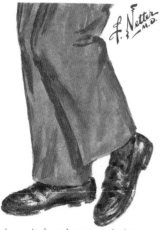

Weak, dragging gait; foot drop or early fatigue on walking

Fig. 62.3 Motor Neuron Disease: Early Clinical Manifestations.

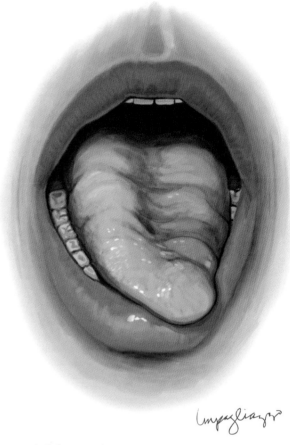

Asymmetric (left greater than right); atrophy, weakness, and fasciculations of the tongue, with deviation to the left on protrusion.

Fig. 62.4 Tongue Atrophy in Amyotrophic Lateral Sclerosis.

likely to have a benign origin, particularly in the absence of weakness or atrophy. The absence of fasciculations does not eliminate the consideration of ALS. They may not be readily visible because of prominent subcutaneous tissue. Physicians often initially recognize fasciculations, although the patient in retrospect may recall that they were present for some time. Muscle cramping is a common, albeit nonspecific, manifestation of motor neuron disease. The initiation of cramps during manual muscle testing is common in ALS.

What constitutes clinical signs of corticospinal or corticobulbar tract pathology may be more ambiguous. Spasticity represents a definite UMN sign; Babinski signs if unequivocal are confirmatory of UMN disease. Unfortunately, Babinski signs may not be elucidated in many ALS patients as a result of LMN toe extensor weakness. The Hoffman sign is generally indicative of UMN involvement of the arms, particularly if asymmetric. Hyperactive deep tendon reflexes, particularly with sustained clonus, indicate UMN involvement. The term relative UMN sign has been used to describe the preservation of a deep tendon reflex in a weak and atrophic muscle. Reflex spread also implicates UMN disease; finger flexion (C8) occurring in response to brachioradialis tendon percussion (C6) and activation of the contralateral thigh adductors when the insertions of the ipsilateral thigh adductors are percussed (crossed adduction) are two notable examples of this phenomenon. Motor impairment in UMN disease typically results in slowness and incoordination. UMN weakness may occur in a specific pattern: the elbow, wrist, and finger extensors are weaker than their flexor

counterparts in the upper extremity; whereas conversely, hip and knee flexors and foot dorsiflexors and evertors are weaker in the lower limb.

Upper motor neuron signs and symptoms in the bulbar region may be more difficult to characterize. The presence of a jaw jerk or snout reflex is considered an indicator of corticobulbar tract dysfunction. An exaggerated gag reflex has a similar implication. One common manifestation of central nervous system involvement in ALS is a pseudobulbar affect; that is, emotional lability with a tendency to readily laugh or cry in the absence of emotion. The pathologic substrate of this phenomenon is not completely understood.

Tongue atrophy, fasciculation, and weakness are perhaps the most frequently occurring and recognized manifestations of LMN involvement of cranial nerves in ALS. It is important to observe for fasciculations when the tongue is relaxed on the floor of the mouth (Fig. 62.4). Tremulousness of the tongue with attempted protrusion may be readily misinterpreted as representing fasciculations. Weakness of both facial and jaw muscles may occur in ALS but they are usually subtle. Weakness of neck extension and neck flexion is common in ALS, and head drop may be a rare presenting feature (Fig. 62.5). Neck drop is commonly associated with posterior neck discomfort and is typically relieved when the neck is supported. Notable for their absence are ptosis and ophthalmoparesis, and symptoms related to sight, hearing, taste, smell, and facial sensation.

Symptoms related to disordered ventilation occur most commonly in the latter stages of ALS but may be the presenting manifestation in

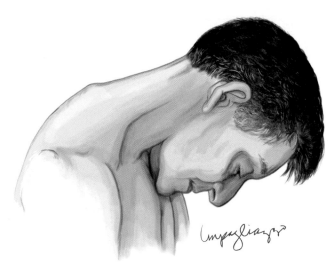

Fig. 62.5 Head Drop in Amyotrophic Sclerosis.

approximately 1% of patients. The inability to generate a robust cough, sniff, or sneeze is due to the inability to generate sufficient intrathoracic pressures due to LMN weakness of the internal intercostal or abdominal muscles. Orthopnea implicates diaphragmatic insufficiency due to anterior horn cell disease in the upper segments (C3–C5) of the cervical cord. Paradoxical abdominal movement; that is, outward (rather than the normal inward) movement of the abdominal wall during inspiration, is a helpful clinical sign. Disordered sleep is probably a common manifestation of impaired nocturnal ventilation, and early morning headache may indicate nocturnal carbon dioxide retention.

Ptosis, abnormal extraocular movements, and urinary and rectal incontinence do not typically occur in ALS. ALS patients with UMN-dominant disease may complain of urinary urgency. Traditionally, ALS is considered to be a painless disease. However, discomfort due to impaired mobility, spasticity, and cramping may be prominent. Immobilized upper extremities commonly result in painful adhesive capsulitis of the shoulders. Back or neck pain may occur as a consequence of paraspinal weakness and lack of spine support. Alteration in gait mechanics from leg weakness may put inordinate stress on the back, hips, and knees, potentially exacerbating preexisting degenerative joint disease.

Behavioral and cognitive abnormalities in ALS have been recognized since the 19th century, but may be obscured by dysarthria or blamed on coexisting depression. These cognitive and behavioral changes are associated with preferential pathologic involvement of the frontal and temporal lobes (frontotemporal lobar degeneration [FTLD] resulting in frontotemporal dementia [FTD]). The FTD associated with ALS may precede, coincide, or follow signs and symptoms of motor neuron disease. It may occur in sALS or fALS, and it is now estimated that 20% of ALS patients will fulfill criteria for FTD. The cognitive changes are most prominent in the domain of executive dysfunction and language. Disorganization, impaired planning, mental inflexibility, nonfluent progressive aphasia (word finding), and fluent semantic dementia (word meaning) may dominate the clinical picture. Tests of verbal fluency provide a sensitive screening method. Normal patients should be able to generate at least 11 words in 1 minute in a defined category (e.g., fruits). Behavioral difficulties are typically displayed in social and interpersonal realms. Patients lose the ability to appreciate nonverbal cues as well as the insight to interpret them. Patients may also become withdrawn, disinhibited, and depressed.

The nosology of ALS and related motor neuron disease remains confusing. Progressive bulbar palsy refers to motor neuron disease that initially exclusively affects bulbar function, typically speech and swallowing. Approximately a quarter of ALS patients, often older women, present in this manner. Identifying ALS as the cause of progressive bulbar palsy is made easier when there are notable LMN findings such as tongue atrophy and fasciculations. Conversely, the diagnosis may be rendered difficult when the more difficult to detect UMN findings predominate. Eventually, the vast majority develop limb involvement and unequivocal ALS.

Of the approximately two-thirds of patients who present with limb-onset disease, about one-third will have predominantly LMN features that may be referred to as LMN dominant ALS. Those cases with exclusive LMN signs have been historically referred to as progressive muscular atrophy (PMA). Most lower motor dominant patients will develop UMN features, leaving little doubt that they have ALS. PMA patients typically progress more slowly than ALS and may never develop UMN signs. Some of these patients, usually men, develop profound weakness that is restricted to either the upper or lower extremities for years before progressing to other regions. These syndromes have been referred to as flail limb syndrome or bibrachial amyotrophic diplegia (BAD) and lower extremity amyotrophic diplegia (LAD), respectively. These designations have little practical value other than to alert clinicians that such atypical presentations exist.

At the opposite end of the phenotypic spectrum is the patient with UMN predominant disease. Five percent or less of MND patients will present in this manner. Signs and symptoms typically begin in the legs but may start in the arms or bulbar regions. Exclusive UMN disease has historically been referred to as primary lateral sclerosis (PLS). PLS often has a much more protracted course than typical ALS. Most series report an average life expectancy of 7–14 years. A percentage of patients with PLS eventually develop clinical and electrodiagnostic evidence of LMN disease, and therefore it would be logical to consider PLS as a subtype of ALS until evidence suggests otherwise. PLS patients who devolve into ALS typically do so within 4 years of onset.

The El Escorial criteria were developed in 1990 in El Escorial, Spain, and were modified in 1998 in Airlie House, Virginia, in the United States, in an attempt to develop consensus criteria for the research diagnosis of ALS. Definite diagnosis according to these criteria requires both UMN and LMN clinical findings in three of the four body regions (cranial, cervical, thoracic, and lumbosacral). In addition to a definite ALS category, there are probable, possible, and laboratory-supported probable ALS categories. The former two are based solely on clinical criteria, whereas the latter allows for consideration of electrodiagnostic evidence of denervation as a surrogate for clinical evidence of LMN disease. In most cases, an experienced neurologist will recognize the inevitability of the ALS diagnosis long before these criteria are fulfilled. Further detracting from the sensitivity of the El Escorial criteria is the recognition that a significant portion of ALS patients will succumb to their disease without fulfilling these criteria. Accordingly, the El Escorial criteria appear to be a more useful research than clinical tool.

In 2006, in an effort to diagnose ALS earlier in patients for clinical trial recruitment and potential therapeutic interventions, a third consensus conference of experts in Awaji, Japan, added two major points to the diagnostic criteria. The Awaji criteria propose that fasciculation potentials may serve as a surrogate for fibrillation potentials/positive waves in muscles with chronic motor unit action potential changes in a patient with clinical features of ALS. The diagnostic utility of the Awaji criteria was assessed in retrospective and prospective studies and established to provide an increased or comparable sensitivity. Whether benign versus malignant fasciculations can be distinguished electrodiagnostically and whether fasciculations represent a surrogate marker for ongoing denervation in ALS remain controversial.

The diagnosis of ALS remains a clinical endeavor. Electromyography, nerve conduction studies, and measurements of ventilatory capacity are routinely obtained in ALS suspects. These tests are done to provide diagnostic support for diffuse LMN and ventilatory muscle involvement, respectively. Other testing is done with the primary intent of identifying or excluding differential diagnostic considerations. Genetic testing may provide the opportunity for diagnostic proof in patients with suggestive family histories; the most frequent mutations associated with fALS, superoxide dismutase (SOD1), and c9orf72 are most commonly tested, but panels of genetic testing in ALS are available (Table 62.1). Current practices regarding genetic testing in ALS are variable, perhaps influenced by geography, provider experience, and financial considerations.

ETIOLOGY, GENETICS, AND PATHOGENESIS

The cause of sALS is unknown. As with other neurodegenerative diseases, it is hypothesized that ALS may result from the dual insult of genetic susceptibility and environmental injury. Attempts to identify predisposing mutations and potential toxic or infectious agents have been unsuccessful to date. There are many proposed mechanisms for motor neuron death in sALS; these include excitotoxicity secondary to glutamate, free radical-mediated oxidative cytotoxicity, mitochondrial dysfunction, protein aggregation, cytoskeletal abnormalities, aberrant activation of cyclo-oxygenase, impaired axonal transport, activation of inflammatory cascades, and apoptosis. However, why the motor neurons and corticospinal/bulbar tracts are vulnerable in a selective manner, and why the disease begins focally and progresses in a regional fashion, remain unknown.

The role of genetic susceptibility in sALS is not well defined. Phenotypically, sALS and fALS are indistinguishable aside from the earlier age of onset in sporadic disease; both are clinically heterogeneous. Estimates of heritability in sALS are variable, ranging from 5% to 28%. The percentage of genetic variants found in patients with sALS that are actually pathogenic is not well understood. It is possible that certain genetic variants may reduce the risk of ALS in an individual.

fALS accounts for approximately 10% of ALS cases and occurs with different modes of inheritance, although an autosomal dominant pattern is by far the most common. Disease mechanisms in fALS are better characterized than in sALS and this has led to clinical therapeutic trials. A major breakthrough in our understanding of fALS took place in 1991 with the identification of cytosolic copper-zinc SOD1 gene mutations on chromosome 21q22.11. SOD1 is a free radical scavenger, leading to the hypothesis that SOD1-fALS was mediated by free radical toxicity. However, SOD1 knock-out mice with no SOD1 protein do not develop motor neuron disease. In contrast, heterozygote mice become symptomatic and die from a paralyzing disorder. It is thought that SOD1 mutations may injure neurons through conformational changes in the SOD1 protein.

Particularly intriguing has been the recognition of the phenotypic heterogeneity in SOD1 fALS (Table 62.2). About 114 pathologic mutations have been identified within the five exons of the SOD1 gene; each of these mutations may produce a distinct phenotype. The most common mutation found in North America is an alanine for valine (A4V) substitution at codon 4; this typically produces a lower motor neuron dominant phenotype (LMN-D) with a life expectancy approximating 1 year. Table 62.2 summarizes the phenotypic heterogeneity that results from different SOD1 mutations. SOD1 mutations are not fully penetrant. It is estimated that individuals carrying the mutation have an 80% chance of developing disease by age 85 years. SOD1 mutations constitute 20%–25% of all individuals with fALS.

More recently, intronic hexanucleotide repeat mutations of c9orf72 were identified as the most common cause of fALS, accounting for 24% of fALS and 4% of sALS in North America. The discovery of GGGGCC

TABLE 62.1   Current Classification of fALS

Name	Genetics	Phenotype
Dominant Inheritance		
ALS1	21q22.1 SOD1	Adult onset—multiple phenotypes (see Table 62.3)
ALS3	18q21	Adult onset
ALS4	9q34 SETX/senataxin	Juvenile onset Slow progression with distal amyotrophy and UMN signs
ALS6	16q11.2 FUS-TLS	Adult onset
ALS7	20p13	Adult onset
ALS8	20q13.3 VAPB/vesicular associated membrane protein	Adult onset
ALS9	14q11.2 ANG/angiogenin	Adult onset
ALS10	1p36.2 TDP-43/TAR DNA binding	ALS ± FTD PSP, PD, chorea
ALS11	6q21 FIG4/polyphosphoinositide phosphatase	
ALS12	10p15-p14 OPTN/optineurin	
ALS13	12q24 ATXN2/ataxin 2	
Not designated	9q21-22 C9ORF72	ALS ± FTD
Not designated	9p13.3 VCP/Valsolin-containing protein	
Not designated	3p11.2 CHMP2B/chromatin-modifying protein 2B	
X-Linked Recessive		
ALSS15	XP11.21 UBQLN2/ubiquilin 2	ALS ± FTD
ALS2	2q33.1 alsin	Juvenile onset—pseudobulbar and UMN
ALS5	15q15.1q21.1	Juvenile onset
ALS12	10p15-p14 OPTN	UMN-D Lower extremities

ALS, Amyotrophic lateral sclerosis; *fALS*, familial ALS; *FTD*, frontotemporal dementia; *PD*, Parkinson's disease; *PSP*, progressive supranuclear palsy; *UMN*, upper motor neuron.

expansions in the c9orf72 gene has transformed our understanding of the disease. Proposed pathogenic mechanisms include loss of function of the c9orf72 protein, and toxic gain of function mechanisms via repeat RNA or from dipeptide repeat proteins (DPRs) produced by repeat associated non-ATG translation. Like the SOD1 model, there has also been translation of this understanding of disease into the development of potential novel therapies.

Known fALS genotypes are listed in Table 62.1. Some of these mutations produce a predominantly LMN or UMN disorder and more closely resemble the phenotypes of spinal muscular atrophy or hereditary spastic paraparesis, respectively.

Mutations that may produce both a frontotemporal lobar degeneration and motor neuron disease can occur in certain proteins identified to date (e.g., c9orf72, TAR DNA-binding protein 43 [TDP-43], valosin-containing protein [VCP], fusion in sarcoma/translated in liposarcoma [FUS-TLS], and ANG/angiogenin proteins). The discovery of TDP-43 was interesting in that non-amyloid, structurally modified TDP-43 has been recognized as a major constituent of the ubiquitinated inclusions found in cortical neurons of patients with both sporadic FTD (sFTD) and familial FTD (fFTD). C9orf72 is relatively common and accounts for 12% of fFTD and 3% of sFTD. Notably, FTLD does not occur in SOD1 fALS.

ALS is pathologically characterized by loss of myelinated fibers in the corticospinal and corticobulbar pathways (see Fig. 62.2) and loss of motor neurons within the anterior horns of the spinal cord and many motor cranial nerve nuclei. Even in individuals in whom UMN or LMN features predominate, pathologic involvement of both systems is seen. Patients with associated FTD have preferential lobar atrophy and neuronal loss from these portions of the brain (Fig. 62.6). As a result of anterior horn cell loss, ventral roots become atrophic in comparison to sparing of their dorsal root counterparts (Fig. 62.7). Anterior horn cell loss occurs within virtually all levels of the spinal cord with selective sparing of the third, fourth, and sixth cranial nerves, and Onuf nucleus within the anterior horn of sacral segments 2–4. There is also cell preservation within the intermediolateral cell columns.

The majority of sALS patients will be found to have ubiquitinated inclusions and Bunina bodies within the central nervous system. The latter are dense granular intracytoplasmic inclusions within motor neurons considered specific for ALS. Additionally in ALS with FTD, spongiform changes of the first and second layers of the frontal cortex have been described.

DIFFERENTIAL DIAGNOSIS

The differential diagnosis of ALS is largely that of other disorders of anterior horn cells, myopathies, disorders of neuromuscular transmission, motor predominant polyneuropathies, and myelopathies

TABLE 62.2 Phenotypic Variation in SOD1 fALS

Phenotype	SOD 1 Mutation
Lower motor neuron predominant	A4V, L84V, D101N
Upper motor neuron predominant	D90A
Slow progression (>10-year survival)	G37R, G41D, G93C, L144S, L144F
Fast progression (<2-year survival)	A4T, N86S, L106V, V148G
Late onset	G85R, H46R
Early onset	G37R, L38V
Female predominant	G41D
Bulbar onset	V148I
Low penetrance	D90A, I113T
Posterior column involvement	E100G

fALS, Familial ALS; *SOD1*, superoxide dismutase.

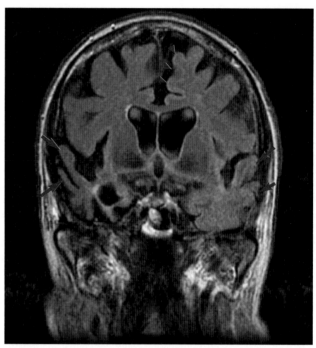

Coronal FLAIR MR image demonstrates ventricular enlargement, especially of the right temporal horn, atrophy of superior and middle temporal gyri (arrow), and prominence of frontal sulci. Notice prominent widening of the interhemispheric fissure (arrowheads). Courtesy of Richard Caselli, MD.

Fig. 62.6 Frontotemporal Atrophy.

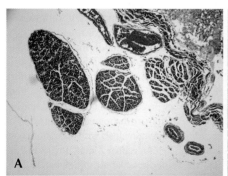 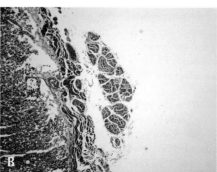 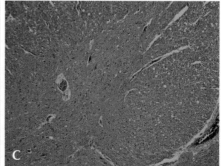

A, Dorsal root (normal), and **B,** ventral root (atrophic due to loss of lower motor neurons) in amyotrophic lateral sclerosis. **C,** Ventral gray matter of lumbar spinal cord showing loss of lower motor neurons. (From Amato AA, Russell JA. Neuromuscular Disorders, McGraw-Hill, New York, 2008, pp. 104-105.)

Fig. 62.7 Dorsal and Ventral Roots and Ventral Horn.

TABLE 62.3   Differential Diagnosis of ALS

UMN and LMN Features	UMN Dominant Limb Onset	LMN Dominant Limb Onset	Bulbar Onset
Spinocerebellar degeneration	Hereditary spastic paraparesis	Multifocal motor neuropathy	Myasthenia gravis
Hexosaminidase deficiency	Compressive myelopathy	Inclusion body myositis	Kennedy disease
Hereditary spastic paraparesis	HTLV 1 infection	Hirayama disease Benign calf amyotrophy	Inclusion body myositis
Copper deficiency	Paraneoplastic	Kennedy disease	Oculopharyngeal MD
Dural vascular malformations		Spinal muscular atrophy	Head and neck neoplasms
Polyglucosan disease		Benign fasciculations	Brainstem pathology
Prion disease		Myasthenia gravis	Multiinfarct state
			Chronic meningitis with multiple cranial nerve palsies

HTLV 1, Human T-cell leukemia virus type 1; *LMV*, lower motor neuron; *MD*, muscular dystrophy; *UMN*, upper motor neuron.

(Table 62.3). With bulbar onset and predominantly LMN features, myasthenia gravis, inflammatory myopathy particularly inclusion body myositis, X-linked bulbospinal muscular atrophy (Kennedy disease), oculopharyngeal muscular dystrophy, multiple cranial neuropathies, or infiltrative head and neck cancers are the primary considerations. Of these, myasthenia gravis (MG) deserves the most attention. Clues favoring a diagnosis of MG include a weak tongue without atrophy or fasciculations, absence of UMN signs, and presence of ptosis or ophthalmoparesis. MuSK myasthenic patients can have atrophy of the tongue, leading to further diagnostic confusion. Dysphagia, usually without dysarthria, may rarely be the initial or most prominent symptom of the inflammatory myopathies. The pattern of limb weakness, the absence of fasciculations, and UMN signs in these disorders provides distinction from ALS. X-linked bulbospinal muscular atrophy or Kennedy disease may have early or prominent weakness of the throat, tongue, or jaw muscles often associated with fasciculation, and may therefore easily be confused with bulbar ALS. A slower evolution of symptoms, the pattern of limb weakness, and the presence of gynecomastia and sensory abnormalities are features that distinguish Kennedy disease from bulbar ALS. Oculopharyngeal muscular dystrophy (OPMD) may be confused with bulbar ALS, although the course of OPMD is typically much longer, with a possible positive family history, prominent ptosis, and a proximal pattern of weakness on examination. Multiple cranial neuropathies (e.g., cancer, sarcoid, facial onset sensory motor neuronopathy [FOSMN]) are commonly accompanied by pain or sensory dysfunction.

The differential diagnosis of head drop includes chronic inflammatory demyelinating neuropathy, radiation injury, MG, and a wide variety of myopathies. The dropped head syndrome may be mimicked by anterocollis resulting from multiple system atrophy and other extrapyramidal disorders. Neuromuscular causes of ventilatory failure in adults include a number of neuropathic disorders. Severe hypophosphatemia and hypokalemia may result in ventilatory muscle weakness. In addition, disorders of neuromuscular transmission and some myopathies may progress to ventilatory insufficiency. Acid maltase deficiency can affect ventilation early in the course. Certain myopathies and myotonic dystrophies may progress to ventilatory failure.

In most series, multifocal motor neuropathy (MMN) is the entity most likely to be confused with LMN presentations of ALS. The distinction is important as MMN represents a potentially treatable disorder. The weakness of MMN occurs in an individual nerve distribution rather than in the myotomal pattern of ALS, and progression is more typically stepwise than the typical insidious course of ALS. In addition, in keeping with its initial demyelinating pathophysiology, MMN often produces weakness in the absence of atrophy. The clinician may have to rely on electrodiagnostic or serologic testing and a therapeutic trial of intravenous immunoglobulin to make a confident diagnosis.

Another disorder that may be mistaken as LMN predominant ALS is sporadic inclusion body myositis (sIBM). sIBM presents with asymmetric painless weakness in older males that may affect distal as well as proximal muscles. The pattern of weakness in sIBM is often distinctive with preferential and asymmetric weakness of wrist and finger flexors and quadriceps, in addition to facial, neck flexor, and foot dorsiflexor muscles. The slow progression and the characteristic pattern of weakness help distinguish sIBM from ALS.

The juvenile segmental form of spinal muscular atrophy (Hirayama disease) may be difficult to initially distinguish from ALS. Hirayama disease is a slowly progressive and self-limited LMN disorder typically affecting young adult men with initial involvement of C7–T1 hand and forearm muscles unilaterally. Benign calf amyotrophy, another focal form of motor neuron disease often with preferential involvement of the calves, is distinct from ALS in that it demonstrates a stable course and predominantly chronic changes on electromyography.

Benign fasciculations tend to occur repetitively in a single region of a single muscle over the course of a few seconds to minutes and then disappear. The calves and the orbicularis oculi tend to be particularly affected. Patients may seek medical attention for fasciculations that they describe as being widespread and pervasive. Their examination demonstrates no pathologic alterations in muscle strength, bulk, or tone, and no reflex abnormalities. In this context, particularly with a normal electromyography (EMG), the patient can be reassured.

UMN presentations of ALS affecting the limbs have a more extensive differential diagnosis. Cervical spondylotic myelopathy is a major differential diagnostic consideration, particularly in individuals presenting with LMN signs in the arms and UMN features in the legs. The presence of sensory and bladder symptoms and imaging should help distinguish this disorder from ALS. Other causes of myelopathy, including ischemic (e.g., dural vascular malformations of the spinal cord), infectious, and inflammatory causes of myelopathy, also remain considerations.

The differential diagnosis of ALS also uncommonly includes a number of hereditary and degenerative disorders. Of these, hereditary spastic paraparesis is potentially the most confounding, particularly in those individuals in whom there is no family history. Slow progression, high arched feet, loss of large fiber sensory perception in the feet, and sparing of upper extremity and bulbar function are distinguishing features. An ALS-like syndrome may occur in certain individuals with hexosaminidase deficiency, typically in compound heterozygotes. A motor neuron syndrome may also accompany the spinocerebellar atrophies, particularly type III (Machado–Joseph disease) or occasionally in prion disorders such as Creutzfeldt–Jakob and Gerstmann–Straussler–Scheinker disease. Polyglucosan disease is a rare heritable disorder of glycogen metabolism that may produce cognitive and genitourinary issues in addition to a motor neuropathy.

Finally, certain toxic, metabolic, infectious, immune-mediated, and paraneoplastic conditions have been reported to mimic ALS. Lead toxicity, hyperthyroidism and parathyroidism, HIV, Lyme disease, and lymphoma are the most notable of these. Serum copper deficiency has been reported as a potential ALS mimic and should receive consideration in anyone with an ALS-like syndrome with unexplained sensory complaints.

DIAGNOSTIC APPROACH

There is no perfect algorithm for the evaluation of an ALS suspect. In a patient with LMN and UMN features that have progressed in a typical pattern and time course, the diagnosis is indisputable. In most cases where ALS is suspected, tests are ordered guided by the clinician's index of suspicion (Table 62.4). In large part, these tests are done to exclude considerations other than ALS.

Virtually every ALS patient undergoes electromyography and nerve conduction studies, collectively referred to as electrodiagnosis (EDX). The goal of EDX in ALS is to confirm a pattern of active denervation, chronic denervation, and fasciculation potentials in multiple muscles innervated by multiple segments in multiple regions. According to the modified El Escorial EDX criteria, a definite diagnosis of ALS requires evidence of active denervation (fibrillation potentials and positive sharp waves) in at least three of the following four body regions: cranial, cervical, thoracic, and lumbosacral. In the limbs, at least two different muscles belonging to different nerve and root innervations need to be affected. Involvement in a single cranial muscle is sufficient to satisfy that region's requirements. Thoracic paraspinal muscles are particularly helpful as they are uncommonly denervated in other neurogenic disorders. Fasciculation potentials are a supportive but not mandatory electrodiagnostic feature. Features that would suggest an alternative diagnosis that might mimic ALS need to be excluded; examples include abnormal sensory conductions in Kennedy syndrome, decremental response to repetitive stimulation consistent with myasthenia, conduction block suggestive of multifocal motor neuropathy, or small motor unit potentials suggestive of a myopathy such as IBM. Finally, EDX may offer insight into the rate of progression, that is, active denervation without chronic denervation and reinnervation, motor unit variability, and a rapid decline in motor unit number estimation predicting a rapidly progressive course.

Magnetic resonance imaging (MRI) of the brain should be strongly considered in any patient with a bulbar presentation without limb involvement to identify brainstem parenchymal, meningeal, or cranial nerve disorders. Imaging of the cervical and/or thoracic cord would be indicated in patients with predominantly UMN limb involvement without bulbar signs. Lumbosacral MRI with gadolinium enhancement is indicated in purely LMN syndromes affecting the lower extremities to evaluate for conus medullaris or cauda equina pathology. MRI, positron emission tomography (PET), or single-photon emission computed tomographic (SPECT) imaging may support preferential atrophy or hypometabolism of the anterior brain in individuals suspected of having FTLD.

Elevated serum creatine kinase levels are not specific for myopathy. Approximately two-thirds of ALS patients will have creatine kinase elevations, typically in the 300 to 500 U/L range but occasionally as high as 1000 or more. Antibodies directed at the GM1 ganglioside are found in high titer in 30%–80% of patients with MMN. They are typically ordered in patients with LMN syndromes without cranial nerve or UMN findings. Serologic tests for myasthenia may be obtained in patients with bulbar presentations. Other tests, listed in Table 62.4, are used more judiciously in the appropriate clinical context. Many patients with ALS inquire about the possibility of Lyme disease, and Lyme serologies are frequently ordered to lessen these concerns. HIV testing is not done in suspected ALS unless the clinical context would suggest an increased probability of infection. Historically, screening for heavy metals, thyroid and parathyroid disorders, and occult neoplasia was emphasized but are currently considered to have limited value. Serum copper, ceruloplasmin, and zinc levels may be considered in any patient with weakness and unexplained sensory symptoms.

Testing for commercially available fALS genetic tests is commonly offered to patients with suspected ALS in whom there have been other affected family members. Practices and attitudes with regard to genetic testing in sALS are variable and influenced by patient and provider factors as well as cost considerations. SOD1 and C9ORF72 are the most commonly tested genes, and panels of genetic testing are available in ALS. C9ORF72 testing may be offered to ALS patients with family history of dementia. Genetic testing in presymptomatic family members is controversial and should only be done after detailed genetic counseling.

TABLE 62.4 Testing Considerations for a Suspected ALS Patient

All Patients	LMN Presentations	UMN Presentations	Bulbar Presentations	Selected Patients
EMG/NCS	Anti-GM1 antibodies	MRI brain, cervical, and thoracic spinal cord	MRI brain	HTLV-1
Pulmonary function	Acetylcholine receptor-binding antibodies	CSF examination	Acetylcholine receptor-binding antibodies	Lyme serology
	Muscle-specific kinase antibodies	HSP genotyping	Muscle-specific kinase antibodies	HIV serology
	MRI lumbosacral spine	Serum copper	CSF examination	Hexosaminidase levels
	Serum CK	Serum B_{12}	Serum CK	Androgen receptor gene mutational analysis
		Mammography		Muscle biopsy
		Amphiphysin antibodies		Nerve biopsy
				C26–C22 long-chain fatty acid ratio
				Survival motor neuron gene mutation
				Paraneoplastic antibodies
				Serum copper and ceruloplasmin
				TSH, calcium, PTH

CK, Creatine kinase; *CSF,* cerebrospinal fluid; *GM1,* ganglioside; *HIV,* human immunodeficiency virus; *HSP,* hereditary spastic paraparesis; *HTLV-1,* human T-cell leukemia virus type 1; *LMN,* lower motor neuron; *MRI,* magnetic resonance imaging; *NCS,* nerve conduction study; *PTH,* parathormone; *TSH,* thyroid-stimulating hormone.

Muscle biopsy is rarely done except to exclude IBM or other myopathies that might mimic ALS. Pulmonary function tests are used to monitor disease progression; forced vital capacity and inspiratory pressure measurements are obtained both in the sitting and supine positions. Forced vital capacity of less than 50% of predicted estimates a 6-month life expectancy and along with a negative inspiratory force of <60 cm H_2O or Pco_2 of >40 mm Hg are indications for the use of positive airway pressure equipment.

MANAGEMENT AND THERAPY

Management of ALS includes disease-specific treatments, symptomatic and supportive treatments, as well as adequate education and counseling. These are summarized in Table 62.5 and are elaborated on in two of the reviews listed in the bibliography. Riluzole was the first US Food and Drug Administration (FDA)-approved and effective pharmacologic agent identified to date. Unfortunately, it prolongs life

TABLE 62.5   Therapeutic Considerations in Amyotrophic Lateral Sclerosis

Problem	Potential Prescription	Problem	Potential Prescription
ALS	Riluzole 50 mg bid	Tripping from foot drop	Ankle–foot orthoses
ALS	IV edavarone (60 mg IV QD 14 days, off 14 days; subsequent cycles of QD 10 of 14 days, off 14 days)	Falling secondary to quadriceps weakness	Canes Crutches Walker Knee–ankle–foot orthoses with mercury switch Wheelchair, manual or power
ALS	Clinical trials	Reduced bed mobility	Hospital bed with side-rails and/or trapeze
Sialorrhea (excessive thin secretions)	Glycopyrrolate Tricyclic antidepressants Robinul Botulinum toxin Atropine Salivary gland radiation Scopolamine Chorda tympani section	Bathroom safety and functionality	Stall shower Shower chair Transfer bench Toilet seat extension Shower and toilet bars
Secretion clearance (thick secretions)	Home suction Cough assist devices Expectorants (e.g., guaifenesin) Beta blockers Nebulized *n*-acetylcysteine and albuterol Tracheostomy	House accessibility	Stair lift Lift chair or chair lift Hoyer lift Elevators Ramps Transfer belt
Pseudobulbar affect	Dextromethorphan hydrobromide and quinidine sulfate Tricyclic antidepressants Selective serotonin reuptake inhibitors Selective serotonin and norepinephrine reuptake inhibitors	Improved ADLs	Velcro for buttons and shoelaces Elastic shoelaces Long-handled grippers Foam collars for pens and utensils
Depression	Tricyclic antidepressants Selective serotonin reuptake inhibitors Selective serotonin and norepinephrine reuptake inhibitors Stimulants	Dysphagia—malnutrition	Neck positioning Change in food consistency Liquid thickeners Percutaneous gastrostomy
Laryngospasm	Antihistamines H_2 receptor blockers Antacids Proton pump inhibitors Sublingual lorazepam drops	Constipation	Bulk and fiber (applesauce–prunes–bran mix) Stool softeners/cathartics Hydration
		Urinary urgency	Tolterodine
Neck drop	Cervical collar (headmaster)	Cramps	Gabapentin Tizanidine or baclofen Benzodiazepines Phenytoin Carbamazepine Mexiletine Primrose oil Brewer's yeast
Communication	AAC devices Pad and pencil or erasable slates		
Hypoventilation	Positive pressure ventilators (e.g., BiPAP) Negative pressure ventilators (e.g., Cuirass) Tracheostomy and mechanical ventilation Morphine sulfate Benzodiazepines	Safety	Lifeline Phone auto dialer Home safety evaluation
Contractures	Night splints Botulinum toxin Range-of-motion exercises		

AAC, Assistive augmentative communication; *ADLs*, activities of daily living; *ALS*, amyotrophic lateral sclerosis; *BiPAP*, bilevel positive airway pressure; *IV*, intravenous; *QD*, once daily.

expectancy on average by 10% without noticeable improvement in function or sense of well-being. Its cost is substantial, and it should be prescribed only after the patient has been informed of its benefits and drawbacks. In 2017, intravenous edaravone, a free radical scavenger, was also FDA approved for ALS after a phase 3 study in Japan demonstrated statistical significance benefit of edaravone over placebo in ALS-Functional Rating Scale (FRS) scores after 6 months in a subgroup of ALS patients who were younger and with mild/early disease. Intravenous edaravone is a daily infusion given for 14 days of the first month, followed by 10 days of each subsequent month. Patients should be made aware of the cost as well as the realistic considerations of how treatment is likely to impact quality of life.

Stem cells continue to be an area of interest in preclinical and clinical trials as they may offer a neuroprotective effect through the delivery of growth factors. Human spinal cord–derived neural stem cell (HSSC) transplantation has been shown to delay motor neuron degenerative in the mouse model of ALS. A small open-label trial of 15 patients suggested that intraspinal transplantation of HSSCs could be relatively safely performed at high doses, although side effects from the procedure and immunosuppression occurred in certain patients. Whether stem cells will provide therapeutic benefits for humans with ALS remains a question.

Patients should be encouraged to participate in clinical trials when available. Many ALS patients utilize alternative health measures. Patients should be informed that any treatment biologically active enough to help is also biologically capable of harm. It is not uncommon for patients to ask for medications that have been touted but are unproven to be effective. If these agents are to be studied in clinical trials, clinicians should discourage their use outside of the trial so as to not subvert the enrollment in and/or the integrity of the trial.

An important aspect of the management of ALS patients and their families is the provision of reliable education. It is important to discuss end-of-life issues with a patient before a ventilatory crisis occurs or the ability to communicate is lost. The primary goals in ALS management are to provide symptom relief and to maintain independent and safe function. In the later stages of disease, the primary goal shifts to the maintenance of comfort (see Table 62.5). In our clinic, we focus on symptoms referable to the following domains: pain, sleep, psychosocial issues, speech and swallowing, ventilation, motor function, and bowel and bladder issues. Pain occurs commonly in ALS. Prophylactic range of motion should be applied to immobilized body parts. Analgesics including opioids may be required. Impaired sleep has many potential causes in an ALS patient, including discomfort secondary to immobility or cramping, depression, impaired ventilation, and bathroom requirements, each of which may have to be identified and addressed separately.

FUTURE DIRECTIONS

Current ALS research is focusing on the identification of biomarkers in ALS that might allow for improved classification of the motor neuron diseases, earlier and more precise identification of ALS patients, and better insights into the biology of the disease. In addition, scientists are currently attempting to identify susceptibility genes that would potentially provide additional clues for disease origins and mechanisms. Although stem cell biology offers the hope of replacing degenerating motor neurons, ultimately identifying the root cause(s) of ALS and eliminating them will provide a realistic means by which to cure this devastating disease.

ADDITIONAL RESOURCES

Amato AA, Russell JA. Neuromuscular disorders. 2nd ed. New York: McGraw Hill; 2016.

Gibson S, Downie J, Tsetsou S, et al. The evolving genetic risk for sporadic ALS. Neurology 2017;89:226–33.

Miller RG, Jackson CE, Kasarskis EJ, et al. Practice parameter update: the care of the patient with amyotrophic lateral sclerosis: drug, nutritional, and respiratory therapies (an evidence-based review): report of the quality standards subcommittee of the American Academy of Neurology. Neurology 2009;73:1218–26.

Miller RG, Jackson CE, Kasarskis EJ, et al. Practice parameter update: multidisciplinary care, symptom management, and cognitive/behavioral impairment (an evidence-based review): report of the quality standards subcommittee of the American Academy of Neurology. Neurology 2009;73:1227–33.

Vajda A, McLaughlin RL, Heverin M, et al. Genetic testing in ALS. Neurology 2017;88:991–9.

63

Other Motor Neuron Diseases and Motor Neuropathies

Doreen T. Ho, James A. Russell

CLINICAL VIGNETTE *A 35-year-old man sought medical attention for leg weakness. He noticed difficulty getting up from low chairs and ascending stairs. Looking back, he reported that 10 years previously he had noticed some difficulty when trying to stand after squatting to paint the baseboard in his dining room; he had to push on his thighs to straighten his knees. He denied weakness in his arms and had no problems with chewing or swallowing. He had no sensory complaints. He reported occasional muscle cramps and twitches in his legs. His examination demonstrated mild weakness in bilateral shoulder abductors and moderate weakness in the proximal legs, mainly hip flexors, hip extensors, and knee extensors. He had normal facial and tongue strength as well reflexes and sensation. Nerve conduction studies were normal, including sensory potentials. Electromyography showed diffuse, predominantly chronic denervation changes and survival motor neuron (SMN) genetic testing revealed a homozygous deletion in the SMN1 gene, with five copies of SMN2, consistent with the diagnosis of spinal muscular atrophy type 4. Ten years later he remained active in his job and ambulated independently.*

In this chapter we address the motor neuron diseases (MNDs) other than amyotrophic lateral sclerosis (ALS). MNDs are disorders that produce painless weakness, atrophy, cramps, and fasciculations; they are a consequence of the degeneration of anterior horn cells and selective cranial motor nuclei. We also address multifocal motor neuropathy (MMN) and hereditary spastic paraparesis (HSP). MMN and HSP are considered separate categories of disorders from MNDs, as MMN and HSP preferentially target motor nerves and corticospinal tracts, respectively, rather than motor nuclei. However, these conditions may have overlapping phenotypes, with MMN sometimes resembling lower motor neuron–dominant ALS and HSP mimicking primary lateral sclerosis (PLS); thus they deserve to be discussed in this chapter.

Many of the disorders discussed in this chapter have known or suspected genetic mechanisms. The spinal muscular atrophies (SMAs) are conceptualized as largely inherited disorders in which there is predominant degeneration of anterior horn cells and selective motor cranial nerve nuclei. In childhood SMAs, mutations of a single gene and derangement of a single gene product are responsible for the majority of cases, and the resultant phenotype is fairly homogeneous. In other disorders, for example, HSP, there are a variety of recognized genotypes associated with a heterogeneous array of phenotypic variations.

SURVIVAL MOTOR NEURON–RELATED SPINAL MUSCULAR ATROPHIES

SMA types I–IV are allelic disorders of the survival motor neuron (SMN) gene 1 located on chromosome 5q12.2–q13.3. When there is more than one affected individual in a given family, the phenotype is typically homogeneous but may be variable in some cases. In normal individuals, there are two copies each of the SMN1 and SMN2 genes. Although both genes produce similar proteins, the SMN2 gene appears to produce an unstable and rapidly degrading protein that compensates to a variable degree for the lack of the SMN1 protein. There are no known clinical consequences from mutations of the SMN2 gene alone.

It is estimated that 95% of SMA I–III patients are homozygous for deletion of exons 7 and 8 of the SMN1 gene. The remainder are thought to be compound heterozygotes with absence of exons 7 and 8 on one allele and a point mutation of the other SMN1 allele. The severity of the SMA phenotype appears to be related to the number of SMN2 copies available to compensate for the deleted SMN1 gene. Homozygotes devoid of SMN1 who harbor two copies of SMN2 tend to manifest as an SMA I phenotype. An increasing number of SMN2 copies correlates with proportionately milder (SMA II–IV) forms of the disease. Individuals homozygous for the SMN1 mutation with five copies of the SMN2 gene have been reported to be asymptomatic. Why motor neurons remain selectively vulnerable to SMN deficiency remains unknown.

SMA is considered to be the most common cause of mortality in infancy among autosomal recessive disorders. The natural history of SMA is variable. For this reason clinical subgroups have historically been defined based on the best motor function attained during development. Type I SMA infants do not sit independently, type II SMA individuals sit at some point but are not able to walk, and type III SMA children and adults are able to walk independently during their childhood.

Of the multiple SMA phenotypes, the infantile and childhood forms are the most prevalent. SMA type I or Werdnig-Hoffman disease is the most severe form (Fig. 63.1). Its incidence is between 4 and 10 in 100,000 lives births depending on the population studied. Clinical manifestations become evident within the first 6 months of life. In some cases recognition of reduced movement occurs in utero or within the first few days of life. Affected infants are hypotonic with symmetric weakness that is either generalized or proximally predominant. As in ALS, facial weakness is typically mild and extraocular muscles are spared. Fasciculations are seen in the tongue but rarely in limb muscles, presumably because of the ample subcutaneous tissue of neonates. Manual tremor, characteristic of SMA types II and III, is rarely present. Deep tendon reflexes are typically absent. Abdominal breathing, a weak cry, and a poor suck are common. Ventilatory difficulties stem primarily from intercostal rather than diaphragmatic weakness. Consequently pectus excavatum and a diminished anteroposterior diameter of the chest are seen. Mild contractures may occur, but arthrogryposis is not part of the classic phenotype. Intellectual development is normal. Without mechanical ventilation, death is inevitable, almost always within a year or two. An earlier age of onset correlates with a shorter life expectancy.

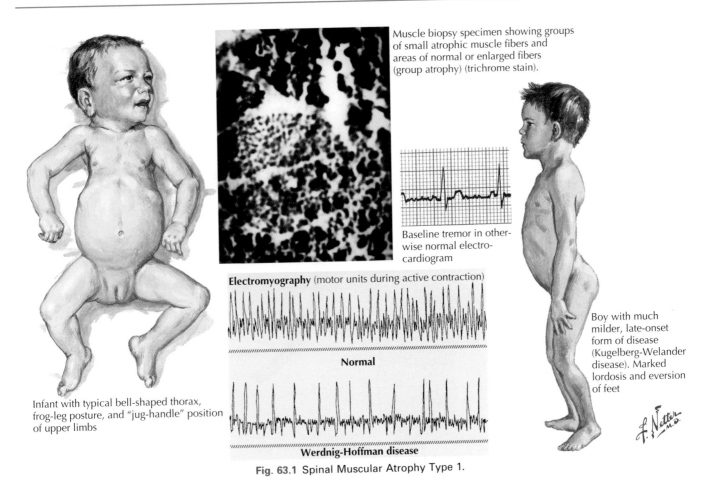

Muscle biopsy specimen showing groups of small atrophic muscle fibers and areas of normal or enlarged fibers (group atrophy) (trichrome stain).

Baseline tremor in otherwise normal electrocardiogram

Electromyography (motor units during active contraction)

Normal

Werdnig-Hoffman disease

Infant with typical bell-shaped thorax, frog-leg posture, and "jug-handle" position of upper limbs

Boy with much milder, late-onset form of disease (Kugelberg-Welander disease). Marked lordosis and eversion of feet

Fig. 63.1 Spinal Muscular Atrophy Type 1.

The intermediate form of SMA II typically begins between 6 and 18 months of age. The disorder is clinically defined by a child who sits independently but never walks. Postural hand tremor is the only significant phenotypic variance from Werdnig-Hoffman disease. Tongue fasciculations, areflexia, and a generalized to proximally predominant and symmetric pattern of weakness mimic the SMA I phenotype. Approximately 98% of these individuals survive to age 5 and two-thirds to age 25. In view of the more protracted course and of wheelchair dependency, SMA II and SMA III patients commonly acquire kyphoscoliosis and joint contractures (Fig. 63.2).

SMA III or the Kugelberg-Welander syndrome differs from the intermediate form only in the age of onset, milestones achieved, and life expectancy. Affected individuals develop the ability to stand and walk. Onset age is typically 18 months or more. Some authors have attempted to divide SMA III into type a and type b, based on age at onset of symptoms, with the intention of better defining the natural history in individual patients. In SMA type IIIa, defined as symptom onset before 3 years, it is estimated that 70% will remain ambulatory 10 years after symptom onset and 20% will still ambulate 30 years after symptom onset. In SMA type IIIb, defined as symptom onset after 3 years, virtually all patients will remain ambulatory at 10 years and 60% at 40 years after symptom onset. Life expectancy extends into the sixth decade and may be normal in many individuals. Initial symptoms are typically related to proximal weakness. Hand tremor, areflexia, and tongue fasciculations are commonplace. Fasciculations in limb muscles are more evident than in SMA types I and II.

Adult-onset SMA IV is a rare genetically heterogeneous disorder. SMA IV children achieve motor milestones at normal ages. Onset of weakness is typically in the third or fourth decade in the recessively inherited cases. Initial symptoms are typically proximal weakness of the lower extremities, particularly the hip flexors, hip extensors, and knee extensors. Shoulder abductors and elbow extensors are the most frequently affected muscles of the arms. Tongue fasciculations, hand tremor, and in some cases calf hypertrophy may occur. Life expectancy in SMA IV is normal. Unlike SMA I-III, SMA IV may be autosomal dominant or recessive.

As in ALS, a multidisciplinary model of care is used in SMA to address socioemotional, nutritional, orthopedic, physical/occupational therapy, and ventilatory issues. Genetic counseling is recommended for families. Comanagement of patients with orthopedic colleagues is important in these patients, particularly in regard to surveillance for spinal curvature and bone health once a patient becomes nonambulatory.

In 2016, the US Food and Drug Administration (FDA) approved the first agent, nusinersen, for SMN-related SMA following multiple studies including a sham-controlled phase 3 trial. Nusinersen is an antisense oligonucleotide that is delivered intrathecally and allows SMN2 to produce full-length protein. It is hoped that ongoing studies will provide insight into its long-term safety and efficacy in children. To date, the evidence of efficacy appears to be highest for treatment of infantile and childhood-onset SMA, and the benefit for older SMA patients remains unclear.

X-LINKED BULBOSPINAL MUSCULAR ATROPHY—KENNEDY DISEASE

In 1968, Kennedy and colleagues first described the syndrome of X-linked bulbospinal muscular atrophy, and in 2001, LaSpada and colleagues

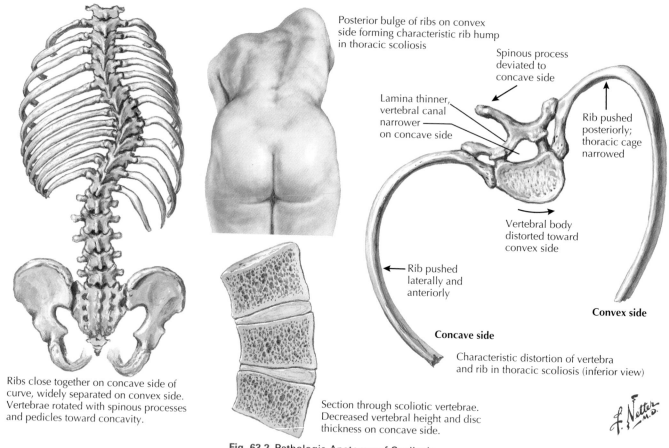

Posterior bulge of ribs on convex side forming characteristic rib hump in thoracic scoliosis

Spinous process deviated to concave side

Lamina thinner, vertebral canal narrower on concave side

Rib pushed posteriorly; thoracic cage narrowed

Vertebral body distorted toward convex side

Rib pushed laterally and anteriorly

Convex side

Concave side

Characteristic distortion of vertebra and rib in thoracic scoliosis (inferior view)

Ribs close together on concave side of curve, widely separated on convex side. Vertebrae rotated with spinous processes and pedicles toward concavity.

Section through scoliotic vertebrae. Decreased vertebral height and disc thickness on concave side.

Fig. 63.2 Pathologic Anatomy of Scoliosis.

identified the associated trinucleotide repeat mutation on exon 1 of the androgen receptor gene. This relatively rare disorder typically affects men in their 40s. Initial symptoms are often nonspecific and consist of muscle cramps, tremor, and subtle weakness of bulbar or proximal muscles; as the symptoms can be slow and insidious, there can be a delay in diagnosis.

As the name implies, the clinical manifestations are largely referable to degeneration of the lower cranial nerve motor nuclei and anterior horn cells of the spinal cord. The weakness progresses insidiously and is proximally predominant and symmetric in pattern. Typically, symptoms referable to the lower extremities have the greatest initial impact. Approximately 10% of the time the initial symptoms pertain to difficulty with swallowing, speaking, or chewing and may include jaw drop. Facial weakness is common. Perioral and tongue fasciculations are common and represent helpful clinical clues. As in the case of virtually all MNDs, ptosis and ophthalmoparesis are absent. As with other SMAs, postural tremor is common. There is an associated but frequently asymptomatic sensory neuropathy that may be recognized only by nerve conduction studies. Clinical heterogeneity exists. Asymmetry of muscle weakness at onset has been emphasized by some authors. Occasionally rapidly progressive weakness occurs. The median age of wheelchair dependency is 61 years, or approximately 15 years after onset of weakness. Women who are heterozygous for the Kennedy disease mutation may rarely be symptomatic.

The effects of X-linked bulbospinal muscular atrophy (BSMA) are not restricted to the neuromuscular system. Affected males suffer the consequences of androgen insensitivity, including gynecomastia, impotence, testicular atrophy, and potential infertility. There is also an increased incidence of diabetes mellitus.

BENIGN FOCAL AMYOTROPHIES

Hirayama Disease

In 1963, Hirayama described a slowly progressive focal MND affecting one upper extremity and sometimes both. Males represent 60% of the cases. Hirayama disease is perhaps best considered a segmental or regional form of MND. Onset is typically between ages 15 and 25. Although most commonly reported in persons of Asian origin, it may occur in individuals of any ethnic background.

Characteristically the disorder causes the insidious development of weakness and atrophy of the C7–T1 muscles of the hand and forearm. It begins unilaterally, typically in the dominant extremity. Over the course of months to years, the weakness may gradually spread to involve more proximal muscles. In one-third of the cases, there is clinical weakness of the opposite limb. An even higher percentage will have bilateral upper extremity involvement on electrodiagnostic studies. Tendon reflexes in the involved limb may be spared, although neither overt pyramidal nor bulbar involvement occurs. Reflex preservation may reflect the restricted nature of the disease and the lack of a reliable C8–T1 muscle stretch reflex. As in the heritable SMAs, tremor may occur. In most cases, there is an arrest of further progression after 6 years or less. Although a significant decline in affected limb function in the cold is common with all MNDs, "cold paresis" is emphasized in this population. Hyperhidrosis of the involved limb has also been described.

Ischemic changes in the cervical spinal cord of a single autopsied case of Hirayama disease led to the hypothesis of a compressive mechanism. In 2000, Hirayama reported the results of dynamic imaging in 73 patients and 20 controls. Ninety-four percent of the patients had significant forward displacement and flattening of the posterior surface

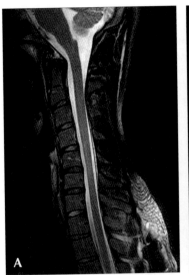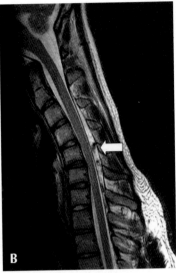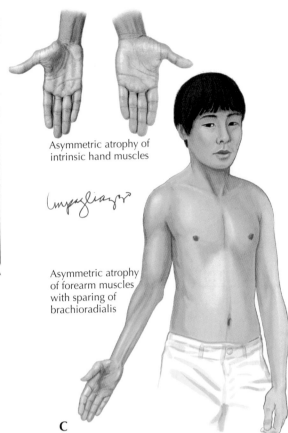

A. and B. Sagittal T2 fast spin echo imaging of cervical spinal cord in (A) neutral and (B) flexion. Note marked expansion of posterior epidural space on flexion with signal voids indicating enlarged veins. **C**, Atrophy of the forearm and intrinsic hand muscles (C7, C8, and T1 myotomes) in Hirayama disease with sparing of brachioradialis.
Courtesy Dr. Devon Rubin, Mayo Clinic.

Asymmetric atrophy of intrinsic hand muscles

Asymmetric atrophy of forearm muscles with sparing of brachioradialis

Fig. 63.3 Hirayama Disease.

of the cervical cord during neck flexion (Fig. 63.3). Anterior shifting of the cervical and thoracic dura was seen, at times with associated engorgement of the venous plexus on dynamic magnetic resonance imaging (MRI) of the cervical spine. The presumptive mechanism is that the blood supply to the spinal cord is mechanically compromised, the anterior horn being a watershed zone particularly vulnerable to ischemic injury. Other observations supporting this hypothesis include the recognition that the spinal cord is often asymmetrically flattened in this disorder with the weaker arm correlating with the side of the greatest spinal cord compression; it is believed that a similar phenotype may occur in individuals with different mechanisms of cervical spinal cord compression. Specifically, a slowly progressive, asymmetric pattern of bibrachial amyotrophy has been reported in individuals with epidural cerebrospinal fluid (CSF) collections associated with chronic spinal CSF leaks.

Scapuloperoneal Syndrome

A scapuloperoneal pattern of weakness may result from either neurogenic or myopathic disorders. The neurogenic form of the scapuloperoneal syndrome has been referred to by the eponym Davidenkow disease. It has been considered to represent a SMA variant even though distal sensory loss was common in Davidenkow's original series. Symptomatic onset typically occurs in late childhood related to asymmetric weakness of scapular fixators or foot dorsiflexors. Weakness typically progresses into a more generalized pattern. Some patients with a neurogenic scapuloperoneal syndrome have been found to have mutations within the *PMP-22* gene. This suggests that the disorder might be more correctly characterized as a hereditary neuropathy.

Benign Calf Amyotrophy

The syndrome of benign calf amyotrophy (BCA) is a disorder that presents as slowly progressive weakness and atrophy in the distal lower extremity, typically the calf. In a small series of 8 patients with BCA, 50% had unilateral symptoms. Symptoms plateaued after 1 to 3 years. Electromyography (EMG) showed mainly chronic reinnervation changes in distal greater than proximal S1 myotomes, particularly in the calves. The mechanism for BCA is not known.

Distal Spinal Muscular Atrophies

Distal spinal muscular atrophies (dSMAs) are dominantly inherited in one-third of cases, with recessive or X-linked inheritance in the remainder. There are numerous genetic loci (Table 63.1). Like HSP, distal SMA can be either "pure" or "complicated" based on other neurologic system involvement. Complicated phenotypes may include diaphragmatic paralysis, vocal cord paralysis, and arthrogryposis.

Harding and Thomas introduced the concept of dSMA in 1980. The dSMAs have been perceived as progressive, hereditary disorders producing distal symmetric weakness in the absence of either clinical or electrodiagnostic evidence of sensory loss. The SMAs' nosology stems from their pure motor phenotype and presumed anterior horn cell localization, but they are frequently and alternatively described as hereditary motor neuropathies in consideration of their length-dependent symmetric manifestations. Distal SMA strongly resembles Charcot–Marie–Tooth (CMT) disease without sensory involvement. In fact, at least three forms of dSMA are allelic to recessively inherited forms of CMT. Weakness in distal SMA typically predominates in ankle dorsiflexors and evertors

TABLE 63.1   Genetics of Spinal Muscular Atrophies

Classification	Chromosome	Gene
SMA I–IV	5q12.2–q13.3	SMN1
SMARD I	11q13.2q13.4	IGHMBP2
SBMA (Kennedy)	X	Androgen receptor gene
Juvenile segmental SMA (Hirayama)	None identified	None identified
Scapuloperoneal (Davidenkow)	17p11.2	PMP 22

and toe extensors. Foot deformities characteristic of CMT are also common. Hand muscles may eventually become involved.

POLIOMYELITIS

Paralytic Polio

Poliomyelitis is a viral infection of the spinal cord and brainstem with tropism for motor nuclei. Historically it was synonymous with paralytic polio, but the syndrome may occur as a consequence of other enteroviral or flaviviral infections. Poliomyelitis resulting from the poliovirus may be either a monophasic or biphasic disease. The initial symptoms are nonspecific, last for 1–2 days, and are predominantly constitutional and/or gastrointestinal in nature. They consist of fever, malaise, pharyngitis, headache, nausea, vomiting, and abdominal cramping (Fig. 63.4). In the majority of infected individuals, the illness is self-limited and ends at this point. In individuals who fall victim to the "major" illness, symptoms of brain or spinal cord involvement develop 3–10 days subsequent to the initial symptoms. The major illness is defined by central nervous system (CNS) involvement with meningoencephalitis with or without an associated paralytic component. Stiff neck, back pain, and fever are prominent; encephalitis with altered mental status can also be seen.

In individuals destined to develop paralytic disease, myalgias and cramping rapidly evolve into muscle weakness. The progression reaches its nadir within 48 hours of onset and the paralysis is typically asymmetric. It is confined to the limbs and trunk in half of the cases. There is a predilection for lumbosacral segments and proximal more than distal muscles (Fig. 63.5). Ten percent of cases have bulbar weakness only. Children are particularly susceptible to bulbar polio. Motor functions of cranial nerves VII, IX, and X are most likely to be affected. Ten percent of patients will manifest both spinal and bulbar weakness; ventilatory failure is more common in this group. Affected limbs are flaccid and areflexic. As in virtually all motor neuron disorders, cranial nerves III, IV, and VI are spared. Sensory signs and symptoms are atypical. In keeping with the known pathologic involvement of the brain stem tegmentum and hypothalamus in cases with encephalitic components, clinical dysautonomia including fluctuating blood pressure, cardiac arrhythmia, and hyperhydrosis may occur.

The natural history of paralytic polio is variable, dependent in large part on the severity and extent of the initial illness. As in Guillain-Barré syndrome (GBS), less than 10% of individuals will die from the acute illness. Acute mortality typically results from ventilatory failure or the complications of immobility. Those who survive typically regain strength in inverse proportion to the severity of the initial illness. The majority of this recovery takes place over the course of weeks to months, presumably due to reinnervation from neighboring motor units not affected by the disease.

The postpolio syndrome (PPS) has been recognized since 1875 but received no more than cursory attention until 1981, when interest escalated in response to the large numbers of people affected by the epidemics of the 1940s and 1950s who were then experiencing new symptoms. Signs and symptoms of PPS have been reported to begin as early as 8 years after the initial illness or as late as 71 years, with an average of 35 years. The likelihood of developing PPS seems to correlate with both the age of the patient at the time of the initial illness as well as with its severity.

Postpolio muscular atrophy (PPMA) is considered to represent a subset of PPS patients where there are signs and symptoms attributable to additional motor neuron loss. Current evidence suggests that patients who develop PPMA do so because of the loss of anterior horn cells that occurs as a consequence of normal aging superimposed on a depleted reserve. There is convincing evidence that some individuals with prior polio may develop slowly progressive weakness (average decline 1% per year) after a protracted period of stability. How frequently PPMA occurs as a manifestation of PPS is a matter of some controversy. In one study, 50 prior polio patients were selected from a cohort of 300 patients and followed for 5 years. Sixty percent of this group developed symptoms. Of this symptomatic group, only one-third had symptoms attributable to musculoskeletal complaints and none of these had measurable evidence of progressive atrophy and weakness. When PPMA occurs, it typically manifests in the regions most severely affected by the initial illness. Ventilatory function may decline, with one study suggesting an approximate 2% loss of vital capacity a year in keeping with the slowly progressive nature of the illness. Criteria have been established to solidify a PPMA diagnosis. These include objective measures of declining strength, muscle atrophy, and fatigue following a documented polio-like illness. This must occur subsequent to a protracted period of stability in absence of an alternative explanation.

West Nile Virus and Others

West Nile virus (WNV) is a mosquito-borne viral pathogen of the Flavivirus family. As in the case of polio, most infected individuals develop a minor nonspecific illness that often includes fever, gastrointestinal complaints, back pain, and rash in addition to potential neurologic manifestations. A number of reports have linked WNV to a poliomyelitis-like phenotype that may affect facial as well as limb muscles with or without an associated meningoencephalitic component. Approximately half of these patients will develop flaccid weakness, which tends to be proximal and asymmetric in distribution, over a 3- to 8-day period. Electrophysiologic and pathologic observations have suggested that this weakness originates from anterior horn cell injury. Confounding these observations are reports that the WNV may produce GBS and transverse myelitis phenotypes. As in the case of the poliovirus, varying degrees of irreversible paralysis may result. Other agents that have been reported to cause poliomyelitis-like illness include enterovirus 71, acute hemorrhagic conjunctivitis, Coxsackie virus group A type 7, echovirus type 6, and the Japanese encephalitis virus. Rabies may also present as a paralytic illness in 20% of cases, with paralysis typically beginning in the inoculated extremity.

Multifocal Motor Neuropathy

The majority of available evidence suggests that MMN is an immune-mediated neuropathy. Elevated serum levels of immunoglobulin M (IgM) antibodies directed against GM1 are detected in 30%–80% of patients with MMN. GM1 ganglioside, a glycolipid found in the paranodal region of the peripheral motor nerve, is theorized to play a role in axonal repair and the maintenance of tight junctions by stabilizing the paranode. Nonetheless, a pathogenic role for GM1 autoantibodies in MMN remains unproven. Reduction in antiganglioside antibody levels does not correlate with disease responsiveness in all

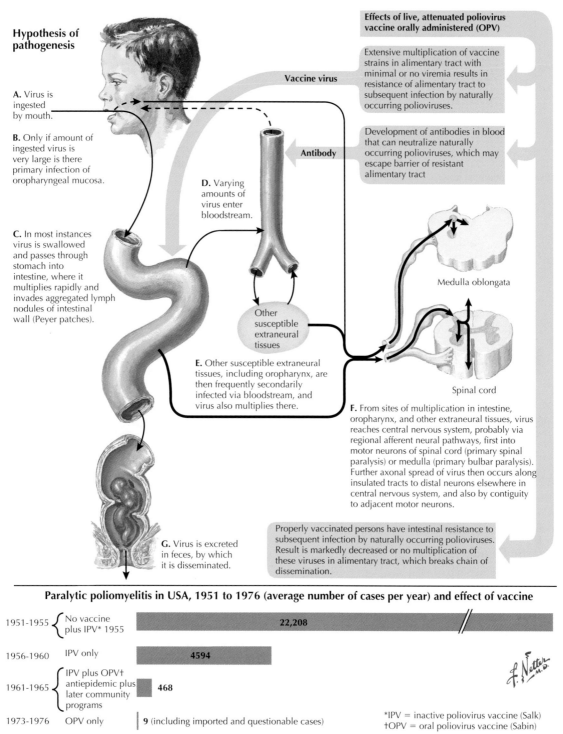

Hypothesis of pathogenesis

A. Virus is ingested by mouth.

B. Only if amount of ingested virus is very large is there primary infection of oropharyngeal mucosa.

C. In most instances virus is swallowed and passes through stomach into intestine, where it multiplies rapidly and invades aggregated lymph nodules of intestinal wall (Peyer patches).

D. Varying amounts of virus enter bloodstream.

E. Other susceptible extraneural tissues, including oropharynx, are then frequently secondarily infected via bloodstream, and virus also multiplies there.

Other susceptible extraneural tissues

G. Virus is excreted in feces, by which it is disseminated.

Vaccine virus

Antibody

Effects of live, attenuated poliovirus vaccine orally administered (OPV)

Extensive multiplication of vaccine strains in alimentary tract with minimal or no viremia results in resistance of alimentary tract to subsequent infection by naturally occurring polioviruses.

Development of antibodies in blood that can neutralize naturally occurring polioviruses, which may escape barrier of resistant alimentary tract

Medulla oblongata

Spinal cord

F. From sites of multiplication in intestine, oropharynx, and other extraneural tissues, virus reaches central nervous system, probably via regional afferent neural pathways, first into motor neurons of spinal cord (primary spinal paralysis) or medulla (primary bulbar paralysis). Further axonal spread of virus then occurs along insulated tracts to distal neurons elsewhere in central nervous system, and also by contiguity to adjacent motor neurons.

Properly vaccinated persons have intestinal resistance to subsequent infection by naturally occurring polioviruses. Result is markedly decreased or no multiplication of these viruses in alimentary tract, which breaks chain of dissemination.

Paralytic poliomyelitis in USA, 1951 to 1976 (average number of cases per year) and effect of vaccine

1951-1955	No vaccine plus IPV* 1955	22,208
1956-1960	IPV only	4594
1961-1965	IPV plus OPV† antiepidemic plus later community programs	468
1973-1976	OPV only	9 (including imported and questionable cases)

*IPV = inactive poliovirus vaccine (Salk)
†OPV = oral poliovirus vaccine (Sabin)

Fig. 63.4 Pathogenesis of Poliomyelitis.

patients. Conversely, patients with the MMN phenotype who are seronegative appear to respond equally well to immunomodulating treatments.

Even though MMN is a nerve disease, it is more likely to be considered in the differential diagnosis of MNDs. Similarly to ALS, it presents with painless weakness in a single limb, often in distal muscles in the upper extremity. Wrist drop, hand weakness, and foot drop can be early symptoms. Sensory symptoms are typically absent, although loss of vibration sense may be present in 20%–25% of patients with MMN.

Cramps and fasciculations may occur, providing an additional phenotypic overlap with ALS. Muscle stretch reflexes are often preserved. The clinical features that are most useful in distinguishing MMN from ALS include slower, often stepwise progression, the absence of unequivocal upper motor neuron signs, weakness without atrophy, a nerve rather than segmental pattern of muscle weakness, and absence of signs attributable to cranial nerve dysfunction. Cases of the latter have been reported only as a rare consequence of MMN. Unfortunately, with disease progression, these diagnostic clues may become obscured. In addition to

Stages in
destruction of
a motor neuron
by poliovirus

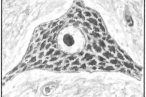

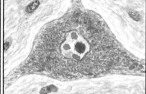

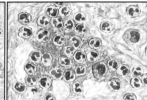

A. Normal motor neuron

B. Diffuse chromatolysis; three acidophilic nuclear inclusions around nucleolus

C. Polymorphonuclear cells invading necrotic neuron

D. Complete neuronophagia

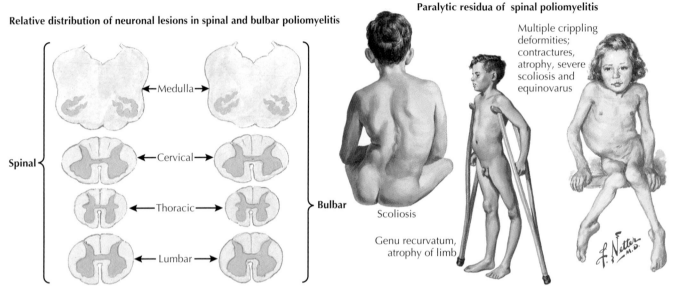

Relative distribution of neuronal lesions in spinal and bulbar poliomyelitis

Spinal

Medulla

Cervical

Thoracic

Lumbar

Bulbar

Paralytic residua of spinal poliomyelitis

Multiple crippling deformities; contractures, atrophy, severe scoliosis and equinovarus

Scoliosis

Genu recurvatum, atrophy of limb

Fig. 63.5 Poliomyelitis.

testing for GM1 autoantibodies, an in-depth electrodiagnostic (EDX) study to assess for conduction block or MRI or ultrasound seeking evidence for focal nerve lesions can be helpful for diagnosis.

Hereditary Spastic Paraparesis

To date, more than 56 HSP loci and 41 HSP-related genes have been associated with the HSP phenotype. Autosomal dominant, recessive, and X-linked modes of transmission are recognized. The multiple genotypes underlying HSP suggest that there is a common mechanism by which mutations of different proteins translate into an identical or nearly identical phenotype. However, a uniform final common pathway has yet to be defined. Proposed mechanisms include disturbances in axon transport, impaired Golgi function, mitochondrial dysfunction, disordered myelin synthesis, and maturational disturbances of the corticospinal tracts. Some of these hypotheses are based on the intracellular positioning of affected proteins. The pathology of HSP would support its conceptualization as a "dying back myelopathy."

HSP is a slowly progressive hereditary disorder in which other affected family members may not be readily identifiable. HSP is classified as "pure" or "uncomplicated" if symptoms are limited to lower extremity spasticity, bladder disturbance, and vibration loss in the lower extremities. In "complicated" forms of HSP, the neurologic deficits of uncomplicated HSP are accompanied by other neurologic or systemic abnormalities such as peripheral neuropathy, dementia, or extrapyramidal findings.

HSP invariably presents with problems related to symmetric lower extremity spasticity. Patients lose the ability to run or hop early in the course because of increased lower extremity extensor tone and the inability to flex the hip or knee in a facile manner. As a result, stride length is reduced. The legs tend to "scissor," that is, cross over each other, because of increased tone of the thigh adductor muscles. Circumduction, that is, advancing the leg in a circular rather than a linear motion, is done for compensatory reasons to avoid tripping on a foot that maintains an inverted and plantarflexed posture. Leg strength may be diminished; if weakness occurs, it does so in an "upper motor neuron" pattern, with hip flexors, knee flexors, and foot dorsiflexors being affected to the greatest extent. Hyperreflexia of the lower extremities is a universal feature, almost always accompanied by extensor plantar responses. Hyperreflexia of the upper extremities with Hoffman signs and reflex spread are common as well. Weakness, increased tone, impaired coordination, or loss of function of the upper extremities as well as cranial nerve dysfunction occur infrequently in pure or uncomplicated HSP and should lead to consideration of an alternative diagnosis. Posterior column involvement with loss of vibratory sense in a length-dependent pattern in the lower extremities may be seen. Urinary frequency, urgency, and urgency incontinence are common symptoms even within the pure forms of the disease. Rectal urgency and incontinence and sexual dysfunction are less common but do occur. High-arched feet and hammer toe deformities, features of a number of chronic neurologic diseases, are common features of the illness. The onset and severity of HSP varies considerably both within and between families. Initial symptoms may be recognized in any decade of life. The reasons for variations of disease onset and severity of affliction, both within and between families of the same genotype, are not currently understood, although other "disease modifying" genes are hypothesized to have a role.

Miscellaneous Causes of Motor Neuron Disease

MND phenotypes have occurred in association with other disorders. Understandably, little is known of the pathogenesis of these disparate and relatively uncommon disorders. Postirradiation neuropathy is frequently a pure motor syndrome; current evidence, including reports of root enhancement on MRI studies in some patients, favors a polyradiculopathy as the proposed mechanism. Radiation injury of the peripheral nervous system is typically delayed in onset with an average latency between exposure and symptoms of 6 years. The range, however, is exceedingly broad, with onset latency varying between 4 months and 25 years. Radiation doses typically exceed 4000 cGY in these patients.

DIFFERENTIAL DIAGNOSIS

Age of onset is an important consideration in the differential diagnosis of MND. The differential diagnosis of infantile SMA I is that of the floppy infant. The majority of these hypotonic neonates will be afflicted with a CNS disorder. An alert and appropriately interactive child with diminished or absent deep tendon reflexes would increase the probability of a neuromuscular cause of hypotonia. Within this category, neonatal or congenital myasthenia; neonatal myotonic dystrophy; Pompe disease; nemaline, myotubular, or other congenital myopathies; infantile botulism; and rare hypomyelinating neuropathies are major considerations.

The differential of MND in childhood includes a wide variety of myopathic disorders: the dystrophinopathies; limb-girdle, myotonic and Emery-Dreifuss muscular dystrophies; dermatomyositis; the congenital myopathies; mitochondrial disorders; and lipid and glycogen storage disorders. Chronic inflammatory demyelinating polyradiculoneuropathy would be the primary neuropathic consideration.

The pattern of weakness also helps to guide the differential diagnosis in certain MNDs. The differential of the bulbar pattern of weakness in Kennedy disease includes ALS, particularly the progressive bulbar palsy variant, and myasthenia gravis. Patients with muscle-specific tyrosine kinase (MUSK) myasthenia may have fixed bulbar weakness. Myopathies such as sporadic inclusion body myositis and oculopharyngeal muscular dystrophy can often display prominent dysphagia. The differential of SMA IV, which has a limb girdle pattern of weakness, is wide and includes the limb girdle muscular dystrophies (LGMDs), other myopathies, myasthenia, Lambert-Eaton myasthenic syndrome, and chronic inflammatory demyelinating polyneuropathy (CIDP).

Focal limb onset presentations of MND are commonly mistaken as mononeuropathies, radiculopathies, or plexopathies. The absence of pain and sensory symptoms should deflect consideration away from these disorders. The age of onset, the speed of disease progression, and the presence or absence of "bulbar" dysfunction and upper motor neuron signs would all aid in the determination of whether ALS, MMN, benign focal amyotrophies, or inclusion body myositis represents the leading consideration.

The distal SMAs are frequently misdiagnosed as the more common CMT disease.

Polio and other "anterior horn cell–tropic" viruses enter into the differential diagnosis of other causes of acute generalized weakness in which weakness predominates over sensory symptoms. GBS, botulism, hypokalemia, and hypophosphatemia and a number of toxic neuropathies are chief considerations in this regard.

The differential diagnosis of HSP includes other causes of spastic paraparesis. Compressive and inflammatory/immune-mediated myelopathies such as multiple sclerosis, neuromyelitis optica, and even stiff-person syndrome deserve consideration. PLS is typically distinguished from HSP by its more rapid progression, its asymmetry, and its frequent upper extremities and bulbar involvement. In addition, cavus foot deformities would not be expected in PLS. Vitamin B$_{12}$ and copper deficiency should be considered as potentially treatable causes of spastic paraparesis. In both cases, these disorders are typically more rapid in their onset as well as dominated by signs of posterior column

involvement. The corticospinal tracts may be affected by retroviral infection, and both the human immunodeficiency virus (HIV) and human T-cell leukemia virus type 1 need to be considered in the appropriate clinical context. Other hereditary neurodegenerative disorders that affect the corticospinal tracts, the leukodystrophies, particularly adrenoleukodystrophy in young adult women, and the spinocerebellar atrophies are considerations.

DIAGNOSTIC APPROACH

As the majority of the disorders discussed in this chapter are heritable, and in consideration of the rapidly evolving nature of genetic testing, the diagnostic approach to these disorders represents a moving target.

In general, when there is a strong correlation between a phenotype and a single gene such as in childhood SMA, mutational analysis of a single gene (SMN1) should be undertaken. Other more invasive tests, such as EMG and muscle biopsy, can be avoided in many cases.

Conversely, when there is poor correlation between a phenotype and single or small-number mutations, for example, HSP, more extensive genetic testing may be required. If genetic confirmation is sought in disorders such as this, targeted panels of known HSP mutations that provide adequate analytic depth are currently suggested. Presumably whole-exome sequencing or whole-genome testing will eventually be utilized in this role when these technologies evolve further.

Whether a clinical diagnosis should be confirmed with the use of genetic testing in an individual where there is no treatment that currently alters the natural history of the disease is a philosophic debate beyond the scope of this chapter.

The majority of tests in clinically suspected MNDs are performed to exclude other diagnostic considerations. EDX serves to identify a pattern consistent with MND and at the same time exclude features that would suggest an alternative localization. This MND pattern would consist of abnormalities of motor nerve conductions and EMG that involve multiple nerve and segmental distributions in one or more body regions. At the same time, features suggesting the possibility of MMN (conduction block or other demyelinating features), myopathy (short duration, low-amplitude motor unit potentials [MUPs]), disorders of neuromuscular transmission (abnormal repetitive stimulation), or Kennedy disease (reduced sensory nerve action potential [SNAP] amplitudes in the context of MND) should be excluded (Fig. 63.6). Electrophysiologic testing in the form of somatosensory evoked potentials (SSEPs) may have a role in distinguishing HSP from PLS.

Imaging in suspected MND is frequently utilized early when signs or symptoms appear to be originating from a singular or limited number of anatomic sites. MRI of the brain is rational in bulbar onset syndromes, as is MRI of the cervical and/or thoracic spine in upper motor neuron syndromes affecting the limbs. As mentioned, MRI or ultrasound imaging of peripheral nerves may be helpful in detecting focal nerve lesions when these are suspected in MMN.

The historical role of histologic analysis in suspected MNDs is diminishing. Muscle biopsy should probably be done only in situations when mutational analysis cannot confirm the diagnosis and myopathy remains within the differential. If muscle biopsy is performed in MND, a typical neurogenic pattern including muscle fiber type grouping and atrophy would be expected. There is little if any role for nerve biopsy in these disorders.

Genetic screening for SMA is a complex issue beyond the scope of this chapter. Preconception, prenatal, and newborn screenings are available owing to advances in whole-genome sequencing and noninvasive prenatal testing. As with any genetic disease, the results should be interpreted with caution and with the support of genetic counseling. As SMAs I to III are recessively inherited, a mutation in one parent in

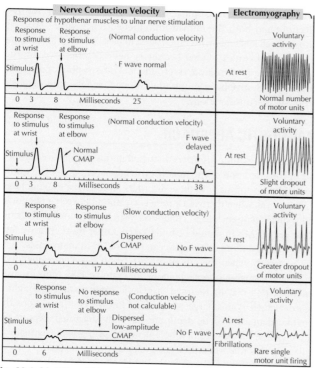

Fig. 63.6 Multifocal Motor Neuropathy: Conduction Block on Nerve Conduction Study.

most cases would not affect offspring, but in rare cases a child with SMA has only one identified heterozygote carrier owing to factors such as spontaneous mutation and false paternity.

MANAGEMENT AND THERAPY

Knowledge of the defective gene product in SMAs I–IV and the correlation between disease severity and functional SMN2 protein has led to the development of nusinersen, the first effective therapy for SMA. In 2016, the FDA approved this intrathecal SMN2-directed antisense oligonucleotide for the treatment of SMA in children and adults based on improvement of motor milestones in phase 3 trials. Cost, accessibility to patients, and pragmatic implications of intrathecal delivery remain significant factors to date. Efficacy and safety in regard to juvenile/adult SMN/SMA patients remain unknown. Other novel therapies, such as viral vector gene therapy and orally available small molecules, are also under investigation.

Supportive care also remains of paramount importance in SMA. Surveillance of bone health is important for immobilized patients. The development of kyphoscoliosis is a common problem in children with SMA who are wheelchair-bound. Spinal stabilization is commonly recommended in individuals whose curves exceed 50 degrees and whose vital capacities exceed 40% of predicted. The goals of this intervention are patient comfort and potential stabilization of restrictive pulmonary deficits. A high index of suspicion is maintained for symptoms of impaired nocturnal ventilation and is, if necessary, treated with application of positive airway pressure. Ventilatory failure in SMA I and II is inevitable; tracheostomy, long-term mechanical ventilation, and insertion of a percutaneous feeding tube are decisions of enormous emotional consequence to the parents of the affected child. Noninvasive positive pressure ventilation may provide an improved quality and duration of life until a decision regarding tracheostomy is required.

In patients with Hirayama disease, decompression of the cervical spinal cord is generally not recommended as it is unclear whether this intervention meaningfully affects the natural history of the disease. Data from a small series of patients suggest that a simple cervical collar may help arrest progression.

Treatment for HSP is supportive. There are a number of different options to reduce spasticity, including oral tizanidine, baclofen, dantrolene, benzodiazepines, intrathecal baclofen, or botulinum toxin injections directly into spastic muscles. The goal of treatment is to improve mobility, augment range of motion, and relieve the discomfort associated with spastic muscles. In an individual who also has considerable underlying weakness, the increased tone of extensor muscles may represent the major source of antigravity resistance. Suppression of this tone may deprive an individual of his or her ability to stand.

The mainstay of treatment for MMN, an immune-mediated neuropathic process, is intravenous immune globulin (IVIG) 2 g/kg given over 2–5 days per month for at least 3 consecutive months. Optimal treatment dosage, intervals, and duration of treatment are not known.

In general, home modification and durable medical equipment are important components of the management of patients with chronic neuromuscular diseases. The goals are to maintain independent mobility and patient safety simultaneously. Ankle-foot orthoses are of great benefit to individual patients. Their primary purpose is to prevent tripping by maintaining the foot in a partially dorsiflexed position. A skilled physical therapist is invaluable in deciding whether a cane, Lofstran crutches, a walker, or a wheelchair is the best solution for an individual patient. Motorized scooters or power wheelchairs are options for patients who lack the ability to propel a manual chair. Although scooters are more attractive to patients, they are often inconvenient as they require a greater degree of upper extremity function to operate, provide less trunk support, and allow for less additional equipment to be mounted on them. In patients who live in multiple-story dwellings, stair lifts provide a safe option. A skilled occupational therapist is also a valuable aid in maintaining independence in activities of daily living.

FUTURE DIRECTIONS

As most of these disorders are heritable, effective treatment may depend on future technologic advances that might allow for the identification and restitution of the affected genes in utero. Truncating the effects of mutated genes pharmacologically and arresting disease progression appears to be another interventional strategy that may be feasible in the near future, at least in certain diseases. Reversal of the established consequences of these mutations will be a more daunting challenge.

ADDITIONAL RESOURCES

Spinal Muscular Atrophy

http://www.mda.org/disease/.
www.nlm.nih.gov/medlineplus/spinalmuscularatrophy.html.
http://www.ncbi.nlm.nih.gov/sites/entrez?db=omim.

Hereditary Spinal Paraparesis

Amato AA, Russell JA. Neuromuscular disorders. 2nd ed. New York: McGraw Hill; 2016.

Bertini E, Burghes A, Bushby K, et al. 134th ENMC international workshop: outcome measures and treatment of spinal muscular atrophy 11-13 February 2005. Naarden, The Netherlands. Neuromuscul Disord 2005;15:802–16.

Chahin N, Klein C, Mandrekar J, et al. Natural history of spinal-bulbar muscular atrophy. Neurology 2008;70:1967–71.

Corey D. Nusinersen, an antisense oligonucleotide drug for spinal muscular atrophy. Nat Neurosci 2017;20:497–9.

Felice K, Whitaker C, Grunnet M. Benign calf amtryotrophy: clinicopathologic study of 8 patients. Arch Neurol 2003;60:1415–20.

Harding AE. Inherited neuronal atrophy and degeneration predominantly of lower motor neurons. In: Dyck PJ, Thomas PK, Griffin JW, et al., editors.

Peripheral neuropathy. 3rd ed. Philadelphia: W. B. Saunders; 1993: 1051–64.

Kumar A, Patwa H, Nowak R. Immunoglobulin therapy in the treatment of multifocal motor neuropathy. J Neurol Sci 2017;190–7.

Irobi J, Dierick I, Jordanova A, et al. Unraveling the genetics of distal hereditary motor neuropathies. Neuromolec Med 2006;8:131–46.

National Ataxia Foundation 2600 Fernbrook Lane Suite 119 Minneapolis, MN 55447 Phone: 763-553-0020 Fax: 763-553-0167 naf@ataxia.org.

Spastic Paraplegia Foundation, Inc. 209 Park Rd. Chelmsford, MA 01824 Phone: 703-495-9261 community@sp-foundation.org sp-foundation.org.

Neuromuscular Hyperactivity Disorders

Jayashri Srinivasan

64

Stiff-Person Syndrome

Michal Vytopil, Jayashri Srinivasan, Ted M. Burns, H. Royden Jones, Jr.[†]

> **CLINICAL VIGNETTE** *A 48-year-old hospital administrator began having difficulties during meetings when her back would stiffen up every time she was asked to get up to speak. Subsequently, she developed episodes of anxiety accompanied by her left leg tightening up. Her internist referred her to a counselor thinking these episodes were "emotionally driven." However, they became more frequent, usually occurring when standing and talking to people at work. She described her legs as feeling like walking "on stilts." On one occasion when she started to laugh, her left leg stiffened and she fell "like a tin soldier." The primary finding on examination was her spontaneous reaction to any sensory stimuli wherein her back stiffened. Other than hyperlordosis and marked hyperreflexia at her knees, her neurologic examination was normal. Magnetic resonance imaging (MRI) of her brain and spine proved normal. A needle electromyography (EMG) study demonstrated cramp discharges in contracting muscles during episodes of stiffness, but was otherwise normal. Immunoprecipitation assay showed a high level of serum glutamic acid decarboxylase 65 (GAD-65) antibodies (47 nmol/L; reference range: ≤0.02 nmol/L). She was diagnosed with stiff-person syndrome (SPS). Diazepam dramatically alleviated symptoms at a daily dose of 40 mg. Treatment with corticosteroids or intravenous immunoglobulin was contemplated, but was ultimately not required thanks to sufficient control with symptomatic therapy. Over the subsequent 5 years, she was successfully tapered off the benzodiazepine.*

Stiff-person syndrome (SPS) is an autoimmune central nervous system disorder with localization primarily to the brainstem and spinal cord. It is characterized by fluctuating muscle stiffness with superimposed spasms and is often accompanied by exaggerated startle response. Possible manifestations include classic SPS, stiff-limb syndrome (SLS), and a rare presentation with some or all components of progressive encephalomyelitis with rigidity and myoclonus (PERM). Also, increasingly recognized are variants of SPS with additional neurologic symptoms of cerebellar ataxia, epilepsy, or limbic encephalitis. The recently introduced term "stiff-person spectrum disorder" (SPSD) reflects this emerging clinical heterogeneity.

SPS is a rare disease with an estimated prevalence of 1 in 1,250,000 people. Women are more often affected than men. SPS generally presents in the fourth through sixth decades. Childhood onset was only recently recognized, with onset as early as 1 year of age. Owing to its rarity and protean symptomatology, SPS is still often misdiagnosed as a psychogenic movement disorder or dystonia. As a result, a delay in diagnosis is not uncommon.

PATHOGENESIS

The current understanding is that SPS is an autoimmune disease targeting proteins associated with gamma-amino-butyric acid (GABA)- or glycine-related inhibitory pathways in the spinal cord and brainstem. Antibodies targeted against GAD-65 (glutamic acid decarboxylase) are found most often in SPS; GlyR (glycine receptor) and amphiphysin are some of the less common antigens, and there are likely others yet to be characterized. The precise pathophysiologic role for the specific antibodies is unclear. The autoimmune basis for SPS is further supported by its frequent association with other autoimmune disorders such as type 1 diabetes mellitus (in almost half of patients), thyroiditis, vitiligo, and pernicious anemia. Rarely, SPS can be a manifestation of paraneoplastic autoimmunity; amphiphysin antibody is detected in some of these cases, most often in older women with breast cancer.

GAD-65 antibodies are found in 60%–80% of patients with classic SPS, and less frequently in other subtypes such as PERM. The antibody titer is typically high (>20 nmol/L). The same antibody, but in low titer, is detected in 90% of patients with type 1 diabetes mellitus. GAD-65 antibody is not specific for SPS; it has been associated with immune-mediated cerebellar ataxia, limbic encephalitis, and temporal lobe epilepsy. Because it is directed against a cytoplasmic antigen, GAD-65 antibody is probably not pathogenic. It is more likely to be a marker for organ-specific autoimmune attack by cytotoxic T-cells. Consequently, the response to GAD-65 antibody-depleting therapy is variable and rarely leads to complete recovery.

Antibodies against glycine receptor (GlyR) are associated with PERM. Unlike GAD-65, GlyR is expressed on the surface of motor neurons in the brainstem and spinal cord. Therefore, GlyR antibodies are more likely to be causative. This may explain why PERM patients, if diagnosed early, may have a better response to antibody-depleting therapy than those with GAD-65 antibodies.

CLINICAL PRESENTATION

Classic Stiff-Person Syndrome

Typically, classic SPS is characterized by spine and leg rigidity with lumbar hyperlordosis as a key feature (Fig. 64.1). Coined "Frankenstein's gait," the patient walks with a wide base and extended legs and tends to fall in a manner similar to a stiff board. Patients experience superimposed painful spasms that may be precipitated by sudden noise, anxiety, or touch. The spasms can be of such abrupt onset and power that these individuals may unexpectedly and precipitously fall. Patients soon recognize that emotional stress often provokes their spasms, and they may develop agoraphobia secondary to the fear of falling in public.

[†]Deceased.

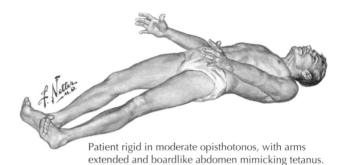

Patient rigid in moderate opisthotonos, with arms extended and boardlike abdomen mimicking tetanus.

Fig. 64.2 Generalized Rigidity Can Be Seen in Advanced Stiff-Person Syndrome or in Progressive Encephalomyelitis With Rigidity and Myoclonus.

Progressive Encephalomyelitis With Rigidity and Myoclonus

PERM is the most severe of SPS subtypes and is often associated with antibodies against glycine receptor (GlyR). In addition to muscle rigidity and stiffness (Fig. 64.2), it is marked by brainstem disturbance with oculomotor and bulbar dysfunction, as well as encephalopathy, seizures, myoclonus, sensory, and autonomic dysfunction. Incomplete presentations are common, and features of myelopathy and lower motor dysfunction may develop. Left untreated, PERM is a relentlessly progressive and fatal disease. A high index of suspicion leading to early diagnosis can be lifesaving; early immunotherapy is effective with often dramatic improvement.

Paraneoplastic Stiff-Person Syndrome

Classic SPS with GAD-65 antibodies is almost never paraneoplastic. Rare paraneoplastic cases with GAD-65 antibodies had overlapping conditions, such as cerebellar ataxia or limbic encephalitis, and often coexisted with other paraneoplastic antibodies. Malignancies described in this setting included small cell lung cancer, thymoma, and lymphoma. In contrast to GAD-65 autoimmunity, antibodies against amphiphysin are typically paraneoplastic and associated with breast cancer or small-cell lung cancer. Compared to typical SPS cases, patients with amphiphysin antibodies have more stiffness in the cervical region and the arms and can have associated myelopathy and sensory neuropathy or neuronopathy. When amphiphysin antibodies are positive, it is important to ensure careful follow-up. One patient had two negative mammograms over a 1-year period only to self-discover a breast mass a short time later.

DIFFERENTIAL DIAGNOSIS

Frequently SPS patients have a history of multiple visits to a variety of physicians, including neurologists. They are often inappropriately labeled as having conversion or somatoform disorders, leading to recurrent psychiatric evaluations.

Ankylosing spondylitis may present with truncal stiffness and pain, particularly in the morning. Unlike SPS, this improves as the day progresses, or simply with warmth. The possibility of a spinal cord disorder is an important consideration in SPS patients with predominant leg symptoms. Basal ganglia disorders, including Parkinson disease, may present with truncal rigidity and gait disorder, but lack the history of painful spasm and exaggerated startle reflex, which is very characteristic for SPS.

In any acute setting, the possibility of tetanus must be considered because of the board-like stiffening of the abdomen and the severity of muscle spasms. Sparing of the jaw muscles and the absence of trismus in SPS make tetanus unlikely.

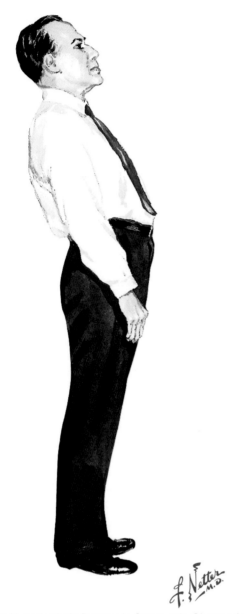

Fig. 64.1 Hyperlordotic Posture Is Commonly Observed in Classic Stiff-Person Syndrome.

Neurologic examination often reveals hyperlordosis, leg rigidity, and "board-like" hardness of paraspinal and abdominal muscles. These findings may not be present until late in the clinical course. Brisk muscle stretch reflexes may be observed.

Stiff-Limb Syndrome

This variant of SPS presents focally with rigidity and spasms involving one or more limbs, often distally. In contrast to the classic SPS, axial involvement is less prominent. However, significant proximal muscle involvement does eventually occur if this focal variant of SPS is not diagnosed and treated early. This was illustrated by one of our patients who had spontaneous quadriceps spasms leading to automobile accidents. These were spontaneous and precipitous contractions that caused him to suddenly apply excess pressure to the accelerator on one occasion and the brake on another. Diagnosis requires high index of suspicion; GAD autoantibody titers are elevated less frequently in these patients compared to classic SPS.

Hereditary hyperekplexia or startle disease with startle-induced spasms is a rare disorder caused by mutations in the GlyR. Startle-induced spasms may also be seen in focal spinal cord lesions such as tumors or syringomyelia.

Patients with psychogenic muscle contraction or spasm usually have an inconsistent and a variable presentation; this diagnosis must only be entertained after long periods of careful observation and recurrent laboratory testing. Other causes of muscular rigidity include disorders of neuromuscular hyperexcitability. Two channelopathies with muscle rigidity—namely myotonia congenita and Isaac syndrome—deserve consideration in the differential diagnosis, but neither of these is associated with the pain typically seen with SPS. Multiple sclerosis, poliomyelitis, Lyme disease, spinal myoclonus, tumors, and even strychnine poisoning are included in the differential diagnosis and might deserve consideration in some cases.

DIAGNOSTIC APPROACH

SPS is primarily a clinical diagnosis, supported by the detection of antibodies and the results of electrodiagnostic testing. Magnetic resonance imaging (MRI) studies are characteristically normal.

The following constellation of clinical features is generally considered necessary for the diagnosis of classic SPS:

1. Stiffness in the axial and limb muscles, often resulting in impaired ambulation and/or abnormal axial posture with increased lumbar hyperlordosis.
2. Superimposed painful episodic spasms precipitated by exaggerated startle or sudden movement.
3. Unequivocal positive response to benzodiazepine.

Serologic studies are important in the evaluation of these patients. High titer of GAD-65 antibodies is seen in the majority of classic SPS cases, but less often in variant cases. Depending on the method of detection, high titer is defined as greater than 20 nmol/L or greater than 2000 IU/mL. Low titers need to be interpreted with caution as they can be present in healthy individuals, type 1 diabetics, and other autoimmune neurologic diseases. In patients with features of PERM, GlyR antibodies can be present. If paraneoplastic context is suspected, one should look for amphiphysin as well as other paraneoplastic antibodies. A significant percentage of SPS cases remain seronegative.

Cerebrospinal fluid (CSF) evaluation is usually normal but can occasionally demonstrate increased protein or oligoclonal bands (OBs). In patients who are seronegative or have only low-titer of GAD antibodies, the presence of CSF-specific OBs provides a helpful clue of central nervous system autoimmunity.

Routine nerve conduction study and needle electromyography (NCS/EMG) are typically normal. In an advanced, diagnostically challenging seronegative case, one can occasionally demonstrate continuous firing of otherwise normal motor units action potentials (MUAPs) in a stiff muscle or simultaneous activation of both agonist and antagonist muscle groups. We have used a simultaneous two-channel recording from quadriceps femoris and biceps femoris, or from lumbar paraspinal and rectus abdominis muscles. Results have to be interpreted with caution; continuous firing of MUAPs is not uncommon in a nervous individual, and simultaneous cocontraction can be produced volitionally.

TREATMENT APPROACH

Most recommendations for the management of SPS are not evidence based; IVIg and rituximab are the only treatments subjected to a randomized trial.

Symptomatic treatment with diazepam, another benzodiazepine, or baclofen is usually the first-line therapy, especially in mild cases. As GABA receptor agonists, these medications are helpful in reducing the symptoms, but they do not address the underlying autoimmune process. Diazepam is typically started at 5 mg two or three times a day. SPS patients may need very high doses, some up to 100–200 mg a day, to control their symptoms. Serious side effects include long-term physical dependence. Much caution is advised if one considers discontinuation of a benzodiazepine; withdrawal reaction can be life-threatening.

Immune therapies are required for patients with more than mild disease or for those with inadequate response to symptomatic treatment. In order to rapidly control the symptoms, *acute therapy* with IVIg is usually initiated. IVIg has been demonstrated to improve stiffness and ambulation in randomized placebo-controlled trial. Pulse intravenous methylprednisolone (IVMP) or plasma exchange can also be considered for acute therapy, but there may be an increased risk of steroid-induced or exacerbated diabetes if corticosteroids are used. In order to rapidly control the symptoms, IVIg has been demonstrated to improve stiffness and ambulation in randomized placebo-controlled trial. If corticosteroids are used, added risk of steroid-induced or exacerbated diabetes in GAD-65 positive patients needs to be considered. If effective, acute therapy can be continued for 6–12 weeks with the goal of inducing long-term remission. In patients with limited or no response to the first therapy tried, one of the other intravenous treatments can be used. For *chronic therapy*, gradual reduction in IVIg or IVMP dose, with or without a long-term immunosuppressant, is required. Azathioprine, mycophenolate mofetil, methotrexate, or oral cyclophosphamide can be used for the maintenance of remission or for reducing dependency on steroids or IVIg. Rituximab or intravenous cyclophosphamide can be considered for refractory cases. Rituximab, an anti-CD-20 monoclonal antibody that attacks B lymphocytes, has been anecdotally reported to lead to clinical improvement in SPS, including in several refractory cases. However, this was not confirmed in a recently published placebo-controlled trial of GAD-65–positive patients. It is possible that only a subset of patients may benefit from rituximab.

ADDITIONAL RESOURCES

Moersch FP, Woltman HW. Progressive fluctuating muscular rigidity and spasm ("stiff-man" syndrome): report of a case and some observations in 13 other cases. Mayo Clin Proc 1956;31:421–7.
The initial and very classic paper with exquisitely detailed patient history.
Murinson BB, Fuarnaccia JB. Stiff-person syndrome with amphiphysin antibodies: distinctive features of a rare disease. Neurology 2008;71(24):1955–8.
Description of paraneoplastic SPS cases associated with amphiphysin antibodies.
Clardy SL, Lennon VA, Dalmau J, et al. Childhood onset stiff-man syndrome. JAMA Neurol 2013;70(12):1531–6.
Case series providing description of pediatric SPS cases.
McKeon A, Tracy J. GAD65 neurological autoimmunity. Muscle Nerve 2017;56:15–27.
Clinically oriented review of conditions associated with GAD autoimmunity.
Martinez-Hernandez E, Arino H, McKeon A, et al. Clinical and immunologic investigations in patients with stiff person spectrum disorder. JAMA Neurol 2016;73(6):714–20.
Clinico-immunologic correlations were studied in this group of 121 patients with SPS spectrum disorders.
Dalakas MS, Rakocevic G, Dambrosia JM, et al. A double-blind, placebo-controlled study of rituximab in patients with stiff person syndrome. Ann Neurol 2017;82:271–7.
The largest controlled trial conducted in SPS patients demonstrated no statistically significant difference between rituximab and placebo.
Dalakas MC, Fujii M, Li M, et al. High-dose intravenous immune globulin for stiff-person syndrome. N Engl J Med 2001;345(26):1870.
In this small randomized placebo-controlled trial, patients who received IVIg had improved measures of stiffness, startle, and ambulation.

65

Other Peripheral Hyperexcitability Syndromes

Michal Vytopil

Peripheral nerve hyperexcitability (PNH) syndromes present with involuntary, continuous muscle overactivity due to hyperexcitability of the motor axon. PNH syndromes are a heterogeneous group of disorders with distinct clinical and electrodiagnostic features. Muscle cramps are the hallmark of these conditions, along with muscle twitching (fasciculations and myokymia) and pseudo-myotonia (delayed relaxation after contraction). Isaac syndrome is the best known of these disorders, whereas cramp-fasciculation syndrome may be more common. Within the PNH spectrum is also Morvan syndrome with its central nervous system (CNS) features of encephalopathy and insomnia.

Needle electromyography (EMG) is marked by continuous firing of motor unit action potentials (MUAPs) in the form of fasciculations and myokymic and neuromyotonic discharges. Neuromyotonic discharges are the defining feature of Isaac syndrome, giving the syndrome one of its many names (acquired neuromyotonia) (Fig. 65.1). They are very high-frequency (100–300 Hz), decrementing, repetitive discharges of a single motor unit that have a characteristic "pinging" sound on EMG. They have the highest interpotential frequency of any discharge.

PATHOGENESIS

Most cases of PNH are acquired, often due to autoimmune causes (e.g., voltage-gated potassium channel [VGKC] antibodies). Paraneoplastic autoimmunity may be present, with thymoma and lung cancer occurring most commonly. Exposure to specific toxins such as that of the rattlesnake, radiation-induced neuropathy, or hereditary motor neuropathy are less frequent mechanisms. Antibodies to VGKCs occur in up to 50% of patients with Isaac syndrome and less frequently in the other PNH forms. These antibodies target various proteins associated with different subtypes of voltage-gated potassium channels. The two best-characterized antigens are *leucine-rich glioma-inactivated protein 1 (Lgi1)* in the CNS and *contactin-associated protein 2 (Caspr2)* in peripheral nerves; the latter is associated with Isaac syndrome.

ISAAC SYNDROME/ACQUIRED NEUROMYOTONIA

Isaac syndrome is characterized by the continuous firing of peripheral motor axons, leading to continuous activity of motor units. Patients complain of muscle cramps worsened by voluntary contraction. Excessive sweating, muscle hypertrophy, and weight loss may also occur. On exam, widespread fasciculations and myokymia are seen. Fasciculations are irregular, spontaneous contractions of a group of muscle fibers belonging to the same motor unit, producing movement of the overlying skin. Myokymia, in contrast, is an undulating wavelike movement visible under the skin. An interesting phenomenon of pseudomyotonia (delayed relaxation after contraction) can be observed. Strength and deep tendon reflexes are usually normal. Diagnosis is suggested when EMG demonstrates continuous firing of normal motor unit potentials (MUAPs), most notably in the form of neuromyotonic discharges. These persist during sleep and are abolished by neuromuscular blockade, suggesting that the generator may be in the motor axon. Autoimmune pathogenesis of Isaac syndrome is suggested by its association with other autoimmune conditions, most notably myasthenia gravis and thyroiditis, and by detection of antibodies against VGKCs in a large proportion of patients. Association with malignancy is well recognized, thymoma and lung in particular.

Various drugs have been used for symptomatic relief, including carbamazepine, phenytoin, gabapentin, and mexiletine, but they do not address the underlying autoimmune process. Various combinations of plasma exchange, corticosteroids, and immunosuppressants such as azathioprine can be effective.

MORVAN SYNDROME

In addition to neuromuscular manifestations identical to Isaac syndrome, patients with Morvan syndrome present with fluctuating encephalopathy, insomnia, and hallucinations. Morvan syndrome shares with Isaac syndrome the same association with VGKC antibodies and thymoma. Plasmapheresis followed by an immunosuppressive agent is usually required.

CRAMP-FASCICULATION SYNDROME

Painful cramps are the hallmark of this syndrome, often accompanied by exercise intolerance and reports of muscle twitching. Needle electromyography (EMG) shows fasciculation potentials but is otherwise normal, and nerve conduction studies may demonstrate afterdischarges on repetitive nerve stimulation. In contrast to Isaac syndrome, the EMG lacks myokymic and neuromyotonic discharges. Some patients have potassium channel antibodies. Treatment of this benign condition, if required, is similar to the symptomatic therapy for Isaac syndrome.

BENIGN FASCICULATION SYNDROME

Patients with this syndrome develop relatively rapid onset of scattered fasciculations. Characteristically these are physicians or medical students who are aware of the ominous association between fasciculations and amyotrophic lateral sclerosis (ALS) and gradually become consumed by the fear of having that disease. However, if there is no concomitant weakness and/or muscle atrophy, this almost always is a benign entity. If both clinical exam and EMG are normal, patients can be reassured that they have no risk of developing ALS.

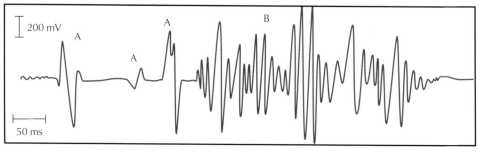

1. A, Fasciculation potential - singular, irregular MUAP discharges; B, Cramp discharge - rapidly but irregularly firing MUAPs, often with abrupt onset and cessation

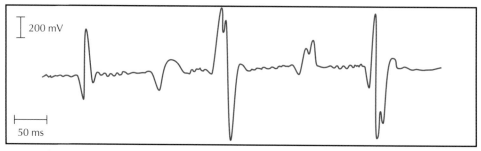

2. Fasciculation potentials

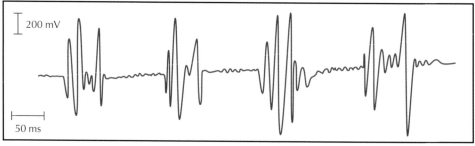

3. Myokymic discharges - rhythmic or semirhythmic discharges of grouped MUAPs

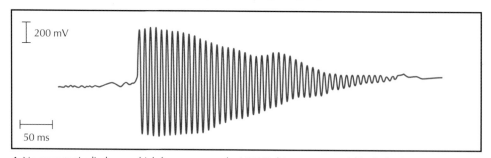

4. Neuromytonic discharge - high-frequency, regular MUAPs firing pattern, quickly dissipating

Fig. 65.1 Electromyographic Discharges in Isaac Syndrome and Other Peripheral Nerve Hyperexcit-ability Disorders. *MUAP,* Motor unit action potential.

MYOKYMIA

Myokymia is characterized by quivering, wormlike muscle activity visible under the skin. Its EMG equivalent—myokymic discharge—consists of semirhythmic firing of grouped discharges of one or more MUAPs, producing a sound likened to soldiers marching. The most common setting is that of a patient with radiation-induced neuropathy. Postradiation brachial plexopathy that emerges in women many years after radiation treatment of breast cancer is the characteristic scenario. Cranial neuropathies following radiation for head/neck cancer, pontine glioma, or even benign Bell palsy are much less common causes of facial myokymia.

ADDITIONAL RESOURCES

Ahmed A, Simmons Z. Isaacs syndrome: a review. Muscle Nerve 2015;52:5–12.
A clinically focused review of Isaac syndrome, including evaluation and management.
Hart IK, Maddison P, Newson-Davis J, et al. Phenotypic variants of autoimmune peripheral nerve hyperexcitability. Brain 2002;125:1887–95.
One of the seminal papers on autoimmune PNH syndromes.
Vernino S, Lennon VA. Ion channel and striational antibodies define a continuum of autoimmune neuromuscular hyperexcitability. Muscle Nerve 2002;26:702–7.
This paper characterized PNH forms as a continuum of conditions defined by autoimmunity against components of voltage-gated potassium channels.

Polyneuropathies

Jayashri Srinivasan

66

Hereditary Polyneuropathies

Obehi Irumudomon, Michal Vytopil

CLINICAL VIGNETTE *A 13-year-old boy presents with frequent tripping. He enjoys playing baseball but has had several falls this season, one resulting in a fractured ankle. Born at term, his early developmental milestones were normal and he walked at 13 months (normal). On examination, he has mild wasting of the distal lower extremities without contractures. He walks well on his toes but cannot walk on his heels. There is mild weakness of ankle dorsiflexion and eversion. The ankle reflexes are absent but other reflexes are preserved. Sensation is intact. There is no family history of neuromuscular disorders. His father, who accompanies him to the appointment, agrees to be examined and is found to have high-arched feet and generalized areflexia. Neurophysiologic testing of the patient and his father reveals marked slowing of ulnar nerve motor conduction (18 m/s), with absent sensory responses. Genetic testing is positive for a duplication of the PMP22 gene on chromosome 17, confirming the clinical diagnosis of Charcot-Marie-Tooth disease type 1A.*

The hereditary sensory and motor neuropathies (HSMNs) are responsible for about one-third of chronic neuropathies. Also known by the eponym Charcot-Marie-Tooth disease (CMT), they affect 1 in 2500 people and are the most common inherited neurologic disorder. CMT1A, the most common form described in the foregoing vignette, is a prototypic hereditary neuropathy responsible for almost half of all CMT cases. CMT is a genetically heterogeneous disease; over 70 genes have been identified and this number is expected to rise.

CLASSIFICATION

Historically, CMTs were divided based on their mode of inheritance and electrophysiologic findings. The majority are autosomal-dominant; whereas X-linked and recessive cases are less common. About two-thirds of CMTs are demyelinating; the rest are primarily axonal. CMT1 refers to dominantly inherited demyelinating neuropathies, whereas type 2 (CMT2) represents dominantly inherited axonal types. Recessively inherited neuropathies are designated as type 4 (CMT4) and can be either demyelinating or axonal. The X-linked form (CMT-X) can be demyelinating or "intermediate."

In CMT disease, both motor and sensory fibers are affected. This contrasts with purely motor or purely sensory forms of hereditary polyneuropathies—distal hereditary motor neuropathies (dHMNs) and hereditary sensory and autonomic neuropathies (HSANs) with prominent autonomic features. Less common inherited polyneuropathies are those associated with systemic genetic degenerative disorders and inborn errors of metabolism (Table 66.1). Of these, peripheral nerve involvement in familial amyloid polyneuropathies (FAPs) can be an early and defining clinical feature. Unique phenotypic features of hereditary neuropathy with liability to pressure palsies (HNPP) and hereditary neuralgic amyotrophy (HNA) place them in separate categories of inherited polyneuropathies.

CLINICAL PRESENTATION

A typical patient with CMT presents in his or her first two decades with foot deformities and abnormal gait (Fig. 66.1). This has been termed the "classical" phenotype. Less frequent presentations include hypotonia and delayed motor milestones in infancy ("infantile-onset" phenotype) or leg weakness in adulthood ("adult-onset" phenotype). Symptom onset is characteristically insidious and cannot be dated with certainty. Patients may recall being called "clumsy" while playing sports as children. Often reported is the history of inability to ice or roller skate, attributed to "weak ankles." Patients rarely report sensory symptoms, and if they do, negative symptoms (i.e., numbness) prevail over positive (e.g., tingling, prickling). On examination, one finds distal weakness and wasting, absent reflexes, and impaired distal sensation. Foot deformities are common; high arches (pes cavus) and curling of the toes (hammertoes) are detected in most cases. Imbalance between weaker anterior muscles (tibialis anterior and peroneus brevis) and stronger posterior muscle group (tibialis posterior, peroneus longus, and extensor digitorum longus) is hypothesized to be responsible for the typical foot appearance in CMT. Some CMT forms come accompanied by skeletal abnormalities such as scoliosis or hip dysplasia, optic atrophy (CMT2A), or tremor (CMT1). An uncommon but interesting presentation is one in which symptoms follow exposure to neurotoxic drugs in a patient with mild or yet undiagnosed CMT; chemotherapy agents paclitaxel and vinca alkaloids are examples.

Charcot-Marie-Tooth Type 1

CMT1—autosomal dominant demyelinating CMT—is the most common form of CMT (Table 66.2). CMT1A—the most common subtype responsible for about 70% of CMT1 and 40%–50% of all CMT cases—is considered a prototypic hereditary neuropathy. Almost all CMT1A patients become symptomatic in their first two decades with characteristic findings of pes cavus and steppage gait due to footdrop. Although sensory loss is not a common presenting complaint, reduced sensation to all modalities is often noted on exam. Nerve conduction velocity is uniformly slowed, most often in 15–35 m/s range. Nerve biopsy is rarely needed; if performed, it shows a hypertrophic "dysmyelinating" neuropathy with "onion bulb" formation. Negative family history is not uncommon; about 10% of CMT1A cases are due to sporadic mutations. In some cases that appear sporadic, one of the parents accompanying the child

TABLE 66.1　Classification of Inherited Polyneuropathies

	Inheritance	Primary Neurophysiology
Charcot-Marie-Tooth Disease and Related Neuropathies		
CMT1	AD	Demyelinating
CMT2	AD or AR	Axonal
CMT3	AD or AR	Demyelinating
CMT4	AR	Demyelinating or axonal
Intermediate CMT	AD or AR	Mixed
CMT-X	X-linked	Mixed
Hereditary sensory and autonomic neuropathies (HSAN)	AD or AR	Axonal
Hereditary motor neuropathies (HMN)	AD, AR, or X-linked	Axonal
Hereditary neuropathy with liability to pressure palsies (HNPP)	AD	Demyelinating
Neuropathies Associated With Inborn Errors of Metabolism		
Lipid Disorders		
Cerebrotendinous xanthomatosis	AR	Mixed
Abetalipoproteinemia	AR	Mixed
Ataxia with vitamin E deficiency	AR	Mixed
Tangier disease	AR	Demyelinating, mixed
Refsum disease	AR	Demyelinating
Adrenomyeloneuropathy (AMN)	X-linked	Axonal
Mitochondrial Cytopathies		
NARP	Mitochondrial	Mixed
MNGIE	AR	Mixed
Leigh disease	AR, mitochondrial or X-linked	Mixed
Lysosomal Storage Diseases		
Globoid cell leukodystrophy	AR	Demyelinating
Metachromatic leukodystrophy	AR	Demyelinating
Fabry disease	X-linked	Axonal
Sphingomyelin Lipidoses		
Niemann–Pick disease type C	AR	Demyelinating
Farber disease (lipogranulomatosis)	AR	Demyelinating
Porphyrias		
Acute intermittent porphyria	AD	Axonal
Hereditary coproporphyria	AD	Axonal
Variegate porphyria	AD	Axonal
Familial Amyloid Polyneuropathies (FAPs)		
FAP I and II (transthyretin-related)	AD	Axonal or demyelinating
FAP III (apolipoprotein A1-related)	AD	Axonal
FAP IV (gelsolin-related)	AD	Axonal
Disorders With Defective DNA Synthesis or Repair		
Ataxia telangiectasia	AR	Axonal
Cockayne syndrome	AR	Demyelinating
Neuropathies Associated With Spinocerebellar Ataxias		
Friedreich ataxia, other SCAs	AR	Axonal
Neuroacanthocytosis	X-linked	Axonal
Other Inherited Neuropathies		
Hereditary neuralgic amyotrophy	AD	Axonal
Giant axonal neuropathy	AD	Axonal
Infantile neuroaxonal dystrophy	AR	Axonal
Andermann syndrome	AR	Axonal

AD, Autosomal-dominant; *AR,* autosomal-recessive; *CMT,* Charcot-Marie-Tooth disease; *MNGIE,* mitochondrial neurogastrointestinal encephalopathy; *NARP,* neuropathy, ataxia, and retinitis pigmentosa; *SCA,* spinocerebellar ataxia.

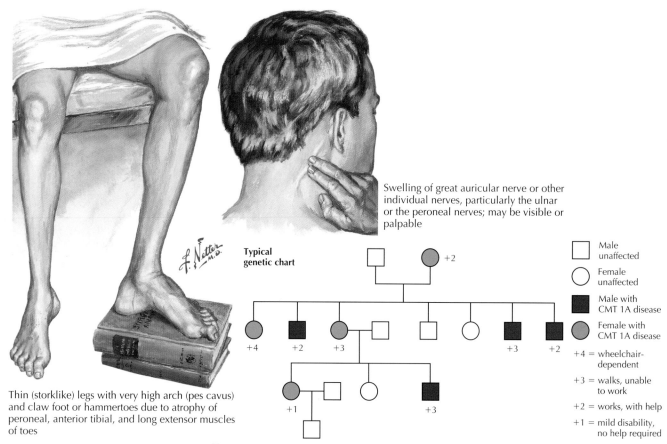

Swelling of great auricular nerve or other individual nerves, particularly the ulnar or the peroneal nerves; may be visible or palpable

Typical genetic chart

Male unaffected

Female unaffected

Male with CMT 1A disease

Female with CMT 1A disease

+4 = wheelchair-dependent

+3 = walks, unable to work

+2 = works, with help

+1 = mild disability, no help required

Thin (storklike) legs with very high arch (pes cavus) and claw foot or hammertoes due to atrophy of peroneal, anterior tibial, and long extensor muscles of toes

Fig. 66.1 Findings in Charcot-Marie-Tooth Disease.

TABLE 66.2	Dominant Demyelinating Forms of Charcot-Marie-Tooth Disease (CMT type 1)			
	% of CMT1	Locus	Gene	Phenotype
CMT1A	60%–70%	17p12	*PMP22 (duplication)*	Classical CMT
CMT1B	10%–15%	1q23.3	*MPZ*	Classical CMT Infantile-onset/DSD Adult-onset
CMT1C	1%–2%	16p13.13	*LITAF/SIMPLE*	Classical CMT
CMT1D	<1%	10q21.3	*EGR2*	Classical CMT Infantile-onset/DSD
CMT1E	1%–2%	17p12	*PMP22* (point mutations)	Associated with deafness Infantile-onset/DSD
CMT1F	<1%	8p21	*NEFL*	Infantile onset/DSD Allelic with CMT2E (axonal, adult-onset)
Roussy-Levy			*MPZ* *PMP22*	CMT1A plus tremor

"Classical CMT" phenotype: onset in first or second decade, normal onset of walking (<15 months); *"Infantile-onset" phenotype:* delayed walking (>15 months), ambulation aids by age 20 years; *"Adult-onset" phenotype:* late onset of leg weakness/sensory loss (often >40 years); *DSS,* Dejerine-Sotas syndrome; *EGR2,* early growth response 2; *LITAF,* lipopolysaccharide-induced tumor necrosis factor alpha; *MPZ,* myelin protein zero; *NEFL,* neurofilament light chain.

may have pes cavus or slow motor conduction, indicating an undiagnosed CMT. The term Roussy-Levy syndrome is applied to those CMT1A patients who have postural tremor. A small minority of CMT1A cases present as Dejerine-Sottas syndrome (DSS), a severe "infantile" phenotype with extreme conduction slowing (MCV < 15 m/s). CMT1A is caused

by duplication of the peripheral protein 22 gene *(PMP22)* on chromosome 17. Interestingly, a heterozygous deletion of the same region causes HNPP, further discussed later. A fraction of CMT1 cases—CMT1E—is caused by point mutations in the *PMP22* gene and can have a severe DSS phenotype. Of the genes associated with CMT1, myelin protein zero *(MPZ)* is the second most common (10%–15% of CMT1s). *MPZ* mutations are associated with a range of phenotypes, from the most severe infantile type (DSS), to classical CMT and milder adult-onset cases with borderline conduction slowing. The remaining CMT1 subtypes are exceedingly rare.

Charcot-Marie-Tooth Type 2

CMT2—the "axonal" dominant form of CMT—is about half as common as CMT1 (Table 66.3). Electrodiagnostic testing is necessary to distinguish CMT2 from CMT1 because the clinical presentation is often similar. In general, however, CMT2 patients are less likely than those with CMT1 to be globally areflexic and they tend to present later in life. In CMT2, nerve conduction studies show normal or near normal motor velocities (>38 m/s) with reduced sensory and motor amplitudes. Unlike CMT1, the number of disease genes for CMT2 is large, all of which are very rare. CMT2A—the most common subtype responsible for 20%–30% of CMT2 cases—is caused by mutation in mitochondrial fusion protein, mitofusin-2 (MFN2). Mutations in MFN2 can be associated with severe early-life weakness, optic atrophy, and/or hearing loss, but it can cause the classical CMT phenotype in other patients. Some of the other CMT2 forms can be associated with vocal cord paralysis (TRPV4), motor deficits in the hands, GARS, or severe sensory loss with mutilating arthropathy RAB7.

Charcot-Marie-Tooth-X

CMT-X1 is the second most common form of CMT, representing 10%–15% of all cases (Table 66.4). Other subtypes of X-linked CMT exist but are exceedingly rare. CMT-X1 is caused by missense mutations in connexin-32 (CX32), also known as the gap-junction beta 1 (GJB1) gene. As in most X-linked diseases, men tend to be affected more severely than women, although one-third of women present similarly to their male counterparts. Typical onset is in the teenage years or early adulthood. As the disease progresses, pronounced atrophy in distal calves and intrinsic hand muscles becomes apparent. Some patients may develop hearing loss, tremor, and CNS pathology marked by white matter and corpus callosum lesions precipitated by exertion or high altitude. Conduction velocities typically fall within the intermediate range (30–45 m/s). Unlike in CMT1, conduction abnormalities can be nonuniform and asymmetric, in some cases producing temporal dispersion and conduction block, mimicking chronic inflammatory demyelinating polyradiculoneuropathy (CIDP).

Hereditary Neuropathy With Liability to Pressure Palsies (HNPP)

> **CLINICAL VIGNETTE** *A 16-year-old boy had broken his right humerus playing soccer and was casted for the entire season. Having to use his left arm to carry a heavy backpack to school, he noted occasional difficulty putting books on high shelves. He noticed similar weakness after rowing 5 miles. He had no pain or numbness. Exam revealed weakness and atrophy of the left deltoid, biceps, supraspinatus, and infraspinatus. The boy's mother had a history of carpal tunnel syndrome and absent ankle reflexes. His maternal uncle was said to have had "neuropathy" since his 20s. Nerve conduction study surprisingly demonstrated evidence of carpal tunnel syndrome in both of the boy's hands as well as slowing of ulnar motor conduction velocity across the elbow. Needle electromyography showed features of denervation and reinnervation in the left infraspinatus and to a lesser degree in the deltoid. Genetic analysis revealed a PMP22 deletion, confirming the diagnosis of HNPP.*

TABLE 66.3 Dominant Axonal Forms of Charcot-Marie-Tooth Disease (CMT type 2)

	Frequency	Gene	Phenotype
CMT2A	20%–30% of CMT2	*MFN2*	Prominent distal weakness Optic atrophy
CMT2B	Multiple families	*RAB7*	Ulcero-mutilating
CMT2C	Multiple families	*TRPV4*	Vocal cord paralysis Diaphragmatic involvement
CMT2D	Multiple families	*GARS*	Hand wasting Allelic with dHMN
CMT2E	Multiple families	*NEFL*	Hearing loss Allelic with CMT1F
CMT2F	Multiple families	*HSPB1*	Motor-predominant/dHMN
CMT2I CMT2J	Multiple families	*MPZ*	Hearing loss/pupillary abnormalities Allelic with CMT1B
CMT2K	Multiple families	*GDAP1*	AD or AR Allelic with CMT4A (vocal cord paralysis)
CMT2L	Multiple families	*HSPB8*	Motor-predominant Allelic with dHMN
CMT2M	Multiple families	*DNM2*	Tremor, ophthalmoplegia
CMT2N	Multiple families	*AARS*	Typical CMT2 Allelic with dHMN
CMT2O	Multiple families	*DYNC1H1*	Learning disability
CMT2P	Multiple families	*LRSAM1*	Mild; sensory-predominant
CMT2Q	One family	*DHTKD1*	Typical CMT2
CMT2U	One family One sporadic	*MARS*	Late-onset
CMT2V	One family	*NAGLU*	Late-onset; painful; sensory-predominant
CMT2W	Multiple families	*HARS*	Typical CMT2 Allelic with dHMN
CMT2Y	One family One sporadic	*VCP*	Typical CMT1 Allelic with ALS14, IBMPFD1
CMT2Z	Multiple families	*MORC2*	Pyramidal signs

AARS, Alanyl-tRNA synthetase; *ALS14*, amyotrophic lateral sclerosis familial 14; *dHMN*, distal hereditary motor neuropathy; *DHTKD1*, dehydrogenase E1 and transketolase domain-containing 1; *DNM2*, dynamin-2; *DYNC1H1*, cytoplasmic dynein-1 heavy chain 1; *GARS*, glycyl-tRNA synthetase; *GDAP1*, ganglioside-induced differentiation associated protein 1; *HARS*, histidyl-tRNA synthetase; *HSPB1*, small heat-shock protein 1; *HSPB8*, small heat-shock protein 8; *IBMPFD1*, inclusion body myositis with Paget disease and dementia; *LRSAM1*, leucine-rich repeats and sterile alpha-motif-containing 1; *MARS*, methionyl-tRNA synthetase; *MFN2*, mitofusin 2; *MORC2*, MORC family CW-type zinc finger protein 2; *MPZ*, myelin protein zero; *NAGLU*, α-N-acetyl-glucosaminidase; *NEFL*, neurofilament light chain; *RAB7*, Ras-related GTP-binding protein 7; *TRPV4*, transient receptor potential cation channel subfamily V, member 4; *VCP*, valosin-containing protein.

TABLE 66.4 X-linked Dominant Forms of Charcot-Marie-Tooth Disease

	Frequency	Gene	Phenotype
CMTX1	10%–15% of CMTs	*GJB1*	Patchy demyelinating
			Hearing loss, CNS demyelination
			Intermediate MCV (35–45 m/s)
			$\frac{1}{3} - \frac{1}{2}$ of females are symptomatic
CMTX6	One family	*PDK3*	Typical CMT2

GJB1, Gap-junction beta 1; *MCV*, motor conduction velocity; *PDK3*, pyruvate dehydrogenase kinase.

HNPP is an allelic disorder with CMT1A. Also inherited dominantly, it is caused by deletion of the same segment of the *PMP22* gene that is duplicated in CMT1A. Clinical features are quite unique—HNPP patients present with reversible painless mononeuropathies that are typically precipitated by minor mechanical compression or stretching of the affected nerve. Crossing one's leg or leaning one's arm against a chair, even for a short while, can result in dropped foot or wrist. Naturally, nerves that have areas of physiologic entrapment (median nerve at wrist or ulnar nerve at elbow) or proximity to a bone (radial nerve at spiral groove or peroneal nerve at fibular head) are more susceptible. Some episodes are preceded by vigorous physical exercise. Proximal arm weakness due to involvement of brachial plexus and its proximal branches, as described in the preceding vignette, can be seen after carrying a heavy bag ("rucksack palsy"). Most patients present in their second or third decade, but childhood onset is not uncommon. Sausage-like structures of excessive myelin folding in paranodal regions—tomacula—are the pathologic hallmarks of HNPP. Electrophysiologic studies typically reveal a diffuse mixed demyelinating and axonal polyneuropathy with features of accentuated demyelination (i.e., slowing, temporal dispersion, or conduction block) at sites of physiologic entrapment. After years of recurrent mononeuropathies, each resulting in additional secondary axonal loss, the pattern of mildly asymmetric and length-dependent "confluent" polyneuropathy emerges.

OTHER CHARCOT-MARIE-TOOTH TYPES

CMT3—or DSS—is also known as congenital hypomyelinating neuropathy. It is a severe "infantile" phenotype with very slow nerve conduction velocities (<15 m/s). DSS manifests at birth or in early childhood and affected infants may be hypotonic. As it progresses, many patients are confined to a wheelchair. Historically believed to be recessive in inheritance because of frequently absent family history, most CMT3 cases are in fact caused by dominant but spontaneous mutations in the *PMP22* (duplication or missense), *MPZ*, *EGR2*, or *SIMPLE/LITAF* genes.

CMT4 encompasses autosomal recessive neuropathies and includes both demyelinating and axonal forms. These neuropathies are rare and usually severe, with childhood onset, and should be considered in the context of consanguinity. Additional features such as vocal cord paralysis, diaphragmatic weakness, and deafness occur in some.

Related to the CMTs are the HSANs, with prominent sensory and autonomic manifestations, and dHMNs. The most common HSAN is caused by mutations in the serine palmitoyltransferase long chain base 1 gene *(SPTLC1)*. Inherited dominantly, the onset is typically in the second to fourth decade, and loss of small fiber–mediated sensation dominates the clinical picture. Weakness and pes cavus can be seen in some patients. Distal HMNs, as the name suggests, are length-dependent purely motor axonal syndromes that are sometimes described as distal spinal muscular atrophies (dSMAs). Considerable genetic and clinical overlap exists between dHMNs and axonal CMTs (CMT2), as mutations in several genes are capable of producing either phenotype. The fact that some dHMNs have minor sensory deficits further underscores this overlap, suggesting that gene-based diagnosis is preferable to the often confusing semantics of classification based on clinical features.

HEREDITARY NEURALGIC AMYOTROPHY (HNA)

Hereditary neuralgic amyotrophy (HNA), also known as hereditary brachial plexopathy, is an autosomal dominant disorder caused by mutation in the *SEPT9* gene on chromosome 17. It presents with pain, weakness, and atrophy in the distribution of the brachial plexus in a patchy pattern similar to the much more common idiopathic brachial plexitis (Parsonage-Turner syndrome). Although recovery is expected, recurrent attacks affecting both sides ultimately lead to some residual permanent weakness. Unlike the idiopathic form, HNA can be associated with dysmorphic features such as hypotelorism, epicanthal folds, or cleft palate.

Another scenario affects a subset of patients with HNPP, children and teenagers in particular, who present with brachial plexopathy or proximal arm mononeuropathy. Unlike HNA, attacks associated with HNPP are usually painless.

FAMILIAL AMYLOID POLYNEUROPATHY (FAP)

Mutations in the transthyretin *(TTR)* gene are responsible for the majority of FAP cases. Early diagnosis is important, since multiple new therapies are now being developed for this otherwise progressive and ultimately fatal disorder. Patients typically present in the third or fourth decade of life with insidious small fiber–predominant sensory neuropathy and autonomic failure. Ultimately deposition of amyloid in the heart leads to death from cardiac failure due to hypertrophic cardiomyopathy. Milder forms of TTR-FAP exist, presenting with carpal tunnel syndrome, mild sensory neuropathy, and mild if any autonomic failure. Careful attention to "red flags" in all polyneuropathy patients is needed to avoid misdiagnosis; TTR-FAP should be suspected if polyneuropathy occurs in the context of a positive family history, systemic involvement (cardiac, gastrointestinal, and renal), autonomic failure, or weight loss. Importantly, TTR-FAP can mimic CIDP with demyelinating electrophysiology, sensorimotor deficits, areflexia, and high CSF protein; it should thus be considered in any CIDP patient who has not responded to adequate immunotherapy. The diagnosis is done by tissue biopsy and/or TTR gene testing. Biopsy typically demonstrates amyloid deposits but is normal in many patients due to patchy involvement. TTR gene testing is therefore warranted if the suspicion is strong. Because the liver produces much of the body's TTR, liver transplant has been used to treat TTR-FAP. A number of exciting and less invasive treatments have recently been studied, such as TTR stabilizers (diflunisal, tafamidis) and gene-modifying approaches including antisense oligonucleotides (inotersen) and small interfering RNAs (patisiran).

Much rarer forms of FAP are associated with mutations in the genes for apolipoprotein 1 and gelsolin. Gelsolin-linked FAP manifests with unique combination of lattice corneal dystrophy, lower cranial neuropathies (CN VII), and abnormally loose skin.

OTHER INHERITED POLYNEUROPATHIES

Of the long list of other hereditary neuropathies (see Table 66.1), only a few can be treated. Lysosomal storage disorders are due to mutations causing enzymatic defects that lead to abnormal accumulations of lysosomal products (sphingolipids, mucolipids, etc.) in neurons. Although CNS manifestations typically dominate, peripheral neuropathy is an important feature in some patients. Fabry disease deserves attention because enzyme replacement therapy (ERT) with recombinant alpha-galactosidase A is available. This X-linked disease typically manifests in young males with lancinating, painful neuropathy in the hands and feet and angiokeratomas. Most morbidity is derived from accumulation of abnormal sphingolipid in vessels, ultimately leading to renal failure and stroke.

Adrenomyeloneuropathy (AMN) and adrenoleukodystrophy are allelic X-linked diseases typically affecting young males and less often manifesting in female carriers. Although this is primarily a CNS leukodystrophy, sensorimotor polyneuropathy, sometimes demyelinating, is also seen in AMN. Bone marrow transplantation has been proposed to treat some patients.

Attacks of acute motor neuropathy in combination with abdominal pain, psychosis, and dysautonomia raise the possibility of porphyria. Attacks are precipitated by drugs and by dietary or hormonal changes. The diagnosis requires demonstration of increased excretion of heme precursors (e.g., porphobilinogen, δ-aminolevulinic acid) in urine or stool and can be confirmed by DNA testing.

DIFFERENTIAL DIAGNOSIS

Hereditary neuropathy from CMT spectrum is distinguished from an acquired process by insidious history often starting in childhood, slowly progressive course, foot deformities, and symmetric weakness without positive sensory phenomena. Patients with acquired neuropathy tend to have a shorter history with well-defined onset and more prominent and often positive sensory symptoms. Severe electrophysiologic abnormalities in a patient with relatively minor symptoms provide a clue that one is dealing with a long-standing, perhaps congenital neuropathy such as CMT. Distal myopathies are exceedingly rare but may be mistaken for CMT; sensory exam and electrodiagnostic studies differentiate the two conditions.

Diagnostic Approach

The diagnosis of inherited neuropathies begins with determining the mode of inheritance and underlying neurophysiology, followed by genetic analysis. Although the number of CMT genes is large and ever-expanding, it is worth remembering that more than half of the cases have one of five genetic mutations (PMP22 duplication, PMP22 point mutation, GJB1, MFN2, and MPZ) (see Tables 66.2–66.4).

A careful family history is critical in determining the inheritance pattern. It is often negative, either because the mutation is sporadic or because mildly affected relatives have escaped clinical attention. It is helpful to remember that no male-to-male transmission should be seen in X-linked diseases and that individuals with recessively inherited disease often have asymptomatic parents. Recessive neuropathies are more likely to be seen in populations in which consanguinity is common.

Nerve conduction studies assist in differentiating demyelinating from axonal processes (Fig. 66.2). Demyelinating disorders will demonstrate slowing of conduction velocities, whereas axonal sensorimotor neuropathies will have decreased amplitudes of both motor and sensory action potentials. Because secondary axon loss is common and occurs in length-dependent fashion, motor conduction velocity from a proximal nerve such as forearm segment of the ulnar nerve is more reliable. Uniform slowing is a hallmark of hereditary demyelinating neuropathy, and nonuniform patchy involvement with temporal dispersion and conduction block is characteristically seen in acquired demyelinating neuropathies such as CIDP. Notable exceptions to this rule include HNPP and sometimes CMT-X1.

Several algorithms have been proposed to guide the selection of genetic tests in diagnosing hereditary neuropathies. Although the advent of next-generation sequencing (NCS), may ultimately render such selective approaches unnecessary, it is still clinically useful for the conceptualization of different CMT categories.

Most algorithms are based on a combination of the patient's phenotype, mode of inheritance, and motor conduction velocity. The majority of CMTs fall into one of three phenotypes: (1) children with the classical phenotype walk at a normal age (at 12–15 months) and their neuropathy manifests within the first two decades; (2) the severe infantile-onset phenotype with delayed walking (>15 months), often requiring ambulation aids by 20 years of age; and (3) the adult-onset phenotype, often after age 40.

Approach to Genetic Testing

1. If a patient has ulnar motor conduction velocity between 15 and 35 m/s and began walking before 15 months of age (classical phenotype), CMT1A with PMP22 duplication is confirmed in the majority of cases. Based on the prevalence of CMT1A, this step should identify nearly half of all CMT patients. The GJB1 and MPZ genes, responsible for CMT-X1 and CMT1B, respectively, account for a small fraction of this group of CMT patients.
2. In patients with intermediate motor conduction velocities (35–45 m/s), GJB1 (CMT-X1) should be assayed first if the inheritance is X-linked and if the patient became symptomatic in the first two decades of life (classical phenotype); in contrast, the MPZ gene (CMT1B) is more likely to be abnormal if the patient presented as an adult.
3. Patients with very slow conduction velocities (<15 m/s) usually present with the severe infantile-onset phenotype and do not walk before 15 months of age. PMP22 duplication (CMT1A), PMP22 point mutation (CMT1E), and MPZ gene defects (CMT1B) are the most often encountered genetic abnormalities in this group.
4. Patients with axonal neuropathy and normal motor conduction velocities (>45 m/s) should be tested for MFN2—the most common form of axonal CMT (CMT2A). Rarely, CMT-X1 and CMT2B due to an MPZ mutation may have normal conduction velocities.

Management and Therapy

There is currently no disease-modifying therapy for CMT. Management is supportive, aimed at maintaining or improving the patient's quality of life. The main cause of morbidity in these patients is related to progressively limited mobility, gait disorder, and the development of contractures.

A carefully designed rehabilitation program can be helpful in preventing joint deformities and falls. Daily stretching exercises, serial casting, and night splints may help to delay ankle contractures. Orthotics, such as ankle-foot orthoses, improve gait by stabilizing the ankles. Orthopedic surgery can be beneficial for severe pes cavus and hammer toe deformity. Soft tissue procedures such as tendon transfers, rebalancing operations, and plantar fascial releases may be required. Osteotomies and arthrodeses may be considered in suitable patients.

CMT patients can develop additional diseases that further threaten peripheral nerves. Careful attention is therefore required to address conditions such as diabetes mellitus, vitamin deficiencies, paraproteinemia, and alcoholism. Exposure of CMT patients to neurotoxins is of particular concern. The peripheral nerves of CMT patients are susceptible to neurotoxic medications such as vincristine or cisplatin. These agents can exacerbate preexisting neuropathy at doses that would be considered nontoxic in patients without CMT. Acute neuropathy after administration of vincristine or another neurotoxic medication can be the first manifestation of yet undiagnosed CMT1A. Other medications that have to be used with caution in CMT patients include colchicine, paclitaxel, thalidomide, and amiodarone.

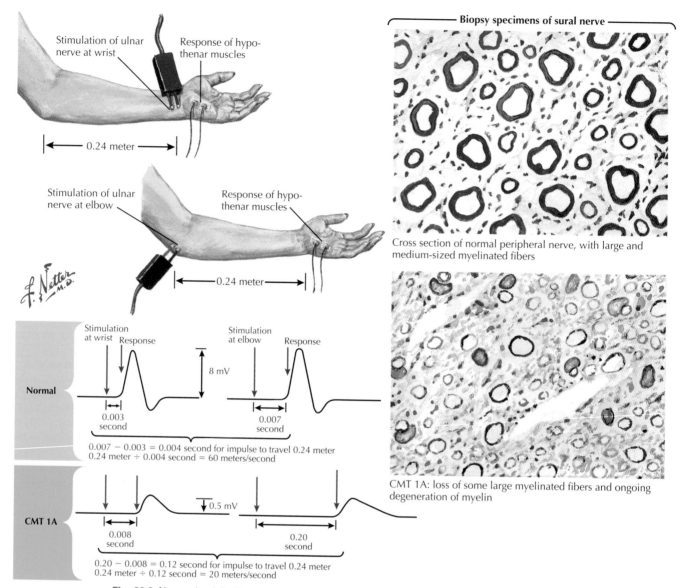

Biopsy specimens of sural nerve

Cross section of normal peripheral nerve, with large and medium-sized myelinated fibers

CMT 1A: loss of some large myelinated fibers and ongoing degeneration of myelin

Stimulation of ulnar nerve at wrist

Response of hypothenar muscles

0.24 meter

Stimulation of ulnar nerve at elbow

Response of hypothenar muscles

0.24 meter

Normal

Stimulation at wrist   Response

Stimulation at elbow   Response

8 mV

0.003 second

0.007 second

0.007 − 0.003 = 0.004 second for impulse to travel 0.24 meter
0.24 meter ÷ 0.004 second = 60 meters/second

CMT 1A

0.5 mV

0.008 second

0.20 second

0.20 − 0.008 = 0.12 second for impulse to travel 0.24 meter
0.24 meter ÷ 0.12 second = 20 meters/second

Fig. 66.2 Neurophysiologic and Pathologic Findings in Type IA Charcot-Marie-Tooth Disease.

ADDITIONAL RESOURCES

Saporta ASD, Sottile SL, Miller LJ, et al. Charcot Marie Tooth (CMT) subtypes and genetic testing strategies. Ann Neurol 2011;69(1): 22–33.

Based on the analysis of clinical, electrodiagnostic, and genetic data from more than 1000 of their CMT patients, the authors determine the frequencies of CMT subtypes and propose cost-effective strategies to guide a parsimonious selection of genetic tests.

Rossor A, Kalmar B, Greensmith L, et al. The distal hereditary motor neuropathies. J Neurol Neurosurg Psychiatry 2012;83:6–14.

The authors provide a review of clinical features of dHMN subtypes to help focus genetic testing for practicing clinician.

Siskind C, et al. A review of genetic counseling for Charcot Marie Tooth disease (CMT). J Genet Counsel 2013;22:422–36.

A comprehensive review of the classification of CMT disease, its clinical features, and molecular genetic testing as well as issues pertaining to genetic counseling.

Rossor AM, Tomaselli PJ, Reilly MM. Recent advances in the genetic neuropathies. Curr Opin Neurol 2016;29(5):537–48.

An update on recent advances in our understanding of CMT genetics and pathogenesis as well as their implications for developing rational therapies.

Plante-Bordeneuve V. Thansthyretin familial amyloid polyneuropathy: an update. J Neurol 2018;265(4):976–83.

A review focused on recent developments in the diagnosis and treatment of TTR-related familial amyloid polyneuropathy.

67

Acquired Polyneuropathies

Michal Vytopil, Ted M. Burns, Michelle Mauermann, Jayashri Srinivasan

DIAGNOSTIC APPROACH

CLINICAL VIGNETTE *A 65-year-old man developed a tingling sensation in the toes, which quickly gave way to painful numbness. Over the next few months, paresthesias ascended to involve his distal thighs and fingertips. Within 6 months, he required a walker to ambulate because of leg weakness. During the review of systems, he commented on the fogginess of vision and light-headedness that he experiences upon standing. He had fainted at least twice, and this was attributed to a newly diagnosed cardiomyopathy. Difficulty passing urine in the previous 2 months led to the placement of a urinary catheter. Prior to this problem the patient had enjoyed good health except for an IgG kappa monoclonal gammopathy of unknown significance (MGUS), which was regularly monitored. Neurologic examination demonstrated diffuse atrophy of the posterior shoulders as well as the hands and thighs. Distal bulk could not be assessed due to edema. Leg weakness was moderate and predominantly distal. Thenar muscles in both hands were atrophic and weak, and the patient was areflexic. Sensation was absent to all modalities up to the distal thighs and also in the median nerve distribution of the hands. Laboratory work demonstrated proteinuria. Nerve conduction study revealed severe length-dependent sensorimotor polyneuropathy, chiefly axonal but with some borderline motor conduction velocities (33 m/s) in the peroneal nerve, which raised the possibility of a demyelinating component. In addition, bilateral carpal tunnel syndrome was demonstrated. Primary amyloidosis with sensorimotor and autonomic neuropathy was strongly suspected. Abdominal fat pad aspiration revealed characteristic amyloid deposits around blood vessels.*

Evaluation of the etiology of a patient's polyneuropathy can be challenging for many reasons, including the fact that there are more than 100 potential etiologies. Ultimately the polyneuropathy is determined to be acquired (i.e., caused by some other disease or exposure) in one-third of cases (Box 67.1), inherited in another one-third, and idiopathic in the remaining one-third. In order to focus on a smaller list of potential etiologies so that the evaluation can be simplified, we believe that it is best for the clinician to first characterize the polyneuropathy. This chapter presents a method for characterizing neuropathy that is easy to remember, based on four simple clinical questions about the neuropathy and the patient: "What?" "Where?" "When?" and in "What setting?"

What?

"What?" refers to what nerve fiber modalities (motor, sensory, autonomic, or a combination) are involved. The identification of sensory nerve involvement, at a minimum, allows the clinician to exclude other neuromuscular diseases not associated with sensory dysfunction, such as disorders of anterior horn cells (e.g., amyotrophic lateral sclerosis), neuromuscular transmission (e.g., myasthenia gravis), or of muscle (myopathy). When sensory symptoms and signs are present, it is useful to characterize neuropathic sensory symptoms into "positive" or "negative" because acquired neuropathies are usually accompanied by positive neuropathic sensory symptoms and inherited neuropathies are usually not. Positive sensory symptoms may be painful (e.g., "burning," "freezing," or "shooting"), usually indicating involvement of small fibers, or symptoms may be painless (e.g., "tingling" or "swelling"). The presence of pain can be a very helpful in differentiating features because it limits the list of possible etiologies (Box 67.2). Positive sensory symptoms and pain are common complaints for patients with diabetic, vasculitic, or alcoholic neuropathy or those with Guillain-Barré syndrome (GBS). Exaggerated discomfort to painful stimuli (hyperalgesia) and to nonpainful stimuli (allodynia) can occur. Painless symptoms, both negative ("numbness," "woodiness") and positive ("socks bunched up under one's feet," "swelling"), are more common in patients with large-fiber involvement. Sensory ataxia from loss of proprioceptive large sensory fibers is another of the negative neuropathic sensory symptoms; patients report imbalance in the dark or after they close their eyes in the shower.

Identification of autonomic nerve involvement can be an important clue because only a small number of neuropathic processes affect both autonomic and somatic nerves (e.g., GBS, paraneoplastic neuropathy, diabetic neuropathy, amyloid neuropathy) (Box 67.3). Autonomic symptoms include light-headedness, syncope, diarrhea, constipation, postprandial bloating, early satiety, urinary complaints, erectile dysfunction, abnormal or absent sweating, and dry mouth and eyes (Fig. 67.1). In the foregoing vignette, our patient's symptoms of burning numbness as well as dysautonomia suggested early involvement of small unmyelinated sensory and autonomic fibers, a pattern commonly seen in neuropathy associated with amyloidosis.

Where?

"Where?" refers to the distribution of nerve damage. An important diagnostic watershed is the determination of whether the process is "length-dependent" (e.g., distal) or not. Length-dependent neuropathies manifest first in the feet and are symmetric. Non–length-dependent neuropathies are not necessarily evident initially in the feet and may be asymmetric, focal, or multifocal. The etiology of length-dependent neuropathies is usually inherited, metabolic/toxic, or idiopathic, whereas a neuropathy that is not length-dependent is often caused by an immune-mediated or infectious process. Some examples of non–length-dependent neuropathies are polyradiculoneuropathies (e.g., GBS), plexopathies (often inflammatory), sensory ganglionopathy (e.g., paraneoplastic subacute sensory neuronopathy in the setting of small-cell lung cancer),

BOX 67.1 Systemic Conditions Associated With Neuropathy

- Diabetes mellitus and impaired glucose tolerance
- Toxins (alcohol, medications, chemotherapeutic agents, heavy metals)
- Metabolic syndrome (obesity, hypertriglyceridemia)
- Nutritional deficiencies (B12, B1, B6, copper)
- Vitamin excess (B6)
- Connective tissue diseases
- Paraproteinemia
- Vasculitis
- Amyloidosis
- Critical illness
- Uremia
- Infection (HIV, Leprosy, VZV, Lyme)
- Malignancy/paraneoplasia
- Sarcoidosis

HIV, Human immunodeficiency virus; *VZV,* varicella zoster virus.

BOX 67.2 Painful Polyneuropathies

Small-Fiber Neuropathy or Length-Dependent Polyneuropathy Pattern

- Diabetes and impaired glucose tolerance
- Metabolic syndrome (obesity and dyslipidemia)
- Alcohol
- Other toxins (including chemotherapeutic agents)
- B-vitamin deficiencies: thiamine, B_{12}, B_6,
- Sjögren syndrome and other connective tissue diseases (length- and non–length dependent)
- Amyloidosis—primary systemic, and inherited
- Hepatitis C and cryoglobulinemia
- HIV neuropathy
- Hereditary (Hereditary sensory neuropathy, Fabry, Tangier)

Multifocal Neuropathy or Length-Dependent Polyneuropathy Pattern

- Vasculitis (25%–30% of cases present as LDPN, multiple mononeuropathy more typical)
- Diabetes mellitus
- Infection (leprosy, Lyme, VZV)
- Infiltrative process (malignancy, sarcoidosis, amyloidosis)
- Lewis-Sumner syndrome (MADSAM)

Polyradiculoneuropathy Pattern

- Guillain-Barré syndrome
- Infiltrative process (malignancy, sarcoidosis)
- Infection (Lyme, VZV, CMV, EBV)

CMV, Cytomegalovirus; *EBV,* Epstein-Barr virus; *HIV,* human immunodeficiency virus; *LDPN,* length-dependent polyneuropathy; *MADSAM,* multifocal acquired demyelinating sensory and motor; *MM,* mononeuritis multiplex; *SN,* sensory neuronopathy; *VZV,* varicella zoster virus.

and multifocal mononeuropathies (e.g., mononeuritis multiplex caused by vasculitis). Our vignette's patient had a combination of two patterns; length-dependent polyneuropathy and focal median neuropathies at the wrist (carpal tunnel syndrome), both produced by infiltration of amyloid fibrils.

BOX 67.3 Polyneuropathies With Autonomic Nervous System Involvement

Length-Dependent Polyneuropathy Pattern

- Diabetes mellitus
- Amyloidosis (hereditary or primary)
- Toxins (chemotherapeutic agents, heavy metals)
- Immune-mediated (Sjögren syndrome, connective tissue disease)
- Immune-mediated/paraneoplasia
- Hereditary sensory and autonomic neuropathies
- HIV-related polyneuropathy

Polyradiculoneuropathy Pattern

- Guillain-Barré syndrome
- Porphyria

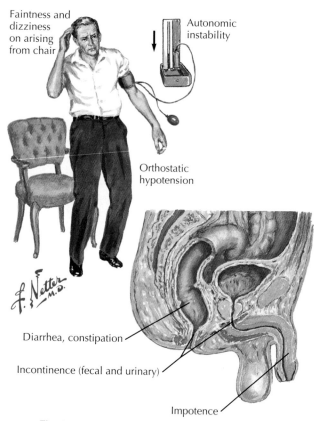

Fig. 67.1 Dysautonomia With Polyneuropathies.

When?

"When?" refers to the temporal evolution of the neuropathy. Because of confusion over what is meant by "acute," "subacute," and "chronic," it is often best to describe symptom onset based on whether or not the neuropathic symptoms had a compelling, definite date of onset. A definite date of symptom onset almost always indicates an acute or subacute onset typical of an immune-mediated or infectious etiology. A less exact date of onset suggests gradual or insidious onset, indicative of inherited, idiopathic, or toxic/metabolic etiologies. The pace of progression following symptom onset is also an important consideration. Symptom onset and pace of progression often correlate in a predictable manner, owing largely to the underlying mechanism. As an example, mononeuritis multiplex caused by systemic vasculitis typically presents with a series of painful mononeuropathies of acute onset, occurring one after the other with the rapid development of significant morbidity. In our patient, on the other hand, the onset was less well defined but the pace of progression was relatively rapid, rendering the patient significantly disabled within several short months. This tempo is too fast for diabetic or inherited neuropathies and too slow for an infectious etiology. It is, however, quite consistent with an immune-mediated or infiltrative process.

What Setting?

"What setting?" refers to an elaboration of the unique clinical circumstance of the individual patient. This is done by determining what in the patient's past medical history, medication list, social history, family history, and the review of systems may be relevant (Fig. 67.2). An understanding of the significance of these clinical factors requires knowledge of the risk factors of neuropathy and of the clinical features of the diseases that may be risk factors for neuropathy. For example, unexplained weight loss raises concern for vasculitis or malignancy (e.g., small-cell lung cancer), both of which cause an immune-mediated neuropathy. The neuropathy secondary to malignancy (e.g., paraneoplastic neuropathy) usually presents differently than vasculitic neuropathy, so it is usually not too difficult to differentiate these two etiologies (Fig. 67.3). A clinical setting of known diabetes mellitus or known kidney disease would elevate those comorbidities on the differential diagnosis. Heavy metal poisoning or other intoxication, although rare, must be considered in the patient with systemic symptoms (e.g., nausea, vomiting) and other manifestations suspicious for poisoning (Fig. 67.4). As in the case of our vignette, known IgG kappa monoclonal gammopathy of unknown significance (MGUS) was an important clue alerting the examiner to the possibility of a neuropathy related to paraproteinemia.

Electrodiagnosis

The fifth step in characterization requires nerve conduction studies (NCSs) and electromyography (EMG). NCS and EMG can contribute to (or rarely refute) the clinical characterization in terms of "what" and "where," as well as provide another view of the temporal evolution ("when"). NCS and EMG can also characterize the neuropathy as being primarily axonal or demyelinating. Neuropathies with axonal injury

are far more common than those with demyelination, but identification of demyelinating features is very important because acquired demyelinating polyneuropathies (e.g., GBS, CIDP, MMN) are often immune-mediated and treatable (Box 67.4). However, our historical concept of dividing neuropathies into disorders of myelin or axon may be too simplistic. It is now recognized that in some immune-mediated neuropathies, the primary targets are proteins and ion channels in the region of the node of Ranvier (Fig. 67.5). Acute motor axonal neuropathy (AMAN), the axonal motor variant of GBS, is the prototypic *nodopathy*; antibodies against GM1 ganglioside—an axolemmal nodal antigen—lead to disruption of sodium channels. The ultimate outcome can be a spectrum ranging from fully reversible conduction failure to irreversible axonal degeneration.

CLINICAL VIGNETTE *A 65-year-old woman reported a 10-month history of painful burning in her toes, particularly at night when her feet came into contact with the bed sheets. She had no symptoms in her hands or face, nor did she have indications of dysautonomia or systemic illness. She was not aware of any weakness. Her medical history included hypertension and hyperlipidemia, and she was taking a diuretic and a multivitamin. Neurologic findings revealed an overweight woman with a body mass index (BMI) of 36. Muscle stretch reflexes were normal in the arms and diminished but present at the knees and ankles. There was a distal stocking-distribution sensory loss to light touch, pinprick, and temperature, but vibration and proprioception were intact. Nerve conduction study (NCS) and electromyography (EMG) were normal. The patient's laboratory tests showed hypertriglyceridemia and mildly elevated hemoglobin A1c (5.7%). Punch skin biopsy with measurement of epidermal nerve fibers was abnormal at the distal side; density at the ankle was 2/1-mm (fifth percentile for gender and age = 3.3), whereas proximal density was normal. She was diagnosed with small-fiber neuropathy (SFN) in the setting of metabolic syndrome. She was referred to medical weight-loss clinic and educated about the benefits of regular aerobic exercise and a low-fat diet.*

Comment: The symmetric pattern of painful burning in the feet with intact reflexes, strength, and normal sensation of large-fiber sensory modalities is consistent with SFN. Many of these conditions are seen in association with prediabetes and other components of metabolic syndrome, mainly obesity and dyslipidemia.

Etiology

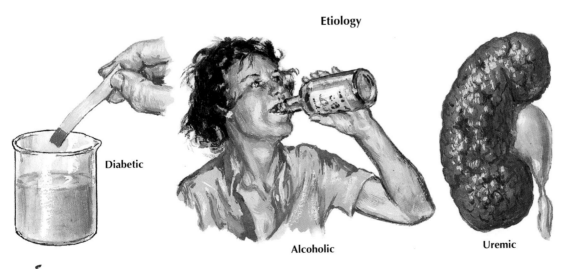
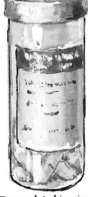

Diabetic — Alcoholic — Uremic — **Drug-related** isoniazid, disulfiram, vincristine, hydralazine, other medications

Fig. 67.2 Peripheral Neuropathies: Metabolic, Toxic, and Nutritional Etiology.

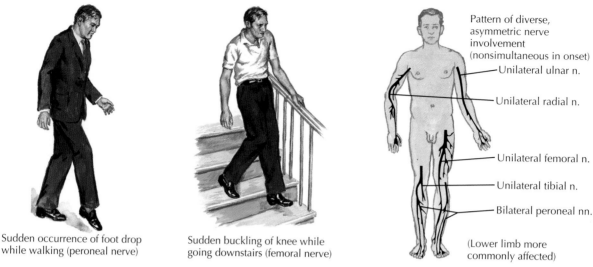

Sudden occurrence of foot drop while walking (peroneal nerve)

Sudden buckling of knee while going downstairs (femoral nerve)

Pattern of diverse, asymmetric nerve involvement (nonsimultaneous in onset)
- Unilateral ulnar n.
- Unilateral radial n.
- Unilateral femoral n.
- Unilateral tibial n.
- Bilateral peroneal nn.

(Lower limb more commonly affected)

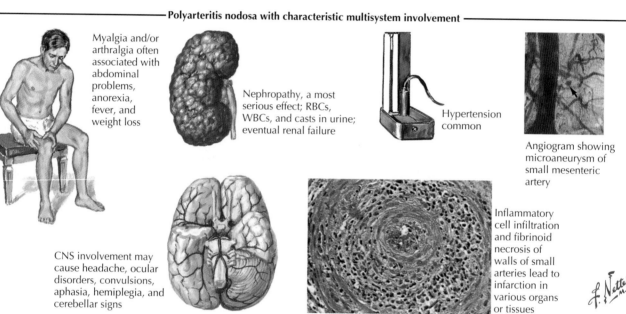

Polyarteritis nodosa with characteristic multisystem involvement

Myalgia and/or arthralgia often associated with abdominal problems, anorexia, fever, and weight loss

Nephropathy, a most serious effect; RBCs, WBCs, and casts in urine; eventual renal failure

Hypertension common

Angiogram showing microaneurysm of small mesenteric artery

Inflammatory cell infiltration and fibrinoid necrosis of walls of small arteries lead to infarction in various organs or tissues

CNS involvement may cause headache, ocular disorders, convulsions, aphasia, hemiplegia, and cerebellar signs

Fig. 67.3 Mononeuritis Multiplex Due to Systemic Vasculitis.

LENGTH-DEPENDENT POLYNEUROPATHIES

Clinical Presentation

Polyneuropathies are among the most common neurologic disorders; the length-dependent pattern is the most prevalent. Also referred to as distal symmetric polyneuropathies (DSPs), the majority of these are axonal, symmetric, and sensory-predominant. Nutrition and other functions of nerve axons rely on metabolic activity of their cell bodies (dorsal root ganglia or anterior horn cells) and on effective axonal transport. When these mechanisms are disrupted, it is the most distal parts of the longest axons (i.e., in the toes) that become most vulnerable and degenerate, leading to the distal-to-proximal gradient of sensory and motor abnormalities ("dying back"). Demonstration of the length-dependent pattern in a patient with polyneuropathy is among the essential exercises in clinical neurology; in a typical patient, the neuropathy does not reach the fingers until lower extremity symptoms have ascended to the knee level. In advanced cases, the scalp vertex and midline trunk are involved. A similar distal-to-proximal gradient applies to the motor exam and muscle stretch reflexes.

Typical patients with length-dependent polyneuropathies (LDPNs) note tingling, numbness, or pain in their toes and feet. They describe a sense of swelling, feeling as though their socks are bunched up under their feet, or a sensation of having cotton between their toes. Motor involvement is often present on EMG but not clinically. If it is seen clinically, big-toe extensors are the first affected muscles. Ankle muscle stretch reflexes can be absent or diminished.

As in the case of our vignette, dissociation of separate sensory modalities may lend valuable clues. A **small-fiber sensory neuropathy (SFN)** is suggested by burning in the feet of patients with impaired pain and thermal sensation and sparing of vibration and proprioceptive sense. The EMG is characteristically normal. Most SFNs do not have identifiable etiologic mechanisms, but careful evaluation for diabetes, prediabetes, and other components of metabolic syndrome is required (see Box 67.2).

Most but not all **sensory LDPNs** have subclinical motor involvement on EMG. Those that are **pure sensory neuropathies** can be seen in the context of diabetes mellitus, renal disease, vitamin deficiencies, various toxins, Sjögren syndrome, and amyloidosis. Some probably represent a

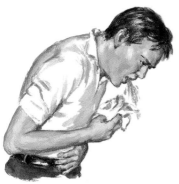

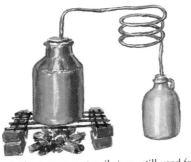

Antique copper utensils (e.g., still used for bootleg liquor) and runoff waste from copper smelting plant may be sources of arsenic poisoning

History of nausea and vomiting may suggest arsenic poisoning in patient with peripheral neuropathy

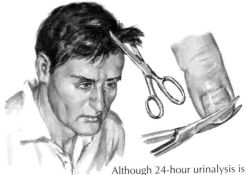

Although 24-hour urinalysis is the best diagnostic test for arsenic, hair and nail analysis may also be helpful

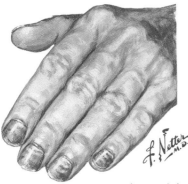

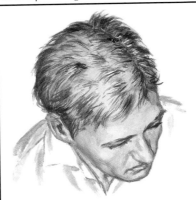

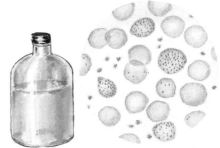

Lead poisoning, now relatively rare, causes baso-philic stippling of red blood cells. 24-hour urinalysis is diagnostic test

Mees lines on fingernails are characteristic of arsenic poisoning

Spotty alopecia associated with peripheral neuropathy characterizes thallium poisoning

Fig. 67.4 Peripheral Neuropathy Caused by Heavy Metal Poisoning.

BOX 67.4 Primary Demyelinating Polyneuropathies

Acquired/Immune-Mediated
- Length-dependent polyneuropathy pattern
  - Anti-MAG neuropathy
- Polyradiculoneuropathy pattern
  - Guillain-Barré syndrome/AIDP variant
  - CIDP
  - Diabetes mellitus
  - POEMS syndrome
- Multifocal neuropathy pattern
  - Multifocal motor neuropathy with conduction block (MMN)
  - Multifocal CIDP (Lewis-Sumner syndrome, MADSAM)

Hereditary
- Length-dependent polyneuropathy pattern
  - Charcot-Marie-Tooth disease (types 1, 3, and 4)
  - Metachromatic leukodystrophy
  - Globoid cell leukodystrophy
- Multifocal pattern
  - Hereditary neuropathy with liability to pressure palsy
  - CMTX

AIDP, Acute inflammatory demyelinating polyradiculoneuropathy; *CIDP,* chronic inflammatory demyelinating polyradiculoneuropathy; *CMT,* Charcot-Marie-Tooth disease; *CMTX,* X-linked CMT; *MADSAM,* multifocal acquired demyelinating sensory and motor neuropathy; *MAG,* myelin associated glycoprotein; *POEMS,* polyneuropathy, organomegaly, endocrinopathy, monoclonal gammopathy, and skin changes.

primary sensory ganglionopathy with distal-predominant presentation. Neuropathic pain and dysautonomia are variably present, depending on the underlying etiology (see Box 67.3).

Motor-predominant LDPNs are primarily genetically determined (i.e., CMT and distal hereditary motor neuropathies [dHMNs]) or, less commonly, immunologically acquired multifocal motor neuropathies presenting in a confluent LDPN-like fashion.

Diagnostic Approach

The differential diagnosis of length-dependent polyneuropathies varies considerably from those that are not length-dependent. In general, non–length-dependent neuropathies, especially those with acute onset and rapid progression, warrant more aggressive testing than typical LDPNs. Approximately 60% of LDPNs have identifiable etiologies; the rest are idiopathic (Box 67.5).

After determining that a neuropathy has an LDPN pattern, the clinician must search for additional clues to the differential diagnosis. Evaluation of a patient's risk-factor profile from personal and family history is important. Diagnosis is often made on an associative basis without absolute proof of causation. Forthright history taking in reference to medications, addictions (including alcohol and tobacco), intravenous (IV) drugs with predilection for hepatitis C and cryoglobulinemia, and occupational or environmental exposure such as glue sniffing or the classic bull's-eye rash of Lyme disease can point to a specific LDPN diagnosis. A thorough physical examination may suggest signs of CMT with pes cavus, Sjögren syndrome with dry eyes and mouth, arsenic poisoning with Mees lines, Raynaud phenomena and purpuric skin eruptions with cryoglobulinemia, pinch purpura with amyloidosis, angiokeratoma in the groin with Fabry disease, and the enlarged yellow-orange tonsils of Tangier disease.

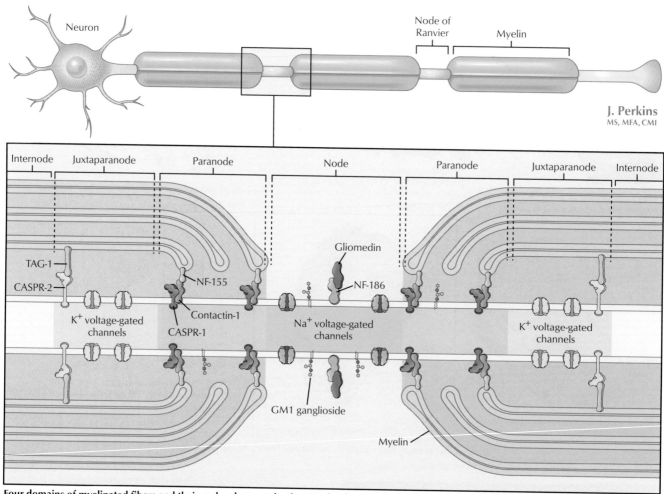

Four domains of myelinated fibers and their molecular organization: *Node of Ranvier* has high density of voltage-gated Na+ channels, the activation of which allows fast "saltatory" propagation of nerve action potential. Na+ channels are anchored to axonal structures and extracellular matrix by Neurofascin-186 (NF-186) and gliomedin complex. Gangliosides such as GM1 are found on nodal and paranodal axonal membrane and can be targets in autoimmune neuropathies such as AMAN. Paranode is surrounded by the loops of uncompacted myelin. Paranodal proteins of the axonal membrane - Contactin-1 and CASPR-1 (Contactin-associated protein-1) - are connected to Neurofascin-155 (NF-155) of paranodal myelin. Septate-like junctions formed by Contactin-1/CASPR-1/NF-155 complex separate nodal Na+ channel clusters from juxtaparanodal K+ channels. Juxtaparanode contains high density of K+ channels. They are anchored by CASPR-2 and TAG-1 (transient axonal glycoprotein-1).

Fig. 67.5 Anatomic Organization of Myelinated Nerve Fibers and Its Subdivisions.

Judicious and targeted use of laboratory testing after exploring these historic and physical findings is encouraged. Premium is placed on identifying treatable etiologies; based on AAN (American Academy of Neurology) guidelines, laboratory testing of all LDPNs should include vitamin B12 (with or without methylmalonic acid), glucose level and serum protein immunofixation. Other features—such as pain, dysautonomia, or systemic disease—can help narrow down the list of etiologies (see Boxes 67.1–67.3).

Electrodiagnostic testing is indicated to confirm the presence of a large-fiber neuropathy, to assess the pattern and severity of the neuropathy, and to distinguish demyelinating from axonal processes. If only small nerve fibers are involved, EMG is normal. Autonomic nervous system testing, quantitative sensory testing, and skin biopsy may be required for diagnostic support. Sural nerve or abdominal fat pad biopsy may be helpful for LDPN patients with suspected amyloidosis, such as those with orthostatic hypotension, where amyloidosis is more likely.

Differential Diagnosis

Acquired metabolic disorders are common causes of LDPN. Diabetes mellitus may produce a number of neuropathic phenotypes, most commonly an LDPN sensory-predominant painful phenotype.

Many potential peripheral **neurotoxins** exist, including alcohol and therapeutic drugs. Chemotherapeutic agents are notorious for causing severe, painful neuropathies. With some medications, neurotoxicity is dose-limiting. Neuropathies resulting from cryptic sources such as heavy metals are uncommon or uncommonly recognized (see Fig. 67.4).

Immune-mediated neuropathies can be associated with monoclonal protein and/or antibodies against peripheral nerve constituents. Monoclonal protein occurs more commonly in patients with polyneuropathy than in age-matched controls without polyneuropathy. However, a precise cause-and-effect relationship is unproven. The strongest association occurs with IgM-κ monoclonal protein with or without the presence of anti–myelin-associated glycoprotein (MAG) antibodies.

Systemic **vasculitis** typically presents as mononeuritis multiplex (MM), but if most lower extremity nerves are involved, the pattern can be indistinguishable from LDPN (confluent MM).

Infection causing LDPN is a rare occurrence; distal symmetric and often painful polyneuropathies are associated with human immunodeficiency virus (HIV) infection or with HIV antiretroviral drug treatments. *Lyme disease* causes polyradiculoneuropathy or mononeuritis multiplex more often than LDPN.

BOX 67.5   Length-Dependent Polyneuropathies

Hereditary
- Charcot-Marie-Tooth disease (hereditary motor sensory neuropathy)
- HSN and HSAN
- DHMN
- FAP
- Mitochondrial disorders

Metabolic
- Diabetes mellitus and impaired glucose tolerance
- Critical illness polyneuropathy
- Celiac disease-associated neuropathy
- Hypothyroidism
- Uremia
- Malnutrition (deficiencies of B12, B1, B6, and others)
- Vitamin excess (B6)

Immune-mediated/Inflammatory
- Primary amyloidosis
- MGUS, including anti-MAG neuropathy
- Connective tissue diseases (including Sjögren syndrome, rheumatoid arthritis, and SLE)
- Sarcoidosis (LDPN most common phenotype, may produce MM, cranial neuropathy, usually occurs in established disease)
- Vasculitis (25%–30% present with LDPN and not with mononeuritis multiplex)
  - Primary (Church-Strauss, polyarteritis nodosa, granulomatosis with polyangiitis)
  - Secondary (connective tissue diseases, drugs, medications, infections)

Idiopathic
Infectious
- HIV
- Lyme disease

Toxic
Alcohol
Pyridoxine (B6) toxicity (sensory neuronopathy mimicking LDPN)
Environmental or industrial exposure
- Arsenic
- Hexacarbons
- Lead
- Mercury
- Organophosphates
- Thallium
Medications
- Chemotherapeutic agents (paclitaxel, thalidomide, vincristine)
- Amphiphilic cationic drugs (amiodarone, chloroquine, perhexiline)
- Colchicine (neuromyopathy)
- Disulfiram
- Hydralazine
- Isoniazid
- Metronidazole
- Nitrofurantoin
- Nitrous oxide
- Nucleosides (ddC, ddI, d4T for AIDS)

AIDS, Acquired immunodeficiency syndrome; *CIDP*, chronic inflammatory demyelinating polyradiculoneuropathy; *CMT*, Charcot-Marie-Tooth neuropathy; *dHMN*, distal hereditary motor neuropathy; *FAP*, familial amyloid polyneuropathy; *GBS*, Guillain-Barré syndrome; *HIV*, human immunodeficiency virus; *HNPP*, hereditary neuropathy with liability to pressure palsy; *HSAN*, hereditary sensory and autonomic neuropathy; *HSN*, hereditary sensory neuropathy; *LDPN*, length-dependent polyneuropathy; *MAG*, myelin-associated glycoprotein; *MGUS*, monoclonal gammopathy of unknown significance; *MM*, mononeuritis multiplex; *MMN*, multifocal motor neuropathy; *SLE*, systemic lupus erythematosus.

Treatment

Specific therapy is available for frustratingly few of these cases. Stabilization or reversal of neuropathy, can occur with treatment of uremia, nutritional deficiencies, and hypothyroidism. Removing neurotoxic drugs may completely reverse mild neuropathies or curtail further progression in more severe cases. A therapeutic trial of prednisone, intravenous immunoglobin (IVIG), or plasmapheresis may have striking results for carefully selected patients with an immune-mediated etiology. Such a trial should be preceded by a careful discussion with the patient about the goals of treatment and specific criteria for its continuation. The importance of diligent foot care to prevent secondary infectious complications of unrecognized wounds, particularly osteomyelitis, cannot be overstated. Medications for neuropathic pain are available and include gabapentin, pregabalin, duloxetine, venlafaxine, and tramadol.

The underlying cause of neuropathy determines the prognosis. Idiopathic sensory-predominant LDPNs usually progress slowly over years and are rarely disabling. In particular, most do not lead to the need for significant ambulatory support or wheelchair, and reassurance by the physician in this regard is often sought by patients and their families.

NEUROPATHIES ASSOCIATED WITH DIABETES

Polyneuropathy is the most common complication associated with diabetes, affecting over 50% of patients during their lifetimes. For an individual patient, diabetic neuropathy often signifies a major reduction in quality of life, particularly if it is associated with pain, gait imbalance, falls, and amputations.

Neuropathy in diabetes is a heterogeneous condition that presents in different forms (Fig. 67.6). Although length-dependent distal symmetric polyneuropathy (DSP) is most common, diabetic neuropathy may occur in proximal as well as distal, large or small, somatic, or autonomic nerve fibers. The classification of diabetic neuropathies that we have found clinically useful is based on the tempo of the disease; chronic forms consist of DSP, small-fiber neuropathy (SFN), and autonomic neuropathy; acute forms include diabetic lumbosacral radiculoplexus neuropathy (DLRPN), treatment-related neuropathy, and diabetic cachexia. The pathogenesis of diabetic neuropathies is far from understood. Multiple pathologic processes are likely at play, including metabolic, microvascular, degenerative, and/or inflammatory. Components of metabolic syndrome other than hyperglycemia—obesity and dyslipidemia in particular—are increasingly recognized as independent factors in the pathogenesis of DSP. Inflammation and microvasculitic changes may be important in some of the acute forms, such as DLRPN.

Distal Symmetric Polyneuropathy (DSP)

The sensory-predominant DSP associated with diabetes constitutes approximately 75% of all diabetic neuropathies. Sensory loss begins in the tips of the toes and gradually progresses proximally in a predictable length-dependent pattern. About 20% of patients report pain, typically of a burning, aching, and shooting quality, most severe in

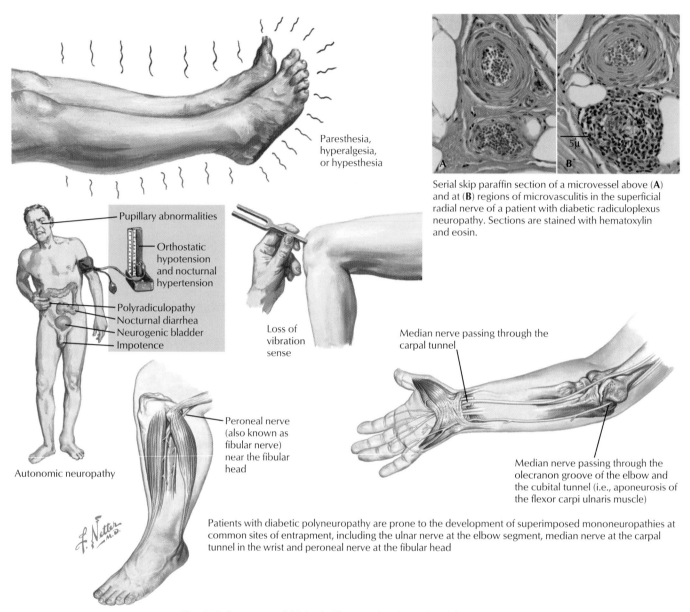

Paresthesia, hyperalgesia, or hypesthesia

Serial skip paraffin section of a microvessel above (**A**) and at (**B**) regions of microvasculitis in the superficial radial nerve of a patient with diabetic radiculoplexus neuropathy. Sections are stained with hematoxylin and eosin.

Pupillary abnormalities

Orthostatic hypotension and nocturnal hypertension

Polyradiculopathy
Nocturnal diarrhea
Neurogenic bladder
Impotence

Loss of vibration sense

Median nerve passing through the carpal tunnel

Autonomic neuropathy

Peroneal nerve (also known as fibular nerve) near the fibular head

Median nerve passing through the olecranon groove of the elbow and the cubital tunnel (i.e., aponeurosis of the flexor carpi ulnaris muscle)

Patients with diabetic polyneuropathy are prone to the development of superimposed mononeuropathies at common sites of entrapment, including the ulnar nerve at the elbow segment, median nerve at the carpal tunnel in the wrist and peroneal nerve at the fibular head

Fig. 67.6 Spectrum of Diabetic Neuropathy–Associated Symptoms.

the evening or at night. Loss of protective sensation combined with diabetic vasculopathy can result in nonhealing ulcers, gangrene of the toes requiring amputations, or joint deformities (Fig. 67.7). Fall risk due to loss of proprioceptive sensation is an underrecognized source of disability in DSP patients. Strength is usually preserved, although weakness of great toe extension is not uncommon. Preserved motor function in diabetic DSP is an important clinical clue; in fact, one should consider etiologies other than diabetes in patients who have significant motor involvement. Electrodiagnostic studies will reveal a length-dependent sensory-predominant axonal process. NCS and EMG are characteristically normal in *small-fiber neuropathy (SFN)*, which can be thought of as a subtype or an early stage of DSP. Preferential injury to unmyelinated small axons within the skin in these patients manifests with severe burning pain and numbness in the feet, sometimes associated with allodynia (a painful response to a nonpainful stimulus such as contact of the feet with the bed sheets). Diagnosis can be confirmed by measurement of intraepidermal nerve fiber density (IENFD) obtained from a punch skin biopsy (Fig. 67.8).

Treatment of DSP and SFN consists of improved control of diabetes and careful attention to other components of metabolic syndrome, such as excess weight and hyperlipidemia. Medications such as gabapentin, pregabalin, tricyclic antidepressants, and others are used for neuropathic pain.

Diabetic Autonomic Neuropathy

Diabetic autonomic neuropathy (DAN) may occur concomitantly with DSP or in isolation; its importance lies in the fact that it is associated with an elevated risk of death. The symptomatology is generally protean but may be subtle. Orthostatic hypotension is readily recognized in a patient who describes orthostatic light-headedness, but it presents a challenge when it masquerades as fatigue, visual blurring, or posterior neck pain (coat-hanger syndrome). Failure to increase heart rate in response to exertion can lead to exertional intolerance, early fatigue, and dyspnea. Erectile dysfunction may be the most frequent symptom, but it is not often volunteered by affected men.

Diabetic Lumbosacral Radiculoplexus Neuropathy (Diabetic Amyotrophy)

DLRPN is an acute, asymmetric, painful condition typically seen in type 2 diabetics who have reasonably good glycemic control (Fig. 67.9). Not infrequently, DLRPN is the first manifestation of diabetes and may even be diagnosed in patients with prediabetes. The classic presentation starts with severe unilateral thigh pain, often worse during the night. Patellar reflex is usually absent on the affected side. The pain subsides within a few days or weeks and is followed by proximal atrophy and weakness. Although proximal muscles are most often involved, distal weakness is not uncommon and can even be seen in isolation. Many patients develop contralateral weakness, but the disease remains asymmetric in most. Most patients experience weight loss. Concurrent thoracic radiculopathy, resulting in severe abdominal or thoracic pain, can be seen. This is a self-limited disease; gradual improvement can be expected to take place over months; however, many patients have residual deficits. Nerve conduction study and EMG will reveal findings suggestive of lumbar root, plexus, and peripheral nerve involvement. Nerve biopsy may reveal perivascular inflammatory infiltrates (microvasculitis) and findings of ischemic nerve injury, suggesting that the pathogenesis is immune-mediated. Immune-modifying treatments such as corticosteroids or IVIG are sometimes tried on an empiric basis but have not been systematically studied.

Treatment-Related Neuropathy

Previously known as "insulin neuritis," this is an acute, painful, small-fiber and autonomic neuropathy that emerges within weeks of tightened glycemic control in a previously poorly controlled diabetic. It is more common in type 1 diabetes and in patients with history of deliberate withholding of insulin for the purpose of weight loss (diabetic anorexia). Spontaneous improvement over weeks can be expected.

TOXIC AND NUTRITIONAL NEUROPATHIES

There are many toxic and nutritional causes of peripheral neuropathy (see Box 67.5). *Alcohol* may be the most common toxin in this category. The prevalence of alcoholic neuropathy correlates with the duration and amount consumed during a lifetime. A direct toxic effect on the nerves appears to be the leading mechanism. Vitamin deficiency may play a role in some cases. The typical phenotype is one of distal, symmetric, sensory-predominant, and often painful neuropathy, sometimes with dysautonomia.

Among neurotoxic medications, *chemotherapeutic agents* deserve special attention. Although most (vincristine, paclitaxel) produce a typical painful, length-dependent polyneuropathy, exceptions exist; platinum-based agents often lead to sensory ganglionopathy and thalidomide can cause proximal involvement.

Common etiologies of *cobalamin (vitamin B₁₂)* deficiency are pernicious anemia, dietary avoidance (vegans), bowel resection, gastric bypass surgeries, and nitrous oxide abuse. Cobalamin deficiency can present with numbness in the feet, suggesting a distal neuropathy similar to other toxic/metabolic etiologies. A non–length-dependent presentation with concurrent myelopathy (neuromyelopathy), however, may be more common; these patients present with sensory symptoms beginning in the hands and with sensory gait ataxia due to impairment of proprioceptive afferents in posterior spinal columns. Extensor plantar responses in a patient with numb feet, particularly if coupled with the complaint of unsteadiness in the dark, should alert the clinician to the possibility of nutritional neuromyelopathy.

Peripheral neuropathy, typically distal, symmetric, painful, sensory or sensorimotor, is one of the many neurologic presentations of *thiamin (B1)* deficiency (dry beriberi). Alcoholics and patients after weight reduction surgeries are at risk.

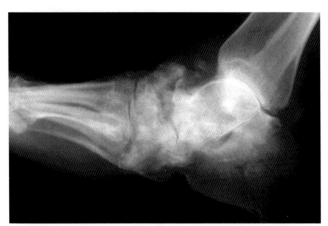

Lateral plain film of ankle and foot demonstrates severe proliferative degenerative changes that are typical of the multiple injuries sustained because of lack of sensation.

Fig. 67.7 Neuropathic Foot (Charcot Arthropathy).

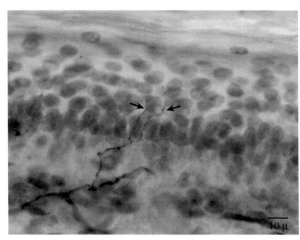

Skin biopsy section immunostained with protein gene product 9.5 showing epidermal nerve fibers (arrows).

Fig. 67.8 Skin Biopsy for Evaluation of Small Fiber Neuropathy.

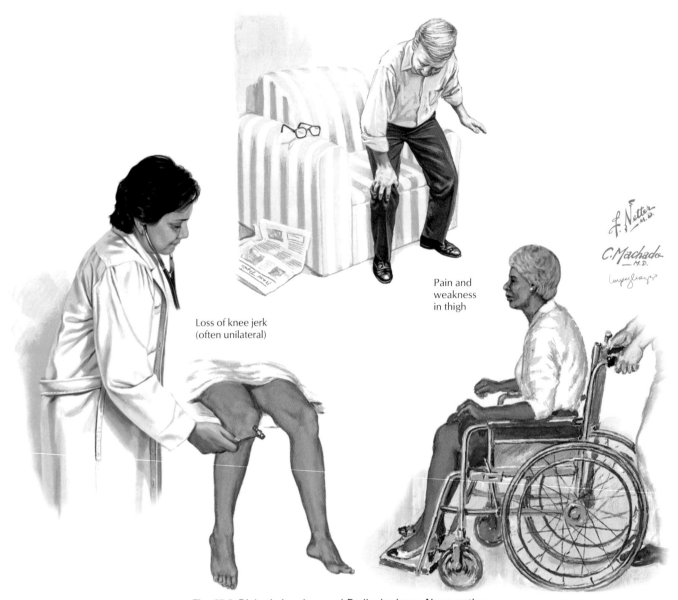

Loss of knee jerk
(often unilateral)

Pain and
weakness
in thigh

Fig. 67.9 Diabetic Lumbosacral Radiculoplexus Neuropathy.

GUILLAIN-BARRÉ SYNDROME AND CHRONIC INFLAMMATORY DEMYELINATING POLYRADICULONEUROPATHY

Guillain-Barre syndrome (GBS) and chronic inflammatory demyelinating polyradiculoneuropathy (CIDP) are autoimmune neuropathies that share the unusual feature of significant widespread peripheral nerve involvement, often including nerve root (Fig. 67.10) and sometimes cranial nerves. Consequently these disorders are categorized as **polyradiculoneuropathies** rather than polyneuropathies. GBS and CIDP share the cardinal feature of predominantly motor symptoms affecting the limbs, with less consistent sensory symptoms. The major clinical difference between GBS and CIDP is the temporal course; GBS is a monophasic illness of acute onset that usually reaches its nadir within 1–4 weeks and then gradually improves (Fig. 67.11). CIDP has a slower onset and more prolonged course that may be progressive or relapsing. Sometimes CIDP can present acutely ("acute CIDP"), mimicking GBS, to be diagnosed correctly only after a clinical relapse or further progression

occur. Because some GBS patients also experience relapse during their recovery (referred to as *treatment-related fluctuation*), the distinction between GBS and acute CIDP can present a diagnostic challenge that is sometimes settled only after a few of careful observation and therapeutic trials. In general, relapses in GBS are expected to occur earlier in the recovery, usually within 4–8 weeks. It is a common misconception that the temporal behavior marks the only difference between GBS and CIDP; there are multiple other differences including pathogenesis and response to therapies. GBS and CIDP are heterogeneous conditions: multiple subtypes exist, as described further on.

Pathogenesis of Guillain-Barré Syndrome and Chronic Inflammatory Demyelinating Polyradiculoneuropathy

Both cellular and humoral immunity seem to be involved in the pathogenesis of GBS and CIDP. The immune attack in both diseases is widespread and occurs proximally at the nerve roots and distally at the motor axon terminal. These two sites are theoretically more vulnerable because of their less complete blood–nerve barriers. Lymphocytes and macrophages are the effector cells involved in damaging myelin and

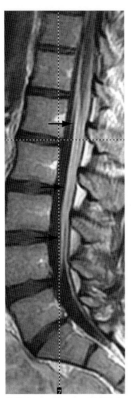

Sagittal T1 post-gadolinium-enhanced MRI demonstrating diffuse enhancement of cauda equina (arrows)

Fig. 67.10 Guillain-Barré Syndrome: Enhancement of Lumbosacral Roots.

the adjacent axons (Fig. 67.12). In some cases, the node of Ranvier and its axolemma is the initial target of autoantibodies, leading to disruption of sodium channels and resultant conduction failure (Fig. 67.5). The weakness and sensory disturbances are due to nerve fiber action potential conduction block (secondary to demyelination) or conduction failure (due to axonal dysfunction).

The pathogenesis of GBS relates to the immune system being first primed as it responds to foreign molecules, such as a virus or bacteria (Fig. 67.13). Subsequently the immune system inappropriately attacks host tissue that shares homologous epitopes—for example, gangliosides found on the cell wall of certain bacteria and the peripheral nerve myelin of the host. This pathologic process has been termed *molecular mimicry*. Approximately two-thirds of GBS patients give a history of antecedent infection 1–3 weeks before the onset of neuropathy. *Campylobacter jejuni* and *cytomegalovirus* are most frequent, usually presenting as gastroenteritis or respiratory infection.

Antecedent infection is observed less commonly in CIDP. Compared with GBS, less is known about the pathogenesis of CIDP. Cellular component may be more important in CIDP; antibody-driven T-cell attack against an unknown peripheral nerve antigen is believed to underlie this chronic disease. As in GBS, antigens from the region of the node of Ranvier (contactin-1 and neurofascins) have been implicated in rare cases.

Clinical Presentation of Guillain-Barré Syndrome and Chronic Inflammatory Demyelinating Polyradiculoneuropathy
Guillain-Barré Syndrome

GBS is a classic acute immune-mediated neuropathy. Characteristically it begins abruptly with relatively symmetric paresthesias and pain in

a previously healthy person. An otherwise innocuous infection, such as diarrhea or an upper respiratory illness, often precedes the onset by 1–3 weeks. Sensory symptoms are accompanied or quickly followed by progressive weakness. Gait ataxia related to the loss proprioceptive sensation or pain can be an important early feature. In early stages of the disease, however, objective abnormalities may be very subtle even in a patient with prominent sensory symptoms and pain; not infrequently is such patient dismissed by multiple physicians, only to be given the correct diagnosis several days later when weakness and areflexia—diagnostic hallmarks of GBS—emerge. Weakness may manifest as trouble climbing stairs, difficulty arising from chairs, unsteadiness, falls, or difficulty with arm use. Cranial nerve involvement is common in GBS; facial weakness occurs in more than half of the patients and is typically bilateral. Ophthalmoplegia, dysarthria, and dysphagia can also occur. Diaphragmatic weakness due to phrenic nerve involvement is common; this, along with weakness of accessory respiratory muscle and oropharyngeal weakness, contributes to the ventilatory dysfunction seen in some. Approximately one-quarter of hospitalized patients require mechanical ventilation. The autonomic nervous system is frequently involved in GBS, especially in severe cases. Cardiovascular dysautonomia most often manifests as sinus tachycardia in the range of 100–120 beats/min with little beat-to-beat variation with respiration. Although this in itself is not a dangerous abnormality, it should alert one to the possibility of other cardiac arrhythmias or labile blood pressure that can be life threatening and warrant close observation. Urinary retention and ileus sometimes occur.

Neurologic examination demonstrates proximal and distal weakness, typically symmetric. Asymmetry can be seen early but is rare in the fully developed syndrome. More subtle proximal weakness should be sought by having the patient rise from a chair, get up from a kneeling position, or walk on his or her heels or toes. The sensory exam is often normal in early stages even in patients with prominent paresthesias, a discrepancy that can mislead a less experienced clinician. Reduced or absent muscle stretch reflexes are the rule, but they may be retained in the first week of the disease.

Guillain-Barré syndrome forms and variants. GBS has several recognized forms. The demyelinating form, *acute inflammatory demyelinating polyradiculoneuropathy (AIDP)*, is the most common form in North America and Europe. The prototypical axonal form of GBS, *acute motor axonal neuropathy (AMAN)*, was originally described during epidemics of *C. jejuni* gastroenteritis in China and is more common in Asia. Patients with AMAN have no sensory symptoms but are otherwise clinically similar to those with the other GBS forms. Molecular mimicry between *C. jejuni* and GM1 gangliosides on axolemma of motor fibers at the node of Ranvier is thought to underlie AMAN. Antibodies against GM1 disrupt sodium channel function, leading to conduction failure or block. Rapid improvement following immunotherapy in some cases of axonal GBS may be explained by the reversal of antibody-mediated conduction failure before axonal degeneration has occurred. *Acute motor and sensory axonal neuropathy (AMSAN)* shares many features with AMAN but includes sensory involvement. *Miller-Fisher syndrome (MFS)* presents with external ophthalmoplegia, ataxia, and areflexia, although all of these components need not be present. Overlapping syndromes consisting of MFS and other features such as facial or limb weakness, are common. Anti-GQ1b antibodies are present in approximately 95% of patients with MFS. A *pharyngeal-cervical-brachial* variant mimicking bulbar myasthenia and *acute dysautonomia* are among other rare GBS variants.

Chronic Inflammatory Demyelinating Neuropathy

The characteristic clinical presentation, also referred to as *classic CIDP*, is one of an individual between 40 and 60 years of age with

Pathogenesis

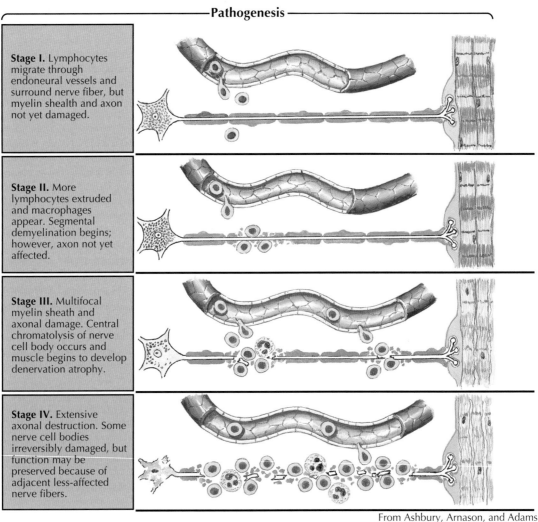

Stage I. Lymphocytes migrate through endoneural vessels and surround nerve fiber, but myelin sheath and axon not yet damaged.

Stage II. More lymphocytes extruded and macrophages appear. Segmental demyelination begins; however, axon not yet affected.

Stage III. Multifocal myelin sheath and axonal damage. Central chromatolysis of nerve cell body occurs and muscle begins to develop denervation atrophy.

Stage IV. Extensive axonal destruction. Some nerve cell bodies irreversibly damaged, but function may be preserved because of adjacent less-affected nerve fibers.

From Ashbury, Arnason, and Adams

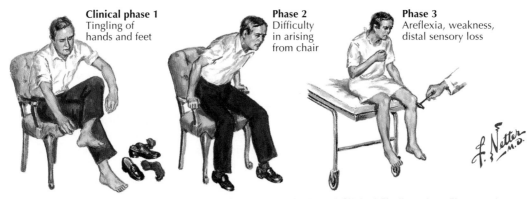

Clinical phase 1
Tingling of hands and feet

Phase 2
Difficulty in arising from chair

Phase 3
Areflexia, weakness, distal sensory loss

Fig. 67.11 Guillain-Barré Syndrome: Electrophysiologic and Clinical Findings (see Fig. 67.12).

symmetric proximal and distal weakness in all limbs (Fig. 67.14). Typically, the weakness has evolved subacutely (i.e., over weeks or a few months). Distal sensory symptoms and weakness are common, but it is the proximal weakness that is usually emphasized by the patient. In contrast to GBS pain and autonomic dysfunction are rare and cranial nerve involvement, usually cranial nerve VII, is seen only in a minority of patients. Progressive, relapsing, and rarely a monophasic course can be observed. Unlike GBS, association with systemic disease has been noted, including HIV, neoplasms such lymphoma and melanoma, MGUS, hepatitis C, or connective tissue disease.

Neurologic examination reveals symmetric proximal and distal weakness. Proximal weakness is among the clues to the diagnosis of classic CIDP even if distal weakness is often more severe.

Reflexes are hypoactive or absent. Sensory symptoms are present in most but are typically overshadowed by motor features. Gait imbalance and tremor, presumably from the dysfunction of myelinated large-fiber proprioceptive sensory fibers, can occur. Confirmation of the clinical diagnosis relies on electrodiagnostic study and CSF analysis, as detailed later. Nerve biopsy is not required in most cases but, if obtained, can reveal features of remyelination (onion bulbs) and inflammatory cells around endoneural vessels.

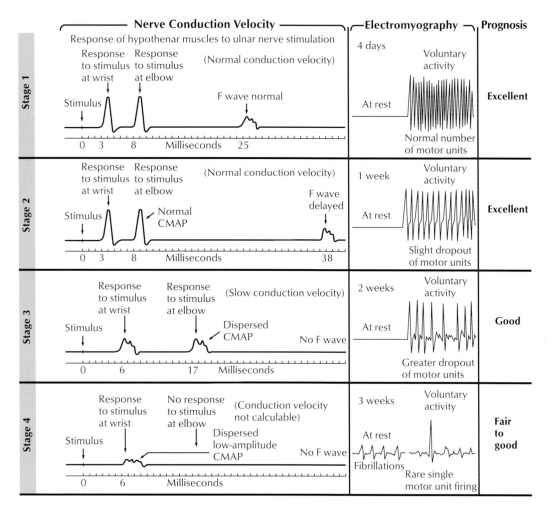

Nerve Conduction Velocity	Electromyography	Prognosis

Fig. 67.12 Guillain-Barré Syndrome: Pathogenesis and Clinical Manifestations (see Fig. 67.11).

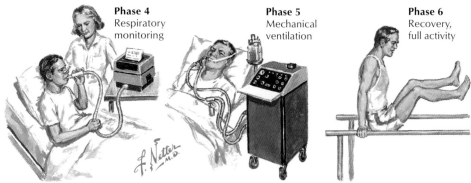

Phase 4 Respiratory monitoring

Phase 5 Mechanical ventilation

Phase 6 Recovery, full activity

CLINICAL VIGNETTE *A 64-year-old otherwise healthy woman presents with a 2-year history of altered sensation in her feet and poor balance. Numbness began in her toes and gradually spread to involve her ankles and distal calves. This has not been painful, only unpleasant, as she often does not know "where her feet are." She initially noticed gait imbalance only in the shower after she closed her eyes, but lately she has started using a cane and now avoids leaving the house. Her neurologic exam was remarkable for impaired proprioception in her toes and ankles and a marked tendency to fall backward when standing with her eyes closed. Areflexia, mild weakness of the toe extensors, pan-modal sensory loss up to her knees, and vibratory loss in her fingers were other notable features. A coarse, irregular tremor with pseudoathetosis was noted in her hands. EMG*

demonstrated very prolonged distal motor latencies. No sensory responses could be elicited in the lower extremities and they were reduced in her upper limbs. Laboratory studies demonstrated a modest amount of IgM lambda paraprotein and a high titer of anti–myelin glycoprotein (MAG) antibodies. The patient was diagnosed with anti-MAG. After unsuccessful trials of IVIG and rituximab, it was decided that she would not receive additional therapeutic trials.

Comment: Impaired proprioception leading to sensory gait ataxia and a Romberg sign (inability to maintain balance without visual input) are core features of neuropathy associated with MAG antibodies. Treatment is disappointing, with only a small subset of patients responding to immune therapies (IVIG, rituximab, corticosteroids, cyclophosphamide).

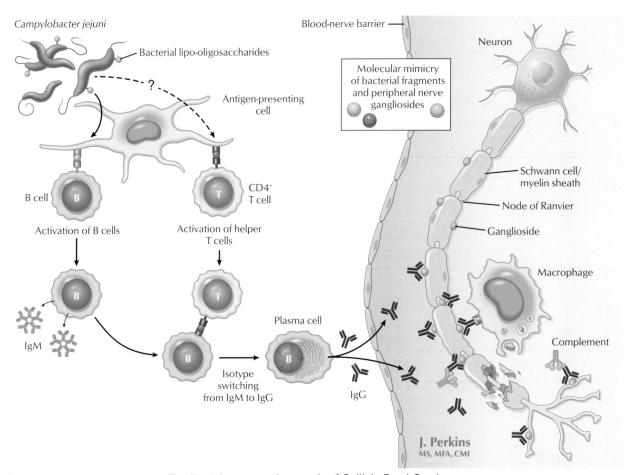

Fig. 67.13 Immunopathogenesis of Guillain-Barré Syndrome.

Chronic inflammatory demyelinating polyradiculoneuropathy: Spectrum and variants. *"Classic" CIDP*, the hallmark of which is symmetric proximal weakness, constitutes more than half of all CIDP cases. Among the rest are regional CIDP variants of distal acquired demyelinating sensory neuropathy (DADS) and multifocal acquired demyelinating sensory and motor neuropathy (MADSAM). Related entities are anti–myelin-associated glycoprotein (MAG) neuropathy; polyneuropathy, organomegaly, endocrinopathy, monoclonal gammopathy, and skin changes (POEMS); and multifocal motor neuropathy.

DADS neuropathy is thought of as a CIDP variant with distal weakness and sensory loss, often producing gait ataxia. Nerve conduction studies reveal markedly prolonged distal motor latencies, confirming distal demyelination. A similar phenotype of distal ataxic neuropathy is often associated with IgM monoclonal protein. About half of these patients have *Anti-MAG neuropathy*, as described in the foregoing vignette, with high titers of antibodies to MAG, a peripheral nerve constituent. *MADSAM*, also known under its eponym Lewis-Sumner syndrome, is an important CIDP variant that clinically resembles multiple mononeuropathies syndromes.

Multifocal motor neuropathy (MMN) is a rare immune-mediated neuropathy manifesting with chronic, slowly progressive, or stepwise weakness without sensory loss. The upper extremities are more involved than the lower, almost always in an asymmetric fashion, with predominantly distal weakness in an individual nerve distribution. Cranial nerves are usually spared. EMG may demonstrate motor conduction blocks, and cerebrospinal fluid protein is often normal. IgM antibody against GM1 is detected in about half the patients. MMN is a very rare but important disorder; as a treatable and nonfatal disease, it must be distinguished from lower motor neuron presentation of amyotrophic lateral sclerosis (ALS), which it can mimic. MMN responds to IVIG and cyclophosphamide, but not to corticosteroid or plasma exchange.

CIDP associated with IgG or IgA MGUS usually presents similarly to CIDP without a monoclonal protein, and treatment response is similar. However, an IgG-λ or IgA-λ (lambda) monoclonal gammopathy suggests the possibility of *POEMS syndrome,* particularly with hyperpigmentation. Polyneuropathy, strikingly similar to CIDP with symmetric proximal and distal weakness and variable sensory loss, can be the presenting symptom. Often an osteosclerotic myeloma, or sometimes an osteolytic bony lesion, is identified by performing a "metastatic bone" radiograph skeletal survey. The level of vascular endothelial growth factor (VEGF) is elevated in the serum in POEMS at least three to four times above normal. Focus-beam radiation therapy of these tumors can dramatically improve the neuropathy. Neither plasmapheresis nor IVIG is helpful. These patients may need allogeneic stem cell transplantation to cure the underlying hematologic malignancy.

Differential Diagnosis of Guillain-Barré Syndrome and Chronic Inflammatory Demyelinating Polyradiculoneuropathy

Presence of sensory symptoms favor GBS or CIDP over muscle or motor unit disorders, including ***myopathies, neuromuscular transmission disorders, or motor neuron disorders.*** Because sensory symptoms also occur with ***myelopathies,*** the possibility of an acute or subacute myelopathy with evolving spinal cord compression must always be considered, especially early in the patient's clinical course. Of noncompressive

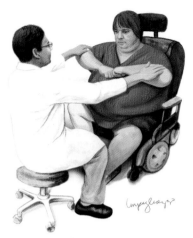

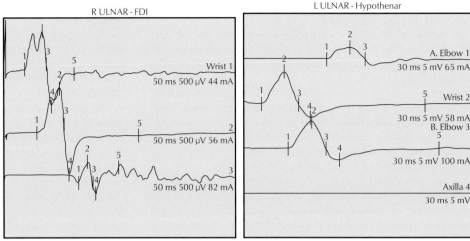

Principal manifestation of CIDP is four-extremity weakness; paresthesias in the feet and hands are also noted. On examination, patient is weak (shoulder abduction testing), areflexic, and demonstrates sensory loss in the feet and hands. NCS/EMG demonstrated a predominantly demyelinating sensorimotor polyradiculoneuropathy.

Motor nerve conduction study of the ulnar motor nerve in a patient with CIDP. The waveform tracings *(left)* illustrate temporal dispersion. On proximal stimulation above the elbow *(lower tracing)*, there is a marked increase in the duration of the CMAP, as well as a significant drop in the amplitude, which is called temporal dispersion. The waveform tracings *(right)* illustrate conduction block. On proximal stimulation above the elbow *(top tracing)*, there is a significant drop in the amplitude compared with CMAPs elicited with more distal stimulation. Temporal dispersion and conduction block are both indicative of acquired demyelination, occurring somewhere in the nerve between the above-elbow and below-elbow stimulation sites.

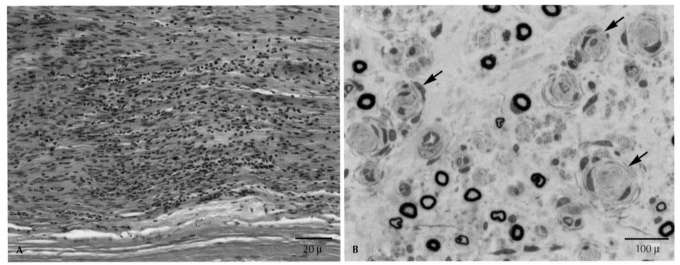

Biopsies of nerves from CIDP. Longitudinal paraffin hematoxylin and eosin preparation of a sciatic nerve biopsy showing endoneurial inflammation (**A**). Methylene blue–stained epoxy section of a sural nerve biopsy showing some fibers with large onion bulbs without myelinated fibers at their centers (**B**, *arrows*), whereas other myelinated fibers do not have onion bulbs (a pattern typical of CIDP).

Fig. 67.14 Chronic Inflammatory Demyelinating Polyradiculoneuropathy *(CIPD)*.

acute myelopathies, ***transverse myelitis (TM)*** is the most common form included in the differential diagnosis of GBS. Important clues to the possibility of a myelopathy include preservation or hyperactivity of muscle stretch reflexes, Babinski signs, sensory spinal cord level, and sphincter dysfunction. Although urinary retention occasionally occurs in early GBS, a myelopathy, conus medullaris, and/or cauda equina disorder must always be considered if sphincter dysfunction is present.

Back pain is common in GBS but not in CIDP. However, when it has a radicular quality, particularly in the thoracic distribution, a **thoracic *spinal mass lesion, dural AVM,* or *TM*** must be considered.

Acute or subacute onset in GBS and CIDP contrasts with many other acquired or ***inherited polyneuropathies*** wherein the onset is so insidious that the patient has no recall as to its precise timing.

Patients with ***mononeuritis multiplex (MM)*** usually have an associated systemic or primary peripheral nervous system vasculitis. The stepwise temporal course and asymmetric distribution are primary diagnostic clues, in direct contrast to CIDP, which has a symmetric evolution. Typically MM patients have sudden acute mononeuropathies, often affecting multiple specific nerves, particularly the peroneal, median, and ulnar, within a 2- to 6-week time period. Subsequently, if many nerves become involved, a confluent clinical picture mimicking a symmetric generalized polyneuropathy can emerge. An increased erythrocyte sedimentation rate or C-reactive protein (CRP), and a peripheral nerve biopsy demonstrating vasculitis provide important diagnostic information. Immediate high-dose immunosuppressive therapy, such as 60–100 mg prednisone daily, is indicated.

In ***tick paralysis,*** an unidentified tick saliva toxin most likely interacts with nerve sodium channels or impairs release of acetylcholine from the presynaptic terminal, producing an acute paralytic illness mimicking GBS. Examiners must always search for ticks in any patient with an acute flaccid paralysis. In the North American variety, the recovery is rapid and complete after the tick is removed.

A number of **toxins,** including some of marine origin (red tide, ciguatoxin), metals (arsenic, thallium), solvents (hexacarbons), insecticides (organophosphates), and native plants such as buckthorn may produce acute generalized weakness.

GBS may be the presenting sign of **HIV.** CSF examination showing excessive pleocytosis is a clue to obtain HIV serology. **Infection of anterior horn cells by neurotropic viruses** (i.e., West-Nile and some enteroviruses) typically has a multifocal and asymmetric pattern and is marked by CSF pleocytosis. EMG demonstrates a segmental distribution of axonal loss consistent with anterior horn cell localization.

Acute intermittent and variegate **porphyria** may produce an acute generalized sensorimotor neuropathy mimicking GBS. Previous attacks, a family history of similar disorders, concomitant abdominal pain, and mental status changes are clinical clues that typify this rare biochemical disorder.

Botulism and **myasthenia gravis** may produce generalized weakness. Botulism is typically acute in onset and myasthenia is usually more indolent, although myasthenia can have a relatively rapid bulbar presentation with ventilatory failure. Neither produces sensory symptoms. Botulism may have prominent manifestations of cholinergic dysautonomia. EMG may be required for distinction from GBS. **Lambert–Eaton myasthenic syndrome (LEMS)** mimics CIDP with a subacute onset of proximal weakness and areflexia. A history of tobacco use and a dry mouth suggest LEMS.

Severe electrolyte disturbances such as hypermagnesemia, **hypokalemia, hyperkalemia,** and **hypophosphatemia** may produce acute generalized weakness. Weakness severe enough to mimic GBS does not usually occur until potassium is less than 2 mEq/mL and phosphate less than 1 mg/mL. Addison disease becomes an important diagnostic consideration in hyperkalemia.

Diagnostic Approach in Guillain-Barré Syndrome and Chronic Inflammatory Demyelinating Polyradiculoneuropathy

Electrodiagnostic study provides a definitive means to assess the presence of a peripheral neuropathic process, ruling out other causes such as disorders of neuromuscular transmission or myopathy. It can demonstrate widespread involvement of spinal roots and peripheral nerves. Defining the process as demyelinating or axonal is straightforward in fully developed cases but can be difficult or even impossible in early stages, sometimes necessitating repeat studies if such differentiation is sought. In demyelinating GBS or CIDP, the motor and sensory conduction velocities are abnormally slow, with prolonged distal motor and F-wave latencies and often absent H reflexes. Nonuniform slowing, conduction block at sites not prone to entrapment, and abnormal temporal dispersion are commonly found in demyelinating GBS and CIDP but not in most inherited demyelinating polyneuropathies. Conduction block is present when there are significant reductions in compound motor nerve action potential amplitude and area with proximal versus distal stimulation. Temporal dispersion is characterized by abnormal prolongation of compound motor nerve action potential duration with proximal but not distal stimulation and is strong sign of acquired demyelination. Conduction velocities on routine nerve conduction studies may be normal when inflammatory lesions are more proximal—for example, in nerve roots or early in the disease course. Documentation of absent F waves is helpful for diagnosis of early GBS, wherein more widespread slowing of conduction is not yet present. It is, however, not uncommon in early GBS for conduction studies to be normal. In such cases one relies on needle EMG to document a dropout of motor

units ("neurogenic" or reduced recruitment) in a clinically weak muscle, a nonspecific but very useful pattern that unequivocally localizes the source of weakness to the peripheral nervous system. Another important feature of electrodiagnostic studies can be the pattern of "sural sparing," which means that there is a normal sural sensory response in the setting of an abnormal median sensory response; this may be seen in CIDP.

CSF analysis in GBS and CIDP characteristically demonstrates increased level of CSF protein (>50 mg/dL) without pleocytosis (<10 cells/mm^3). CSF examination is often normal within the first week of GBS (about 50% of patients); however, by the end of the second week, more than 90% of GBS patients have an increased level of CSF protein. The same CSF profile is seen in more than 90% of CIDP patients. Although 10–50 cells/mm^3 in the CSF may occur in GBS, more than 50 cells/mm^3 must arouse suspicion of an alternate diagnosis, including Lyme neuroborreliosis, HIV-associated polyradiculoneuropathy, poliomyelitis, or lymphomatous meningoradiculitis.

The role of magnetic resonance imaging (MRI) and other imaging studies in GBS and CIDP is limited; it mainly serves to rule out mimicking conditions such as myelopathy. In some cases smooth and symmetric enhancement of multiple roots is seen in a pattern distinct from the multifocal and nodular enhancement of malignant meningitis (see Fig. 67.10).

Treatment and Prognosis
Guillain-Barré Syndrome

Care of patients with GBS varies from watchful waiting to emergency intervention, but initially always in a hospital because of the potential for rapid respiratory compromise. Patients with mild GBS who are able to ambulate are often cared for without specific treatment. Those individuals who are unable to walk, who develop respiratory compromise, or who exhibit rapid progression are treated with plasmapheresis (PE) or IVIG. Treatment within 2 weeks from onset appears to be of the greatest benefit. IVIG is given at a total dose of 2.0 g/kg over 2–5 days. PE is done as five plasma exchanges of one plasma volume each over 9–10 days. IVIG after PE provides no additional benefit. The combination of PE after IVIG has not been studied but is not advised on the basis that PE would probably wash out the IVIG previously administered. Corticosteroids are not effective for GBS. On occasion the IVIG or PE treatment is repeated on an empiric basis in patients with severe disease who have failed to improve and in those who experience a relapse.

Respiratory failure is common in GBS; 20% of patients require mechanical ventilation. Early in the course of GBS, negative inspiratory force and vital capacity must be closely monitored in all patients. Attention to autonomic dysfunction, mainly labile hypertension and arrhythmias, is critical, often prompting observation and management in the intensive care unit. Supportive care—including emotional and nutritional support, judicious pain management, and prophylaxis for common complications of hospitalized, immobile patients (e.g., deep venous thrombosis and decubitus ulcers)—is important.

Most patients with GBS recover within a few months, particularly those without significant axonal degeneration. Up to 20% report significant residual symptoms 12 months after their diagnosis. Some are left with weakness and numbness, whereas others may have chronic pain. Fatigue is common and can last for years after substantial motor improvement. The etiology of the fatigue appears to be multifactorial; intensive physical therapy seems to be beneficial.

Chronic Inflammatory Demyelinating Polyradiculoneuropathy

First-line treatment for CIDP is with corticosteroids, IVIG, or PE. Predetermined neurologic endpoints—such as strength, gait, and reflexes—must be monitored closely to assess the therapeutic response.

Corticosteroids are effective in 60%–70% of patients, but adverse effects associated with their use, particularly long-term use of oral prednisone, must be considered. Oral prednisone can be started at 1 mg/kg per day, continued until remission is achieved, and then tapered based on the individual's response. Pulse oral dexamethasone or pulse intravenous methylprednisolone (IVMP) may also be effective and may have fewer side effects than oral prednisone. Oral dexamethasone at 40 mg is given on 4 consecutive days once a month for 6 months. A reasonable regimen of IVMP consists of 500–1000 mg daily for 3–5 days, followed by 500–1000 mg weekly for 6–12 weeks, with individualized taper afterward.

Overall, IVIG is often the first-line treatment used by many clinicians given its efficacy and low risk of adverse effects. High cost, thromboembolic complications, and the need for administration at an infusion center are the main disadvantages. A common initial regimen is 2 g/kg over 2–5 days, followed by 1g/kg in 1 day every 3 weeks for several months. The maintenance dose and interval between treatments vary widely and are typically individualized. Subcutaneous immunoglobulin is emerging as a promising alternative.

PE is not used as frequently as oral steroids or IVIG for CIDP because it is more invasive and not any more efficacious. Nonetheless, PE remains an option if rapid improvement is required—for example, in a severely affected hospitalized patient.

Patients who do not respond to one of the first-line treatments may still respond to the other modalities. Long-term immunosuppression may, however, be necessary in refractory patients, or in those who are in need of a steroid-sparing agent. Azathioprine, mycophenolate mofetil, methotrexate, cyclophosphamide, and rituximab have been used in this setting.

The long-term outcome varies for patients with CIDP who are treated with conventional therapy. Most return to normal strength, although some require intermittent IVIG or long-term immunosuppression to maintain improvement. Unfortunately patients may progress despite aggressive immunotherapy.

SENSORY NEURONOPATHIES

> **CLINICAL VIGNETTE** *A 69-year-old lifelong smoker noted difficulty passing urine. Two weeks later he developed numbness over his anterior abdomen. Clumsiness with his arms use became frustrating even during simple tasks such as putting on his glasses. Increasing difficulty in maintaining balance followed, and within 8 days he was too unsteady to walk on his own. He had no pain but did complain that he had not had a bowel movement in 10 days. A weight loss of 16 pounds was attributed to "poor appetite."*
>
> *Examination revealed a man who initially seemed to give incomplete effort during manual muscle testing. This was corrected by having him directly visualize tested body parts. Muscle stretch reflexes were absent throughout. He had pan-modal sensory loss, including proprioception in his fingers and below the knees. Marked pseudoathetosis in the arms was evident. No nystagmus was noted, and his speech was normal. He was mildly inattentive. While being examined by a medical student, a 25-second episode of expressive aphasia was observed. EMG revealed absent sensory nerve action potentials throughout. Motor conduction and needle electrode examination results were normal. Subsequently anti-Hu antibodies returned positive. Computed tomography (CT) of the chest did not show any concerning masses, but whole body positron-emission tomography (PET) CT revealed a small hypermetabolic lesion within a left mediastinal node. Biopsy confirmed small-cell lung cancer.*
>
> *Comment: An acute and rapidly disabling sensory and autonomic neuropathy developed in this patient. Non–length-dependent sensory loss with profound proprioceptive loss manifesting with pseudoathetosis in the arms and early*

*loss of ambulation are indicative of a sensory neuronopathy. The explosive temporal evolution in a smoker was a particularly ominous sign suggestive of **paraneoplastic sensory neuronopathy (PSN)** associated with anti-Hu antibody and small-cell lung cancer (SCLC). Concurrent development of bladder atonia, intestinal obstruction, and possibly also limbic encephalitis with aphasic seizures suggested a more widespread paraneoplastic syndrome. Tumor diagnosis can be challenging; PSN often develops when SCLC is in its earliest stages and cannot be proven on initial radiologic studies. In these patients, as in the case of this vignette, whole-body PET CT can be revealing. Unfortunately this is a devastating disease that often leads to death from complications related to patients' bedridden state rather than from cancer progression.*

Clinical Presentation and Differential Diagnosis

Some individuals presenting with sensory symptoms have a pathologic process that primarily targets the sensory neuron cells within the dorsal root ganglion (DRG) (in contrast to more common length-dependent neuropathies such as LDPN, affecting the distal nerve axon) (Fig. 67.15). Such patients are described as having a primary **sensory neuronopathy or ganglionopathy.** Distinguishing sensory neuronopathy from sensory LDPN is important because it allows for a focused differential diagnosis (Box 67.6).

Sensory neuronopathy is typified by a non–length-dependent distribution of sensory loss and sometimes pain. Acute or subacute onset is frequently seen, particularly in autoimmune cases, and contrasts with the indolent course of most LDPNs. A disproportionate loss of position sense occurs when large sensory fibers are affected, resulting in pseudoathetoid limb movements with eye closure. Severe sensory ataxia frequently presents and is distinguished from cerebellar pathology by the absence of nystagmus and dysarthria. Complete absence of sensory responses on nerve conduction study often confirms the clinically suspected diagnosis.

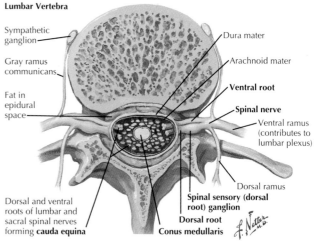

Fig. 67.15 Spinal Nerve Origin: Sensory Components.

> **BOX 67.6 Sensory Neuronopathy**
>
> Paraneoplastic autoimmunity (small-cell lung cancer most common)
> Connective tissue disease (Sjögren syndrome, scleroderma)
> Toxicity (platinum-based drugs, pyridoxine excess)
> Hereditary (Friedreich ataxia)
> Idiopathic

In **paraneoplastic sensory neuronopathy (PSN),** it is proposed that similar antigenic components in DRG and cancer cells, most often small-cell lung carcinoma (SCLC), set the stage for molecular mimicry. PSN typically has an acute to subacute presentation and progresses relentlessly. As was the case in foregoing vignette, it is not unusual for the patient to be bed-bound within a few weeks. Most patients develop more widespread involvement including limbic encephalitis and autonomic dysfunction. SCLC is the most frequently associated tumor; these patients usually have anti-Hu antibodies. Treatment is disappointing; anticancer treatment is more effective than immunomodulation. An occasional patient can stabilize with early treatment of the cancer combined with immunologic therapies.

Sjögren syndrome is an autoimmune process associated with several neuropathy phenotypes. The classic sensory neuronopathy form is uncommon. It is clinically similar to other DRG lesions, particularly paraneoplastic sensory neuronopathy. Trigeminal and autonomic involvement can occur. Diagnostic findings include the sicca complex with dry eyes and mouth, presence of anti-Ro and anti-La antibodies (also known as SS-A and SS-B) inflammatory involvement of salivary glands on lip biopsy, or a combination of these. Sensory neuronopathy can also be associated with other inflammatory conditions such as scleroderma or lupus erythematosus.

Sensory neuronopathy due to **cisplatin and carboplatin toxicity** is well recognized. **Pyridoxine** in large doses (>200 mg daily) is neurotoxic and may cause irreversible sensory neuronopathy.

Friedreich ataxia is an autosomal recessive neurodegenerative disease that can present with clinical and electrodiagnostic findings of sensory neuronopathy. Additionally, a varying degree of pyramidal, extrapyramidal, and spinocerebellar involvement is present.

Some of the sensory neuronopathies remain **idiopathic** even after careful exclusion of occult cancer, rheumatologic disease, and toxins. It is possible that some may involve a yet undiscovered malignancy.

Vitamin B$_{12}$ deficiency and **tabes dorsalis** are important in the differential diagnosis of sensory ataxia. Both have a predisposition to affect the posterior columns and/or dorsal (sensory) roots.

Diagnostic Approach

EMG provides a means to differentiate between LDPN and sensory neuronopathy. Many patients with LDPNs, even those without clinical weakness, have EMG evidence of motor involvement on motor conduction studies or needle EMG. Patients with a primary sensory neuronopathy have only sensory nerve conduction abnormalities, and these do not follow a length-dependent pattern.

When sensory neuronopathies are confirmed, subsequent ancillary testing is limited to disorders known to cause such patterns (see Box 67.6). Testing for serum anti-Hu antibodies is important, particularly for patients with a smoking history. In patients with positive anti-Hu antibody and in those without a definable etiology, chest CT or whole-body PET CT may be indicated to rule out occult malignancy. Patients with suspected Sjögren syndrome require a combination of serologic tests, particularly SSA and SSB antibodies, Schirmer test of lacrimation, and minor salivary gland (usually lip) biopsy. Vitamin B$_{12}$ levels and syphilis serology should be routinely done. A nerve biopsy is usually not indicated in sensory neuronopathies.

Treatment and Prognosis

Treatment of sensory neuronopathy is tailored to the underlying cause but is generally disappointing. In sensory neuronopathy associated with Sjögren syndrome, IVIG, plasmapheresis, or rituximab have been effective in some cases. Paraneoplastic forms are generally resistant to therapy; specific treatment of the underlying neoplasm combined with intense immunotherapy has led to neurologic stabilization in rare cases. Unfortunately these individuals usually have an inexorably progressive course. Neurotoxins, including vitamin B$_6$, require identification and subsequent elimination.

Prognosis varies depending on the underlying cause of the neuropathy and the extent of axonal damage before treatment initiation. Severe cases may prevent independent ambulation, even with gait aids.

ADDITIONAL RESOURCES

Mauermann ML, Burns TM. The evaluation of chronic axonal neuropathies. Semin Neurol 2008;28:133–51.

Lauria G, Hsieh ST, Johansson O, et al. EFNS/PNS guideline on the use of skin biopsy in the diagnosis of small fiber neuropathy. Report of a joint task of the European Federation of Neurological Societies and the Peripheral Nerve Society. J Neurology 2010;17:903–12.
Review of guidelines focusing on use of skin biopsy to diagnose small fiber neuropathy. Normative data for age and gender are proposed.

Gibbons CH, Freeman R. Treatment-induced neuropathy of diabetes: an acute, iatrogenic complication of diabetes. Brain 2015;138:43–52.
Description and definition of the clinical entity previously known as "insulin neuritis."

Uncini A, Kuwabara S. Nodopathies of the peripheral nerve: an emerging concept. JNNP 2015;86:1186–95.
A discussion of anatomic, pathophysiologic, and clinical features of nodopathies.

Callaghan BC, Xia R, Banerjee M, et al. Metabolic syndrome components are associated with symptomatic polyneuropathy independent of glycemic status. Diabetes Care 2016;39(5):801–7.
One of many papers supporting emerging evidence for the role of metabolic syndrome components other than hyperglycemia on the development and progression of polyneuropathy.

Gwathmey KG. Sensory neuronopathies. Muscle Nerve 2016;53(1):8–19.

Verboon CH, Van Doorn PA, Jacobs BC. Treatment dilemmas in Guillain-Barre syndrome. JNNP 2017;88:346–52.
A clinically oriented discussion and review of available evidence with respect to treatment controversies in Guillain-Barre syndrome (e.g., how to treat patients who do not improve or relapse, among others).

Lewis RA. Chronic inflammatory demyelinating polyneuropathy. Curr Opin Neurol 2017;30(5):508–12.

Mauermann ML. The peripheral neuropathies of POEMS syndrome and castleman disease. Hematol Oncol Clin North Am 2018;32(1):153–63.

Russell JA. General approach to peripheral nerve disorders. Continuum (Minneap Minn) 2017;23(5):1241–62.

Van Shaik IN, Bril V, Van Geloven N, et al. Subcutaneous immunoglobulin for maintenance treatment in chronic inflammmatory demyelinating polyneuropathy (PATH): a randomised, double-blind, placebo-controlled, phase 3 trial. Lancet Neurol 2018;17:35–46.
In this well-designed trial, subcutaneous immunoglobulin administered weekly at doses of 0.2 g/kg or 0.4 g/kg, showed that both doses were efficacious for maintenance treatment of CIDP.

Neuromuscular Transmission Disorders

Jayashri Srinivasan

68

Myasthenia Gravis

Allison Crowell, Ted M. Burns, Kelly G. Gwathmey

CLINICAL VIGNETTE *A 65-year-old previously healthy man presented to the emergency department for several months of progressive upper extremity weakness and blurry vision. He reports that over the past 3 months, playing the violin and mowing the lawn have become more difficult because the longer he does these activities, the weaker his arms become. His hands and forearms still feel strong. His brother accompanies him and has noticed that in the evenings his eyelids seem to droop more. The drooping worsens the more he blinks. He also feels short of breath when lying flat. He was admitted to the neurology service for further workup. Respiratory parameters were monitored throughout his hospital course and remained stable. Neurologic exam was significant for asymmetric, right greater than left ptosis, significant eye closure and cheek puff weakness, and fatigable weakness of proximal upper and lower extremities. On electromyography, repetitive stimulation of the spinal accessory muscle demonstrated a reproducible, 30% decrement in compound muscle action potential amplitudes.*

He was treated with intravenous immunoglobulins for presumed myasthenia gravis with improvement in his ptosis and proximal muscle weakness. Chest computerized tomography (CT) did not reveal a thymoma or thymic hyperplasia. He was started on prednisone and pyridostigmine. He presented to clinic 1 month later in follow-up at which point his acetylcholine receptor antibodies had returned to positive. His prednisone dose was increased due to continued symptoms and he was started on a steroid-sparing immunosuppressive therapy with mycophenolate mofetil.

ETIOLOGY AND PATHOPHYSIOLOGY

Myasthenia gravis (MG) is caused by autoantibodies directed against components of the postsynaptic neuromuscular junction (NMJ). The loss of large numbers of functional acetylcholine receptors (AChRs) decreases the number of muscle fibers that can depolarize during motor nerve activation, resulting in reduced muscle fiber action potentials and muscle fiber contraction. Failure of neuromuscular transmission results in clinical weakness when it affects large numbers of muscle fibers (Fig. 68.1). The most common cause of acquired MG (approximately 85%) results from the development of autoantibodies directed to the nicotinic AChR on the postsynaptic membrane. AChRs are composed of five protein chains (2 α, β, ϵ, and δ) that are arranged in a transmembrane ion channel that crosses the postsynaptic cell membrane (Fig. 68.2). Anti-AChR autoantibodies target the α subunit, which has binding sites for acetylcholine. Another target for autoantibodies in MG is the muscle-specific tyrosine kinase (MuSK) postsynaptic protein. MuSK anchors the AChR to the postjunctional membrane. Anti-MuSK antibodies are found in approximately 5%–7% of all MG patients. Several more antibody targets have been recently discovered in MG patients who are seronegative to both AChR and MuSK. These include autoantibodies against low-density lipoprotein receptor-related protein 4 (LRP4), agrin, and cortactin. LRP4 is a receptor for agrin and MuSK. The binding of LRP4 to agrin increases agrin's affinity for MuSK. This protein complex in turn activates and clusters AChRs at the NMJ. Additionally, MuSK anchors acetylcholinesterase at the synaptic basal lamina. Cortactin acts downstream of the agrin/MuSK complex to promote AChR clustering. Antibodies to titin and ryanodine receptors have also been identified; their clinical significance is still under investigation (Fig. 68.3).

The AChR autoantibodies disrupt neuromuscular transmission in one of three ways: (1) complement-mediated activation that leads to destruction of the postsynaptic membrane, (2) endocytosis of the AChR, and (3) less commonly, direct blockage of the ACh binding site. The loss of functional AChRs in this way decreases the number of muscle fibers that can depolarize, resulting in decreased generation of muscle fiber action potentials and subsequent muscle contraction. This leads to functional muscle weakness.

The thymus gland is an immune system organ that generates many naive T cells and clearly plays a role in the pathogenesis of MG. Patients can have follicular hyperplasia or thymomas, and the presence of either has implications for the progression and treatment of the disease. Thymomatous MG is typically more severe and requires thymectomy (Fig. 68.4).

CLINICAL PRESENTATION

MG is classified as generalized, ocular, neonatal, congenital, or drug-induced based on the distribution of clinical symptoms, serology, thymic status, and age of onset. The most common initial presentation of MG is diplopia and/or ptosis. Within 1–2 years, more generalized weakness develops in 85%–90% of patients. If bulbar or generalized weakness does not develop during the first 2 years, further progression to generalized MG is significantly less likely, and these patients are classified as having ocular MG (OMG). The hallmark of MG is fluctuating and fatigable weakness that is worse at the end of the day and during or following exercise (Fig. 68.5). Patients will improve with rest, and symptoms often worsen throughout the day. Proximal muscle groups are most commonly affected and patients have increasing difficulty lifting their arms overhead or climbing stairs as the disease progresses. Neck extension weakness can lead to difficulty in holding one's head upright. Facial weakness manifests as weakness of eye and mouth closure, resulting in an expressionless face. Clinically, ptosis often begins asymmetrically and can be elicited with sustained upgaze. With sustained horizontal gaze, ocular weakness manifests as disconjugate eye movements and reported diplopia. Pupillary responses are always normal, in contrast to other disorders of neuromuscular transmission such as botulism. Bulbar symptoms manifest as swallowing weakness (dysphagia) that may not be present at the beginning of the meal but may develop during the course of the meal, particularly when eating foods that are

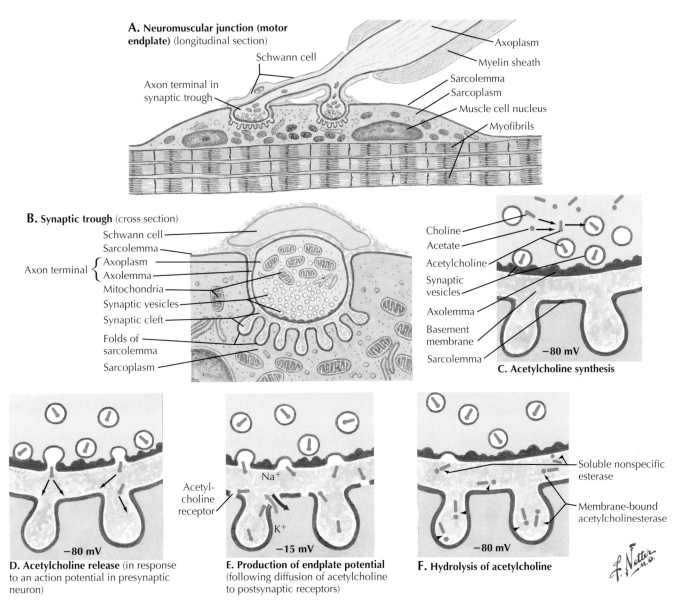

A. Neuromuscular junction (motor endplate) (longitudinal section)

Schwann cell

Axon terminal in synaptic trough

Axoplasm

Myelin sheath

Sarcolemma

Sarcoplasm

Muscle cell nucleus

Myofibrils

B. Synaptic trough (cross section)

Schwann cell

Sarcolemma

Axon terminal { Axoplasm / Axolemma

Mitochondria

Synaptic vesicles

Synaptic cleft

Folds of sarcolemma

Sarcoplasm

Choline

Acetate

Acetylcholine

Synaptic vesicles

Axolemma

Basement membrane

Sarcolemma

−80 mV

C. Acetylcholine synthesis

Acetylcholine receptor

Na⁺

K⁺

−80 mV

D. Acetylcholine release (in response to an action potential in presynaptic neuron)

−15 mV

E. Production of endplate potential (following diffusion of acetylcholine to postsynaptic receptors)

Soluble nonspecific esterase

Membrane-bound acetylcholinesterase

−80 mV

F. Hydrolysis of acetylcholine

Fig. 68.1 Somatic Neuromuscular Transmission.

difficult to chew. Other bulbar symptoms include nasal dysarthria or slurred speech, in which the patient's voice becomes softer with a breathy "twang" with prolonged talking. Respiratory failure is rare in isolation and often accompanies other bulbar signs and symptoms. Respiratory muscle involvement can lead to hypoventilation and is potentially life threatening. When a patient develops respiratory failure, he or she is considered to be in "crisis."

Weakness may progress over weeks to months. MG exacerbations are common and can be precipitated by a number of factors. Hot weather, concurrent infection or illness, and pregnancy are all potential exacerbating factors. Many medications that function at the NMJ (e.g., antibiotics such as aminoglycosides) may exacerbate and even precipitate incipient MG. Myasthenic crisis, the frequency of which is higher in MuSK-positive patients, may lead to respiratory failure, requiring ventilation and aggressive treatment with plasmapheresis, intravenous immunoglobulin (IVIg), and corticosteroids. Although mortality from MG used to be common (40%–50%), the development of immunomodulatory therapies and more effective respiratory support has decreased the mortality rate to 5%–14%. Most patients will improve after the first 1–2 years and only 4% of patients worsen.

The various underlying autoantibodies that cause MG can have implications in the clinical presentation. For instance, MuSK-positive MG can look indistinguishable from AChR-positive MG or can have a craniobulbar distribution with weakness, atrophy, and fasciculations that predominantly affects the neck, shoulders, and tongue.

CLINICAL VIGNETTE *A 35-year-old African American woman presented to the clinic for a second opinion regarding her long-standing history of dysarthria and diplopia. Her symptoms first began in her 20s and fluctuate throughout the day but are primarily worse in the evening hours. Her speech has developed a nasal tone and she often develops blurry or double vision later in the day. She has previously had negative acetylcholine receptor antibody testing but repetitive nerve stimulation testing of the ulnar nerve demonstrated a compound muscle action potential amplitude decrement greater than 10%. Her neurologic exam is significant for fatigable ptosis, diplopia after prolonged lateral gaze, primarily lower facial weakness, and neck flexion weakness.*

Over the course of several years, she has been admitted to the hospital for worsening respiratory distress and dysarthria, consistent with myasthenia

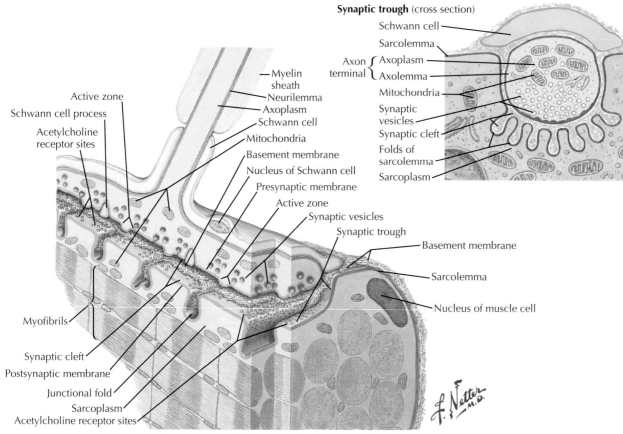

Synaptic trough (cross section)

Schwann cell
Sarcolemma
Axon terminal — Axoplasm
Axolemma
Mitochondria
Synaptic vesicles
Synaptic cleft
Folds of sarcolemma
Sarcoplasm

Active zone
Schwann cell process
Acetylcholine receptor sites

Myelin sheath
Neurilemma
Axoplasm
Schwann cell
Mitochondria
Basement membrane
Nucleus of Schwann cell
Presynaptic membrane
Active zone
Synaptic vesicles
Synaptic trough

Basement membrane
Sarcolemma
Nucleus of muscle cell

Myofibrils
Synaptic cleft
Postsynaptic membrane
Junctional fold
Sarcoplasm
Acetylcholine receptor sites

Fig. 68.2 Neuromuscular Neurotransmission.

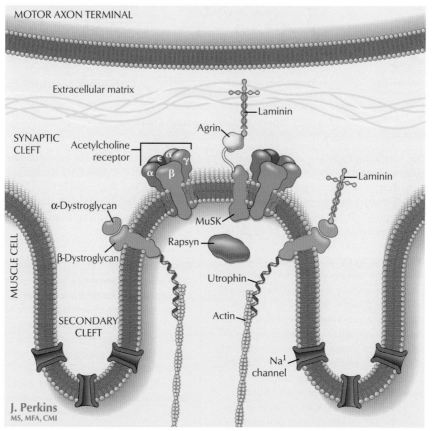

MOTOR AXON TERMINAL

Extracellular matrix
Laminin
Agrin
SYNAPTIC CLEFT
Acetylcholine receptor
ε α α
α β γ
Laminin
α-Dystroglycan
MuSK
Rapsyn
β-Dystroglycan
MUSCLE CELL
Utrophin
Actin
SECONDARY CLEFT
Na^1 channel

J. Perkins
MS, MFA, CMI

Schematic representation of the normal neuromuscular junction, adult acetylcholine receptor in the postsynaptic muscle membrane and other important associated proteins.

Fig. 68.3 Acetylcholine Receptor and Neuromuscular Junction. *MuSK,* Muscle-specific tyrosine kinase.

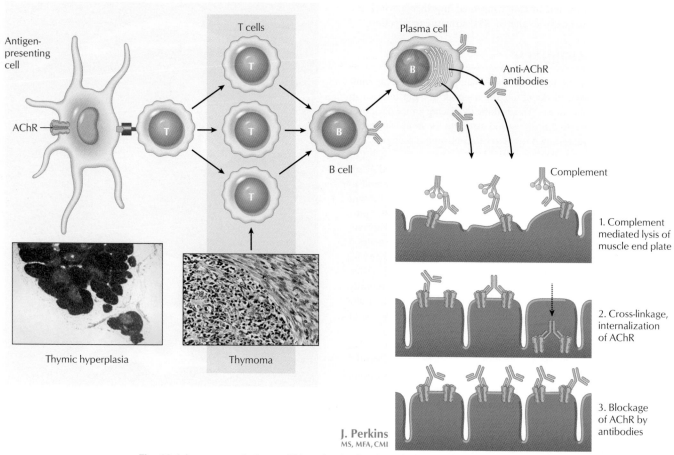

Fig. 68.4 Immunopathology of Myasthenia Gravis. *AChR,* Acetylcholine receptors

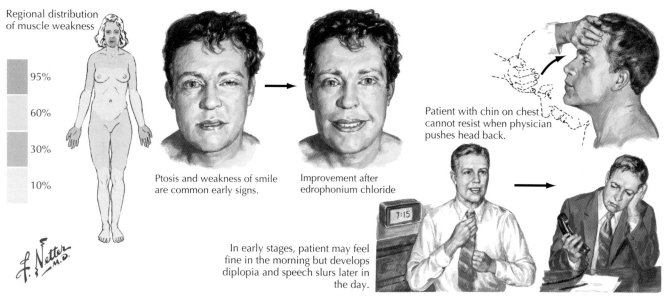

Fig. 68.5 Myasthenia Gravis: Clinical Manifestation.

gravis (MG) crisis. She was treated with plasma exchange with good response. Prednisone was initially very effective but had to be discontinued due to side effects of worsening anxiety and suicidal ideations. Muscle-specific tyrosine kinase (MuSK) antibody testing was eventually performed and confirmed the diagnosis of MuSK-positive MG. Given her MuSK positivity, she was started on rituximab with excellent response.

Overall, women are more likely to develop the disease than men. Peak symptom onset in women develops in the second or third decade; symptoms in men more commonly present in the fifth or sixth decade. Women with MG have a 15%–20% chance of having a child with neonatal MG. The infant has transient weakness, poor suck, and respiratory compromise that lasts for a few months and is due to transplacental transfer of AChR antibodies. Transient neonatal myasthenia should be differentiated from the uncommon congenital myasthenia, which is a genetic condition arising from altered NMJ structure or function.

DIAGNOSTIC APPROACH

The patient's history and neurologic examination should raise the clinical suspicion for MG. In the clinic, the ice pack test can be used in patients with fatigable ptosis. This is done by placing an ice pack over the affected eye for 2 to 5 minutes and assessing for improvement in the ptosis. Additional testing is necessary to confirm the diagnosis. The first step in confirming the diagnosis is by testing for serum AChR or MuSK antibodies. Some seronegative patients will have clustered AChR antibodies detectable only on cell-based assay. These patients tend to be younger and have a milder form of the disease. Eighty-five percent of patients with generalized MG will have positive serum AChR antibodies. Approximately 50% of purely ocular MG patients will have positive AChR antibodies. Another 5%–7% of patients with generalized MG have MuSK antibodies. Notably, 15% of initially seronegative MG patients will have AChR antibodies upon repeat testing 12 months later. The LRP4 antibody is now commercially available. The other recently discovered antibodies (agrin and cortactin) do not yet have commercially available testing and may account for many of the remaining 8% of generalized MG patients who are "seronegative."

The hallmark electrodiagnostic finding of MG is the presence of an electrodecremental response of the compound muscle action potential (CMAP) amplitude during slow (i.e., 2- or 3-Hz) repetitive motor nerve stimulation. In unaffected individuals, inherent functional reserve in neuromuscular transmission usually enables preservation of the CMAP amplitude during repetitive stimulation. However, in MG, the loss of functional AChRs can result in a decrement of at least 10% between the first and fourth CMAP amplitudes on repetitive stimulation. Repetitive stimulations of the ulnar, spinal accessory, and occasionally facial nerve are conducted. If these studies are normal, then proceeding to single-fiber electromyography (EMG) may be indicated. Single-fiber EMG is a technically more demanding test of NMJ function that records single muscle fiber discharges. The patient is asked to voluntarily activate the muscle until a suitable pair of muscle fiber action potentials belonging to the same motor unit is found. In MG, the variation in time interval between individual muscle fibers firing, or jitter, is increased. If neuromuscular transmission is significantly impaired, there may be intermittent blocking of neuromuscular transmission. Single-fiber EMG has a sensitivity of more than 90% in the diagnosis of both ocular and generalized MG.

Once MG is diagnosed, all patients should undergo imaging of the mediastinum to evaluate for the presence of a thymoma or thymic hyperplasia. A computerized tomography (CT) scan with contrast is the imaging modality of choice. Ten to 15% of MG patients have thymomas; these may be benign (75%–90%) or malignant thymic tumors (Fig. 68.6). Of those patients without thymomas, 70% have thymic lymphoid follicular hyperplasia.

TREATMENT

The treatment of MG is an ever-expanding field, and new developments have led to improved outcomes and longer-term survival for patients. With more and more therapeutic options, the treatment approach should be tailored to the individual patient. The first breakthrough in the treatment of MG came in the mid-1930s with the discovery and widespread use of the anticholinesterase (AChE) inhibitor, pyridostigmine. Pyridostigmine works by decreasing the rate of breakdown of ACh at the NMJ. It is usually started at 30–60 mg orally every 6–8 hours and can be titrated up to clinical effectiveness. However, doses of more than

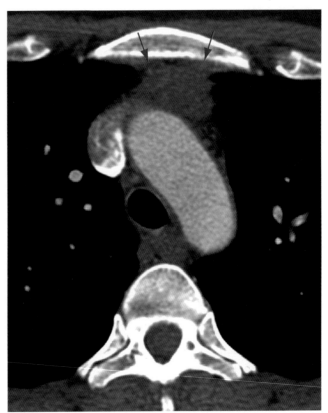

Axial CT scan of upper chest demonstrates a soft tissue mass anterior to the enhancing aorta (arrows).

Fig. 68.6 Thymoma.

120 mg every 3–4 hours can cause a paradoxical cholinergic crisis, in which patients develop worsening weakness, salivation, abdominal cramping, diarrhea, and muscle fasciculations. AChE inhibitors are typically less effective in MuSK-positive patients. AChE therapy does not treat the underlying autoimmune mediated process, and thus, most patients with MG require some form of immunosuppressive or immunomodulatory therapy to adequately treat the disease.

Corticosteroids are the initial immunosuppressant of choice. Oral prednisone is often effective in achieving remission or, at the very least, considerably improving symptoms. However, oral steroids can lead to a paradoxical worsening of MG symptoms several days after the initiation of therapy. Therefore, the initial titration of steroids has to be dictated by the patient's current clinical status. In critically ill patients who are hospitalized, it is reasonable to start higher doses (40–60 mg daily) because they can be closely monitored for deterioration. In patients who are clinically stable and being treated as an outpatient, neurologists tend to start at low doses (10–20 mg daily) and gradually increase by 10 mg every 3–4 days until reaching maximal doses (40–80 mg). Once MG patients achieve remission for 1–2 months, prednisone is gradually tapered to reduce the deleterious effects of long-term corticosteroid use, such as aseptic necrosis of the femoral head, osteoporosis, diabetes mellitus, cataracts, depression, and emotional lability. The mean response time to maximum benefit is 5 to 9 months. Successful dose reduction correlates with a slower rate of taper and higher final dose of steroid.

There are several steroid-sparing agents that are used in the treatment of MG to target the underlying abnormal immune response. These include azathioprine, mycophenolate mofetil, methotrexate, cyclophosphamide, cyclosporine, tacrolimus, and rituximab. They serve as steroid-sparing agents but have a significant latency for therapeutic effect. Therefore, they are introduced in addition to corticosteroids so that eventually the corticosteroids can be gradually decreased while long-term immunosuppression is maintained with these agents.

Azathioprine and mycophenolate mofetil have long been used as first-line immunosuppressive therapy in MG. Azathioprine works by nonspecifically preventing B- and T-cell proliferation by reducing nucleic acid synthesis. Typical dosing is 100–150 mg/day. It is generally a well-tolerated medication and common side effects include leukopenia and flulike reaction. Mycophenolate mofetil works by impairing purine synthesis and thereby suppressing B- and T-cell proliferation. It is typically prescribed as 1000–1500 mg twice daily and is also generally well tolerated. Clinical effectiveness is delayed with the use of either medication and optimal benefit may require up to 1 year of continued administration.

Other immunosuppressive medications that are used in MG include cyclosporine, tacrolimus, methotrexate, and cyclophosphamide. There is some retrospective and limited clinical trial evidence to support the efficacy of each of these and this is an active area of research. Tacrolimus is considered an alternative second-line choice for patients with moderate to severe MG but the benefit seems to be less robust in patients with relatively stable disease. Cyclophosphamide and cyclosporine are typically reserved for third-line therapy as they both have significant side-effect profiles. A recent prospective, randomized controlled trial did not demonstrate any steroid-sparing benefit of methotrexate after 12 months. This study and the mycophenolate mofetil trials have emphasized that study design in MG is challenging. Patients improve on prednisone alone, outcome measures must be standardized, and an understanding of responsiveness across outcome measures is mandatory.

Both plasma exchange and IVIg are used for the acutely ill patient with MG exacerbation or crisis. They are also used for symptom optimization prior to thymectomy or other planned surgical procedures. Rarely, they can be used as maintenance therapy in patients with refractory disease. Both therapies are thought to be equally effective; therefore, the decision between the two is made based on the patient's comorbidities, cost, and potential side effects. Plasma exchange removes AChR antibodies from blood and produces rapid but transient clinical improvement. It is classically prescribed as alternate day dosing for four to six exchanges. Potential side effects include hypotension, infection, thrombotic complications, and bleeding tendencies. IVIgs are pooled polyclonal IgG from donors and have antiinflammatory and immunomodulatory effects with demonstrable clinical improvement in 5–10 days after the start of therapy. Patients typically receive 2 g/kg in divided doses over 2 to 5 days. Common side effects are related to infusion reactions and include fever, nausea, and headache but more serious adverse effects, including aseptic meningitis, thrombotic events, and renal failure, are also possible.

In those patients with refractory disease, rituximab has been shown in a meta-analysis of observational studies to provide significant benefit. Rituximab is a chimeric monoclonal antibody that targets the B-cell–surface CD20 antigen, which interferes with B-cell activation, differentiation, and growth. Although it has been suggested that rituximab is more effective in MuSK-positive MG, the immunomodulatory effect has been demonstrated in a meta-analysis of observational studies to provide efficacy in more than 80% of patients with MG, regardless of which antibody was positive. Although the onset of action is slower than IVIg or plasma exchange, the effect can last anywhere from 6 months to 5 years. The most common side effects are infusion reactions (nausea, fever, or hypotension). Progressive multifocal leukoencephalopathy (PML) is also a potential complication. Additional prospective, randomized studies of rituximab in MG are ongoing. In 2017, the US Food and Drug Administration approved a new medication, eculizumab,

for use in patients with refractory, generalized, AChR antibody-positive MG who have failed first-line treatments. Eculizumab is a humanized monoclonal antibody directed against the terminal complement protein C5, disrupting the terminal complement cascade. Though meningococcal disease is a potential, severe risk, appropriate pretreatment vaccination has mitigated this risk greatly. Cost is one of the biggest barriers in the use of eculizumab.

The use of thymectomy for MG dates back to the late 1930s. In the 10%–15% of patients with identified thymoma, the recommendation is to undergo thymectomy regardless of age because up to 25% of thymomas are malignant. In nonthymomatous AChR-positive patients, thymectomy is now recommended in those under age 65 and can lead to higher rates of symptomatic improvement, pharmacologic remission, and survival, particularly in patients with moderate to severe disease burden. The role of thymectomy in seronegative and MuSK- or LRP4-antibody–positive MG remains uncertain. Symptomatic improvement after thymectomy may take up to 1 to 2 years.

The treatment approach to OMG is generally more cautious than that of generalized MG because the symptoms of OMG are not life threatening. However, OMG can cause significant disability and should be weighed against the risks and benefits of medications. When symptoms are manageable, it may be best to defer treatment until they become functionally debilitating. It is reasonable to try pyridostigmine, though this is often ineffective in OMG. Prednisone is often very effective and a low starting dose with a slow titration can successfully achieve the lowest effective dose, thereby minimizing side effects of long-term corticosteroid use. If prednisone alone does not provide optimal benefit, other steroid-sparing immunosuppressants, with or without steroids, can be considered.

FUTURE DIRECTIONS

The future of research in the field of MG lies in the identification of other autoantibodies that can be implicated in the disease process. This will primarily have consequences for those few patients with refractory disease that is less amenable to current immunomodulatory strategies. In this way, we can better understand the exact mechanism of disease for individual patients and use this information to tailor the modulation of the immune system in more specific ways. This will lead to more effective long-term treatment strategies and will hopefully reduce exacerbations, episodes of crisis, and the potential for negative consequences related to systemic immunosuppression.

ADDITIONAL RESOURCES

Howard JF Jr. Electrodiagnosis of disorders of neuromuscular transmission. Phys Med Rehabil Clin N Am 2013;24(1):169–92.

Iorio R, Damato V, Alboini PE, et al. Efficacy and safety of rituximab for myasthenia gravis: a systematic review and meta-analysis. J Neurol 2015;262(5):1115–19.

Oger J, Frykman H. An update on laboratory diagnosis in myasthenia gravis. Clin Chim Acta 2015;449:43–8.

Sanders DB, Wolfe GI, Benatar M, et al. International consensus guidance for management of myasthenia gravis: executive summary. Neurology 2016;87(4):419–25.

This is an international consensus statement created by 15 myasthenia experts to guide clinicians who care for myasthenia gravis patients.

Silvestri NJ, Wolfe GI. Treatment-refractory myasthenia gravis. J Clin Neuromuscul Dis 2014;15(4):167–78.

Wolfe GI, Kaminski HJ, Aban IB, et al. Randomized trial of thymectomy in myasthenia gravis. N Engl J Med 2016;375(6):511–22.

69

Other Neuromuscular Transmission Disorders

Allison Crowell, Ted M. Burns, Kelly G. Gwathmey

LAMBERT-EATON MYASTHENIC SYNDROME

CLINICAL VIGNETTE *A 61-year-old woman with no remarkable past medical history developed, over a few months, weakness of her legs with difficulty getting in and out of chairs and climbing stairs. She also experienced significant fatigue. This persisted for 6 months, and then, she developed dysarthria, mild dysphagia, blurred vision, and mild proximal upper extremity weakness. She also endured dry eyes and dry mouth for nearly 1 year.*

Examination was remarkable for normal cranial nerves. On motor exam, she had moderate weakness of neck flexion and hip flexion. Reflexes were trace and symmetric at the biceps, triceps, brachioradialis, patella, and Achilles bilaterally, and became easier to elicit after 10 seconds of maximal contraction of the muscle. Gait exam was normal.

Repetitive nerve stimulation testing of the right median and ulnar nerves demonstrated low-amplitude compound muscle action potential amplitudes, which was facilitated following 10 seconds of isometric exercise. Acetylcholine receptor and muscle specific tyrosine kinase antibodies were negative. Voltage-gated calcium channel antibodies were found to be elevated. Computed tomography (CT) of the chest was unremarkable. ^{18}F-fluorodeoxyglucose positron-emission tomography (FDG-PET) was normal.

The patient is now 3 years out from her symptom onset and has not developed any malignancy. She has been receiving 3,4-diaminopyridine and has improved dramatically. Her examination is now normal.

Lambert-Eaton myasthenic syndrome (LEMS) is the most common presynaptic neuromuscular transmission disorder in adults with an annual incidence of approximately 0.5×10^{-6}. It has a 10 times lower annual incidence rate than myasthenia gravis, the most common postsynaptic neuromuscular transmission disorder. Roughly 50% of LEMS patients will have an underlying malignancy, which is usually small cell lung cancer (SCLC). Those without malignancy are presumed to have a sporadic autoimmune etiology. Both paraneoplastic and nonparaneoplastic forms are associated with the P/Q type voltage-gated calcium channel (VGCC) antibodies. Other antibodies to presynaptic proteins that have been associated with LEMS include ERC1, synaptotagmin I, laminin β2, and presynaptic muscarinic acetylcholine receptor. SOX-1 antibodies have been identified in the majority of paraneoplastic LEMS patients, but are not associated with nonparaneoplastic LEMS. The age of disease onset varies between the paraneoplastic and nonparaneoplastic LEMS. In the paraneoplastic form, the average age of onset is 60 years. There is a bimodal peak of incidence for the nonparaneoplastic form with one peak at approximately 35 years and a second peak around 60 years. LEMS often precedes tumor detection in the paraneoplastic form.

The immune response producing LEMS begins early in the tumor evolution.

Etiology and Pathophysiology

The neuromuscular junction is composed of the presynaptic nerve terminal, junctional cleft, and the postsynaptic muscle endplate, which houses the acetylcholine receptors (Fig. 69.1). When an action potential propagates down the motor axon to the motor nerve terminus, depolarization opens the VGCC, resulting in an influx of calcium into the presynaptic membrane. The VGCC are heteromeric multisubunit complexes that are composed of Ca^{2+} selective pore-forming α1 subunit, a largely extracellular α2δ subunit, an intracellular β subunit, and sometimes a γ subunit. The autoantibodies target multiple VGCC subunits including α and β subunits. Sometimes the α2δ subunit is also targeted but not in isolation. The intracellular calcium binds to calmodulin and activates calcium-dependent signaling pathways, which mobilizes acetylcholine vesicles from "active zones" into the synaptic cleft. The acetylcholine binds to the acetylcholine receptors, which causes sodium and potassium movement across the endplate membrane. When the endplate potential depolarizes and reaches the threshold, a muscle fiber action potential is initiated causing muscle contraction. In LEMS, antibodies block the P/Q subtype of VGCC preventing calcium influx and less acetylcholine vesicles are released from motor and autonomic cholinergic nerve terminals. There is a lower probability of reaching the endplate depolarization threshold and generating a muscle fiber action potential.

VGCCs are expressed on SCLC and other cancer cells in addition to the presynaptic motor nerve terminal membrane. These channels present in SCLC tumor cells have antigenic potential and stimulate autoantibody production. In nonparaneoplastic LEMS patients, nearly 65% will have the HLA-B8-DR3 haplotype. Ten to 15% of patients with LEMS do not have detectable P/Q-type VGCC antibodies. These seronegative patients have clinical and electrophysiologic features that are indistinguishable from seropositive patients.

Clinical Presentation

LEMS has a similar presentation regardless of the presence of an underlying malignancy (Fig. 69.2). The clinical triad in LEMS is proximal muscle weakness, autonomic dysfunction, and areflexia. The most common presenting symptom is leg weakness followed by generalized weakness, muscle pain or stiffness, and dry mouth. Rarely, patients present with arm weakness, diplopia, or dysarthria. Some patients have no detectable weakness on exam on manual motor testing. The physician must rely on history of impaired function or evidence of difficulty rising from a chair or climbing stairs. Patients often have severe fatigue. The majority of patients with LEMS will develop autonomic dysfunction

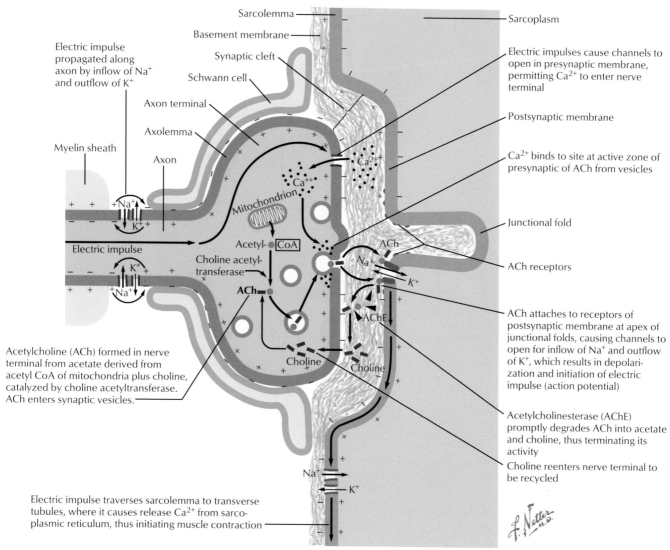

Sarcolemma — Sarcoplasm

Basement membrane

Synaptic cleft

Schwann cell

Axon terminal

Axolemma

Myelin sheath

Axon

Electric impulse propagated along axon by inflow of Na+ and outflow of K+

Electric impulse

Mitochondrion

Acetyl-CoA

Choline acetyltransferase

ACh

Ca++

Ca2+

Na+

ACh

K+

AChE

Choline

Choline

Electric impulses cause channels to open in presynaptic membrane, permitting Ca2+ to enter nerve terminal

Postsynaptic membrane

Ca2+ binds to site at active zone of presynaptic of ACh from vesicles

Junctional fold

ACh receptors

ACh attaches to receptors of postsynaptic membrane at apex of junctional folds, causing channels to open for inflow of Na+ and outflow of K+, which results in depolarization and initiation of electric impulse (action potential)

Acetylcholinesterase (AChE) promptly degrades ACh into acetate and choline, thus terminating its activity

Choline reenters nerve terminal to be recycled

Acetylcholine (ACh) formed in nerve terminal from acetate derived from acetyl CoA of mitochondria plus choline, catalyzed by choline acetyltransferase. ACh enters synaptic vesicles.

Na+

K+

Electric impulse traverses sarcolemma to transverse tubules, where it causes release Ca2+ from sarcoplasmic reticulum, thus initiating muscle contraction

Fig. 69.1 Physiology of the Neuromuscular Junction.

including dry mouth, blurred vision, hypohidrosis, constipation, and orthostatic hypotension. Dry mouth is the most common autonomic symptom. Deep tendon reflexes are classically diminished. In nearly half of patients, diminished reflexes will facilitate and become more pronounced following brief exercise. Respiratory symptoms are unusual but may occur later in the disease course. Interestingly, some patients with LEMS will complain of vague sensory symptoms such as numbness and tingling.

The primary diagnosis considered in the differential for LEMS is myasthenia gravis. In contrast to LEMS patients who present with leg weakness, most myasthenic patients will first develop ocular symptoms, including diplopia and ptosis. In LEMS, the weakness typically spreads rostrally, whereas weakness in myasthenia spreads caudally. The reduction in reflexes and autonomic dysfunction are also distinctive features of LEMS. Because LEMS typically presents with proximal weakness, this may simulate a myopathy. Myopathic patients would not typically have areflexia or autonomic dysregulation. LEMS may mimic chronic inflammatory demyelinating polyradiculoneuropathy (CIDP) given the weakness and areflexia. The absence of sensory involvement and presence of autonomic dysfunction differentiates LEMS from CIDP.

Diagnostic Approach

Serologic testing in LEMS includes a creatine kinase and a paraneoplastic panel, which includes P/Q-type VGCC antibodies. Although nearly 90% of patients with LEMS will have P/Q-type VGCC antibodies, 10%–15% will remain seronegative. Up to 40% of SCLC patients will have P/Q-type VGCC antibodies without clinical or electrophysiologic evidence of LEMS. An evaluation for underlying malignancy is necessary with postcontrast computed tomography (CT) or magnetic resonance imaging (MRI) of the chest. Should these be negative, then an ^{18}F-fluorodeoxyglucose (FDG) positron emission tomography (PET) is recommended. Follow-up chest imaging is recommended for cancer surveillance in those patients with LEMS and a smoking history. Antibodies to SOX-1, which is a transcription factor in the SRY family of high-mobility group box proteins, has high specificity for SCLC. SOX-1 antibodies have been described in 67% of patients with paraneoplastic LEMS and only 5% of nonparaneoplastic LEMS.

Electrophysiologic testing is critical in the diagnosis of LEMS. There are three key findings: low-amplitude compound muscle action potentials (CMAPs) at rest, decrement of CMAP amplitude on slow (2–3 Hz) repetitive nerve stimulation, and postactivation facilitation

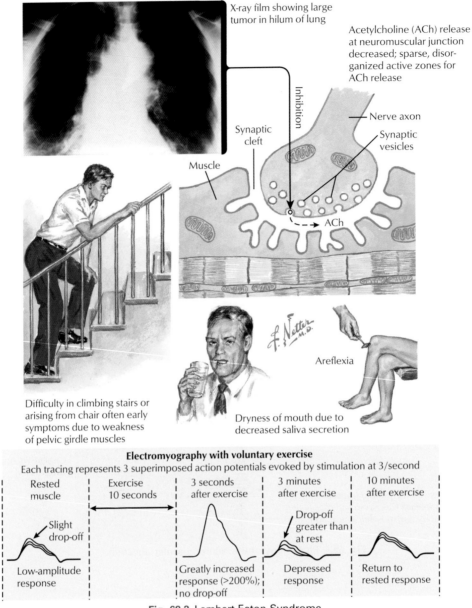

X-ray film showing large tumor in hilum of lung

Acetylcholine (ACh) release at neuromuscular junction decreased; sparse, disorganized active zones for ACh release

Inhibition

Nerve axon

Synaptic cleft

Synaptic vesicles

Muscle

ACh

Areflexia

Difficulty in climbing stairs or arising from chair often early symptoms due to weakness of pelvic girdle muscles

Dryness of mouth due to decreased saliva secretion

Electromyography with voluntary exercise
Each tracing represents 3 superimposed action potentials evoked by stimulation at 3/second

| Rested muscle | Exercise 10 seconds | 3 seconds after exercise | 3 minutes after exercise | 10 minutes after exercise |

Slight drop-off

Low-amplitude response

Greatly increased response (>200%); no drop-off

Drop-off greater than at rest

Depressed response

Return to rested response

Fig. 69.2 Lambert-Eaton Syndrome.

with an increase in CMAP amplitude by more than 100% following either high-frequency repetitive nerve stimulation or 10 seconds of voluntary isometric contraction. The electrophysiologic difference between a presynaptic and postsynaptic neuromuscular junction transmission disorder is the lack of facilitation of CMAP amplitude in those with postsynaptic disease (myasthenia gravis). The low-amplitude CMAPs on routine nerve conduction studies would also not typically be seen in myasthenia gravis. In both LEMS and myasthenia gravis, one would expect to see a decrement of the CMAP amplitude with low-frequency repetitive nerve stimulation testing. In myasthenia gravis, the decremental pattern decreases during a train of CMAPs, whereas in LEMS, the decremental pattern becomes progressively greater. Two or three muscles may be screened for facilitation, including abductor pollicis brevis, abductor digiti minimi, and extensor digitorum brevis muscles. Single-fiber EMG demonstrates increased jitter and blocking. Symptomatic management should be withdrawn 12 hours before electrophysiologic studies.

Treatment

The treatment of SCLC-associated and other paraneoplastic LEMS will differ from treatment of nonparaneoplastic LEMS. Treatment of the underlying malignancy with chemotherapy, radiation, and surgery will often result in symptomatic improvement of the LEMS. It is possible that using immunosuppressive therapies to treat paraneoplastic LEMS will allow the tumor to avoid normal immune-mediated suppression and promote its growth. In general, however, immunosuppressant medications are not contraindicated in LEMS patients.

Symptomatic treatment of LEMS is focused on improving neuromuscular transmission. Pyridostigmine, which is an anticholinesterase medication, blocks the breakdown of acetylcholine at the neuromuscular junction. Pyridostigmine is not as useful for LEMS as it is for myasthenia gravis, but is often initiated given that it is relatively benign. 3,4-Diaminopyridine (3,4-DAP), a potassium channel blocker, promotes the release of acetylcholine from the presynaptic nerve terminus by prolonging the time that the VGCC is open. Patients improve with regard to strength and autonomic dysfunction. The typical dose is 10 mg three times daily and the maximum response to treatment occurs 23 days after its initiation. The duration of effect lasts 4 hours. 3,4-DAP is available at present through Treatment Investigational New Drugs (IND) studies and carries an orphan drug designation. It is also available through expanded access programs and continues to be studied in phase 3 clinical trials. Amifampridine (3,4-DAP), which is a salt form of 3,4-DAP, has been demonstrated to have superior stability compared to the 3,4-DAP base, whose drug content is variable. Amifampridine has recently been demonstrated in a phase 3, double-blind randomized study of 38 patients to be efficacious in LEMS. One of the major side effects is central nervous system complications including seizures. 3,4-DAP and pyridostigmine, when used together, may have a synergistic effect.

Immunotherapy is used to modulate or suppress the immune system's response directed at the presynaptic neuromuscular junction. Various immunotherapies that have been used include corticosteroids, intravenous immunoglobulins, and plasmapheresis. These treatments are often used in those with sporadic autoimmune (nonparaneoplastic) LEMS. The treatment benefit of intravenous immunoglobulins and plasmapheresis is short-lived. Rituximab, which is a monoclonal antibody against B-lymphocytes, has also been used with short-term benefit. A combination of prednisone and azathioprine has been described as a long-term treatment approach.

Certain medications that impair neuromuscular transmission may exacerbate LEMS symptoms. These include aminoglycoside antibiotics, magnesium citrate, lithium, and quinine. Cardiac drugs including calcium channel blockers and antiarrhythmic agents such as procainamide and quinidine should be avoided.

The prognosis for paraneoplastic LEMS is worse than for nonparaneoplastic LEMS and depends on the stage of the malignancy. Most patients live only a few years. That said, as LEMS is often the initial manifestation of the malignancy, its identification may prompt earlier diagnosis and initiation of treatment. Those with nonparaneoplastic LEMS will often survive for more than 20 years out from diagnosis. They typically respond positively to immunomodulatory and symptomatic therapy.

Future Directions

In patients with nonparaneoplastic LEMS, the pathologic mechanism is not well understood. Further research in this area is needed to pave the way for discovery of effective symptomatic treatments. Because 10%–15% of patients with LEMS do not have identifiable P/Q-type VGCC antibodies, one must assume that other yet-to-be-discovered autoantibodies exist. Other nonpathogenic antibodies to neurotransmission-related molecules such as synaptotagmin have already been discovered. A novel Ca^{2+} channel agonist, GV-58, has been described as a possible alternative treatment strategy for LEMS. Its combination with 3,4-DAP in mouse models had a supra-additive effect that reversed the deficit in neurotransmitter release from the presynaptic junction. Compared to using either GV-58 or 3,4-DAP alone, the combination had a much more robust effect.

BOTULISM

Botulism is a rare and potentially lethal disease that is caused by release of the neurotoxin produced by the bacterium *Clostridium botulinum*. This toxin blocks the release of acetylcholine from the presynaptic junction, resulting in symmetric oculobulbar weakness followed by descending skeletal muscle weakness, respiratory compromise, and autonomic dysfunction. Infantile botulism is much more common than adult-onset botulism. Given the severity of disease, early identification can result in expedited treatment and improved outcomes.

CLINICAL VIGNETTE *A previously healthy 5-month-old girl was admitted to the hospital for hypotonia, dysphagia, and constipation. She had one loose stool 4 days prior and has had no stools since. Her mother denied exposure to honey, canned goods, or construction sites. Two days prior to symptom onset, she went to an indoor water park and played in the water. She presented to her pediatrician 3 days ago for difficulty swallowing, weak cry, and somnolence. Because she had noisy breathing and a hoarse voice, she was treated with ibuprofen and dexamethasone for possible croup and sent home. When she did not improve, she went to the emergency department for intravenous hydration. There she was noted to have low tone throughout her extremities, weak cry, and weak suck. She had diminished movement of her extremities and diminished reflexes. She was admitted to the pediatric intensive care unit given the potential for respiratory failure in the setting of possible infantile botulism. She was started on high-flow nasal cannula to maintain open airways. She was treated with intravenous human botulism immune globulin (BabyBIG). She slowly improved, regaining normal tone and cry. Her stools became more frequent. She was on nasogastric tube feeds for 9 days, and then, the nasogastric tube was removed the day before discharge. Stool test eventually resulted positive for Clostridium botulinum type B toxin.*

Etiology and Pathophysiology

The Centers for Disease Control and Prevention (CDC) has four categories of transmission of the botulinum toxin. They include infant, food-borne, wound, and other. The other category includes adult intestinal colonization and bioterrorism threat of aerosolized toxin via inhalation. Infantile botulism comprises about 75% of cases, food-borne botulism 15%, wound botulism 5%, and botulism from another or unknown causes 5%. Seven different serotypes of botulinum toxin (A–G) are known. The ubiquitous spores are found in the soil and water. In infantile botulism, the vast majority are caused by type A or type B toxin. The bacteria's propensity for infants is thought to be due to immature gut flora and inability to prevent colonization of *C. botulinum*. Food-borne botulism is typically in the setting of home-canned foods and fermented fish and other marine animals. There are numerous cases of food-borne botulism reported in Alaska on an annual basis. Usually, ingested spores of *C. botulinum* are excreted from the human intestine without germination or toxin production. Food-borne botulism is caused most often by toxin A (50%) and toxins B or E (each 25%). *C. botulinum* forms spores that resist regular cooking and food processing techniques. The toxin denatures at temperatures greater than 80° C but the spores can only be destroyed when exposed to temperatures greater than 120° C for several minutes. Wound botulism occurs most often in injection drug users and particularly in black tar heroin users. It occurs when traumatized tissue is contaminated by clostridial spores. Wound abscesses often form. Eighty percent of wound botulism is caused by toxin A and 20% by toxin B. The incubation period is between 4 and 14 days from the time of injury. Adults who are prone to developing botulism from gastrointestinal colonization often have disruption of their normal gut flora as a result of Crohn's disease, gastrointestinal surgery, or antibiotic treatment. There are approximately 110 cases of botulism reported to the CDC annually.

The pathophysiology of botulism is dysfunction at the presynaptic junction. When acetylcholine-filled vesicles fuse with the presynaptic terminal membrane, they rely on the fusion complex, which is made up of three soluble *N*-ethylmaleimide–sensitive factor attachment protein receptor (SNARE) proteins: syntaxin, synaptosomal-associated protein 25 (SNAP-25), and vesicle-associated membrane protein (VAMP, otherwise known as synaptobrevin). After the botulinum toxin is taken up in the presynaptic terminal, it cleaves to one of the SNARE proteins, disrupts formation of the fusion complex, and prevents acetylcholine release into the synaptic cleft. The toxin is then distributed by retrograde neuronal transport or hematogenously. The heavy chain of the toxin binds to either synaptotagmin-II or another protein resulting in endocytosis of the toxin into the presynaptic vesicles. Within the vesicles the disulfide bond, which connects the heavy and light chain, breaks. The light chain leaves the vesicle and enters the nerve terminal causing irreversible disruption of acetylcholine release by interacting with the SNARE complex of proteins. For function to be restored, a new terminal and synapses must form.

Clinical Presentation

The mechanism of transmission dictates the clinical presentation. Infantile botulism, the most common form of botulism, occurs in children between 1 and 6 months of age (Fig. 69.3). The classic exposures are contaminated soil (construction sites) or honey. Only 20% of US cases of infant botulism are caused by honey ingestion. All major pediatric

and public health organizations recommend against feeding honey to infants less than 12 months of age. The incubation period of infantile botulism is between 3 and 30 days following time of exposure. California has the highest reported incidence of infantile botulism. The clinical symptoms include bulbar symptoms (weak cry, difficulty feeding), sluggish pupillary reflexes, and weakness of extremity muscles. Fever is typically absent. Over days, children lose control of their head, become hypotonic, and have diminished spontaneous movements. Fatigability appreciated during repeated examinations is nearly pathognomonic. Similar to LEMS, autonomic dysfunction, in the form of urinary retention, dry mouth, tachycardia, and labile blood pressure, can occur. Constipation is a key clinical feature.

Food-borne botulism occurs following a 12- to 48-hour incubation period. Patients complain of blurred vision due to pupillary dilation. Half of all patients will have pupillary dilation. Similar to myasthenia gravis, they complain of ocular symptoms (diplopia and ptosis) and bulbar dysfunction (dysphagia and dysarthria). Symmetric descending weakness develops next. Gastrointestinal symptoms such as nausea,

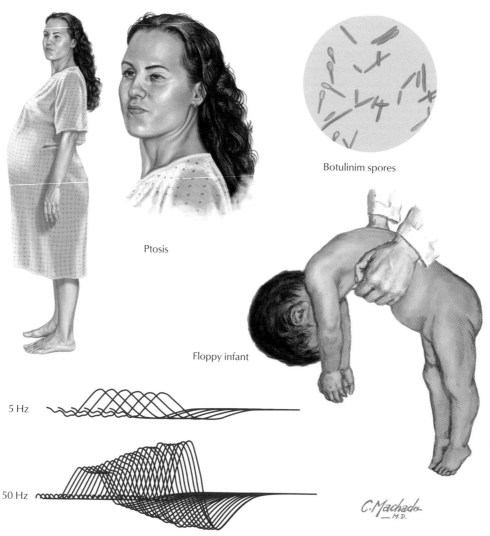

Botulinim spores

Ptosis

Floppy infant

5 Hz

50 Hz

Repetitive stimulation at 5 Hz of a hypotonic baby's ulnar nerve; recording at the hypothenar eminence demonstrates no facilitation or decrement in the response, whereas 50-Hz stimuli promotes an almost 100% facilitation in the eventual size of the recorded response. Facilitation on 50-Hz stimulation is the characteristic and diagnostic finding of a presynaptic defect in neuromuscular transmission as occurs with infantile botulism.

Fig. 69.3 Infantile Neuromuscular Junction (NMJ) Disorder.

vomiting, and diarrhea may be present. Autonomic dysfunction with decreased tearing and salivation are often present. Patients will have fluctuating heart rate and blood pressure. Intestinal dysmotility and bladder atony are common. As *C. botulinum* toxin does not cross the blood-brain barrier, mentation is preserved. In severe intoxication, respiratory weakness ensues and mechanical ventilation is often necessary. Early detection can result in supportive treatment, administration of the antitoxin, and decreased mortality. Food-borne botulism is fatal in 10% of all worldwide cases.

Diagnostic Approach

A thorough clinical history including timing of progression of neurologic symptoms and change in bowel habits should alert the physician to the possibility of botulism. In infantile botulism, stool samples are sent for identification of spores. These spores take at least 6 days to grow, and it takes another 1 to 4 days to detect the toxin. In infantile botulism, the serum toxin is only detectable early in the course of the illness. Therefore, stool samples are preferred specimens for culture and toxin assay. Given that many infants have constipation, a sterile water enema can be used to collect the sample. With food-borne botulism, the toxin can be detected in the serum using a mouse neutralization assay, which remains the most sensitive and specific test available. The serum and stool can also be cultured for bacteria. All specimens should be collected and tested before the antitoxin is administered.

Electrodiagnostic studies may help to confirm the diagnosis. The motor nerve conduction studies will be abnormal with low-amplitude CMAPs, a decremental response to slow repetitive nerve stimulation testing, and facilitation of at least 20% following either high-frequency repetitive nerve stimulation testing or 10 seconds of isometric exercise. In contrast to LEMS, the facilitation will persist for up to 40 minutes. Single-fiber EMG demonstrates increased jitter and blocking.

Treatment

Close monitoring with intensive supportive care is necessary as respiratory failure is a primary cause of death. For patients older than 1 year, there is an equine-derived antitoxin available. For children younger than 1 year, there is human-derived botulism immunoglobulin (BabyBIG). The antitoxin should be administrated immediately. The use of these antitoxins shortens hospitalization, length of mechanical ventilation, and duration of parenteral or tube feeding and results in improved outcomes. The equine-derived antitoxin is not administered to infants because of the risk of serum sickness, anaphylaxis, and possible sensitization to equine proteins. The antitoxins neutralize the toxins circulating in the blood but do not reverse the damage at the neuromuscular junction. Nerve terminal regeneration is necessary for recovery. Most infants recover fully, although it may occur over many months. In contrast to other forms of botulism, antibiotics should be used in wound botulism. Additionally the wound should be debrided.

Future Directions

At present, there are new in vitro assays to detect the presence of botulinum toxin that are in development to replace the mouse neutralization bioassay. In one method, human induced pluripotent stem cell–derived neurons and the enzyme-linked immunosorbent assay (ELISA) technique are used to determine SNAP-25 cleavage by botulinum toxin following toxin exposure. Another novel botulinum toxin detection assay uses mouse embryonic stem cell–derived neurons cultured on multielectrode arrays.

ADDITIONAL RESOURCES

Antoine JC, Camdessanché JP. Treatment options in paraneoplastic disorders of the peripheral nervous system. Curr Treat Options Neurol 2013;15(2):210–23.

This is a nice review of the medications used to treat paraneoplastic neurologic syndromes including Lambert-Eaton myasthenic syndrome. The dosage, contraindications, and drug interactions are discussed.

Oh SJ, Shcherbakova N, Kostera-Pruszczyk A, et al. Amifampridine phosphate (Firdapse®) is effective and safe in a phase 3 clinical trial in LEMS. Muscle Nerve 2016;53(5):707–25.

Phase 3 clinical trial demonstrating efficacy of amifampridine, a salt form of 3,4-DAP, in Lambert-Eaton myasthenic syndrome.

Rosow LK, Strober JB. Infant botulism: review and clinical update. Pediatr Neurol 2015;52(5):487–92.

Excellent review article on infantile botulism.

Sabater L, Titulaer M, Saiz A, et al. Sox1 antibodies are markers of paraneoplastic Lambert-Eaton myasthenic syndrome. Neurology 2008;70(12):924–8.

Article discussing that the presence of SOX-1 antibodies in patients with Lambert-Eaton myasthenic syndrome predicts the presence of small cell lung cancer.

Schoser B, Eymard B, Datt J, et al. Lambert-Eaton myasthenic syndrome (LEMS): a rare autoimmune presynpatic disorder often associated with cancer. J Neurol 2017;264(9):1854–63

An up-to-date detailed review of Lambert-Eaton myasthenic syndrome including a diagnostic and oncologic screening algorithm.

Myopathies

Jayashri Srinivasan

70

Hereditary Myopathies

Doreen T. Ho, Jayashri Srinivasan

In this chapter, we discuss a group of hereditary, often progressive, muscle disorders. These can be categorized as channelopathies, metabolic and mitochondrial myopathies, muscular dystrophies, and congenital myopathies (Table 70.1).

CHANNELOPATHIES

Periodic Paralyses and Congenital Myotonic Disorders

> **CLINICAL VIGNETTE** *A 56-year-old man sought medical attention for recurrent attacks of stiffness and weakness. He recalls that when he was a child and attended summer camp, he had a spell of weakness after drinking grapefruit juice. For the past 10 years, he has had weakness triggered by certain foods, activities in the cold such as shoveling snow, and exercise. He reports stiffness, with difficulty relaxing his grip when he shakes hands. At the time of diagnosis, genetic testing was not available and he was diagnosed with hyperkalemic periodic paralysis (HyperKPP) by a potassium challenge test. Subsequent genetic testing showed a mutation in the voltage-gated skeletal muscle sodium channel Nav1.4 (encoded by the SCN4A gene on chromosome 17q23–25). He was treated with acetazolamide for the prevention of attacks and mexiletine for his myotonia; he has remained in good health overall, although recently he has developed fixed proximal weakness in his hands and legs. More recently he has started taking dichlorphenamide, which had been approved for this condition, instead of acetazolamide; in addition to its lower efficacy, acetazolamide had also caused kidney stones.*
>
> *Comment: This patient is a classic example of periodic paralysis; symptoms typically begin in midchildhood. The use of a carbonic anhydrase inhibitor initially protected him from frequent attacks of weakness; however, as he reached his fifth and sixth decades, he developed a fixed proximal weakness that limited his activities of daily living (ADLs).*

The various genetically determined hyperkalemic or hypokalemic channelopathies are phenotypically similar disorders related to abnormal ion passage within the muscle membrane ion channels. Their clinical picture is often stereotypical, as illustrated by the previous vignette. It is often difficult to document the occurrence of transient serum hyperkalemia or hypokalemia as it is unusual to evaluate a patient during an episode when the abnormal values typically occur.

Variable mutations within genes encoding muscle membrane ion channels are responsible for the different forms of periodic paralyses as well as other myotonic disorders (Table 70.2). Most of these patients have an autosomal dominant inheritance. During the episodic paralyses, the skeletal muscle membrane's excitability transiently disappears. The degree of weakness may vary from one family member to another.

HyperKPP and paramyotonia are sodium channel disorders, whereas hypokalemic periodic paralysis (HypoKPP) is due to voltage-gated

calcium channel dysfunction. The congenital myotonias are chloride channel disorders inherited in either a dominant (Thomsen disease) or recessive (Becker disease) fashion.

Clinical Presentation

Although most instances of weakness related to periodic paralysis have a symmetric distribution, occasionally a patient may have a focal or asymmetric distribution of weakness. The latter occurs when a few specific muscles are overutilized; for example, a jeweler who developed symptoms confined to his dominant hand or the patient in the clinical vignette who developed weakness in his dominant arm when shoveling snow. Hypokalemic patients may also have paralytic events precipitated by rest after exercise as well as occurring subsequent to significant carbohydrate intake, alcohol ingestion, or cold weather. Bulbar and respiratory muscles are typically not affected. However, by midlife, the periodic events usually cease and some individuals may develop a fixed weakness, as illustrated in the vignette.

HyperKPP, unlike HypoKPP, can be associated with clinical or electrical myotonia (impaired muscle relaxation) or with paramyotonia. Clinical myotonia can be seen on exam in the eyelids, finger extensors, or thenar eminence by percussing the muscle or by activity. We find that the finger extensors are particularly helpful in eliciting percussion myotonia. Myotonia congenita (MC), a chloride channelopathy, is especially aggravated by immobility and ameliorated by exercise and warming; in MC, the myotonia is generally elicitable on examination. Fixed weakness is not usually present in dominant MC (Thomsen disease). A rather unique characteristic of Thomsen disease is the pseudo-hypertrophy of the skeletal muscles, providing the patient with a pseudo-herculean habitus (Fig. 70.1). It may be so profound that athletic coaches enthusiastically encourage these individuals to participate in sports activities. Unfortunately some of these individuals may develop mild progressive weakness. Transient episodes of true weakness precipitated by sudden movements after rest that are relieved by exercise are characteristic of MC. Interesting examples include a baseball player who cannot run after hitting the ball or a subway rider who wishes to get off when the train stops but is frozen in place or falls when he arises to leave the train.

Paramyotonia congenita (PMC) is an even more uncommon hyperkalemic disorder often associated with periodic paralysis. Similar to MC, cold weather exacerbates muscle stiffness in paramyotonia. In contrast to MC, where rest promotes weakness, exercise exacerbates the stiffness in PMC patients.

Malignant Hyperthermia

Malignant hyperthermia (MH) is a heterogeneous syndrome mentioned with the channelopathies in that it may be caused by mutations in the ryanodine receptor *(RYR1)* gene located on chromosome 19q13.1, leading to abnormalities in the release of calcium from the sarcoplasmic

TABLE 70.1 Hereditary Myopathies

Myopathy	Type	Locus	Gene Product
Dystrophies			
Myotonic			
Classic distal	1[a]	AD 19q13	Myotonin protein kinase
Proximal (PROMM)	2[a]	AD 3q21	ZNF9 (zinc finger protein)
Limb-girdle	1A	AD 5q22–34	Myotilin
	1B	AD 1q11–21	Lamin A/C
	1C	AD 3p25	Caveolin-3
	1D	AD 7q36	DNAJB6
	1E	AD	Desmin
	1F	AD	Transportin-3
	1G	AD 4q21	?
	1H	?	?
	2A	AR 15q15	Calpain-3
	2B[b]	AR 2p13	Dysferlin
	2C[b]	AR 13q12	γ-Sarcoglycan+
	2D[b]	AR 17q12	α-Sarcoglycan+ (adhalin)
	2E[b]	AR 4q12	β-Sarcoglycan+
	2F[b]	AR 5q33	δ-Sarcoglycan+
	2G	AR 17q11	Telethonin
	2H	AR 9q31–33	E3 ubiquitin ligase (Trim 32)
	2I	AR 19q13.3	Fukutin-related protein
	2J	AR 2q31	Titin
	2K	AR 9q34.1	POMT1
	2L	AR	Anoctamin-5
	2M	AR	Fukutin
	2N	AR	POMT2
	2O	AR	POMGnT1
	2P	AR	Alpha dystroglycan
	2Q	AR	Plectin-1
	2R	AR	Desmin
	2S	AR	TRAPPC11
Dystrophinopathies			
	Duchenne	XR Xp21	Dystrophin
	Becker		
Facioscapulo-humeral	[b]	AD 4q35	?
Scapuloperoneal		AD 12	?
Emery-Dreifuss	1[b]	X Xq28	Emerin
	2	AD 1q11–q21	Lamin A/C, nesprin-1 and -2
Oculopharyngeal	[b]	AD 14q11.2–q13	Poly (A) binding protein 2
Bethlem		AD 21q22, 2q37	Collagen type VI Subunit α1 or α2
		AD 2q37	Collagen type VI Subunit α3
Congenital Muscular Dystrophy			
	Classic CMD[b]	AR 6q22–23	Laminin-α2 chain of merosin
	α7 Integrin CMD	AR 12q13	Integrin α7
	Fukuyama	AR 9q31–33	Fukutin
	Walker-Warburg	AR ?	?
	Muscle-eye-brain	AR 1p32–34	*O*-mannose β-1,2-*N*-acetylglucosaminyl transferase
	Rigid spine	AR 1p35–36	Selenoprotein N1
Congenital Myopathies			
	Central core	AD 19q13.1	Ryanodine receptor
	Nemaline	AD 1q21–23	α-Tropomyosin
	Nemaline	AR 2q21.2–22	Nebulin
	Nemaline	AR 1q42	α-Actin
	Nemaline	AD 9p13	β-Tropomyosin
	Nemaline	AR 19q13	Troponin T

Continued

TABLE 70.1   Hereditary Myopathies—cont'd

Myopathy	Type	Locus	Gene Product
	Centronuclear	AD 19p13.2	Dynamin-2
	Myotubular	X Xq28	Myotubularin
	Myotubular	AR?	?
	CFTD	?	?
	Myofibrillar	AD 11q22	α,β-Crystallin
	Myofibrillar	AD 2q35	Desmin
	Myofibrillar	AR?	?
Metabolic *Glycogen Storage*			
	II–Acid maltase deficiency[c]	AR 17q21–23	α1,4-Glucosidase
	III–Debrancher deficiency[c]	AR 1p21	Amylo-1,6-glucosidase
	IV–Branching enzyme deficiency[c]	AR 3	Branching amylo-1,4-1,6-transglucosidase
	V–Myophosphorylase deficiency		
	VII–Phosphofructokinase		
Lipid storage	Carnitine deficiency	AR/AD	

[a]DNA mutational analysis commercially available.
[b]Immunostain commercially available.
[c]Biochemical analysis available.
AD, Autosomal dominant; *AR*, autosomal recessive; *CFTD*, congenital fiber–type disproportion; *CMD*, congenital muscular dystrophy; *nesprin*, nuclear envelope spectrin repeat proteins; *PROMM*, proximal myotonic myopathy; *X*, X linked; *?*, unclear mode of transmission.

TABLE 70.2   Channelopathies Affecting Skeletal Muscle

	Age at Onset	Duration of Episodes	Weakness	Myotonia	Precipitants	Alleviating Factors	Gene Mutation/Inheritance and Cation
Hyperkalemic periodic paralysis (HyperKPP)	Infancy–early childhood	Minutes–hours	Episodic, possibly permanent later in life	Possibly (between episodes of weakness) EMG (+)	Potassium loading, cold, fasting, rest, after exercise	Carbohydrate loading, exercise	CN4A 17q23: AD Sodium channel
Paramyotonia congenita (PMC)	Infancy	Minutes	Very uncommon	Present EMG (+)	Repeated exercise, cold, fasting	Warming	SCN4A 17q23: AD Sodium channel
Sodium channel myotonia	Childhood–adolescence	Variable	Very uncommon	Present (often painful)	Rest after exercise, potassium loading, fasting	—	SCN4A 17q23: AD Sodium channel
Hypokalemic periodic paralysis (HypoKPP)	Puberty	Hours–days	Episodic, possibly permanent later in life	Absent	Cold, rest after exercise, carbohydrate loading	Potassium loading, exercise	CACNLA3, SCN4A 17q23: AD Calcium channel
Myotonia congenita	Infancy–early childhood	Minutes	Uncommon	Present EMG (+)	Exercise after rest, cold	Repeated exercise	CLC-1 7q: AD (Thomsen), AR (Becker) Chloride channel
Anderson-Tawil syndrome	Childhood–adolescence	Variable	Episodic, can have cardiac arrythmias and distinctive skeletal abnormalities	No	Usually hypokalemia but can be normo or hyperkalemic during attacks	—	KCJN2 (ATS1) encoding for Kir2.1

AD, Autosomal dominant; *AR*, autosomal recessive.

reticulum. In MH (see Fig. 70.3, bottom), patients can have severe life-threatening episodes of hyperthermia following inhaled anesthetics and muscle relaxants; such episodes are characterized by stiffness, myoglobulinuria, cardiac complications, and even death if there is a delay in diagnosis and treatment.

Differential Diagnosis

The differential diagnosis of a patient with periodic paralysis includes disorders of neuromuscular transmission, notably myasthenia gravis (MG). MG classically has fluctuating symptoms, often with diurnal variation, predominantly confined to ocular bulbar muscles and typically proximal

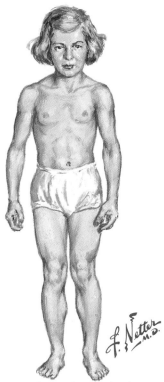

Myotonia and muscular overdevelopment.
Disease affects both males and females.

Fig. 70.1 Myotonia Congenita (Thomsen Disease).

extremity musculature. Acquired myopathies can occasionally present with stiffness and myalgias as well as weakness (e.g., dermatomyositis).

Addison disease requires urgent consideration during the evaluation of any acute, generally weak patient presenting with hyperkalemia. Thyrotoxicosis can be associated with periodic paralysis in some patients, particularly young Asian men; therefore such patients must also be screened for clinical signs and laboratory findings of thyroid dysfunction.

Diagnostic Approach

The clinical history is the best means to diagnose a channelopathy. This may be relatively simple in patients with a positive family history examined while symptomatic and documented to have an abnormal serum potassium level or found to have demonstrable myotonia clinically or electrodiagnostically. In sporadic cases, diagnosis may be more difficult, especially when clinical examination results are normal and provocative testing does not demonstrate any biochemical or neurophysiologic abnormalities.

Regardless of whether the underlying channelopathy leads to hyperkalemia or hypokalemia, the serum potassium is normal between attacks. The clinician rarely has the opportunity to obtain a serum specimen during an event. However, during episodes of HyperKPP, the serum potassium is elevated. It is between events that the cold-induced and electromyography (EMG)-defined myotonia occurs. Similarly, the HypoKPP patient has low serum potassium findings, also confined to the precise time of paralysis. Measurement of the serum potassium level is indicated in any patient observed during spontaneous episodes of weakness or, if recurrent, an attack of periodic paralysis.

Genetic testing has greatly enhanced the specificity of the diagnostic evaluation of a patient with a question of periodic paralysis. These include DNA testing for the skeletal muscle sodium channel as seen in HyperKPP and the skeletal muscle calcium channel specific for HypoKPP.

The previously used provocative studies, such as carbohydrate loading to make the patient hypokalemic, are therefore no longer used today because of the availability of genetic testing.

Nerve conduction studies sometimes demonstrate decreased compound motor action potential amplitudes in the rare instance when a clinician has the opportunity to examine a patient during an episode of periodic paralysis; otherwise these are normal. In the EMG laboratory, having the potential periodic paralysis patient exercise for prolonged periods may lead to progressive diminution in compound motor action potential amplitudes. Much more rarely, when a patient is being evaluated during individual episodes of periodic paralysis, needle EMG will demonstrate that affected muscles are electrically inactive when they are fully depolarized. Myotonic discharges occur on EMG in the sodium channelopathy HyperKPP as well as in the chloride channelopathies. This electrophysiologic finding is particularly useful in the differential diagnosis of hyperkalemic and paramyotonic varieties from the nonmyotonic hypokalemic variety. Clinical myotonia is often not evident in HyperKPP, although it may be so in paramyotonia when the patient is exposed to the cold.

Serum creatine kinase levels are usually normal or minimally increased in the periodic paralyses and myotonic disorders. Muscle biopsy is normal early in the course of periodic paralyses. However, after patients develop persistent weakness, biopsy may demonstrate vacuolar myopathy with tubular aggregates. Muscle biopsy is, however, rarely necessary for diagnosis.

Treatment and Prognosis

The treatment of choice for a patient having an acute attack of periodic paralysis is by the correction of abnormal potassium levels. Severe hyperkalemia necessitates emergency treatment with intravenous (IV) glucose and insulin. Inhaled β-adrenergic agents or ingestion of carbohydrates is fine for less severe episodes. With any patient experiencing his or her first episode of hyperkalemia-associated paralysis, Addison disease is always a diagnostic possibility; therefore the administration of IV corticosteroids is indicated after a serum cortisol level is obtained. IV potassium or, in the milder case, oral supplementation is the best means of caring for the patient with a hypokalemic episode. Such episodes are prevented by avoiding dietary carbohydrate loads.

Maintenance therapy with acetazolamide, hydrochlorothiazide, or dichlorphenamide is usually indicated to prevent attacks. When the treatment of myotonia is also required, therapy with mexiletine or other membrane stabilizers is usually effective.

Generally a diminution in the frequency and severity of periodic paralysis attacks occurs in middle age. However, in some patients with periodic paralysis, as in the initial vignette of this chapter, fixed, progressive, typically proximal weakness develops over time and independent of attacks.

Metabolic Myopathies

CLINICAL VIGNETTE *A 14-year-old female high school student was seen in the emergency room for evaluation of muscle pain and dark urine occurring subsequent to track-and-field practice. Her creatine kinase (CK) level was found to be 50 times normal. Myoglobin was demonstrated in her urine. The patient was admitted to the hospital and treated with vigorous IV hydration. Her symptoms resolved within several days.*

The exercise forearm test failed to demonstrate the normally expected postexercise increase in lactate but did show significant and normal elevations of venous ammonia levels. The latter demonstrated that the patient had successfully stressed her muscle metabolism. The combination of no change in lactate and appropriate rise in ammonia levels was classic for the presence of a glycogen storage disease. On muscle biopsy, subsarcolemmal blebs seen on a periodic acid-Schiff–stained muscle biopsy specimen was consistent with glycogen excess. Biochemical analysis demonstrated decreased levels of myophosphorylase, confirming the diagnosis of McArdle disease.

Comment: This is a classic example of myophosphorylase deficiency (McArdle disease) (Fig. 70.2), the most common GSD.

GSDs are relatively uncommon clinical entities. Myophosphorylase deficiency is the most common of them. The classic picture of the GSDs is one of exercise-induced painful muscle cramps associated with myoglobinuria. However, not all patients will have myoglobinuria and not all attacks are related to exertion. Generally GSDs may demonstrate dynamic symptoms (e.g., exertional cramps, myalgias, and myoglobinuria) and/or static symptoms (fixed progressive weakness). Very rarely, prolonged use of one extremity in isolation will uncover the presence of a previously unsuspected GSD. The concomitant laboratory documentation of profoundly elevated serum CK levels and myoglobinuria

suggests either a carbohydrate or lipid enzymatic deficiency of inborn metabolism (Fig. 70.3 and Table 70.3).

Pathophysiology

Skeletal muscle function is energy-dependent. Normal muscle metabolism requires the presence of both circulating glucose and free fatty acids (Figs. 70.4 and 70.5). At rest, muscles use fatty acids for basal metabolic demands. When one first begins to exercise vigorously, usually within the first 10 minutes, the glycolysis of glycogen, already stored within muscle tissues, is the primary energy source. Its breakdown produces glucose, but only for a relatively short time. However, when the vigorous exercise is prolonged past these first few minutes, the body shifts to anaerobic glycolysis. This is manifested clinically by the second-wind phenomenon. Here lipid stores in the form of free fatty acids are mobilized as the primary source of energy. Effective glycolysis is blocked in the various muscle glycogenoses. This essentially deprives muscle of the initial need for glucose; consequently an accumulation of under-utilized glycogen occurs within muscle. These muscles are inappropriately stressed by what is considered normal exercise in healthy individuals.

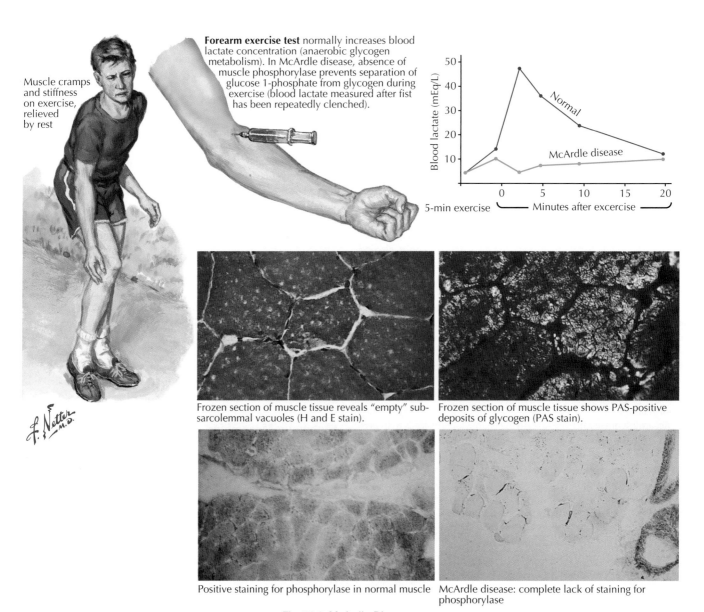

Muscle cramps and stiffness on exercise, relieved by rest

Forearm exercise test normally increases blood lactate concentration (anaerobic glycogen metabolism). In McArdle disease, absence of muscle phosphorylase prevents separation of glucose 1-phosphate from glycogen during exercise (blood lactate measured after fist has been repeatedly clenched).

Frozen section of muscle tissue reveals "empty" subsarcolemmal vacuoles (H and E stain).

Frozen section of muscle tissue shows PAS-positive deposits of glycogen (PAS stain).

Positive staining for phosphorylase in normal muscle

McArdle disease: complete lack of staining for phosphorylase

Fig. 70.2 McArdle Disease.

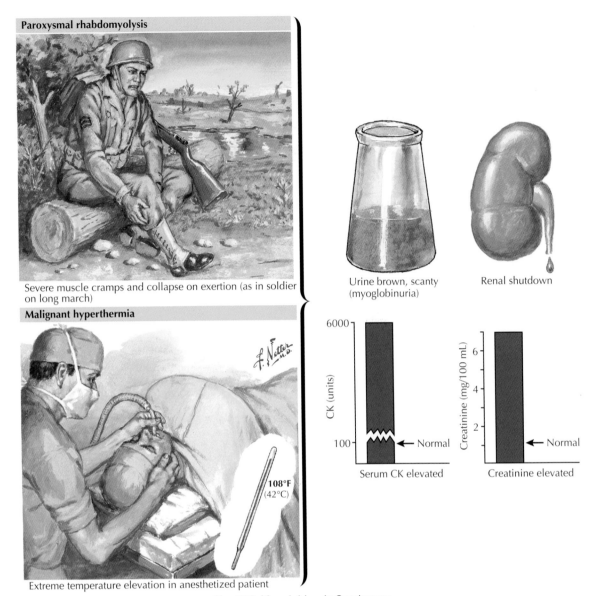

Paroxysmal rhabdomyolysis

Severe muscle cramps and collapse on exertion (as in soldier on long march)

Malignant hyperthermia

Extreme temperature elevation in anesthetized patient

Urine brown, scanty (myoglobinuria)

Renal shutdown

108°F (42°C)

CK (units) — 6000, 100 ← Normal — Serum CK elevated

Creatinine (mg/100 mL) — 6, 4, 2 ← Normal — Creatinine elevated

Fig. 70.3 Myoglobinuric Syndromes.

TABLE 70.3 Myopathies Presenting With Exercise Intolerance

Glycogenoses	Respiratory Chain Defects	Lipid Metabolism Disorders
Myophosphorylase deficiency (McArdle disease)—Type V	Complex 1 deficiency	Carnitine deficiency
Phosphofructokinase deficiency (Tauri disease)—Type VII	Coenzyme Q_{10} deficiency	Carnitine palmitoyltransferase deficiency
Phosphorylase B kinase deficiency—Type VIII	Complex III deficiency	Very long chain, long-chain, medium-chain, or short-chain acyl-CoA dehydrogenase deficiency
Phosphoglycerate kinase deficiency—Type IX	Complex IV deficiency	3-Hydroxy acyl-CoA dehydrogenase deficiency protein deficiency
Phosphoglycerate mutase deficiency—Type X	Complex V deficiency	Glutaric aciduria type II (electron-transferring flavoprotein and CoQ oxidoreductase deficiencies)
Lactate dehydrogenase deficiency—Type XI	Combination of I–V	Neutral lipid storage disease with myopathy; neutral lipid storage disease with ichthyosis
Beta enolase deficiency—Type XII		

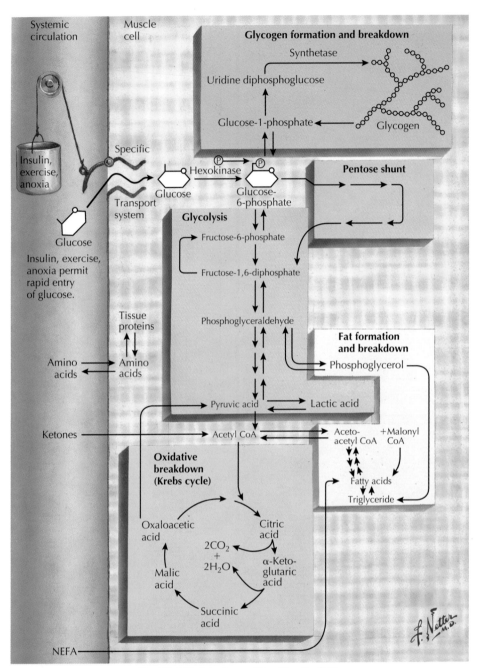

Fig. 70.4 Metabolism of the Muscle Cell.

Genetics

Myophosphorylase deficiency is an autosomal recessive disorder caused by the glycogen phosphorylase, muscle associated *(PYGM)* gene, which encodes myophosphorylase. In contrast, the much more rare phosphoglycerate kinase deficiency is usually X-linked. The remaining other glycogenoses, as well as the various disorders of lipid metabolism, the respiratory chain defects, and muscle adenylate deaminase deficiency are usually recessively inherited. As based on the specific enzyme deficiency, there are 15 different types (0-XV) of GSDs. Type V, McArdle disease, is the most common, presenting with classic exercise-induced painful symptomatology (see Fig. 70.2). Similar phenotypes occur with types VII, IX, X, and XI GSDs.

Clinical Presentation

Severe painful muscle cramping and stiffness occurring after exertion are the hallmark of an enzymatic deficiency glycogen or lipid storage disorder. There may be a characteristic second-wind phenomenon, where brief periods of rest at the onset of myalgia alleviate symptoms and enable prolonged exercise. Symptomatic relief may come with rest (see Fig. 70.3). Recurrent myoglobinuria is common, and permanent weakness may develop in older patients. Patients with myalgias and exercise intolerance with or without hypercalemia are commonly evaluated by neuromuscular specialists. The exercise-induced symptomatology with the subsequent myalgia (in contrast to joint or soft tissues), muscle stiffness, and myoglobinuria provides the primary diagnostic criteria for investigating the possibility of a metabolic myopathy. Specific defects of muscle energy metabolism, as described in this chapter, are sometimes precisely defined; however, more commonly and very frustratingly, specific enzymatic defects cannot be identified in this setting.

A few patients with a GSD, particularly acid maltase deficiency in the adult, present with fixed, often progressive weakness. These individuals have no typical history of episodic symptomatology.

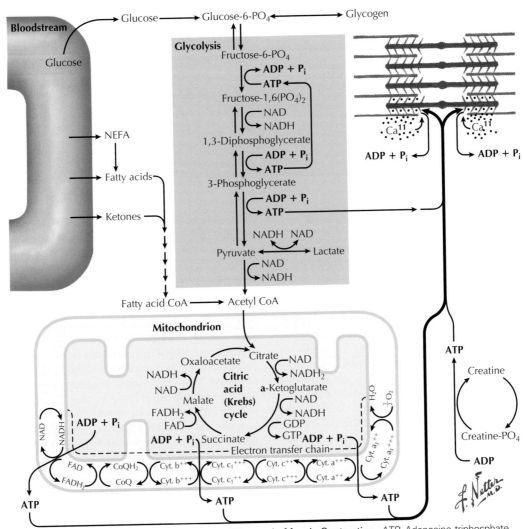

Fig. 70.5 Regeneration of ATP for Source of Energy in Muscle Contraction. *ATP,* Adenosine triphosphate.

Myoadenylate deaminase (MAD) deficiency is a controversial "disorder" because it is not clear whether this is a discrete biochemical disorder. These patients also experience exertional muscle cramping, stiffness, weakness, and pain; the relation between the MAD deficiency and the symptoms is not clear. However, in contrast to a GSD, such individuals do not demonstrate an appropriate increase in serum ammonia levels after forearm exercise but do have the normal increase in serum lactate, indicating normal glycogen metabolism. Myoglobinuria can occur, although it is relatively rare in muscle adenylate deaminase deficiency, which may represent a disorder of defective purine metabolism. Neuromuscular examination is typically normal.

Carnitine palmitoyltransferase II deficiency is the most common disorder of lipid metabolism. Dynamic symptoms include myalgia without muscle cramping. Most commonly, young men present with recurrent myoglobinuria after prolonged but not necessarily strenuous exercise. Brief periods of exercise are usually well tolerated. Episodes may also be triggered by fasting, cold, or stress. Unlike the GSDs, no second-wind phenomenon is seen, fixed weakness does not develop, and serum CK values may normalize between episodes.

Diagnostic Approach

Precise diagnosis of a GSD requires biochemical findings manifested by an abnormal exercise forearm test. Baseline measurements of plasma lactate, pyruvate, and ammonia are obtained. The patients then vigorously exercise their hands for 1–2 minutes (see Fig. 70.5). Subsequently serial lactate and ammonia determinations are made immediately after exercise and 1, 3, 6, and 10 minutes thereafter. Normally there is a fivefold rise in serum lactate and a tenfold rise in the serum ammonia level. Glycogen metabolism storage disorders are suspected where there is failure to achieve the normal increase of serum lactate. MAD deficiency is entertained when there is a lack of the expected increase in plasma ammonia after exercise and the normal increase in serum lactate. The test's sensitivity is dependent on patient effort.

Muscle tissue histochemical analysis may also be important in the workup of metabolic myopathies. A muscle biopsy may be obtained and then specific stains looking for the presence or absence of the enzyme myophosphorylase are performed. When this is normal, then other GSDs or, even more rarely, inborn errors in muscle lipid metabolism must also be assessed. Genetic testing for CPT2 is available, so biopsy can be avoided if clinical suspicion is high and the exercise forearm test is normal.

Idiopathic HyperCKemia

It is common to find moderate postexercise hyperkalemia in normal, healthy individuals. Typically, this CK elevation is less than five times the upper limit of normal after moderately vigorous exercise. These elevated CK levels return to normal levels within 3–8 days postexercise. The range of "normal" CK in most laboratories is likely too strict and

TABLE 70.4 Biochemical Analyses Available for Specific Metabolic Myopathies

Glycogen Storage	Lipid Storage	Mitochondrial	Purine
Acid maltase	Carnitine	NADH dehydrogenase	Myoadenylate deaminase
Neutral maltase	Carnitine palmitoyltransferase	NADH cytochrome-c reductase	Adenylate kinase
Phosphofructokinase		Succinate dehydrogenase	
Phosphorylase		Succinate cytochrome-c reductase	
Phosphorylase β kinase		Cytochrome-c oxidase	
Phosphoglycerate kinase		Citrate synthase?	
Phosphoglycerate mutase		Fumarase	

?, Unclear mode of transmission.

certain demographic groups may display mild elevations in CK even without exercise.

The evaluation of patients who have nonspecific symptoms or who are serendipitously found to have increased CK is often frustrating in the absence of clinically demonstrated weakness or specific EMG abnormalities. The yield of muscle biopsy in search of glycogen or lipid storage changes is relatively low, even with extensive histochemical staining and DNA tests. Abnormalities found on the routine analysis of muscle biopsy specimens do not accurately predict abnormalities on biochemical testing. Some metabolic myopathies are specific to skeletal muscle. Here one needs to specifically study the involved muscles. Other metabolic disorders of muscle are more systemically distributed and can be detected on enzymatic testing of fibroblasts or leukocytes.

EMG generally is not a useful diagnostic tool as it is usually normal in these various energy metabolic defects. The one exception is if one has the opportunity to perform the EMG while the patient is actually experiencing an active and often painful contracture, when there will be total electrical silence. This finding is unique to GSDs. GSD type II, also known as acid maltase (alpha glucosidase) deficiency, is the one other exception where there are classic EMG findings of a very active myopathy mimicking polymyositis; the findings here are frequently most profound in the paraspinal musculature. Overall the primary utility of EMG in this group of metabolic skeletal muscle disorders is to provide a means to exclude other motor unit processes before moving on to other studies.

Lymphocyte or cultured skin fibroblast analysis supersedes the need for muscle biopsy in certain metabolic myopathies. Testing is available for many glycogenoses and disorders of lipid metabolism.

Muscle Biopsy

Abnormal accumulation of glycogen or lipid may be detected in a muscle biopsy specimen using periodic acid–Schiff or Oil Red O staining, respectively. Muscle phosphorylase, phosphofructokinase, and MAD deficiency are the primary enzyme-specific stains available for metabolic myopathies. Lipid stains may be normal or show mild lipid accumulation in carnitine palmitoyltransferase II deficiency. Biochemical testing of muscle is available for some myopathies (Table 70.4).

Treatment and Prognosis

Most patients with metabolic myopathies learn to adapt to limited exercise tolerance. No specific treatments are available for most of these conditions. Isolated reports attribute clinical benefit in the glycogenoses to aerobic training, high-protein diets, and creatine supplementation. However, none are proven as reliable therapies. Patients with carnitine palmitoyltransferase II deficiency can often prevent attacks by increasing dietary carbohydrate intake before prolonged exercise or during febrile illness.

Myoglobinuria is always a major concern; it is a major risk for acute renal failure because there is deposition of myoglobin within renal tubules potentially leading to renal shutdown. This is a significant problem with the various muscle metabolism glycogenoses and lipid storage disorders. As many as 50% of patients with recurrent myoglobinuria experience episodes of acute renal insufficiency. Patients who are at risk for myoglobinuria are advised to seek prompt medical attention if such occurs. Treatment includes forced diuresis and alkalinization. A complete recovery is expected if the episodes are appropriately managed.

Metabolic myopathies are generally nonprogressive disorders, although fixed weakness develops with increasing age in some patients who have a glycogenosis. This is particularly the case with acid maltase deficiency, which can mimic polymyositis or a limb girdle muscular dystrophy in phenotype. When acid maltase deficiency presents in middle age, there is early potential for significant respiratory compromise. In a few patients with the very rare carnitine palmitoyltransferase II deficiency, respiratory muscle involvement also occurs. This may require ventilatory support during episodes of severe weakness. Generally these episodes are reversible with appropriate supportive care.

MUSCULAR DYSTROPHIES

These are genetically determined myopathies distinguished from congenital myopathies by their generally progressive clinical course and characteristic dystrophic histology profile of myofiber degeneration, regeneration, and fibrotic and fatty replacement of muscle (Fig. 70.6, bottom panel). The milder dystrophies, for example, oculopharyngeal muscular dystrophy, may lack some of these classic histologic features.

CLINICAL VIGNETTE *A 32-year-old chef presented with weakness that had developed gradually over 5 years. She noticed reduced strength in her lower extremities with difficulty climbing stairs and fatigue. She was not sure how long ago her symptoms had started, and this was the first time she had sought medical attention for them. On examination, she had bilateral ptosis, temporalis wasting, mild proximal weakness, and bilateral foot drop. Reflexes were reduced throughout. Sensory examination was normal. Forced handgrip revealed slow relaxation (clinical myotonia). Electrodiagnostic studies revealed normal nerve conduction studies. EMG showed evidence of myotonic discharges with small myopathic units in all muscles tested. Genetic testing revealed 1200 CTG repeats on chromosome 19q13 for the myotonin protein kinase (DMPK). Upon questioning, she replied that her father had the same hatchet appearance to his face, but he had died in his early 50s. Examination of a photograph of her father at the subsequent clinic visit confirmed this.*

Comment: This vignette portrays a young patient with type 1 myotonic muscular dystrophy (DM1). Myotonic muscular dystrophies are the most common adult forms of muscular dystrophy and are discussed in the following section. The myotonic dystrophies can occur as type DM1 or type 2 myotonic dystrophy (DM2), also called proximal myotonic myopathy (PROMM).

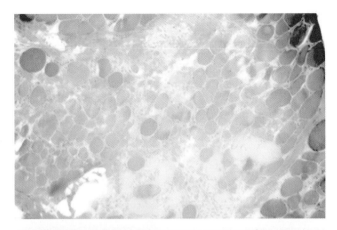

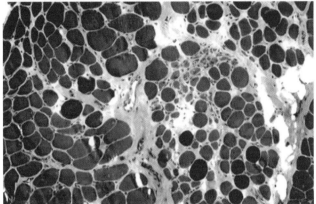

Muscle biopsy specimens showing necrotic muscle fibers being removed by groups of small, round phagocytic cells (**top,** trichrome stain) and replaced by fibrous and fatty tissue (**bottom,** H and E stain).

Fig. 70.6 Duchenne Muscular Dystrophy: Muscle Biopsy Specimens.

Myotonic Muscular Dystrophy, Type 1

The classic autosomal dominant form usually presents in early adulthood but may be recognized from the neonatal period, presenting as a floppy infant as in the case of some of the congenital myopathies and congenital dystrophies (Fig. 70.7). This condition presents with distal weakness that progresses to involve proximal muscles. Myotonia is delayed skeletal muscle relaxation and is best demonstrated with a forceful handgrip or by thenar eminence or extensor forearm compartment percussion. Temporalis, masseter, and sternocleidomastoid wasting; frontal balding; and ptosis contribute to the characteristic myotonic facies (Fig. 70.8). Facial, pharyngeal, tongue, and neck muscles are also weak. Limb weakness predominantly affects distal extensor muscle groups and then progresses proximally.

Various systemic problems occur concomitantly with DM1: impaired gastrointestinal dysmotility, alveolar hypoventilation, cardiac conduction defects, and cardiomyopathy. The last three often shorten life expectancy. Neurobehavioral manifestations include hypersomnolence, apathy, depression, personality disorders, and cognitive impairment. Premature posterior subcapsular cataracts are common and may sometimes provide the essential clue leading to the initial diagnosis of DM1. Testicular atrophy and impotence occur in men. Pregnant women have a high rate of fetal loss.

Laboratory investigations demonstrate that the CK may be mildly elevated. Nerve conduction studies are normal. Needle EMG predominantly demonstrates myotonic potentials. Muscle biopsy is characterized by an increase in internalized nuclei, atrophy, pyknotic clumps, and

ring fibers. Genetic testing for the myotonin protein kinase (DMPK) will reveal more than 37 CTG repeats on chromosome 19q13.2. Greater repeat lengths are associated with more severe disease. Amplification of repeat size occurs in newborn babies of mothers with DM1, resulting in congenital dystrophy.

Proximal Myotonic Myopathy (Type 2 Myotonic Dystrophy)

Type 2 myotonic dystrophy (DM2), also called proximal myotonic myopathy (PROMM), is another autosomal dominant myotonic disorder that typically presents in adulthood. Patients present with myotonia, myalgia, and proximal weakness. Weakness begins in the legs and is slowly progressive. Patients may describe episodic fluctuation in their weakness and may experience severe muscle pain. Ptosis, facial weakness, and weakness of the respiratory muscles are uncommon in DM2. Associated systemic abnormalities include cataracts, cardiac arrhythmias, and testicular atrophy. The proximal weakness and absence of signature features make DM2 a more difficult clinical diagnosis than DM1.

Serum CK may be mildly increased. EMG demonstrates myotonia, which often provides an important diagnostic clue when evaluating patients with typical clinical pictures of proximal myopathies. In DM2, genetic studies for zinc finger protein 9 on chromosome 3 will reveal more than 177 base pairs of CCTG expansion.

Limb-Girdle Muscular Dystrophies

Limb-girdle muscular dystrophies (LGMDs) are a genetically heterogeneous group of disorders wherein the precise classification is rendered more complicated by the frequency of variable phenotypes resulting from mutations of the same gene. It is difficult to distinguish clinically the various subtypes of LGMD, although patterns of weakness or other clinical features may suggest various genotypes. The nosology of LGMDs was historically determined by mode of inheritance (1 for dominant and 2 for recessive inheritance) and letter (usually in the order of discovery of the chromosomal locus) (see Table 70.1); more recently, LGMDs are most easily identified by the genetic mutation, acknowledging the phenotypic heterogeneity associated with many known mutations.

Weakness in these individuals typically has a symmetric limb-girdle pattern, usually affecting the proximal leg muscles before the shoulder girdle. There is relative sparing of facial, oculomotor, pharyngeal, and neck muscles. Certain clinical clues may be helpful. Scapular winging may occur in the calpainopathies and sarcoglycanopathies, with facioscapulohumeral dystrophy (FSHD) on the differential as an alternative diagnosis. Contractures may occur in laminopathies and calpainopathies, with Bethlem and Emery-Dreifuss muscular dystrophy (EDMD) and dystrophinopathies as considerations in the differential of such a patient. Hypertrophy of muscles can be seen in the sarcoglycanopathies and fukutinopathies; in these patients, dystrophinopathies may also be on the differential. Cardiomyopathy may be present in dystrophinopathies, laminopathies, and fukutinopathies. Onset is usually before the age of 20 years, although LGMD is frequently unrecognized until early middle life, and women and men are affected with equal frequency in most LGMDs. Systemic involvement is uncommon.

CK increases in range from normal to 20 times normal in LGMDs. A normal CK is quite unusual for an autosomal recessive LGMD and should raise suspicion of an alternative diagnosis. Dysferlinopathies and anoctaminopathies are more likely to have very high CKs. Magnetic resonance imaging (MRI) of the calf or thigh, muscle biopsy, EMG, and genetic testing are often parts of the workup. Genetic testing is available for some of the LGMDs. Anoctomin 5 mutations are interestingly more common in males. The frequency of the different LGMDS seems to vary by the geographic region studied.

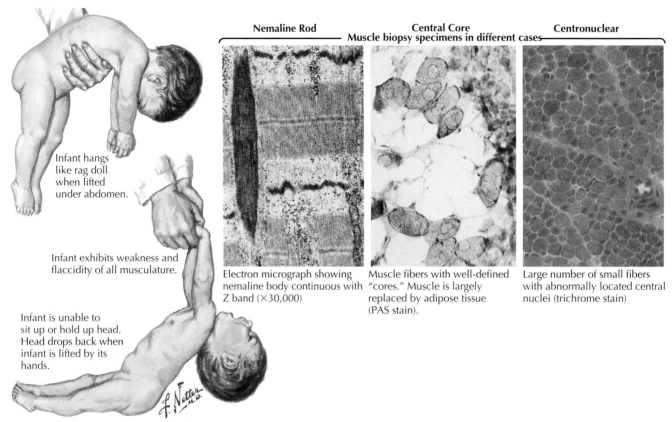

Nemaline Rod — **Central Core** — **Centronuclear**
Muscle biopsy specimens in different cases

Infant hangs like rag doll when lifted under abdomen.

Infant exhibits weakness and flaccidity of all musculature.

Infant is unable to sit up or hold up head. Head drops back when infant is lifted by its hands.

Electron micrograph showing nemaline body continuous with Z band (×30,000)

Muscle fibers with well-defined "cores." Muscle is largely replaced by adipose tissue (PAS stain).

Large number of small fibers with abnormally located central nuclei (trichrome stain)

Fig. 70.7 Congenital Myopathies: Floppy Infant.

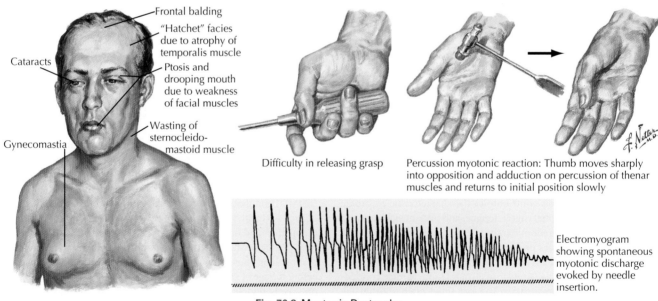

Frontal balding

"Hatchet" facies due to atrophy of temporalis muscle

Cataracts

Ptosis and drooping mouth due to weakness of facial muscles

Wasting of sternocleido-mastoid muscle

Gynecomastia

Difficulty in releasing grasp

Percussion myotonic reaction: Thumb moves sharply into opposition and adduction on percussion of thenar muscles and returns to initial position slowly

Electromyogram showing spontaneous myotonic discharge evoked by needle insertion.

Fig. 70.8 Myotonic Dystrophy.

Dystrophinopathies

The dystrophinopathies are the most common muscular dystrophies occurring during childhood and in some adults. Dystrophin is a subsarcolemmal protein present in skeletal and cardiac muscle. Dystrophin along with the sarcolemmal proteins forms the dystrophin-sarcoglycan complex (Fig. 70.9).

Duchenne Muscular Dystrophy

Duchenne muscular dystrophy (DMD) is a primarily X-linked recessive dystrophinopathy; however, in one-third of patients, this occurs sporadically, presenting in early childhood with proximal weakness and difficulty walking (Fig. 70.10). Untreated patients, usually boys, become wheelchair-dependent by midadolescence. Calf hypertrophy, heel cord

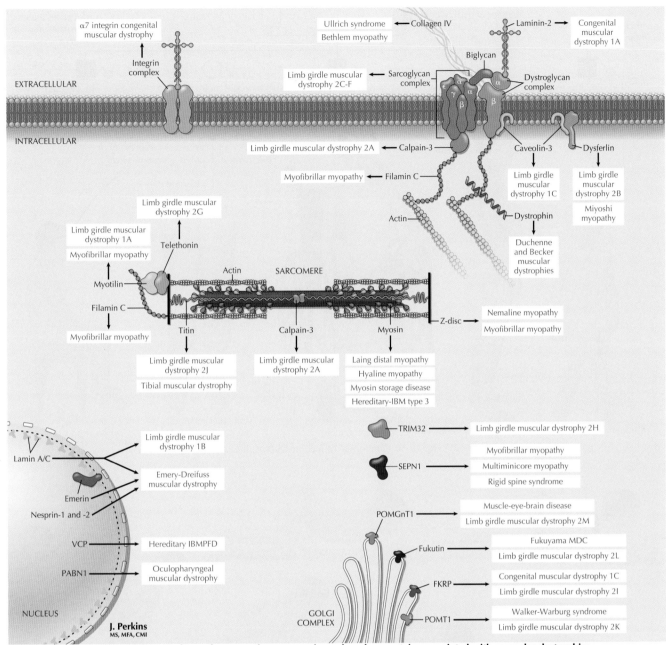

Schematic representation of the sarcolemmal, enzymatic, sarcomeric, and nuclear proteins associated with muscular dystrophies.

Fig. 70.9 Sarcoglycan Complex and Sarcomere Proteins.

shortening, and blunted intellect help to differentiate this disorder from other myopathies. Common initial signs are a clumsy gait, frequent falls, and proximal lower extremity weakness. Children cannot rise from a squatting position on the floor and use their hands to push off on their legs (Fig. 70.11). Most patients are wheelchair-bound by 12 years of age.

An associated cardiomyopathy is common and can cause arrhythmias or congestive heart failure. Respiratory failure due to neuromuscular weakness may be exacerbated by the development of kyphoscoliosis and contractures. Most patients die of respiratory or cardiac complications in the second or third decade of life unless they choose long-term mechanical ventilation. Smooth muscle involvement may occur, manifesting as an ileus or gastric atony.

CK levels are significantly elevated in DMD to approximately 30–50 times normal. Serum molecular genetic testing for mutations in the

dystrophin gene is the first step in children in whom a dystrophinopathy is suspected. When DNA analysis is negative, a muscle biopsy may be necessary for dystrophin immunostaining, immunoblotting, or Western blot analysis. Immunostaining demonstrates that most fibers are devoid of dystrophin in DMD. Electrodiagnostic studies and muscle biopsy, once the mainstays of diagnosis, are no longer necessary in most cases. Needle EMG demonstrates myopathic-appearing motor units as well as profuse fibrillation potentials. The main differential includes the LGMDs.

Becker Muscular Dystrophy

Becker muscular dystrophy (BMD) is another X-linked dystrophinopathy that is allelic to DMD. This usually presents with a milder phenotype. Patients present with difficulty walking in the late first or

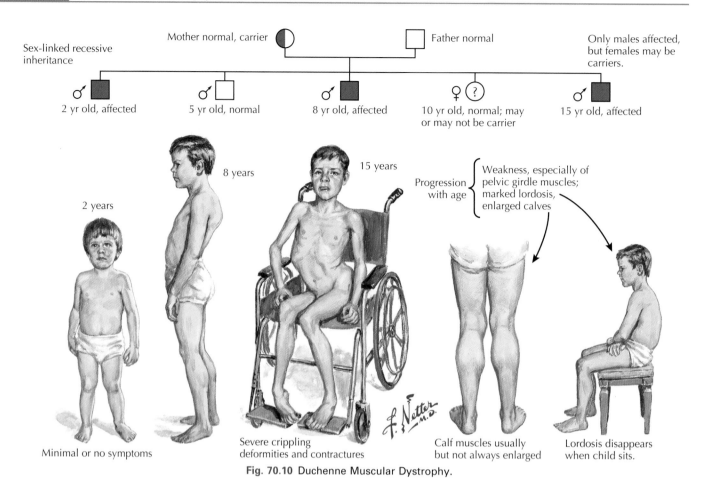

Sex-linked recessive inheritance

Mother normal, carrier   Father normal

Only males affected, but females may be carriers.

2 yr old, affected   5 yr old, normal   8 yr old, affected   10 yr old, normal; may or may not be carrier   15 yr old, affected

2 years

8 years

15 years

Progression with age { Weakness, especially of pelvic girdle muscles; marked lordosis, enlarged calves

Minimal or no symptoms

Severe crippling deformities and contractures

Calf muscles usually but not always enlarged

Lordosis disappears when child sits.

Fig. 70.10 Duchenne Muscular Dystrophy.

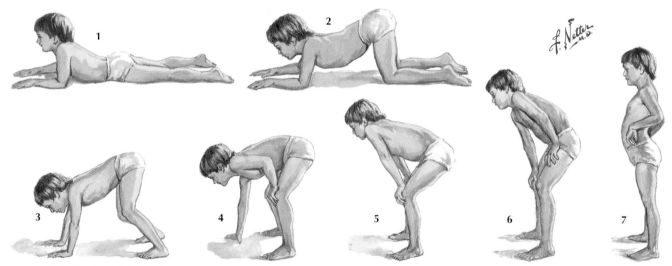

Characteristically, the child arises from prone position by pushing himself up with hands successively on floor, knees, and thighs, because of weakness in gluteal and spine muscles. He stands in lordic posture.

Fig. 70.11 Duchenne Muscular Dystrophy: Gowers Maneuver.

early second decade of life. BMD is sometimes manifest by exertional myalgias, cardiomyopathy, or asymptomatic increased serum CK levels. Increased CK may not occur early on; some patients have normal values in childhood, developing increased serum CK levels later in their 20s. Life expectancy is still reduced but is usually significantly longer than in DMD. Diagnosis is similar to that of DMD. In-frame mutations are more likely to present with the BMD phenotype.

Female carriers (i.e., daughters of patients with BMD) can present with asymptomatic hyperkalemia and very rarely with symptomatic myopathies as adults. CK can, however, be normal. Genetic testing is important for the detection of carrier status, and counseling is recommended. Prenatal testing is available.

In both BMD and the rare female carrier, muscle biopsy demonstrates a mix of dystrophin staining and nonstaining fibers. Both immunoblotting and immunostaining results for dystrophin in muscle biopsies are quantitatively and qualitatively abnormal in BMD.

Treatment of Dystrophinopathies

Long-term corticosteroid therapy in ambulatory patients may help to ameliorate the course of DMD. Corticosteroids may be associated with significant side effects and patients will need to be monitored for weight gain, stunted growth, osteoporosis, and mood changes. Ataluren, available in Europe, promotes ribosomal read-through of nonsense mutations; this may be an option for boys with DMD who ambulate and have nonsense mutations (10%–15% of DMD boys). Eteplirsen was approved by the US Food and Drug Administration (FDA) in 2016 for a subset of patients with DMD with out of frame deletions amenable by exon 51 skipping (13%–15% of DMD deletions). Further clinical trials are under way as are studies of biomarkers in DMD and BMD. Aggressive treatment of heart failure and consideration for cardiac transplant in patients is also recommended; this is especially important in patients with BMD presenting with cardiomyopathy. A multidisciplinary approach with supportive treatment—including physiatry, cardiology, pulmonology, psychology, and genetic counseling as well as physical, occupational, speech, and respiratory therapy—is an important aspect in the care of these patients and their families.

Facioscapulohumeral Muscular Dystrophy

Facioscapulohumeral (FSH) muscular dystrophy is a dominantly inherited disorder with variable penetrance. Patients may present with facial weakness and scapular winging in the second to fifth decades of life (Fig. 70.12). Atrophy and weakness of biceps and triceps muscles typically occur; paradoxically, there is relative sparing of deltoid and forearm

strength. In the lower extremity, ankle dorsiflexors are usually first affected. An asymmetric pattern of weakness is a common feature. Abdominal muscle weakness and a Beevor sign (caudal or rostral movement of the umbilicus with head flexion) may be present. Variations in phenotype include the rare absence of any demonstrable facial weakness. An infantile form presents with a rapidly progressive course, leading to wheelchair dependency by the age of 10 years.

Electrodiagnostic studies demonstrate myopathic findings. Genetic testing (a D4Z4 repeat contraction on chromosome 4q35) reveals mutations on the 4q35 chromosomal region in patients with FSHD1, which accounts for 95% of patients with FSHD. FSHD2 patients do not have a D4Z4 contraction but instead have mutations on the *SMCHD1* gene on chromosome 18p11.32 and display the same downstream effects of hypomethylation of the D4Z4 region. Treatment is supportive for patients with FSHD. Scapular fixation (fixation of the scapula to the chest wall) is not commonly utilized in our practice and only considered for patients with good muscle bulk and strength in the deltoid muscles.

Scapuloperoneal Syndromes

These various disorders need consideration in the differential diagnosis of FSHD. The genetic pattern in scapuloperoneal syndromes may be autosomal dominant or recessive, sometimes X-linked, or even sporadic. Usually these children present with arm weakness before a foot drop is recognized. Most patients have normal longevity with relatively mild disability.

Emery-Dreifuss Muscular Dystrophy

This is inherited in either an X-linked or autosomal dominant manner. Distinctive features include a humeroperoneal (elbow flexion and

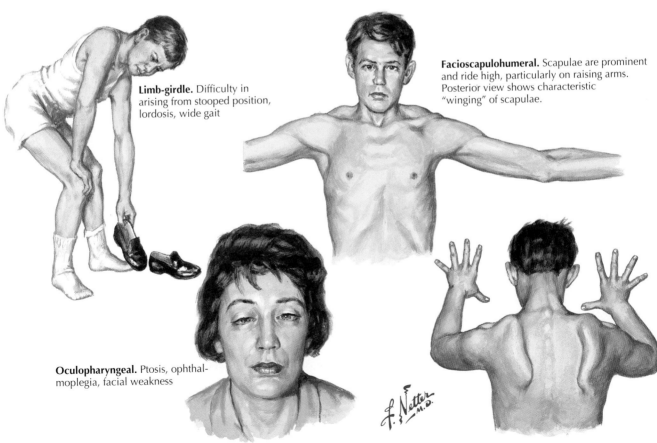

Fig. 70.12 Other Types of Muscular Dystrophy.

extension, foot dorsiflexion) pattern of weakness and early contractures (especially of the Achilles tendons, elbows, and posterior cervical muscles). Most patients present with contractures causing difficulty extending the elbows and dorsiflexing the ankles.

Cardiac conduction defects are common causes of stroke and life-threatening arrhythmias and are sometimes the clinically presenting feature of this disorder. Genetic tests will reveal mutations in the Emerin gene on chromosome Xq28 (X-linked form), lamin A/C gene on chromosome 1q11–23 (autosomal dominant form), or the nesprin-1 and nesprin-2 genes (autosomal dominant or sporadic cases).

Bethlem Myopathy

This is an autosomal disorder similar to Emery-Dreifuss muscular dystrophy, with early childhood onset. It is an indolent myopathy also including prominent elbow flexion contractures but without cardiac complications.

Oculopharyngeal Muscular Dystrophy

This autosomal dominant myopathy is particularly prevalent in North America among individuals of French-Canadian ancestry. Most patients present in middle to late adulthood with prominent ptosis and dysphagia. Mild proximal weakness may also develop. Genetic testing for the presence of a GCG repeat in the *PABN1* gene on chromosome 14q11.1, if positive, will confirm the diagnosis (see Fig. 70.12, bottom right panel).

Myofibrillar Myopathy

Genetically and phenotypically heterogeneous, myofibrillary myopathy (MFM) is characterized by desmin or other protein accumulation within the muscle. Electron microscopy (EM) findings demonstrate the presence of myofibrillar disruption, probably due to Z-disk disruption. The clinical phenotype is varied. Diagnosis is made by the presence of the characteristic histologic features. It can present at any age with proximal or distal weakness. Surveillance for associated cardiomyopathy, cardiac arrhythmia, ventilatory insufficiency, or both is required. Mutations have been identified in *myotilin, ZASP, filamin-C, desmin, selenoprotein n, alphabeta crystallin, FHL-1, titin, transportin-3, and bag-3*. The pattern of inheritance is variable.

Congenital Muscular Dystrophies

These are a heterogeneous group of recessively inherited neonatal disorders commonly confused with congenital myopathies, particularly when infants are hypotonic, often presenting as floppy babies. Children with congenital muscular dystrophy often have joint contractures or arthrogryposis. Some forms are associated with associated brain or ocular abnormalities. These clinical features coupled with increased CK values and dystrophic muscle histology distinguish congenital muscular dystrophies from congenital myopathies and other infantile neuromuscular disorders.

Distal Myopathies or Muscular Dystrophies

The distal myopathies are rare and present with progressive distal weakness; they may be sporadic or inherited. The distal myopathies are classified based on the inheritance, pattern of weakness, and histopathologic findings (Table 70.5). It is important to remember that other myopathies can present with a distal pattern of weakness, for example, DM1, EDMD, FSHD, scapuloperoneal, nemaline myopathy, and centronuclear myopathy due to a dynamin-2 mutation.

Congenital Myopathies

These disorders are usually evident at birth or in infancy. They may be severe but often tend to be only minimally progressive if the child survives infancy. Affected children are often limited in their physical capacities, but many live to adulthood. These myopathies are typically named for key histologic features, for example, nemaline (threadlike) rods.

The most common congenital myopathies are centronuclear (myotubular) myopathy, central core disease, and nemaline myopathy (see Fig. 70.7, *bottom panel*). These are relatively well-defined clinically and genetically heterogeneous disorders. Concomitant congenital skeletal changes such as high-arched palates and kyphoscoliosis are commonplace and are suggestive of these genetically determined disorders. Although the presentation is usually that of a floppy infant, some individuals are mildly affected and may not present until early to middle adulthood. Babies surviving infancy tend to have minimal progression and a reasonable life expectancy.

Centronuclear myopathy, previously called myotubular myopathy, is a disorder associated with characteristic muscle biopsy findings of central nuclei. It is seen as an X-linked recessive neonatal disorder frequently causing death from respiratory insufficiency in infancy; rarely it presents indolently in childhood or early adulthood. Ptosis and ophthalmoparesis help to distinguish this from other congenital myopathies. Muscle biopsy demonstrates nuclei in the center of the fiber, sometimes forming longitudinal chains. Mutations in myotubularin or dynamin-2 are linked to this condition.

Central core myopathy presents in infancy or childhood with generalized weakness. Muscle biopsies demonstrate cores that appear in type 1 fibers and are seen on NADH stains as nonstaining regions. Z-band streaming and myofibrillar disruption may result in the formation of cores. This condition is associated with an increased risk for MH; it is particularly seen on exposure to volatile anesthetics or depolarizing neuromuscular blockers.

Nemaline myopathy can present at any age from infancy to adulthood and is phenotypically and genetically heterogeneous. Affected children have delayed motor milestones, but those surviving past infancy eventually achieve some degree of functional independence. On muscle biopsy there is type 1 predominance, with the presence of nemaline rods in the subsarcolemmal region best seen on Gomori trichrome stain. EM is useful to confirm the presence of the rods. The rods are thought to represent disrupted Z-disk structure.

The diagnosis of congenital myopathies is usually confirmed with routine histochemical staining of muscle in concert with the appropriate phenotype. A few metabolic myopathies can be diagnosed by histochemical staining, but many require biochemical analysis of the muscle biopsy specimen or other tissue.

Hereditary Inclusion Body Myopathy

The hereditary inclusion body myopathies (h-IBMs) are difficult to classify. They manifest in the second or third decade of life and are histologically identical to sporadic IBMs but without inflammation. They can be autosomal dominant or recessive. Two forms are allelic to distal myopathies. In h-IBM2, or GNE myopathy, the genetic basis relates to a mutation in the gene encoding the enzyme complex UDP-*N*-acetylglucosamine-2-epimerase-*N*-acetylmannosamine kinase (GNE), which catalyzes the rate-limiting step in sialic acid production. An autosomal dominant form of hereditary IBM associated with frontotemporal dementia and Paget disease of the bone has been linked to mutations in the gene encoding for valsolin containing protein (VCP). Another form presents with congenital arthrogryposis and has been linked to mutations in the *MYH2* gene. Finally, a rare recessive form of h-IBM can be associated with cerebral hypomyelination.

Diagnostic Approach to Genetic Myopathies

The diagnostic testing required in patients with generalized chronic myopathies varies depending on clinical presentation (Table 70.6), as provided in guidelines for routinely and selectively ordered tests. Many

TABLE 70.5 The Distal Myopathies

| | Age at Onset | INITIAL MUSCLE | | | CHROMOSOME | | |
		Group Involved	Serum CK	Muscle Biopsy	Inheritance	Linkage	Gene
Nonaka (h-IBM type 1)	Early adulthood	AC legs	N or sl ↑	Rimmed vacuoles	AR	9p1–q1	GNE
Miyoshi	Early adulthood	PC legs	↑ × 10–150	Myopathic changes, occasional inflammation	AR	2p13	Dysferlin
Laing	Childhood–adulthood	AC legs, neck flexors	↑ × 1–3	Myopathic changes	AD	14q11	MYH7
Myofibrillar myopathy (desmin)	Childhood–adulthood	Hands or AC legs	N or sl ↑	Myopathic changes with vacuoles or cytoplasmic inclusions	AD, sporadic, ? AR, ? X-linked	2q35, 11q21–23, 12q, 10q22.3	Various genes
Welander	Late adulthood	Finger and wrist extensors	N or sl ↑	Myopathic changes, vacuoles	AD	2p13	
Udd	Late adulthood	AC legs but can be highly variable	N or ↑ CK	Dystrophic, can have rimmed vacuoles	AD/AR		2q31 mutation in gene for titin
Markesbury-Griggs	Late adulthood	AC legs	N or ↑ CK	Myofibrillar myopathy and rimmed vacuoles	AD		ZASP (Z-band alternatively spliced PDZ motif-containing protein)
Distal myopathy with vocal cord and pharyngeal weakness	Late adulthood	AC legs, finger extensors, late vocal cord and pharyngeal weakness	N or ↑ × 3–6	Vacuolar myopathy	AD	5q31[a]	

AC, Anterior compartment; *AD*, autosomal dominant; *AR*, autosomal recessive; *CK*, creatine kinase; *N*, normal; *PC*, posterior compartment; *sl*, slight; ↑, increased; *?*, unclear mode of transmission.
[a]Previously thought localized to 5q31 but now thought of as linked to *MATR3* gene on X chromosome.

diagnostic tools are available for evaluating a patient with an apparent myopathy. Extensive analyses of muscle should be undertaken only when warranted by a reasonable index of clinical suspicion.

Treatment

General goals for the management of chronic myopathies are largely supportive (Box 70.1).

Corticosteroids are often used in ambulatory patients with DMD or BMD. There is evidence suggesting that these drugs may delay wheelchair dependency by years in afflicted males. This benefit occurs despite the potential drawbacks of steroids in individuals who have not grown to full stature and who are prone to complications of immobility. Side effects must be monitored carefully. Ataluren is considered for boys with DMD who ambulate and have nonsense mutations; eteplirsen is considered for a subset of patients with DMD with out of frame deletions amenable by exon 51 skipping. The impact of treatment on quality of life as well as cost considerations may be factors. A multidisciplinary approach with supportive treatment is used in patients with DMD and BMD.

Carnitine supplementation in lipid-storage myopathies is effective in few patients, presumably those with primary rather than secondary causes of carnitine deficiency.

Symptomatic myotonia can occur in DM1 and DM2. Mexiletine is the most effective treatment but requires caution in relation to possible side effects of cardiac conduction problems.

BOX 70.1 Management Goals in the Chronic Proximal/Generalized Myopathies

- *Maintenance of optimal, independent neuromuscular function* for as long as possible, with particular attention to ambulation, via durable medical equipment and occupational therapy evaluation and intervention
- *Reduction in the risk of falls and injury* through home modification, durable medical equipment, or physical therapy instruction
- *Patient comfort* maintenance:
- *Prevention or correction of joint contractures,* particularly spine deformities and kyphoscoliotic cardiopulmonary disease
- *Appropriate nutrition* maintenance of (adequate calories in those with feeding difficulties; caloric restrictions in those with a propensity to obesity)
- *Genetic counseling* where needed
- Prenatal diagnosis when needed
- *Aspiration pneumonia prevention* or prompt treatment (when appropriate)
- *Cardiac/pulmonary support:* Recognition and treatment of associated congestive heart failure, symptomatic cardiac conduction defects, and pulmonary hypertension
- *Malignant hyperthermia* prevention: Patient should alert anesthesiologist prior to surgery of the potential for this life-threatening disorder
- *Identification of patient (or parental) goals* in situations in which the severity of the illness may be anticipated to significantly shorten the patient's life expectancy (with provision of adequate counseling)

TABLE 70.6 Evaluation of a Patient With Suspected Muscle Disease

Primary Studies	Studies That May Be Indicated in Some Patients
• EMG • CK	• Muscle biopsy • Potassium (serum) • Aldolase • Lactate (serum) • Thyroid function tests, electrolytes • Anti–acetylcholine receptor antibodies • Exercise forearm testing (lactate, ammonia) • Exercise forearm testing (venous O_2) • Total eosinophil count • Immunofixation (serum) • DNA mutational analysis for dystrophinopathy • DNA mutational analysis for FSH muscular dystrophy • DNA mutational analysis for oculopharyngeal muscular dystrophy • DNA mutational analysis for specific mitochondrial disorders • DNA mutational analysis for myotonic muscular dystrophy types I and II • Myositis specific antibodies (e.g., anti-Signal Recognition Particle, Anti-Jo1) • Forced vital capacity • Electrocardiogram, echocardiogram • Slit-lamp examination

CK, Creatine kinase; *EMG,* electromyography; *FSH,* facioscapulohumeral.

Cardiomyopathies, with or without cardiac conduction abnormalities, occur in several of these disorders. Serial electrocardiographic surveillance and echocardiographic screening are important if the natural disease history or the patient's symptoms raise the possibility of accompanying cardiac dysfunction. Cardiac transplantation is rarely considered in BMD or other myopathies wherein congestive heart failure is the dominant symptom.

Prognosis

Accurate diagnosis remains important for counseling, prognosis, and treatment considerations. Precise definition of inheritance patterns is particularly important in myopathic disorders wherein the ADLs and life expectancy are diminished, especially where prenatal testing may be available. Affected patients and sometimes their families must be made aware of all implications of their diagnoses as tactfully and honestly as possible. The issues are even more compelling when dealing with an affected child. Many patients and their families have the misconception that all muscle diseases have a natural course similar to that of DMD. Those with more indolent disorders including certain congenital myopathies and milder forms of muscular dystrophy can often be reassured that the expected natural history is one of mild progression and normal life expectancy.

ADDITIONAL RESOURCES

Amato AA, Russell JA. Neuromuscular disorders. 2nd ed. New York: McGraw-Hill; 2016.

Domingos J, Sarkozy A, Scoto M, et al. Dystrophinopathies and limb-girdle muscular dystrophies. Neuropediatrics 2017;48:262–72.

Moxley R. Channelopathies affecting skeletal muscle in childhood. In: Jones HR, De Vivo D, Darras BT, editors. Neuromuscular disorders of infancy, childhood, and adolescence. Philadelphia, PA: Butterworth-Heinemann; 2003:783–812.

North K, Goebel HH. Congenital myopathies. In: Jones HR, De Vivo D, Darras BT, editors. Neuromuscular disorders of infancy, childhood, and adolescence. Philadelphia, PA: Butterworth-Heinemann; 2003:601–32.

North K, Jones K. Congenital muscular dystrophies. In: Jones HR, De Vivo D, Darras BT, editors. Neuromuscular disorders of infancy, childhood, and adolescence. Philadelphia, PA: Butterworth-Heinemann; 2003:633–48.

Snyder R. Bioethical issues. In: Jones HR, De Vivo D, Darras BT, editors. Neuromuscular disorders of infancy, childhood, and adolescence. Philadelphia, PA: Butterworth-Heinemann; 2003:1279–86.

71

Acquired Myopathies

Doreen T. Ho, Jayashri Srinivasan

CLINICAL VIGNETTE *A 55-year-old female with a recent history of interstitial lung disease reported weakness in her arms and legs. Recently she had noticed that she could not climb the 10 steps up from her basement. She had also developed difficulty picking up jars from the shelves of tall cabinets, as well as an inability to keep her hands over her head to brush her hair. She had no problems with swallowing. Her examination was significant for bilateral weakness of her hip flexors (iliopsoas), deltoids, biceps, and triceps. Muscle stretch reflexes were diminished but present. Sensory examination was normal.*

Serum creatine kinase (CK) was increased to 1200 U/L (six times normal). Electromyography (EMG) demonstrated normal nerve conduction studies. However, needle examination was abnormal, with large numbers of short-duration, low-amplitude, polyphasic motor unit potentials associated with scattered fibrillation potentials and complex repetitive discharges.

Comment: This patient's presentation is typical for a myopathic process with the clinical picture of evolving proximal weakness, elevated serum CK, and abnormal EMG.

The common acquired myopathies are classified into those having a primary inflammatory process, an underlying endocrinopathy, a toxic pathophysiology, or an underlying associated systemic disorder. Much less commonly, a few infectious agents, such as trichinosis, may lead to a primary myopathy. Myopathies typically present with symmetric symptoms and signs of muscle weakness affecting the proximal limbs and paraspinal musculature (Fig. 71.1). Asymmetric, distal, generalized, or regional patterns of weakness also occur in certain distinct myopathies such as sporadic inclusion body myositis (sIBM). Less commonly, ventilatory muscles or cardiac muscles are primarily affected. Myopathies occasionally present with periodic weakness, exercise-induced muscle pain, or stiffness.

Certain other neuromuscular disorders may mimic myopathies. Myopathies are included in the same differential diagnosis as neuromuscular transmission disorders, motor neuron disease, and rarely chronic inflammatory demyelinating polyneuropathies (CIDPs). Muscle stretch reflexes are generally normal or reduced, and sensation is usually unaffected in primary myopathies. The presence of certain distinguishing clinical features may help in the diagnosis of a myopathy. These include the pattern of weakness (e.g., presence of ptosis, ophthalmoparesis, ventilatory muscle weakness, scapular winging, head drop, symmetry, and proximal vs. distal weakness) or other clinical features (e.g., contractures, skeletal dysmorphisms, calf hypertrophy, myotonia, cardiac involvement, or subtle to marked dermatologic changes). Another very important diagnostic determinant is an assessment of the clinical temporal profile (e.g., the rate of progression), any history of a relapsing (periodic) weakness, diurnal variation, and symptoms that occur only with exertion. Other important factors include genetic predisposition, medication and toxin exposure, and other organ system involvement.

DIAGNOSTIC APPROACH

Patients who present with symptoms of myalgia and muscle weakness with a normal muscle strength examination and with normal or mildly elevated serum creatine kinase (CK) levels are common in clinical practice. Such patients are diagnostically and therapeutically challenging. Definable myopathic disorders are uncommon in patients who present with muscle pain, fatigue, or exercise intolerance in the absence of objective clinical, laboratory, or electrophysiologic abnormalities.

Laboratory Evaluation

Serum CK is characteristically increased in many myopathies; this may vary from a 2- to 50-fold increase, although in most myopathies CKs are usually in the 500–5000 IU/mL range (Fig. 71.2). When this enzyme is abnormally elevated, its serum levels do not closely parallel disease severity or activity. Serum aldolase levels are also frequently elevated in myopathies; its increase generally parallels the increase in CK; therefore many clinical neuromuscular specialists do not routinely order an aldolase level. CK levels may be helpful in distinguishing certain muscle conditions. For instance, CK in necrotizing myopathy is typically significantly elevated (>10× normal). CK is typically elevated (up to 5–10× normal) in sIBM but may be normal.

An increased CK level is a nonspecific finding. Other motor unit disorders (amyotrophic lateral sclerosis or spinal muscular atrophy) and systemic processes (particularly myxedema) are commonly associated with increased CK of two to five times normal levels. Conversely, serum CK can be normal in certain patients with dermatomyositis (DM) and sIBM. Certain demographic groups tend to have higher CKs, and CK tends to be slightly higher in men than women.

Patients with persistently increased CK levels, sometimes associated with muscle pain but without clinically demonstrable weakness, family history, or exposure to potentially myotoxic substances, are classified as having hyperCKemia. Despite thorough clinical and laboratory examination, it is often difficult to assign a specific pathophysiologic mechanism to this finding. Patients with hyperCKemia are at increased risk of malignant hyperthermia, and they need to be aware of this rare complication with certain anesthetic agents.

Serum aspartate and alanine aminotransferases (AST and ALT) are frequently elevated in many myopathies because these enzymes are released by diseased muscle. Rarely, some patients with clinically unsuspected myopathies undergo unnecessary evaluation for liver disease when AST and ALT elevations are found and CK has not been checked. Other liver function studies (e.g., gamma glutamyl transpeptidase and

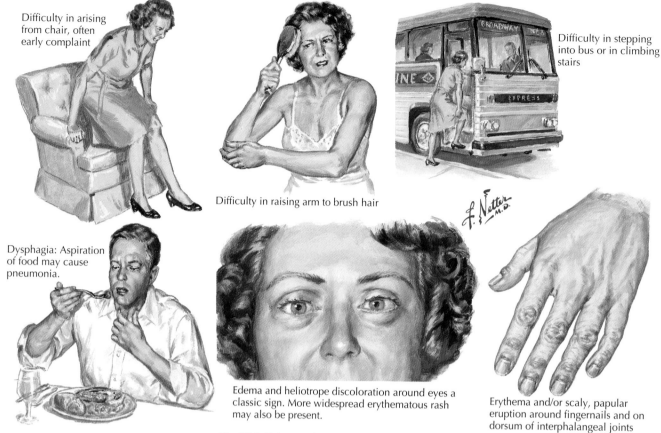

Difficulty in arising from chair, often early complaint

Difficulty in raising arm to brush hair

Difficulty in stepping into bus or in climbing stairs

Dysphagia: Aspiration of food may cause pneumonia.

Edema and heliotrope discoloration around eyes a classic sign. More widespread erythematous rash may also be present.

Erythema and/or scaly, papular eruption around fingernails and on dorsum of interphalangeal joints

Fig. 71.1 Polymyositis and Dermatomyositis.

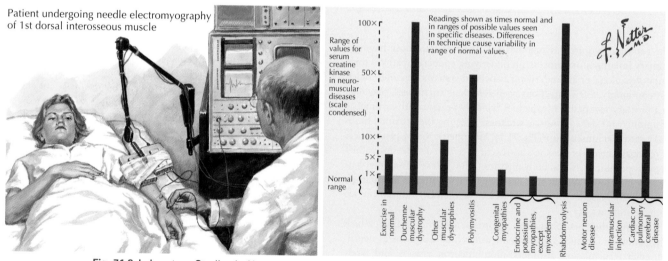

Patient undergoing needle electromyography of 1st dorsal interosseous muscle

Range of values for serum creatine kinase in neuro-muscular diseases (scale condensed)

Readings shown as times normal and in ranges of possible values seen in specific diseases. Differences in technique cause variability in range of normal values.

Normal range

Exercise in normal

Duchenne muscular dystrophy

Other muscular dystrophies

Polymyositis

Congenital myopathies

Endocrine and potassium myopathies, except myxedema

Rhabdomyolysis

Motor neuron disease

Intramuscular injection

Cardiac or pulmonary cerebral disease

Fig. 71.2 Laboratory Studies in Neuromuscular Diseases: Electromyography and Serum Enzymes.

prothrombin time) are normal in myopathies, providing another clue to the probability of a primary skeletal muscle rather than a hepatic disorder.

Routine biochemistry and hematologic laboratory tests are usually normal in patients with myopathy. Serum potassium levels should be checked to exclude Addison disease with hyperkalemia. Various muscle disorders characterized by episodic periodic paralysis may sometimes have either hypokalemia or hyperkalemia if they are tested during the overt period of paralysis. However, these patients most often have normal potassium values if tested between episodes of weakness. Serum markers of inflammation such as the erythrocyte sedimentation rate (ESR) and C-reactive protein (CRP) may be elevated in some acute myopathies. Thyroid function evaluation (serum thyroid-stimulating hormone [TSH] levels) must be considered in all patients presenting with an acute or chronic myopathy. Both hypothyroidism and rarely hyperthyroidism may present with primary muscle involvement. Appropriate endocrine evaluation is necessary in myopathic patients when a more obvious diagnosis is not apparent. These also include pituitary adrenal disorders such as

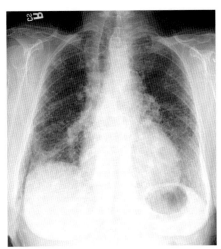

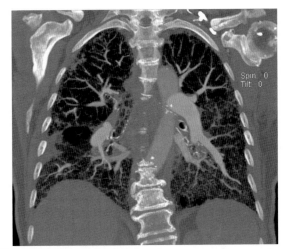

A. Posterioranterior chest film shows extensive pulmonary fibrosis with typical honeycomb pattern.

B. Coronal reconstruction of chest from computed tomography angiography shows extensive interstitial thickening, cystic changes, and honeycombing bilaterally with cystic changes involving more the upper than lower lungs. Confluent pleural thickening is seen laterally on the right.

Fig. 71.3 Severe Pulmonary Fibrosis.

Cushing syndrome or Addison disease, and very rarely hyperparathyroidism. In certain ethnic groups, thyrotoxicosis may be associated with hypokalemia and a proximal myopathy resembling periodic paralysis.

Serum myositis-specific and myositis-associated antibodies are other testing parameters that are useful in the evaluation of some patients with a myopathy. The presence of anti-Jo-1 (antibody to histidyl t-RNA synthetase) antibodies suggests potential end organ comorbidity, for example, interstitial lung disease (ILD; Fig. 71.3). In these patients, use of methotrexate is therefore not recommended. Signal recognition particle (SRP) antibodies are most often associated with necrotizing myopathies and may suggest a refractory course. Antibodies against cytosolic 5′ nucleotidase 1a (cN1a) may be helpful in the diagnosis of sIBM. Anti-3-hydroxy-3-methylglutaryl-coenzyme A reductase (anti-HMGCR) has been described in patients with a necrotizing myopathy that responds to immunosuppression and may be associated with statin use.

Sometimes polymyositis (PM) is associated with an underlying connective tissue disorder. In those patients, serologic markers for the underlying disease may be positive. These include antinuclear antibody (ANA) and/or rheumatoid factor. On occasion, the presence of these antibodies can aid in the diagnosis of the occasional patient for whom the history is not definitive. This is especially so when there is diagnostic confusion between the possibility of an acquired inflammatory myopathy and a genetically determined dystrophy. When PM and, less commonly, DM are associated with other collagen-vascular diseases, the combination is referred to as an overlap syndrome. Systemic lupus erythematosus (SLE), systemic sclerosis, rheumatoid arthritis, and Sjögren syndrome may have weakness as a component of their myriad symptoms and signs. In these cases, muscular weakness exceeds what arthritis alone can account for. They are characterized by elevated titers of anti–U1/U2-ribonucleoprotein antibodies, PM-Scl antibodies, or anti-Sjögren's-syndrome-related antigen A (SSA) antibodies in scleroderma, Sjögren syndrome, SLE, or mixed connective tissue disease. DM is rarely associated with other collagen-vascular diseases, with the exception of scleroderma. sIBM is associated with underlying autoimmune disorder (e.g., SLE, Scleroderma, Sjögren) in up to 15% of cases.

Paraneoplastic antibody evaluation may occasionally be helpful in the differential diagnosis of proximal weakness. This is particularly so in patients with Lambert-Eaton myasthenic syndrome (LEMS) who often present with symptoms mimicking a myopathy. These individuals have elevated levels of voltage-gated calcium channel antibodies. This finding, in addition to the classic EMG nerve conduction studies typically seen in LEMS, is very specific for this diagnosis. In addition, anti-Hu antibodies may be positive in patients with myopathy associated with small cell lung cancer.

Immunofixation to look for the presence of serum monoclonal protein is necessary in certain instances if either amyloid myopathy or sporadic late-onset nemaline myopathy (SLONM) is in the differential diagnosis. Approximately 20% of patients with sIBM also have a monoclonal gammopathy of uncertain significance (MGUS). Appropriate endocrine evaluation is necessary in myopathic patients when a more obvious diagnosis is not apparent.

Vitamin D levels are also important. Rarely, hypovitaminosis D may present with a myopathy. Similarly, patients with primary or secondary osteomalacia may present with proximal weakness. Elevated serum alkaline phosphatase and low serum calcium values may point toward these under recognized disorders.

Electromyography

EMG evaluation of patients with suspected myopathies is important (Fig. 71.4, and see Fig. 71.2). Results of routine nerve conduction studies are normal in myopathies, with the exception of diminished compound muscle action potential amplitudes in more severe disorders. The primary EMG abnormalities in the myopathies are classically found at the time of the needle examination. Classic findings of a myopathy include the presence of abnormally low amplitude, short duration, and polyphasic motor unit potentials (MUPs). In myopathies, patients have both an early recruitment and increased numbers of MUPs early on in the muscle activation for a given effort. However, adding to diagnostic confusion, patients with chronic myopathies (e.g., sIBM) can sometimes have needle examination findings resembling that of a chronic neurogenic process. Destruction of myofibrils or muscle membrane results in abnormal insertional activity, particularly fibrillation potentials and complex repetitive discharges. Inflammatory myopathies, dystrophies, and myotonic disorders may be distinguished from neurogenic disorders by the presence of myotonic potentials on needle EMG.

Concomitantly, EMG helps to exclude disorders that affect other anatomic sites within the peripheral motor unit, particularly those with symmetric proximal weakness mimicking a myopathy. These include

A. Electromyography

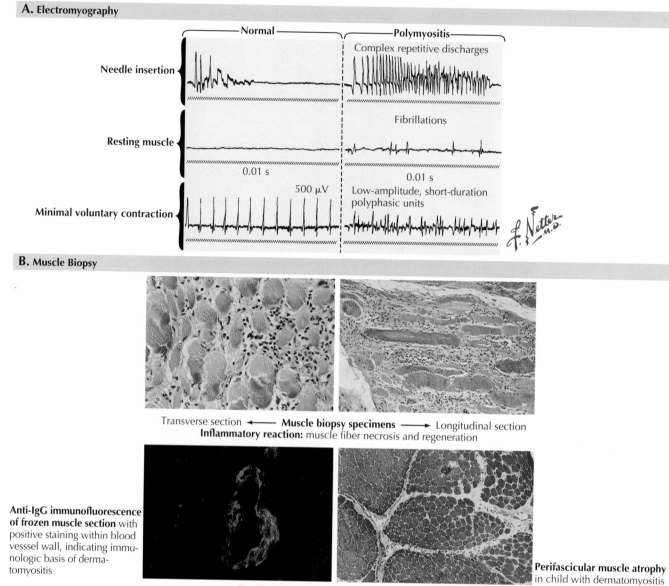

Fig. 71.4 Polymyositis/Dermatomyositis.

motor neuron disorders, such as amyotrophic lateral sclerosis and spinal muscular atrophy type 3 and 4, CIDP, neuromuscular transmission disorders (particularly LEMS), and myasthenia gravis. Results of EMG are often normal in the various endocrine, mitochondrial, and congenital myopathies.

Imaging Studies

Magnetic resonance imaging (MRI) of muscles, in addition to EMG to look for signal change abnormalities, is useful in patients with inflammatory myopathies because it may highlight the pattern of preferential involvement (e.g., the quadriceps in sIBM) and may help in the selection of a diseased muscle that can be a potential biopsy site. MRI of muscles may also be helpful in certain patients in whom muscle biopsy is contraindicated.

Muscle Biopsy

Muscle biopsy is the definitive diagnostic tool for many myopathies (Fig. 71.5). The selection of the biopsy site is important; muscles that are unaffected, that are severely affected and therefore likely to only show end-stage changes, or that have been recently subjected to needle EMG evaluation should be avoided. Muscles commonly biopsied include the vastus lateralis, deltoid, rectus femoris, and biceps brachii. The gastrocnemius muscle is often avoided due to the possibility of incidentally discovered neurogenic atrophy. The upper lumbosacral muscles, thoracic paraspinal muscles, such as the multifidus, and much less commonly the cervical paraspinal muscles provide alternative sites for biopsy.

The muscle biopsy specimen is divided into separate aliquots for formalin fixation, paraffin embedding, and immediate freezing in isopentane cooled in liquid nitrogen. The formalin-fixed piece is stained with hematoxylin and eosin (H and E) because this permits a rapid means for initial evaluation. This is especially useful for identifying inflammatory myopathies where such a diagnosis offers the potential for successful therapeutic intervention. Frozen specimens are best for other stains, including nicotinamide adenine dinucleotide dehydrogenase (NADH), modified Gomori trichrome, adenosine triphosphatase, and lipid and glycogen stains (Fig. 71.6 and see Fig. 71.4).

Muscle biopsy specimens are also subjected to biochemical analysis, mutational analysis, and electron microscopy (EM) when these

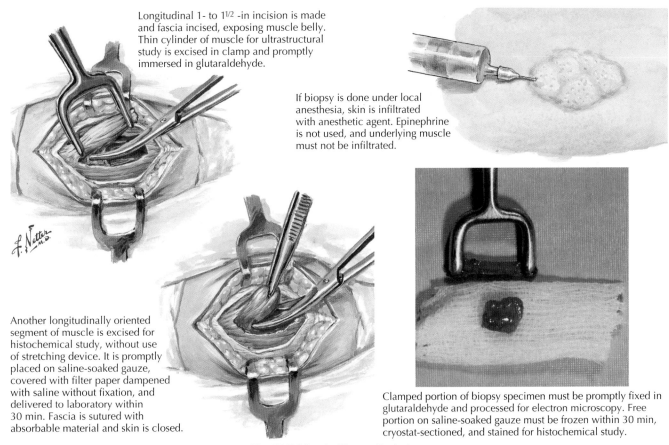

Longitudinal 1- to 1½ -in incision is made and fascia incised, exposing muscle belly. Thin cylinder of muscle for ultrastructural study is excised in clamp and promptly immersed in glutaraldehyde.

If biopsy is done under local anesthesia, skin is infiltrated with anesthetic agent. Epinephrine is not used, and underlying muscle must not be infiltrated.

Another longitudinally oriented segment of muscle is excised for histochemical study, without use of stretching device. It is promptly placed on saline-soaked gauze, covered with filter paper dampened with saline without fixation, and delivered to laboratory within 30 min. Fascia is sutured with absorbable material and skin is closed.

Clamped portion of biopsy specimen must be promptly fixed in glutaraldehyde and processed for electron microscopy. Free portion on saline-soaked gauze must be frozen within 30 min, cryostat-sectioned, and stained for histochemical study.

Fig. 71.5 Muscle Biopsy: Technique.

techniques are indicated. Inherited myopathies, such as the various muscular dystrophies, are evaluated by immunohistochemical stains and immunoblotting; testing is available for calpain, caveolin, dysferlin, the dystroglycans, dystrophin, laminin-2 (formerly merosin), and the sarcoglycans.

SPECIFIC INFLAMMATORY MYOPATHIES

There are three acquired inflammatory myopathies: PM, DM, and sIBM. Necrotizing myopathies are often classified with the inflammatory myopathies because they are immune mediated; however, they lack inflammation or have minimal inflammation on muscle biopsy.

Polymyositis

This relatively uncommon inflammatory myopathy is seen mainly in adults and presents subacutely usually over a period of several weeks to a few months. Clinically, an important means for distinguishing PM from DM is the absence of skin involvement in PM. However, DM may also rarely present without skin involvement (sine dermatitis). Various criteria have been proposed to make a definitive diagnosis of PM. Usually PM patients present with symmetric proximal weakness, involving the upper and lower extremities. Mild dysphagia, myalgia, and systemic symptoms, such as polyarthritis, may accompany the weakness. Rarely, patients may present with either a clinically isolated head drop or respiratory muscle weakness. Acid maltase deficiency (glycogen storage disease type II) needs to be considered in those individuals presenting primarily with respiratory symptoms. The proximal and symmetric pattern of weakness in PM distinguishes it from the classic asymmetric regional pattern of weakness in sIBM. Historically, certain

patients with sIBM were likely misdiagnosed as having PM; sIBM is more common than PM.

EMG is often abnormal and may show characteristic findings of myopathic motor units and increased insertional activity, with fibrillation potentials and complex repetitive discharges. Laboratory studies reveal an elevated CK level. Muscle biopsy demonstrates perimysial and endomysial inflammatory infiltrate with CD8+ T cells invading nonnecrotic muscle fibers (see Fig. 71.4). ILD can be seen in 10%–20% of patients with PM and may be associated with positive anti-Jo-1 antibody. Cardiac involvement (cardiomyopathy and congestive heart failure) is common, although the incidence of these associated conditions is unknown.

Dermatomyositis

DM is seen in both children and adults. Proximal weakness develops insidiously over weeks. The characteristic rash may accompany or precede the myopathy (see Fig. 71.1). The rash is present over the exposed areas of the face, neck, and arms. Other dermatologic manifestations include heliotrope rash over the eyelids and erythematous rash over the knuckles, known as Gottron papules (Fig. 71.1, *bottom*). Nail bed examination will often demonstrate capillary telangiectasia. Occasional DM patients never develop this classic rash; here the differential diagnosis from PM is made on the classic pathologic findings of perifascicular atrophies in the muscle biopsy. In contrast, some patients present with the classic DM rash but have no signs of a clinical myopathy (i.e., amyopathic DM). Other systemic manifestations include calcinosis, dysphagia, cardiomyopathy, and ILD (see Fig. 71.3). As in PM, ILD may be associated with positive anti-Jo-1 antibodies in some patients.

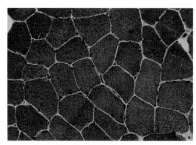

Cryostat section of normal adult muscle stained with hematoxylin and eosin. Muscle fibers are uniform in size and stain pink with eosin; their sarcolemmal nuclei are peripherally located and stain blue with hematoxylin.

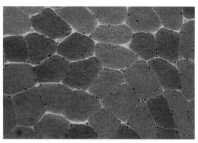

Cryostat section of normal adult muscle treated with modified Gomori trichrome stain, which stains muscle fibers greenish blue and sarcolemmal nuclei dark red.

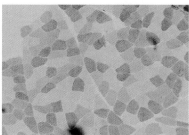

Cryostat section of normal muscle from adult male (ATPase stain, pH 4.6). Type II fibers, which contain low amounts of acid-stable ATPase, are subtyped into IIA (lightest) and IIB (intermediate) fibers. Type I (darkest) fibers contain largest amount of acid-stable ATPase. Each of these 3 fiber types amounts to about 1/3 of total number.

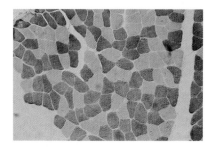

Cryostat section of normal muscle from adult male (ATPase stain, pH 9.4), showing typical checkerboard pattern with about twice as many type II fibers, which are high in alkali-stable ATPase and hence stain darkly.

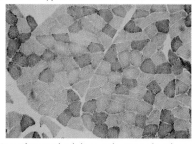

Cryostat section of normal adult muscle stained with NADH, an oxidative enzyme that reacts with mitochondria, sarcoplasmic reticulum, and T tubules. Type I fibers stain more darkly.

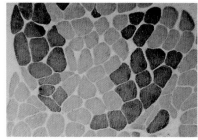

Cryostat section of reinnervated skeletal muscle stained with ATPase (pH 9.4), showing grouping of 2 fiber types: type I (lighter), type II (darker). Compare with normal section stained with ATPase (pH 9.4) above.

Fig. 71.6 Sections From Muscle Biopsy Specimens.

DM in adults may be associated with underlying malignancy. The cumulative incidence rate of malignancy varied from 20% at 1 year post-DM diagnosis to approximately 30% 5 years after the diagnosis of DM. Adult patients should undergo evaluation for a possible underlying malignancy. The intensity of diagnostic evaluation for a potential occult cancer is determined individually. Factors that point to a higher likelihood of an associated malignancy include age at diagnosis older than 45 years, a rapid onset of skin and/or muscular symptoms, the presence of skin necrosis or periungual erythema, high levels of inflammatory markers, and certain myositis specific antibodies (e.g., anti-p155/140). This association with malignancy is not seen in juvenile DM and much less commonly in PM. A general physical examination, a thorough review of systems, a chest radiograph or computed tomography (CT), a mammogram (in women), a complete blood count (CBC), urinalysis, and stool guaiac, colonoscopy, Pap smears in women, CT scan of abdomen and pelvis, and tumor markers are considered reasonable screening protocols.

Laboratory tests typically demonstrate elevated CK, although CK may be normal in DM. ANA and anti-Jo-1 antibodies may be elevated. EMG will reveal characteristic myopathic changes in established disease.

The characteristic histopathology in DM is perifascicular atrophy, although this may not be seen in early disease (see Fig. 71.4). Inflammation is not prominent; when present it is seen in the perimysial and perivascular regions.

The pathogenesis of DM is thought to be a microangiopathy. A membrane attack complex (MAC) can be demonstrated on capillaries. EM may reveal tubuloreticular inclusions in endothelial cells.

Specific Pharmacologic Therapies

PM and DM respond to immunomodulation treatments. Prednisone is the "gold standard," although its efficacy has never been confirmed in a well-designed prospective study; typically, prednisone equivalents of 1–1.5 mg/kg/day are started. To diminish the severity of the corticosteroid side effects, alternate-day dosing and/or appropriate dose tapers must be considered as soon as symptoms are adequately controlled. Second-line agents, such as azathioprine, methotrexate, mycophenolate mofetil, or rituximab, may be used as a steroid-sparing agent. Sequential CK measurements may be useful because a rise in CK may herald a clinical relapse while on treatment. Previous tuberculosis exposure should be excluded before initiation of steroid treatment. Vitamin D and calcium are regularly supplemented in patients on prednisone, particularly in women. Bone densitometry is indicated for patients at risk of osteopenia. Serum glucose and potassium levels need to be monitored at regular intervals and treated or supplemented when needed. Other immunomodulation options include intravenous immunoglobulin (IVIG) or plasma exchange.

Inclusion Body Myosotis

> **CLINICAL VIGNETTE** *A 61-year-old woman reported a 5-year history of weakness in her legs and hands. She noticed that when getting down on the ground to play with her grandchildren, she could not get up. More recently, she had several falls in the past 6 months, all of them due to "knee buckling and legs giving out." Lately she had noted difficulty flossing her teeth because of weakness in her fingers. When questioned, she did admit to choking on salads more frequently.*
>
> *Neurologic examination revealed significant weakness of the finger flexors bilaterally, as well as severe asymmetric weakness of the knee extensors with atrophy of both ventral forearms and quadriceps. There was also mild weakness of the right wrist, ankle dorsiflexors, and neck flexors, as well as mild bilateral facial weakness. Ankle jerks were diminished; the remainder of muscle stretch reflexes and sensory examination results were normal.*
>
> *Serum CK was increased to 900 IU/L. Nerve conduction studies were normal. EMG revealed a mixed myopathic-neuropathic pattern of motor units with increased insertional activity and fibrillation potentials. Muscle biopsy of the left quadriceps demonstrated endomysial inflammation and atrophic and hypertrophic fibers. Rimmed vacuoles were identified with a modified Gomori trichrome stain. Electron microscopy revealed tubofilament inclusion bodies in affected fibers.*

sIBM is the most common inflammatory myopathy occurring in patients older than age 50. It is often an indolent, progressive condition presenting after years of subtle symptoms. Because the onset is quite insidious, the mean interval from symptom onset to diagnosis may be 5–10 years. Men are more commonly affected (2 : 1 to 3 : 1 ratio). sIBM is frequently characterized by the finding of an asymmetric weakness that typically affects the finger and wrist flexors in the upper extremities as well as knee extensors and foot dorsiflexors in the lower extremities (Fig. 71.7). Much less commonly, patients with sIBM may present with a limb girdle pattern of weakness. Dysphagia is common in sIBM (up to 60% of patients). Approximately 30% of patients have facial weakness. An associated sensory neuropathy may occur in sIBM patients and may be detected on EMG as a mild axonal sensory neuropathy. Usually there is no involvement of the other systems. Unlike that in PM or DM, there is no associated ILD, myocarditis, or malignancy. However, patients may have concomitant autoimmune disease (e.g., Sjögren, SLE). Approximately 20% of patients with sIBM have an MGUS.

Laboratory tests reveal a normal to elevated CK (usually up to 10 times normal). Nerve conductions may show an associated sensory neuropathy. EMG will classically reveal myopathic units with muscle membrane irritability. However, needle EMG may show chronic neurogenic-appearing motor unit action potentials (large polyphasic motor unit action potentials) or mixed myopathic and neurogenic units, due to the chronic course of the disease. Muscle biopsy may demonstrate endomysial inflammation and the characteristic rimmed vacuoles, although sampling error may occur and the absence of rimmed vacuoles does not exclude the possibility of sIBM. Ragged red fibers may be present. Intranuclear and intracytoplasmic tubulofilament inclusions may be demonstrated by EM. Antibodies against cytosolic 5′-nucleotidase 1A may be present in approximately two-thirds of patients with sIBM.

The pathogenesis of IBM is unknown. Muscle biopsy may demonstrate an inflammatory component, and myopathic changes appear chronic. sIBM may be autoimmune. However, despite therapeutic trials of a number of various immunosuppressive pharmacologic agents, none of the traditional immunomodulation therapies are beneficial and treatment to date is supportive. sIBM could be a degenerative disorder.

The general prognosis for an sIBM patient is of a slowly indolent course with typically normal life span. However, patients with sIBM have various significant limitations, particularly due to finger flexor weakness, that impairs fine manipulations such as buttoning clothes, handwriting, and putting keys into locks. Dysphagia may be a progressive issue over time and lead to complications. Esophageal dilation and botulinum toxin of lower esophageal sphincter may be considered based on largely anecdotal evidence. For some patients, dysphagia progresses to the point that they have required percutaneous endoscopic gastrostomy. Physical and occupational therapy and braces are important aspects of supportive care for these patients.

Immune-Mediated Necrotizing Myopathies

Immune-mediated necrotizing myopathies (IMNMs) are often classified with the acquired inflammatory myopathies due their suspected autoimmune mechanism; however, notably, IMNMs lack inflammation on muscle biopsy. Patients have proximal weakness and very high CKs (e.g., >10× the upper limit of normal). IMNM may be paraneoplastic in origin, and thorough workup for malignancy is recommended. IMNM may also be rarely triggered by a statin medication and require long-term immunosuppression even when the statin is withdrawn. Patients with immune-mediated necrotizing myopathy associated with statins have anti-HMGCR autoantibodies (see later).

The workup for IMNM tends to be similar to that of PM or DM, with a high degree of surveillance for malignancy. Treatment of IMNM tends to involve both steroids, IVIG, and a steroid-sparing agent (e.g., azathioprine, mycophenolate mofetil). In refractory cases rituximab may be another option.

OTHER ACQUIRED MYOPATHIES

Toxic Myopathies

Many pharmacologic agents may cause myopathies as rare adverse effects of their use (Box 71.1). The almost ubiquitously used 3-hydroxy-3-methyl-glutaryl-coenzyme A (HMG-CoA) reductase inhibitor (statin) class of lipid-lowering agents may trigger an IMNM in a very small percentage of these patients. Muscle biopsies in severely affected patients demonstrate necrosis without inflammation. These patients tend to require immunosuppressive treatment for their IMNM because symptoms do not remit even after withdrawal of the statin medication.

More commonly, a slightly larger percentage of patients on statin medications develop an asymptomatic hyperCKemia. This is thought to be related to subclinical muscle inflammation. On other occasions, some patients taking statins present with myalgias and/or proximal weakness. Very rarely a rhabdomyolysis may develop in this setting. The risk for muscle toxicity increases in patients simultaneously exposed to multiple potentially myotoxic drugs. Fibric acid derivatives and niacin also occasionally demonstrate myotoxic properties. Typically in these patients, symptoms improve with withdrawal of the offending agent and treatment is supportive.

Chloroquine may cause an amphiphilic neuromyopathy. These patients classically demonstrate both a peripheral neuropathy and a myopathy. The serum CK level is often modestly increased in this setting. Muscle biopsy characteristically reveals an autophagic vacuolation, with markedly increased staining for acid phosphatase.

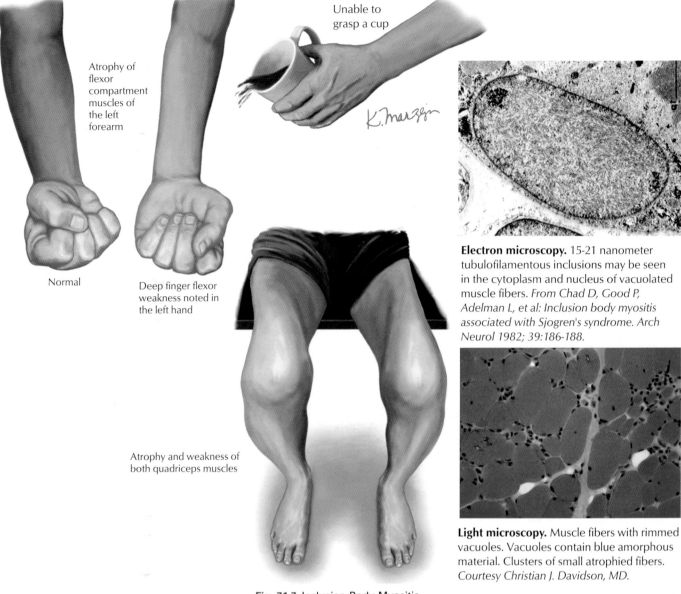

Atrophy of flexor compartment muscles of the left forearm

Unable to grasp a cup

Normal

Deep finger flexor weakness noted in the left hand

Atrophy and weakness of both quadriceps muscles

Electron microscopy. 15-21 nanometer tubulofilamentous inclusions may be seen in the cytoplasm and nucleus of vacuolated muscle fibers. *From Chad D, Good P, Adelman L, et al: Inclusion body myositis associated with Sjogren's syndrome. Arch Neurol 1982; 39:186-188.*

Light microscopy. Muscle fibers with rimmed vacuoles. Vacuoles contain blue amorphous material. Clusters of small atrophied fibers. *Courtesy Christian J. Davidson, MD.*

Fig. 71.7 Inclusion Body Myositis.

BOX 71.1 **Toxic Myopathies**	
Alcohol	Leuprolide
Aminocaproic acid	Lithium
Amiodarone	L-Tryptophan
Chloroquine/hydroxychloroquine	Neuromuscular blocking agents
Cholesterol-lowering agents	Omeprazole
Cimetidine	Penicillamine
Colchicine	Procainamide
Corticosteroids	Propofol
Cyclosporine	Rifampin
Emetine	Tacrolimus
Illicit drugs (intramuscular injections)	Toluene (inhalation)
Ipecac	Vincristine
Labetalol	Vitamin E
Lamotrigine	Zidovudine

Chronic administration of steroids, typically at doses higher than 30 mg/day, can also cause a myopathy. Steroid myopathy can present acutely or subacutely, classically with preferential involvement of the proximal lower extremities. Bulbar and distal muscles, sensation, and reflexes are typically spared. Importantly, CK is normal. Nerve conduction and needle EMG are typically normal, and muscle biopsy may demonstrate atrophy of type II (especially IIB) fibers, lipid droplets within type I fibers, and rarely abnormal mitochondria on EM.

Amiodarone is an antiarrhythmic drug that causes a neuromyopathy similar to that produced by chloroquine. It can also cause myopathy indirectly by inducing hypothyroidism.

Colchicine may also cause either a myopathy or neuropathy, which may be related to colchicine-induced alteration of microtubular function. CK is usually increased, and muscle biopsies demonstrate autophagic vacuoles. Symptoms improve with drug discontinuation.

Immunosuppressive agents, including cyclosporine and tacrolimus, may cause generalized myalgias and proximal muscle weakness within months after starting therapy. The pathogenic basis for this effect is still

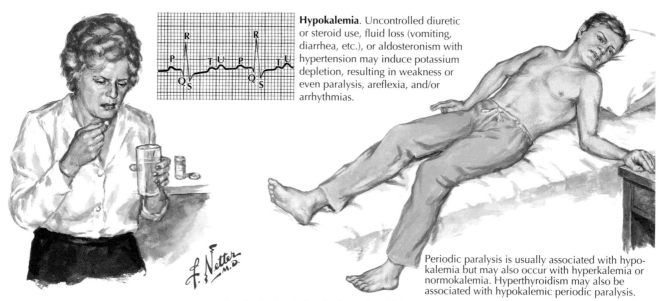

Hypokalemia. Uncontrolled diuretic or steroid use, fluid loss (vomiting, diarrhea, etc.), or aldosteronism with hypertension may induce potassium depletion, resulting in weakness or even paralysis, areflexia, and/or arrhythmias.

Periodic paralysis is usually associated with hypokalemia but may also occur with hyperkalemia or normokalemia. Hyperthyroidism may also be associated with hypokalemic periodic paralysis.

Fig. 71.8 Hypokalemia Associated Myopathy.

unknown; there is some suggestion that cyclosporine myotoxicity may have a pathogenesis similar to that of statins. There is a further increased risk of developing a myopathy when patients take both cyclosporine and statins.

Labetalol is an antihypertensive drug that has been associated with rare reports of necrotizing myopathy. Symptoms improve after discontinuation of the drug.

Propofol is a relatively newer anesthetic agent increasingly used in sedating ventilated patients. There have been reports of rhabdomyolysis and myoglobinuria described in children but not in adults. Vincristine, a chemotherapeutic agent, acts by disrupting the polymerization of tubulin into microtubules. It is classically associated with a severe sensorimotor axonal neuropathy, but occasionally it can also cause proximal muscle weakness accompanied by myalgias.

Zidovudine (AZT), a primary therapy for human immunodeficiency virus (HIV) infection, can induce a myopathy related to mitochondrial dysfunction. The myopathies caused by zidovudine and by HIV infection are clinically indistinguishable. CK values are usually increased. EMG does not distinguish between toxic AZT and HIV myopathies. Muscle biopsies demonstrate endomysial inflammation. Prominent ragged red fibers suggest AZT-induced mitochondrial abnormalities. AZT myopathies usually improve on drug cessation.

Critical Illness Myopathy

Critical illness myopathy (CIM) is also referred to as acute quadriplegic myopathy or myopathy associated with thick filament (myosin) loss. It is probably the most common cause of generalized weakness identified for patients having a prolonged stay in the intensive care unit (ICU). CIM is commonly seen in patients treated with high doses of corticosteroids or neuromuscular blocking drugs. Often these patients were initially septic and developed multiorgan failure. It may be associated with a sensorimotor axonal polyneuropathy (critical illness neuropathy), and certain patients may have features of a neuromyopathy due to critical illness.

In CIM, the weakness in these patients develops over several days. It is often not recognized until there is an attempt to wean the patient from the ventilator. Clinical examination reveals a profound, occasionally asymmetric, weakness with reduced muscle stretch reflexes but a normal sensory examination. Serum CK is increased in less than half of these patients. Muscle biopsies may demonstrate muscle fiber necrosis,

atrophy of type 1 and 2 fibers, and patchy loss of uptake with adenosine triphosphatase stains; the latter correlates with electron microscopic demonstration of thick filament (myosin) loss. The pathogenesis of this entity is not known.

Hypokalemic Myopathies

Hypokalemia is a rare metabolic cause of an acute myopathy (Fig. 71.8). The presentation may mimic Guillain-Barré syndrome. ICU observation is recommended because of potential serious cardiac arrhythmias that the severe hypokalemia may induce. The differential diagnosis includes various potassium-losing diuretics and corticosteroids and other medications (e.g., laxatives, lithium, or amphotericin). Chronic alcoholism, rarely hyperaldosteronism or a villous adenoma of the colon, and excessive intake of licorice are other important causes of hypokalemia-induced weakness.

Endocrine Myopathies

CLINICAL VIGNETTE *A 41-year-old woman had reported weakness in arms and legs. Her husband noted that her emotions were more labile. Neurologic examination demonstrated moderate proximal weakness. Serum CK was normal, but aldolase was mildly elevated. When she returned for her EMG, the neurologist noted generalized bruising that resembled that of patients taking corticosteroids, although she was not taking any; also, there was no other common stigmata of Cushing syndrome apparent. The patient's EMG demonstrated myopathic motor unit potentials with fibrillation potentials.*

Because of her obvious classic dermatologic stigmata, Cushing syndrome was considered in the differential of this slowly evolving myopathy. Serum cortisol and particularly urinary free cortisol levels, as well as 24-hour 17-OH corticosteroids, were increased. An endocrinologist also found evidence of recent-onset hypertension; exam demonstrated mild increase in facial hair, slight mooning of her facies, but no abdominal striae or shoulder hump. Elevated adrenocorticotropic hormone (ACTH) levels led to the diagnosis of a corticotrophin-producing pituitary tumor.

Comment: This patient's clinical picture was suggestive of a proximal myopathy, and the easy bruising on examination led to the suspicion of Cushing syndrome. Clinically the typical features of Cushing syndrome were quite subtle. Her EMG findings were surprising because most endocrine myopathies, including corticosteroid-induced myopathies, are not associated with myopathic MUPs or abnormal insertional activity. Despite such, laboratory tests confirmed the diagnosis of Cushing disease.

Disorders of the adrenal, thyroid, parathyroid, and pituitary glands can result in subacute or, less commonly, acute myopathies. Interestingly, muscle involvement in such conditions may be apparent before patients develop typical clinical findings of their primary endocrinopathy. This is well illustrated by the prior vignette.

Cushing syndrome due to hyperadrenocorticism is either primary, iatrogenic, or rarely secondary to excessive pituitary secretion of ACTH (Fig. 71.9). This is one of the more common causes of an endocrine myopathy. Patients with Cushing syndrome, irrespective of etiology, experience proximal muscle weakness with atrophy usually starting in the hip girdles. Distal, bulbar, and ocular muscles are usually unaffected. Women seem to be more susceptible than men. Alternate-day corticosteroid dosing schedules and enriched protein diets may reduce susceptibility to iatrogenic-induced Cushing syndrome. The serum CK level is usually normal. EMG is normal in iatrogenic steroid myopathy but is occasionally "myopathic" in patients with true Cushing syndrome. Muscle biopsy demonstrates a nonspecific type II muscle fiber atrophy. The pathogenesis of the myopathy is poorly understood but may be related to increased protein catabolism.

Primary adrenocortical insufficiency or Addison disease may be associated with a myopathy. Addison disease is characterized by weight loss, bronzing of the skin, hypotension, and hyperkalemia (see Fig. 71.9). Muscle weakness may be an early symptom of this disease and may be due to the associated hyperkalemia.

Thyroid dysfunction is another important consideration in the differential diagnosis of adult-onset myopathies. Hypothyroidism-associated myopathy is characterized by proximal weakness, fatigue, slowed movements and reflexes, stiffness, myalgia, and muscle cramps (Fig. 71.10). An elevated CK, sometimes up to 10 times normal, is a common finding in hypothyroid patients.

Hyperthyroidism-induced myopathy may also present with weakness, and the incidence of weakness in patients with thyrotoxicosis is high (up to 82%). Patients with thyrotoxicosis tend to have proximal muscle weakness and fatigue as prominent complaints (Fig. 71.11). Serum enzyme levels, including creatine kinase (CK) and AST, tend to be normal.

In addition to typical myopathic features, hyperthyroid patients have brisk muscle stretch reflexes, thyroid eye disease with proptosis, and impairment of extraocular muscle function. Furthermore, myasthenia gravis occurs in approximately 5% of thyrotoxic patients. Asian males with hyperthyroidism also have a propensity to hypokalemic periodic paralysis. Serum CK and routine electrodiagnostic study results are usually normal.

Hyperparathyroidism may be associated with a painful myopathy. This most likely relates to the effect of hyperparathyroidism on vitamin D metabolism and resultant osteomalacia.

Osteomalacia, Hypovitamin D Myopathy

Lack of vitamin D can lead to decreased calcium and phosphorus absorption and secondary hyperparathyroidism with eventual osteomalacia. This is associated with an unusual but very treatable myopathy with associated bone pain, loss of appendicular height, and kyphoscoliosis.

Although usually considered in chronic renal failure, osteomalacic myopathy may also occur in patients receiving long-term treatment with phenytoin or with various malabsorptive syndromes. Individuals taking statins are more prone to developing symptomatic myositis secondary to hypovitaminosis D. Supplementation of same may totally relieve the symptoms of a painful myopathy while continuing to use the statin medication. Serum vitamin D levels may be very low while CK and electrodiagnostic studies are normal. Muscle biopsy, if performed, demonstrates type II fiber atrophy. Vitamin D and calcium supplementation can lead to excellent improvement.

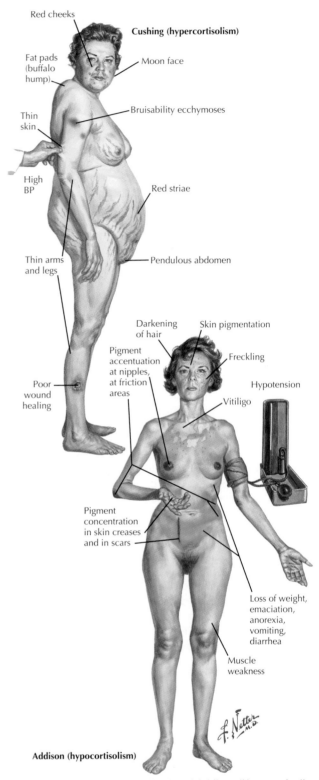

Fig. 71.9 Cushing (Hypercortisolism) and Addison (Hypocortisolism) Syndrome.

Granulomatous Myopathies

Although patients with sarcoidosis often have granulomas in muscle tissue, most commonly these patients have no clinical evidence of a myopathy. However, when these are symptomatic, focal pain, atrophy, or generalized proximal weakness may be seen. Diagnosis usually requires

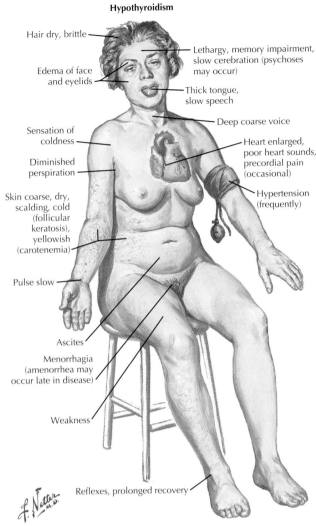

Hypothyroidism

Hair dry, brittle

Lethargy, memory impairment, slow cerebration (psychoses may occur)

Edema of face and eyelids

Thick tongue, slow speech

Deep coarse voice

Sensation of coldness

Heart enlarged, poor heart sounds, precordial pain (occasional)

Diminished perspiration

Hypertension (frequently)

Skin coarse, dry, scalding, cold (follicular keratosis), yellowish (carotenemia)

Pulse slow

Ascites

Menorrhagia (amenorrhea may occur late in disease)

Weakness

Reflexes, prolonged recovery

Fig. 71.10 Hypothyroidism.

involvement of other end organs typically involved by sarcoidosis, particularly the liver or lungs. Nonspecific inflammatory granulomatous myopathies are rare, although they may be seen with underlying myasthenia gravis and thymoma. Ocular and bulbar symptoms attributable to myasthenia may accompany proximal weakness. Rarely, patients may have distal weakness.

Eosinophilic Myopathy

This myopathy is usually present as a component of the hypereosinophilic syndrome. The pattern of weakness is indistinguishable from that of the inflammatory myopathies. Systemic features of hypereosinophilic syndrome involve the heart, lungs, skin, kidneys, and gastrointestinal tract.

Infectious Myopathies

HIV infection may produce a primary inflammatory myopathy with subacute or chronic proximal weakness and myalgia. Typically seen in patients with CD4 counts of less than 200/mm^3, HIV myopathy may be difficult to distinguish from PM.

Nonspecific viral syndromes, particularly in relation to the enteric and influenza viruses, often cause significant myalgia in their prodromal phases. An acute relatively specific viral myositis occasionally occurs in children. It presents with prominent calf pain and toe walking. The CK

level is usually increased; EMG may demonstrate myopathic changes, and muscle biopsy reveals scattered necrotic and regenerating fibers. The course is self-limiting. Rarely, there may be severe muscle rhabdomyolysis with significant increase of CK, myoglobinuria, and consequent metabolic derangement.

Trichinosis, typically caused by the ingestion of inadequately cooked pork, is the most common parasitic infection of muscle. Some patients have a prodrome of nausea, vomiting, and periorbital edema within days after exposure. Strikingly severe myalgia, weakness, fever, and sometimes encephalopathy then develop. Occasionally, trichinosis causes a chronic myopathy. Typically there is an associated eosinophilic leukocytosis. The serum CK level may be increased. Muscle biopsy sometimes demonstrates organisms and eosinophilic infiltration.

Pyomyositis is a rare primary bacterial infection characterized by a focal myopathy. This is primarily seen in the tropics. It is more common in immunodeficient individuals. A variety of gram-positive and gram-negative organisms have been associated with this. Muscle pain, tenderness, and fever are prominent. Neutrophilic leukocytosis and bacteremia also occur. CT and MRI of muscle may demonstrate muscle abscesses.

TREATMENT OF MYOPATHIES

PM, DM, and necrotizing myopathies typically respond to immunosuppressive agents. To date, there is no known treatment for sIBM, and treatment is supportive. Most toxic myopathies and CIM commonly resolve within weeks to months of withdrawal of the offending agent. In this setting, treatment is supportive, and most patients recover muscle strength. However, in IMNM triggered by statin medications, withdrawal of the statin does not lead to improvement; one or more immunosuppressive agents is often used.

Endocrine myopathies are responsive to treatment of hormonal excess or deficiency. Corticosteroid-induced endocrine myopathies usually respond to cessation of steroid therapy or treatment of primary pituitary or adrenal lesions. Some infectious myopathies, such as trichinosis, may respond to antimicrobial agents, corticosteroids, or both. Treatment of pyomyositis consists of appropriate antibiotics and surgical drainage of abscesses.

Supportive Therapies

The goal of all treatments is maximization of patient function. Many patients with myopathies may benefit from the involvement of physiatrists, physical therapists, and occupational therapists early in the course of their illness. Rehabilitation specialists are best able to decide what form of support aids, including braces, canes, crutches, walkers, wheelchairs, lift chairs, stair lifts, elevators, bed rails, and lifting devices, are best suited for the individual patient. Lift chairs are beneficial to ambulatory patients with proximal weakness that precludes them from independently rising from a chair. Elevators and stair lifts are valuable when accessing more than one floor. Speech and swallow therapists are helpful in patients with myopathies associated with swallowing dysfunction.

Prognosis

Control rather than immediate cure is often the most realistic initial management goal. DM and PM eventually stabilize or achieve a good to excellent remission, but drug therapy may be required for months or years. Patients with sIBM usually have a normal life span, but some require a wheelchair or scooter within 10–15 years after diagnosis. Patients with endocrine, metabolic, infectious, toxic, and vitamin D deficiency myopathies that are usually amenable to treatment generally have an excellent prognosis. The prognosis of paraneoplastic necrotizing myopathies is dependent on that of the underlying malignancy.

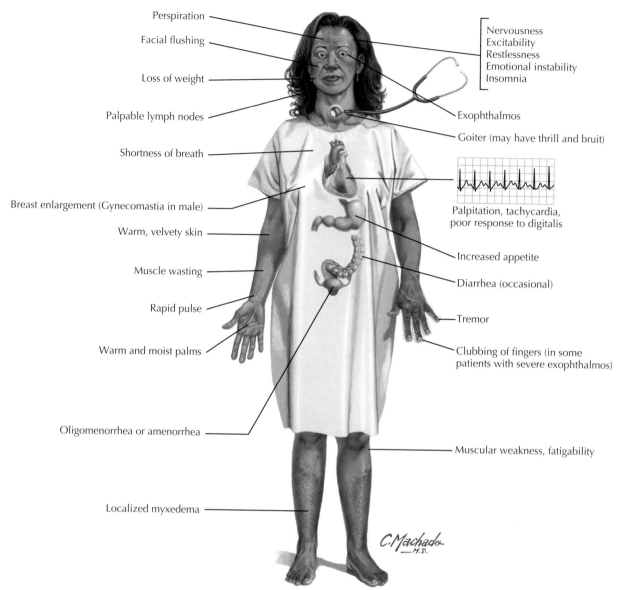

Perspiration

Facial flushing

Loss of weight

Palpable lymph nodes

Shortness of breath

Breast enlargement (Gynecomastia in male)

Warm, velvety skin

Muscle wasting

Rapid pulse

Warm and moist palms

Oligomenorrhea or amenorrhea

Localized myxedema

Nervousness
Excitability
Restlessness
Emotional instability
Insomnia

Exophthalmos

Goiter (may have thrill and bruit)

Palpitation, tachycardia, poor response to digitalis

Increased appetite

Diarrhea (occasional)

Tremor

Clubbing of fingers (in some patients with severe exophthalmos)

Muscular weakness, fatigability

Fig. 71.11 Hyperthyroidism (Graves Disease).

ADDITIONAL RESOURCES

Ahmed W, Khan N, Glueck CJ, et al. Low serum 25 (OH) vitamin D levels (<32 ng/mL) are associated with reversible myositis-myalgia in statin-treated patients. Transl Res 2009;153(1):11–16.

Al-Said YA, Al-Rached HS, Al-Qahtani HA, et al. Severe proximal myopathy with remarkable recovery after vitamin D treatment. Can J Neurol Sci 2009;36(3):336–9.

Amato AA, Barohn RJ. Inclusion body myositis: old and new concepts. J Neurol Neurosurg Psychiatry 2009;80:1186–93.

Amato AA, Russell JA. Neuromuscular disorders. 2nd ed. New York: McGraw-Hill; 2016.

Davies NP, Hanna MG. The skeletal muscle channelopathies: distinct entities and overlapping syndromes. Curr Opin Neurol 2003;16:559–68.

DiMauro S, Lamperti C. Muscle glycogenoses. Muscle Nerve 2001;24:984–99.

Engel AG. Metabolic and endocrine myopathies. In: Walton NJ, editor. Disorders of voluntary muscle. 5th ed. Edinburgh: Churchill-Livingstone; 1988.

Engel AG, Banker BQ, editors. Myology. New York: McGraw-Hill; 1986.

Fardet L, Dupuy A, Gain M, et al. Factors associated with underlying malignancy in a retrospective cohort of 121 patients with dermatomyositis. Medicine (Baltimore) 2009;88(2):91–7.

Felice KJ, Schneebaum AB, Jones HR. McArdle's disease with late onset symptoms. J Neurol Neurosurg Psychiatry 1992;55:407–8.

Ferrante MA, Wilbourn AJ. Myopathies. In: Levin KH, Luders HO, editors. Comprehensive clinical neurophysiology. Philadelphia, PA: WB Saunders; 2000:268–81.

Griggs RC, Engel WK, Resnick JS. Acetazolamide treatment of periodic paralysis. Ann Int Med 1970;73:39–48.

Griggs RC, Mendell JR, Miller RG. Evaluation and treatment of myopathy. Philadelphia, PA: FA Davis Co; 1995.

Haller RG, Knochel JP. Metabolic myopathies. In: Johnson RT, Griffin JW, editors. Current therapy in neurologic disease. St. Louis, MO: Mosby-Year Book; 1993:397–402.

Jones HR, Darras B, De Vivo DC. Neuromuscular disorders of infancy, childhood, and adolescence: a clinician's approach. Elsevier Health Sciences; 2002.

Kassardjian C, et al. Clinical features and treatment outcomes of necrotizing autoimmune. JAMA Neurology 2015;72(9):996–1103.

Moxley RT III. Channelopathies affecting skeletal muscle in childhood: myotonic disorders including myotonic dystrophy and periodic paralysis. In: Jones HR, De Vivo DC, Darras BT, editors. Neuromuscular disorders of infancy, childhood, and adolescence. Philadelphia, PA: Butterworth-Heinemann; 2003:1017–35.

Simmons A, Peterlin BL, Boyer PJ, et al. Muscle biopsy in the evaluation of patients with modestly elevated creatine kinase levels. Muscle Nerve 2003;27:242–4.

Page numbers followed by *f* indicate figures; *t*, tables; *b*, boxes.